General Practice
The Integrative Approach

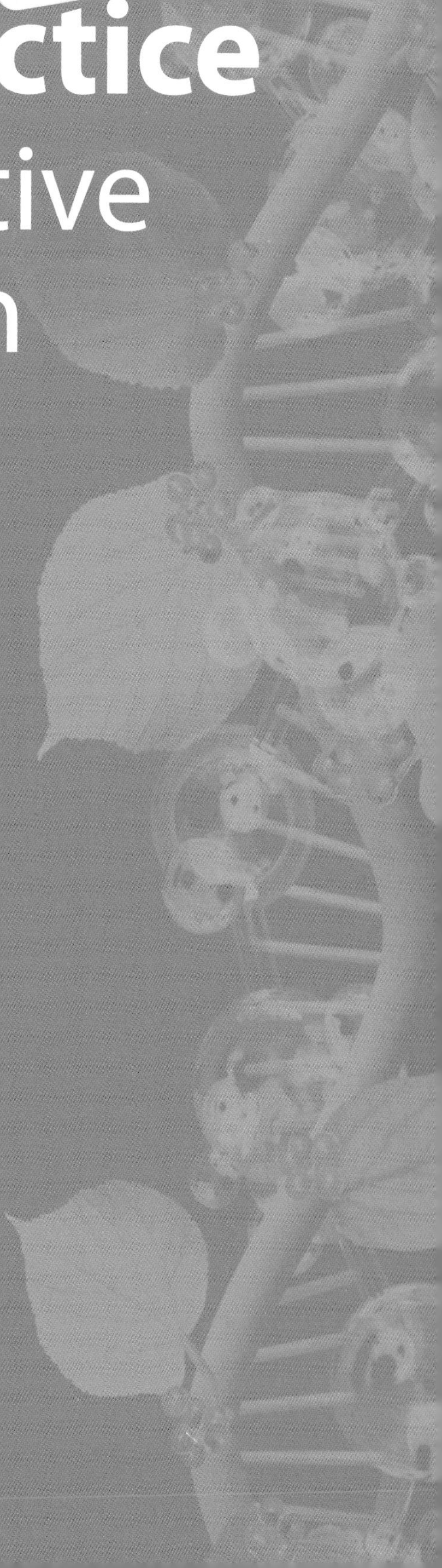

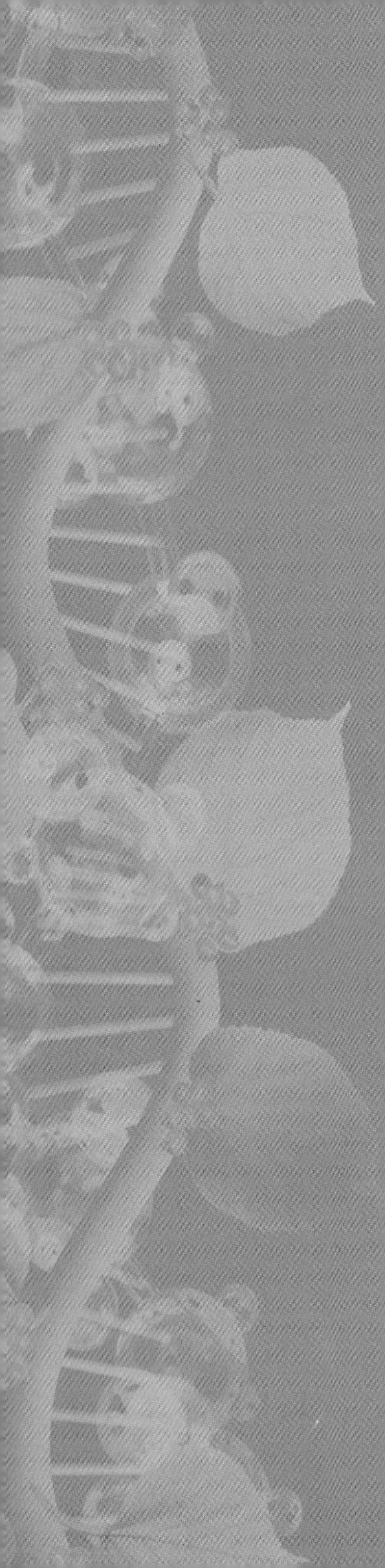

General Practice
The Integrative Approach

Kerryn Phelps
MBBS(Syd), FRACGP, FMA
Adjunct Professor, Sydney Medical School,
University of Sydney, Sydney, New South Wales

Craig Hassed
MBBS, FRACGP
Deputy Head, Department of General Practice,
Monash University, Melbourne, Victoria

CHURCHILL LIVINGSTONE
ELSEVIER

Sydney Edinburgh London New York Philadelphia St Louis Toronto

ELSEVIER

Churchill Livingstone is an imprint of Elsevier

Elsevier Australia. ACN 001 002 357
(a division of Reed International Books Australia Pty Ltd)
Tower 1, 475 Victoria Avenue, Chatswood, NSW 2067

National Library of Australia Cataloguing-in-Publication Data

---

Phelps, Kerryn.

General practice: the integrative approach / Kerryn Phelps, Craig Hassed.

9780729538046 (pbk.)

Physicians (General practice)
Family medicine

Hassed, Craig.

601

Publisher: Sophie Kaliniecki
Developmental Editor: Neli Bryant
Publishing Services Manager: Helena Klijn
Project Coordinator: Karen Griffiths
Edited by Kay Waters
Editorial coordination by Teresa McIntyre
Proofread by Tim Learner
Illustrations by TNQ
Cover and internal design by Darben Design
Index by Michael Ferreira
Typeset by Pindar NZ
Printed by C & C Offset Printing Co. Ltd.

Contents

Contributors

Based on their respective expertise, the following people have contributed content to the book and we would like to extend our gratitude to them for dedicating their time, knowledge and input to ensure the success of this project.

Kerryn Phelps and Craig Hassed have added integrative content to each of the chapters in the book.

Suzanne Abraham, MSc, PhD (Medicine)
Associate Professor, University of Sydney, NSW, Australia
Co-Director, Eating Disorder Unit, The Northside Clinic

Stuart Aitken, MBBS, Dip Ven, FAChSHM
Sexual Health Physician, Gold Coast Sexual Health Clinic, Queensland, Australia
Assistant Professor, Health Sciences and Medicine, Bond University
Senior Lecturer, Medicine and Oral Health, Griffith University

A/Prof Kristine Barlow-Stewart, PhD, FHGSA (Genetic Counselling)
Director, The Centre for Genetics Education, Royal North Shore Hospital, St Leonards, NSW, Australia
Clinical A/Professor, Northern Clinical School, Faculty of Medicine, University of Sydney

David Bennett, MBBS, FRACP, FSAHM
Clinical Professor, University of Sydney, Senior Staff Specialist, Department of Adolescent Medicine and Head, NSW Centre for the Advancement of Adolescent Health, Sydney Children's Hospitals Network, Sydney, NSW, Australia

Laura Brass, BSc, ND
Naturopath, Uclinic, Sydney, NSW, Australia

Lesley Braun, PhD, BPharm, DipAppSci (Naturopathy), GradDip Phytotherapy
Research Fellow, Cardiothoracic Surgical Research Unit, Monash University (Alfred Hospital)
Research Pharmacist, Alfred Hospital
Lecturer at RMIT and Monash Universities, Melbourne, Victoria, Australia
Vice President of the National Herbalists Association of Australia

Elizabeth Brophy, PhD, MSW (Hons), LLB, Dip Social Studies
Barrister/Mediator, The Victorian Bar, Victoria, Australia

Ian Chenoweth, MBBS, FRACGP, MFM
Part-time senior lecturer, Department of General Practice, School of Primary Health Care, Faculty of Medicine, Nursing and Health Sciences, Monash University, Australia

Warren N Chin, MBBS, DM (Urol)
Urology Fellow, Monash Medical Centre, Victoria, Australia

Jacqui Conomos, MBBS
Registrar, Gold Coast Sexual Health Clinic, Queensland, Australia

David Colquhoun, MBBS, FRACP
Associate Professor of Medicine University of Queensland
Cardiologist, Wesley and Greenslopes Private Hospitals, Queensland, Australia

Grant Cracknell, BSc, MBBS
Advanced Trainee in Endocrinology, Princess Alexandra Hospital, Brisbane, Queensland, Australia

Dr John Eden, MBBS, MD, FRCOG, FRANZCOG, CREI
Associate Professor of Reproductive Endocrinology, University of NSW, Sydney, NSW, Australia
Director Barbara Gross Research Unit Royal Hospital for Women
Director Sydney Menopause Centre Royal Hospital for Women
Director Women's Health and Research Institute of Australia

Susan Evans, MBBS, FRANZCOG, FFPMANZCA
Private practice, Adelaide
University of Adelaide, South Australia, Australia

Dr H John Fardy, MBBS (UNSW), DRCOG (London), FRACGP
General practitioner, Gerringong
Regional Hospital Academic Coordinator
University of Wollongong Graduate School of Medicine
The Wollongong Hospital, NSW, Australia

Mark Frydenberg, MBBS, FRACS
Associate Professor, Department of Surgery, Faculty of Medicine, Nursing and Health Sciences, Monash University
Chairman, Department of Urology, Southern Health, Melbourne, Victoria, Australia

Peter Gates, MBBS, FRACP
Associate Professor of Neurology, University of Melbourne
Director of Stroke, Director of Neuroscience and a Director of Physician Training at Barwon Health, Geelong, Victoria, Australia

Michelle Gold, MBBS, FRACP, FAChPM, PG Dip Palliative Medicine
Director, Palliative Care Service, Alfred Health, Victoria, Australia

Ivan Goldberg, MBBS (Sydney), FRANZCO, FRACS
Clinical Associate Professor, University of Sydney, NSW, Australia
Head, Glaucoma Unit, Sydney Eye Hospital
Director, Eye Associates, Sydney

Mark Hardy, BSc (Med), MBBS, FRACGP
Fellow in Addiction Medicine, Royal North Shore Hospital, St Leonards, NSW, Australia

Kelsey Hegarty, MBBS, FRACGP, Dip RACOG, PhD
Associate Professor, University of Melbourne, Victoria, Australia

Anne Howard, MBBS, FRACP, FACD
Senior dermatologist, Royal Melbourne Hospital, Western Hospital, Royal Women's Hospital, Royal Children's Hospital, Victoria, Australia

Jennifer Hunter, BMed, MScPH, DipLSHTM
Integrative General Practitioner, Uclinic, Sydney, NSW, Australia

Rohan Jayasinghe, MBBS (Hons Class 1, Sydney), MSpM, PhD, FRACP, FCSANZ
Director of Cardiology, Gold Coast Hospital, Queensland
Professor of Cardiology, Griffith University, Queensland, Australia

Dr David Joske, MBBS, FRACP, FRCPA
Head, Department of Haematology, Sir Charles Gairdner Hospital, Western Australia, Australia
Clinical Professor of Medicine, University of Western Australia
Executive Chairman, SolarisCare Foundation

Melissa Kang, MBBS, MCH
Senior Lecturer, Department of General Practice, University of Sydney, NSW, Australia

Kelvin Kong, BSc, MBBS, FRACS
ENT VMO, John Hunter Hospital, NSW, Australia

Leon Lack, PhD, MAPS
Professor in Psychology, Flinders University, Adelaide, South Australia, Australia
Director of Insomnia Treatment Program, Adelaide Institute of Sleep Health, Repatriation General Hospital, Daw Park, South Australia

Peter A Leggat, MD, PhD, DrPH, FAFPHM, FACTM, FFTM ACTM, FFTM RCPSG, FACRRM
Professor and Head of School, School of Public Health, Tropical Medicine and Rehabilitation Sciences
Associate Dean for Faculty Affairs, Faculty of Medicine, Health and Molecular Sciences, James Cook University, Townsville, Queensland, Australia

Dr Michael Lowy, MBBS, MPM, FAChSHM
Sexual Health Physician, Sydney Men's Health, Bondi Junction, NSW, Australia

Ciaran Lynch, MD, FRCS (Urol)
Urology Fellow, Department of Urology, Monash Medical Centre, Melbourne, Victoria, Australia

Stuart MacKay, BSc (Med), MBBS (Hons), FRACS
Clinical Senior Lecturer, Otalaryngology Head and Neck Surgeon, Woollongong Hospital, Wollongong, NSW, Australia

Dr Scott Masters, MBBS, FRACGP, FAFMM, Dip MSM
Director Caloundra Spinal and Sports Medicine Centre, Caloundra, Queensland, Australia

Katy Melrose, BMedSci, MBBS (Hons), FRACP
Geriatrician, Austin Health and Northern Health, Victoria, Australia

Robert Newton, PhD, AEP, FAAESS, FNSCA
Director, Vario Health Institute, Edith Cowan University, Western Australia, Australia

Tuan Nguyen, PhD
Senior Research Fellow, Group Leader, Bone Research Program, Garvan Institute of Medical Research
Professor, Faculty of Medicine, University of New South Wales, NSW, Australia

John Orchard, MBBS, BA, MD, PhD, FACSP, FACSM, FASMF, FFSEM (UK)
Sports physician; Adjunct Associate Professor, School of Public Health, University of Sydney, NSW, Australia

Dzung Price, MBBS (Hons), FRACGP, Master NLP Pract
Integrative Medical Doctor, Queensland, Australia

Graham J Reynolds, MBBS, FRACP, DCH, MHP, MHEd
Associate Professor, Australian National University Medical School
Department of Paediatrics and Child Health, The Canberra Hospital, ACT, Australia

Kathryn Robertson, MBBS, FRACGP, MEd
General Practitioner and Faculty Member, Cognitive Institute and The Medical Protection Society, Australia

George Rubin, FRACP, FAFPHM, FAChAM
Director, Clinical Governance, South Eastern Sydney Illawarra Area Health Service
Professor of Public Health, Universities of Sydney and NSW, NSW, Australia

Professor Avni Sali, MBBS, PhD, FRACS, FACS, FACNEM
Medical practitioner
Founding Director, National Institute of Integrative Medicine
Honorary Professor, School of Medicine, University of Queensland, Queensland, Australia
President, International Council of Integrative Medicine

Philip Sambrook, OAM, MBBS, MD, LLB, FRACP
Professor of Rheumatology, Kolling Institute of Medical Research and Sydney Medical School
Royal North Shore Hospital, St Leonards, NSW, Australia

Penelope Sheehan, MBBS, RANZCOG, GDEB
Staff specialist obstetrician, Maternity Unit Head, Royal Women's Hospital, Melbourne, Victoria, Australia
Senior Clinical Research Fellow, Department of Perinatal Medicine Pregnancy Research Centre

Philip Siddall, MBBS, Grad Dip Ac, MM (Pain Mgt), PhD, FFPMANZCA
Senior Principal Research Fellow and Visiting Medical Officer, Pain Management & Research Centre, Royal North Shore Hospital, St Leonards, NSW, Australia

Phillip D Stricker, MBBS (Hons), FRACS
Chairman Department Urology, St Vincents, Sydney, NSW, Australia
Associate Professor of Urology, University of NSW

Michael Talbot, MB ChB, FRACS
Conjoint Senior Lecturer, University of NSW, NSW, Australia
Conjoint Senior Lecturer in Surgery, St George Hospital

Ruban Thanigasalam, MBBS, MS (Urol)
Urology Advanced Trainee, Royal North Shore Hospital, St Leonards, NSW, Australia

Dr Julie Thompson, MBBS, Grad Dip Ed
Senior Clinical Advisor, National Breast and Ovarian Cancer Centre, NSW, Australia

Lily Tomas, MBBS, BSc (Med)
Integrative Medical Practitioner, Pambula, NSW, Australia
Vice President of Australasian Integrative Medical Association
Medical author and journalist

Associate Professor Luis Vitetta, PhD, GradDip NutrEnvironMed, GradDip IntegrMed
Director, Centre for Integrative Clinical and Molecular Medicine, School of Medicine, University of Queensland, Queensland, Australia

John Walters, MBBS, DPDerm Distn, FASEM, FACRRM, FRACGP
GP Clifton Hill, Victoria, Australia

Sanjiva Wijesinha, MBBS (Ceylon), MSc (Oxford), FRCS (Edinburgh), FRCS (Ireland), FACS, FRACGP
Associate Professor of General Practice, Monash University, Melbourne, Victoria, Australia

Michael Woodward, MBBS, FRACP
Head, Aged Care Services, Austin Health, Victoria, Australia

Helen Wright, PhD, MPsych(Clin), MAPS
Research Fellow/Psychologist, School of Psychology, Flinders University, South Australia, Australia

Alina Zeldovich, MBBS, BSc (Med), FRANZCO
Eye Associates and Sight Foundation Theatre, NSW, Australia

Dr Helen Zorbas, MBBS, FASBP, MAICD
CEO Cancer Australia and National Breast and Ovarian Cancer Centre, Australia

HERBAL RESEARCH REFERENCE DATABASE CONTRIBUTORS

This team provided an extensive database of herbal research which acted as a reference for some of the therapeutics in the book.

Eshaifol Azam Omar, MBBS, M Herb Med (Hon)
PhD candidate, Faculty of Pharmacy, University of Sydney, NSW, Australia
Cluster of Integrative Medicine, Advanced Medical and Dental Institute, Universiti Sains, Malaysia

Karen E Bridgman, PhD, MSci (Hons), MEd (Higher Ed), MAppSci, ND, DBM, Dip Hom
Part-time Lecturer, Faculty of Pharmacy, University of Sydney, NSW, Australia
Director, Starflower Pty Ltd and Starflower Herbals

Tom Hsun-Wei Huang, BPharm (Hons Class 1), PhD, MBA, MACP
Part-time Lecturer, Faculty of Pharmacy, University of Sydney, NSW, Australia

Yuk Lan Liew, MB, BS, DTPH, DFM, MFM, M Herb Med
Part-time Lecturer, Faculty of Pharmacy, University of Sydney, NSW, Australia

George Q Li, BSc, MSc, PhD, GCertEdStud (Higher Ed), MRACI, MACS
Sesquicentenary Lecturer in Herbal Medicines, Faculty of Pharmacy, University of Sydney, NSW, Australia

Srinivas Nammi, BPharm, MPharm, PhD
Lecturer in Pharmaceutical Sciences, Faculty of Health, University of Canberra, ACT, Australia
Honorary Associate, Faculty of Pharmacy, University of Sydney, NSW, Australia

Indu Narayan, BSAM, BAMS (Integ Modern Med), GCertEdStud (Higher Ed)
Accredited member, Australian Medicine Society Ltd (ATMS)
Professional Member & NSW State Representative, Australasian Association of Ayurveda (AAA)
Associate member, Australian Integrative Medicine Association (AIMA)
Part-time Lecturer in Herbal Medicines, Faculty of Pharmacy, University of Sydney, NSW, Australia

Lily Yingmin Li, BMed, PhD
Part-time Lecturer, Faculty of Pharmacy, University of Sydney, NSW, Australia

Reviewers

Bianca Cannon, MBBS, FRACGP
General practitioner, private practice, Sydney, NSW, Australia

Tana Fishman, FRNZCGP (Dist), DO, MS
Senior Lecturer, Department of General Practice and Primary Health Care, University of Auckland, New Zealand
Executive Board, Royal New Zealand College of General Practitioners
General practice, Greenstone Family Clinic, Manurewa, Auckland

Dr Tim Francis, BSc (HMS) (UQ), MBBS (UQ), FRACGP
Medical Educator, North Coast NSW General Practice Training
VMO, Macksville District Hospital, NSW
General Practitioner, Nambucca Heads, NSW, Australia

Dr Geoff Mitchell, MBBS, PhD, FRACGP, FAChPM
Professor of General Practice and Palliative Care and Head, MBBS Program Ipswich, University of Queensland, Ipswich, Queensland, Australia

George Ostapowicz, BMedSc, BMed (Ncle), MD (Melb), FRACP
Director of Gastroenterology, Gold Coast Health Service District, Queensland, Australia
Associate Professor, Faculty of Health Sciences and Medicine, Bond University, Queensland

Dr Elen ApThomas, MBBS, DRANZCOG
Integrative medicine general practitioner, Gold Coast, Queensland

Dr Emma Warnecke, MBBS (Hons), FRACGP
Associate Head, Student Affairs
Senior Lecturer, Discipline of General Practice School of Medicine, University of Tasmania, Australia
General Practitioner, Tasmania

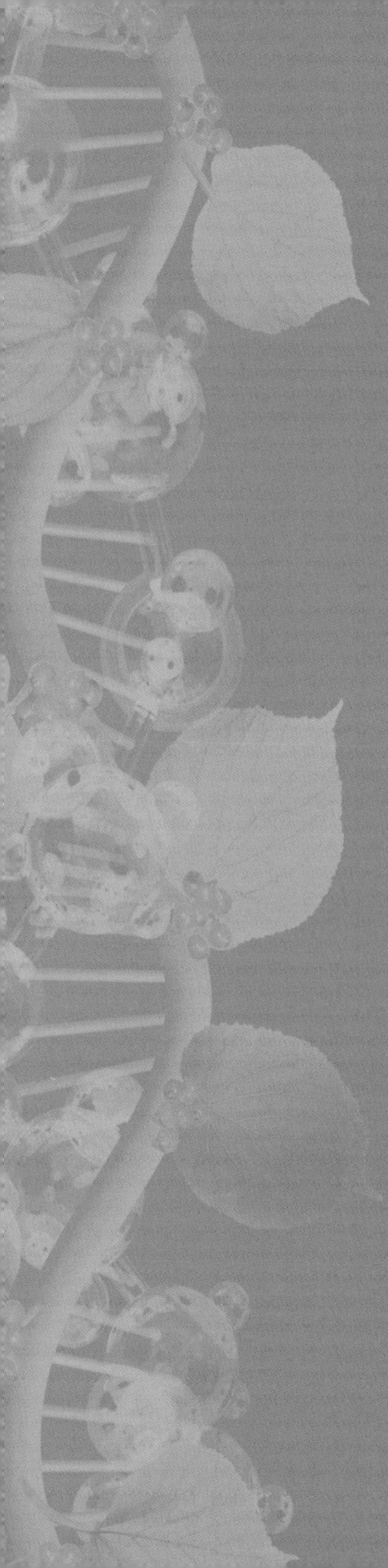

Foreword

As general practitioners we are skilled at balancing the art and the science of medicine. We practise holistic medicine, providing comprehensive care that considers the physical, social, emotional and spiritual needs of each of our patients. We are aware of the impact of lifestyle and wellbeing on the way many conditions manifest in our patients and their response to our treatments and advice.

We also know that medical wisdom changes over time. Many of the lessons we learned in medical school no longer apply. The rise of evidence-based medicine over recent years has hastened some of this change, often in ways which we can see provide great benefit to our patients.

We are also aware that our scientific knowledge has its limitations and that there are some challenges in the care of our patients which traditional Western medicine is yet to meet.

As we strive to do the best for our patients, we are open to new ways of thinking. We know that our best teachers are often our individual patients who may teach us about what it is like to live with a certain condition and new ways of coping with the challenges of ill-health.

We are also aware that many of our patients favour additional or alternative treatments to what we may recommend and prescribe. And, if we are wise, we create a situation where our patients can discuss these treatment options with us, and perhaps we can learn together as we explore the boundaries of contemporary medical knowledge.

Integrative medicine as a concept should therefore not come as a surprise to most experienced general practitioners. In this book it is described as having a focus on the whole person and a commitment to using all appropriate evidence-based therapeutic approaches, in partnership with other healthcare professionals, to achieve optimal health and healing.

My own introduction to this style of medicine was in the early 1990s when I was working as a general practitioner providing care to people with HIV. This was before effective treatments were available and when HIV was an inevitably terminal condition for many people. Using the best evidence available I provided advice to my patients about their treatment options, using emerging antiretroviral medications while at the same time working with my patients and other healthcare providers to do all we could to support each person's health and wellbeing. I worked as part of a multidisciplinary team which included other medical practitioners, nurses, counsellors, nutritionists, acupuncturists, massage therapists, traditional Chinese medicine practitioners and dedicated carers, all with one aim—to deliver the best care we could to the people who were trusting us for their healthcare and advice.

And so I came to this book with an open mind. Kerryn Phelps, Craig Hassed and colleagues have written a general practice textbook with a difference, and provide their views on ways general practitioners might adopt an integrative approach. Some of the recommendations I agree with, while others grate against what I have been taught but also make me stop and consider if there could be additional or alternative ways of approaching management and care.

At its heart this is a book which embraces many of the principles of general practice. Yet it has the capacity to change the way you think about general practice.

Professor Michael Kidd, AM
President-elect, World Organization of Family Doctors

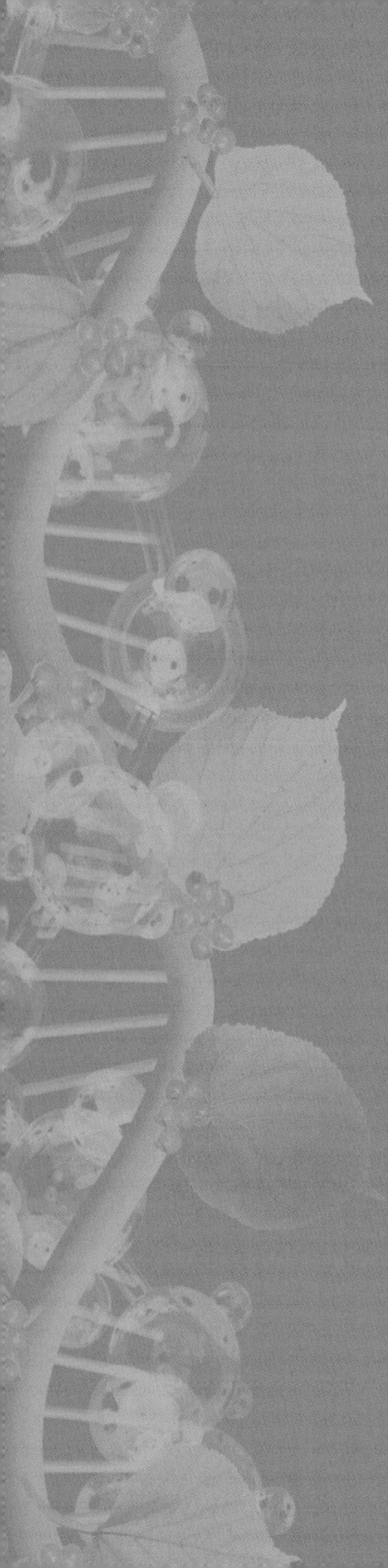

Preface

With a first-edition textbook such as this, it is important to reflect for a moment on its evolution.

We have been medical practitioners since the early 1980s. In that time we have seen the common, the rare and the esoteric. We have seen patients suffer and die from diseases that may or may not have been preventable.

There were times when we were asked the question, 'Is there anything else I can do, Doctor?' Not wanting to admit defeat, a doctor needs to realise that we need more tools in our kit than medical school and our orthodox training have prepared us for. Doctors need to open their eyes, ears and minds to the stories our patients are telling us—that they had tried a supplement or herb, seen a naturopath, been treated by a chiropractor, had acupuncture and felt better … after medicine had told them there was no more to offer. We observed patients with cancer who seemed to tolerate their treatment much better than others, and wanted to know why.

Over a period of time we felt a sense of the metaphorical brick wall breaking down. We had always followed what we thought was a 'holistic' approach, but there are levels and degrees of engagement with this concept, both professionally and personally.

Then Kerryn had her own health crisis. Yes, doctors have them too; we are not immune. Far from it. 'I was flying around the continent, working ridiculous hours as President of the Australian Medical Association, and trying to run a practice and a family. I was in my early 40s and my cycle became erratic. Rather than take the time to look at the underlying cause of the problem, I spoke to my gynaecologist who prescribed a hormone treatment. A few weeks later I noticed I was having trouble walking up hills. The next day I couldn't get up the stairs without stopping. A day later I couldn't make it across the consulting room without losing my breath.

'I called in to see a specialist in respiratory medicine at St Vincent's Hospital in Sydney. Within an hour I was in intensive care with a confirmed, life-threatening pulmonary embolism. It was time for a reality check.

'Apart from the cause of the embolism, the treatment similarly needed a broad view. We could clear the clots with anticoagulant injections—but what next? What changes did I need to make to my life to find perspective, look after the fundamentals like exercise, diet, sleep and stress management? How could I overcome the fatigue and recover my fitness? And how could I plan my later years knowing that hormone replacement was off the agenda if menopause struck with a vengeance? My professional interest in integrative approaches to health problems had become very personal.

'In my search for more evidence and clinically relevant material, I looked for papers and books to support my quest for information specific and relevant across the whole spectrum of general practice. Here was the genesis of this book.'

For Craig, the move towards integrative medicine has been a life-long journey. 'For me it was an intuitive experience when I noticed that how I lived and thought had subtle, cumulative but noticeable effects on my physical wellbeing, as if the body was a mirror of the inner state. It always seemed best to prevent illness, and recognising and following simple and natural principles of wellness were the best way of doing that. This starts with the mind and living consciously, and then living the lifestyle follows from that. In wanting what seemed best for myself, later when I became a doctor I could not want anything better for my patients. I also recognised in my medical education that the mind of the medical profession can sometimes be closed or at least narrow in its perspective, not always listening to patients' experiences nor being as respectful of the evidence-based approach as it espoused. For me, what I noticed gave rise to a calling to contribute towards the education of a new generation of medical practitioners who will apply a wellness approach in conjunction with the judicious use of the best that modern medicine has to offer. Being invited to co-author this book has been an honour and is a significant step towards meeting that goal.'

We realised that GPs like us with a curiosity to explore the boundaries of health and disease really needed a reference book written specifically for the generalist; a practical approach to the diagnosis, investigation and integrative management of the vast range of problems presented to GPs.

Over four years the content came together, drawing from the clinical experience and expert knowledge of a superb panel of contributors. There is some clinical judgment and opinion in the therapeutic strategies where official guidelines are lacking. Such is the art of medicine.

Like medical knowledge itself, we expect the content of this textbook to be organic, to grow and develop in the future as evidence and the study of integrative medicine itself grows and develops.

Professor Kerryn Phelps
Dr Craig Hassed
November 2010

Acknowledgements

Compiling a textbook like this is a massive task. It has taken years of conceptualising, researching, reflection, writing and editing. I am indebted to a number of remarkable people who have made this possible.

First my wife Jackie Stricker, who has impelled me to question and probe beyond the outer reaches of my professional and intellectual boundaries in my quest to help redefine Western medical practice, and who enabled the creative space I needed at home to produce the book.

I am also enormously grateful to my patients who have taught me so much about the broader meaning of health and illness, and challenged me to help them find solutions to their problems.

I am indebted to my co-author Dr Craig Hassed. His calm presence and sharp intellect have made him the perfect writing partner for a project such as this.

This textbook draws on the expertise and opinions of my colleagues, some of the great minds in clinical medicine and healthcare practice in Australia. Their contributions to this text are invaluable and I am grateful for their support of this project.

Thank you to my colleagues and staff at Uclinic in Sydney who have all taken the 'leap of faith' to help establish our multidisciplinary integrative medicine clinic, and every day challenge the dominant medical paradigm.

Thanks also to the editorial and production team at Elsevier for their persistence and commitment to this project from the outset and throughout the entire process.

Professor Kerryn Phelps

Appendix 1, pages 906–966 is reproduced with permission from *Herbs and Natural Supplements: an evidence-based guide*, 3rd edn © 2010 Elsevier Australia. This is a National Pharmacy Board 2010 recommended evidence-based reference on complementary medicines. The authors are:

Lesley Braun, PhD, BPharm, DipAppSci Naturopathy, GradDip Phytotherapy; Senior Reseach Fellow, Cardiothoracic Surgical Research Unit, Monash University (Alfred Hospital), Melbourne; Research Pharmacist, Alfred Hospital Melbourne; Lecturer at RMIT and Monash Universities, Melbourne; Vice President of the National Herbalists Association of Australia

Marc Cohen, MBBS (Hons), PhD (TCM), PhD (Elec Eng), BMedSc (Hons), FAMAC, FICAE; Professor of Complementary Medicine and Program Leader, Master of Wellness, School of Health Sciences, RMIT University, Melbourne.

The book presents evidence-based information on the 130 most popular herbs, nutrients and food supplements used across Australia and New Zealand. Organised alphabetically by common name, each herb or nutrient listed includes information such as daily intake, main actions/indications, adverse reactions, contraindications and precautions, safety in pregnancy and comprehensive herb–drug interaction charts.

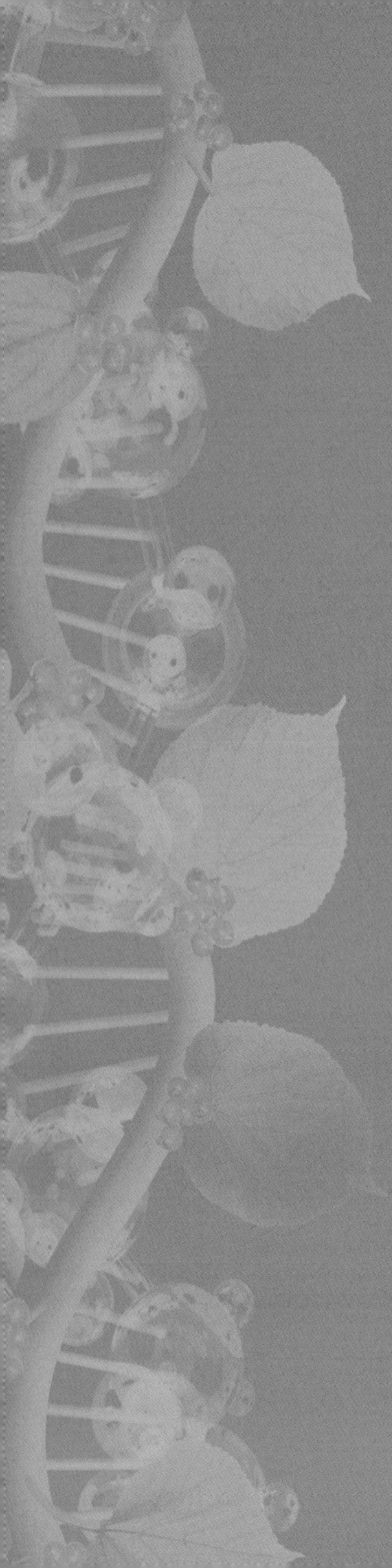

part ONE

Principles of integrative medicine

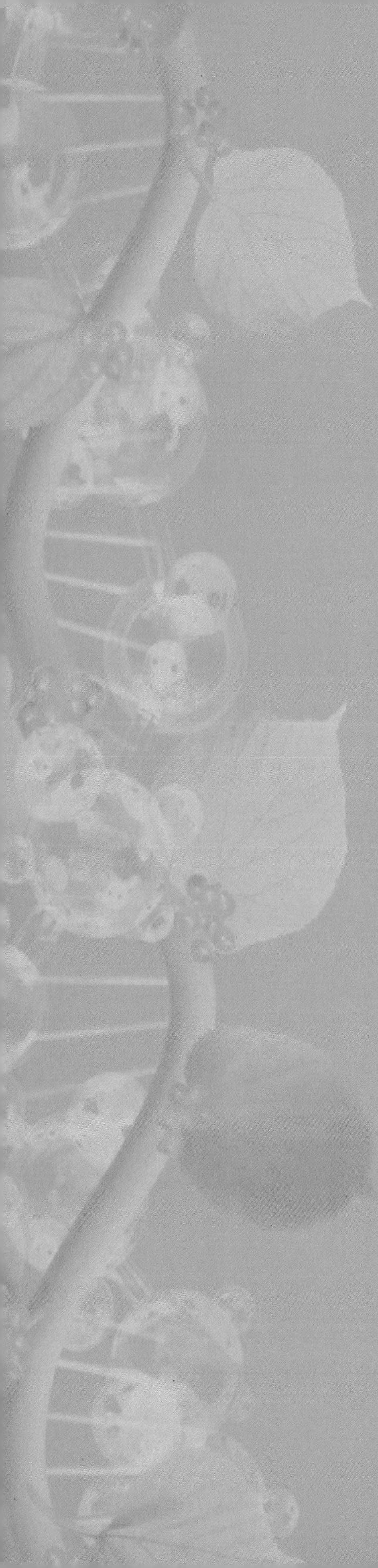

chapter 1

Introduction to the concept of integrative medicine

This is a general practice textbook with a difference. It is designed to be a practical guide to integrative general practice.

We have been general practitioners (GPs) for over two decades. In that time a GP will have seen and heard just about every clinical scenario. We have also seen many medical fads come and go, such as the fashion for prescribing hormone replacement therapy to every perimenopausal woman because it was supposed to improve her future health, the rise and fall of non-steroidal anti-inflammatory drugs for managing arthritis pain, and the passing epidemic of repetitive strain injury. We have similarly seen many natural therapy and dietary fads come and go. Many experienced practitioners will remember the era when every other patient arrived with the news that they had 'hypoglycaemia', and then there was the 'systemic candida' phase.

We have experienced the intellectual excitement of the 'clever' diagnosis, the sadness of delivering bad news to a patient, the delight of guiding a patient back to health, and the frustration of hitting a brick wall when our Western medical training left us feeling there was nothing further we could offer.

The emergence of evidence-based medicine and, more recently, evidence-based complementary medicine is challenging many previously held notions of best practice. As evidence emerges, many Western medical therapies are being confirmed as correct, or challenged as ineffective or harmful. Similarly, many complementary therapies are being confirmed as correct, while others are being found ineffective or harmful. Such is the inevitable evolution of healthcare.

It is also important that evidence-based healthcare at every level be considered a 'work-in-progress', whether it is in the discovery of the genetic basis of disease, the development of previously untested technology or the clinical application of a treatment. The nature of scientific research is such that new information becomes available at a great rate, and that knowledge often changes the status quo.

It is in the GP's consulting room that patients ideally have the opportunity to explore what is likely to be the best option for their healthcare. We see the gamut of health concerns, from a person wanting a check-up and interested in doing more to maintain good health, to a patient who is symptomatic and wanting a diagnosis and treatment, or a patient with an established diagnosis who is looking for either a cure or a way of optimising their wellbeing as they live with their illness.

Like that of our colleagues, our medical training was in the allopathic model. Through a combination of professional and personal experience and further study, our practice paradigm has gradually evolved into an integrative model of healthcare.

We do not expect to become proficient in every modality of therapy. However, we do believe that patients should expect their doctor to be familiar with a comprehensive range of therapies likely to work in their circumstances, and what the risks and benefits are likely to be. In this way general practice will be enriched and patient outcomes enhanced. Patients are increasingly looking for an integrated model of healthcare and much prefer it to be delivered, or at least coordinated and supervised, by their family doctor rather than having to fly blind, often without their doctor's knowledge or approval.

Western medical practice coexists with many other healing traditions, whether doctors are aware of it or not. And just as GPs work in partnership with other medical specialties, so we can also work more effectively with appropriately qualified complementary and alternative healthcare providers.

One of the impediments to working in an integrative model is the lack of a common language between practitioners of different persuasions. For example, the concepts of 'yin and yang' and 'chakra' are not easily explained in medical school language. However, the fact that we may not understand the language, mechanisms or concepts of these therapies and modalities does not mean that they do not have a great deal to offer. As doctors become more familiar with different therapeutic options, so their familiarity with these terms will increase. Similarly, as doctors and other healthcare practitioners increasingly work together in teams or 'virtual teams', a common form of communication is emerging.

WHAT IS INTEGRATIVE MEDICINE?

Integrative medicine is the practice of medicine that reaffirms the importance of the relationship between practitioner and patient, focuses on the whole person, is informed by evidence, and makes use of all appropriate therapeutic approaches, healthcare professionals and disciplines to achieve optimal health and healing.

(Developed and adopted by the Consortium of Academic Health Centers for Integrative Medicine, May 2004, edited May 2005)

Integrative medicine, as defined by the US National Center for Complementary and Alternative Medicine, combines conventional medical treatments and alternative treatments for which there is some high-quality scientific evidence of their safety and effectiveness. Integrative medicine also implies a greater emphasis on patient empowerment and choice, holism, lifestyle interventions and, wherever possible, using the safest and simplest option available.

The term 'integrative medicine' is *not* interchangeable with 'complementary or alternative medicine' (CAM), although many people confuse them. Integrative medicine is about incorporating a range of modalities of healthcare into practice so that practitioners can expand the options available to patients, with healthcare providers from different paradigms ideally working in cooperation rather than competition.

In addition to providing best-practice medical care, integrative medicine focuses on prevention of illness, treatment of illness and maintenance of health, by incorporating all factors that may affect health outcomes, including lifestyle—diet, exercise, stress management—and emotional and spiritual wellbeing. It requires patients to be active participants in their own healthcare. The medical practitioner's role in the integrative model is a combination of advisor, role model, patient advocate and source of reliable recommendations for therapeutic options. Therapeutic options might include nutritional changes, exercise prescription, nutritional supplements, herbal remedies, bodywork, acupuncture, psychological counselling, prescription medication, surgery and more.

THE HEALTHCARE REVOLUTION

Healthcare is about to come full circle. From its beginnings as an integrated and holistic art, through the epochs of allopathic–scientific practice, it is evolving back to its roots as an integrative system of health maintenance and disease management.

THE PAST

Dis-integration and reductionism

Hippocrates, Plato and Aristotle were among the first proponents of the holistic model of healthcare in Western history, believing in the combination of the physical and spiritual elements of the human condition.

In the early 1600s, Rene Descartes philosophically split the mind and body, and some time after that the reductionist movement sought to find simple explanations for the function of the human body.

The Flexner report of 1910 ensured that medical training was based strictly on a materialist interpretation of the scientific model, maintaining the principle of the Cartesian split or the mind/body duality, and teaching core disciplines as if they were unrelated to each other. The focus was squarely on illness and little attention was given to wellness and prevention.

Subspecialisation of medical care followed and, philosophically, further fragmented the human body into its composite organs and systems. Rather than subspecialisation, the term 'partialisation' could be used.

While there is undoubtedly merit in the concentration of knowledge and expertise in specialised areas, this fragmentation simply does not account for complex or chronic diseases, or for the significant effects of psychological, social, environmental and spiritual factors in the health and healing of the whole person.

An 'us and them' mentality

There is still a prevailing, though gradually dwindling, 'us and them' mentality in the practice of healthcare, with 'orthodox' medical practitioners in one corner and CAM proponents in the other. This mistrust between practitioners in different fields is based on complex historical factors. Non-medical practitioners often see people who have been mistreated, or are disillusioned, disappointed or unable to be helped by traditional Western medicine. Medical practitioners often see patients who have tried alternative treatments unsuccessfully or for whom diagnoses were missed or wrong. With the human tendency to generalise from personal experience, these encounters influence how we view other paradigms. 'Alternative' is often held to be synonymous with 'unproven'. 'Allopathic' is often held to be synonymous with 'soul-less'.

The history of medical science has created a deliberate lack of integration of mind, body and spirit in the pursuit of one possibly narrow interpretation of the scientific model. Many doctors remain unaware of the evidence for CAM. This is partly due to scientific evidence for some modalities being relatively recent or published in other languages and so not readily available to doctors trained in the English language. There is often a false sense of confidence that all allopathic treatments are all strongly evidence-based. Past failed experiments like MUA (spinal manipulation under anaesthesia) for back pain, or bone marrow transplantation for metastatic breast cancer, are examples of non-evidence-based treatments that have since been abandoned. Most antibiotic prescriptions have little evidence to support them. Even the evidence for commonly prescribed antidepressants is under question. The impact of commercialisation on medical research and practice is such that patients and non-medical practitioners are questioning the foundations of conventional medical care.

The integration of CAM modalities into general practice has not been helped by the perception of a 'lunatic fringe' making claims that have not or cannot be substantiated and may do harm or delay effective treatments, or of unqualified and unregulated practitioners adversely affecting the reputations of highly trained and skilled practitioners.

NOW

The practice of healthcare is in a state of rapid transition. Technological and pharmaceutical advances have been accompanied by an increasing desire for natural and holistic healing. In this information age, patients are more empowered by knowledge and this has resulted in a change in the balance of power in the therapeutic relationship. Along with the explosion in information and the increased availability of complex technological solutions has come an increase in the expectations of patients and less tolerance of uncertainty. The emergence of evidence-based medicine has created an increased demand for evidence of efficacy for all modalities of treatment.

Ideally, integrative medicine combines the best of allopathic medicine and the best of CAM practices into comprehensive treatment plans, working with the body's natural healing potential and based on the individual patient's needs and preferences. Integrative healthcare is not just about procedures or substances. It is about a philosophy of living, helping to create optimum environments for good health.

This may sound like common sense but historically, and still today, there are impediments to achieving this balance in the health field in a way that focuses solely on the wellbeing of the patient.

Stories from our student days were valuable learning experiences for us. From Kerryn's experience comes the following story:

I had just completed my surgery exams. During the exam, I was given a problem that involved a group of symptoms that made no sense to me. It was clear that this had not been in the syllabus for that term. Shortly after I left the exam, I encountered my surgery professor on the ward. He asked me how the exam had gone, and I told him how annoyed I had been that there was a question I could not answer because the condition described had not been taught to us. He nodded and smiled, then he gave me some advice I have carried with me throughout my clinical career. He said, 'Any condition of the human body, any problem that could ever present itself to you in practice requiring diagnosis and management ... that is the syllabus for medical training.'

Craig remembers being in a cardiology lecture at the beginning of his first clinical placement in fourth year:

The head of cardiology stood up at the beginning of the first lecture and commenced to tell us about all the foolish and naive things doctors used to believe 100 years ago about the causes and treatments for heart disease. We laughed. Then he said, 'What do you think they will say about what I am about to teach you 100 years from now?' I stopped laughing and reflected on how impermanent so-called 'scientific knowledge' is. Much of what we as students and doctors take to be fact is really just opinion, fiction or fashion. Times change and we learn from improved evidence and our mistakes, but always through the prism of our culture and upbringing.

And so it is with the story of everyday clinical practice. For most of us, medical training cannot prepare us for every possible clinical problem or for the expectations of today's consumers or the consumers of the future. We are regularly presented with problems, some of which cannot be solved with the tools of our particular trade as we originally learnt it. This is no reflection on us as individual practitioners, or on our profession. Just as we do not have the training or the skills to remove a cerebral aneurysm or perform an anterior resection, we may not practise acupuncture or hypnotherapy, but we do see patients who will benefit from those treatments and happily refer them to skilled practitioners when it is appropriate.

Through expanding our own awareness and skill, we can expand the options available to our patients, by looking at the evidence for an integrative approach and by working in cooperation with other practitioners.

Professor Kerryn Phelps
Dr Craig Hassed

chapter 2

Evidence-based healthcare

INTRODUCTION AND OVERVIEW

This chapter covers some of the generic issues related to evidence-based medicine (EBM), with particular emphasis on how these apply to integrative general practice and complementary therapies. Although EBM principles are a vital part of the armamentarium of the modern doctor, they are a two-edged sword.

MEDICAL OPINION VERSUS EVIDENCE

Traditionally, doctors in training have looked to 'expert opinion' from senior medical staff as their primary source of guidance on clinical decision-making. Their long experience and learning from prior generations of medical experts was deemed sufficient authority and was rarely questioned. Then the general practitioner (GP) would also add their personal clinical experience as it was gathered over the years to formulate and adapt their particular approach to clinical problems.

As simple and intuitive as this approach is, it has always had deficiencies. Our perceptions, attitudes and range of options can be informed by expert opinion, but equally they can be limited or biased by them. A recent study concluded that:

> The vast majority of exotic expert opinions expressed by senior staff members during grand rounds are not evidence-based. Thus, great care must be taken to ensure that exotic expert opinion is not accepted as factual without careful review. Furthermore, this study shows that … seniority is … negatively associated with reviewing the merits of such opinion.[1a]

Put another way, when we are confident of our opinions, and have had them handed down to us from respected authorities without question, and when we are not questioned about the validity of our opinions, we are less likely to determine whether they are based on evidence.

POTENTIAL AND LIMITATIONS OF EBM

As history is written, the exponential growth in EBM gained momentum in the late twentieth century. Published data increasingly revealed:

- effective medical treatments not being widely used
- ineffective treatments continuing to be used, and
- unacceptable adverse effects going unrecognised.

The Cochrane Collaboration was formed out of this movement, and its systematic reviews follow a transparent process 'intended to minimise bias'. We accept this as almost a motherhood statement, but the processes inherent in EBM contain a number of major flaws.

In recent decades, EBM has rightly assumed a leading role in informing medical practice. Stratifying and analysing the results of all published trials for a disease or an intervention provides some guidance on the three pillars—quality, safety and efficacy—and allows for comparisons to be made. To make clinical decisions and formulate clinical guidelines that are contrary to evidence is at best ineffectual and wasteful of resources, and at worst harmful to the patient.

However, a bland statement that the clinician should make decisions that are evidence-based is not as simple as it seems, for a number of reasons.

- In many areas of medicine, there is little evidence with which to make an informed decision one way or the other.
- Evidence can be and often is ambiguous.
- Evidence will often give a guide to what might work overall but may not be relevant or adapted to suit an individual patient.

- Interpretation of evidence can be influenced by factors such as researcher bias or predominant opinion.
- The evidence available to clinicians can be heavily influenced by publication bias and the marketing agenda of pharmaceutical companies.
- The research agenda can be influenced by what is popular or patentable, and many important topics or interventions therefore receive little funding for research.
- Lack of evidence of an effect is not evidence of a lack of effect.

EBM can provide answers to the following questions.

- *Can it work? (efficacy)*
  - Some things look like they should work in principle, but do not work so well in practice.
- *Does it work? (effectiveness)*
  - Some things produce the expected effect, but it can be clinically inconsequential.
- *Is it worth it? (efficiency)*
  - The financial or time-related costs may be so considerable, and the benefits so marginal, that the therapy is not worth the trouble. Health economists are constantly looking at medical practice from this perspective.
- *Is it harmful? (safety)*
  - Harmful effects being common, or uncommon but major, may preclude the therapy from being desirable for doctor or patient.
- *How does it work? (mechanisms)*
  - Often we know something works, such as acupuncture for pain, but we know little about the mechanisms by which those effects are produced. Alternatively, we might understand the mechanism whereby a therapy should work, such as shark cartilage for cancer, but the outcomes do not support the expectation.

Some particular limitations of EBM in the general practice setting are summarised by Stephenson:[2]

- In general practice, questions are not always easy to define—for example, multiple and ill-defined problems, complex psychosocial issues, diagnosis not always established.
- Many problems are poorly researched in general practice—data from hospital studies and tertiary centres may not be applicable to the general practice situation.
- GPs may not have the time or expertise to evaluate the literature.

It is for these reasons that the best approach to clinical decision-making will combine knowledge of the best available evidence with:

- the individual clinical circumstances of the patient
- associated comorbidities
- the experience and skills of the practitioner
- the clinician's informed judgment and intuition.

Many complementary therapies are particularly affected by the points raised above. Naturally occurring products, for example, are not patentable, and so they don't attract the large research budgets that patentable pharmaceuticals do. Even where there is mounting evidence that a particular complementary therapy is safe and effective, it is often treated with scepticism by the medical mainstream because it falls outside the imaginary boundary of conventional medical practice. As clinicians we need to be interested in what is safe, works and is cost-effective regardless of which side of an artificially created demarcation line between complementary and conventional therapies it comes from.

LEVELS OF EVIDENCE

EBM experts tend to refer to the 'level of evidence' for or against a particular therapy or intervention. Broadly speaking there are four main levels of evidence, although there are subdivisions within these:

- *Level 1* Systematic review or meta-analysis of rigorous randomised controlled trials (RCTs)
- *Level 2* At least one RCT
- *Level 3* Non-randomised controlled trials
- *Level 4* Descriptive studies or accepted medical opinion.

Obviously, level 1 evidence is considered the highest; the relative weight given to each of the others diminishes as you go down the levels. In reality, however, it is not as simple as this. For various reasons, some interventions or issues do not lend themselves to RCTs or cannot attract the necessary funding for high-quality RCTs and will therefore never have level 1 evidence supporting them. This does not mean that they are invalid, but simply that one needs to be flexible in interpreting evidence and that EBM needs to be supported by common sense and clinical experience.

Meta-analyses also rely on the publication of all available studies. Because publication bias is more likely to exclude negative findings, meta-analyses of published studies tend to skew to positive findings.

EBM reviews sometimes provide challenging findings. For example, a meta-analysis published in *The Lancet* gave surprising results on the efficacy of homeopathy, finding that the odds ratio for positive trial results was 2.45 in favour of homeopathy.[3] Though more high-quality RCTs are required, either homeopathy is clinically effective for a range of conditions or there is a publication bias in favour of homeopathy. Thus, even with 'level 1 evidence' a clinician still needs to interpret the findings and decide what to make of them.

Patients and the general public are often not aware of levels of evidence, and nor can they easily interpret evidence for themselves. Furthermore, they can be significantly affected by misleading marketing. The GP therefore has a vitally important role in helping people to:

- access quality information
- sift and interpret that information
- apply it to that person's particular clinical circumstances.

The evidence that most patients regard first and foremost is the evidence from their own personal experience or the experience of people close to them. The question most relevant to them is, 'Does it work for me?' A doctor telling a patient that a therapy, such as a herbal treatment, is not supported by evidence when it is clearly providing benefit for them will not convince them and could alienate them from the doctor. It may be more useful to say that it has been little researched but that the person's experience is also a valid form of evidence. It is also unconvincing for the patient to be told that a therapy is well supported by evidence when it is not working or they are experiencing side effects that are worse than the condition for which they are being treated. Thus the findings and recommendations arising from EBM need to be interpreted and communicated with sensitivity and in a way that is appropriate to the individual patient.

CAM RESEARCH

For many complementary therapies it is difficult to attract research dollars. From a marketing perspective, products that are not patentable are a less desirable topic of investigation. Independent research funds are therefore often the only avenue available for CAM researchers. Without such research data, clinicians and patients are making less-informed decisions. In Australia, independent funds for CAM research were provided for the first time in 2008. With the establishment of the National Center for Complementary and Alternative Medicine (NCCAM) in the USA there was a rapid rise in research funds and competitive grants won for CAM research.

By and large, there are too few studies of most complementary therapies, and those that are done are often of poor quality, due to limited funds or inexperienced researchers. Nevertheless, the number of CAM citations in the medical literature has grown exponentially in recent years.

EVIDENCE AND COMPLEX INTERVENTIONS

Another problem with CAM research is that many therapies are practised 'holistically', with the therapy being individualised to the patient, and some therapies—such as acupuncture, lifestyle interventions and counselling—present difficulties with placebo trials and blinding. This means that it is much harder to perform RCTs on many CAM modalities in the Western paradigm.

Another question that arises around whether EBM is the only arbiter of quality, safety and efficacy is whether the RCT is as applicable to complex interventions as it is to single-substance pharmaceutical interventions. Compared with drug trials or trials of surgical procedures, the design and development of a trial of an integrated intervention or therapy is far more complex. Randomised trials alone may not be able to tell us why an intervention was or was not successful, or which part might have been.

This is not an argument against providing evidence for CAM but is an argument for being more flexible and creative in the way that CAM research is carried out. Even when there is useful evidence available, it is not always easy for doctors to become aware of this evidence or to have it reported in an unbiased way.

A SYSTEMATIC APPROACH TO EVIDENCE

Because of limited time and skills in searching the medical literature, many GPs look to educational seminars and conferences, or up-to-date review articles in general practice or family medicine journals that are tailored to GP management of various conditions. It is assumed that the speaker or author has reviewed the evidence in an objective and unbiased way and is able to clearly summarise it. Such articles and talks can be a simple, helpful and time-efficient way to get an overview of a topic, but there are potential limitations. The material may be presented by a specialist who does not understand the particulars of general practice mentioned above, or it may be less objective and unbiased than we would hope for.

Exploring a clinical question or decision for oneself can be very informative and excellent practice in critical thinking. Box 2.1 gives an outline of a systematic approach to exploring an issue through EBM.

Having skills and knowledge about how and where to find reliable evidence is a prerequisite for the above-mentioned approach. (Some resources are listed at the end of this chapter.) It takes time to learn to search the medical literature in an efficient and targeted way. Using the right search words and strategy can mean the difference between a long, fruitless search and a short, fruitful one.

PUBLICATION BIAS

A clinician can only make decisions based on the quality of evidence or advice that is available. We generally trust

BOX 2.1 An approach to evidence-based medicine

Step 1 Identify the need for information to inform a decision and then frame the question.
Step 2 Find the best evidence to answer the question.
Step 3 Critically appraise the evidence for *validity* (is it true), *impact* (effect size) and *applicability* (relevance to your practice).
Step 4 Integrate the results of the appraisal with your clinical judgment, the circumstances and the patient's values.
Step 5 Evaluate your performance and reflect on ways to improve performance.

(from Sackett et al[4])

that when we consult a medical database or the opinion of an expert body we will receive unbiased and objective information. Unfortunately, this is often not the case. All evidence is not equal.

Retail spending on prescription drugs in the USA climbed from $US78.9 billion to $US154.5 billion between 1997 and 2001.[5] With such amounts at stake, market forces commonly influence research, publication and the interpretation of research data. Thus, even with the best intentions, the basis upon which clinicians make decisions will often be biased as a result. For example, pharmaceutical companies have an interest in promoting antidepressant prescribing. Not only is it advantageous to increase the potential market—for example, prescribing for younger patients—but it is also advantageous to lower the threshold for prescribing. However, although most of the antidepressant trials published show a positive effect, in many of these trials the data have been interpreted in a way that makes the findings look more positive than they really are, and almost none of the negative trials are published.[6] The actual effect size of antidepressants is more than 30% lower than published trials would have one believe. A fuller analysis of both the published and the unpublished data suggests that antidepressants actually have no more than a placebo effect for mild to moderate depression and only a marginal effect for severe depression,[7] with approximately 80% of the clinical effect being attributable to the placebo response.[8] Concerns about the effect of publication bias on other medication categories such as chemotherapy also exist.[9]

For systematic reviews to be meaningful, there needs to be an assessment of all trials, positive and negative, and complete honesty and transparency about findings. Although we like to think that drugs which make it to market have been intensively scrutinised, researchers from the University of California, San Francisco, found troubling evidence of suppression and manipulation of data in studies published in (or often withheld from) peer-reviewed medical journals.[10] They compared the information that companies shared with the USA's Food and Drug Administration (FDA) about those drugs on application for approval to market, with what was eventually published in medical journals. Only three-quarters of the original trials were ever published, and those with positive outcomes were nearly five times as likely to be published as those that were negative. There may be many reasons for this—commercial reasons for the pharmaceutical companies, professional or academic issues for the researchers who want to be associated with a 'successful' drug development, decisions by the editors of peer-reviewed journals who may feel that positive results make better reading and give them headlines in the mainstream press.

The huge investment in getting pharmaceuticals to market also brings with it a reluctance to reveal adverse outcome data, as we saw in the case of Celebrex and Vioxx (the COX 2 inhibitors), as well as the wholesale prescription of hormone replacement therapy (HRT) to perimenopausal and menopausal women prior to the release of the Million Women Study and the Women's Health Initiative Study showing the relationship between HRT and increased rates of breast cancer and myocardial infarction.

MEDICAL PRACTICE, MARKETING AND EBM

The entanglement of clinical medicine with the pharmaceutical industry is widespread and has almost infinite potential to influence practice.[11] Many expert bodies that determine therapeutic guidelines have multiple members with conflicts of interest due to their association with pharmaceutical companies. Sponsors of medical educational seminars and conferences are also known to influence the speaker list and content. Many of the medical stories promoted by the media are industry-driven, although this is rarely transparent to consumers or doctors.[12] Transparency is therefore a vital part of a doctor's ability to make an informed decision about how much weight to give to a particular guideline or opinion.

Many common medical practices that had been accepted for decades have been found to be contrary to evidence when tested by studies. For example:

- Most antibiotic prescriptions, even for conditions such as childhood otitis media, have little evidence to support their use.[13]
- Routine admissions of uncomplicated twin pregnancies produce worse outcomes for mothers and babies than women with uncomplicated twin pregnancies staying at home.[14,15]
- Arthroscopic knee surgery in osteoarthritis is no better than placebo.[16]

- Antidepressants are probably no better than placebo for all but severe depression.[7]
- The improvement in 5-year survival for the 22 major adult malignancies that can be attributed to chemotherapy is approximately 2%.[17]

Well-supported, safe and effective therapies such as omega-3 fatty acids in the management of hyperlipidaemia, glucosamine for osteoarthritis and exercise for improving cancer survival should be considered first-line therapy options. Rapidity in adopting newly approved pharmaceutical treatments, slowness in rationalising or ceasing use of a conventional therapy or practice that is unfounded, or slowness in adopting an unconventional therapy that is well founded, points to factors other than evidence affecting clinical decisions. These factors could include such things as marketing, peer expectations, medico-legal concerns, political forces, complacency and habit.

There are other CAM modalities for which there is no convincing evidence, such as iridology or Vega machines as diagnostic tools. These may waste resources but be harmless enough unless the advice given about their use misleads the patient or delays important diagnosis and treatment. Patient concerns, fears and expectations can have a significant impact on a doctor's clinical decisions, for better or worse. For example, in some countries pharmaceutical companies can market drugs directly to patients. Advertising aimed at encouraging patients to request a drug from a doctor will increase many-fold the likelihood that the doctor will prescribe the medication even in the absence of any clinical indication. Similar concerns can arise about the inappropriate use of CAM, particularly where patient fears are greatest, such as in cancer patients.

What lessons can we glean from the abovementioned examples? First, even with the best intentions, standard medical practice is often contrary to guidelines, and guidelines can be contrary to evidence. Sometimes the continued use of unproven therapies can be costly or produce adverse events. Unfortunately, industry rather than good evidence often drives practice, leading to inappropriate practice and over-prescribing. This, combined with a lack of healthy scepticism about therapies, whether conventional or complementary, can have significantly negative effects for doctors, patients and the healthcare system.

'THERE IS NO EVIDENCE'

When someone such as a medical colleague or authority states that 'there is no evidence' for a particular therapy, it is useful to stop and reflect upon the fact that this statement could mean a number of things. It could, for example, mean that:

- studies suggest that the evidence is negative—that is, the therapy is not helpful or is possibly harmful
- studies suggest that the evidence is inconclusive
- studies suggest that the evidence is positive, but the doctor is unaware of the evidence and so concludes that there is no evidence
- there is evidence, but only from empirical studies or from studies using a different paradigm
- the therapy has not been studied yet.

Healthy scepticism and an enquiring and open mind are vital for the doctor who wishes to practise an informed form of EBM.

RESOURCES

Carefully chosen textbooks and subscription to peer-reviewed journals can help to provide ready access to quality information. For more specific questions or issues, medical and psychological databases can provide published studies and review articles, and some also have consumer databases that are useful to recommend to patients. Learning how to search a medical database efficiently takes practice and some guidance from experienced peers. Some of the most authoritative databases include:

- Medline
- PubMed
- Cochrane Library
- Psychinfo.

Databases and websites with information specifically on CAM

Alternative and Complementary Medicine Centre, www.healthy.net/clinic/therapy/index.asp

Alternative and Complementary Therapies, http://www.liebertpub.com/act (a Medline-listed journal)

Alternative Medicine Foundation, HerbMed, http://www.herbmed.org (valuable information about herbs and drug–herb interactions)

National Cancer Institute, http://www.cancer.gov/cancertopics/factsheet/therapy/CAM (US site with useful oncology information)

NHS Evidence, http://www.library.nhs.uk/cam/ (comprehensive and easy to use, with good links)

National Institutes of Health, National Center for CAM, http://www.nccam.nih.gov/health/

Research Council for Complementary Medicine, http://www.rccm.org.uk/cameol/Default.aspx (excellent source of information and easy to navigate)

REFERENCES

1 Linthorst G, Daniels J, Van Westerloo D. The majority of bold statements expressed during grand rounds lack scientific merit. Med Educ 2007; 41(10):965–967. a p 965.

2 Stephenson A. A textbook of general practice. 2nd edn. London: Arnold; 2004.
3 Linde K, Clausius N, Ramirez G et al. Are the clinical effects of homeopathy placebo effects? A meta-analysis of placebo controlled trials. Lancet 1997; 350(9081):834–843.
4 Sackett D, Straus S, Richardson W et al. Evidence-based medicine: how to practise and teach EBM. 2nd edn. Edinburgh: Churchill Livingstone; 2000.
5 National Institute for Health Care Management Research and Educational Foundation. Report on drug prices. 2002:2. Online. Available: http://www.nihcm.org/spending2001.pdf
6 Turner EH, Matthews AM, Linardatos E et al. Selective publication of antidepressant trials and its influence on apparent efficacy. N Engl J Med 2008; 358(3):252–260.
7 Kirsch I, Deacon BJ, Huedo-Medina TB et al. Initial severity and antidepressant benefits: a meta-analysis of data submitted to the Food and Drug Administration. PLoS Medicine 2008; 5(2):e45 doi:10.1371/journal.pmed.0050045
8 Kirsch I, Moore TJ, Scoboria A et al. The emperor's new drugs: an analysis of antidepressant medication data submitted to the US Food and Drug Administration. 2002; Prev Treat 5 article 23. Online. Available: http://journals.apa.org/prevention/volume5/pre0050023a.html.
9 Peppercorn J, Blood E, Winer E et al. Association between pharmaceutical involvement and outcomes in breast cancer clinical trials. Cancer 2007; 109(7): 1239–1246.
10 Rising K, Bacchetti P, Bero L. Reporting bias in drug trials submitted to the food and drug administration: review of publication and presentation. PLoS 2008; 5(11):e217. doi:10.1371/journal.pmed.0050217. Online. Available: http://medicine.plosjournals.org/perlserv/?request=get-document&doi=10.1371/journal.pmed.0050217&ct=1
11 Moynihan R. Who pays for the pizza? Redefining the relationships between doctors and drug companies. 1: Entanglement. BMJ 2003; 326(7400):1189–1192.
12 Moynihan R, Bero L, Ross-Degnan D et al. Coverage by the news media of the benefits and risks of medications. N Engl J Med 2000; 342(22):1645–1650.
13 Thompson PL, Gilbert RE, Long PF et al. Has UK guidance affected general practitioner antibiotic prescribing for otitis media in children? J Pub Health (Oxf) 2008; 30(4):479–486.
14 MacLennan A, Green R, O'Shea R et al. Routine hospital admission in twin pregnancy between 26 and 30 weeks gestation. Lancet 1990; 335(8684):267–269.
15 Andrews W, Leveno K, Sherman M et al. Elective hositalisation in the management of twin pregnancy. Obstet Gynecol 1991; 77(6):826–831.
16 Nutton RW. Is arthroscopic surgery a beneficial treatment for knee osteoarthritis? Nat Clin Pract Rheumatol 2009; 5(3):122–123.
17 Morgan G, Ward R, Barton M. The contribution of cytotoxic chemotherapy to 5-year survival in adult malignancies. Clin Oncol 2005; 16(8):549–560.

chapter 3

Therapeutic modalities in integrative medicine

INTRODUCTION

In general practice, time and training can limit us to using only a narrow range of modalities in order to promote wellbeing or manage a patient's illness. This could be likened to using only one or two octaves of a keyboard. The medical and surgical options are like one octave that we are familiar with, and lifestyle factors may be another, but a range of other modalities can be made available, given time, training and some rearranging of the practice.

This chapter examines some of the language and the main modalities used in integrative medicine. Many of these are outlined in more detail in other chapters, in the context of particular conditions and systems. One important distinction in the mind of the GP will be to determine which are effective and, even more importantly, which are safe and which are not. It is vital to help patients make informed decisions that will increase their wellbeing wherever possible, or at least not to cause them harm. There are legitimate concerns if patients forgo effective medical therapies in order to use complementary therapies that might be unsafe or of lesser efficacy.

DEFINITIONS

This section explains the following terms, which are commonly used in integrative medicine and complementary therapies:

- integrative medicine
- orthodox (conventional) medicine
- unorthodox medicine
- alternative medicine
- complementary medicine
- complementary and alternative medicine
- natural medicine
- holistic medicine.

INTEGRATIVE MEDICINE

As has been discussed previously, *integrative medicine* (IM) refers to the practice of medicine that incorporates evidence-based and safe therapies, whatever their origin. There is particular emphasis on safety, holism and complementarities. IM uses conventional medical care, but lifestyle interventions and evidence-based complementary medicine are also given a significant level of attention and may be used as a range of possible alternatives or as adjuncts. Used properly, IM is not 'alternative practice' but 'best practice'.

ORTHODOX (CONVENTIONAL) MEDICINE

The term *orthodox medicine* (OM) (also called *conventional medicine*) is used to denote what is widely taught in medical schools, and is accepted clinical practice by most practitioners. Definitions of OM generally link it with being 'scientific' or 'evidence-based' but this is not always a good distinguishing factor between orthodox and unorthodox therapies. One would not have to search too far to find instances of widely used and promoted orthodox therapies not being based on science or evidence, or examples of therapies that have been shown by long-term follow-up studies to have caused more harm than anticipated.

UNORTHODOX MEDICINE

The term *unorthodox medicine* is sometimes used to denote those therapies that are not generally taught in medical schools or widely accepted in clinical practice. They are also sometimes referred to as *unconventional medicine.* By definition, unorthodox therapies are 'non-scientific' or not based on credible science or evidence, because if they were then they would be orthodox. However, this is not always the case, as there are an increasing number of examples of treatments that are not widely accepted or practised but are well supported by evidence. The boundary between orthodox and unorthodox therapies is shifting and often indistinct. For example, acupuncture would have been outside the boundary 30 years ago, but today, with a significant evidence base and approximately 90% of Australian GPs referring patients for acupuncture, it could no longer be considered an unorthodox therapy.

ALTERNATIVE MEDICINE

Alternative can have a number of meanings. It can mean that there are a number of potentially useful approaches to treatment which could be employed, such as whether to use a benzodiazepine, meditation or melatonin for insomnia, or taking glucosamine instead of NSAIDs for osteoarthritis. It can also denote that a patient wishes to reject conventional healthcare and prefers instead to use an alternative approach to therapy. This latter situation may or may not be a problem. It is certainly a problem when the conventional treatment being offered is clearly efficacious and the preferred alternative treatment is not, such as wishing to reject primary surgery for malignant melanoma and preferring ozone therapy instead. In such a case, patient autonomy is going beyond the bounds of safety and reason—after having fully and respectfully listened to the patient's point of view, the doctor needs to clearly inform the patient about the evidence, costs, benefits, risks and safety issues.

COMPLEMENTARY MEDICINE

The term *complementary medicine* (CM) is in far more common usage than 'alternative medicine' because it better reflects the attitude of most patients wishing to seek out such therapies. Most patients do not wish to reject conventional medical care but simply feel that it is incomplete and needs to be enhanced or broadened by other approaches. CM therefore denotes therapies that are used to complement, or be adjuncts to, conventional treatments so as to:

- enhance outcomes—e.g. a man taking pomegranate juice as a part of his management for prostate cancer
- minimise side effects—e.g. using acupuncture to help control nausea, or meditation to control stress
- reduce costs—e.g. using the Ornish lifestyle programs to minimise progression of heart disease.

COMPLEMENTARY AND ALTERNATIVE MEDICINE

Complementary and alternative medicine (CAM) is a less specific but widely used term, particularly in the United States. It encompasses both alternative medicine and CM.

NATURAL MEDICINE

Natural medicine generally relies on the use of naturally derived products such as herbs, diet or vitamins but can also encompass lifestyle and environmental issues. It can be seen as a philosophy as much as a form of medicine. These therapies are generally aimed at enhancing nature's ability to heal (e.g. using diet to improve immunity) or boosting the body's defences. It does not always distinguish well between conventional medicine and CM, because many therapies used in conventional medicine are 'natural' and some therapies used by CM practitioners may not be natural. Although most natural therapies do well in terms of safety, being 'natural' does not necessarily mean being safe. Some herbs or high doses of vitamins have interactions and side effects that can be problematic.

HOLISTIC MEDICINE

Holistic medicine generally denotes a philosophy that informs therapies or approaches to practice. The holistic approach encompasses body, mind, social, spiritual, lifestyle and environmental factors. It might be delivered by one therapist or a number of therapists working together. It does not necessarily distinguish between conventional medicine and CM, as many conventional therapies and practitioners are holistically oriented and some therapies used by CM practitioners may not be.

GP USE OF CAM

Primary care physicians in the developed world are integrating a range of complementary therapies into their practices either by delivering the therapy themselves or by referring patients to practitioners (Table 3.1). The therapies most integrated tend to be those that the doctor believes are based on good evidence and/or are safest.[1] Four therapies with particularly high referral rates are acupuncture, meditation, hypnosis and chiropractic. Herbal medicine, naturopathy and osteopathy also have referral rates of close to 30%. In terms of doctors practising complementary therapies, vitamin therapy is most frequently used, followed by acupuncture, meditation and hypnosis. Despite the increasing prevalence of use of CM, medical education has been slow to incorporate these topics into the curriculum.

MODALITIES OF CAM

There are five categories of CAM, according to the most widely accepted classification from the National Center for Complementary and Alternative Medicine (NCCAM) in the United States:[3]

- alternative medical systems
- mind–body therapies

TABLE 3.1 Rates of practice and referral for complementary therapies by Australian GPs

	Ever referred (%)	Have practised (%)
Acupuncture	89.6	19.0
Meditation	79.6	15.3
Hypnosis	81.6	8.7
Chiropractic	68.5	5.0
Herbal medicine	29.1	4.8
Naturopathy	29.7	3.2
Vitamin therapy	16.9	25.1
Homeopathy	19.2	2.5
Osteopathy	29.6	2.8
Aromatherapy	17.5	1.1
Spiritual healing	19.5	2.1
Reflexology	10.1	0.5

Source: Pirotta et al[2]

- biologically based therapies
- manipulative and body-based therapies
- energy-based therapies.

ALTERNATIVE MEDICAL SYSTEMS

Alternative medical systems are generally comprehensive healthcare systems, often embedded within a culture. They are holistic in focus and are underpinned by a philosophy of healthcare as much as by therapeutic techniques. These philosophies are naturalistic and generally metaphysical, with bioenergetic explanations for physical phenomena. Indigenous medicine, Ayurveda and traditional Chinese medicine are examples of such systems. Some would also classify naturopathy as an example of an alternative system. Embedded within them are generally a range of techniques including herbal medicine, contemplative practices, approaches to exercise, body-based therapies such as acupuncture, and even moral codes. These systems often have a long tradition with a strong emphasis on respect for the healing power of nature, including fostering the body's defences, integration with the environment and the use of natural products. Their descriptions of the origin of and cures for diseases are often significantly at variance with conventional Western biomedicine. Regardless of whether we accept these explanations for the causes of and cures for diseases, undoubtedly these systems incorporate a wide range of effective therapies and strategies.

Ayurveda (from the Sanskrit *ayur* = life, *veda* = knowledge) is the traditional Indian healing system and incorporates lifestyle advice, herbs, meditation, body typing (doshas) and yoga. The yoga system is said to have eight 'limbs' or branches incorporating physical, psychological, mental, social and spiritual health, as well as disciplines such as meditation and lifestyle modification, and the more widely known postures and breathing techniques. Traditional Chinese medicine (TCM) is, again, more than just acupuncture and Chinese herbs. It also incorporates movement therapies (e.g. t'ai chi), breathing and meditation. Naturopathy can be seen by some as just the use of herbs but in its fullest sense it is underpinned by a 'naturalistic' philosophy. Patients will often use aspects of these alternative systems without adopting the underlying philosophy—such as using acupuncture for chronic pain—although in a purist sense, this would be seen as less congruent and less effective.

MIND–BODY THERAPIES

Many mind–body therapies are now considered largely mainstream and are used by the majority of doctors. They include stress management, relaxation therapies, meditation, imagery, biofeedback, prayer, humour, mindfulness, journal keeping and hypnosis. Support groups, family therapy and cognitive behaviour therapy can also be used to facilitate healing or for coping with physical illnesses and so these are also classified as mind–body therapies. Of all the modalities, mind–body probably has the most sound evidence base. A review of mind–body therapies found that:

> Drawing principally from systematic reviews and meta-analyses, there is considerable evidence of efficacy for several mind–body therapies in the treatment of coronary artery disease, headaches, insomnia, incontinence, chronic low back pain, disease and treatment-related symptoms of cancer and improving post-surgical outcomes.[4a]

This is not reflective of the limitations of mind–body therapies, but an indication of how far the research has progressed.

BIOLOGICALLY BASED THERAPIES

Biologically based therapies include those that use biologically active compounds, most of which are naturally occurring. These would most often include food, herbs, vitamins and supplements, but could also include things such as homeopathic remedies and essential oils used in aromatherapy. Much of the rationale for herbal therapies comes from the philosophy that whole-plant compounds include a range of co-factors, vitamins and nutrients that would not be available if one biologically active ingredient were isolated, measured and administered. Such an approach is said to improve efficacy and minimise side effects. Many pharmaceuticals, of course, are derived from plants, including aspirin, digoxin, penicillin, quinine and metformin, to name a few. Although most biologically based therapies are safer than their pharmacological counterparts, they are biologically active and can interact with drugs, and so it is important to know what patients are taking and to check potential interactions.

MANIPULATIVE AND BODY-BASED THERAPIES

These physical therapies are, like other categories, diverse and widely used. They include:

- *chiropractic* and *osteopathy*—both use spinal manipulation of high or low impact. Although these approaches can be effective for a wide range of back and neck complaints (disc prolapse would be considered a contraindication) as well as headache, it is less certain whether the chiropractic explanation—that the origin of most illnesses is related to spinal malalignment—is accurate, or whether chiropractic and osteopathy are effective for many other conditions for which they are commonly used
- *massage*—the many varieties can be broadly categorised into therapeutic massage and relaxation massage. Massage can be beneficial for a wide range of physical and psychological conditions and symptoms
- *reflexology* and *shiatsu*—these therapies rely on a combination of massage and pressure, and incorporate acupressure points and energy flow
- *acupuncture*—this is part of TCM and is said to work with changing 'energy flow' throughout the body, and therefore is also sometimes classified as an 'energy' therapy. It is clearly effective for many conditions, but not all for which it is used. Its mechanism of action is still not well understood.

ENERGY-BASED THERAPIES

There are two main types of energy therapies:

- *biofield therapies*—such as qi gong, reiki and therapeutic touch; these use the body's own energy flow
- *bioenergetic therapies*—these generally involve the use of pulsed electromagnetic fields, such as pulsed fields, magnetic fields, or alternating-current and/or alternating and direct-current fields.

Energy therapies are probably the least researched and hardest to validate, although some positive outcomes have been found, mostly in controlling symptoms. The mechanisms of action are difficult to explain. Other philosophical systems that have 'bioenergetic' explanations include qi gong, acupuncture, TCM and yoga.

RESOURCES

Alternative and Complementary Therapies and Journal of Alternative and Complementary Medicine, http://www.liebertpub.com/act (main Medline-listed journals focusing on CAM)

Alternative Medicine Center, http://www.healthy.net/clinic/therapy/index.asp (has a workable database and searches for practitioners)

Australasian Integrative Medicine Association, http://www.aima.net.au (peak umbrella body for integrative medicine in Australasia)

Cochrane reviews, Medline, PubMed

IMgateway, http://www.imgateway.net/page.jsp?p_name=Home (Australian organisation that collates data and networks people)

National Foundation for Alternative Medicine, http://www.nfam.org

US government, National Center for CAM, http://www.nccam.nih.gov (a good place to start, with guidance for therapists considering adopting CAM)

REFERENCES

1 Cohen MM, Penman S, Pirotta M et al. The integration of complementary therapies in Australian general practice: results of a national survey. J Altern Complement Med 2005; 11(6):995–1004.

2 Pirotta MV, Cohen MM, Kotsirilos V et al. Complementary therapies: have they become accepted in general practice? Med J Aust 2007; 172(3):105–109.

3 National Center for Complementary and Alternative Medicine (NCCAM). What are the major types of complementary and alternative medicine? Online. Available: www.nccam.nih.gov

4 Astin JA, Shapiro SL, Eisenberg DM et al. Mind–body medicine: state of the science, implications for practice. Am Board Fam Pract 2003; 16(2):131–147. a p 131.

chapter 4

Principles of herbal medicine

INTRODUCTION

Throughout human history, people have relied on nature to provide their basic needs. Plants in particular have been a source of clothing, shelter, food, flavours and fragrances. Importantly, plants have also formed the basis of numerous traditional medicinal systems around the world, including Ayurveda (Indian), traditional Chinese medicine, Unani (Persian) and European. Herbs used within these healing systems have given rise to many of the drugs used in contemporary Western medical practice and continue to be a source of therapeutic medicines for many people (see Table 4.1). While many of the time-honoured attributes of herbal medicines have been confirmed with scientific testing and have proved to be significant and still extremely useful, others have proved to be erroneous.

Today, herbal medicine (or phytomedicine) can be broadly defined as both the science and the art of using botanical medicines to prevent and treat illness, and the study and investigation of these medicines.[1] The term *phytotherapy* is used to describe the therapeutic application of herbal medicines, and was first coined by the French physician Henri Leclerc (1870–1955), who published numerous essays on the use of medicinal plants.[2] Herbal medicine has come a long way since the days of ancient 'herbalism', especially in regards to growing and manufacturing techniques, quality control and the steady accumulation of scientific evidence to elucidate mechanisms of action, efficacy and safety.

TABLE 4.1 Examples of pharmaceutical drugs derived from plants

Drug	Herb
Aspirin	Meadowsweet
Atropine	*Atropa belladonna*
Caffeine	*Camellia sinensis*
Cocaine	*Erythroxylum coca*
Colchicine	Autumn crocus
Digoxin	*Digitalis purpurea*
Ephedrine	*Ephedra sinica*
Morphine	*Papaver somniferum*
Pilocarpine	*Pilocarpus* species
Paclitaxel	Pacific yew
Theophylline	*Theobroma cacao* and others
Vincristine	Madagascar periwinkle

HERBS, DRUGS AND PHYTOCHEMICALS

Botanical medicines are chemically complex substances with many different constituents. For example, a herbal medicine may contain mucilage, essential oils, macro- and micronutrients such as fats and carbohydrates, proteins and enzymes. They also contain many other phytochemicals such as secondary metabolites, which form the plant's natural defence against herbivores, pathogens, insect attack and microbial decomposition, or are produced in response to injury or infection or used for signalling and growth regulation. Secondary metabolites are important in herbal medicine as they are often the constituents responsible for producing the herb's main therapeutic effects. Examples of secondary metabolites are tannins, isoflavones, saponins, flavonoids, glycosides, coumarins, bitters and phyto-oestrogens.[3]

It can be tempting to adopt a reductionist approach and attribute a herb's activity to one particular active constituent; however, this is rarely the case as the herb's pharmacological activity depends on the composition of the whole extract. Other constituents, even those with no direct physiological effect, may influence the uptake, distribution, metabolism and excretion of other components. Furthermore, this background matrix may affect the solubility, stability and bioavailability of any given compound.

CHEMICAL DIVERSITY

As herbal medicines are not produced synthetically and contain a myriad naturally occurring components, chemical diversity is always present. In herbal medicine, it is essential to use the correct species and type of plant, and plant part, and understand the growing, harvesting and manufacturing processes involved that influence the chemical make-up of the final product.

Interestingly, the wine and beer industries manipulate these same factors to achieve the multitude of variations available for their products. And as any wine drinker knows, wine produced one year from a particular vineyard will be different from one produced the following year, and wines of the same grape variety will also differ between vineyards.

Many commercial herbal medicine manufacturers are also using sophisticated methods of evaluating the influence of various growing, harvesting and extracting techniques as a means of producing consistently high-quality herbal medicines. In order to detect variations between batches, manufacturers use laboratory techniques such as thin layer chromatography (TLC) and high-performance liquid chromatography (HPLC), both of which provide a visual characterisation of the presence of different chemical constituents within the herb. The graphs produced from TLC and HPLC testing are often referred to as 'fingerprints' and used to determine the identity of herbal material and the integrity of the extraction process, as well as to measure quantities of individual constituents.

CLINICAL RELEVANCE

Having an appreciation of the chemical diversity of herbal medicines is vital when interpreting findings from clinical trials.

Readers should identify the particular herbal extract used, because the composition of products varies between manufacturers, and evidence of efficacy (and safety) should be considered extract specific. At best, evidence can be extrapolated only to preparations of the same herb with a very similar phytochemical profile, although even this is not completely accurate.

Unfortunately, many early trials did not provide sufficient details about the herb or extract used and some did not test samples to confirm the identity of the plant or that samples actually contained sufficient active constituents. This is a critical oversight. Clinical trials using herbal extracts that have not been adequately defined in phytochemical terms are of questionable value because we cannot know whether a negative result was because the herb was lacking in activity or because the extract was of inadequate quality. This requires a shift of thinking in Western research, which is used to dealing with pharmaceutical drugs that tend to consist of only one standardised chemical entity and need relatively little description.

Phytochemical analysis is also important when case reports of adverse events are evaluated, to ensure the authenticity of the herbal medicine and identify whether confounding influences such as contamination or adulteration are present. Until testing is performed, conclusions regarding herbal medicines are open to error.

The herb St John's wort is a useful example of the clinical relevance of chemical diversity, the importance of intra-herbal interactions and the accumulating evidence base surrounding phytomedicines.

St John's wort has been used as a treatment for neuralgic conditions since the time of Ancient Greece and as a treatment for psychiatric disorders since the time of Paracelsus.[4] It was traditionally used as a tea, an aqueous extract, and it is included in the national pharmacopoeias of many European countries. In 2005 a Cochrane systematic review of 37 clinical trials, including 26 comparisons with placebos and 14 comparisons with synthetic antidepressant drugs, confirmed its effectiveness for mild to moderate depression, thereby providing strong support for one of its main traditional uses.[5]

St John's wort contains several active constituents, but it is generally accepted that the hyperforin and hypericin constituents are chiefly responsible for its antidepressant and anxiolytic effects.[1] In the past 5 years, researchers have identified that an extract devoid of both hypericin and hyperforin still has antidepressant effects, suggesting that other constituents in the extract are also pharmacologically active.[6] Current research has identified several new active constituents, but others remain elusive. In addition, several other components previously considered devoid of activity have been found to alter the pharmacokinetics of key active constituents. For example, procyanidin B_2 and hyperoside increase the oral bioavailability of hypericin by 58% and 34% respectively.[7] Therefore, current scientific knowledge has demonstrated that the total extract has to be considered the active substance, and that the herb's pharmacological effects cannot be described as simply due to one or two active constituents.

In the late 1990s, the extraction method used by some commercial producers was modified, resulting in higher hyperforin concentrations than previously seen.[8] A St John's wort extract known as LI 160 is one of these higher-hyperforin types. Since this time, numerous reports and studies have identified pharmacokinetic drug interactions with St John's wort based on its ability to induce cytochromes and P-glycoprotein, and the hyperforin constituent has been identified as the key constituent responsible for these induction effects.[1] Meanwhile, studies with low-hyperforin St John's wort preparations, such as Ze 117, have not found evidence of the same interactions.[8] Unfortunately, the distinction between preparations is not well appreciated in the literature and many reference texts fail to mention this important point.

QUALITY CONTROL AND PRODUCT REGULATION

There are considerable differences in the classification and regulation of herbal products in the world market. Regulation tends to be influenced by ethnological, medical and historical factors. Because herbal medicines do not fall easily into the legal categories of food or drug, they often inhabit a grey area between the two.

In Australia there is an international best-practice, risk-based regulatory system for both complementary and pharmaceutical medicines.[1] The Commonwealth Department of Health and Aged Care delegates responsibility for the regulation of complementary medicines to the Therapeutic Goods Administration (TGA), which has an office dedicated to this role (Office of Complementary Medicines). The TGA is responsible for product quality, safety, claims, registration, post-marketing monitoring and setting standards for manufacturing. All herbal products manufactured commercially in Australia must be produced according to the code of Good Manufacturing Practice (GMP). In 1997, the Parliamentary Secretary to the Minister for Health and Family Services established a new ministerial advisory committee, the Complementary Medicines Evaluation Committee (CMEC), which advises the TGA and government on the regulation of complementary medicines.

All complementary medicines imported into, supplied in or exported from Australia are entered onto the Australian Register of Therapeutic Goods (ARTG) and allocated an AUST L number if considered low risk and generally safe (most herbal products) or AUST R number if considered high risk (most prescription drugs). For both AUST L and AUST R products, there are statutory guidelines, stringent labelling requirements and regulations regarding advertising and compliance of the manufacturing process with a recognised code of good manufacturing practice. Penalties are imposed for manufacturers found to be in breach of these regulations.

In 2004, Health Canada officially added a new term to the global list of synonyms for dietary supplements: natural health products (NHP), with the release of its *Natural Health Products Regulations* (the NHP regulations). The regulations are applicable to the sale, manufacture, packaging, labelling, importation, distribution and storage of NHP, and are administered by the recently formed Natural Health Products Directorate (NHPD) within Health Canada. Herbal medicines fall into the NHP category. One of the main components of the NHP regulations is product licensing. Under the new regulations, all NHP are required to undergo pre-market review to obtain a product licence and a corresponding Natural Product Number (NPN). In addition to providing data on the safety, efficacy and quality of NHP ingredients, each manufacturer applying for a product licence must provide information regarding the site of manufacture, packaging, labelling, distribution or importation, with corresponding site licence (SL) numbers, acquired through the submission of a site licence application (SLA). A site licence provides some assurance that current good manufacturing practice is being undertaken.[9]

In the United States, the Food and Drug Administration (FDA) has treated dietary supplements, such as herbal medicines, as foods since 1994 with the enactment of the Dietary Supplement Health Education Act (DSHEA). The DSHEA resulted from a grassroots campaign protesting against the ongoing efforts of the FDA to regulate dietary supplements as drugs, not foods. The DSHEA led to the existence of two sets of regulatory standards, one for foods (including dietary supplements) and the other for drugs (medicines). It also transferred to manufacturers the responsibility for ensuring product safety and the requirement that any therapeutic claims be substantiated by adequate evidence.[10]

Regulation of herbal products differs substantially between Australia, Canada and the United States in that, under the DSHEA, a manufacturer is not required to obtain approval from the FDA prior to marketing its product, although other provisions must be satisfied to ensure a reasonable expectation of safety. Because the FDA has no regulatory control over what products are on the market, it can only remove a dietary supplement from the market if it can prove that the product has violated the regulations governing product safety, information and labelling, or claims after the product reaches the market. To withdraw a product, the FDA must also prove that the product places the consumer at 'significant or unreasonable risk'.[10]

Unlike Australia, Canada and the United States, in several European countries botanical medicines have always been part of mainstream medicine and therefore have been included in the regulations of each country from the beginning. Herbal medicines fall within the scope of the European Directive 2001/83/CE, but there is still little harmonisation between countries in regards to regulation.[11] In some European Union (EU) countries, herbal products are sold as foods, or incorporated in functional/fortified foods or as food supplements, meaning that no medicinal claims are made, whereas in other EU countries these preparations are registered by full or simplified registration procedures. In some countries, the medicinal product status is automatically linked to pharmacy-only status.[12] For example, in Germany, almost all botanical medicines are considered medicinal agents and require medical authorisation. In the United Kingdom, some herbal medicines require registration under the Traditional Herbal Medicinal Products Directive or full medicines authorisation, whereas others considered not medicinal by function are permitted in supplements and foods.[12]

The classification of *Ginkgo biloba* in different countries provides a further example: in the United Kingdom and the Netherlands, *Ginkgo biloba* can be sold as a food supplement; in Germany and France it is a registered OTC medicine; in Ireland it is available as 'prescription only'.[12]

HERBAL SAFETY AND ADVERSE REACTIONS

The World Health Organization (WHO) defines an adverse drug reaction (ADR) as a 'response to a medicine which is noxious and unintended that occurs at doses normally used in humans'. When two medicines interact in a way that produces an unwanted effect, this is also referred to as an adverse drug reaction. Factors associated with an increased likelihood of developing an ADR to a drug or herbal medicine include: advanced age, polypharmacy, dementia or confusion, history of atopic disease, prolonged and frequent therapy, and compromised hepatic and/or renal function.[1]

ADRs can arise due to an intrinsic or an extrinsic effect. An *intrinsic effect* refers to the active ingredient itself, such as the herbal medicine present within a product. An *extrinsic effect* relates to product characteristics resulting from poor manufacturing and quality control, such as contamination or adulteration.

Herbal adverse effects can be categorised in a similar way to pharmaceutical medicines and are mainly type A or type B reactions. *Type A reactions* are anticipated and predictable reactions and tend to be dose related. A herbal example is halitosis and dyspepsia caused by garlic, and a pharmaceutical example is bleeding caused by warfarin or hepatotoxicity from paracetamol. *Type B reactions* are idiosyncratic and uncommon, difficult to predict and not dose related. They tend to have higher morbidity and mortality than Type A reactions and are often immunologically mediated.[13] A herbal example is hepatotoxicity caused by black cohosh, and a pharmaceutical example is interstitial nephritis with the use of NSAIDs.

When manufactured, prescribed and used appropriately, the safety of over-the-counter herbal medicines is high. Serious adverse effects and dangerous interactions are rare, particularly when one considers the millions of doses taken around the world each year. Even so, practitioners should consider the likelihood and potential consequences of an adverse reaction for each patient before prescribing any herbal medicine.

EVIDENCE AND SCIENTIFIC VALIDATION

Over the centuries, empirical knowledge about herbal medicines has slowly accumulated to form a body of evidence commonly referred to as 'traditional evidence'. This form of evidence is based on the basic tenets of good clinical practice: careful observation of people, their environment and the diseases they acquire. While there is now a stronger focus on scientific evidence in Western countries, the accumulation of traditional evidence continues today in many parts of the world.

Over the past 40 years, scientific evidence has extended the traditional evidence base and enabled a better understanding of phytomedicines to emerge. Research has been conducted to isolate and identify key active constituents in botanical medicines and their mechanisms of action. This field of enquiry is appropriately termed *phytochemistry*. Efficacy and safety studies have also been conducted and there is now good evidence from systematic reviews and meta-analyses (including Cochrane reviews) of randomised controlled trials for the efficacy of certain standardised herbal extracts. Three examples are provided in Table 4.2.

Although these studies have been useful in broadening our knowledge of herbal medicine, randomised trials using a standard 'one size fits all' treatment approach do not accurately reflect 'real world' practice. Phytotherapy relies on individual diagnosis and treatments, which often comprise multiple-ingredient formulations together with diet and lifestyle advice. Investigation of a single extract in a poorly defined population (by phytotherapy standards) will only go part of the way towards supporting or disputing the clinical significance of this approach.

Until recently, most phytomedicine research was conducted in Europe and Asia, where there is a rich tradition of use. Research in this area in the United States remained stagnant until the 1990s, when rapid growth and public interest in phytotherapy motivated the government to start dedicating more funds to research. Interestingly, by 1997, the Office of Alternative Medicine in the United States was renamed the National Center for Complementary and Alternative Medicine

TABLE 4.2 Examples of three botanical medicines supported by meta-analyses

Medicinal substance	Use	Evidence and comments	Safety
Hawthorn *(Crataegus laevigata)*	Chronic heart failure (NYHA classes I–II)	A meta-analysis of eight rigorous clinical trials involving 632 subjects with chronic heart failure (NYHA classes I to III) concluded that treatment with standardised hawthorn extracts produced significant improvement in maximal workload, pressure–heart rate product, as well as symptoms such as dyspnoea and fatigue compared with placebo.[14]	Treatment is considered well tolerated; mild, transient side effects have been reported, such as headache, sweating, dizziness, palpitations, sleepiness, agitation and gastrointestinal symptoms.[15]
Kava kava *(Piper methysticum)*	Anxiety	Cochrane review was a meta-analysis of seven placebo-controlled studies and concluded that kava kava significantly reduced anxiety as measured by the Hamilton Anxiety Scale ($n = 380$).[16] A more recent meta-analysis of trials with high methodological standards using kava extract WS 1490 confirmed these results.[17]	Cochrane review concluded that adverse events reported in the reviewed trials were mild, transient and infrequent.[16] Currently, the TGA has advised Australian manufacturers to place a cautionary statement on product labels due to the rare incidence of hepatic side effects. The risk-to-benefit ratio of kava extracts nevertheless remains good compared with that of other drugs used to treat anxiety.[18]
Saw palmetto *(Serenoa repens)*	Benign prostatic hypertrophy	Cochrane review of 21 randomised trials ($n =$ 3139) lasting 4–48 weeks concluded that Saw palmetto provides mild to moderate improvement in urinary symptoms and flow measures compared with placebo, which is similar to finasteride.[19]	Cochrane review concluded that Saw palmetto is associated with fewer adverse treatment events than finasteride.[19]

NHYA: New York Heart Association

(NCCAM), indicating greater acceptance of therapeutic approaches such as phytotherapy.[20] Notwithstanding these efforts, a relative lack of resources, infrastructure, government funding and financial incentives for investment in non-patentable medicines research has impeded herbal research worldwide.

Phytomedicine research in Australia continues to struggle due to a severe lack of funds despite its enormous public popularity. In 2007 the Australian Government earmarked $5 million for complementary medicine research via a National Health and Medical Research Council special call. Over 140 submissions were made, indicating enormous interest among researchers. In the same year, the National Institute of Complementary Medicine (NICM) was created using seed money provided by the Commonwealth Department of Health and Ageing together with the New South Wales Office for Science and Medical Research (OSMR) (www.nicm.org.au). The aim of the NICM was to build the capacity of complementary medicine research across Australia, effectively connecting complementary medicine researchers and professionals with the broader research community, industry and other stakeholders, to provide strategic focus and foster excellence in research. However, funding was suspended in 2009.

THE PRACTICE OF WESTERN HERBAL MEDICINE

Western herbal medicine is the main form of phytotherapy practised today by herbalists in the United States, Europe, Canada, Australia and New Zealand. It is built on European and Greco-Roman healthcare traditions and can be traced back to prominent physicians such as Dioscorides, Hippocrates and Galen. Over the past century, with greater cross-cultural exchange, the European influence in Western herbal medicine practice has lessened and there has been some adoption of herbal medicines and practices from other continents. The popular immune-modulating herb *Echinacea* and the menopausal treatment black cohosh are two examples of this cross-cultural exchange, having emanated from the North American Indians. With today's increased ease of global communication and transport, the continued exchange of ideas and medicines with other cultures keeps broadening the practice of Western phytotherapy. It is now commonplace to find herbs such as Korean ginseng from Asia, *Echinacea* from North America, tea tree from Australia, chamomile from Germany and *Andrographis* from India sitting together in a herbalist's dispensary.

PHILOSOPHY AND THE HERBALIST'S APPROACH

The practice of phytotherapy is based on a synthesis of traditional and modern philosophies of health and disease. The person-centred approach is standard practice and highly individualised treatment plans are the norm. Attention is paid to a patient's individual presentation, their diet and lifestyle choices, past history, general constitution, overall vitality and particular environmental circumstances.

Medical herbalists are trained in basic sciences such as anatomy, physiology and biochemistry, basic pharmacology and clinical diagnosis in order to enable a comprehensive history to be taken, identifying symptoms and underlying disease. According to an Australian workforce survey, 85% of naturopaths and Western herbalists also hold first aid certification and approximately 90% regularly attend continuing education seminars.[21] The same survey identified that nearly 40% of practitioners use Western diagnostic tests such as pathology and radiology to guide their clinical practice and nearly two-thirds perform physical examinations. In addition, most use traditional naturopathic diagnostic assessments.

Therapy is aimed at addressing the cause of disease, reducing the influence of exacerbating factors and providing symptomatic relief in an overall attempt to achieve deeper and longer-lasting healing. As a result, herbal combinations are prescribed rather than single herbs, and treatments can vary significantly between individual patients who present with outwardly similar symptoms. Preparations such as tinctures, fluid extracts, syrups, capsules and creams are all part of the treatment armoury. Education about pharmacognosy, herbal materia medica, manufacturing and botany provide Western herbalists with the foundation knowledge on which to base treatment choices.

In most cases, liquid herbal preparations are dispensed on site and commercially prepared oral dose forms are used. In recent years, awareness of drug–herb interactions has meant that practitioners are now being trained to take a full medication history and understand how to avoid inducing a negative interaction.

The herbalist's wholistic approach also encourages patient responsibility and enlists them as a key partner in the healing process. This is a common theme in all traditional healing systems and is central to the practice of phytotherapy.

In Australia, the knowledge and practice of herbal medicine has been preserved and nurtured mainly by Western herbalists. In fact, the National Herbalists Association of Australia (NHAA) has represented medical herbalists since 1920. Today, the association is widely recognised as setting industry standards for education in medical herbalism. It has a constitution and a code of ethics, liaises with private health funds to ensure reimbursement of patient fees for its accredited practitioners and continues to advocate professional registration by government bodies. Clinicians are encouraged to check whether herbal practitioners to whom they refer have undergone accredited courses. Further information can be found by contacting the association or accessing the website (www.nhaa.org.au).

Source: NHAA[22]

HOW PHYTOTHERAPY INTEGRATES WITH GENERAL PRACTICE

Surveys conducted in the Western world consistently report on the popularity of herbal medicines.[23–26] This means that general practitioners are coming into contact with an increasing number of patients taking or enquiring about herbs. From this perspective, it is important for clinicians to become familiar with commonly used botanical medicines so they can provide an informed opinion on their safety and efficacy. In addition, the practice of evidence-based medicine demands that treatment decisions be based on the best available evidence. As a consequence, when there is evidence to support the efficacy and safety of a herbal extract, it should also be considered in the treatment plan. As a starting point, Table 4.3 provides a list of 20 over-the-counter (OTC) herbal medicines that GPs should become familiar with. The list is based on popularity and does not include all OTC phytomedicines supported by evidence.

TALKING WITH PATIENTS ABOUT HERBAL MEDICINES

Studies indicate that most patients using complementary medicines (including herbal medicines) do not routinely disclose this information to their medical practitioner. In the United States, Eisenberg and colleagues identified that, in 1990, only 39.8% of complementary medicine users disclosed their use to physicians, and in 1997 this figure was 38.5%, suggesting that disclosure had remained poor.[25] Many other surveys have had similar findings. One review of patients attending medical clinics identified non-disclosure rates of 23–72%.[27] In all 12 studies reviewed, the same three themes were consistently reported as barriers to communication: patient concern about eliciting a negative response from the physician; the patient's perception that their

TABLE 4.3 Popular phytomedicines that all GPs should become familiar with

Common name of herb (Latin name)	Indications/uses
Bilberry (*Vaccinium myrtillus*)	Ocular symptoms/disease: preventing and treating diabetic retinopathy, poor night vision, light adaptation and photophobia
Black cohosh (*Cimicifuga racemosa* or *Actea racemosa*)	Menopausal symptoms, premenstrual syndrome
Chaste tree (*Vitex agnus-castus*)	Premenstrual syndrome, menstrual irregularities
Cranberry (*Vaccinium macrocarpon*)	Prevention of urinary tract infection
Devil's claw (*Harpagophytum procumbens*)	Symptomatic relief in osteoarthritis, non-specific lower back pain
Echinacea (*Echinacea angustifolia* and *Echinacea purpurea*)	Immune modulation, viral upper respiratory tract infections, wound healing (topical)
Feverfew (*Tanacetum parthenium*)	Migraine prophylaxis
Ginger (*Zingiber officinalis*)	Prevention and treatment of motion sickness, morning sickness
Ginkgo (*Ginkgo biloba*)	Dementia, intermittent claudication and poor peripheral circulation
Guarana (*Paullinia cupana*)	Central nervous system stimulant
St John's wort (*Hypericum perforatum*)	Mild to moderate depression
Hawthorn (*Crataegus oxycantha*)	Heart failure (NYHA classes I–III)
Horse chestnut (*Aesculus hippocastanum*)	Chronic venous insufficiency
Kava kava (*Piper methysticum*)	Anxiety
Peppermint (*Mentha piperita*)	Irritable bowel syndrome, dyspepsia
Saw palmetto or serenoa (*Sabal serrulata* or *Serenoa repens*)	Symptomatic relief in benign prostatic hypertrophy
Slippery elm (*Ulmus rubra*)	Symptomatic relief of gastritis, dyspepsia, gastric reflux, peptic ulcers, irritable bowel syndrome and Crohn's disease
St Mary's thistle (*Silybum marianum*)	Prevent liver injury
Tea tree oil (*Melaleuca alternifolia*)	Topical infections
Valerian (*Valeriana officinalis*)	Anxiety, insomnia

NHYA: New York Heart Association

medical practitioner did not need to know about complementary medicine use because they would be unable to contribute useful information; and lack of clinician enquiry.

Lack of patient disclosure combined with lack of practitioner enquiry results in a 'don't ask, don't tell' culture in which communication barriers are continually reinforced.[28] Not only is this situation potentially dangerous, it is also a missed opportunity for practitioners to learn from patients about their reasons for using herbal medicines, whether the treatment has been effective or ineffective, and other details about their healthcare beliefs.

Clear and open communication is essential for the delivery of high-quality, safe patient care. General practitioners must be able to talk with patients about a variety of healthcare and treatment options, especially those that are commonly used by the public, such as herbal medicines. Asking a few open-ended questions in a non-judgmental way will help the clinician to assess whether a patient is taking any herbal medicines and enable a discussion to begin.

NEXT STEPS

Asking patients about their use of botanical medicines is relatively easy, but interpreting their answers can be far more difficult. The following steps are recommended:

- Record the patient's responses in their record so anyone can consult it and check for potential safety concerns, such as drug interactions.
- Advise the patient about the safety and effectiveness of the botanical medicines they are taking or considering taking. If you are unable to answer all the patient's questions, be prepared to refer them to an evidence-based information source or an accredited medical herbalist or other appropriate

expert. Most naturopaths and some pharmacists have received additional phytotherapy training and are also good sources of information. If Chinese medicines are involved, consider referral to a registered or accredited traditional Chinese medicine practitioner.

- If you suspect an adverse reaction, you have a professional responsibility to report it. In Australia, notifiy the Adverse Drug Reactions Advisory Committee (ADRAC)—reporting is confidential, open to everyone and is now possible online (www.tga.gov.au).
  Ideally, you should also notify the following:
  - the relevant herbal and natural medicine associations—such as the National Herbalists Association of Australia (www.nhaa.org.au)
  - the relevant manufacturer—manufacturers keep their own records and are formally obliged to inform the TGA
  - the prescriber, if applicable.

PRESCRIBING HERBAL MEDICINES

Botanical medicines can play an important role in general practice and provide practitioners with many additional therapeutic tools. While the fully fledged practice of phytotherapy requires several years of specialised training, general practitioners can successfully integrate some simple, pre-prepared herbal treatments into their practice.

Once it has been determined that a herb is efficacious and safe for a specific patient, the patient should be encouraged to choose a high-quality product. Practitioners are advised to become familiar with their local regulations and herbal manufacturing companies, to ascertain which products present the best quality. For example, in Australia, it is important that products contain an AUST L or AUST R number on the label together with an expiry date, and any product without these should not be used. Practitioner-only companies in Australia pride themselves on producing higher-quality products which are only available in clinics under supervision.

Once the correct herbal extract has been chosen, the choice of dose follows. Doses used in clinical trials provide a useful guide but they are sometimes difficult to interpret. Doses provided by manufacturers on product labels also provide a general guide, but can be conservative and may need to be increased to reach full therapeutic effect. For more specific information, refer to reputable texts or even ring the product manufacturer about dosing schedules, as many have dedicated enquiry phone lines.

Patients should be provided with instructions about where they can find the particular product prescribed, how to take and store the medicine, and what they should expect. It is worth discussing a sensible time frame for trialling a herbal medicine so that expectations are realistic and management can be modified if the treatment is not effective. Once again, information about this can be found in clinical trials and good reference texts. For example, herbs such as *Ginkgo biloba* for mild dementia require a trial of at least 3 months, whereas ginger treatment should alleviate nausea within 1 hour. Box 4.2 provides a summary of these steps.

BOX 4.1 Reasons to consider using herbal medicines in practice

- *Efficacy*—herbal medicines with demonstrated efficacy should be adopted as part of standard practice
- *Safety*—when the herbal treatment option is safer than other therapies
- *Cost*—when herbal treatments are a lower-cost option
- *Adjunct*—if the effectiveness and/or safety of other interventions can be improved by combining with herbal medicine
- *Prevention*—when herbal medicine provides a safe prevention strategy in an at-risk population
- *Enhanced health*—if a safe herbal medicine can increase a patient's sense of wellbeing and quality of life
- *Patient involvement*—the patient is involved in their own healthcare

adapted from Braun & Cohen[1]

BOX 4.2 Rational use of herbal medicines: the prescribing steps

1. Know the benefits and risks associated with popular and evidence-based herbal medicines, including potential drug interactions. If in doubt, refer to a credible resource or trained expert.
2. Choose quality products—if an Australian product, check that an AUST L or AUST R number and expiry date are on the label; if the product comes from overseas, make sure it is manufactured according to the Code of Good Manufacturing Practice.
3. Choose the correct herbal extract and dose—use clinical trials, reference texts and manufacturer information for guidance.
4. Provide the patient with instructions on where to buy the product—supermarket, pharmacy, health-food store, medical herbalist's dispensary, other.
5. Select a sensible time frame for trialling the herbal treatment—some herbs provide symptomatic relief within 1 hour; others can take several months. This also ensures that the patient does not keep taking a herbal treatment when it is ineffective.

As with good food and good wine, the quality of commercially prepared herbal medicines will vary, as will the price. Learning about different company philosophies and products takes time but will help clinicians to become more confident prescribers. Most importantly, look for opportunities to learn more about herbal medicines from credible sources and become familiar with accredited medical herbalists and pharmacists who have additional herbal medicine training.

If a patient is keen to start using a herbal medicine but as their practitioner you lack confidence or knowledge about it, consider referring the patient to an accredited medical herbalist. A standard referral letter should be sufficient, and should include the names of all medications being used by the patient. If you would like the practitioner to provide correspondence about their phytotherapeutic approach, ensure that this is stated in the referral letter.

RESOURCES

Blumenthal M (ed). Herbal medicine: expanded commission E monographs. American Botanical Society Publishers; 2000. The English translation of the official German herbal monographs, with some additional information and commentary.

Blumenthal M. ABC clinical guide to herbs. Austin: Amercian Botanical Council; 2003.

Bone K, Mills S. Principles and practice of phytotherapy. Churchill Livingstone; 2000. Detailed information about phytotherapeutics, herbal philosophy and phytochemistry, with additional monographs.

Braun L, Cohen M. Herbs and natural supplements: an evidence-based guide. 3rd edn. Sydney: Elsevier Australia; 2009. Comprehensive, evidence-based information about 130 complementary medicines popular in Australia and New Zealand, and detailed drug–herb interaction charts.

Gurib-Fakim A. Medicinal plants: traditions of yesterday and drugs of tomorrow. Mol Aspects Med 2006; 27(1): 1–93.

Murray M. The healing power of herbs. 2nd edn. California: Prima Press; 1995.

National Herbalists Association of Australia, http://www.nhaa.org.au

Therapeutic Goods Administration, http://www.tga.gov.au

REFERENCES

1 Braun L, Cohen MM. Herbs and natural supplements: an evidence-based guide. 3rd edn. Sydney: Elsevier; 2009.

2 Weiss R. Herbal medicine. Stuttgart: Beaconsfield; 1991.

3 Mills S, Bone K. Principles and practice of phytotherapy. Sydney: Elsevier; 2000.

4 Blumenthal M, Goldberg A, Brinckmann J. Herbal medicine: expanded commission E monographs. American Botanical Council; 2000.

5 Linde K, Mulrow CD, Berner M et al. St John's wort for depression. Cochrane Database Syst Rev 2005; 2:CD000448.

6 Butterweck V, Christoffel V, Nahrstedt A et al. Step by step removal of hyperforin and hypericin: activity profile of different *Hypericum* preparations in behavioral models. Life Sci 2003; 73(5):627–639.

7 Butterweck V, Lieflander-Wulf U, Winterhoff H et al. Plasma levels of hypericin in presence of procyanidin B_2 and hyperoside: a pharmacokinetic study in rats. Planta Med 2003; 69(3):189–192.

8 Madabushi R, Frank B, Drewelow B et al. Hyperforin in St John's wort drug interactions. Eur J Clin Pharmacol 2006; 62(3):225–233.

9 Nestmann ER, Harwood M, Martyres S. An innovative model for regulating supplement products: natural health products in Canada. Toxicology 2006; 221(1): 50–58.

10 Brownie S. The development of the US and Australian dietary supplement regulations: what are the implications for product quality? Complement Ther Med 2005; 13(3):191–198.

11 Silano M, De Vincenzi M, De Vincenzi A et al. The new European legislation on traditional herbal medicines: main features and perspectives. Fitoterapia 2004; 75(2):107–116.

12 Gulati OP, Berry Ottaway P. Legislation relating to nutraceuticals in the European Union with a particular focus on botanical-sourced products. Toxicology 2006; 221(1):75–87.

13 Myers SP, Cheras PA. The other side of the coin: safety of complementary and alternative medicine. Med J Aust 2004; 181(4):222–225.

14 Pittler MH, Schmidt K, Ernst E. Hawthorn extract for treating chronic heart failure: meta-analysis of randomized trials. Am J Med 2003; 114(8):665–674.

15 Rigelsky JM, Sweet BV. Hawthorn: pharmacology and therapeutic uses. Am J Health Syst Pharm 2002; 59(5):417–422.

16 Pittler MH, Ernst E. Kava extract for treating anxiety (Cochrane Review). Cochrane Database Syst Rev 2003; 1:CD003383.

17 Witte S, Loew D, Gaus W. Meta-analysis of the efficacy of the acetonic kava-kava extract WS 1490 in patients with non-psychotic anxiety disorders. Phytother Res 2005; 19(3):183–188.

18 Clouatre DL. Kava kava: examining new reports of toxicity. Toxicol Lett 2004; 150(1):85–96.

19 Wilt T, Ishani A, Mac DR. *Serenoa repens* for benign prostatic hyperplasia. Cochrane Database Syst Rev 2002; 3:CD001423.

20 Marwick C. Alterations are ahead at the OAM. Office of Alternative Medicine. JAMA 1998; 280(18):1553–1554.

21 Bensoussan A, Myers SP, Wu SM et al. Naturopathic and Western herbal medicine practice in Australia: a workforce survey. Complement Ther Med 2004; 12(1):17–27.

22 National Herbalists Association of Australia (NHAA). Online. Available www.nhaa.org.au 3 January 2008.

23 MacLennan AH, Myers SP, Taylor AW. The continuing use of complementary and alternative medicine in South Australia: costs and beliefs in 2004. Med J Aust 2006; 184(1):27–31.

24 Xue C, Zhang L, Lin V et al. Current usage of complementary and alternative medicine in Australia: a national population-based study. J Altern Complement Med 2007; 13(6):643–650.

25 Eisenberg DM, Davis RB, Ettner SL et al. Trends in alternative medicine use in the United States, 1990–1997: results of a follow-up national survey. JAMA 1998; 280(18):1569–1575.

26 Harris P, Rees R. The prevalence of complementary and alternative medicine use among the general population: a systematic review of the literature. Complement Ther Med 2000; 8(2):88–96.

27 Robinson A, McGrail MR. Disclosure of CAM use to medical practitioners: a review of qualitative and quantitative studies. Complement Ther Med 2004; 12(2/3):90–98.

28 Giveon SM, Liberman N, Klang S et al. A survey of primary care physicians: perceptions of their patients' use of complementary medicine. Complement Ther Med 2003; 11(4):254–260.

chapter 5

Herb–drug interactions

INTRODUCTION

Complementary medicines such as herbal medicines are available through a variety of channels such as supermarkets, pharmacies, health-food stores, clinic rooms, internet sites and mail order companies. Many people self-select their products and do not receive professional advice about their safe and appropriate use.[1,2] When using a complementary medicine, many do not discuss its use with their medical practitioner, either in the community or in the hospital setting.[1,3–14] Importantly, people using complementary medicines tend to have poorer health than the general community[15] and are not generally dissatisfied with conventional medicine but use complementary medicines as an adjunct to conventional medical care.[1,4,16,17] This raises the possibility of dual care from both complementary and conventional practitioners and the concomitant use of herbs and pharmaceutical medicines. Widespread use, self-selection and poor disclosure suggest that many people feel sufficiently confident that over-the-counter (OTC) herbal medicines are beneficial and that their safety is assumed. This assumption is supported by several Australian studies.[1,18]

The assumed safety of herbal medicines is sometimes attributed to the fact that they are considered 'natural' and therefore inherently safe. This view is encouraged by some in the health-food industry and is too simplistic. Nature provides us with many examples of unsafe substances, such as the naturally occurring poisons hemlock, jimsonweed and oleander. Also, the concept of safety is a complex one and is ultimately determined by two main variables: 'likelihood' and 'consequence'. For each individual and their particular circumstances, the concept of safety has to be redefined.

Australia's risk-based regulatory process for therapeutic goods (including herbal medicines) provides some safeguard. Clinicians can feel reassured that OTC herbal medicines allocated an AUST L number have been produced according to the Code of Good Manufacturing Practice (GMP) and their ingredients assessed for safety. Alternatively, potentially unsafe herbal medicines have warning labels and may even be restricted from sale via the scheduling system, much like pharmaceutical medicines (more information about the regulation of herbal products can be found in Ch 4).

Despite this, it has become apparent over the past decade that some commonly used OTC herbal medicines are capable of causing significant drug interactions, which must be identified and managed to optimise patient safety. Open communication, familiarisation with the most commonly used complementary medicines and understanding the interaction mechanisms involved are vital first steps in promoting patient safety. This chapter provides an introduction to herb–drug interactions; detailed information about specific herb–drug interactions is beyond the scope of this chapter. Comprehensive drug–herb interaction charts and further information are available in *Herbs and natural supplements—an evidence-based guide* by Braun & Cohen.[19]

INTERACTIONS

Herbs contain a chemically complex cocktail of naturally occurring ingredients. In this way, they are very different from pharmaceutical medicines. The pharmacological effect of a herbal medicine is the end result of an interplay between various interactions. There are intra-herbal interactions between constituents, interactions between the herb and the vehicles it is mixed with during processing and manufacture, and then the final interaction between the product and person receiving it. Interactions can also occur between the foods, drugs and other herbal medicines being taken by that individual. As you can see, interactions are unavoidable and should not present any clinical problem unless they are unanticipated.

In medicine, a pharmacological interaction is an alteration of the usual predicted effect of one substance when used at the same time as another. Usually the term 'interaction' has a negative connotation when referring to therapeutic agents, as interactions can lead to adverse effects, drug toxicity or a loss of drug effect, and clinical outcomes can be difficult to predict. Interactions need not have negative outcomes; when manipulated skilfully they can be harnessed to produce beneficial outcomes, and managed or avoided to reduce harm. In clinical practice, this occurs every day.

THE MAIN INTERACTION MECHANISMS: OVERVIEW

Considering the great variation in physical properties and pharmacological effects of the numerous substances used as medicines, together with the variable nature of herbal medicines, a virtually endless number of interactions is possible. Interaction mechanisms can be broadly categorised as pharmacodynamic or pharmacokinetic interactions (Fig 5.1). Regardless of the interaction mechanism at work, there are three possible outcomes:

- increased therapeutic or adverse effects
- decreased therapeutic or adverse effects
- a unique response that does not occur when either agent is used alone.

PHARMACOKINETIC INTERACTIONS

A *pharmacokinetic interaction* occurs when substance A alters the absorption, distribution, metabolism or excretion of substance B, causing a change in the amount and persistence of the available substance B at receptor sites or target tissues. The interaction causes a change in the strength or duration of effect, but not the type of effect.

Absorption

Most absorption of orally administered medicines occurs in the small intestine, which has a larger surface area than the stomach and greater membrane permeability. If a slow-release dosage form is taken and it continues to release the drug for more than 6 hours, then absorption will also occur in the large intestine. The absorption of oral dose forms is influenced by differences in pH along the gastrointestinal tract, surface area per luminal volume, blood perfusion, the presence of bile and mucus, and the nature of epithelial membranes. Changes to gastrointestinal flora, transport systems, chelation and ion exchange also influence absorption. Ultimately, a change to any of these processes can alter the rate and/or extent of absorption.

A reduced *rate* of absorption can lead to a 'sustained release' effect, whereas a reduced *extent* of absorption is particularly problematic for drugs with a narrow therapeutic index (NTI). Gums and mucilages (such as guar gum and psyllium) are examples of substances known or thought to affect drug absorption. For example, a double-blind study found that guar gum

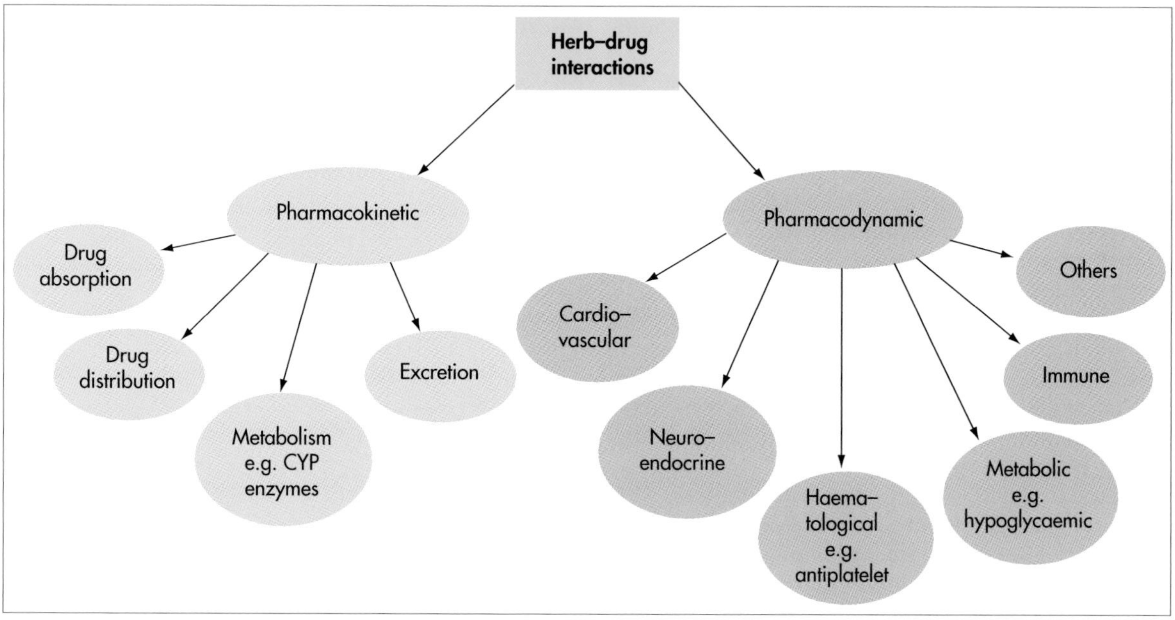

FIGURE 5.1 The main classes of interactions

slowed the absorption rate of digoxin but did not alter the extent of absorption, whereas penicillin absorption was both slowed and reduced.[20] This brings into question the effects of other gums and highly mucilaginous herbal medicines such as *Ulmus fulvus* (slippery elm), *Althea officinalis* (marshmallow) and *Plantago ovata* (psyllium). Poorly lipid soluble, the mucilaginous content forms an additional physical barrier that needs to be traversed before the medicine can enter systemic circulation. Whether this will have clinically significant effects on the rate and/or extent of absorption of other medicines is uncertain and remains to be tested.

More research has been conducted on the way in which nutrients interact and alter the absorption of other medicines. The interactions between iron and mineral-based antacids are a useful example. Separating the intake of iron and the last antacid dose by at least 2 hours reduces the risk of interaction.[19]

Metabolism

Drug metabolism involves a wide range of chemical reactions, including oxidation, reduction, hydrolysis, hydration, conjugation, condensation and isomerisation. These processes largely determine the duration of a drug's action, elimination and toxicity.

Metabolism can occur prior to and during absorption, thereby limiting the amount of drug reaching systemic circulation; however, most drug metabolism occurs in the liver in two apparent phases, known as phase 1 and phase 2.

Phase I reactions involve the formation of a new or modified functional group or a cleavage (oxidation, reduction, hydrolysis), whereas phase 2 reactions involve conjugation with an endogenous compound (e.g. glutathione, amino acids, sulfates, glycine). The metabolites produced after phase 1 metabolism are often chemically reactive and may even be more toxic or carcinogenic than the initial drug. A well-known example is paracetamol, whose phase 1 metabolite is chiefly responsible for its toxicity. Metabolites produced after phase 2 reactions are usually inactive.

Although there are many enzymes responsible for phase I reactions, the most important enzyme group is the cytochrome P-450 system (CYP). Many factors can interfere with CYP activity, such as the ingestion of environmental contaminants, certain food constituents, beverages, herbs and pharmaceutical medicines. Some of these factors induce CYP enzymes, whereas others have an inhibitory effect.

Enzyme *inhibition* is an immediate response, with effects seen rapidly.[21] It can be reversible, quasi-reversible or irreversible. In practice, most inhibition is reversible, ceasing when use of the inhibitor agent is discontinued. The result of CYP enzyme inhibition is elevated serum levels of those drugs chiefly metabolised by the affected enzyme. Medicines with narrow therapeutic margins, such as digoxin, are of particular concern as small elevations in serum levels have the potential to produce toxic effects. In practice, enzyme inhibition is not always harmful and has been manipulated to raise serum drug levels without the need to increase the dose administered. The result has obvious cost advantages when expensive drugs are involved and has been used in some hospitals for medicines such as cyclosporin. Grapefruit is one example of a natural product having significant enzyme inhibition effects.

Unlike enzyme inhibition, enzyme *induction* is a relatively slow process and results in reduced serum levels of the drugs chiefly metabolised by the affected CYP enzyme. Many different medicines and everyday substances have been found to be capable of inducing CYP enzymes—examples are broccoli, brussel sprouts, chargrilled meat, high-protein diets and alcohol.[19]

St John's wort is a good example of a herbal substance capable of interacting with a variety of drugs through this mechanism. Clinical studies have confirmed that long-term administration of St John's wort has significant CYP inducer activity, particularly CYP3A4.[22–25] This is significant because CYP3A4 is responsible for the metabolism of many pharmaceutical drugs. Studies have isolated the hyperforin component as a potent ligand for the pregnane X receptor, which regulates expression of CYP3A4 mono-oxygenase. In this way, hyperforin increases the availability of CYP3A4, resulting in enzyme induction.[26] Examples of CYP3A4 substrates are alprazolam, codeine, erythromycin and simvastatin. Importantly, low-hyperforin St John's wort extracts such as Ze 117 do not significantly induce CYP3A4, 2D6, 2C9, 1A2 or 2C19, according to human pharmacokinetic studies.[27–29] As such, the Ze 117 extract may present a safer treatment option for patients taking multiple drugs at the same time.

Excretion

Drug excretion occurs chiefly via the kidney but also to a lesser extent via the colon, saliva, sweat, breast milk and lungs. If a medicine is eliminated chiefly by one pathway, then alterations to that particular pathway can theoretically have a significant influence on its excretion. In the case of urinary excretion, factors that alter urinary pH are of prime importance. For example, the half-life of an acidic medicine, such as a salicylate, can be increased with the acidification of urine, such as with high-dose ascorbic acid ingestion, because less is eliminated.

PHARMACODYNAMIC INTERACTIONS

A *pharmacodynamic interaction* occurs when one substance alters the sensitivity or responsiveness of tissues to another substance. This type of interaction results in additive, synergistic or antagonistic drug effects. Pharmacodynamic interactions can also occur when therapeutic substances with overlapping side effects or toxicities are used together, leading to more serious side effects than when either substance is used alone. A good understanding of the pharmacological activity of the therapeutic substances involved can help to theoretically predict potential interactions and optimise therapy.

In practice, clinicians of every variety frequently use additive or synergistic pharmacodynamic interactions to improve clinical outcomes. For example, medical practitioners prescribe combination therapy to eradicate *Helicobacter pylori* infection or several antihypertensive agents at once if response to a single agent has not been satisfactory. Herbal medicine practitioners widely prescribe combinations of herbs with similar actions to strengthen clinical effects, and naturopaths may combine nutritional and herbal supplements in a similar way.

Although pharmacodynamic interactions involving herbal and pharmaceutical medicines have not been well investigated, it is easy to make theoretical predictions based on the known pharmacological actions of the medicines involved. For example, kava kava, a herbal central nervous system (CNS) sedative, could be reasonably assumed to interact with benzodiazepines, causing additive or synergistic sedative effects. Alternatively, the herbal CNS stimulant guarana may cause antagonistic effects when used together with benzodiazepines, so that less sedation results. Although predictions such as these are easy to make, this does not mean we can accurately predict the clinical significance of such interactions.

EVALUATING HERB INTERACTIONS

Most studies investigating herb–drug interactions have used in vitro testing of herbal constituents in microsomal systems, supersomes, cytosols, expressed enzymes or cell culture systems such as transfected cell lines, primary cultures of human hepatocytes and tumour-derived cells. There has also been some in vivo investigation in normal, transgenic and humanised animals and, increasingly, in humans. Although these studies are useful, they have limitations. Table 5.1 presents a summary of the limitations of different types of research. Most interaction studies conducted to date have focused on herbal constituents and their effects on cytochrome (CYP) enzymes and, increasingly, P-glycoprotein (P-gp), with few studies investigating effects on drug transport or phase 2 metabolism.

TABLE 5.1 Advantages and limitations of herb–drug interaction studies

Study type	Advantages	Limitations
In vitro	• Provides information about mechanisms • Relatively simple to conduct compared with clinical studies • Relatively cheap to conduct compared with clinical studies • Relatively quick to conduct	• May use higher doses than can be achieved in clinical practice • Does not account for poor bioavailability of the test compound • May use one isolated constituent, whereas herbal extracts contain multiple constituents • Does not account for human genetic polymorphism
In vivo using animal models	• Can address some of the issues relating to bioavailability • Can produce results more quickly than clinical studies • Can provide information when clinical studies cannot be conducted	• Species variations require different interpretation of results • Selection of appropriate dosage can be difficult, and often very large doses are used • Does not account for human genetic polymorphism
Clinical studies	• Provide the most relevant information and are the most definitive	• Most studies are conducted in healthy male subjects, but the most relevant results are obtained when conducted in the population who will be using the product • Inter-product variability in constituent ratios means the tested product may not accurately represent the effects of other products • Cannot differentiate between gut and liver effects (e.g. cytochromes) • Does not provide information about mechanisms • Costly to produce • Time consuming • May never be done, due to ethical reasons (e.g. safety studies in pregnancy)

PROBLEMS IN EXTRAPOLATING DATA

A review of the peer-reviewed literature reveals that there is a lack of clinical data and research regarding interactions between herbs and drugs, and it is apparent that much remains untested. Despite this, several OTC herbal medicines have demonstrated pharmacodynamic and pharmacokinetic interactions with drugs in clinical studies. One major concern is those herbal medicines that interact with transporters such as P-gp or cytochromes such as CYP3A4 which are responsible for the transport or metabolism respectively of many drugs commonly used in clinical practice.

In some instances, results obtained in vitro or with animal models about interactions do not accurately predict clinically significant effects in humans. This makes predicting the clinical significance of a possible interaction problematic, and a reliance on evidence other than clinical data is bound to lead to inaccuracies. To illustrate this point, the herbs *Ginkgo biloba* and saw palmetto will be used here as examples.

In vitro tests and/or tests with animal models have shown both CYP induction and inhibition for *Ginkgo biloba*.[30–44] In contrast, four clinical studies have failed to identify a clinically significant effect on a variety of cytochromes. In one clinical study, Gurley and colleagues demonstrated that *Ginkgo biloba* had no significant effect on CYP1A2, CYP2D6 or CYP3A4 activity.[45] Markowitz and colleagues also conducted a human study and found no significant effects on CYP2D6 or CYP3A4 activity.[46] Two further clinical studies found no significant effect for *Ginkgo biloba* on CYP2C9 activity.[47,48]

In the case of saw palmetto, the herb has shown potent inhibition of CYP3A4, CYP2D6 and CYP2C9 in vitro,[49] but no significant effect was observed on CYP2D6 or CYP3A4 activity in a clinical study by Markowitz et al.[50] Gurley et al. also found no significant effect for saw palmetto on CYP1A2, CYP2D6, CYP2E1 or CYP3A4 activity in healthy subjects.[51]

To add to the complexity of the problem, in some instances researchers have tested individual herbal components or different forms of a herb, and found different effects on CYPs. For example, one study of different constituents of garlic used animal models and showed that diallyl sulfide (100 μmol/kg) slightly but significantly increased cytochrome CYP2E1 activity (1.6-fold *vs* control), whereas diallyl disulfide and diallyl trisulfide did not affect CYP2E1 activity or the hepatic total CYP level or CYP1A1/2 activity.[52] The significance of these results in clinical practice is difficult to determine, as the overall effect on CYP activity will depend on the concentrations of these various constituents present in a garlic product. The example also highlights the general difficulty of extrapolating results for one herbal extract to another, as there may be significant chemical variations between batches of the same herbal product and between different products of the same herb produced by various manufacturers.

PUTTING THEORY INTO PRACTICE: CLINICAL CONSIDERATIONS

In clinical practice, not every patient who takes potentially interacting substances will experience an adverse effect. It is difficult, however, to predict which person is at greater risk. Some of the characteristics of both patients and drugs that appear to increase the risk of harmful interactions are:

- drugs with a narrow therapeutic index
- older and frailer patients
- patients with renal or hepatic disease
- patients already taking multiple medications
- multiple practitioners involved in patient care
- poor communication between patient and practitioner
- poor communication between complementary and medical practitioners
- use of products not manufactured under strict Code of GMP
- self-selection of OTC products without professional assistance.[19]

In addition, factors such as dose, timing of herbal intake, dosing regimen and route of drug administration are other influences.

METOPIA ALGORITHM

The METOPIA algorithm provides clinicians with a framework for making rational decisions about the possibility of a herb–drug interaction.[19] The acronym METOPIA refers to:

- **M**edication and mechanisms
  - Understanding the medicines involved is essential. For example, when drugs with a NTI are being used, extra care is required.
  - An understanding of the pharmacokinetic parameters and pharmacodynamic effects of the medicines involved is fundamental to predicting the likelihood of a proposed interaction occurring. In the case of herbal medicines, this information might not be available and much will be speculative.
- **E**vidence available
  - A review of the literature is required, to determine what evidence is available and its strengths and limitations. As illustrated, in vitro studies are poor indicators of the clinical significance of an anticipated interaction, but may be the only evidence available.

- Timing and dose—introducing which, when and for how long?
  - For physicochemical interactions in particular, the scheduled administration times of the medicines are important.
  - This step also includes considering the chronicity of use of the medicinal agents, as interaction mechanisms may only develop over several days or weeks (such as CYP induction) or may occur rapidly.
- Outcomes possible
  - The time of onset and severity of the possible clinical consequence may be predicted from the available evidence, although in the case of herbal medicines, where much remains untested, this is likely to be speculative.
- Practitioner considerations
  - The ability and willingness of the practitioner to monitor and manage a potential interaction that is clinically significant can depend on the practitioner and the patient's setting. For example, in a hospital setting an interaction may be considered important if something needs to be done in order to relieve the patient's symptoms, or if it will have a significant impact on critical therapy. Practitioners and nursing staff are in an ideal position to detect and manage interactions if necessary. In a community setting, general practitioners, pharmacists and CM practitioners are well placed to advise on interactions and ensure adequate patient self-monitoring.
- Individual considerations—these include:
  - individual patient risk factors that may be present and may increase the likelihood of an adverse reaction
  - the patient's individual treatment preferences
  - the patient's ability to self-monitor a potential interaction and seek professional advice if they are concerned.
- Action required—having considered the previous steps to predict the 'likelihood' and 'consequence' of an interaction, five actions are possible:
  - *Avoid the new medicinal agent*—a relatively high likelihood and/or severity of the consequence make it an unacceptable risk, so an alternative treatment should be considered.
  - *Avoid unless adequate medical monitoring is possible*—a relatively high likelihood and/or severity of the consequence may be acceptable if professional help is available to manage the outcome and supervise treatment.
  - *Caution*—the likelihood of an adverse effect is relatively lower and/or a more minor consequence is possible than the previous level, making it an acceptable risk if the patient is made aware of the possibility and seeks professional advice if concerned.
  - *Observe*—there is a relatively low likelihood and/or negligible clinical consequence of a predicted interaction, making it an acceptable risk.
  - *Prescribe*—there is a relatively high likelihood of a beneficial consequence, making the interaction clinically useful.

If you suspect an interaction, what are the next steps?

1 **Case reporting**
   - A detailed case report should be written, to alert authorities to the possible interaction.
   - All suspected adverse reactions should be reported to the relevant authority(ies):
     - the local government agency responsible for post-marketing surveillance and collecting adverse drug reaction case reports (in Australia this is the Adverse Drug Reactions Advisory Committee (ADRAC)—reporting is confidential, open to everyone and can be done online, www.tga.gov.au)
     - local herbal and natural medicine associations
     - the relevant product manufacturer—in some countries, manufacturers keep their own records and are obligated to inform the relevant government authorities; they may also need to recall suspected faulty products
     - the prescriber—if applicable.

2 **Analysis of the medicine**
   - Ask the patient to bring in a sample of the medicine. If an interaction involving a herbal or natural medicine is highly likely, then it must be authenticated and botanically verified, and analysed for the presence of contaminants. These essential steps will establish whether the interaction is due to an intrinsic property of the medicine itself and therefore reproducible, or due to extrinsic factors such as poor manufacturing processes.

CONCLUSION

The evidence on the safety of herbal medicines is incomplete, complex and confusing. As with pharmaceutical medicines, their use is associated with both risks and benefits. As more people take herbal medicines, the pressure increases on healthcare professionals such as doctors, pharmacists, naturopaths and herbalists to be well informed about the subject, and on researchers to fill the many and somewhat embarrassing gaps in our current knowledge. It could be argued that failing to do (and fund) this work constitutes the true risk associated with herbal medicines.

RESOURCES

Adverse Drug Reactions Advisory Committee (ADRAC), http://www.tga.gov.au

Braun L, Cohen M. Herbs and natural supplements: an evidence-based guide. 3rd edn. Sydney: Elsevier; 2009.

Brinker F. Herb contraindications and drug interactions. 3rd edn. USA: Eclectic Medical Publications; 2001.

Bone K, Mills S. The essential guide to herbal safety. Sydney: Elsevier; 2005.

Natural Standard, http://www.naturalstandard.com/

Natural Medicines Comprehensive Database, http://www.naturaldatabase.com/(S(frcdl52p5bn02uqyb2buvg33))/home.aspx

REFERENCES

1 MacLennan AH, Wilson DH, Taylor AW. The escalating cost and prevalence of alternative medicine. Prev Med 2002; 35(2):166–173.

2 Jamison JR. Herbal and nutrient supplementation practices of chiropractic patients: an Australian case study. J Manipulative Physiol Ther 2003; 26(4):242.

3 Barraco D, Valencia G, Riba AL et al. Complementary and alternative medicine (CAM) use patterns and disclosure to physicians in acute coronary syndrome patients. Complement Ther Med 2005; 13(1):34–40.

4 Eisenberg DM, Davis RB, Ettner SL et al. Trends in alternative medicine use in the United States, 1990–1997: results of a follow-up national survey. JAMA 1998; 280(18):1569–1575.

5 Norred CL, Zamudio S, Palmer SK. Use of complementary and alternative medicines by surgical patients. AANA J 2000; 68(1):13–18.

6 Kaye AD, Clarke RC, Sabar R et al. Herbal medicines: current trends in anesthesiology practice—a hospital survey. J Clin Anesth 2000; 12(6):468–471.

7 Leung JM, Dzankic S, Manku K et al. The prevalence and predictors of the use of alternative medicine in presurgical patients in five California hospitals. Anesth Analg 2001; 93(4):1062–1068.

8 Norred CL. Complementary and alternative medicine use by surgical patients. AORN J 2002; 76(6):1013–1021.

9 Adusumilli PS, Ben Porat L, Pereira M et al. The prevalence and predictors of herbal medicine use in surgical patients. J Am Coll Surg 2004; 198(4):583–590.

10 Norred CL. A follow-up survey of the use of complementary and alternative medicines by surgical patients. AANA J 2002; 70(2):119–125.

11 Tsen LC, Segal S, Pothier M et al. Alternative medicine use in presurgical patients. Anesthesiology 2000; 93(1):148–151.

12 Wang SM, Caldwell-Andrews AA, Kain ZN. The use of complementary and alternative medicines by surgical patients: a follow-up survey study. Anesth Analg 2003; 97(4):1010–1015.

13 Skinner CM, Rangasami J. Preoperative use of herbal medicines: a patient survey. Br J Anaesth 2002; 89(5):792–795.

14 Vaabengaard P, Clausen LM. Surgery patients' intake of herbal preparations and dietary supplements. Ugeskr Laeger 2003; 165(35):3320–3323.

15 MacLennan AH, Myers SP, Taylor AW. The continuing use of complementary and alternative medicine in South Australia: costs and beliefs in 2004. Med J Aust 2006; 184(1):27–31.

16 Astin JA. Why patients use alternative medicine: results of a national study. JAMA 1998; 279(19): 1548–1553.

17 Eisenberg DM, Kessler RC, Van Rompay MI et al. Perceptions about complementary therapies relative to conventional therapies among adults who use both: results from a national survey. Ann Intern Med 2001; 135(5):344–351.

18 Siahpush M. Why do people favour alternative medicine? Aust NZ J Public Health 1999; 23(3):266–271.

19 Braun L, Cohen MM. Herbs and natural supplements—an evidence-based guide. 3rd edn. Sydney: Elsevier; 2009.

20 Huupponen R, Seppala P, Iisalo E. Effect of guar gum, a fibre preparation, on digoxin and penicillin absorption in man. Eur J Clin Pharmacol 1984; 26(2):279–281.

21 Rodrigues AD, Lin JH. Screening of drug candidates for their drug–drug interaction potential. Curr Opin Chem Biol 2001; 5(4):396–401.

22 Roby CA, Anderson GD, Kantor E et al. St John's Wort: effect on CYP3A4 activity. Clin Pharmacol Ther 2000; 67(5):451–457.

23 Ruschitzka F, Meier PJ, Turina M et al. Acute heart transplant rejection due to Saint John's wort. Lancet 2000; 355(9203):548–549.

24 Durr D, Stieger B, Kullak-Ublick GA et al. St John's wort induces intestinal P-glycoprotein/MDR1 and intestinal and hepatic CYP3A4. Clin Pharmacol Ther 2000; 68(6):598–604.

25 Wang Z, Gorski JC, Hamman MA et al. The effects of St John's wort (*Hypericum perforatum*) on human cytochrome P450 activity. Clin Pharmacol Ther 2001; 70(4):317–326.

26 Moore LB, Goodwin B, Jones SA et al. St John's wort induces hepatic drug metabolism through activation of the pregnane X receptor. Proc Natl Acad Sci USA 2000; 97(13):7500–7502.

27 Madabushi R, Frank B, Drewelow B et al. Hyperforin in St John's wort drug interactions. Eur J Clin Pharmacol 2006; 62(3):225–233.

28 Mueller SC, Uehleke B, Woehling H et al. Effect of St John's wort dose and preparations on the pharmacokinetics of digoxin. Clin Pharmacol Ther 2004; 75(6):546–557.
29 Arold G, Donath F, Maurer A et al. No relevant interaction with alprazolam, caffeine, tolbutamide, and digoxin by treatment with a low-hyperforin St John's wort extract. Planta Med 2005; 71(4):331–337.
30 Zhao LZ, Huang M, Chen J et al. Induction of propranolol metabolism by *Ginkgo biloba* extract EGb 761 in rats. Curr Drug Metab 2006; 7(6):577–587.
31 Mohutsky MA, Anderson GD, Miller JW et al. *Ginkgo biloba*: evaluation of CYP2C9 drug interactions in vitro and in vivo. Am J Ther 2006; 13(1):24–31.
32 Chang TK, Chen J, Teng XW. Distinct role of bilobalide and ginkgolide A in the modulation of rat CYP2B1 and CYP3A23 gene expression by *Ginkgo biloba* extract in cultured hepatocytes. Drug Metab Dispos 2006; 34(2):234–242.
33 Chang TK, Chen J, Yeung EY. Effect of *Ginkgo biloba* extract on procarcinogen-bioactivating human CYP1 enzymes: identification of isorhamnetin, kaempferol, and quercetin as potent inhibitors of CYP1B1. Toxicol Appl Pharmacol 2006; 213(1):18–26.
34 Chatterjee SS, Doelman CJ, Noldner M et al. Influence of the *Ginkgo* extract EGb 761 on rat liver cytochrome P450 and steroid metabolism and excretion in rats and man. J Pharm Pharmacol 2005; 57(5):641–650.
35 von Moltke LL, Weemhoff JL, Bedir E et al. Inhibition of human cytochrome P450 by components of *Ginkgo biloba*. J Pharm Pharmacol 2004; 56(8):1039–1044.
36 Sugiyama T, Kubota Y, Shinozuka K et al. *Ginkgo biloba* extract modifies hypoglycemic action of tolbutamide via hepatic cytochrome P450 mediated mechanism in aged rats. Life Sci 2004; 75(9):1113–1122.
37 Gaudineau C, Beckerman R, Welbourn S et al. Inhibition of human P450 enzymes by multiple constituents of the *Ginkgo biloba* extract. Biochem Biophys Res Commun 2004; 318(4):1072–1078.
38 He N, Edeki T. The inhibitory effects of herbal components on CYP2C9 and CYP3A4 catalytic activities in human liver microsomes. Am J Ther 2004; 11(3):206–212.
39 Sugiyama T, Kubota Y, Shinozuka K et al. Induction and recovery of hepatic drug metabolizing enzymes in rats treated with *Ginkgo biloba* extract. Food Chem Toxicol 2004; 42(6):953–957.
40 Kuo I, Chen J, Chang TK. Effect of *Ginkgo biloba* extract on rat hepatic microsomal CYP1A activity: role of ginkgolides, bilobalide, and flavonols. Can J Physiol Pharmacol 2004; 82(1):57–64.
41 Kubota Y, Kobayashi K, Tanaka N et al. Pretreatment with *Ginkgo biloba* extract weakens the hypnosis action of phenobarbital and its plasma concentration in rats. J Pharm Pharmacol 2004; 56(3):401–405.
42 Ohnishi N, Kusuhara M, Yoshioka M et al. Studies on interactions between functional foods or dietary supplements and medicines. I. Effects of *Ginkgo biloba* leaf extract on the pharmacokinetics of diltiazem in rats. Biol Pharm Bull 2003; 26(9):1315–1320.
43 Ryu SD, Chung WG. Induction of the procarcinogen-activating CYP1A2 by a herbal dietary supplement in rats and humans. Food Chem Toxicol 2003; 41(6): 861–866.
44 Shinozuka K, Umegaki K, Kubota Y et al. Feeding of *Ginkgo biloba* extract (GBE) enhances gene expression of hepatic cytochrome P-450 and attenuates the hypotensive effect of nicardipine in rats. Life Sci 2002; 70(23): 2783–2792.
45 Gurley BJ, Gardner SF, Hubbard MA et al. Cytochrome P450 phenotypic ratios for predicting herb–drug interactions in humans. Clin Pharmacol Ther 2002; 72(3):276–287.
46 Markowitz JS, Donovan JL, Lindsay DC et al. Multiple-dose administration of *Ginkgo biloba* did not affect cytochrome P-450 2D6 or 3A4 activity in normal volunteers. J Clin Psychopharmacol 2003; 23(6):576–581.
47 Greenblatt DJ, von Moltke LL, Luo Y et al. *Ginkgo biloba* does not alter clearance of flurbiprofen, a cytochrome P450-2C9 substrate. J Clin Pharmacol 2006; 46(2): 214–221.
48 Mohutsky MA, Anderson GD, Miller JW et al. *Ginkgo biloba*: evaluation of CYP2C9 drug interactions in vitro and in vivo. Am J Ther 2006; 13(1):24–31.
49 Yale SH, Glurich I. Analysis of the inhibitory potential of *Ginkgo biloba*, *Echinacea purpurea*, and *Serenoa repens* on the metabolic activity of cytochrome P450 3A4, 2D6, and 2C9. J Altern Complement Med 2005; 11(3):433–439.
50 Markowitz JS, Donovan JL, Devane CL et al. Multiple doses of saw palmetto (*Serenoa repens*) did not alter cytochrome P450 2D6 and 3A4 activity in normal volunteers. Clin Pharmacol Ther 2003; 74(6):536–542.
51 Gurley BJ, Gardner SF, Hubbard MA et al. In vivo assessment of botanical supplementation on human cytochrome P450 phenotypes: *Citrus aurantium*, *Echinacea purpurea*, milk thistle, and saw palmetto. Clin Pharmacol Ther 2004; 76(5):428–440.
52 Fukao T, Hosono T, Misawa S et al. The effects of allyl sulfides on the induction of phase II detoxification enzymes and liver injury by carbon tetrachloride. Food Chem Toxicol 2004; 42(5):743–749.

chapter 6

The essence of good health

INTRODUCTION AND OVERVIEW

As community attitudes evolve, healthcare costs spiral and evidence accumulates, the community and general practitioners are steadily recognising the importance of moving towards more holistic and wellness-based models of healthcare. Models such as Dean Ornish's lifestyle program for heart disease have been shown to significantly reduce costs while also leading to better therapeutic outcomes.[1]

Among the great advances in healthcare in the twentieth century were antibiotics, anaesthetics and immunisation, with the genetic revolution just beginning to gain momentum. Despite these significant discoveries, the greatest burden of illness in affluent countries is due to lifestyle-related illnesses.[2] Cardiovascular disease is still the leading cause of death, followed closely by cancer. It is predicted that by 2030 depressive illnesses will be the leading burden of disease.[3] The trends in obesity, inactivity, drug use and mental illness are far from encouraging, and the long-term impact of these determinants of health may be far greater than expected. They all interact synergistically to predispose towards illness; and conversely, positive strategies to enhance health also act synergistically.

An important aspect of a holistic or wellness approach is to empower the patient and their carers as much as is practicable. Responsible patient empowerment accords with most patients' wishes and is also associated with better clinical and economic outcomes.

Initiatives instigated by health promotion organisations make a significant contribution to reversing the trends mentioned above, but for these initiatives to be effective they need to be targeted at, and reinforced by, various sectors in the healthcare community, spanning policy makers, individual therapists and consumer groups. The potential role that GPs and other primary health practitioners can play is enormous, although the economic and legislative systems in which doctors work do not always make this approach as easy to instigate as it should be.

THE ESSENCE MODEL

This chapter gives an outline of the ESSENCE model of healthcare. ESSENCE is a mnemonic:

E Education
S Stress management
S Spirituality
E Exercise
N Nutrition
C Connectedness
E Environment

ESSENCE extends and gives further structure to the biopsychosocial and environmental models of healthcare. Some brief comments about the relevance and application of each aspect are made below, along with some examples of how they are applied in practice.

The ESSENCE approach is a comprehensive framework to assist in the prevention and management of illness as well as promoting wellness. It is holistic in its focus, designed to complement conventional medical care and is eminently applicable to the primary care setting.[4] ESSENCE has been the basis for the Health Enhancement Program (HEP) taught as core curriculum for all medical students at Monash University, Melbourne. It serves to enhance the personal wellbeing of the practitioner as well as to foster patient wellbeing and provide clinical knowledge and skills.[5]

The ESSENCE model forms a useful structure upon which educational, preventive and therapeutic approaches can be built and is readily adaptable for health professionals, individual patients, targeted groups suffering chronic illness, practice populations and public health campaigns.

For lifestyle interventions to be optimally effective, a structured, systematic and comprehensive approach to dealing with a range of relevant variables needs to be used. This helps the planning, implementation and evaluation of lifestyle and healthcare plans. This chapter gives an overview of the model and its relevance to a condition such as cardiovascular disease, and illustrates its application to a case of multiple sclerosis.

EDUCATION

In its broadest sense, education is at the core of what it means to be a doctor, for no condition could be said to be adequately treated without educating the patient, and their carers, about relevant aspects of their condition and its management. Education can therefore include:

- knowledge about the condition and its management, which, for chronic conditions especially, is beneficial in a number of ways—it improves cost-effectiveness, adjustment to the illness, perceived self-competence and compliance, and it reduces the use of medical services[6]
- information about the effects of lifestyle factors on health, and about reducing or ceasing relevant behaviours such as smoking or alcohol use
- behaviour-change, motivational and self-mastery strategies, which are vital in activating knowledge so it is more than just information. Simple information about the ill-effects of various cardiac risk factors, for example, has little effect on reducing cardiac risk. If, however, this information is supported by strategies that improve 'control' or 'autonomy', such as stress management, behaviour change, self-mastery and motivational strategies, then the information can be acted upon and health benefits follow.[7,8]

In the conventional sense, education is also protective of health, and a lack of formal education by itself is a risk factor for poor health.[9] Indeed, one of the most powerful ways to improve health in developing countries is to improve literacy rates among women.

STRESS MANAGEMENT

In the ESSENCE model, 'stress' refers not just to stress in the common sense of the word, but also mental health in the broadest sense. Good mental health is central to being able to make and maintain other lifestyle improvements. This is illustrated in the Ornish lifestyle program for heart disease, in which stress management was the vital factor in ensuring that all the other lifestyle factors could be implemented and maintained.[1,10] We well know that making healthy lifestyle changes while stressed, anxious or depressed is difficult, if not impossible.

The need to cultivate positive mental and emotional health is an issue for everyone, not just those with significant mental illness. In our thinking and terminology, healthcare practitioners draw an imaginary line below which a person has mental illness and above which they don't. A wellness model, on the other hand, acknowledges that health is a continuum. Although we draw arbitrary lines to assist us in defining and diagnosing various conditions, we are all moving in one direction or another towards more or less wellbeing. It follows therefore that all can benefit from applying positive mental health strategies. The benefits are both direct, in providing greater quality of life, and indirect, in providing improvements in lifestyle.

Mental health has a profound and direct effect upon physical health and recovery from illness. To illustrate, it is well known that depression is a major independent risk factor for cardiovascular disease (Fig 6.1)[11]—chronic severe depression increases the risk of cardiovascular disease fivefold—but less well known is the evidence that the addition of a comprehensive psychologically based stress-management plan to conventional cardiac rehabilitation nearly halves the risk of subsequent cardiac events.[12] One effective stress-management program reduced cardiac events by 74% over a 5-year follow-up compared with usual care alone.[13] So improving mental health is important for quality of life, to facilitate other healthy lifestyle changes and for its direct physiological health benefits.

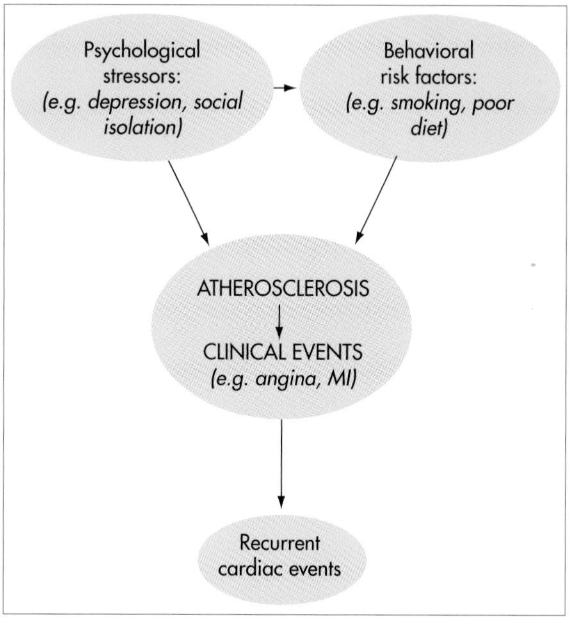

FIGURE 6.1 Psychosocial factors contributing to cardiovascular disease

SPIRITUALITY

'Spirituality' is not confined to being 'religious'. It can, depending on the individual's view, be explored through an active search for 'meaning' or 'purpose', or it can denote a belief in something greater than oneself. Each individual explores and expresses spirituality in a way which is relevant to themselves and their cultural background. For some, spirituality is explored and expressed through science, or through altruism and philanthropy, or in art and creativity, or through a commitment to environment and ecology.

The influence of spirituality on health is not always easy to determine, and yet evidence clearly points to it having an important role in the prevention and management of a range of psychological and physical diseases[14,15] as well as helping the individual to cope, especially with chronic and life-threatening disease.[16]

Although some doctors may believe that spirituality is not the domain of the medical practitioner, evidence suggests that approximately 80% of patients wish to discuss spiritual matters with their doctors in certain circumstances, such as when confronting a life-threatening illness.[17] If doctors are to incorporate spiritual and religious issues where the need arises, then patient-appropriate language, an attitude of cultural and religious tolerance, and appropriate referral sources, will be essential in underpinning that conversation. These issues will be discussed in more depth in the chapter on spirituality (Ch 12).

EXERCISE

Exercise in itself is a therapeutic tool[18] and lack of exercise ranks second to smoking as a cause of disability and death in Australia.[19] There is an enormous amount of evidence on the beneficial effects of exercise in preventing and managing virtually any condition, and yet exercise is not a central part of the management plan as often as it should be. Obviously the type, duration and intensity of exercise needs to be tailored to an individual's needs, tastes, health and abilities.

The important role of exercise can be illustrated using an example of cardiovascular disease (CVD). Apart from reducing all-cause mortality,[20] regular exercise also decreases disease-specific mortality from CVD.[21–23] This is through a variety of effects, such as improvements in lipid profile, reduced thrombogenesis, improvement in insulin resistance and reduction of blood pressure. If exercise is prescribed for CVD it has positive side effects, such as benefits for osteoporosis and diabetes,[24] and reduced cancer risk (including lung, colon, breast and prostate).[25–27] Exercise also has an important role in mental health for old and young—for example, it is therapeutic for depression[28] and anxiety.[29] These issues will also be explored in a subsequent chapter.

NUTRITION

The prevalence of unhealthy diet and obesity is escalating in most affluent countries. Nutritional advice can mean providing guidelines about things such as the amount of fat or salt to eat in the diet, but it also includes the use of 'food as medicine'.

Deficient diets are a more major source of illness than tends to be acknowledged in medical education and this no doubt is reflected in clinical practice. Carefully chosen supplements may play a role in some circumstances, but they are not a replacement for a healthy diet. For example, beta-carotene supplements are probably not effective in preventing cancer,[30] whereas beta-carotene-rich foods are.[31,32] Research has shown that:

> Women in the highest quartile of plasma total carotenoid concentration (marker of intake of vegetables and fruit) had significantly reduced risk for a new breast cancer event (HR 0.57) [that is, a 43% reduction in risk of recurrence].[33]

and that:

> Vegetable and, particularly, fruit consumption contributed to the decreased risk ... These results indicate the importance of diet, rather than supplement use, in concert with endogenous antioxidant capabilities, in the reduction of breast cancer risk.[34]

A similar picture is seen in CVD. Fish oils, due to their high concentration of omega-3 fatty acids, for example, produce benefits for triglyceride[35] and very low-density lipoprotein (VLDL) profiles,[36] prevention of arrhythmias,[37,38] reduction of blood pressure[39] and reduction of atherogenesis,[40] and they have antithrombotic and antiplatelet activity.

For the greater part of clinical practice, the dietary advice given by doctors tends to be non-specific. Perhaps this is a reflection of the level of attention given to the topic in medical education and literature, but if the effects attributable to healthy nutrition were attributable to a pharmaceutical product, then a doctor would probably be negligent in not knowing about it in detail and prescribing it widely. The important role of nutrition will also be explored in Chapter 10.

CONNECTEDNESS

'Connectedness' or social support is important at any age or situation in life. For children and adolescents, connectedness at home and at school is strongly protective against comorbidities such as depression, suicide, drug and alcohol abuse, teenage pregnancy, crime and violence.[41] The presence of 'functional relationships' is associated with a better recovery from depression. Social marginality or isolation has been shown to predispose to heart disease, cancer, depression, hypertension, arthritis, schizophrenia, tuberculosis and overall mortality.[42] All-cause mortality in socially isolated males was 2–3 times higher and in women was 1.5 times higher over a 12-year follow-up than in people who were more socially connected.[43] With regard to heart disease, socioeconomic and occupational factors are independent risk factors,[44,45] but even when a person has well-established heart disease, their social context has a profound effect on recovery. There was a fourfold increased in the death rate following acute myocardial infarction (AMI) for people who were socially isolated and experiencing high levels of stress.[46] Those over 65 years of age were three times more likely to die following an AMI if they had poor social support, as measured by the simple question: 'Can you count on anyone to provide you with emotional support (talking over problems or helping you to make a difficult decision)?'[47] So connectedness plays an important role in the prevention and management of any disease and at any stage of the life cycle. The GP is well placed to provide emotional support, to encourage patients to seek out sources of social support, and in some settings to facilitate support in the form of support groups.

ENVIRONMENT

'Environment' means much more than air, water and earth, as important as these are. It includes the number and types of chemicals we are exposed to, domestically and occupationally. It includes the radiation and electromagnetic fields to which we are exposed.[48] Importantly, it includes the social and sensory environment we create for ourselves. An overly noisy medical environment, for example, is associated with poorer health and higher stress.[49]

Sunlight can play both a positive and a negative role for health, depending on the amount and type of sun exposure. Although sunburn increases the incidence of malignant melanoma, regular moderate doses of sunlight help to reduce the incidence of a range of illnesses including depression, heart disease, a number of cancers including melanoma, multiple sclerosis and osteoporosis, to name a few.[50]

Obviously it is beyond the power of the doctor to change most types of environmental exposure, but nevertheless they can help to give practical advice about environmental issues and exposure. Furthermore, some doctors play an important role as community advocates, policy makers or researchers.

USING ESSENCE IN PRACTICE

The ESSENCE model is designed to give a structure to lifestyle and holistic management. Without structure it is often difficult for doctors and patients to set systematic, specific and achievable goals. When confronted by a number of potential goals it can be prudent to work on one goal at a time. As improvement is established with regard to one goal, another can be tackled according to the patient's motivation and priorities. Many aspects of ESSENCE, such as making healthy dietary changes, may well need the support and engagement of relevant others such as family members. An example of applying ESSENCE to a case is provided here.

CASE STUDY

Helen is a 37-year-old woman with a past history of multiple sclerosis (MS) diagnosed when she was 32 years old. She has recently moved from interstate with her husband and two children and now presents to you with a view to finding a new GP. At the initial consultation you find that she has only mild ongoing neurological impairment by way of some weakness in her left leg and numbness in the right leg. She is interested in taking an active part in the management of her MS and wants to take a holistic approach to her illness.[51] You encourage her in her endeavour and make a long appointment for next week for her to come back to discuss the ESSENCE approach. In the meantime you explore further background information about lifestyle factors and MS to help inform yourself more fully. At the follow-up consultation you discuss the following issues with her.

Education

You provide the patient with education in the following information and self-help strategies, as well as by suggesting a readable and authoritative text on the subject of lifestyle factors and MS.[52]

Stress management

Psychological health has a significant impact on the progression of MS and on how a person copes with it.[53–55] You inform Helen about the basic principles of how stress affects immune function and autoimmune conditions, and suggest that stress management is a vital part of improving psychological wellbeing and of assisting her in making and maintaining other lifestyle changes. Helen expresses interest in joining the evening stress management classes being held in your practice.

Spirituality

Helen states that although she is not overly religious, looking for meaning in dealing with her illness has helped her to cope. You encourage her to continue to explore this area of her life.

Exercise

For MS patients, regular exercise can increase general fitness and strength, reduce disability,[56] improve mood and coping, reduce the number of falls and fractures, enhance social interaction and improve immune function. You discuss and agree on an 'exercise prescription', which includes attending her local fitness centre and walking regularly with her husband, in the morning and late afternoon sun where possible. You also encourage Helen to explore the MS Society's hydrotherapy program.

Nutrition

Studies of dietary interventions for the management of MS[57–59] have suggested that MS patients on a low-fat diet (less than 20 g/day) may have lower death rates, disability and numbers of MS exacerbations than those not on a low-fat diet. Supplements with omega-3 fatty acids may also be associated with significant reductions in the frequency and severity of relapses.[60] Fish and flaxseed oils, high in omega-3 fatty acids, have significant anti-inflammatory properties in a range of conditions including MS, and fish oils are also an excellent source of vitamin D. Vitamin D enhances immune function, and seems to reduce the incidence and progression of MS.[61] Potentially protective nutrients for MS patients include vegetable protein, dietary and cereal fibre, other vitamins (C, thiamin and riboflavin), calcium and potassium.[62] You inform Helen of these findings, and she is keen to start including these dietary changes in her diet and will also explore using some selected dietary supplements under your guidance.

Connectedness

Stressful life events and an unsupportive social life are associated with the onset and exacerbation of a variety of autoimmune diseases.[63] Helen says that she gets great support from her family, although moving interstate has been a source of potential concern. She also finds that going to the MS Society has given her great support and that attending the hydrotherapy classes will enhance this even further.

Environment

Countries with lower levels of sunshine have significantly higher incidences of MS. Within countries, those regions with more sunlight also have a substantially lower incidence.[64,65] The progression of MS over an 11-year period was nearly halved (odds ratio (OR) 0.53) for those with higher residential sun exposure.[66] High residential exposure and occupational exposure combined was associated with an OR of 0.24, that is, a quarter chance of dying over that 11-year period compared to those with low sun exposure. The benefits of sunlight may be due to the direct effects of sunlight on immune function, melatonin levels[67] and vitamin D.[68] Helen says that she has tended to avoid sunshine and will make an effort to get at least 20 minutes of sun exposure daily and that linking it to her exercise times will be a sensible way of doing that.

You make plans to review Helen's progress in two weeks.

Acknowledgment

This chapter is adapted from Hassed C. The essence of health. Sydney: Random House; 2008.

RESOURCES

Hassed C. The essence of health. Sydney: Random House; 2008.

Jelinek G. Taking control of MS. Melbourne: Hyland House; 2005.

Also see other chapters on individual elements such as nutrition, exercise, mind–body and connectedness.

REFERENCES

1 Ornish D, Brown SE, Scherwitz LW et al. Can lifestyle changes reverse coronary heart disease? Lancet 1990; 336:129–133.
2 Lopez AD, Mathers CD, Ezzati M et al. Global and regional burden of disease and risk factors, 2001: systematic analysis of population health data. Lancet 2006; 367(9524):1747–1757.
3 Mathers CD, Loncar D. Projections of global mortality and burden of disease from 2002 to 2030. PLoS Med 2006; 3(11):e442.
4 Hassed C. The ESSENCE of healthcare. Aust Fam Physician 2005; 34(11):957–960.
5 Hassed C, de Lisle S, Sullivan G et al. Enhancing the health of medical students: outcomes of an integrated mindfulness and lifestyle program. Adv Health Sci Educ 2009; 14(3):387–398.
6 Lehrer PM, Sargunaraj D, Hochron S. Psychological approaches to the treatment of asthma. J Consult Clinical Psychol 1992; 60(4):639–643.
7 Syme SL, Balfour JL. Explaining inequalities in coronary heart disease. Lancet 1997; 350(9073):231–232.
8 Syme SL. Mastering the control factor. The Health Report, ABC Radio. Health Report transcript, 9 November 1998. Online. Available: www.abc.net.au/rn
9 Eckert JK, Rubinstein RL. Older men's health. Sociocultural and ecological perspectives. Med Clin North Am 1999; 83(5):1151–1172.
10 Ornish D, Scherwitz L, Billings J et al. Intensive lifestyle changes for reversal of coronary heart disease. JAMA 1998; 280:2001–2007.
11 Bunker SJ, Colquhoun DM, Esler MD et al. 'Stress' and coronary heart disease: psychosocial risk factors. Med J Aust 2003; 178(6):272–276.
12 Linden W, Stossel C, Maurice J. Psychosocial interventions for patients with coronary artery disease: a meta-analysis. Arch Int Med 1996; 156(7):745–752.

13 Blumenthal J, Jiang W, Babyak MA et al. Stress management and exercise training in cardiac patients with myocardial ischaemia. Arch Int Med 1997; 157:2213–2223.
14 Koenig HG. Religion and medicine II: religion, mental health, and related behaviors. Int J Psychiatry Med 2001; 31(1):97–109.
15 Townsend M, Kladder V, Ayele H et al. Systematic review of clinical trials examining the effects of religion on health. South Med J 2002; 95(12):1429–1434.
16 Sullivan MD. Hope and hopelessness at the end of life. Am J Geriatr Psychiatry 2003; 11(4):393–405.
17 McCord G, Gilchrist VJ, Grossman SD et al. Discussing spirituality with patients: a rational and ethical approach. Ann Fam Med 2004; 2(4):356–361.
18 Bauman A. Updating the evidence that physical activity is good for health: an epidemiological review 2000–2003. J Sci Med Sport 2004; 7(1 Suppl):6–19.
19 Australian Institute of Health and Welfare. Heart, stroke and vascular diseases—Australian facts 2001. National Heart Foundation of Australia, National Stroke Foundation of Australia (Cardiovascular Disease Series No 14). AIWH Cat. No. CVD 13. Canberra: AIWH; 2001.
20 Kampert J, Blair S, Barlow C et al. Physical activity, fitness and all cause and cancer mortality. Ann Epidemiol 1996; 6: 542–547.
21 Maiorana A, O'Driscoll G, Cheetham C et al. Combined aerobic and resistance exercise training improves functional capacity and strength in CHF. J Appl Physiol 2000; 88:1565–1570.
22 Berlin J, Colditz G. A meta-analysis of physical activity in the prevention of coronary heart disease. Am J Epidemiol 1990; 132: 612–628.
23 Tanasescu M, Leitzmann MF, Rimm EB et al. Exercise type and intensity in relation to coronary heart disease in men. JAMA 2002; 288:1994–2000.
24 Helmrich S, Ragland D, Paffenbarger R. Prevention of non-insulin dependent diabetes mellitus with physical activity. Med Sci Sports Exerc 1994; 26:649–660.
25 Colditz G, Cannuscio C, Grazier A. Physical activity and reduced risk of colon cancer. Cancer Causes Control 1997; 8:649–667.
26 Thune I, Lund E. The influence of physical activity on lung cancer risk. Int J Cancer 1997; 70:57–62.
27 Friedenreich CM, McGregor SE, Courneya KS et al. Case-control study of lifetime total physical activity and prostate cancer risk. Am J Epidemiol 2004; 159(8): 740–749.
28 Dunn AL, Trivedi MH, Kampert JB et al. Exercise treatment for depression. Efficacy and dose response. Am J Prev Med 2005; 28(1):1–8.
29 Byrne A, Byrne DG. The effect of exercise on depression, anxiety and other mood states: a review. J Psychosom Res 1993; 13(3):160–170.
30 Hennekens CH et al. Lack of effect of long-term supplementation with beta carotene on the incidence of malignant neoplasms and cardiovascular disease. N Engl J Med 1996; 334(18):1145–1149.
31 Omenn GS, Goodman GE, Thornquist MD et al. Effects of a combination of beta carotene and vitamin A on lung cancer and cardiovascular disease. N Engl J Med 1996; 334(18):1150–1155.
32 Shekelle RB, Lepper M, Liu S et al. Dietary vitamin A and the risk of cancer in the Western Electric study. Lancet 1981; 2(8257):1186–1190.
33 Rock CL, Flatt SW, Natarajan L et al. Plasma carotenoids and recurrence-free survival in women with a history of breast cancer. J Clin Oncol 2005; 23(27):6631–6638.
34 Ahn J, Gammon MD, Santella RM et al. Associations between breast cancer risk and the catalase genotype, fruit and vegetable consumption, and supplement use. Am J Epidemiol 2005; 162(10):943–952.
35 Jeppesen J, Hein HO, Suadicani P et al. Triglyceride concentration and ischemic heart disease: an eight-year follow up in the Copenhagen Male Study. Circulation 1998; 97(11):1029–1036.
36 Vanschoonbeek K, de Maat MP, Heemskerk JW. Fish oil consumption and reduction of arterial disease. Nutrition 2003; 133:657–660.
37 de Lorgeril M, Salen P. Alpha-linolenic acid and coronary heart disease. Nutr Metab Cardiovasc Dis 2004; 14(3):162–169.
38 McLennan PL, Abeywardena MY, Charnock JS. Dietary fish oil prevents ventricular fibrillation following coronary artery occlusion and reperfusion. Am J Heart 1988; 116(3):709–717.
39 Geleijnse JM, Grobbee DE. Blood pressure response to fish oil supplementation: meta regression analysis of randomised trials. J Hypertension 2002; 20(8): 1493–1499.
40 von Schacky C. The role of omega-3 fatty acids in cardiovascular disease. Curr Atherocler Rep 2003; 5(2):139–145.
41 Resnick MD, Bearman P, Blum R et al. Protecting adolescents from harm; findings from the National Longitudinal Study on Adolescent Health. JAMA 1997; 278(10):823–832.
42 Pelletier K. Mind–body health: research, clinical and policy applications. Am J Health Promot 1992; 6(5):345–358.
43 House J, Landis K, Umberson D. Social relationships and health. Science 1988; 241:540–545.
44 Lantz PM, House JS, Lepkowski JM et al. Socioeconomic factors, health behaviours, and mortality: results from a nationally representative prospective study of US adults. JAMA 1998; 279(21):1703–1708.

45 North FM, Syme SL, Feeney A et al. Psychosocial work environment and sickness absence among British civil servants: the Whitehall II study. Am J Public Health 1996; 86(3):332–340.
46 Ruberman W, Weinblatt E, Goldberg JD et al. Psychosocial influences on mortality after AMI. N Engl J Med 1984; 311:552–559.
47 Berkman LF, Leo-Summers L, Horwitz RI. Emotional support and survival after AMI: a prospective, population-based study of the elderly. Ann Intern Med 1992; 117:1003–1009.
48 Henshaw DL. Does our electricity distribution system pose a serious risk to public health? Med Hypotheses 2002; 59(1):39–51.
49 Topf M. Hospital noise pollution: an environmental stress model to guide research and clinical interventions. J Adv Nurs 2000; 31(3):520–528.
50 Hassed C. Are we living in the dark ages? The importance of sunlight. Aust Fam Physician 2002; 31(11):1039–1041.
51 Jelinek G, Hassed CS. Managing multiple sclerosis in primary care: are we forgetting something? Qual Prim Care 2009; 17(1):55–61.
52 Jelinek G. Taking control of multiple sclerosis. Melbourne: Hyland House; 2000.
53 Mohr DC, Hart SL, Julian L et al. Association between stressful life events and exacerbation in multiple sclerosis: a meta-analysis. BMJ 2004; 328(7442):731. Epub 19 March 2004.
54 Martinelli V. Trauma, stress and multiple sclerosis. Neurol Sci 2000; 21(4 Suppl 2):S849–S852.
55 Ackerman KD, Stover A, Heyman R et al. Relationship of cardiovascular reactivity, stressful life events, and multiple sclerosis disease activity. Brain Behav Immun 2003; 17(3):141–151.
56 Patti F, Ciancio MR, Cacopardo M et al. Effects of a short outpatient rehabilitation treatment on disability of multiple sclerosis patients—a randomised controlled trial. J Neurol 2003; 250(7):861–866.
57 Swank RL, Dugan BB. Effect of low saturated fat diet in early and late cases of multiple sclerosis. Lancet 1990; 336(8706):37–39.
58 Swank RL. Multiple sclerosis: fat–oil relationship. Nutrition 1991; 7(5):368–376.
59 Swank RL, Goodwin JW. How saturated fats may be a causative factor in multiple sclerosis and other diseases. Nutrition 2003; 19(5):478.
60 Nordvik I, Myhr KM, Nyland H et al. Effect of dietary advice and omega-3 supplementation in newly diagnosed MS patients. Acta Neurol Scand 2000; 102(3):143–149.
61 Hayes CE. Vitamin D: a natural inhibitor of multiple sclerosis. Proc Nutr Soc 2000; 59(4):531–535.
62 Ghadirian P, Jain M, Ducic S et al. Nutritional factors in the aetiology of multiple sclerosis: a case control study in Montreal, Canada. Int J Epidemiol 1998; 27:845–852.
63 Homo-Delarche F, Fitzpatrick F, Christeff N et al. Sex steroids, glucocorticoids, stress and autoimmunity. J Steroid Biochem Mol Biol 1991; 40(4–6):619–637.
64 O'Reilly MA, O'Reilly PM. Temporal influences on relapses of multiple sclerosis. Eur Neurol 1991; 31(6):391–395.
65 McMichael AJ, Hall AJ. Does immunosuppressive ultraviolet radiation explain the latitude gradient for multiple sclerosis? Epidemiology 1997; 8:642–645.
66 Freedman DM, Dosemeci M, Alavanja MC. Mortality from multiple sclerosis and exposure to residential and occupational solar radiation: a case-control study based on death certificates. Occup Environ Med 2000; 57(6):418–421.
67 Hutter CD, Laing P. Multiple sclerosis: sunlight, diet, immunology and aetiology. Med Hypotheses 1996; 46(2):67–74.
68 Green MH, Petit-Frere C, Clingen PH et al. Possible effects of sunlight on human lymphocytes. J Epidemiol 1999; 9(6 Suppl):S48–S57.

chapter 7

Behaviour change strategies

INTRODUCTION AND OVERVIEW

It is increasingly being acknowledged that lifestyle factors contribute significantly to virtually all the common chronic conditions encountered in affluent countries. Changing people's health behaviours, however, is easier said than done, particularly with behaviours that have been ingrained for a long time, or where the motivation for change is mixed. The challenge of behaviour change can also be compounded by addiction, where a person's upbringing has not fostered responsible or balanced lifestyle choices and where the environment in which one is living works against healthy behaviour change.

AUTONOMY

Being able to successfully change and maintain healthy behaviours relies on more than just receiving health information from a healthcare professional.

> Helping people change high-risk behavior will be the key to prevention. To develop more effective prevention programs, we will have to train a new generation of experts who can not only provide people with risk information but also work with them as partners in achieving mutually agreed upon goals.[1]

Much of the early research into cardiovascular risk factors suggested that, independently of other lifestyle factors, a learned or perceived lack of control or autonomy is a central factor in the development of an illness. Gaining autonomy, on the other hand, is consistently associated with better health outcomes. Control is also intimately linked with stress, because when a person goes through a stressful life-event, having some control over either the event or their attitude to it will buffer the person from the potential for stress in response to the event. This is indicated in many ways, from changes in immune function, blood pressure and gut function to important changes in brain activity. When a perceived lack of control is a consistent state, it has a cumulative effect on emotional wellbeing, allostatic load and behaviour.

To illustrate this point, a study on the association between work stress (job strain and effort–reward imbalance) and the risk of death from cardiovascular disease found a strong association. Over 800 employees were followed up for 25 years. It was found that high job strain (high demands, low job control) led to more than a doubling of the risk of dying from heart disease compared with those with low job strain.[2] An effort–reward imbalance (low salary, lack of social approval and few career opportunities relative to efforts required at work) produced a similar effect. Noting the association is interesting. Intervening to mitigate its effects, though, is far more useful.

The 'control' associated with higher levels of stress and illness is an uneasy balance between tensions and counter-tensions. The control associated with greater health and self-determination is closely related to self-awareness, mindfulness, emotional regulation and emotional intelligence.

ENABLING STRATEGIES

Behaviour is deeply rooted in attitudes, biology and neurology. It is, however, modifiable when one learns appropriate skills and changes are made to the social environment which are conducive to healthy lifestyle change. Strategies that are aimed at enabling a person to be more autonomous and able to make desired behaviour change are known as 'enabling strategies'. Having information but not being enabled to translate it into action means that the information is inert.

Much of the time a healthcare practitioner can think it is enough to provide health information and let the case for behaviour change rest on that. Saying, for example, that smoking is bad for one's health and providing some medical reasons for that will increase the smoking cessation rate over the next year from about 1% to 2%. When enabling strategies are included with the information it is far more effective and, in the case of smoking cessation rates, quit rates can be improved to around 30% or higher. Examples of enabling strategies that will help to facilitate healthy change include: behaviour change skills, motivation, empowerment, health coaching principles, the behaviour change cycle and goal setting. The ESSENCE model (see Ch 6) may also help to give structure to a total lifestyle plan.

MOTIVATION

The first step in enablement is to examine insight and motivation. Nothing happens without insight and motivation—this is just as relevant for the clinician as it is for the patient—and so, for the skilled clinician, the first factor is to raise awareness and enhance motivation.

Our reasons for acting the way we do are often unseen and therefore unexamined. Habits, biases and assumptions are far more influential when we are less conscious. Being aware of our competing motivations for various behaviours is an important first step in being able to understand and change them. Often we don't consciously examine the pros and cons of continuing to follow a particular path of action. If we eat an unhealthy diet, for example, consciously or unconsciously we will probably be doing so for a variety of reasons. We might, for example, have assumed that:

- diet is not an important health issue
- an unhealthy diet is less expensive than a healthy one
- unhealthy food tastes better
- it would take too much effort to change our eating pattern
- unhealthy food is far more convenient.

If we examined such assumptions more closely, they might not stand up to scrutiny. For example, we might not:

- know how much we are increasing our chances of getting cancer or heart disease by not eating healthy food
- realise that healthy food can cost less than buying 'fast' or prepackaged food
- have been creative in using recipes that bring out the good tastes in healthy food
- have realised what it will cost us not to change until we become ill
- have considered that healthy food can be very 'fast' to prepare. If in a hurry it can take a lot more time to heat a prepackaged pizza than it takes to pick up a piece of fruit, a handful of walnuts or some dip and rice crackers.

One way of clarifying and galvanising motivation is to use the cycle of behaviour change model, which is described in more detail later in this chapter. Another way is for the patient to write down on a piece of paper all the costs and benefits of making or not making a particular change. An example is given in Table 7.1.

Having done this, the next step is to look at the things standing in the way of healthy change and then to consider how valid or fixed they are. Take cost as an example. The preferred form of exercise might be skiing, but this is not very accessible and has a high financial cost. But exercise can also be relatively inexpensive—walking is an example. Furthermore, exercise can reduce a significant financial and time burden by reducing the

TABLE 7.1 Costs and benefits of changing or not changing behaviour to include regular exercise

	Changing	Not changing
Benefits	• More vitality • Better mood and less anxiety • Weight control • Less likely to become ill (infections, heart disease, cancer, dementia etc) • Social interaction • Sustainable performance • Sense of achievement	• Comfortable • Easy • Time for other things
Costs	• Takes money • Out of comfort zone • Requires effort • Time taken from other things • Might injure oneself	• Low vitality • Lowered mood and greater anxiety • Weight problems • More likely to become ill (infections, heart disease, cancer, dementia etc) • Have to take time away from other things for being ill • The cost of being ill • Less social interaction • Poorer performance • Sense of not taking on challenges

likelihood of becoming ill and needing time off work. Rather than costing money, it is likely to save money. In truth, being sedentary may be the far more expensive option. A similar process can be followed for each factor, such as tiredness—exercise increases energy and vitality. If there is a concern about injury then it will be important to choose a form of exercise suitable for the person's current age and level of fitness—what is appropriate for a 20-year-old may not be appropriate at age 50.

The aim of such an exercise is to help remove the influence of inhibitors of the behaviour and to emphasise the enhancers. If such an exercise is undertaken in a creative and unbiased way, it is likely that there will be far fewer barriers to healthy change.

EDUCATION

In the healthcare setting, education can be enormously empowering. Having an education is protective against a whole range of illnesses, not just because a person has factual health information they would not otherwise have had, but because a person who has had an education often feels more confident, is able to weigh up options and make decisions, and can ask questions and seek alternatives. Therefore, one of the most enabling things that can be done for a person is not just to educate them in the form of providing information but also to foster their self-empowerment, self-governance and problem-solving abilities. This can be implemented by the general practitioner, and also through community-based programs.

ENVIRONMENT

Enabling strategies also need to be supported by an environment that is conducive to healthy change. Providing someone with information and skills related to smoking cessation will help them to quit, but if that person is subjected to a constant barrage of pro-smoking marketing messages, if they are regularly exposed to passive smoking in the workplace, and if their family and friends are not supportive of the change, then that person's ability to remain a non-smoker will be seriously undermined. Similarly, if a person wanted to increase their level of exercise, then having a safe environment to exercise in, access to adequate facilities and parks, and supportive people to help maintain the change, will make them much more likely to maintain the new behaviour. Thus, no matter what behaviour change we wish to make, choosing and enhancing our social and physical environments carefully is an important part of the change process.

PSYCHOLOGICAL FACTORS

A number of psychological factors are important enabling strategies. These factors include stress management, attention regulation and emotional regulation. These will be dealt with in the mind–body chapter (Ch 8).

PROCHASKA DICLEMENTE CYCLE OF BEHAVIOUR CHANGE

The Prochaska DiClemente cycle of behaviour change is a model initially developed to explain the steps we go through in changing a behaviour. It has been used widely in health and psychology settings for various behaviours, although it was initially applied to smoking cessation. It is applicable to almost any behaviour and can be adapted as such. The steps in the process are outlined in Figure 7.1 and below.

The model simply acknowledges the fact that we go through different stages in making any change in behaviour. The cycle begins even before we first think about the behaviour, and continues until the new behaviour eventually becomes established or maintained. It also embraces the fact that behaviour often relapses.

The stages are self-explanatory but there are some important points to remember when implementing the process. Early in the process it is important to determine which stage a person is in. Knowing the stage helps one to tailor questions, direct information, enhance motivation and provide skills relevant to that stage. Trying to encourage action, for example, before a person has clarified their motivation will be inappropriate and

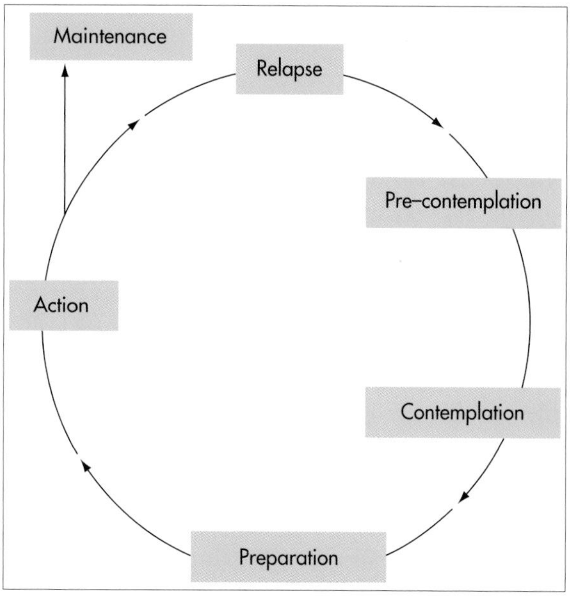

FIGURE 7.1 Prochaska DiClemente cycle of behaviour change

is almost certain to fail. The art is to move through the stages from where the person is currently and in a way that is suitable for their needs and motivation.

PRE-CONTEMPLATION

Pre-contemplation is the time before a person has even begun to think about changing a behaviour. For example, a smoker presents to a doctor with a cold but has not yet thought of giving up, and may not have made many connections between their smoking and their tendency to get upper respiratory tract infections. Obviously, no change is possible until the person has begun to think about change, and so the doctor might help the patient to make the link between their smoking and the acute illness they have presented with. Many anti-smoking advertisements are also aimed at making people think about their habit. They are motivating people to consider the next stage by raising awareness and modulating emotion and attitude.

CONTEMPLATION

Contemplation is when the person first starts to think about changing the behaviour. Contemplation can take a short time (seconds) until the behaviour changes, or it can be long (years or even decades). In our example above, the GP may mention that smoking is contributing to the person's tendency to get colds as well as putting them at risk of other illnesses. This is 'opportunistic'—that is, waiting for the opportunity to present itself rather than being proactive. Such prompts can also be included in a more structured way, for example by using computer prompts or medical guidelines about screening all patients for smoking. In the contemplation phase it is important to examine what motivates the behaviour. Motivation is always particular to the individual, and so exploring this needs to be done in a patient-centred way. For example, for a young professional, having a cold may be relevant because time off work is a major inconvenience. Concern about lung cancer or heart disease may not be important for a 20-year-old, but saving money, sporting performance, attractiveness to the opposite sex and accelerated ageing of the skin might be. If the patient is interested in proceeding, then this process can be supported with further discussion, information, reading materials and other aids.

PREPARATION

The preparation stage is when a person takes steps to put things in place to help ensure that the behaviour change is more likely to be successful. This can include accessing information about how to stop smoking by phoning the QUIT Line, or informing the family that a 'quit date' has been set, or planning which places to avoid once having stopped smoking. At this time the person may also be developing the enabling strategies that will help them to maintain the desired behaviour after action has taken place. Care needs to be taken in this stage, and failure to recognise this can lead to a lack of success.

ACTION

In the action stage, the person is implementing the new behaviour. For example, they have thrown away the cigarettes and are not smoking. A supportive environment is very important in this stage if the behaviour is to be maintained, and this includes avoiding situations and places that are likely to activate the old behaviour. The tendency to revert to the old unhealthy behaviour is strongest in the initial stages. Like going uphill, it takes effort and it is easy to roll down again if one loses focus.

RELAPSE

With some habits, relapse can occur a number of times until lasting change is finally achieved. It is very useful not to see 'relapses' as 'failures' but to reframe them as learning opportunities. If a person has reverted to the old behaviour then it will be for a reason. Stress, overwork and emotional upsets are the most common reasons for relapse but other factors can also come into play. Perhaps they may have lost focus, or become complacent that the old behaviour wasn't an active issue any longer, or perhaps they didn't pay attention to the environmental issues. The important thing is not to dwell on a perceived failure but, rather, to learn what brought about the relapse in order to make future attempts more likely to succeed. Dwelling on failure saps energy and disheartens. To learn a useful lesson is to make something good out of an otherwise negative situation. Although relapse takes the person back to the start of the cycle, they will generally move through the preliminary stages a lot more quickly and easily than was the case the first time around.

MAINTENANCE

The maintenance stage is where change, having been made, becomes long-term. The initial establishment of the behaviour has been passed and the new behaviour takes relatively little effort to maintain. Provided the motivation remains clear and the benefits of the new behaviour pattern are obvious, there will tend to be few problems. Again, complacency and stress are common reasons for relapse. For example, 'I'll just have one cigarette' can quickly become a full-blown reactivation of the old habit. Reactivation of dormant thought patterns and neural pathways can take place quite quickly. An old behaviour pattern can return with surprising force, even after many years.

SMART GOAL-SETTING

If one decides to make a healthy change, it is worth considering a way of setting goals that will help them to be realised. Setting unrealistic goals, for example, can be discouraging and can perpetuate negative patterns of thought. Being SMART about setting goals can be very helpful. The SMART approach is widely used and can be applied for setting goals related to any behaviour. The SMART acronym stands for:

Specific
Measurable
Attractive
Realistic
Time dependent.

Often, goals are not achieved because one or other of these issues was not attended to. A goal is harder to attain and progress is harder to measure if it is vague or ill-defined. For example, one might aspire to the goal of 'exercising more', but what does that mean? How much exercise? How often? What type of exercise? If a goal is not specific then the person never really knows whether they are achieving it. It is easy to think that we are doing better or worse than we really are. A specific goal would be something along the lines of, 'I plan to walk around the park (three kilometres) four evenings per week'. This is specific—it gives the type, duration and frequency of exercise. With a specific goal set, the person can then measure how well they are doing in relation to it. As one goal is attained, a new and more ambitious goal can be set.

Measurable

If a specific goal is set, it can be measured much more easily. Measuring progress towards attaining goals helps one to gauge progress in an objective fashion. Measuring progress can also provide encouragement by recognising progress towards the goal, or it can provide a reality check. It can also help us to modify a goal, if appropriate, by either stepping it up or cutting it back. In the exercise example above, a person might find that they have been able to walk around the park only three times per week, not four. On that basis they can decide whether they need to increase their effort or perhaps reduce the goal if it is unrealistic.

Attractive

If a goal is not attractive or enjoyable, it won't be maintained in the long term. If, for example, the person does not enjoy the form of exercise they have chosen, they will not maintain it for long, certainly not past the point where their initial enthusiasm has died down. In this case, they would either need to find a way of making that form of exercise attractive—for example, by running with friends or in beautiful parks, or playing a team sport—or choose a different form of exercise. With the right form of exercise a number of goals can be realised within one activity—increasing social interaction at the same time as doing exercise, for example. It is best to choose exercise that we enjoy, is appropriate to our age and fitness and suits our life situation. A noisy gymnasium might not be appropriate for an older person, or an expensive sport might not be right for someone with limited income. It is also useful to consider that a number of things can make a goal 'attractive'. A goal can be attractive because the activity is pleasurable, but equally it can be the end-product, rather than the means of achieving it, that is attractive. For example, a person may wish to pursue a certain career but may not find the effort, sacrifice and study along the way all that pleasant. Persevering, however, may help them develop a great deal of character and resilience in a way that taking the pleasant option would never have done.

Realistic

If a goal is unrealistic, or not achievable, then a sense of discouragement and failure may arise when the goal is not realised. This may even be despite the fact that an enormous amount of progress has been made. So, for example, a plan to quickly go from no exercise to running every day is unlikely to be achievable or sustainable. If there has been a recurrent attitude of thinking of oneself as a failure, then that attitude will have been reinforced. So a modest but achievable goal is often a far better foundation upon which to build than a more far-reaching goal. Realistic goals can certainly be built upon steadily as they are achieved. The initial goal may be modest, and revised a month later, at which time a slightly higher goal is set. A month later it can be revised again. In this way a goal that might have seemed unrealistic at an early stage can be achieved in the longer term via a series of smaller, realistic goals. Some people intentionally set very high goals in order to extend their performance because they thrive on the challenge. As long as the goal is not dangerous, that can also be a valid way of working towards a goal for those with high confidence and a resilient sense of self. For such people, not meeting a high goal is not a sign of defeat but is a motivator to rise to a challenge or make further effort.

Time dependent

It is useful for a goal to have a specific time frame rather than being too open-ended. This can increase focus and maintain motivation. For example, a person may aim to be fit enough to compete in a fun run in 6 months' time. As such it can help a person to stay focused and not become complacent. This helps us to make our goals specific, map our progress, provide incentive and keep goals realistic.

SMART goal-setting activity

In using the above model, a patient might like to set a SMART goal for themselves. It can be done as an intellectual exercise but in order for it to have more meaning it needs to be related to a goal that really matters, a goal that the person has a desire to implement. The goal could be anything—it could, for example, relate to:

- exercise
- change of diet
- weight control
- study
- learning a skill
- getting over a phobia
- renovating the house.

BASK

Any educational intervention relates to behaviours, attitudes, skills and knowledge. As has been mentioned, simply thinking that knowledge or information is going to change behaviour is generally a false assumption. The most powerful way to change behaviour is through a shift in emotion and attitude, supported and directed by knowledge. BASK is an acronym:

- ***B**ehaviour* is what a person *does.*
- ***A**ttitudes* are what a person *believes.*
- ***S**kills* are what a person *can do.*
- ***K**nowledge* is what a person *understands.*

Interventions can be directed at any or all of the above dimensions. The Ornish program (which will be described in detail in the chapters on heart disease (Ch 25) and cancer (Ch 24)) is a good example of a program that contains all these aspects contained in BASK. That is largely why the program is so successful.

Interventions directed at the wrong aspect of BASK will tend to be ineffective. For example, it is little use giving knowledge where there is an attitudinal problem preventing change. In such a case the attitude needs to be dealt with first. The knowledge will not translate into action while that barrier is in place. In advertising aimed at smoking cessation, increasing knowledge is only a secondary aim, whereas the primary aim is to make a negative emotional and attitudinal association between smoking and wellbeing. Put another way, most of the time a person already knows the basic principles of what is healthy and what isn't, but reasons other than knowledge are maintaining the unhealthy behaviour. Doctors too often interpret patient education as only giving factual information, and this is one of the main reasons that giving advice on behaviour change frequently does not result in action.

JOURNAL KEEPING

Keeping a journal is a powerful way of following progress, gaining insight and reinforcing change. A variety of studies suggest that keeping a journal about important issues is therapeutic in itself, particularly for dealing with emotional issues. For a journal to be of real use it needs to be about events and issues that are important to the person.

HEALTH PROMOTION[3]

Health promotion is powerful, effective, and cheap! (Dr Rob Moodie)

The health of individuals and communities depends on many determinants. Health is affected not only by our genetic endowment and physical risk factors, but also by such things as:

- socioeconomic status
- social supports
- level of education
- employment (or lack of it)
- culture
- mental health
- physical environment.

As already mentioned, simply providing information without attending to the social, economic, cultural and physical environment will be ineffective and potentially wasteful of resources.

An example will help to put this into a practical context. The road toll among young males is a major health issue and is largely contributed to by alcohol abuse, speeding and other risk-taking behaviours. To help young males avoid binge drinking, drink-driving and speeding requires that attention be paid to the attitudes and skills of young males. Young males, for example, are prone to impulsivity, a feeling of immortality and over-confidence, all at a time of gaining newfound freedom. This confluence of circumstances and psychological factors predisposes them to risk. To succeed in reducing the road toll among this group requires legislation (laws on speeding, alcohol consumption and drink-driving), changes to alcohol advertising, increasing the price of alcohol, and social marketing aimed at changing attitudes to drink-driving. It also requires the providing of alternatives to drinking excess alcohol (e.g. making water available in clubs and pubs) as well as adequate public transport. Such strategies work, and save a huge amount of social, emotional and economic waste.

The individual practitioner has an important role to play in reinforcing key health messages, whether it be opportunistically or in a systematic way.

A population approach to health promotion is far more cost-effective than treating individuals. This is well illustrated in the reduced rates of many infectious diseases through immunisation. Illnesses such as measles are uncommon now. Polio is rare. Smallpox has been eradicated. Other examples of major health promotion successes include:

- tobacco control
- reducing road trauma
- HIV/AIDS control
- skin cancer prevention.

Now fewer than 17% of adults smoke, whereas the figure was around 72% among males in the middle of the twentieth century.[4,5] The effects of this change will be increasingly felt in coming generations as the rates of smoking-related illnesses decline. In developed countries, road tolls have more than halved over the past 30 years.[6] This is despite a doubling of the population and an even larger increase in the number of cars on the road. The number of new HIV/AIDS cases diagnosed per year has dropped significantly in most developed countries, due largely to public campaigns promoting safe sex and harm minimisation among drug users being strongly reinforced by healthcare practitioners. Skin cancer rates—most importantly the rates of malignant melanoma—have plateaued in recent years in places where sunburn rates have been reduced. In Victoria, Australia, for example, there has been a 60% decline in weekend sunburn rates over the past 20 years.[7] Sun-smart campaigns have been implemented not just through medical practices but also in schools and via social marketing.

VicHealth figures suggest that, per life year gained, the cost of smoking prevention is approximately 1/500th that of treating lung cancer. In Australia, the treatment for AIDS in the early 1990s cost over $46 000 per life year gained, whereas it only costs $185 per life year gained when the money is spent on preventing HIV infection.[8]

Effective health promotion depends on a number of factors, and these are outlined below.[9]

- *Good background data and information*—not only do we need to know such things as which health problems are prevalent and who they affect, but also how effective any interventions or programs are. Good epidemiological data, unbiased research and evidence are therefore vital in helping guide community initiatives as well as clinical practice.
- *Clear and sensible policy, legislation and regulation*—the policies of organisations and political parties can support or undermine any attempts to implement effective strategies. Positive examples of using legislation to enhance health include laws on the promotion of tobacco, drink-driving laws, enforcing speed limits, and laws promoting the wearing of seatbelts. Other topical areas being considered include such things as limiting the marketing of unhealthy foods to children, drug harm minimisation strategies and genetic testing.
- *Quality communication*—communication and advocacy can make or break health promotion initiatives. This can include education, enhancing motivation, changing attitudes, improving cooperation, and providing practical information about available services.
- *Well-trained and diverse professionals*—well-trained healthcare professionals are essential in ensuring that health promotion initiatives are well planned and effectively delivered in the community. Those involved with implementing health promotion can include doctors, nurses, counsellors and services providing screening, marketing, education and business support, as well as sporting bodies, arts bodies, police, media and local government. General practitioners are a vital link in the chain, and health promotion activities can be informed by up-to-date guidelines and screening schedules produced by the professional colleges.
- *Community involvement*—health promotion is implemented through the community, by the community and for the community. Without community engagement, inspiration and support, any initiative will be far less effective and will waste resources. General practitioners can play an important role through program development, implementation and evaluation. They can reinforce health messages, act as advocates and become involved in research.
- *Political support and funding*—without ongoing political support and funding, health promotion programs and organisations have a tenuous future. It is important for the success of health promotion initiatives that the political and financial support for them does not become politicised.

RESOURCES

Australian Federation of AIDS Organisations, http://www.afao.org.au

Australian Health Promotion Association, http://www.healthpromotion.org.au.

Cancer Council of Victoria, http://www.accv.org.au

International Union for Health Promotion and Education, http://www.iuhpe.org

Public Health Association of Australia, http://www.phaa.net.au

Quit Program, http://www.quit.org.au

Transport Accident Commission, http://www.tac.vic.gov.au

VicHealth, http://www.vichealth.vic.gov.au

REFERENCES

1 Syme SL. Psychosocial interventions to improve successful aging. Ann Intern Med 2003; 139(5/2):400–402.
2 Kivimaki M, Leino-Arjas P, Luukkonen R et al. Work stress and risk of cardiovascular mortality: prospective cohort study of industrial employees. BMJ 2002; 325(7369):857.
3 This section draws upon principles outlined in the Monash University Health Promotion course in 2007 by Dr Rob Moodie, the then CEO of VicHealth.
4 State Government, Victoria. Quit Victoria. Smoking rates in Victoria. Online. Available: http://www.quit.org.au/article.asp?ContentID=7241
5 State Government, Victoria. Quit Victoria. Smoking rates in Australia. Online. Available: http://www.quit.org.au/article.asp?ContentID=7240
6 State Government, Victoria. Transport Accident Commission. Online. Available: http://www.tacsafety.com.au/jsp/content/NavigationController.do?areaID=12
7 Davis KJ, Cokkinides VE, Weinstock MA et al. Summer sunburn and sun exposure among US youths ages 11 to 18: national prevalence and associated factors. Pediatrics 2002; 110(1):27–35.
8 VicHealth (Victorian Health Promotion Foundation). Online. Available: www.vichealth.vic.gov.au
9 Moodie R, Hulme A. Hands on health promotion. Melbourne: IP Communications; 2004.

chapter 8

Mind–body medicine

INTRODUCTION AND OVERVIEW

The father of Western medicine, Hippocrates, said that 'the human being can only be understood as a whole'. Such sentiments are reflected in many cultures. Generally speaking, ancient approaches to health are essentially holistic, with wellbeing, illness and healing considered to be strongly connected to the mind, society, morality, spirituality and ecology. In this view, nature is imbued with intelligence, consciousness and order, and it is the role of the healer to observe, understand and follow these laws. Furthermore, any understanding of the universe or the creatures existing within it is metaphysical in nature—that is, mind or intelligence governs physical phenomena.

To the ancient Greeks, as with other ancient Eastern and Western healing systems, the 'whole person' encompasses the body, the mind—including thought and emotion—and the spirit or consciousness. The physical body, viewed as the most superficial aspect, is 'moved' or enlivened by the deeper aspects of the 'self'. It is analogous to the driver of a car being the mind and the car being the body. Consciousness is the primary substance of our being and also the source of energy. The mind gives form and direction to consciousness. Thus, what affects one level of our being also affects all the others. This interrelationship as defined by ancient healing systems is echoed in the WHO holistic definition of health as:

> a state of complete physical, mental and social well-being and not merely the absence of disease or infirmity[1]

In the nineteenth and twentieth centuries, with the rise of a more reductionist and materialist approach to science, this ancient and holistic view has been supplanted. As a consequence, explanations for phenomena have become far more mechanistic in nature. Human development can be explained by genes, thought and emotion by neurotransmitters, and even love by evolutionary biology.

More recently, however, this mechanistic and materialistic view of science has again been questioned, not so much from initiatives started by religious institutions, but from within the scientific establishment itself. Much of this is due to collaborative research between psychologists, sociologists, immunologists, physiologists and neuroscientists. The broad term given to these new scientific disciplines is 'mind–body medicine' (MBM). Essentially, although we now have a complex understanding of the mechanisms underpinning the mind–body interaction, it is clear that the principles were well understood in ancient times. These principles are extremely simple and, as such, they have enormous application to modern clinical practice although, of course, this integration needs to take place alongside sound clinical practice and the best available evidence.

WHAT IS MIND–BODY MEDICINE?

The main premise of MBM is that the mind (intelligence) governs or regulates the body. Although mind is non-physical—and therefore MBM is in essence a metaphysical explanation for physical phenomena—mind uses the body to execute its purposes. More particularly, the mind, powered by consciousness, thinks and feels through the agency of the brain. Mind, brain and body are inseparable. Mind and intelligence make themselves evident by observable results in the physical world.

A practical way of expressing this principle is to say that psychological states such as chronic stress, depression, anxiety and fear produce profound and clinically relevant effects upon the body. These effects have implications for health and illness. Psychological states and social context can have both positive and negative effects that manifest on many different levels, all the way from muscle tension to genetic expression. Over time the cumulative effects of negative mental and emotional states can take a heavy toll on the body. Conversely, research also suggests that psychosocial interventions can play an important part in ameliorating these negative effects and can assist in promoting healing.

Despite the enormous scope and clinical potential of MBM, it has been relatively slow to enter mainstream medical education and practice. This lack of awareness among clinicians tends not to be reflected in the general community, which has a strong interest in and intuitive appreciation of MBM principles, although expectations are sometimes unrealistic. The desire for a 'holistic philosophy' to underpin healthcare is a major reason that many people search out complementary therapies.[2]

The relative slowness of the medical community to integrate MBM may be the result of a number of things, including a lack of access to current research findings, bias against explanations that do not fit assumed scientific paradigms, and lack of economic interest in non-patentable and non-technological therapies. This will no doubt change as medical practice evolves to encompass changing community values, the growing evidence base behind MBM, and the need for more cost-effective and less invasive approaches to therapy.

This chapter provides a broad overview of the medical literature on MBM and explores some of its clinical implications. Subsequent chapters on various systems also include content on MBM where relevant. Without paying attention to the mind, we may be dealing only with the manifestations of diseases, not their causes.

Acknowledging the role of the mind's effect on the body does not deny the important role of physical risk factors and treatments. Indeed, the approach recommended in this textbook is to use the best that conventional medicine has to offer, but within a holistic context. Recognising, for example, that stress and emotion can exacerbate asthma does not ignore the importance of pharmacological therapy, careful monitoring and occasional emergency care.

THE CAUSE AND EFFECTS OF STRESS

It is best not to take the label 'stress' at face value without exploring what a person means by it. 'Stress' is a commonly used term covering, often imprecisely, a wide range of human experiences. Some describe stress as a 'perceived inability to cope', others as when 'demands exceed means'. Patients may use the word 'stress' in these contexts, but often it is used to describe psychological and emotional states such as fear, anger, indecisiveness, distractibility, depression or rumination. Stress can also be used by many to describe the physical effects of increased sympathetic nervous system (SNS) activity such as increased muscle tension, tremulousness, clamminess or rapid heartbeat. These manifestations of the 'fight-or-flight response' can lead to tiredness and other symptoms associated with chronic stress.

Most affluent countries around the world are observing significant increases in the rates of stress, depression and suicide. Evidence suggests that stress hormones play an important role in the development of psychiatric disorders[3] as well as having direct effects on serotonergic pathways.[4] Serotonin is the principal neurotransmitter implicated in depression, and antidepressant medications are largely aimed at modulating serotonin.

Chronic stress and the accumulation of a number of minor stresses is a contributor to many illnesses. When appropriately activated, the fight-or-flight response is a natural, necessary and life-preserving physiological response to a threatening situation. For example, if you are about to be chased by a lion, you need to:

- respond quickly
- exert a significant amount of energy
- potentially deal with tissue damage.

The fight-or-flight response, when based on a clearly perceived and real threat, is physiologically encoded to preserve life, and therefore the changes associated with it make sense. These changes include:

- secretion of adrenaline, leading to elevation of blood pressure and heart rate
- diversion of blood flow to muscles and away from the gut and skin
- increased platelet adhesiveness, allowing the blood to clot more effectively in case of blood loss
- short-term mobilisation of white blood cells and a surge in white cell numbers in case of a breach of tissue defences
- activation of inflammatory mediators such as cytokines and interleukins, in case of tissue damage
- mobilisation of energy stores for fuel, leading to increased blood glucose and fats
- perspiration, in anticipation of significant exertion
- increased respiration and metabolic rate.

These changes, designed to help the body cope with demands and potential injury, will mobilise according to whatever we perceive as a threat. When the situation is over, the physiology should return to rest if the situation is mentally left in the past. Even one's own doctor can be perceived as a threat. The prospect of having one's blood pressure measured is enough to elevate it to a point where approximately 25% of patients are inappropriately diagnosed with hypertension.[5] This is known as 'white-coat hypertension' and is just another example of the clinical implications of the mind–body response.

The activation of the fight-or-flight response is not detrimental to health, provided it is mobilised only when it needs to be, is deactivated when it is no longer required, and is not prolonged. Unfortunately, in the vast majority of occasions on which this response is mobilised, it is done so unnecessarily and is maintained long after the event is passed, and the person is unable to deactivate it. Much of the inappropriate activation of the response has to do with the imagination of future and past events taken to be real. The word 'anxiety' comes from a Latin word, *anxius*, meaning to 'anticipate some future event'. Furthermore, mentally replaying an event can reproduce the stress response many times even though the event is over and happened only once. In the most extreme cases this replaying can be so vivid that a person's present experience is all but totally overlaid with the past, leading to what is called 'post-traumatic stress disorder'. Here, through neuron plasticity, the memory, emotion and physiological response have become wired into the neural circuitry of the brain, principally through the limbic system, which mediates memory and emotion.

The chronic or long-term inappropriate activation of the stress response, mediated through the SNS, leads to a significant level of physiological wear and tear. This is called 'allostatic load'.[6] It is much like a car being driven so hard that the heavy demands placed upon it will lead to failure of its parts. High allostatic load is associated with both anxiety and depression and will lead to, among other things:

- impaired immunity
- acceleration of atherosclerosis
- increased risk of metabolic syndrome (type 2 diabetes, central obesity, hyperlipidaemia, hypertension)
- bone demineralisation or osteoporosis because of chronically high cortisol levels
- atrophy of nerve cells in the hippocampus and prefrontal cortex of the brain.

These effects are logical sequelae of the prolonged activation of the SNS. Stress and inflammatory mediators, such as cytokines, also have important effects on mood, behaviour and emotion.[7] Activation of the immune system via these immune mediators, such as takes place during an acute infection, induces sickness behaviour (apathy, lethargy, lack of motivation and appetite). This behaviour is the body's way of ensuring that one takes the rest required to assist the body in recovering from an infection. Many of these symptoms are also seen in depression and a significant part of the reason may be because of the high levels of cytokines associated with high allostatic load. Some cytokines activate cerebral noradrenergic and serotonergic systems and so anxiety and depression are often seen as a mixed picture. It may also be part of the reason that depression occurs more frequently in people with medical disorders associated with immune dysfunction. From a therapeutic perspective it is important to remember that every investment in reducing anxiety, improving coping and enhancing wellbeing is a step towards reducing suicide risk.

MENTAL HEALTH INDICATORS

Measures of mental health in developed countries have not been heading in a positive direction in recent decades:

> In spite of recent clinical and research advances, an increased burden of mortality and morbidity related to stress and mental ill health can be noted, especially in European societies and populations undergoing stressful transitions and dramatic changes. A societal syndrome, consisting of depression, suicide, abuse, risk-taking and violent behaviour as well as vascular morbidity and mortality, can be observed.[8]

Evidence suggests that the stress associated with modern life has been increasing at a surprisingly rapid rate: 45% over the past 30 years in some surveys.[9] Depression currently 'causes the largest amount of non-fatal burden, accounting for almost 12% of all total years lived with disability worldwide'[10] and it is estimated that in Australia mental health issues, principally depression, will be the major cause of morbidity within the next two decades.[11] Among affluent countries around the world it is estimated that, by the year 2030, unipolar depression will account for over 1.5 times the burden of disease that will be accounted for by cardiovascular disease.[12] This is independent of the secondary effects of depression, such as it being an independent risk factor for heart disease and associated co-morbidities such as substance abuse.

The higher prevalence of poor mental health could be explained in part by an increased awareness of mental health issues. Aside from this it is apparent that many people have more pressured and stressful lives. The rapid increase in the amount of social change, job insecurity, the speed of life, escalating competitiveness, higher expectations and many other factors all contribute.

Today, higher rates of depression are occurring at younger ages. Suicidal ideation is surprisingly common in adolescents. Data suggest that 1 in 2 young people report experiencing high levels of psychological stress and as many as 25% of 15–24 year-olds presenting to a GP for any reason reported experiencing recent suicidal thoughts[13] despite the fact that most did not present for psychological reasons.

Evidence suggests that antidepressant medications in children and adolescents, although widely used, are not effective and that such approaches have to be questioned.[14,15] Part of their overuse may be driven by marketing forces and parental anxiety. Particularly in this group of patients it is important for attention to be paid to the social and domestic causes of stress and to the fostering of protective factors and resilience through education and community programs.

The causes of declining adolescent mental health are contributed to by a wide range of factors, including physical inactivity, poor nutrition, substance abuse and social influences. Some elements of youth culture and excessive pleasure-seeking behaviour may also be contributing factors. Although adolescents will 'self-medicate' for depression by using substances and promiscuous sexual behaviour, recent studies also suggest that substance abuse and promiscuous sexual behaviour precede and predict the later development of depression: 'Engaging in sex and drug behaviors places adolescents, and especially girls, at risk for future depression.'[16a]

Some groups on the fringe of society, such as the Goth subculture, seem to be at very high risk for self-harm and attempted suicide.[17] Music is also a powerful modulator of emotion and behaviour and can significantly increase risk-taking behaviour.[18] The assessment and management of mental health issues among adolescents therefore requires attention to such issues.

DOPAMINE AND REWARD SYSTEMS

Different brain pathways accord with differing approaches to pursuing fulfillment. Dopamine is a neurotransmitter with multiple actions at each level of the mesocorticolimbic reward pathway—it is intimately associated with the ability to experience pleasure and motivation.[19] The pursuit of pleasure is a vital activity associated with survival. For example, we would not eat or reproduce unless it was pleasurable. Some people are, however, more genetically at risk of developing addictive behaviours, and the over-activation of the mesolimbic system can trigger addictions of various kinds. In such situations it requires increasingly intense and frequent stimuli to produce the same pleasure response; over time, this 'tires' the reward system, predisposing to anhedonia and depression. Dysfunction of dopamine transmission in the reward circuit is associated with symptoms such as anhedonia (inability to experience pleasure), apathy and dysphoria (disturbed mood). It is found in various neuropsychiatric disorders, including Parkinson's disease, depression and drug addiction. Prolonged and significant stress early in life can also affect one's dopamine pathways for life.[20] What begins as a pursuit of pleasure eventually becomes an uneasy retreat from the pain and anxiety associated with withdrawal. This has implications for the development of impulsivity and reactivity.

Increased dopamine release is also seen in the brain during the relaxation response. This is associated with reduced impulsivity or reactivity,[21] which may have something to do with the development of emotional and impulse regulation associated with long-term meditation practice. This may also help to facilitate healthy lifestyle change.

Mood, neurochemistry and behaviour are intimately entwined. Mood affects behaviour and is a common reason for relapse into unhealthy behaviours.[22] Major depression, for example, triples the risk of progression to daily smoking[23] but, conversely, a history of daily smoking nearly doubles the risk of major depression. In adolescents, experimental smoking very significantly increases the risk of taking up smoking as a habit. Depression, anxiety and peer smoking strongly predict the risk of experimental smoking, and depression and anxiety increase susceptibility to peer influence to establish risk-taking behaviours. Building resilience and emotional intelligence in adolescents, particularly boys, may therefore produce a number of benefits including the ability to avoid unhealthy behaviours. It also goes part of the way towards explaining why CBT and antidepressant medications both reduce relapse rates for smokers.[24,25]

Brain scans show that mental anticipation can have as significant an effect upon brain activity as physical stimulation. The thought of eating activates areas of the brain associated with rewards and pleasure.[26] As these centres are important in addictions it is likely that potential forms of therapy for treating addictions will be developed that target these biochemical reactions pharmacologically[27] and behaviourally.

STRESS AND PERCEPTION

> Man is not disturbed by events but by the view he takes of them.[28]
>
> Epictetus

That stress is intimately related to perception is not a new concept. The mind has a key role in eliciting the stress response through its functions of perception, cognition, interpretation and conditioning. When perceptions are distorted or cognitions are irrational, this leads to a consequent inappropriate activation of the stress response.

Learned patterns of coping and personality styles are generally more influential than the situation in activating the stress response. By understanding the basic mechanisms that underlie this process, it is possible to use strategies to deactivate it. Such strategies can include:

- meditation
- relaxation therapy

- cognitive-behaviour therapy (CBT)
- mindfulness-based cognitive therapy (MBCT)
- acceptance commitment therapy (ACT)
- dialectic behaviour therapy (DBT)
- rational-emotive therapy (RET).

These help to reverse the effects of inappropriate stress by attacking it at its cause—thought. Reviews of the literature suggest that cognitive and relaxation-based forms of stress management are the most effective strategies in general practice settings, and that working in groups potentiates outcomes.[29] A certain amount of stress can be useful in enhancing motivation. Furthermore, the fight-or-flight response can be entirely necessary in extreme situations. Aside from this, however, most of the stress experienced in daily life is neither necessary nor helpful in improving our ability to deal with a challenge. Most of the unhelpful stress experienced is associated with an agitated and unfocused mind that also has a limited capacity at the time to distinguish between present-time reality and imagination. Mental projections and anticipation are given a reality they do not deserve. Examples might include projecting fears into the future about upcoming exams or interviews or habitually recreating past anxieties and conflicts. Here the stressors are in the mind, not in reality, but the body will nevertheless faithfully translate this mentally generated stressor into the stress response. It will not stop until it is told to, regardless of whether the stressor is real or imagined. If one imagines a rope to be a snake, the body will react to the perception, not the reality. Even events that are actually happening at the time will only cause stress depending on the mental interpretation of them. To attribute our stress solely to the events around us and to ignore our own role in generating stress is disempowering and will lead to less than favourable therapeutic outcomes.

GENDER AND THE STRESS RESPONSE

Much of the early stress research focused on men, and hence the fight-or-flight response, which is largely a male response, has become the predominant paradigm in stress medicine. But there is good evidence to suggest that women do not respond to stressful situations in entirely the same way as men, emotionally, socially, behaviourally or physiologically. Reviews of the literature 'suggest that the female stress response of tending to offspring and affiliating with a social group is facilitated by the process of "befriending", which is the creation of networks of associations that provide resources and protection for the female and her offspring under conditions of stress'.[30]

Both males and females have the capacity to activate the fight-or-flight response if required, but men are especially built for this response. Testosterone contributes significantly to this[31] and also has a role in the development of 'rough- and-tumble play' and sporting interests among boys. Excessive testosterone levels are implicated in excessive physical aggression and crime among men. Female aggression, on the other hand, is more 'cerebral'—that is, it seems more likely to be expressed 'in the form of gossip, rumour-spreading and enlisting the cooperation of a third party in undermining an acquaintance'.[32]

The females of most species are more involved in tending the young because they have the biological or behavioural disposition to 'tend-and-befriend'. In humans this effect is largely mediated through female hormones such as oxytocin and oestrogen.[33] Levels of these hormones are highest during activities like breastfeeding as well as in social interaction, massage and caring physical contact. These hormones have a calming or settling effect on stress and down-regulate the fight-or-flight response.[34] Women therefore have less of a tendency to become overly aggressive. None of this suggests that men cannot tend and befriend, or that women cannot elicit the fight-or-flight response when required, but it does suggest that each gender is more or less adapted for one or other response. This is an example of the complementarity of nature but equally it is part of the reason that men and women will respond in different ways to life events and therapies. Women, for example, will tend to feel more comfortable with talking-based therapies, especially dealing with emotional content, whereas men will more often wish to approach problems in an action-based way.

STRESS AND PERFORMANCE

One of the reasons that many people value stress is that they use it as a motivator to enhance performance. It is an assumption for many that if there were no stress there would be no performance. Inertia is, initially at least, a low-stress state but as stress increases, perhaps before an exam or a deadline, stress will often stimulate an increase in performance (Fig 8.1). If the

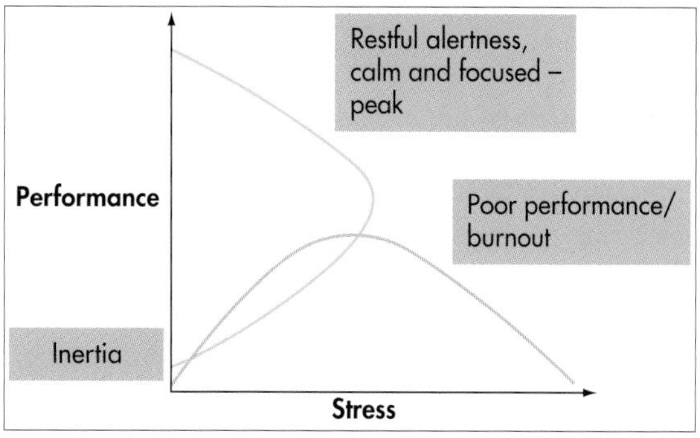

FIGURE 8.1 Stress–performance curve

stress remains manageable and is not too prolonged, then there tends not to be a significant problem. If, however, the stress escalates due to rising demands on performance, and stress is the only motivator being used to drive performance, then the person goes over the top of the stress-performance curve (red line) and finds that, despite high stress and energy consumption, performance drops. If this situation goes on for long, burnout soon eventuates.

There is another option (green line). We will have had experiences when we functioned at our peak. In athletic circles this is called 'the zone'; it is also called a 'flow state'. In such a state there is an increased focus of attention and this has two significant effects. First, because attention is less monopolised by anxieties and fears there is a reduction in stress, leading to a sense of being inwardly calm. Secondly, because of the high level of focus or 'restful alertness', the resulting perceptiveness is associated with a high level of performance and efficiency. A hallmark of this state is a sense of effortlessness.

Unfortunately, burnout is common, particularly among doctors. A study of medical interns found a steady increase in the point prevalence of burnout, which peaked at a prevalence of 75%, 8 months into the intern year. Seventy-three per cent of interns met the criteria for psychiatric morbidity—that is, an anxiety or depressive disorder—on at least one occasion throughout the year.[35] For this reason, an increasing number of medical schools are introducing self-care skills into medical education to foster resilience for later careers. Burnout is measured by levels of things such as depersonalisation, lack of motivation and low sense of achievement.

Even in the absence of burnout, living and working in a 'hyperkinetic environment' encourages a lower level of focus, which some call 'attention deficit trait' (ADT).[36] In dealing with so much input coming at such a speed, a person tends to become increasingly reactive, adopts 'black-and-white thinking', has difficulty staying organised and setting priorities, and manages time poorly. It is often associated with a constant low level of panic and guilt. The management of ADT is through learning to focus or regulate attention, lifestyle maintenance, changing the environment to be less frenetic and learning how to stop at the end of the day.

Studies of learning styles indicate that certain motivation and learning styles need stress to drive performance, and others don't. Biggs' model describes three learning approaches: surface learning, achievement learning and deep learning.[37] Deep learners are driven by interest, not stress, and do not need stress to perform well. They integrate what they learn and tend to enjoy it far more. Surface learners tend to learn by rote and the main motivation is to avoid failure. Achievement learners often study hard but are motivated by ego-enhancement, that is, wishing to achieve well in order to earn respect or look good. Surface and achievement learners tend to need stress to perform. The highest achievers all use deep approaches, while third-class honours students tend to use surface approaches.[38]

MIND AND BRAIN

In the field of MBM, there is much debate about the distinction, if any, between mind and brain. Are they the same, or does the mind communicate through the brain? In this view, mind is non-physical and is constituted by thought and emotion. The brain, on the other hand, is the physical organ that translates thought and emotion into biological and electrical activity and thereby regulates the body. The statement that an illness, pain or stress is 'in the mind' is correct, but it is also in the body.

Depression is an emotional state that is also associated with a range of other symptoms and somatic effects. These are mediated via the neurotransmitter and hormonal changes associated with depression and the rich interconnections between emotional and cognitive centres in the brain. Although there are undoubtedly changes in neurotransmitter profiles in the brain associated with depression, serotonin being the most important, sophisticated brain-imaging techniques are making it clear that thought and belief have a major role in driving brain activity. Functional MRI (fMRI), for example, can show that changes in brain activity associated with the placebo response when a person receives a mock antidepressant is biologically similar to that in people who receive the active drug. Such observations are impossible to explain with the view that the cause of recovery from depression is purely a chemical one. The same is also seen in people who receive placebo analgesics by mapping regional metabolic changes in parts of the brain that modulate the pain response.[39,40] Interestingly, brain scans mapping the recovery from depression associated with cognitive approaches demonstrate that it is via different pathways than those associated with pharmacological therapies.[41,42]

In various chronic pain syndromes, the changes in the brain associated with stress and sympathetic nervous system reactivity sensitise the pain pathways in the brain to register pain messages even with relatively low-level stimuli and in the absence of tissue damage. To the person experiencing the chronic pain syndrome, the experience of pain feels real. This is part of the reason that chronic pain and other manifestations of somatisation are such common accompaniments to emotional states such as depression, anxiety and burnout. It also explains, at least in part, why it is often difficult to demonstrate tissue damage associated with pain in various conditions such as chronic musculoskeletal pain, chronic low back pain, chronic fatigue syndrome and fibromyalgia.[43] Sustained attention and arousal are crucial in creating and sustaining the neural loops associated with chronic pain.[44] In other words, when a person becomes highly vigilant and reactive to pain messages, the brain will fire off pain messages with fewer and fewer stimuli. From a therapeutic perspective, this may be part of the reason that attention regulation exercises, such as mindfulness meditation, help in chronic pain syndromes. It is likely that the reduced reactivity to sensations may actually help to 'rewire' the brain in a way that minimises these effects.

Depression, stress and other psychological and emotional states are undoubtedly associated with physical sequelae. For instance, it has been shown that chronic severe depression is associated with a fivefold-increased risk of coronary heart disease independent of other risk factors.[45] These effects are not just the result of changes to one neurotransmitter—serotonin. There is a huge variety of biochemical, physiological and hormonal changes relevant to the cardiovascular system that are associated with depression. It therefore follows that treating depression with antidepressants does not significantly reduce the risk of cardiovascular disease. If, however, thought changes biology, then changing thought for the better among depressed patients should have a more significant effect in reducing the risk of cardiovascular disease, which it does. A meta-analysis of 23 studies clearly showed major reductions in ongoing morbidity and mortality for cardiac patients who received, as part of their rehabilitation, psychosocial interventions aimed at improving coping and emotional health.[46] The increased risk for those with no psychosocial treatment as a part of their on-going management was 1.70 for mortality and 1.84 for recurrence. The conclusions drawn from this study were unambiguous: 'The addition of psychosocial treatments to standard cardiac rehabilitation regimens reduces mortality and morbidity, psychological distress, and some biological risk factors … It is recommended to include routinely psychosocial treatment components in cardiac rehabilitation.'

The above discussion has given some indication of the scope and potential of MBM.

MAPPING MIND AND BRAIN

The vast and rapidly expanding field of neuroscience is providing plausible ways of understanding the mind–body connection. Mapping of the brain began in the early twentieth century. Specific functions could be attributed to specific regions of the brain, although this early work led to some naive and simplistic approaches to managing mental illness and behavioural problems. Psychosurgical techniques such as the frontal lobotomy have understandably been relegated to history, although other techniques such as electroconvulsive therapy (ECT) remain in use, and newer techniques such as transcranial magnetic stimulation (TMS) are being developed. The mainstay of the management of mental illness since the 1960s has been pharmaceutical. In more recent times, psychotherapies have accumulated more evidence supporting their use.

Many long-held myths about the brain have recently been challenged, particularly since the rise of neuron-imaging techniques. It was once thought that, after initial development, the CNS changes very little for the rest of the lifespan, but it is now becoming increasingly obvious that major modification of the brain takes place in response to experience, memory, attention and emotion. This is called 'neuroplasticity'. It suggests that although maladaptive reactions and ways of coping can become 'wired' into the circuitry of the brain, from a therapeutic perspective these reactions can also be wired out again, given the right strategies and persistence. The adaptability of the brain is exemplified by experiments on the effects of stress on the animal brain.[47] It was demonstrated that remodelling, particularly of the amygdala, which is associated with emotions and anxiety states, took place over a few weeks. This 'rewiring' is reversed if the animal is allowed to return to a stress-free environment. Such modelling and remodelling is more rapid in younger animals than in older animals. From a developmental perspective, it has significant implications for the long-term development of anxiety and depression. Memory of emotionally traumatic events with a high level of emotional reactivity reinforces the pairing of the thought with the emotion and accompanying physiological response. In its most extreme form it leads to post-traumatic stress disorder.

There are a number of changes to the brain associated with persistently high allostatic load. The brain is biochemically and structurally very responsive to stress hormones. The hippocampus, important for learning and memory, tends to atrophy and is vulnerable to the effects of stress and trauma. This has implications for the later development of dementia. The prefrontal cortex is important for working memory, and executive functions such as reasoning, emotional regulation, immune modulation and extinction of learning. The prefrontal cortex also plays a key role in modulating the stress response[48] but it too tends to atrophy through stress. The amygdala, on the other hand, which mediates the physiological and behavioural fear response, shows growth in response to persistent stress. Other parts of the brain have also been shown to be involved in the stress and fear responses.

States of mind such as those induced by mindfulness meditation are associated with changes in brain activity, specifically activation of the left frontal lobe, which is associated with better mood and improved immunity.[49] A predominance of left-sided anterior prefrontal activation is associated with positive affect and optimism. Other studies also link meditation to specific changes in brain activity associated with attention regulation and control of the autonomic nervous system.[50] Long-term meditation is now thought to have effects on brain structure and to slow age-related neuronal loss,[51] particularly in brain regions associated with attention, interoception and sensory processing. These were significantly thicker in meditators than in matched controls. Meditation 'might offset age-related cortical thinning' and provide 'evidence for ... cortical plasticity', probably a result of down-regulation of the stress hormones associated with allostatic load and implicated in acceleration of brain ageing.

THE PLACEBO RESPONSE

The placebo response is probably the most widely known example of the mind–body interaction. It refers to when a clinically significant effect is derived from the use of a chemically inert substance that the subject believes to be an active compound. In drug trials it is the most consistent confounding factor. Apart from the difficulty of identifying the mechanisms by which it is mediated, the placebo effect also makes it difficult to determine the effectiveness of medications, and can produce unwanted 'side effects'—this is called the 'nocebo effect'.

Harnessing the clinical potential of the placebo response raises ethical issues, as it is held to be unethical to mislead a patient. On the other hand, demystifying the placebo response has the potential to negate a significant part of the clinical response for many treatments.

Conditions that seem to be most subject to the placebo effect are those most influenced by emotion, perception and interpretation. Hence, the placebo effect for antidepressants, anxiolytic agents and analgesics is extremely high. To illustrate, reviews of the published research data suggest that the level of placebo effect of antidepressants is 60–80%; that is, only 20–40% of the clinical effect can be attributed to the chemical. More recent reviews, which include unpublished as well as published data, suggest that antidepressants are no better than placebo for mild–moderate depression and only marginally better than placebo even for severe depression.[52,53] This is not surprising if one considers that fMRIs on patients receiving antidepressants show that brain activation in those receiving the drug is almost identical to that of those who receive a placebo.[39] Recovery from depression through cognitive therapies is via different neurological pathways than those activated by drugs. In the future it may be possible to use patients' brain scans to identify those who are more likely to respond to drug or cognitive therapies.[42,54] fMRI also shows that giving a placebo to a person in pain leads to a different cascade of neuron-chemical changes than those associated with mood regulation—rather, one associated with pain pathways.[55] Explanations for such phenomena are difficult unless one takes a more metaphysical view of the relationship between mind, brain and biology.

Surgical techniques are rarely subjected to placebo-controlled trials but when they are, the results are interesting. For example, a trial on arthroscopic knee surgery for osteoarthritis found that 'the outcomes after arthroscopic lavage or arthroscopic debridement were no better than those after a placebo procedure'.[56]

THE EXPERIENCE OF PAIN

The experience of pain is 'holistic' in the sense that the mental, emotional and physical are all involved. Pain is not localisable to any one centre of the brain, but is dependent on the interaction of many centres that register, modify or amplify pain signals. Such pain pathways can be affected by attention, mood, emotion, fear and cognition.

Empathy, or experiencing another's pain, has biological correlates. Again, under fMRI, empathy has been shown to be associated with similar changes in brain activity to those in the loved one actually experiencing the pain. Although the body is not registering physical pain, in empathy a person 'suffers' emotionally as they would if they were experiencing physical pain.[57] 'Stress' also affects acute and chronic pain perception. Chronic pain syndromes are very common in individuals with anxiety, depression, poor coping and high levels of helplessness and hopelessness. Equally, it is often difficult to identify somatic disease in such conditions as burnout, multiple chemical sensitivity, chronic musculoskeletal pain, chronic low back pain, chronic fatigue syndrome and fibromyalgia. In chronic pain syndromes, evidence suggests that neural loops become sensitised to register the experience of pain with minimal stimuli. They are maintained by 'sustained attention and arousal' in that the person is constantly vigilant for, and reactive to, pain messages.[58,59] It may be through the reversal of such effects that practices such as mindfulness, which reduce arousal and reactivity and refocus attention, have excellent long-term effects in the management of chronic pain.[60]

The comorbidity of chronic pain and depression may be partly explained by the fact that pain alters the hippocampus and gene expression, and reduces neurogenesis. In total, this adds up to the sensitisation of the nervous and limbic systems, in depressed patients.[61]

Chronic pain conditions are responsive to a range of mind–body interventions. For example, a study[62] of irritable bowel patients found that 71% initially responded to hypnosis and, of these, 81% maintained their improvement in the longer term. This correlated with improvements in quality of life, anxiety or depression scores, and led to a reduction in consultation rates and medication use. These benefits were still demonstrable after 5 years.

No management of a chronic pain syndrome should be considered complete without attention to the mind–body interaction. Taking a mind–body approach, however, will require a patient to have both insight and motivation.

THE EFFECTS OF STRESS REDUCTION

Psychological stress affects every system of the body. For example, there are effects on cardiac risk factors such as:

- increased blood pressure
- increased cholesterol
- increased platelet adhesiveness
- poor diet and sedentary behaviour
- addictive behaviours, including smoking.

BOX 8.1 Physiological benefits of relaxation and stress reduction

- Marked decrease in oxygen consumption, respiratory and metabolic rate and economy, and lower catechol receptor sensitivity[67–69]
- Reduction in blood pressure and heart rate[70]
- Reduction in serum cholesterol[71]
- Better control and lower rate of complications for diabetics[72]
- Increase in skin resistance and decrease in blood lactate[73]
- Changes in EEG patterns, including an increase in alpha and theta waves and EEG coherence[74]
- Reduction in epileptic seizure frequency[75]
- Changes in neurotransmitter profile, including high serotonin[76]
- Selective increase in cerebral blood flow[77]
- Reduction in cortisol levels[78]
- Reduced TSH and T_3 levels[79]
- Improved response time and reflexes[80]
- Improvement in proprioception, perceptiveness of hearing and other senses[51,81]
- Immune regulation—improved immune function, reduced inflammation and better response to immunisation[82]
- Neuroplasticity—increased left prefrontal lobe activity, thicker grey matter (prefrontal lobes)[51]
- Reduced calcium loss associated with high cortisol[83]
- Adjunct to therapy for a variety of illnesses such as heart disease, cancer, chronic pain,[84] asthma,[85] diabetes[86]
- Reduced mortality (cardiac, cancer and all-cause mortality)[87]

BOX 8.2 Psychological benefits of stress reduction

- Decreased anxiety[88,89]
- More optimism, decreased depression[90,91]
- Improved coping capabilities[92]
- Improved wellbeing[93]
- As an adjunct to psychotherapy[94]
- Reduced reliance upon drugs (prescribed and non-prescribed) or alcohol[95]
- Improved sleep—more restful, less insomnia and, in time, less sleep needed[96]
- Reduced aggression and criminal tendency[97]
- Improved IQ and learning capabilities, including the aged and intellectually impaired[98,99]
- Greater efficiency and output and reduced stress at work[100]
- Reduced 'attentional blink' and greater ability to absorb information[101]
- Better time management and improved concentration, academic performance and memory[102–104]
- Reduction in personality disorders and ability to change undesired personality traits[105,106]
- Greater emotional intelligence and emotional regulation[107]

Stress affects immune function (see section on psychoneuroimmunology, later in this chapter), slows wound healing[63,64] and alters genetic function, damage and repair (see section on genetic expression, later in this chapter). The implications are enormous.

The relaxation response, on the other hand, reverses the harmful effects of the inappropriate activation of the stress response. The 'relaxation response' was first coined by Professor Herbert Benson of Harvard University.[65] Although it can be fostered in a variety of ways, the effects are similar: a relaxed physical condition and a focused and alert mental state. This state of body and mind is sometimes called 'restful alertness'.

Some of the physical and psychological effects of stress that can be reversed through stress reduction techniques are listed in Boxes 8.1 and 8.2.[66] Overall there is a restoration of physiological balance or homeostasis. This movement towards balance, efficiency and health is natural and will take place automatically if it is not interfered with. Similarly, the mind will return to happiness and contentment if it is allowed.

Meditation is possibly the most powerful way of eliciting the relaxation response. Physiological and psychological benefits are cumulative when such exercises are practised over time. They work largely by reversing the unwanted effects of high allostatic load as well as helping to facilitate healthy behaviour change.

Some insurance companies are interested in the health benefits of stress reduction and meditation. This interest is based on the findings of some large audits. One compared 600,000 non-meditators to 2000 meditators.[108] The findings demonstrated reduced illness rates and medical care utilisation in every disease category. For example, there was an 87% reduction in heart disease and a 55% reduction in tumours among those who meditated compared with those who didn't. Follow-up over an 11-year period showed further improvements, with an overall 63% reduction in healthcare costs (that is, 63 cents in the health dollar saved), with less than one-eleventh the number of hospital admissions for cardiovascular disease, one-third the number for cancer and one-sixth the number for mental disorders and substance abuse, in meditators compared with non-meditating controls.[109] These studies did not control for all lifestyle and personality factors, and so self-selection and healthy lifestyle change would have contributed to the results along with direct physiological benefits. On the strength of the evidence, some insurance companies in the United States and Europe offer substantial reductions in life insurance premiums of up to 30% for those who regularly practise an approved form of meditation, in this case transcendental meditation (TM).

PSYCHONEUROIMMUNOLOGY

> The mind in addition to medicine has powers to turn the immune system around.[110]
>
> Jonas Salk (discoverer of the polio vaccine)

In recent decades there has been an explosion of research into how psychological factors affect the immune system. Put simply, psychoneuroimmunology (PNI) means that the mind is connected to the immune system via the nervous and endocrine systems. These effects have major implications for susceptibility to infections and cancer, response to allergens, and the modulation of autoimmune and inflammatory conditions. As it would be hard to find a disease process that is not influenced by immune function, PNI should be considered an important factor in the development of any illness.

Although the notion that the mind affects our resistance to disease dates back thousands of years, PNI began to gain credence in the mid-1970s. Communication between the CNS and the immune system takes place via 'hard wiring' (nerves) and a 'postal system' (blood-borne hormones and neurotransmitters). By these two means the CNS communicates with every element of our immune defences in a bi-directional feedback system.[111,112] Over 70 neurotransmitter receptors have been found on the surface of white blood cells. Especially important in the feedback loop are the limbic system in the brain, primarily concerned with emotion, and the prefrontal lobes. A predominance of left-prefrontal lobe activity is associated with better mood, optimism, intense positive emotion response to emotionally positive stimuli and an ability to minimise negative affect in daily life.[113–115] This correlates with greater natural killer (NK) cell activity. Predominantly right-brain active people experience lower mood, more pessimism and intense negative emotion in response to emotionally negative stimuli. The right prefrontal lobe is more important for antibody and immunoglobulin response.[116]

The 'chemistry of thought' is not localised to the brain, because the same neurotransmitter receptors are found in virtually every tissue in which they are sought. This goes a long way to explaining how emotional states such as stress, anxiety and depression cause distant physiological effects and affect susceptibility to disease. Also important is the fact that drugs that have psychoactive properties are also found to affect immune function and have clinically relevant side effects on immunity. Furthermore, the blood–brain barrier is made more porous by stress[117] and PNI mechanisms may play a role in the development of psychiatric disorders.[3]

There are many ways of measuring immune status. The commonly used measures of immunity are simply the number and types of immune cells—this indicates 'how large the army is' but tells us little about how well it is functioning. Tests of immune cell function are more specialised and expensive but are designed to give a more important indicator of how well the cells are performing their designated roles.[118] Such tests include measuring white blood cell 'proliferation' in response to an antigenic challenge and measuring how well NK cells kill tumour cells through a cytotoxic activity assay. These tests are performed in vivo. Other tests are performed in vitro by measuring the body's ability to stimulate antibodies or the delayed-type hypersensitivity response (allergic response). Negative emotional states have a negative effect on immunity largely by affecting how well immune cells carry out their core functions, such as lymphocyte proliferation in response to infection[119] or by inhibiting NK cell activity,[120] rather than having major effects on cell numbers. In terms of day-to-day health, the size of the army, though important, may be of secondary importance to how well that army is performing. For these reasons compromised immune function due to stress is harder to pick up on standard blood tests, which give cell counts but tell us little about how well those cells are functioning.

Immune cells discriminate 'self' from 'non-self' and do not attack self unless that cell has become a threat, as in cancer, or it has become infected by a virus. Immune dysfunction occurs when immune cells lose their ability to discriminate between self and non-self, attacking healthy tissue inappropriately or not attacking things that should be attacked. The former, through inflammatory mechanisms, leads to autoimmune and inflammatory diseases, and the latter, through immunosuppression, predisposes to infections and cancer. During high-stress periods there is a shift towards the type-2 immune response and type-2-mediated conditions (infections, latent viral expression, allergic conditions and autoimmune conditions).[121] This inappropriate response is called immune 'dysregulation' and partially explains the increased incidence or relapse of such illnesses during high-stress periods (Box 8.3).

Immune cells mirror emotional states[122] and emotional states are associated with a variety of disease states, whether as a result of an accumulation of many small stressors or the impact of large ones. An accumulation of small daily stressors can be as detrimental to health as major stressors, if not more so.[123] Changes in immune cell numbers and function start to occur within five minutes of an event that is perceived to be stressful.[124] Depending on the reaction to the stressor, that effect can remain for up to 72 hours afterwards.[125] If a person perceives that they have some control over the situation or control over their response to the situation, then they are partially protected from the stress and its consequent immunosuppressive effects. People who perceive that they have no control over the event or their response to it, especially if they are anxious to be in control, experience prolonged negative effects on immune function.

Acute stress alters quantitative and functional components of cellular immunity, and individuals vary markedly in the magnitude of their response. These differences can be predicted by individual variability in perception and consequent stress-induced hypothalamic-pituitary-adrenal-axis (HPA-axis) and SNS activation. Those who have higher SNS reactivity to stress (increased blood pressure, heart rate, catechol secretion) have the greatest disturbance to immunity

BOX 8.3 Clinical effects of poor emotional and social health on immunity

- Immune dysregulation
- Lowered immune markers
- Increased susceptibility to infections
- Increased severity and progression of infections
- Increased relapse of chronic and latent infections
- Slower wound healing
- Increased activity of inflammatory illnesses
- Increased activity of autoimmune conditions
- Poor response to immunisation
- Aggravation of allergic conditions
- Poorer immune response to some cancers

and susceptibility to infection in response to stressful events. These variations are of clinical significance.[126] High cortisol reactors with high levels of life events have approximately double the incidence of verified upper respiratory infection than high reactors with low levels of life events and low reactors irrespective of their life event scores.[127] This has been further illustrated in studies measuring the stress levels of medical interns and their correlation with immunity.[128]

Salivary immunoglobulin A (S-IgA) is the first line defence against infection in the respiratory gastrointestinal and urinary systems, and is one of the easiest markers of immune competence to measure. Low levels of S-IgA are associated with increased risk of infection[129,130] and have been found to be reduced by stressful life events such as exam pressure, social isolation,[131] grief,[132] anxiety[133] and the 'need to have power and to influence others'.[134] Positive emotional states, however, are associated with immunoenhancement.[135,136] S-IgA can be increased or decreased for 4–5 hours even by inducing positive (e.g. care and compassion) or negative (e.g. anger and frustration) emotions for only 5 minutes.[137] Mental and emotional states also influence the speed of wound healing due to the effects on interleukins and cytokines.[138]

In response to 'standardised stressors' some people experience immunoenhancement and others immunosuppression, depending on the person's perception of the event. Studies of life stress and its impact on cancer incidence have had similar findings. In determining the impact of stress upon health it is important to take into account the individual's perception and coping style. Those with positive perceptions and coping styles consistently experience immunoenhancement, including improved NK cell activity and S-IgA, and those with negative perceptions and coping styles consistently experience immunosuppression.[139–141] Furthermore, those who have higher SNS reactivity to stress as measured by increased blood pressure, heart rate and catechol secretion also seem to have the greatest disturbance to immunity when under stress.[142] Immune change is also predicted by brain activity.[143]

Lifestyle factors can also influence immune function significantly (see Table 8.1).[144] A healthy lifestyle helps our immune function to operate at an optimal level. No lifestyle factor is innately 'good' unless it is at the right level. For example, exercise prior to infection can enhance immunity and be protective against becoming ill, but high-intensity exercise after infection can worsen the infection and the symptoms. Very intense or prolonged exercise, because of the effects on allostatic load, can reduce immunity and predispose to infections. Elite athletes, for example, tend to have poor immunity.[145] So too much and too little exercise are

TABLE 8.1 Lifestyle and effect on natural killer cell activity[144]

Behaviour	Advantage in NK activity (%)
Exercise	47
Managing stress	45
Enough sleep	44
Balanced meals	37
Not smoking	27
Eating breakfast	21
Working moderate hours	17
Avoiding alcohol	0

both associated with poor immunity, as are too much and too little sleep. Being employed is good for health but too little or too much work is associated with poor health.[146]

An unhealthy lifestyle is promoted by stress[147] and depression,[148] and therefore effective stress management is a prerequisite for sustained healthy lifestyle change.[149] Meditation,[150] psychological interventions such as CBT,[151,152] a positive attitude and humour[153] are all powerful immune system stimulants in that they help to reverse the immunosuppressive effect of stress.

The abovementioned fluctuations in immune function are significant factors in susceptibility to infection.[154] The likelihood of contracting a clinical infection when exposed to a virus is directly proportional to the level of stress that the host was experiencing not just at the time of exposure but during the preceding months. The severity of a viral illness, such as influenza, is greater with higher stress levels.[155] There is also a strong link between high stress and relapse for chronic infections such as herpes viruses,[156] HIV and shingles. Such viruses lie dormant and are more able to reactivate when the immune system is depleted. Data show that stress and social connectedness are important factors affecting the rate of progression of HIV to AIDS.[157] Those who were experiencing above-average levels of stress and had below average levels of social support were 2–3 times more likely to progress to AIDS over a 5-year follow-up. For every one severe stressor per 6-month study interval, the risk of early disease progression to AIDS was doubled.[158] Such observations indicate the importance of offering psychological interventions as a part of standard care. For example, giving CBT to HIV-positive men reduced depression and anxiety, and these changes were paralleled by reductions in stress hormones, improvements in white cell counts[159] and elevation of DHEA (dehydroepiandrosterone),[160] which is also an important hormone in patients with chronic fatigue syndrome.

Studies of medical students[152] during the exam period reveal profound immunosuppression, with lowered NK-cell activity, a 90% reduction in gamma interferon and lowered response of T-cells, which corresponds with the tendency to succumb to illness during or just after exams. Students who learn and practise relaxation techniques show significantly better immune function and less illness in exam periods. Even keeping a journal about significant life events is associated with improved immune function and fewer doctor visits for infectious disease.[161] Carers have been found to exhibit immune suppression proportional to the level of distress they feel.[162] The degree of immunosuppression observed in those going through a stressor such as marital separation is proportional to the amount of negative emotion and difficulty the person experiences in letting go.

AUTOIMMUNE AND INFLAMMATORY ILLNESSES

Mediators of inflammation play an important role in many illnesses. Cytokines can be typed as type 1 (e.g. γ-interferon) or type 2 (e.g. interleukin-10). A high ratio of type 1 to type 2 leads to what is called a 'type-1 response' and a low ratio leads to a 'type-2 response'. It has been shown that during high-stress periods there is a shift towards the type-2 response, which partially explains the increased incidence of type-2-mediated conditions including infections, latent viral expression, allergic conditions and autoimmune conditions during high-stress periods.[163] Thus, psychological state not only regulates the level of immune response but also the type of response. This inappropriate immune response is called immune 'dysregulation'. Autoimmune diseases are associated with immune dysregulation, whether the response is directed to the joints in rheumatoid arthritis or the myelin sheath in multiple sclerosis. Even coronary heart disease has a significant inflammatory component. PNI offers potential explanations of the mechanisms by which stressful life events and unsupportive social environments can trigger and exacerbate a variety of autoimmune diseases.[164–166]

For example, stress is associated with increased inflammation, pain and disease activity in rheumatoid arthritis patients.[167] Those with supportive relationships and better coping skills are noted to have lower levels of inflammatory hormones such as interleukins.[168] 'Irrational beliefs [that are stress-inducing] are associated with increased inflammation process, among apparently healthy individuals.'[169] There are also established links between major depression, early life stress and adverse health outcomes in inflammatory diseases.[170] Systemic lupus erythematosus (SLE) is also significantly affected by life stress,[171] as is multiple sclerosis.[172] From a clinical perspective, the important point is that the comprehensive treatment of any inflammatory or autoimmune illness requires the management of life stress, but unfortunately such interventions are too often ignored or seen as being of peripheral importance. Innovative studies, such as the following, have shown significant promise:

- clearing psoriasis twice as quickly when orthodox medical treatment is combined with meditation[173]
- improving outcomes for rheumatoid arthritis and asthma patients by enhancing positive emotional adjustment with journal writing as a form of stress release[174]
- including CBT in the management of rheumatoid arthritis.[175]

ALLERGIES

As with immunosuppression, it is possible to classically condition allergies by pairing a stimulus with exposure to the allergen.[176] At present it is not known whether they can be un-conditioned. Unhealthy lifestyle and poor physical and mental health practices have been implicated in the aggravation of allergies.[177] The reverse hypothesis—that stress reduction reduces allergies—is still to be comprehensively tested, but some evidence suggests that it can play a role. For example, the treatment of atopic dermatitis was more successful and required fewer topical steroids when it was combined with relaxation therapy, CBT and an education program.[178] It has been further demonstrated that stress is an important prognostic factor for response to immunotherapy.[179]

STRESS AND IMMUNISATION

The efficacy of vaccination such as with the hepatitis B or influenza vaccines is affected by stress. Those who are stressed prior to vaccination have significantly worse antibody and T-cell response,[180,181] and reducing stress has been demonstrated to improve response to flu vaccination.[49]

PSYCHOGENETICS

The DNA or genetic code contains the blueprint for the whole body. Each human shares 99.9% of their genes with other humans, which means that the other 0.1% account for all the differences between humans. Until recently, genes and genetic expression were looked upon as largely fixed but now, as with the neurosciences, this thinking is being revised.

Genotype is the information coded into the genes, whereas *phenotype* is what the genes express. Many genes contained within a genotype may lie dormant or not be expressed at any given time. The activation and deactivation of various genes trigger the onset and progression of many diseases.

Studies on animals and humans[182,183] have revealed that psychological stress can induce DNA damage and chromosomal aberrations. Mental state can not only increase the number of genetic mutations, but can also impair the body's ability to repair damage.[184] DNA damage is particularly important in the genesis of cancer,[185] which is also affected by genetically modulated cell replication, cell death (apoptosis) and cancer suppressor genes. Damage to these genes can lead to cancer.

DNA repair capacity (DRC) is a measure of the cell's ability to repair damage. Stresses, such as coping with trauma, while increasing oxidative damage to DNA, also stimulate compensatory DNA repair mechanisms.[186] During periods of high stress, such as during exams, compared to periods of low stress, such as after vacations, there is an increase in DRC in most people,[187] implying an adaptive response to increased DNA damage. Those with higher and more consistent stress and mood disturbance have high DNA damage but no increase, or even a reduction, in DRC in high-stress periods, suggesting that the response has been impaired in some way. The implications may be significant. For example, studies comparing DRC in women with and without breast cancer showed that the DRC of those with cancer was lower than that in the control group.[188] A 1% decrease in DRC corresponded to a 22% increase in breast carcinoma risk, with younger breast cancer patients having a more significant reduction in DRC. Thus, DRC may be a useful marker in predicting susceptibility.

Psychological state affects genetic expression in other ways. A genetic predisposition to an illness—such as addictive behaviours,[189] cardiovascular reactivity,[190] depression,[191] schizophrenia[192] and asthma[193]—is commonly activated by stress. Rather than saying that stress is the cause of the illness, it might be more accurate to say that it is a common trigger for many disease processes. In schizophrenia, for example, the 'normal ingrowth of dopamine fibres during late adolescence and their formation of aberrant connections with abnormal intrinsic cortico-limbic circuits could "trigger" the onset of symptoms in those who carry the constitutional vulnerability for schizophrenia'. In terms of genetic tendency to addictive behaviours, 'stresses, such as drug use and social adversity, in adolescence or early adult life may propel the neuro-developmentally impaired individual over a threshold into frank psychosis'.[194] Drug-seeking behaviour can be triggered by various factors, including 'priming injections', drug-associated environmental stimuli and stress. Drug-associated stimuli and stress may activate this system via neural circuits from the prefrontal cortex, amygdala and HPA-axis.

Psychological and social factors also significantly affect the rate of genetic ageing. Telomeres can be used as a marker of genetic age. A study of healthy premenopausal women found that psychological stress, in terms of both perception and chronicity, is significantly associated with higher oxidative stress, lower telomerase activity (the enzyme that repairs telomeres) and shorter telomere length. Women with the highest levels of perceived stress compared with low-stress women had telomeres shorter on average by the equivalent of 9–17 years of additional ageing.[195] This has many implications for understanding how stress promotes earlier onset of age-related diseases. Mental illness is a major risk factor for CVD. Part of this may be associated with accelerated genetic ageing. Telomere shortness and low telomerase activity are associated with exaggerated autonomic reactivity (allostatic load) to acute mental stress and elevated nocturnal catechol secretion. Low telomerase activity is also associated with risk factors for CVD—smoking, lipids, high blood pressure, high fasting glucose and greater abdominal adiposity (metabolic syndrome).[196]

The inherited disposition to depression can be activated by the interaction between heredity and upbringing. Developmentally, this is crucial for risk later in life. Childhood trauma (CT) and genetic factors contribute to the pathophysiology of depression, and experience of at least one type of CT is reported by 80% of adults with depression. The common traumas include physical neglect, emotional abuse and emotional neglect. There is an earlier age of onset of depression in those with CT and earliest onset in those with highest CT.[197] Children raised in deprived environments can consequently have severe cognitive and behavioural difficulties and poor response to stress lasting into adulthood. These changes are associated with ongoing alterations in gene expression, 'environmental programming' and downstream effects on the HPA axis.[198]

From a research perspective, the new field of psychogenetics has the potential to explain the mechanisms of illness and recovery. From a therapeutic perspective, it is important to give attention to mental and emotional health in the prevention and management of any chronic health condition.

PERSONALITY AND ILLNESS

The notion that personality directly affects our physical health has a long history. For example, mythology and religion have long related moral and emotional character to health and healing. A relationship between personality and illness undoubtedly exists, but the depth of that relationship is unknown, imprecise and hard to determine because of the interrelation between psychology, upbringing, environment and health behaviours. This having been said, care needs to be taken in discussing this issue, for a number of reasons.

- Although objective self-examination and a sense of personal responsibility for behaviour is useful, one should avoid the tendency towards self-blaming or fatalism, which are common reactions.
- Giving information on the role of personality and emotional style in leading to illness can do more harm than good if it is not delivered with the skills and support to modify unhelpful traits.
- Personality is just one causal factor, albeit an important one, interplaying with others, such as environment, lifestyle and genetic predisposition.
- Much modern mythology concerning the relationship between personality and illness—for example, the idea that a lack of communicativeness will express itself through specific forms of cancer such as laryngeal cancer—cannot be supported by evidence.
- Personality is not fixed, although it takes persistent and conscious effort to change a long-held personality trait.

Any emotional 'state', even anger, has its place if it is appropriate to the situation, is not 'over-expressed' or 'under-expressed' and is left in the past once the situation is over. A person will generally know if the expression is appropriate or inappropriate by the after-effects. A personality 'trait', on the other hand, will tend to reflect a conditioned or 'default' response to situations. A tendency to experience and express anger, regardless of its appropriateness and usefulness, will rarely be helpful for oneself or others. It is such traits that are associated with poor mental and physical health.

Research in this field is inherently difficult due to the varying personality classifications and interpretations. Classifying personality types by clustering groups of traits together can be simplistic and risks ignoring the infinite variation and subtlety of human character and psychology. For example, studies of type A (hard-driving, ambitious, aggressive etc) personalities give inconsistent findings. Some suggest it is a risk factor for heart disease, but others do not.[199] More recent and decisive studies have concentrated more on individual traits, such as anger or hostility, rather than combining a number of traits. This may make more sense, as personality traits are blended differently in every individual and traits can be interpreted differently. One person might be ambitious or hard-driving, for example, but in a very compassionate and altruistic way, whereas another may be self-centred. Assertiveness can be useful or destructive, depending on which aspect of our nature is asserting itself. A person with emotional intelligence may experience anger but will be able to determine whether it is worth expressing or not.

Be that as it may, some research has demonstrated that particular personality types may be predisposed to particular types of illnesses. For example, the personality types listed below have been implicated, with differing incidences, in cancer, coronary heart disease (CHD) and overall mortality when individuals with these personality types were followed over 10 years.[200]

- *Type 1:* Cancer-prone individuals tended to hopelessness, helplessness and suppression of emotion.
- *Type 2:* CHD-prone individuals tended to anxiety, aggression and ambition, and express emotion inappropriately.
- *Type 3:* A mixture of the other types were intermediate in terms of amount and type of illness.
- *Type 4:* These people suffered far less illness. They tended to live more in harmony with themselves and others, communicated better, tended to optimism, were more self-aware and remained calmer under stress.

Establishing an unambiguous causal relationship between personality and illness is inherently difficult. Other lifestyle factors may not be controlled. Testing the hypothesis that altering personality traits alters future risk of disease is also difficult. Some research has suggested that minimising unhelpful personality traits and communication patterns and enhancing better ones has a positive long-term effect on physical and psychological health.[201,201] Cancer-prone and heart-disease-prone individuals given 'autonomy training' over 6 months had far lower all-cause and cause-specific mortality than the control group. This suggests that as personality markers change, so too does the disease profile.

Other studies on patients with established and severe CHD[202] show that those with a 'type D' personality are nearly five times more likely to have another acute myocardial infarction (AMI) in the next 6–10 years. Type D personality is made up of two main elements: a high level of negative affect (anxiety, anger, worry etc) and a tendency to withhold the expression of these emotions. Emotional stress and its suppression have also been found to increase the number of ischaemic episodes by a factor of 2.2, even when controlled for other factors.[203] Among emotions, chronic anger and hostility seem to be most unhealthy, not just for CHD risk but also possibly for cancer risk[204,205] and survival.[206] Other studies have given conflicting results.[207] Part of the discrepancy is explained by the fact that many studies do not control as stringently for individual perception and coping style. People perceive the same events differently. For example, two people undergoing divorce will respond differently. For one it may be a relief of stress and for another a trauma, and in each case the physiological, endocrine and immune response will react to the perception of the event rather than the event itself. Therefore, the former is at minimal increased risk of illness, whereas the latter has a much higher risk.

Personality traits are far more malleable than they are often assumed to be, given the right support and motivation. Personality is in part genetic (nature) and in part 'learned' (nurture). It can be learned, and unlearned. Important elements in autonomy training, which is a behavioural approach, are self-awareness, relaxation, improved communication and behavioural strategies such as practising new ways of dealing with stressful situations. It is delivered within a support group setting and shows a lot of overlap with other approaches like mindfulness, positive psychology and emotional intelligence. Without awareness, insight and motivation it is all but impossible to change personality traits, except by the less conscious path of consistent conditioning and reinforcement.

In conclusion, advising a patient that the mind has an important role in the genesis, experience and progression of an illness is not to tell them that it is 'all in the mind'. Rather, it is to emphasise that the state of the mind affects the body. The two are not separate. The body expresses what is happening on deeper emotional levels. As Plato would have said, prevention and therapy, therefore, must include help on the psychological as well as the physical level, if it is to achieve its potential.

MIND–BODY INTERVENTIONS

You ought not to attempt to cure the body without the soul.

Plato (Charmides)

Almost any therapy that affects a person's mental and emotional states, because it will have consequent effects on their physical state, could be considered a mind–body therapy. For example, various meditative techniques have been found to be helpful for a range of conditions as diverse as epilepsy, premenstrual syndrome, menopausal symptoms, mood and anxiety disorders, and coping with serious illnesses, with few or no significant adverse events reported.[208] Yoga therapy also has a range of benefits.[209] Mind–body techniques will be helpful as adjuncts or alternatives in a far wider range of illnesses and symptoms but evidence on their efficacy sometimes lags behind community and practitioner experience. It is important that a GP who wishes to use mind–body strategies in the consulting room has adequate training. Although largely safe, their efficacy can be diminished and the potential for adverse events increased when used by inexperienced practitioners.

Techniques that can be included in the classification of mind–body therapies are described below.

Cognitive behaviour therapy

Cognitive behaviour therapy (CBT) is widely used for a range of mental health problems. It is easily learned by medical practitioners with adequate training and has a solid evidence base supporting its use.

Autonomy training

Autonomy training assists patients in self-expression and awareness. It incorporates relaxation and communication skills and has a body of evidence supporting its use.

Mindfulness-based therapies

A range of therapies use mindfulness principles, including *mindfulness-based stress reduction* (MBSR),[210] *mindfulness-based cognitive therapy* (MBCT),[211] as well as *acceptance commitment therapy* (ACT) and *dialectic behaviour therapy* (DBT). There is a high level of clinical and research interest in mindfulness-based therapies because of promising outcomes in mental health[212] and neurosciences. Mindfulness uses meditative practices in conjunction with a range of cognitive strategies.[213]

Meditation

Broadly speaking, meditation exercises are mental disciplines that involve attention regulation. They vary in the focus of the attention. There are many varieties of meditative practices, and many have a long tradition. The two most widely investigated varieties are *transcendental meditation*™, which uses a mantra, and *mindfulness meditation*, which largely uses the senses, breath and body. Meditation can be used for general wellbeing, as a form of therapy or as a discipline for spiritual development. Relaxation is a side effect rather than the central aim of these practices. Meditation can be used on its own or as an adjunct to other therapies.

Relaxation training

Physical relaxation is the central aim of these practices. *Progressive muscle relaxation* (PMR) is the most widely studied and used variety. The techniques generally involve progressively giving attention to particular muscle groups and relaxing them with or without tensing them first. They are clearly useful strategies but do not have as many useful effects on the mind as meditative practices do.

Autogenic training and hypnosis

Autogenic training and hypnosis are often associated with trance states. Like meditation training, they also involve focal awareness—for example, concentrating on a swinging pendulum. Unlike meditative practices, they involve the induction of a condition in which critical faculties are suspended and the 'limits of … a person's … usual frame of reference and beliefs temporarily altered … making him/her … receptive to other patterns of association and modes of mental functioning'.[214] It can also use concentration on 'heaviness' or 'warmth' and uses power of suggestion. It can be induced by others or self-induced. There is clear evidence that these techniques can be useful for a variety of conditions.

Conditioning

Classical conditioning can be used to induce a relaxation or other response when paired with a stimulus. There is clear experimental evidence supporting the hypothesis, although it is not often used in therapeutic settings.

Biofeedback

Biofeedback techniques have a sound evidence base, although they require specialised technical equipment. Patients can be trained to induce a relaxation response by following a physiological marker, like blood pressure or pulse, and learning how to lower it.

Prayer

Prayer has been used in various forms in virtually every culture and religious tradition for millennia. There is obvious overlap between some forms of prayer and meditative practices. There is less research evidence on prayer as a therapeutic modality but it is clearly beneficial for patients from appropriate cultural and religious backgrounds.

Visualisation techniques and mental imagery

Visualisation and imagery approaches use the mind's ability to project—thinking of a peaceful scene, for example. They have some overlap with self-hypnosis and often combine relaxation. These strategies can help to shift attention from distressing thoughts and can include focus on goals, behaviour change, 'inner guide', symbolic meaning and unlocking the unconscious. As most stress is related to 'mental imagery', because pleasant mental images do not last, and because these approaches may or may not help to improve focus in daily life, they are probably not as therapeutic as meditative practices.

Affirmations

Affirmations use a statement to 'un-condition' an unhelpful thought pattern and replace it with a more positive one. They are specific and goal-directed. The statement works best if it is short, true and repeated many times a day until it becomes automatic.

Affirmations can be incorporated with deep relaxation, but to be effective the thought needs to be supported and reinforced by action.

Movement-based therapies

Strategies such as t'ai chi, yoga and the Alexander technique are primarily movement- or body-based. Because of their reliance on focus and awareness, they also overlap with meditative practices and can have a range of benefits for stress and other mental health issues as well as physical benefits.

There is not scope within this textbook to include in-depth instruction on a range of mind–body strategies, but a mindfulness practice that will be useful for clinicians is provided below. As with any approach, a note of caution should be sounded: it is advisable to be experienced in any practice and to have had adequate instruction before using it.

PRACTISING MINDFULNESS MEDITATION

Mindfulness is about raising awareness and as such it is also about learning to concentrate, in a restful way. There are few contraindications to mindfulness-based practices but acute psychosis and intoxication are probably two. There is, however, some recent evidence that mindfulness-based approaches taught during remission may be useful in improving functioning and reducing some symptoms in patients with psychosis.[215] Caution should also be exercised for the inexperienced, to avoid moving on to intensive practice too soon.

There are different approaches to the amount of time that one should take to practise mindfulness. In the following program it is recommended that the meditation be practised initially for 5 minutes twice daily. Before breakfast and dinner are good times, because after eating is a low point for the metabolism and sleep can predominate more easily then. The duration of practice can be built up to 10, then 15, 20 and even up to 30 minutes or longer if required, depending on one's time availability, motivation, needs and commitment. Many people may find that starting with a regimen of longer practice times is too onerous and makes it difficult to get the practice established. Some very well respected and widely used programs such as MBSR and MBCT do start with longer periods of practice but this is generally in the context of people dealing with major illness or pain, where the motivation is already very high.

If longer practices of meditation can be compared to 'full stops' punctuating the day, then regular short pauses of 30 seconds to 2 minutes might be compared to commas. These commas during the day can help to reinforce our ability to be mindful for the whole day. Even pausing only for long enough to take a couple of deep breaths can help break the build-up of tension and mental activity throughout the day.

PREPARATION

It is helpful, wherever possible, to have a quiet place to practise without interruption. This is not to say that mindfulness cannot be practised anywhere, at any time—indeed, it is important for the practice to be as 'portable' as possible. We can practise on trains. We can pause while waiting at a red light (eyes open, preferably) or before a meal. If interruptions do occur then it helps not to be concerned, but rather just to deal with them mindfully and then, if possible, go back to the practice.

POSITION

The sitting position is generally preferred, as one is less likely to go to sleep in an upright position. In sitting for meditation it is best if the back and neck are straight and balanced, requiring a minimum of effort or tension to maintain the position. Lying down can also be useful, particularly if relaxation is the main aim of the practice, or if the body is extremely tired, in pain or ill. The ease of going to sleep while lying down may not always be desirable unless it is late at night. Having settled into the preferred position, it would be usual to let the eyes gently close. Meditation can also be practised with open eyes, in which case they would generally be cast gently down, resting on a point a metre or two in front of the body.

From here, one can move on to practise mindfulness using the sense of touch focused on the body (body scan) or breath, or another sense such as hearing can be used. One can also practise using a combination of these. The important thing about the body and the senses is that they are always in the present moment. In Jon Kabat-Zinn's MBSR program developed at the UMass Medical Center in Worcester, Massachusetts, the first mindfulness practice is to investigate a raisin, slowly and deliberately with each of the senses—this is the so-called 'raisin exercise'. Contact with any of the senses will automatically draw the attention away from the mental distractions that otherwise monopolise our attention.

THE BODY SCAN

Initially, be conscious of the whole body and let it settle. Now, progressively become aware of each individual part of the body, starting with the feet and then moving to the legs, stomach, back, hands, arms, shoulders, neck and face. Take your time. The object of this practice is to let the attention rest with each part, simply noticing what is happening there, what sensations are taking place, moment by moment. Practise cultivating an attitude of impartial awareness, that is, not having to judge the experiences as good or bad, right or wrong. Simply accept them as they are. There is no need to change your experience from one state to another or to 'make something happen'. Observing the mind judge, criticise or become distracted, for example, are simply mental experiences to observe non-judgmentally as they come and go. As often as the attention wanders from an awareness of the body, simply notice where the attention has gone and gently bring it back to an awareness of the body. It is not a problem if thoughts come in or the mind becomes distracted.

BREATHING

The attention can be rested with the breath as it passes in and out of the body. The point of focus could be right where the air enters and leaves through the nose, or it could be where the stomach rises and falls with the breath. Again, no force is required, and in mindfulness there is no need to try and regulate the breath—let the body do that for you. Again, if distracting thoughts and feelings come to your awareness, carrying your attention away with them, just be aware of them but let them come and go by themselves, letting go of any notion that one needs to 'battle' with them or 'get rid' of them. There is no need to try and stop these thoughts coming into your mind, or to try and force them out. Notice that trying to force thoughts and feelings out just feeds them with attention, makes them stronger and increases their impact. Try practising being less reactive to them, even if the thought is about the meditation itself and how well or poorly you think it might be going. It sometimes helps to just see mental activity as images on a movie screen or passing trains with which one does not need to get involved, be they pleasant or unpleasant.

LISTENING

When using listening, the practice of restful attentiveness is similar to the body scan and breathing. Here we are simply practising being conscious of the sounds in the environment, both near and far. As we listen, we let the sounds come and go and in the process also let any thoughts about the sounds—or anything else for that matter—come and go. Keep gently bringing your attention back to the present when it wanders. The value of listening is that your attention is not being used to feed the usual mental commentary that runs so much of the time in our minds. It is this commentary that is so full of habitual and unconscious rumination, and is almost constantly reinforcing ideas about ourselves and the world.

FINISHING

After practising for the allotted time, gently come back to an awareness of your whole body and then slowly allow your eyes to open. After remaining settled for a few moments, move into the activities of the day that need your attention. The mindfulness practice is not finished when you get out of the chair: it has just begun!

RESOURCES

Websites

Benson-Henry Institute for Mind Body Medicine, http://www.massgeneral.org/bhi/default.aspx

Center for Mindfulness in Medicine, Health Care and Society, University of Massachusetts Medical School, http://www.umassmed.edu/content.aspx?id=41252

Centre For Mindfulness Research And Practice, Bangor University, http://www.bangor.ac.uk/mindfulness/

Mind and Life Institute, http://www.mindandlife.org/

What is complementary and alternative medicine? NCCAM background on mind-body medicine, http://nccam.nih.gov/health/whatiscam/mind-body/mindbody.htm

Books

Ader R. Psychoneuroimmunology. Burlington: Elsevier; 2007.

Doige N. The brain that changes itself. New York: Penguin; 2007.

Harrington A. The cure within: a history of mind-body medicine. New York: Random House; 2008.

Hassed C. Know thyself: the stress release program. Melbourne: Michelle Anderson Publishing; 2002.

Hassed C. The essence of health: the seven pillars of wellbeing. Sydney: Ebury Press; 2008.

Segal Z, Williams M, Teasdale J. Mindfulness-based cognitive therapy for depression: a new approach to preventing relapse. New York: Guilford Press; 2002.

Siegal D. The mindful brain. New York: WW Norton; 2007.

Watkins A. Mind-body medicine: a clinician's guide to psychoneuroimmunology. Churchill Livingstone, New York; 1997.

Williams M, Teasdale J, Segal Z et al. The mindful way through depression: freeing yourself from chronic unhappiness. New York: Guilford Press; 2007.

REFERENCES

1 World Health Organization. Online. Available: www.who.int/en/

2 Astin J. Why patients use alternative medicine: results of a national study. JAMA 1998; 280(9):784–787.

3 Muller N, Ackenheil M. Psychoneuroimmunology and the cytokine action in the CNS: implications for psychiatric disorders. Prog Neuropsychopharmacol Biol Psychiatry 1998; 22(1):1–33.

4 Porter RJ, Gallagher P, Watson S et al. Corticosteroid-serotonin interactions in depression: a review of the human evidence. Psychopharmacology (Berl) 2004; 173(1/2):1–17.

5 Brown MA, Buddle ML, Martin A. Is resistant hypertension really resistant? Am J Hypertens 2001; 14(12):1263–1269.

6 McEwen BS. Protection and damage from acute and chronic stress: allostasis and allostatic overload and relevance to the pathophysiology of psychiatric disorders. Ann NY Acad Sci 2004; 1032:1–7.

7 Dunn AJ, Swiergiel AH, de Beaurepaire R. Cytokines as mediators of depression: what can we learn from animal studies? Neurosci Biobehav Rev 2005; 29(4/5):891–909.

8 Rutz W. Rethinking mental health: a European WHO perspective. World Psychiatry 2003; 2(2):125–127.

9 Miller M, Rahe R. Life changes scaling for the 1990s. J Psychosom Res 1997; 43(3):279–292.

10 Ustun TB, Ayuso-Mateos JL, Chatterji S et al. Global burden of depressive disorders in the year 2000. Br J Psychiatry 2004; 184:386–392.

11 Mathers CD, Vos ET, Stevenson CE et al. The Australian Burden of Disease Study: measuring the loss of health from diseases, injuries and risk factors. Med J Aust 2000; 172(12):592–596.

12 Mathers CD, Loncar D. Projections of global mortality and burden of disease from 2002 to 2030. PLoS Med 2006; 3(11):e442.

13 McKelvey R, Pfaff J, Acres J. The relationship between chief complaints, psychological distress, and suicidal ideation in 15–24-year-old patients presenting to general practitioners. Med J Aust 2001; 175:550–552.

14 Jureidini JN, Doecke CJ, Mansfield PR et al. Efficacy and safety of antidepressants for children and adolescents. BMJ 2004; 328(7444):879–883.

15 Vitiello B, Swedo S. Antidepressant medications in children. N Engl J Med 2004; 350(15):1489–1491.

16 Hallfors DD, Waller MW, Bauer D et al. Which comes first in adolescence—sex and drugs or depression? Am J Prev Med 2005; 29(3):163–170. a p 163.

17 Young R, Sweeting H, West P. Prevalence of deliberate self-harm and attempted suicide within contemporary Goth youth subculture: longitudinal cohort study. BMJ 2006; 332(7549):1058–1061.

18 Martino SC, Collins RL, Elliott MN et al. Exposure to degrading versus nondegrading music lyrics and sexual behavior among youth. Pediatrics 2006; 118(2): e430–e441.

19 Bressan RA, Crippa JA. The role of dopamine in reward and pleasure behaviour—review of data from preclinical research. Acta Psychiatr Scand Suppl 2005; 427:14–21.

20 Brake WG, Zhang TY, Diorio J et al. Influence of early postnatal rearing conditions on mesocorticolimbic dopamine and behavioural responses to psychostimulants and stressors in adult rats. Eur J Neurosci 2004; 19(7):1863–1874.

21 Kjaer TW, Bertelsen C, Piccini P et al. Increased dopamine tone during meditation-induced change of consciousness. Brain Res Cogn Brain Res 2002; 13(2):255–259.

22 Covey LS, Glassman AH, Stetner F. Depression and depressive symptoms in smoking cessation. Compr Psychiatry 1990; 31:350–354.

23 Breslau N, Peterson EL, Schultz LR et al. Major depression and stages of smoking. A longitudinal investigation. Arch Gen Psychiatry 1998; 55:161–166.

24 Hurt RD, Sachs DP, Glover ED et al. A comparison of sustained-release bupropion and placebo for smoking cessation. N Engl J Med 1997; 337(17):1195–1202.

25 Hall SM, Muñoz RF, Reus VI. Cognitive-behavioral intervention increases abstinence rates for depressive-history smokers. J Consult Clin Psychol 1994; 62:141–146.

26 Small DM, Zatorre RJ, Dagher A et al. Changes in brain activity related to eating chocolate: from pleasure to aversion. Brain 2001; 124(9):1720–1733.

27 Kim SW, Grant JE, Adson DE et al. Double-blind naltrexone and placebo comparison study in the treatment of pathological gambling. Biol Psychiatry 2001; 49(11):914–921.

28 Epiquote. Epictetus. Online. Available: http://en.wikiquote.org/wiki/Epictetus

29 Sims J. The evaluation of stress management strategies in general practice: an evidence-led approach. Br J Gen Pract 1997; 47(422):577–582.

30 Taylor SE, Klein LC, Lewis BP et al. Biobehavioural responses to stress in females: tend-and-befriend, not fight-or-flight. Psychol Rev 2000; 107(3):411–429.

31 Girdler SS, Jamner LD, Shapiro D. Hostility, testosterone and vascular reactivity to stress: effects of sex. Int J Behav Med 1997; 4:242–263.

32 Holstrom R. Female aggression among the great apes: a psychoanalytic perspective. In: Bjorkqvist K, Niemela P eds. Of mice and women: aspects of female aggression. San Diego, CA: Academic Press; 1992; 295–306.

33 Uvans-Moberg K. Oxytocin-linked antistress effects—the relaxation and growth response. Acta Psychiatr Scand 1997; 640 (Suppl):38–42.

34 Altemus M, Deuster A, Galliven E et al. Suppression of hypothalamic-pituitary-adrenal axis response to stress in lactating women. J Clin Endocrinol Metab 1995; 80:2954–2959.

35 Willcock SM, Daly MG, Tennant CC et al. Burnout and psychiatric morbidity in new medical graduates. Med J Aust 2004; 181(7):357–360.

36 Hallowell EM. Overloaded circuits: why smart people underperform. Harv Bus Rev 2005; 83(1):54–62, 116.

37 Biggs J. Student approaches to learning and studying. Australian Council for Educational Research: Melbourne; 1987.

38 Bullimore D. Study skills and tomorrow's doctors. WB Saunders: Edinburgh; 1998.
39 Mayberg HS, Arturo Silva J, Branna SK et al. The functional neuroanatomy of the placebo effect. Am J Psychiatry 2002; 159(5):728–737.
40 Wager TD, Rilling JK, Smith EE. Placebo-induced changes in FMRI in the anticipation and experience of pain. Science 2004; 303(5661):1162–1167.
41 Goldapple K, Segal Z, Garson C. Modulation of cortical–limbic pathways in major depression: treatment-specific effects of cognitive behavior therapy. Arch Gen Psychiatry 2004; 61(1):34–41.
42 Mayberg HS. Modulating dysfunctional limbic-cortical circuits in depression: towards development of brain-based algorithms for diagnosis and optimised treatment. Br Med Bull 2003; 65:193–207.
43 Eriksen HR, Ursin H. Subjective health complaints, sensitization, and sustained cognitive activation (stress). J Psychosom Res 2004; 56(4):445–448.
44 Ursin H, Eriksen HR. Sensitization, subjective health complaints, and sustained arousal. Ann NY Acad Sci 2001; 933:119–129.
45 Rugulies R. Depression as a predictor for coronary heart disease. a review and meta-analysis. Am J Prev Med 2002; 23(1):51–61.
46 Linden W, Stossel C, Maurice J. Psychosocial interventions for patients with coronary artery disease: a meta-analysis. Arch Int Med 1996; 156(7):745–752.
47 Pawlak R, Margarinos AM, Melchor J et al. Tissue plasminogen activator in the amygdala is critical for stress-induced anxiety-like behaviour. Nat Neuroscience 2003; 6(2):168–174.
48 Wang J, Rao H, Wetmore GS et al. Perfusion functional MRI reveals cerebral blood flow pattern under psychological stress. Proc Natl Acad Sci USA 2005; 102(49):17804–17809.
49 Davidson RJ, Kabat-Zinn J, Schumacher J et al. Alterations in brain and immune function produced by mindfulness meditation. Psychosom Med 2003; 65(4):564–570.
50 Lazar SW, Bush G, Gollub RL et al. Functional brain mapping of the relaxation response and meditation. Neuroreport 2000; 11(7):1581–1585.
51 Lazar SW, Kerr CE, Wasserman RH et al. Meditation experience is associated with increased cortical thickness. Neuroreport 2005; 16(17):1893–1897.
52 Kirsch L, Moore TJ, Scoboria A et al. The emperor's new drugs: an analysis of antidepressant medication data submitted to the US Food and Drug Administration. Prev Treat 2002; 5(1):ArtID 23. Online. Available: http://journals.apa.org/prevention/volume5/pre0050023a.html
53 Kirsch I, Deacon BJ, Huedo-Medina TB et al. Initial severity and antidepressant benefits: a meta-analysis of data submitted to the Food and Drug Administration PLoS Medicine 2008; 5(2):e45. doi:10.1371/journal.pmed.0050045
54 Goldapple K, Segal Z, Garson C et al. Modulation of cortical–limbic pathways in major depression: treatment-specific effects of cognitive behavior therapy. Arch Gen Psychiatry 2004; 61(1):34–41.
55 Wager TD, Rilling JK, Smith EE et al. Placebo-induced changes in FMRI in the anticipation and experience of pain. Science 2004; 303(5661):1162–1167.
56 Moseley JB, O'Malley K, Petersen NJ et al. A controlled trial of arthroscopic surgery for osteoarthritis of the knee. N Engl J Med 2002; 347(2):81–88.
57 Singer T, Seymour B, O'Doherty J et al. Empathy for pain involves the affective but not sensory components of pain. Science 2004; 303(5661):1157–1162.
58 Eriksen HR, Ursin H. Subjective health complaints, sensitization, and sustained cognitive activation (stress). J Psychosom Res 2004; 56(4):445–448.
59 Ursin H, Eriksen HR. Sensitization, subjective health complaints, and sustained arousal. Ann NY Acad Sci 2001; 933:119–129.
60 Kabat-Zinn J, Lipworth L, Burney R. The clinical use of mindfulness meditation for the self-regulation of chronic pain. J Behav Med 1985; 8(2):163–190.
61 Duric V, McCarson KE. Persistent pain produces stress-like alterations in hippocampal neurogenesis and gene expression. J Pain 2006; 7(8):544–555.
62 Gonsalkorale WM, Miller V, Afzal A et al. Long-term benefits of hypnotherapy for irritable bowel syndrome. Gut 2003; 52(11):1623–1629.
63 Glaser R, Kiecolt-Glaser J, Marucha P et al. Stress-related changes in pro-inflammatory cytokine production in wounds. Arch Gen Psychiatry 1999; 56(5):450–456.
64 Kiecolt-Glaser J, Marucha PT, Malarkey WB. Slowing of wound healing by psychological stress. Lancet 1995; 346:1194–1196.
65 Benson H. The relaxation response. New York: HarperCollins; 2000.
66 Murphy M, Donovan S. The physical and psychological effects of meditation. A review of contemporary research with a comprehensive bibliography 1931–1996. Institute of Noetic Sciences. Sausalito, California; 1997.
67 Kesterton J. Metabolic rate, respiratory exchange ratio and apnoeas during meditation. Am J Physiol 1989; 256(3):632–638.
68 Benson H. The relaxation response and norepinephrine: a new study illuminates mechanisms. Aust J Clin Hypnotherapy Hypnosis 1989; 10(2):91–96.
69 Mills P, Schneider R, Hill D et al. Beta-adrenergic receptor sensitivity in subjects practicing TM. J Psychosom Res 1990; 34(1):29–33.

70 Delmonte M. Physiological responses during meditation and rest. Biofeedback Self-regulation 1984; 9(2):181–200.

71 Vyas R, Dikshit N. Effect of meditation on respiratory system, cardiovascular system and lipid profile. Indian J Physiol Pharmacol 2002; 46(4):487–491.

72 Surwit RS, van Tilburg MA, Zucker N et al. Stress management improves long-term glycemic control in type 2 diabetes. Diabetes Care 2002; 25(1):30–34.

73 Bagga O, Gandhi A, Bagga S. A study of the effect of TM and yoga on blood glucose, lactic acid, cholesterol and total lipids. J Clin Chem Clin Biochem 1981; 19(8):607–608.

74 Echenhofer F, Coombs M. A brief review of research and controversies in EEG biofeedback and meditation. J Transpers Psychol 1987; 19(2):161–171.

75 Deepak KK, Manchanda SK. Maheshwari MC. Meditation improves clinico-electroencephalographic measures in drug-resistant epileptics. Biofeedback Self-regulation 1994; 19:(1)25–40.

76 Bujatti M, Riederer P. Serotonin, noradrenaline, dopamine metabolites in TM technique. J Neural Transm 1976; 39:257–267.

77 Jevning R, Anand R, Biedebach M et al. Effects on regional cerebral blood flow of TM. Physiol Behav 1996; 59(3):399–402.

78 Doraiswamy PM, Xiong GL. Does meditation enhance cognition and brain longevity? Ann NY Acad Sci 2007; 28 Sep. [Epub ahead of print]

79 Werner OR, Wallace RK, Charles B et al. Long-term endocrine changes in subjects practicing the TM and TM-siddhi program. Psychosom Med 1986; 48(1/2): 59–65.

80 Jedrczak A, Toomey M, Clements G et al. The TM–siddhi program, age, and brief tests of perceptual motor speed and non-verbal intelligence. J Clin Psychol 1986; 42(1):161–164.

81 Brown D, Forte M, Dysart M et al. Visual sensitivity and mindfulness meditation. Percept Mot Skills 1984; 58:775–784.

82 Carlson LE, Speca M, Patel KD et al. Mindfulness-based stress reduction in relation to quality of life, mood, symptoms of stress, and immune parameters in breast and prostate cancer outpatients. Psychosom Med 2003; 65(4):571–581.

83 Coehlo R, Silva C, Maia A et al. Bone mineral density and depression: a community study in women. J Psychosom Res 1999; 46(1):29–35.

84 Kabat-Zinn J, Lipworth L Burney R. The clinical use of mindfulness meditation for the self-regulation of chronic pain. J Behav Med 1985; 8(2):163–190.

85 Wilson AF, Honsberger R, Chiu JT et al. Transcendental meditation and asthma. Respiration 1975; 32:74–80.

86 Cerpa H The effects of clinically standardised meditation on type 2 diabetics. Dissertation Abstr Int 1989; 499(8b):3432.

87 Schneider RH, Alexander CN, Staggers F et al. Long-term effects of stress reduction on mortality in persons ≥ 55 years of age with systemic hypertension. Am J Cardiol 2005; 95(9):1060–1064.

88 Kabat-Zinn J, Massion AO, Kristeller J et al. Effectiveness of a meditation-based stress reduction program in the treatment of anxiety disorders. Am J Psychiatry 1992; 149:936–943.

89 Eppley KR, Abrams AI, Shear J et al. Differential effects of relaxation techniques on trait anxiety: a meta-analysis. J Clin Psychol 1989; 45(6):957–974.

90 Teasdale J, Segal Z, Williams J. How does cognitive therapy prevent depressive relapse and why should attention control (mindfulness) training help? Behav Res Ther 1995; 33(1):25–39.

91 Bujatti M, Riederer P. Serotonin, noradrenaline, dopamine metabolites in TM technique. J Neural Transm 1976; 39(3):257–267.

92 Kornfield J. Intensive insight meditation: a phenomenonological study. J Transpers Psychol 1979; 11(1):48–51.

93 Baer RA, Smith GT, Lykins E et al. Construct validity of the five facet mindfulness questionnaire in meditating and nonmeditating samples. Assessment 2008; 15(3):329–342.

94 Kutz I, Lerserman J, Dorrington C et al. Meditation as an adjunct to psychotherapy. An outcome study. Psychother Psychosom 1985; 43(4):209–218.

95 Gelderloos P, Walton KG, Orme-Johnson DW et al. Effectiveness of the TM program in preventing and treating substance misuse: a review. Int J Addict 1991; 26:293–325.

96 Mason L, Alexander C, Travis F et al. Electrophysiological correlates of higher states of consciousness during sleep in long-term practitioners of the TM program. Sleep 1997; 20(2):102–110.

97 Simpson TL, Kaysen D, Bowen S et al. PTSD symptoms, substance use, and vipassana meditation among incarcerated individuals. J Trauma Stress 2007; 20(3):239–249.

98 Gaylord C, Orme-Johnson D, Travis F. The effects of the transcendental meditation technique and progressive muscle relaxation on EEG coherence, stress reactivity, and mental health in black adults. Int J Neurosci 1989; 46(1/2):77–86.

99 Wallace RK, Orme-Johnson DW, Mills PJ et al. Academic achievement and the paired Hoffman reflex in students practicing meditation. Int J Neurosci 1984; 24(3/4):261–266.

100 Carrington P, Collings G, Benson H et al. The use of meditation and relaxation techniques for the

management of stress in a working population. J Occup Med 1980; 22(4):221–231.
101 Slagter HA, Lutz A, Greischar L et al. Mental training affects distribution of limited brain resources. PLoS Biology 2007; 5(6):e138. Online. Available: doi:10. 1371/journal.pbio.0050138
102 Paul G, Elam B, Verhulst SJ. A longitudinal study of students' perceptions of using deep breathing meditation to reduce testing stresses. Teach Learn Med 2007; 19(3):287–292.
103 Verma IC, Jayashankarappa BS, Palani M. Effect of transcendental meditation on the performance of some cognitive psychological tests. Indian J Med Res 1982; 77(Suppl):136–143.
104 Shah AH, Joshi SV, Mehrotra PP et al. Effect of Saral meditation on intelligence, performance and cardiopulmonary functions. Indian J Med Sci 2001; 55(11):604–608.
105 Delmonte M, Kenny V. Conceptual models and functions of meditation in psychotherapy. J Contemp Psychother 1987; 17(1):38–59.
106 Hansen E, Lundh LG, Homman A et al. Measuring mindfulness: pilot studies with the Swedish versions of the Mindful Attention Awareness Scale and the Kentucky Inventory of Mindfulness Skills. Cogn Behav Ther 2009; 38(1):2–15.
107 Baer RA, Smith GT, Allen KB. Assessment of mindfulness by self-report: the Kentucky inventory of mindfulness skills. Assessment 2004; 11(3):191–206.
108 Orme-Johnson D. Medical care utilisation and the transcendental meditation program. Psychosom Med 1987; 49:493–507.
109 Orme-Johnson D, Herron R. An innovative approach to reducing medical care utilisation and expenditures. Am J Manag Care 1997; 3:135–144.
110 Salk J. In: Dossey L. Meaning and medicine. New York: Bantam; 1991.
111 Bovberg DH. Psychoneuroimmunology: implications for oncology? Cancer 1991; 67:828–832.
112 Ader R. Psychoneuroimmunology. Sydney: Elsevier; 2007.
113 Wheeler RE, Davidson RJ, Tomarken AJ. Frontal brain asymmetry and emotional reactivity: a biological substrate of affective style. Psychophysiology 1993; 30(1):82–89.
114 Tomarken AJ, Davidson RJ. Frontal brain activation in repressors and nonrepressors. J Abnorm Psychol 1994; 103(2):339–349.
115 Tomarken AJ, Davidson RJ, Wheeler RE et al. Psychometric properties of resting anterior EEG asymmetry: temporal stability and internal consistency. Psychophysiology 1992; 29(5):576–592.
116 Kang DH, Davidson RJ, Coe CL et al. Frontal brain asymmetry and immune function. Behav Neurosci 1991; 105(6):860–869.
117 Covelli V, Maffione AB, Nacci C et al. Stress, neuropsychiatric disorders and immunological effects exerted by benzodiazepines. Immunopharmacol Immunotoxicol 1998; 20(2):199–209.
118 Cohen S, Herbert T. Health psychology: psychological factors and physical disease from the perspective of human psychoneuroimmunology. Ann Rev Psychol 1996; 47:113–142.
119 Knapp P, Levy E, Giorgi R et al. Short-term immunological effects of induced emotion. Psychosom Med 1992; 54:133–148.
120 Jemmott J, Hellman C, McClelland D et al. Motivational syndromes associated with natural killer cell activity. J Behav Med 1990; 13:53–73.
121 Marshall G, Agarwal SK, Lloyd C et al. Cytokine dysregulation associated with exam stress in healthy medical students. Brain Behav Immun 1998; 12(4): 297–307.
122 Hassed C. Psychoneuroimmunology: a Platonic view of the immune system. Aust Fam Physician 1999; 28(9):950–951.
123 Jandorf L, Deblinger E, Neale J et al. Daily vs major life events as predictors of symptom frequency: a replication study. J Gen Psychol 1986; 113:205–218.
124 Herbert T, Cohen S, Marsland A et al. Cardiovascular reactivity and the course of immune response to an acute psychological stressor. Psychosom Med 1994; 56:337–344.
125 Sieber W, Rodin J, Larson L et al. Modulation of human natural killer cell activity by exposure to uncontrollable stress. Brain Behav Immun 1992; 6:141–156.
126 Marsland AL, Bachen EA, Cohen S et al. Stress, immune reactivity and susceptibility to infectious disease. Physiol Behav 2002; 77(4/5):711–716.
127 Cohen S, Hamrick N, Rodriguez MS et al. Reactivity and vulnerability to stress-associated risk for upper respiratory illness. Psychosom Med 2002; 64(2):302–310.
128 Tendulkar AP, Victorino GP, Chong TJ et al. Quantification of surgical resident stress 'on call'. J Am Coll Surg 2005; 201(4):560–564.
129 Rossen R, Butler W, Wladman R. The protein in nasal secretion. JAMA 1970; 211:1157–1161.
130 Jemmot J, McClelland D. Secretory IgA as a measure of resistance to infectious disease. Behav Med 1989; 15:63–71.
131 Jemmott J, Magloire K. Academic stress, social support and S-IgA. J Pers Soc Psychol 1988; 55:803–810.
132 He M. A prospective controlled study of psychosomatic and immunologic changes in recently bereaved people. Chin J Neurol Psychiatry 1993; 24:90–93.
133 Annie C, Groer M. Childbirth stress—an immunology study. J Obstet Gynecol Neonatal Nurs 1991; 20: 391–397.

134 McClelland D, Floor E, Davidson R et al. Stressed power motivation, sympathetic activation, immune function and illness. J Hum Stress 1980; 6:11–19.
135 Labott S, Ahleman S, Wolever M et al. The physiological and psychological effects of the expression and inhibition of emotion. Behav Med 1990; 16:182–189.
136 Dillon K, Minchoff B, Baker K. Positive emotional states and enhancement of the immune system. Int J Psychiatry Med 1986; 15(1):13–16.
137 Rein G, Atkinson M, McCraty M. The physiological and psychological effects of compassion and anger. J Advancement Med 1995; 8(2):87–105.
138 Christian LM, Graham JE, Padgett DA et al. Stress and wound healing. Neuroimmunomodulation 2006; 13(5/6):337–346.
139 Jemmott J, Borysenko J, Borysenko M et al. Academic stress, power motivation, and decrease in secretion rate of salivary secretory immunoglobulin A. Lancet 1983; 1(8339):1400–1402.
140 Marsland A, Manuck S, Fazzari T et al. Stability of individual differences in cellular immune response to stress. Psychosom Med 1995; 57:295–298.
141 Boyce WT, Chesney M, Alkon A et al. Psychobiologic reactivity to stress and childhood respiratory illnesses: results of two prospective studies. Psychosom Med 1995; 57(5):411–422.
142 Manuck S, Cohen S, Rabin B et al. Individual differences in cellular immune response to stress. Psychol Sci 1991; 2:111–115.
143 Liang SW, Jemerin JM, Tschann JM et al. Life events, frontal electroencephalogram laterality, and functional immune status after acute psychological stressors in adolescents. Psychosom Med 1997; 59(2):178–186.
144 Kusaka Y, Londou H, Morimoto K et al. Healthy lifestyles are associated with higher natural killer cell activity. Prev Med 1992; 21:602–615.
145 Malm C, Celsing F, Friman G. Immune defense is both stimulated and inhibited by physical activity. Lakartidningen 2005; 102(11):867–868, 870, 873.
146 Sokejiana S, Kagamimori S. Working hours as a risk factor for acute myocardial infarction in Japan: case control study. BMJ 1998; 317(7161):775–780.
147 Pelletier KR. Mind–body health: research, clinical, and policy applications. Am J Health Promot 1992; 6(5):345–358.
148 Glassman A, Helzer J, Covery L et al. Smoking, smoking cessation, and major depression. JAMA 1990; 264: 1546–1549.
149 Sutherland JE The link between stress and illness: do our coping methods influence our health? Postgrad Med 1991; 89(1):159–164.
150 Magarey C. Meditation and health. Patient Management 1989; May:89–101.
151 Crepaz N, Passin WF, Herbst JH et al. Meta-analysis of cognitive-behavioral interventions on HIV-positive persons' mental health and immune functioning. Health Psychol 2008; 27(1):4–14.
152 Kiecolt-Glaser JK, Glaser R. Psychoneuroimmunology: can psychological interventions modulate immunity? J Consult Clin Psychol 1992; 60(4):569–575.
153 Kiecolt-Glaser JK, McGuire L, Robles TF et al. Psychoneuroimmunology and psychosomatic medicine: back to the future. Psychosom Med 2002; 64(1):15–28.
154 Cohen S, Tyrrell DA, Smith AP. Psychological stress and the common cold. N Eng J Med 1991; 325:606–612.
155 Cohen S, Doyle WJ, Skoner DP. Psychological stress, cytokine production, and severity of upper respiratory illness. Psychosom Med 1999; 61(2):175–180.
156 Glaser R, Kiecolt-Glaser J, Speicher C et al. Stress, loneliness and changes in herpes-virus latency. J Behav Med 1985; 8(3):249–260.
157 Leserman J, Jackson E, Petitto J et al. Progression to AIDS: the effects of stress, depressive symptoms and social support. Psychosom Med 1999; 61(3): 397–406.
158 Evans D, Leserman J, Perkins D et al. Severe life stress as a predictor of early disease progression in HIV infection. Am J Psychiatry 1997; 154:630–634.
159 Antoni MH, Cruess DG, Cruess S et al. Cognitive-behavioral stress management intervention effects on anxiety, 24-hr urinary norepinephrine output, and T-cytotoxic/suppressor cells over time among symptomatic HIV-infected gay men. J Consult Clin Psychol 2000; 68(1):31–45.
160 Cruess DG, Antoni MH, Kumar M et al. Cognitive-behavioral stress management buffers decreases in dehydroepiandrosterone sulfate (DHEA-S) and increases in the cortisol/DHEA-S ratio and reduces mood disturbance and perceived stress among HIV-seropositive men. Psychoneuroendocrinology 1999; 24(5):537–549.
161 Kiecolt-Glaser J, Glaser R. Stress and the immune system: human studies. Ann Rev Psychiatry 1991; 11:169–180.
162 Kiecolt-Glaser J, Dura J, Speicher C et al. Spousal caregivers of dementia victims: longitudinal changes in immunity and health. Psychosom Med 1991; 53: 345–362.
163 Marshall G, Agarwal S, Lloyd C et al. Cytokine dysregulation associated with exam stress in healthy medical students. Brain Behav Immun 1998; 12(4): 297–307.
164 O'Leary A. Stress, emotion, and human immune function. Psychol Bull 1990; 108(3):363–382.
165 Homo-Delarche F, Fitzpatrick F, Christeff N et al. Sex steroids, glucocorticoids, stress and autoimmunity. Steroid Biochem Molec Biol 1991; 40:619–637.

166 De Vellis R, De Vellis B, McEvoy H et al. Predictors of pain and functioning in arthritis. Health Educ Res: Theory Pract 1986; 1:61–67.
167 Zautra A, Hoffman J, Potter P et al. Examination of changes in interpersonal stress as a factor in disease exacerbations among women with rheumatoid arthritis. Ann Behav Med 1997; 19(3):279–286.
168 Zautra AJ, Hoffman JM, Matt KS et al. An examination of individual differences in the relationship between interpersonal stress and disease activity among women with rheumatoid arthritis. Arthritis Care Res 1998; 11:271–279.
169 Papageorgiou C, Panagiotakos DB, Pitsavos C et al. Association between plasma inflammatory markers and irrational beliefs: the ATTICA epidemiological study. Prog Neuropsychopharmacol Biol Psychiatry 2006; 30(8):1496–1503.
170 Pace TW, Mletzko TC, Alagbe O et al. Increased stress-induced inflammatory responses in male patients with major depression and increased early life stress. Am J Psychiatry 2006; 163(9):1630–1633.
171 Da Costa D, Dobkin P, Pinard L et al. The role of stress in functional disability among women with systemic lupus erythematosus: a prospective study. Arthritis Care Res 1999; 12(2):112–119.
172 Coyle P. The neuroimmunology of multiple sclerosis. Adv Neuroimmunol 1996; 6(2):143–154.
173 Kabat-Zinn J, Wheeler E, Light T et al. Influence of a mindfulness meditation-based stress reduction intervention on rates of skin clearing in patients with moderate to severe psoriasis undergoing phototherapy (UVB) and photochemotherapy (PUVA). Psychosom Med 1998; 60(5):625–632.
174 Smyth JM, Stone AA, Hurewitz A et al. Effects of writing about stressful experiences on symptom reduction in patients with asthma or rheumatoid arthritis. A randomised trial. JAMA 1999; 281: 1304–1309.
175 Young LD. Psychological factors in rheumatoid arthritis. J Consult Clin Psychol 1992; 60(4):619–627.
176 Gauci M, Husband A, Saxarra H et al. Pavlovian conditioning of nasal tryptase release in human subjects with allergic rhinitis. Physiol Behav 1994; 55(5): 823–825.
177 Shirakawa T, Morimoto K. Lifestyle effect on total IgE. Lifestyles have a cumulative impact on controlling total IgE levels. Allergy 1991; 46(8):561–569.
178 Ehlers A, Stangier U, Gieler U. Treatment of atopic dermatitis: a comparison of psychological and dermatological approaches to relapse prevention. J Consult Clin Psychol 1995; 63(40): 624–635.
179 Ippoliti F, De Santis W, Volterrani A et al. Psychological stress affects response to sublingual immunotherapy in asthmatic children allergic to house dust mite. Pediatr Allergy Immunol 2006; 17(5):337–345.
180 Glaser R, Kiecolt-Glaser JK, Bonneau RH et al. Stress-induced modulation of the immune response to recombinant hepatitis B vaccine. Psychosom Med 1992; 54:22–29.
181 Kiecolt-Glaser JK, Glaser R, Gravenstein S et al. Chronic stress alters the immune response to influenza virus vaccine in older adults. Proc Nat Acad Sci 1996; 93:3043–3047.
182 Adachi S, Kawamura K, Takemoto K. Oxidative damage of nuclear DNA in liver of rats exposed to psychological stress. Cancer Res 1993; 53(18):4153–4155.
183 Fischman H, Pero R, Kelly D. Psychogenic stress induces chromosomal and DNA damage. Int J Neurosci 1996; 84(1/4):219–227.
184 Kiecolt-Glaser J, Glaser R. Psychoneuroimmunology and immunotoxicology: implications for carcinogenesis. Psychosom Med 1999; 61(3):271–272.
185 Levine A. The tumour suppressor genes. Ann Rev Biochem 1993; 62:623–651.
186 Oldham KM, Wise SR, Chen L et al. A longitudinal evaluation of oxidative stress in trauma patients. J Paren Enteral Nutr 2002; 26(3):189–197.
187 Cohen L, Marshall G, Cheng L et al. DNA repair capacity in healthy medical students during and after exam stress. J Behav Med 2000; 23(6):531–545.
188 Ramos JM, Ruiz A, Colen R et al. DNA repair and breast carcinoma susceptibility in women. Cancer 2004; 100(7):1352–1357.
189 Self D, Nestler E. Relapse to drug seeking: neural and molecular mechanisms. Drug Alcohol Depend 1998; 51(1/2):49–60.
190 Cui Y, Gutstein W, Jabr S et al. Control of human vascular smooth muscle cell proliferation by sera derived from 'experimentally stressed' individuals. Oncol Rep 1998; 5(6):1471–1474.
191 Lopez J, Chalmers D, Little K et al. Regulation of serotonin 1A, glucocorticoid, and mineralocorticoid receptor in rat and human hippocampus: implications for the neurobiology of depression. Biol Psychiatry 1998; 43(8):547–573.
192 Benes F. The role of stress and dopamine-GABA interactions in the vulnerability for schizophrenia. J Psychiatr Res 1997; 31(2):257–275.
193 Mrazek DA, Klinnert M, Mrazek PJ et al. Prediction of early-onset asthma in genetically at-risk children. Pediatr Pulmonol 1999; 27(2):85–94.
194 Howes OD, McDonald C, Cannon M et al. Pathways to schizophrenia: the impact of environmental factors. Int J Neuropsychopharmacol 2004; 7(Suppl 1):S7–S13.
195 Epel ES, Blackburn EH, Lin J et al. Accelerated telomere shortening in response to chronic stress. Proc Natl Acad Sci USA 2004; 101(49):17312–17315.

196 Epel ES, Lin J, Wilhelm FH et al. Cell aging in relation to stress arousal and cardiovascular disease risk factors. Psychoneuroendocrinol 2006; 31(3):277–287.

197 Moskvina V, Farmer A, Swainson V et al. Interrelationship of childhood trauma, neuroticism, and depressive phenotype. Depress Anxiety 2007; 24(3):163–168.

198 Meaney MJ, Szyf M. Maternal care as a model for experience-dependent chromatin plasticity? Trends Neurosci 2005; 28(9):456–463.

199 Rozanski A, Blumenthal J, Kaplan J. Impact of psychosocial factors on the pathogenesis of cardiovascular disease and implications for therapy. Circulation 1999; 99(16):2192–2217.

200 Eysenck HJ, Grossarthy-Maticek R. Creative novation behaviour therapy as a prophylactic treatment for cancer and coronary heart disease: Part 2 Effects of treatment. Behav Res Ther 1991; 29:17–31.

201 Eysenck HJ. Psychological factors, cancer and ischaemic heart disease. BMJ 1992; 305:457–459.

202 Denollet J, Brutsaert DL. Personality, disease severity, and the risk of long-term cardiac events in patients with a decreased ejection fraction after myocardial infarction. Circulation 1998; 97:167–173.

203 Gullette EC, Blumenthal JA, Babyak M et al. Effects of mental stress on myocardial ischaemia during daily life. JAMA 1997; 277:1521–1526.

204 Kune G, Kune S, Watson LF et al. Personality as a risk factor in large bowel cancer: data from the Melbourne Colorectal Cancer Study. Psychol Med 1991; 21:29–41.

205 Chen C, David A, Nunnerley H et al. Adverse life events and breast cancer: a case control study. BMJ 1995; 311:1527–1530.

206 Watson M, Haviland J, Greer S et al. Influence of psychological response on survival in breast cancer: a population-based study. Lancet 1999; 354: 1331–1336.

207 Protheroe D, Turvey K, Horgan K et al. Stressful life events and difficulties and onset of breast cancer: case control study. BMJ 1999; 319:1027–1030.

208 Arias AJ, Steinberg K, Banga A et al. Systematic review of the efficacy of meditation techniques as treatments for medical illness. J Altern Complement Med 2006; 12(8):817–832.

209 Khalsa SB. Yoga as a therapeutic intervention: a bibliometric analysis of published research studies. Indian J Physiol Pharmacol 2004; 48(3):269–285.

210 Kabat-Zinn J. Full catastrophe living: using the wisdom of your body and mind to face stress, pain, and illness. New York: Delacorte; 1990.

211 Segal ZV, Williams JMG, Teasdale JD. Mindfulness-based cognitive therapy for depression: a new approach to preventing relapse. New York: Guilford Press; 2002.

212 Teasdale JD, Segal ZV, Williams JMG et al. Prevention of relapse/recurrence in major depression by mindfulness-based cognitive therapy. J Consult Clin Psychol 2000; 68:615–623.

213 Hassed C. Know thyself. Melbourne: Michelle Anderson Publishing; 2002.

214 Erickson M, Rossi E. Experiencing hypnosis. New York: Irvington; 1981.

215 Chadwick P, Hughes S, Russell D et al. Mindfulness groups for distressing voices and paranoia: a replication and randomized feasibility trial. Behav Cogn Psychother 2009; 37(4):403–412.

chapter 9

Exercise as therapy

INTRODUCTION

Exercise science is a large and growing body of knowledge about the acute and chronic effects of physical activity on health, structure and function. A Medline search for 'exercise' in the title returns 57,000 scientific journal articles. This discipline has truly come of age and is a key component of any integrative approach to patient care.

EXERCISE DEFINED

Physical exercise involves the voluntary movement of the body, incorporating large muscle groups, with the goal of enjoyment, relaxation and physical exertion to improve the body's structure and function. The different types of exercise will be discussed shortly, but the avenues for exercise include sport participation, recreational activities such as bushwalking, fitness training such as resistance training, aerobic classes, yoga, Pilates, occupational and recreational work such as gardening, and incidental exercise such as walking to the shops or cycling to work.

WHY IS EXERCISE ESSENTIAL FOR HEALTH?

The renowned exercise biologist, Professor Frank Booth, described in great detail the importance of exercise for maintaining normal function and health, in his extensive review of the research literature.[1] The basic tenet is that the human genome has not changed appreciably in the past 45,000 years and developed in an environment of high levels of physical activity. While our lifestyles have become predominantly sedentary in our working and leisure environments, our underlying biology expects stimuli involving physical work for extended periods, possibly dawn until dusk, as well as high-force and high-power activities such as would have been required to carry water, children, food, construction materials and tools as well as to run after animals that we sought to kill, or run away from animals desiring to eat us.

Contemporary humans are flying in the face of our genome, which dictates every biochemical process in our bodies. The result is progressive disease and disability from early adulthood, or even earlier in the case of sedentary and often overweight children. Our physical health, apart from injury or infection, is dictated by four interacting factors: genetic predisposition, physical activity, nutritional intake, and environmental factors such as toxins and sun exposure.

Chronic disease is now being described as an epidemic currently accounting for some 70% of our total health burden. This is being driven principally by the three most significant risk factors for chronic disease: tobacco use, inappropriate nutrition and physical inactivity.

EXERCISE TRENDS IN AUSTRALIA AND ELSEWHERE

Despite the strong research evidence indicating that regular physical exercise is essential for human health, rates of sedentary and low exercise levels in Australia remain very high, at around 70% of the population over 15 years of age.[2] This has not changed appreciably in the past 10 years despite the best efforts of government and organisations such as the Cancer Council and Heart Foundation to address this societal problem. The rate of no or low physical exercise is higher in females (73%) than in males (66%), and higher in the oldest age group of 75 years and over, at 83%. The rate is lowest in people aged 15–24 years but still frighteningly high at 62%.

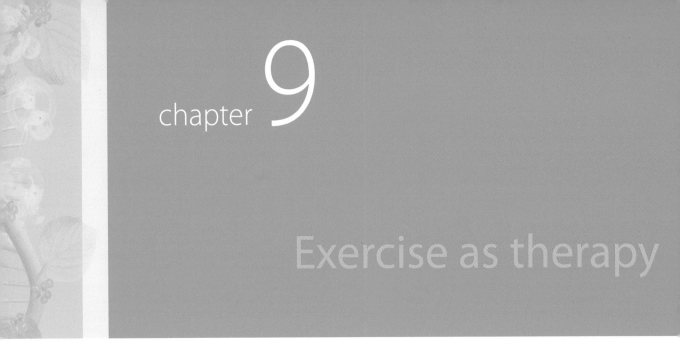

The 2007 Australian National Children's Nutrition and Physical Activity Survey is one of the most extensive investigations of exercise patterns in children aged 2–16 years conducted to date, with some 4487 participants. It was encouraging that most children aged 9–16 years met the Department of Health and Ageing recommendation that children aged 5–18 years accumulate at least 60 minutes, and up to several hours, of moderate to vigorous physical activity every day. According to the survey, there was a 69% chance that any given child would achieve this recommendation. With regard to gender, girls met the guidelines less frequently than boys, both boys and girls were less likely to meet the requirement as they got older, and this drop-off was much higher in older girls.[3]

Internationally the data are similar for the developed nations; however, physical inactivity levels appear to be increasing markedly in developing countries with modernisation. One trend that is clear throughout the world is the increasing use of screen-based technologies such as television, computers and mobile phones, which appears to have the direct effect of reducing physical activity.

GENERAL HEALTH, QUALITY OF LIFE AND LONGEVITY

The application of exercise for prevention and management of some specific health problems will be described later in this chapter. To establish the importance of exercise for general health, quality and quantity of life, the overall effects of exercise are summarised in Table 9.1.

With such beneficial effects one would expect active people to live longer and better-quality lives, and this is certainly borne out in the research.

TYPES OF EXERCISE

AEROBIC EXERCISE

Cardiorespiratory capacity or fitness relates to the ability to perform large-muscle-group, dynamic, moderate-to-high intensity exercise such as walking or cycling for prolonged periods.[4] Exercise prescription for cardiovascular fitness is based on mode, intensity, duration and frequency of the activity. The activities prescribed most frequently are walking, cycling, jogging, running, rowing, swimming and hiking. It is suggested that individuals should choose activities that they enjoy and are enthusiastic about continuing, as this will increase program compliance.

ANABOLIC EXERCISE

The other major form of exercise critical to long-term health is anabolic exercise, which is also termed 'resistance training' or 'weightlifting'. This form of exercise involves performing movements against resistance such as barbells, dumbbells, resistance machines or elastic resistance, such that the number of repetitions that can be completed is limited to 12 or less. This is a very important stipulation of intensity. If the movement can be completed more than 10–12 times then the

TABLE 9.1 Effects of regular exercise on health

Health parameter	Effect of regular exercise	Preferred exercise mode
Hypertension	Reduction of systolic and diastolic blood pressure	Aerobic predominantly but some research indicates anabolic also effective
Cardiac function	Increased stroke volume and maximum cardiac output	Aerobic exercise
Cardiorespiratory fitness	Increased efficiency and maximum capacity	Aerobic exercise
Haemoglobin	Increased	Aerobic exercise
Cholesterol	Reduces LDL, elevates HDL, lowers total cholesterol and triglycerides	Aerobic exercise
Glucose metabolism	Glucose tolerance and insulin sensitivity improved	Aerobic and anabolic exercise
Bone density	Increased bone mineral density, bone mineral content, cortical thickness and fracture threshold	Anabolic and ground-based impact exercises (e.g. skipping, bounding, jumping)
Body fat	Reduced percentage body fat	Aerobic and anabolic combined
Muscle mass	Increased muscle cross-sectional area, increased fibre size	Anabolic exercise
Strength	Increased	Anabolic exercise
Physical functioning	Gait speed, stair climb, sit to stand, balance, falls risk all improved	Anabolic and aerobic exercise
Quality of life	Improvement in both general and disease-specific QOL measures	Anabolic and aerobic exercise

HDL: high-density lipoprotein; LDL: low-density lipoprotein; QOL: quality of life.

resistance is too light and must be increased. Without such resistance the positive anabolic effects on muscle and bone will not be realised and the hormonal changes that are so neuro-protective will not result.

This concept may seem a little 'out there' for people who have not exercised previously or even lifted weights before but the research evidence in support of regular anabolic exercise is huge, demonstrating marked improvements in muscle mass, bone strength, functional capacity and positive effects on mental health and cognitive function. The recommendation of the American College of Sports Medicine is for people aged over 65 years to complete resistance training two to three times per week. The precise prescription is presented in Boxes 9.1 and 9.2.

For healthy adults over age 65 or adults aged 50–64 with chronic conditions, the physical activity guidelines in Box 9.1 are recommended.

FLEXIBILITY EXERCISE

Maintaining range of motion about our joints is also critical at all stages of life, and even more so as we age. Flexibility training involves taking the joints to a position which places the muscles on stretch—that is, they are at or near their maximal length. Holding the muscle at this stretched position when repeated over time causes the muscle to grow longer, which increases its length and results in increased joint range of motion.

MODE AND DOSAGE

The American College of Sports Medicine and the American Heart Association released a combined position stand in 2007. The recommendation on physical activity for healthy adults under 65 years of age is shown in Box 9.2.

BOX 9.1 Physical activity guidelines for healthy adults over 65 years, or those aged 50–64 with chronic conditions

Do moderately intense aerobic exercise 30 minutes a day, 5 days a week
or
Do vigorously intense aerobic exercise 20 minutes a day, 3 days a week
and
Do 8–10 strength-training exercises, 10–15 repetitions of each exercise 2–3 times per week
and
If you are at risk of falling, perform balance exercises
and
Have a physical activity plan

Source: Nelson et al 2006[5]

BOX 9.2 Physical activity guidelines for healthy adults under 65 years

Do moderately intense cardio 30 minutes a day, 5 days a week
or
Do vigorously intense cardio 20 minutes a day, 3 days a week
and
Do 8–10 strength-training exercises, 8–12 repetitions of each exercise, twice a week

Source: Haskell et al 2007[6]

ACCUMULATION OF EXERCISE IS THE KEY

One of the most common excuses people provide for their low level of physical activity is that they simply do not have the time. As can be seen in Boxes 9.1 and 9.2, the total commitment required is only 150 minutes of aerobic exercise per week and 90 minutes of strength training. This is less than 4% of a person's total waking minutes per week. The key is to be flexible in how this is scheduled. Exercise can be undertaken at any time of day or night, and organised into any preferred blocks of effort, with little decrement in health benefit. So whether the patient completes a single bout of 30 minutes of aerobic exercise in a given day or three blocks of 10 minutes, the effect is essentially the same.

INCIDENTAL EXERCISE

While structured exercise sessions are very important in assisting people to meet the minimum recommended physical activity guidelines and in ensuring that all aspects of exercise modes are addressed, the importance of physical activity accumulated during a normal day should also be recognised. Such physical activity is termed 'incidental exercise' and recent research has demonstrated considerable benefit for weight control and diabetes management. The overall goal is to accumulate as many minutes each day of non-sedentary time and in particular to reduce the time spent sitting. Importantly, recent research indicates that increasing the time spent standing rather than sitting increases the overall energy usage through the day. Another effective strategy to increase physical activity is to take 5–10 minutes break each hour, stand up and take a walk. This provides benefit by increasing metabolic rate, and work efficiency will probably be improved overall.

There are a myriad ways to increase one's incidental exercise each day. For example, instead of desperately trying to find a car park close to the bank or shopping centre, park a couple of hundred metres away and walk. Take the stairs instead of the lift or escalator. Walk to your next meeting if it is only down the road, rather than driving or catching a taxi.

GETTING STARTED

The first step on any great journey is often the hardest, and initiating an exercise program can also be daunting. If a person has never been involved in an ongoing exercise program, how to begin, what to expect, whether one is overdoing it or not working hard enough, are all questions the new exerciser faces. For many of us the experience of our bodies responding to exercise with increased heart rate, increased breathing, body temperature rising, muscles aching and the discomfort that can accompany exercise, is foreign and unsettling. For the vast majority these experiences are not harbingers of illness or death. They are the normal adjustments that the body makes automatically to help us perform exercise. Of course if the discomfort is excessive then this is a warning sign, and the person experiencing it should consult their doctor or exercise specialist. Habitual exercisers come to enjoy these changes in their physiology—the sweat, heat and exertion—because they are often associated with positive changes in the brain chemistry and a feeling of exhilaration and success.

If the patient is over 35 years of age or has any primary risk factors for cardiovascular disease such as a family history of heart attack or stroke, high blood pressure, high cholesterol or existing cardiovascular disease, or is overweight, then it is important that they consult their doctor before starting an exercise program.

To begin, it is a good idea to consider seeking expert advice or joining a supervised exercise program. Some insurers provide limited cover for visits to many of these professionals and programs. General practitioners can provide referral to an exercise physiologist as these are the recognised allied health professional for the prescription and monitoring of exercise programs, particularly for people with existing chronic disease.

No matter which option the patients selects, if it has been a while since they have been active it is important to start slowly. Find a routine that suits them. If the person enjoys the activity they are much more likely to stick with it. Whenever possible they should exercise with a friend or relative. Many people find the social aspects of exercise the most enjoyable, and having someone else along also increases safety.

EXERCISE EQUIPMENT

Physical activity, or exercise, does not need expensive equipment. Exercise equipment is big business but it is not necessary to have all the latest gear.

Appropriate shoes are vital and help prevent injury. A podiatrist or reputable shoe shop can help the patient select the right shoes. It is also important that they wear flexible, comfortable clothes, such as shorts and a t-shirt, when exercising. If heat or cold are significant factors then clothing should be adjusted accordingly.

Other equipment, such as heart rate monitors and home-gym systems, can certainly be useful, but are definitely not necessary. Most exercises can be done without the need for any additional equipment.

SELECTING AN EXERCISE PROGRAM

There are many ways to be physically active without too much cost or inconvenience. A person might choose to exercise at home or they might prefer the structure and safety of a supervised exercise program. For many people the best option is a mix of exercising at home and a supervised exercise program.

If the patient chooses a supervised exercise program, ask about the level and quality of the supervision provided. Look for a program run by a qualified exercise physiologist. If it is convenient for the patient to exercise in a fitness centre or community facility, try to contact a local exercise physiologist to assess the patient's level of risk and design an exercise program specifically for them.

Wherever the patient chooses to be physically active, it is important that the GP and the patient consider comfort, health and safety.

WHO TO TALK TO

Exercise physiologists are healthcare professionals specifically trained to give advice on exercise. An exercise physiologist will work with the patient and/or the doctor to ensure an appropriate exercise prescription. Many structured exercise programs will require the patient to seek a medical clearance before starting, and this is advisable.

Before taking part in any exercise program, particularly if the patient has been diagnosed with a chronic illness, it is important for the patient's GP to discuss the exercise plan with the exercise physiologist. The GP should ensure that they convey any concerns and advise on additional precautions.

WHAT IS A PHYSIOTHERAPIST?

Physiotherapists are trained to assess the underlying causes of joint, muscle and nerve injuries and provide treatment to ensure that people can resume their normal lifestyle as soon as possible.

WHAT IS AN EXERCISE PHYSIOLOGIST?

An exercise physiologist specialises in the delivery of exercise, lifestyle and behavioural modification programs for the prevention and management of chronic diseases. Exercise physiologists are the most appropriate allied healthcare professionals for:

- exercise prescription and management
- prevention and wellness
- secondary management of chronic disease.

Many medical insurers and government-funded programs around the world include exercise physiologists and may require referral from the GP to the exercise physiologist for the patient to receive a medical insurance rebate, depending on the particular nationalised insurance system. Most private health insurers now cover exercise physiologist services.

COMPONENTS OF AN EXERCISE SESSION

Warm-up

Warm-up facilitates the transition from rest to exercise; it may reduce susceptibility to musculoskeletal injury by improving joint range of motion, and reduce the risk of adverse cardiovascular events.[4] Regardless of training mode, exercise sessions should start with 5–10 minutes of low-intensity exercise incorporating stretching exercises and/or progressive lower-intensity aerobic activity. For example, participants who use 20 kg in a chest press exercise for 12 repetitions might have a warm-up set using 5–10 kg for 15 repetitions before initiating this particular exercise. Similarly, participants who use brisk walking or jogging might conduct a warm-up phase using a slow walk before initiating the training program. Implementing a gradual transition from rest to intense exercise is critical in reducing the risk of an adverse event, such as muscle strain or even a cardiovascular event. The body is much more comfortable with gradual changes in exercise intensity.

Specific phase

Cardiorespiratory training includes 20–60 minutes of continuous or intermittent (minimum of 10-minute bouts accumulated during the day) of aerobic activity training at 60–90% maximum heart rate (MHR) or 50–85% MHR reserve.[7] Anabolic resistance exercises include performing 1–4 sets per muscle group training at 50–80% of 1 RM (repetition maximum) or 6–12 RM.[7] Flexibility or range-of-motion training includes performing 2–4 sets per muscle group at 30–60 seconds stretching time.[7]

Exercise order

The ordering of anabolic exercises should generally follow these rules:

- large muscle groups first (e.g. legs)
- multi-joint exercises (e.g. bench press) before single-joint (e.g. elbow extension)
- abdominal and lower-back exercises after whole-body ground-based exercises such as squat, dead lift, bench press and so on.

This is to avoid pre-fatiguing the muscle groups that stabilise and support the trunk. However, it is also important *not* to program abdominal and lower-back exercises last, as the person may often be getting tired or bored and drop them from the program. These exercises are very important for posture and protecting the lower back and so must be completed during each session.

Cool-down

This phase provides a gradual recovery from the specific activity performed and includes exercises using lower intensities. For example, participants can use slow walking when completing higher-intensity aerobic activity or lower-intensity stretching when completing a resistance training session. The cool-down allows appropriate circulatory adjustment of heart rate and blood pressure to near-resting values, facilitates dissipation of heat, reduces potential post-exercise hypotension and promotes removal of lactic acid.[4]

BASIC PRINCIPLES OF EXERCISE

The aim of this section is to provide knowledge of the basic principles of exercise and in particular aerobic and anabolic exercise. Exercise programs may be implemented in a range of settings and may not always have personnel with qualifications and experience in exercise physiology. The following discussion provides a very basic level of knowledge necessary to understand the principles underlying the exercise programs presented in the later sections of this chapter.

EXERCISE PROGRAM VARIABLES

Adaptation

If a lift in a building were required to lift its maximum capacity from the ground floor to the rooftop each day, it would not increase in its performance and be able to carry more people. It would be more likely to deteriorate—its bearings would wear, the electric motor would become less efficient and performance overall would decline. The human body is a very different machine because it has the ability to respond to a stimulus, such as the work of running or the stress of lifting weights, by altering its structure and function in order to better perform that activity in future. This is termed 'adaptation' and is the basis of physical training. A number of points about adaptation must be considered.

First, the body must have a biological mechanism enabling it to make the adaptation. For example, shortening the length of the bones of the upper arm and forearm would greatly increase the amount of weight that could be lifted in the bench press due to increased mechanical advantage, but the body is not capable of this process. Increasing the size of the muscles that perform the bench press would also allow the body to lift more weight and this is certainly an adaptation that is within our capabilities.

Second, the adaptation is very specific to the stimuli—resistance training tends to produce an increase in muscle size, whereas swimming produces an increase in the heart's ability to pump blood. The concept of specificity will be discussed in more detail later in this chapter.

Overload

A training adaptation occurs in response to an overload. A situation in which the body is required to perform work beyond that which it is accustomed to or which is normal will result in an overload. In strength training this overload is the requirement of the neuromuscular system to exert forces that are more than that required during the activities of daily living. In aerobic training it involves exercising to maintain the heart rate at a higher level for longer than the body is accustomed to. In general, the extent of the training adaptation is related to the degree of overload—greater overload results in more rapid and larger biological changes. However, there is a limit beyond which the body cannot adapt. This limit can be exceeded through either too high intensity or excessive volume, or a combination of both. It is important for the person to listen to signs of the body—excessive or persistent pain, sleep disruption, tiredness and predisposition to infection are signs of overtraining. In practice this is rare, except in elite athletes who train at high intensity for several hours per day, a time luxury that most of us cannot afford.

Repetitions, sets, rest and sessions

Many program variables can be manipulated to provide various forms of overload and, thus, specific training adaptations. To understand the training program design and goals it is important for us to define and understand these program variables.

The basic unit of a resistance training session is the repetition. For a given training movement, a repetition is the completion of one complete cycle from the starting position, through the end of the movement and back to the start. When strength training, a series of repetitions is normally completed and this is termed a 'set'. During the set, the neuromuscular system will fatigue, and performing the exercise will become more difficult. At the completion of the required number of repetitions or when the person is no longer able to complete any more repetitions, the set is completed. The person then waits until the neuromuscular system recovers and then completes further sets of exercise. The period between sets is called 'rest' or 'recovery' and is another important program variable that can be altered to achieve specific training goals.

During an exercise session, a series of sets of different exercises is completed. The term 'session' refers to the block of time devoted to the training.

For aerobic exercise sessions it is usual to complete a continuous bout of exercise and so we speak more in terms of session duration or distance covered. In quantifying the load of an aerobic session, the distance covered, whether it be swum, walked, run or biked, is the best indicator of the volume of work. Interval training involves successive repetitions of work and rest intervals. The same principles as for anabolic exercise apply. Interval training of aerobic capacity creates variation from continuous exercise and some research indicates that it is more effective for fat loss.

Exercise intensity

The intensity of an exercise session refers to how hard someone must push themselves to get benefits from the activity. Intensity and duration of exercise determine the total caloric expenditure of a training session. Similar improvements in the cardiovascular training component may be derived from higher-intensity and short-duration activity or lower-intensity and longer-duration programs.[4]

Monitoring exercise intensity

Training heart rate

Heart rate (HR) is used extensively as a guide to monitor exercise intensity due to its relationship between heart function and consumption of oxygen by the working body. The most simple and often-used HR assessment is the percentage of maximal HR (maxHR), which can be estimated as 220 – age. The proposed maxHR intensity range for older people during cardiovascular activities is 60–90% of maxHR.[4] For example, if an individual is 40 years of age, their maxHR is 180. Their target training heart rate for 60–90% of the maxHR is 108–162 beats per minute.[4]

It is important to monitor heart rate during the exercise sessions to ensure adequate intensity but without working so hard as to induce excessive fatigue. The simplest method is to measure the pulse rate at the wrist, counting the number of beats for, say, 15 seconds and then multiplying by four to calculate beats per minute. However, electronic heart monitors available from any sports store are relatively inexpensive and very convenient.

Rating of perceived exertion

Rating of perceived exertion (RPE) is a valuable instrument in controlling exercise intensity in individuals who have difficulty with HR palpation and especially in cases where medication can alter the HR response to exercise (e.g. beta-blockers).[4] The best known and established RPE scale is the Borg scale. This scale was developed to allow the participant to subjectively rate their feelings during exercise, taking into account fitness level, fatigue and environmental factors.[4] More recently, Robertson and colleagues (2003)[8] developed the OMNI scale, which uses verbal and pictorial descriptors along a numerical scale of 0–10 to rate an individual's perceived exertion. This scale has been successfully validated with children and young adults from both sexes during cardiovascular[9] and resistance exercise,[8] and may also be an option for exercise sessions with older people and patients. RPE can be taken at different points during an exercise session—following each set of an exercise, for example. It can also be taken after the end of the session, which provides a global rating of the exercise session intensity. This measure of session RPE provides essentially the same information as taking multiple measures throughout the session. A sample RPE scale suitable for older people exercising is contained in Figure 9.1.

The talk test

As a method of making exercise prescription more simple, an informal guideline, widely referred to as the talk test, has arisen within the exercise community. This guideline suggests that if the exercise intensity is such that the patient can just respond to conversation, then it

6	
7	Very, very light
8	
9	Very light
10	
11	Fairly light
12	
13	Somewhat hard
14	
15	Hard
16	
17	Very hard
18	
19	Very, very hard
20	

This scale is used to indicate the self-assessed level of exertion for the individual performing exercise.

FIGURE 9.1 RPE scale for older people

may be just about right (that is, within accepted ranges of exercise training intensity). The ability to converse during exercise (that is, to pass the talk test) has been shown to produce exercise intensities consistently within the parameters suggested in clinical guidelines for exercise training in a variety of populations.[10] The talk test appears to be a practical way for people to monitor their intensity during exercise, and an advantage of this method is that it does not require any equipment and no training is needed to understand your ability to speak based on how hard you are working. Because research has shown this method to be very consistent, people can use it in their everyday lives, in gyms or when working out at home, to meet their health and fitness goals while reducing the risk of injuries or other complications that can happen with over-exertion.

Intensity during resistance training

Intensity when resistance training refers to the relative load or resistance that the muscle is working against—or, looking at it another way, the percentage of the muscle's maximum strength that is exerted during the training movement. This is often expressed as '% 1RM', the load lifted as a percentage of the maximum that the individual can lift only once. Another common method for describing intensity is in terms of repetition maximum—that is, how many repetitions can be completed before muscular failure occurs and the load cannot be lifted again. Thus, a 6 RM load is a higher intensity than a 10 RM load. For the older population, the intensity must be sufficient to produce the structural and functional changes required or at least stem functional and structural decline. For resistance training, the intensity should be no lighter than 12 RM. For a person who has not performed resistance training in the past 12 weeks, the intensity in the initial few weeks should be kept low, to reduce muscle soreness. For this person an initial intensity of 8–12 RM is appropriate, increasing over the first 4 weeks to 6–10 RM.

FREQUENCY

The number of training sessions completed each week is termed 'frequency'. For resistance training, one session per week, while better than none, is sub-optimal. The target should be at least two sessions per week and the ideal is three sessions per week.

An optimal training frequency for cardiorespiratory fitness in healthy adults has been proposed as three to five times per week, depending on the intensity of the exercise (see Boxes 9.1 and 9.2). However, deconditioned individuals are likely to improve their condition with lower training frequencies.[4]

VOLUME

Volume indicates the total amount of work completed while training. For resistance training, it is usually weight × repetitions × sets. For the older population, each session should consist of 3–4 sets of 6–9 different exercises. However, lower training volumes (e.g. 1–2 sets) are more appropriate in the initial stages of training (e.g. the first few training sessions).

With regard to cardiorespiratory training, the combined duration and intensity of an exercise bout result in the expenditure of energy and calories, giving health benefits from the activity. The duration of cardiovascular activities recommended by the ACSM[4] for healthy older adults is 20–60 minutes of continuous or intermittent (minimum of 10-minute bouts accumulated during the day) of aerobic activity training.

MINIMUM INTENSITY

When training for strength there appears to be a load below which no training adaptation will result. This may vary depending on training state, muscle group and the individual; however, the lifting of very light loads without maximal effort seems to be ineffective for increasing maximal strength and muscle power. Reiterating the comments above, the intensity should be at least 12 RM and within the first 2–3 weeks progress to a load of 6–10 RM.

In terms of cardiovascular exercise, the minimum intensity for useful benefit is most likely 60% of maxHR.

PROGRESSIVE RESISTANCE TRAINING

In order to stimulate the neuromuscular system towards adaptations conducive to increased muscle strength and power, the training performed must place the system under a greater load than it is accustomed to. As previously defined, this is termed 'overload' and in strength development translates into using the muscles of the body to exert forces at or near their maximum potential. The neuromuscular system adapts to the training with increases in muscle size, improved coordination, better motor unit recruitment and at higher firing frequencies, and the result is an increase in strength. However, as strength increases, the initial overload becomes progressively less relative to the increased maximal strength capability, and thus the stimulus to adapt declines if the person continues to train with the same absolute loads. This brings us to the very important concept of progressive resistance training. To continue to elicit gains in muscle strength and power, the loads must be progressively increased so the relative intensity remains high enough to provide an adequate overload. By expressing intensity as % 1RM or specifying a load which can only be lifted a given number of times, the overload is progressive because as strength increases, so do the training loads and thus relative intensity is maintained.

REVERSAL

Just as the body adapts to overload by increasing performance, it also modifies capacity in response to a decrease in physical activity—this is known as 'detraining'. For example, when a person stops regular resistance training, their strength level gradually returns to what it was prior to the commencement of the program. Importantly, the higher the level of strength attained through training, the longer it takes to return to pre-training levels. Further, one can reduce the amount of resistance training performed each week and still maintain strength at or near the level attained through training. In other words, the volume of training required for maintenance of strength is much less than that required to achieve a given strength level. Similar effects occur with aerobic fitness.

VARIATION IN TRAINING

Two foremost factors when designing training programs are: the principle of overload (already discussed); and variation in training. To provide an overload and thereby continue to stimulate the body to adapt, the training must be novel—it must change in character. The more novel the task, the greater will be the changes in performance capacity towards the new task.

Designing a resistance training program which involves performing, say, three sets of 6 RM with six different exercises is relatively straightforward. As strength increases, the 6 RM load lifted increases and the overload is maintained. However, such a program involves no variation and will not prove as effective as a program with greater variation in exercise selection, intensity and volume. The principle of variation relates to changes in program characteristics to match changing program goals as well as to provide a changing target for the body to adapt to. The careful planning and implementation of this variation is known as periodisation.

The importance of variation in training for maintaining motivation should not be underestimated either. Making the program novel and varying the program parameters is important to avoid boredom, staleness and over-training. It will also increase compliance with the program and help avoid people dropping out of the training program.

All program parameters can be modified to achieve variation in the training. Intensity and volume are obvious choices and it is well accepted that within a week there should be heavy and light days, and the volume should undulate over longer periods of 4–12 weeks or more. However, subtle changes to exercise may include:

- varying the depth of the squat or leg press exercise
- performing explosive exercises
- slowing the tempo down and using 'super slow' training
- combining supersets, pre-fatigue, and upper and lower body combinations
- heavy eccentric training, which involves using a heavier resistance during the lowering portion of an exercise
- performing circuit training rather than traditional resistance training
- multi-sport aerobic training, swapping between cycling, running, swimming, paddling and rowing exercise
- swapping sessions between continuous aerobic exercise and interval-type training.

The key is to alter the nature of the overload to encourage the neuromuscular and cardiorespiratory systems to continue to adapt. This becomes more critical as the person becomes more experienced with this mode of exercise.

PLANNING AN EXERCISE SCHEDULE

Maintaining an exercise habit throughout life can be difficult, especially when so many aspects of work and family life compete for our time. For this reason it is helpful to develop an exercise plan for the long-term with realistic goals in mind. This might be as simple as a calendar for the week listing the exercise sessions, start and end times, and the activity. Longer-term planning might entail preparing for a particular event such as a fun run, milestone birthday or the check-up with the family doctor. A 12-week plan is a workable strategy because it is long enough to allow variation in volume, intensity and activity type while also being sufficient to produce significant and observable improvements in health and fitness. This plan can then be repeated or modified according to the season, exercise opportunities and increasing fitness.

The exercise schedule in Table 9.2 provides sufficient exercise to meet the recommended guidelines for someone under 65 years of age. The intensity should be specific to the individual but within the range previously prescribed.

BARRIERS TO EXERCISE

No one said it was easy to start an exercise program and then stick to it. There are many barriers to exercise that must be overcome. The greatest by far is lack of motivation to change one's behaviour. The GP can be a powerful influence in taking the patient through the stages of change necessary to make exercise a lifelong habit. Convincing the patient of the importance of exercise for their health and even instilling some fear of the consequences of a sedentary lifestyle can be all it takes to start the process. Other personal, financial, environmental and societal barriers can make it difficult to exercise. However, these can all be overcome if the motivation of the patient and the support of their family and friends is sufficient. Regardless of a patient's illness or injury, there is still the potential to perform some form of physical activity. For example, research in patients with various cancers indicates that exercise can be tolerated, is effective for improving physical and mental health and may even be enjoyable. Lack of financial means is often cited as limiting exercise opportunities but effective exercise programs do not necessarily require expensive equipment and specialist trainers. A quality exercise program meeting the minimum recommended requirements can be achieved in the home with little or no equipment if the patient is given specialist advice to enhance their motivation to exercise. It has been demonstrated that the environment in which the patient lives can affect their opportunities for exercise. For example, a neighbourhood that appears to be unsafe, and has graffiti and broken and dangerous pathways is clearly not conducive to pursuing a walking program. Societal influences can also reduce a patient's willingness to maintain an active lifestyle. Teenage girls are less likely to exercise, because of peer pressure.

TABLE 9.2 Example of an exercise schedule for a person under 65 years of age

	am	lunch	pm
Monday	Stretch for 15 min		Resistance exercise @ gym
Tuesday	10 min walk		Walk dog for 20 min
Wednesday	10 min walk before work	10 min walk	10 min walk after work
Thursday	Stretch for 15 min		Resistance exercise @ home
Friday	10 min walk		Walk dog for 20 min
Saturday	Beach swim 30 min		
Sunday	Cycle 20 min to and from breakfast cafe		Walk dog for 20 min

Certain religious and cultural groups devalue exercise or actively discourage it. Many children believe that their elderly parents should rest, not exercise, especially when ill. Exercise research indicates that this strategy is counterproductive.

All these barriers to physical activity can be overcome with education and support.

SAFETY AND AVOIDING INJURY

The most effective strategy for reducing injury risk is to seek appropriate expert advice prior to embarking on a new exercise program. For people under 35 years of age and with no cardiovascular risk factors or prior history, exercise can be performed with relative safety. If not, then a medical consultation with a GP is recommended to check family history and current health status, and assess possible risk. If risk is deemed low then the patient might join a health and fitness centre or take up a sport or recreational activity of their choosing. However, if there are issues of concern, a consultation with an exercise physiologist is recommended. The exercise physiologist will perform a more detailed assessment of exercise risk, perform various tests to determine the person's fitness capacity and then design an appropriate exercise prescription. For individuals with existing chronic disease, consultation with an exercise physiologist is advisable to obtain safe and effective exercise guidelines. Patients with existing musculoskeletal or neuromuscular injuries should be treated initially by a physiotherapist and their exercise program modified.

Exercise can be performed in two broad categories of environment:

- *controlled environments*—conditions are relatively stable, appropriately qualified personnel are on hand, emergency equipment such as automatic defibrillation, oxygen and first aid are available, and emergency procedures are in place and effective, with immediate contact with ambulance or medical personnel if required; includes most health and fitness centres, exercise clinics and some sporting facilities
- *uncontrolled environments*—the listed facilities and personnel are not all available; includes exercise at a park or beach, sporting field or any other facility which does not have emergency procedures in place.

Millions of people in Australia exercise each day in 'uncontrolled' environments without incident. The issue is ameliorating risk, such that high-risk patients should either exercise only in controlled environments or reduce exercise intensity to lower the possibility of adverse events.

INJURY

The incidence of injury is relatively low, especially in controlled environments with a patient undertaking a program designed and delivered by an exercise physiologist. People often get injured when they begin exercising after being sedentary with no planning or gradual return to exercise volume. For example, lifting weights at home alone can be dangerous. Doing high-intensity exercise without warm-up and cool-down and building gradually in fitness to this level can be dangerous.

A final word on injury and safety: the consequences of being sedentary far outweigh the risks of exercise. It is a matter of a responsible and planned approach with appropriate support from medical and allied healthcare practitioners where required.

OVER-EXERCISING

Above a certain volume and intensity of chronic exercise, the body is not able to recover and repair sufficiently, resulting in 'over-training' syndrome. This is relatively rare in non-athlete populations, and even in athletes it is usually due to over-zealous coaches or parents rather than being volitional on the athlete's part. In people who are not competitive athletes there are instances of excessive exercising to the point of ill health and injury. Exercise can become addictive and obsessive in certain individuals, to their detriment, but this is a very small minority. Signs include increased incidence of injury, very low body fat or sudden weight loss, increased incidence of upper respiratory infections, anaemia, sleep problems, increased resting heart rate, persistent muscle soreness, depression, irritability and decreased appetite.

The ACSM/AHA guidelines presented earlier[5] are recommended exercise to maintain health. The volume of exercise can be increased considerably before over-training becomes an issue, but some simple strategies to avoid the syndrome include:

- making one day each week exercise-free or very light recovery (e.g. walking, water exercise)
- avoiding repeating the same type of exercise on consecutive days
- allowing at least 48 hours between resistance training on the same muscle group
- measuring resting heart rate each morning on waking, to detect increases
- keeping exercise sessions to less than 60 minutes.

EXERCISE AND DISEASE

Meeting the recommended guidelines for physical activity has been demonstrated to markedly reduce the risk of most chronic diseases and so has a strong prophylactic benefit. Once chronic disease progression has produced clinical signs and symptoms there are other key roles for exercise in:

- slowing progression
- alleviating symptoms
- preventing or at least delaying the onset of other chronic diseases.

DON'T SUFFER THE SIDE EFFECTS

Treatment side effects are of concern to patient and doctor, and decisions have to be made regarding the relative risks and benefits. In some instances, exercise prescription as adjuvant therapy can alleviate some side effects and improve tolerance of pharmaceutical, radiation and other treatments. For example, testosterone suppression for prostate cancer results in muscle and bone loss and fat gain.[11] Fracture risk is increased and recent reports indicate a high incidence of cardiovascular disease and metabolic syndrome.[12] It is now well established that exercise can alleviate all these side effects (Figure 9.2).[13] Muscular strength is strongly and inversely associated with incidence of metabolic syndrome and the effect is independent of age and body size. Potential benefits of resistance exercise training to increase muscular strength should be considered in primary prevention of metabolic syndrome.[14]

CANCER

Much of the research to date on exercise and cancer has focused on cancer prevention, and there is strong benefit particularly for colorectal and breast cancers. Recently, research has begun to examine the effectiveness of exercise programs for patients undertaking therapy. All the evidence collected so far suggests that exercise plays a beneficial role for most patients during cancer treatment. The evidence also shows that there is very little risk of harm when precautions are taken and professional exercise advice is followed closely.[16]

Regular and vigorous physical exercise has been scientifically established as providing strong preventative effect against cancer, with the potential to reduce incidence by 40%. The effect is strongest for breast[17] and colorectal cancer,[18] but evidence is accumulating for the protective influence on prostate cancer, although predominantly for more advanced disease and in older men.[19]

Following cancer diagnosis, exercise prescription can have very positive benefits in improving surgical outcomes, reducing symptom experience, managing side effects of radiation and chemotherapy, improving psychological health, maintaining physical function, reducing fat gain and reducing muscle and bone loss

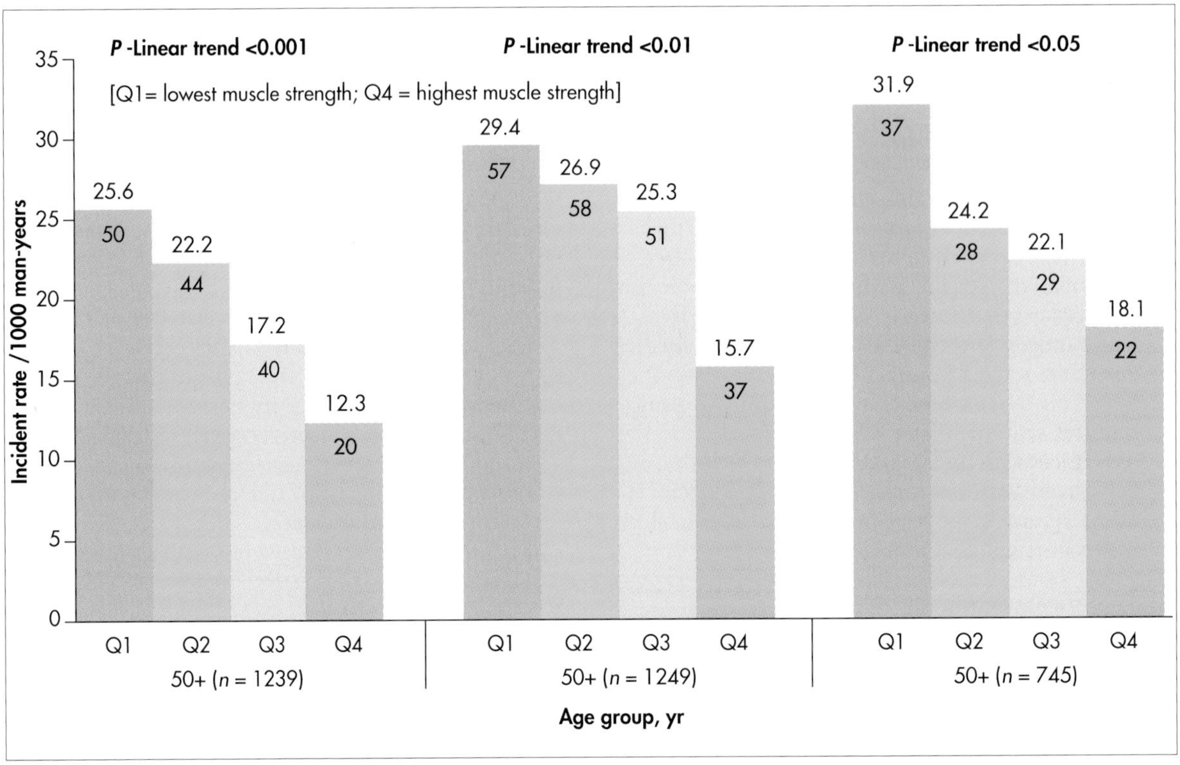

FIGURE 9.2 Potential benefits of exercise for metabolic syndrome (from Jurca et al[15])

TABLE 9.3 Summary of exercise-induced changes in cancer patients reported in 26 research papers reviewed by Galvão and Newton 2005[7]

Increased	Decreased
Muscle mass	Nausea
Muscle strength and power	Fatigue
Cardiorespiratory fitness	Symptom experience
Maximum walk distance	Lymphocytes and monocytes
Immune system capacity	Duration of hospitalisation
Physical functional ability	Heart rate
Flexibility	Resting systolic blood pressure
Quality of life	Psychological and emotional stress
Haemoglobin	Depression and anxiety
	Body fat

(see Table 9.3). There is now irrefutable evidence from large prospective studies that regular exercise post diagnosis actually increases survivorship by 50–60%, with the strongest evidence currently for breast[20] and colorectal cancers,[21] over follow-up periods varying from 5 to 18 years (see Ch 24, Cancer).

OSTEOPOROSIS

It has been suggested that the most effective way to avoid osteoporosis is to build as large a 'bone bank' as possible during life so as to be able to make 'withdrawals' as we age without depleting to an osteoporotic level.[22] Physical activity is the most effective lifestyle factor to stimulate bone accretion but the activity needs to be ground-based and with higher loads and impacts. For example, bone mineral density in weightlifters is higher than for active controls and this continues into later life.[23] The effect is persistent, with one study showing that competitive sport early in life is associated with higher bone mineral density in 75-year-old men.[24] Swimming, which lacks impacts and the effects of gravity, does not appear to have a protective effect, and swimmers may actually have a lower bone mineral density than people participating in land-based physical activity.[25]

Physical activity in later life can improve or at least slow bone loss with ageing, and the most effective activity appears to be anabolic exercise. Walking and similar exercises appear to be too low-intensity, with several studies reporting superior results from high-intensity resistance training,[26] and it is significantly more effective than calcium and vitamin D supplementation alone.[27]

SARCOPENIA

Affecting 60% of people over 80 years old, sarcopenia is a major cause of disability and loss of independence for the elderly. Nutrition (under-nutrition and lack of vitamin D) and decreased hormone levels (growth hormone, testosterone) precipitate some of the muscle loss and the ageing process per se; however, it is clear that reduced physical activity, particularly anabolic exercise, is a major factor. The condition is reversible even in the very old, with appropriate anabolic exercise resulting in large increases in lean muscle mass, fibre cross-sectional area and strength.[28] It is well known in athlete and healthy populations that there are optimal combinations of anabolic exercise and nutrition. Specifically, glucose and amino acid intake can be manipulated before, during and after the exercise session to produce much stronger anabolic effects. Supplements such as creatine monohydrate are also effective when combined with anabolic exercise, and more research is being done on their application to patient populations.

ALZHEIMER'S DISEASE

It has now come to light that the genetic and lifestyle risk factors for Alzheimer's disease are very similar to those for cardiovascular disease. This is encouraging in one respect in that exercise is beneficial; however, it is problematic in that the various populations of the world are becoming less active, or at least a high percentage are already sedentary, and obesity is increasing markedly. As a result of these lifestyle choices and an ageing demographic, the incidence of Alzheimer's disease is predicted to increase greatly in the future. Exercise has several roles to play here. First, lifelong physical activity can delay the onset of Alzheimer's even in those with high genetic predisposition. For example, in one population based-study (n = 1740) with 6.2 years follow-up, the reported incidence rate of dementia was 13.0 per 1000 person-years (exercise three or more times per week) compared to 19.7 per 1000 person-years (exercise fewer than three times per week).[29] In the early stages, regular exercise slows the progression of the disease, helping to maintain both physical and cognitive capacity. Interestingly, even a single bout of exercise results in an acute improvement in memory and cognitive function in patients with existing disease.

OBESITY

The evidence is clear that the only effective way to lose body fat when overweight or obese is a combination of habitual physical activity and reduction in energy intake. It appears that increased physical activity alone is not as effective as reduced caloric intake, but it is far easier to stick to a lifestyle in which a negative energy balance is achieved 50% through increased exercise and 50% through diet modification. But the application of exercise for weight management has other important benefits. Any fat-loss diet is also a muscle and bone loss diet as these tissues are also affected. Exercise, and in particular anabolic exercise, is critical for preventing these catabolic effects. Second, exercise increases muscle mass, which concomitantly increases resting metabolic rate, enhancing fat reduction. Finally, in terms of patient health, 'fitness rather than fatness' should be the focus, as research indicates that a person can be overweight but if they are physically fit then their risk of death is no greater than a person of normal weight.[30] The same cannot be said of someone who is of normal weight but sedentary.

ANXIETY AND DEPRESSION

A number of trials have reported reduced risk of anxiety and depression in children who exercise, compared with inactive controls.[31] The evidence in adults is less convincing due to a lack of clinical trials, but there are indications of a positive effect.[32] However, in older people diagnosed with clinical depression, certain types of exercise have been demonstrated to be more effective than routine GP care.[33] This was a single blind control trial which indicated that high-intensity resistance training could produce a 50% reduction in depression rating in 61% of the group. This compared to a similar drop in only 21% of patients in the GP-care group. A 29% reduction was observed in a low-intensity resistance training group, indicating that social interaction was not the only stimulus but the lifting of heavier weights produces some physiological effect benefiting the depressed elderly.

The effects of exercise build gradually but are sustainable throughout life. Initiating exercise in the acute stage will permit a transition to long-term control of depression, hopefully with reduced requirements for medication.

TYPE 2 DIABETES

Exercise improves glucose tolerance and insulin resistance, and is considered very beneficial for preventing and treating type 2 diabetes. In fact, it is estimated that appropriate levels of physical activity could prevent 30–50% of new cases of type 2 diabetes.[34] However, benefits for preventing and treating diabetes occur only with regular sustained physical activity patterns. Aerobic exercise is often hindered in older, obese, comorbid patients, and anabolic exercise has been demonstrated in several studies to be safe and more effective.[35]

OSTEOARTHRITIS

Osteoarthritis can be severely debilitating and limit participation in physical activity. However, reduced movement will exacerbate the disease. Strong research has demonstrated that exercise, in particular anabolic, can result in increased function as assessed by stair climbing and descending, chair rising, walking, reduced ratings of pain and reduced stiffness. These studies report exercise to be 'safe, effective and well tolerated in patients with osteoarthritis'.[36] Exercise frees joint movement, increases joint lubrication, and slows or even reverses muscle atrophy, resulting in better joint support and improved function.[36]

CARDIOVASCULAR DISEASE

Habitual exercise provides a strong protective effect against cardiovascular disease. This is due to a range of positive physiological effects already mentioned, but principally:

- reduced body fat
- improved blood lipids
- reduced blood pressure
- improved heart and vascular function—for example, a mean 2 mmHg reduction in diastolic blood pressure across the population is relatively easy to achieve through targeted exercise, and has been predicted to reduce prevalence and risk of development of hypertension (17%), coronary heart disease (6%) and stroke (15%).[37]

How strong a predictor physical exercise is in reducing mortality is summarised in Figure 9.3.

Some decades ago, the medical advice for patients post stroke or heart attack was rest; however, research revealed that the outcomes were quite poor with this strategy. It is now recognised that exercise is a critical therapy for recovery from such events, especially when it is applied at the early stage recovery in the long-term management plan. Both aerobic and anabolic exercise modes are used and have been demonstrated to significantly reduce mortality and morbidity.[38]

SUMMARY

Human physiology expects and requires regular exercise for normal health and maintenance of physical and psychological function. Despite this overwhelming evidence, two-thirds of the population are sedentary

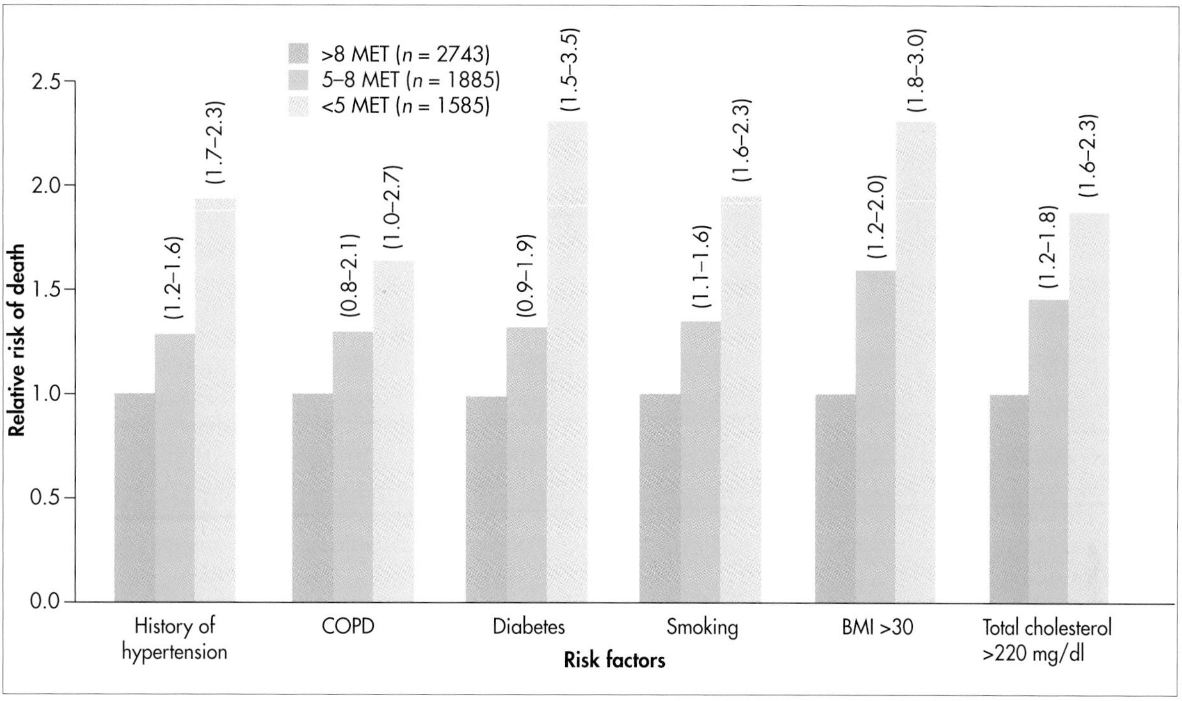

FIGURE 9.3 Exercise capacity is a more powerful predictor of mortality among men than other established risk factors for cardiovascular disease.[14] MET: metabolic equivalent tasks.

or have low physical activity levels despite the best efforts of health promotion. This behaviour is driving a catastrophic rise in chronic disease incidence across the world, such that by 2020 it is predicted that 80% of the health burden will be due to these largely preventable illnesses. For all patients with chronic disease, illness or injury, exercise plays a role as a primary or adjuvant therapy. Exercise physiologists are the most qualified and appropriate allied healthcare professionals for the assessment, prescription and monitoring of exercise programs for chronic disease management. Exercise should form a component of all patient management plans as a critical aspect of integrative medicine.

RESOURCES

Australian Association for Exercise and Sports Science, http://www.aaess.com.au.

Heart Foundation, www.heartfoundation.com.au.
Companion readings from this website:

National Heart Foundation of Australia, Physical Activity Policy

Promoting physical activity – ten recommendations from the Heart Foundation

Physical activity and children: a statement of importance and call to action

VicFit in Victoria / Kinect Australia, www.vicfit.com.au.
Companion readings from this website:

The Active Script Program in Victoria

Physical activity and heart disease and type 2 diabetes

REFERENCES

1 Booth FW, Gordon SE, Carlson CJ et al. Waging war on modern chronic diseases: primary prevention through exercise biology. J Appl Physiol 2000; 88(2):774–787.

2 Australian Bureau of Statistics. Australian snapshots. Physical activity in Australia: a snapshot, 2004/05. Online. Available: http://www.abs.gov.au/ausstats/abs@.nsf/mf/4835.0.55.001

3 Australian Government Department of Health and Ageing. 2007 Australian National Children's Nutrition and Physical Activity Survey. Online. Available: http://www.health.gov.au/nutritionmonitoring

4 American College of Sports Medicine. ACSM's guidelines for exercise testing and prescription. Philadelphia: Lippincott Williams & Wilkins; 2000.

5 Nelson ME, Rejeski WJ, Blair SN et al. Physical activity and public health in older adults: recommendation from the American College of Sports Medicine and the American Heart Association. Med Sci Sport Exer 2007; 39(8):1435–1445.

6 Haskell WL, Lee IM, Pate RR et al. Physical activity and public health: updated recommendation for adults from the American College of Sports Medicine and the

American Heart Association. Med Sci Sport Exer 2007; 39(8):1423–1434.
7 Galvão DA, Newton RU. Review of exercise intervention studies in cancer patients. J Clin Oncol 2005; 23(4):899–909.
8 Robertson RJ, Goss FL, Rutkowski J et al. Concurrent validation of the OMNI perceived exertion scale for resistance exercise. Med Sci Sport Exer 2003; 35(2): 333–341.
9 Robertson RJ, Goss FL, Dube J et al. Validation of the adult OMNI scale of perceived exertion for cycle ergometer exercise. Med Sci Sport Exer 2004; 36(1):102–108.
10 Persinger R, Foster C, Gibson M et al. Consistency of the talk test for exercise prescription. Med Sci Sports Exerc 2004; 36(9):1632–1636.
11 Galvão DA, Spry NA, Taafe DR et al. Changes in muscle, fat, and bone mass after 36 weeks of maximal androgen blockade for prostate cancer. Brit J Urol Int 2008; 102:44–47.
12 Keating NL, O'Malley AJ, Smith MR et al. Diabetes and cardiovascular disease during androgen deprivation therapy for prostate cancer. J Clin Oncol 2006; 24(27):4448–4456.
13 Galvão DA, Nosaka K, Taaffe DR et al. Resistance training and reduction of treatment side effects in prostate cancer patients. Med Sci Sport Exer 2006; 38(12):2045–2052.
14 Myers J, Prakash M, Froelicher V et al. Exercise capacity and mortality among men referred for exercise testing. N Engl J Med 2002; 346(11):793–801.
15 Jurca R, Lamonte MJ, Barlow CE et al. Association of muscular strength with incidence of metabolic syndrome in men. Med Sci Sport Exer 2005; 37(11):1849–1855.
16 Newton RU, Galvao DA. Exercise in prevention and management of cancer. Curr Treat Opt Onc 2008; 9(2/3):135–146.
17 Friedenreich CM, Cust AE. Physical activity and breast cancer risk: impact of timing, type and dose of activity and population sub-group effects. Br J Sports Med 2008; 42:636–647.
18 Samad AK, Taylor RS, Marshall T et al. A meta-analysis of the association of physical activity with reduced risk of colorectal cancer. Colorectal Dis 2005; 7(3): 204–213.
19 Nilsen TIL, Romundstad PR, Vatten LJ et al. Recreational physical activity and risk of prostate cancer: A prospective population-based study in Norway (the HUNT study). Int J Cancer 2006; 119:2943–2947.
20 Holmes MD, Chen WY, Feskanich D et al. Physical activity and survival after breast cancer diagnosis. JAMA 2005; 293(20):2479–2486.
21 Demark-Wahnefried W. Cancer survival: time to get moving? Data accumulate suggesting a link between physical activity and cancer survival. J Clin Oncol 2006; 24(22):3517–3518.
22 Bailey DA, Faulkner RA, McKay HA et al. Growth, physical activity, and bone mineral acquisition. Exerc Sport Sci Rev 1996; 24:233–266.
23 Karlsson MK, Hasserius R, Obrant KJ et al. Bone mineral density in athletes during and after career: a comparison between loaded and unloaded skeletal regions. Calcif Tissue Int 1996; 59(4):245–248.
24 Nilsson M, Ohlsson C, Eriksson AL et al. Competitive physical activity early in life is associated with bone mineral density in elderly Swedish men. Osteoporosis Int 2008; 19(11):1557–1566.
25 Bellew JW, Gehrig L. A comparison of bone mineral density in adolescent female swimmers, soccer players, and weight lifters. Pediatr Phys Ther 2006; 18(1): 19–22.
26 Humphries B, Newton RU, Bronks R et al. Effect of exercise intensity on bone density, strength, and calcium turnover in older women. Med Sci Sport Exer 2000; 32(6):1043–1050.
27 Kemmler W, Engelke K, Weineck J et al. The Erlangen Fitness Osteoporosis Prevention Study: a controlled exercise trial in early postmenopausal women with low bone density—first-year results. Arch Phys Med Rehab 2003; 84(5):673–682.
28 Fiatarone MA, Marks EC, Ryan ND et al. High-intensity strength training in nonagenarians. Effects on skeletal muscle. JAMA 1990; 263(22):3029–3034.
29 Larson EB, Wang L, Bowen JD et al. Exercise is associated with reduced risk for incident dementia among persons 65 years of age and older. Ann Intern Med 2006; 144(2):73–81.
30 Sui X, LaMonte MJ, Laditka JN et al. Cardiorespiratory fitness and adiposity as mortality predictors in older adults. JAMA 2007; 298(21):2507–2516.
31 Larun L, Nordheim LV, Ekeland E et al. Exercise in prevention and treatment of anxiety and depression among children and young people. Cochrane Database Syst Rev 2006; 3:CD004691.
32 Mead GE, Morley W, Campbell P et al. Exercise for depression. Cochrane Database Syst Rev 2008; 4:CD004366.
33 Singh NA, Stavrinos TM, Scarbek Y et al. A randomized controlled trial of high versus low intensity weight training versus general practitioner care for clinical depression in older adults. J Gerontol A Biol Sci Med Sci 2005; 60(6):768–776.
34 Manson JE, Spelsberg A. Primary prevention of non-insulin-dependent diabetes mellitus. Am J Prev Med 1994; 10(3):172–184.

35 Willey KA, Singh MA. Battling insulin resistance in elderly obese people with type 2 diabetes: bring on the heavy weights. Diabetes Care 2003; 26(5):1580–1588.

36 Bennell KL, Hunt MA, Wrigley TV et al. Muscle and exercise in the prevention and management of knee osteoarthritis: an internal medicine specialist's guide. Med Clin North Am 2009; 93(1):161–177.

37 Cook NR, Cohen J, Hebert PR et al. Implications of small reductions in diastolic blood pressure for primary prevention. Arch Intern Med 1995;155(7):701–709.

38 Taylor RS, Brown A, Ebrahim S et al. Exercise-based rehabilitation for patients with coronary heart disease: systematic review and meta-analysis of randomized controlled trials. Am J Med 2004; 116(10):682–692.

chapter 10

Introduction to clinical nutrition: food and supplements

INTRODUCTION AND OVERVIEW

A healthy diet and lifestyle are prerequisites for wellness and the prevention of many chronic diseases. Identifying specific components in the diet that promote health remains a challenge, as the relationships are complex and often multifactorial. Nutritional epidemiology and interventional research with specific food components and nutritional supplements provide evidence that helps us to better understand the role of nutrition in health promotion and disease and provide patients with better advice.

Early studies in nutrition originated from observations of deficiency and its signs and symptoms. Probably the best known of these is the identification of scurvy as a diet-related disease with a potentially fatal outcome, sometime in the fifteenth century. Approximately 200 years later, James Lind identified citrus fruits as both a preventative treatment and a cure; however, it wasn't until the 1920s that vitamin C was isolated and identified as the true source of the treatment's success.

Contemporary research using more sophisticated methodologies has allowed new approaches to be used in nutritional studies. These include large prevalence and community studies, cohort and case-control studies and randomised trials. Generally, food intake diaries and surveys, biomarkers (e.g. vitamin C in urine), clinical indicators (e.g. cholesterol) and anthropometry are used as key measurements. Although these measures are useful, they are not without limitations, and research is still being conducted to identify new and more accurate measures and methods of assessment.

Clinical nutrition is the use of this information in diagnosis, disease prevention and treatment, and health promotion. Treatment consists of dietary manipulation and using food and nutritional supplements as medicine, based on individual assessment.

INADEQUATE NUTRITIONAL INTAKE

Many factors can affect an individual's nutritional status. The most obvious factors are human biological factors and physiological phases, such as age, gender and the stages of growth, pregnancy, lactation and older age. Less obvious but just as influential can be system factors such as the healthcare system, the education system and the food supply system (industry, agriculture and institutions).

Factors affecting nutritional status can be divided into three broad categories: external, internal and food factors. These are listed in Table 10.1.

One factor that tends to be overlooked is the effect of medication use on nutritional status and the possibility of inducing deficiency with long-term use. Table 10.2 gives examples of some commonly used drugs and the nutrients that can be affected. In particular, clinicians should consider the nutritional result of chronic medication use in individuals who have a barely adequate diet, take multiple drugs or are elderly and frail.

RDAs AND RDIs

The concept of recommended daily allowances (RDAs) originated in the United States in the 1940s as a basis for setting the poverty threshold and food stamp allotments for the military and civilian populations during times of war and/or economic depression.[2] At this time, the first RDAs were determined for vitamins A, C, D, E, thiamine, riboflavin, niacin, energy, protein and the minerals calcium and iron. These levels were established by observing a healthy population's usual dietary intakes and extrapolating from this information.

Over the subsequent 50 years, new ideas about and scientific research into health and nutrition emerged, and as a result the original concept of RDAs required modification. The key ideas to emerge were as follows:

TABLE 10.1 Factors affecting food choices and nutritional status

External factors	Internal factors	Food factors
Educational system: nutrition and health knowledge	Age, gender and genetics affecting nutritional requirements	Food supply chain: • availability • nutritional quality • affordability • clean and uncontaminated
Peer beliefs and practices	Physiological phases affecting nutritional requirements, e.g. growth, pregnancy, lactation, older age	Quantity of food consumed
Family beliefs and practices	Altered organ function or metabolism, e.g. malabsorption syndromes, intolerances	Flavour and palatability of food
Ethnicity and cultural influences	Personal attitudes, beliefs and behaviours, e.g. following a fad diet, vegetarianism	Texture of food
Religious beliefs and practices	Appetite, e.g. poor appetite due to disease or disease treatment	Appearance of food
Occupation	Dental health, e.g. ill-fitting dentures, sensitive teeth, gum disease	Odour of food
Media and advertising	Physical disabilities making it difficult to shop for fresh produce, prepare food, self-feed, chew and/or swallow food	Availability of nutrients in foods, e.g. binding to other food components
Economic influences, e.g. household finances, economy of community/country	Gastrointestinal symptoms, e.g. nausea, vomiting	
Medication use (see Table 10.2)	Psychosocial factors, e.g. isolation, confusion, loneliness	
Cooking techniques, e.g. up to 100% of vitamin C can be lost through cooking	Everyday moods and emotions, e.g. comfort eating	

Source: adapted from Braun & Cohen (2007)[1]

TABLE 10.2. Examples of drugs and their interactions with nutrients

Drug or drug class	Nutrient(s) affected
Loop diuretics	Increased urinary excretion of vitamin B_1, magnesium and zinc
Oral contraceptive pill	Reduced levels of folate, vitamins B_2, B_3, B_5, B_6, B_{12} Increased serum levels of vitamin A
Corticosteroids	Reduced calcium, vitamin D, calcium and iron
Antibiotics	Reduced endogenous synthesis of vitamins B_1, B_5
Proton pump inhibitors and H_2 antagonists	Reduced dietary absorption of folate, iron, vitamin B_{12}
Orlistat	Reduced dietary absorption of vitamins A, D, E, K
L-thyroxine	Insoluble complexes formed with iron, magnesium, calcium and zinc, resulting in reduced drug and nutrient absorption

Source: Braun & Cohen 2007.[1]

- Many other nutrients and food components are important for health, so the list of substances with recommended levels needed to be expanded.
- There was a need to delineate the appropriate uses of the derived nutrient standard recommendations—that is, nutrient intake levels specified for a variety of uses.
- Clearer endpoints by which to set adequacy levels were required.
- Nutritional intake levels were required to prevent not only deficiency, but also future disease.
- Risk assessment was needed.

As a result of these developments, a new framework was set up in the mid-1990s. It aimed to establish new nutrient intake recommendations to meet a variety of uses and to base nutrient requirements on the reduction of chronic disease risk, with a clear rationale for the endpoints chosen. The new guidelines still contain RDAs but have been expanded to include three new intake recommendations: estimated average requirements (EARs), adequate intake (AI) and upper level (UL) intake.

Revisions were also afoot in Australia and New Zealand, and in 2006 the National Health and Medical Research Council (NHMRC) published its newly adjusted nutritional guidelines.[3] These new guidelines are far more comprehensive than previous versions and have incorporated some of the new initiatives developed in the United States.

The guidelines are for healthy people and have been differentiated into gender and age requirements, assuming an average body weight for the adult male as 76 kg and female as 61 kg. Four key terms used in the document are defined here:

- *estimated average requirement (EAR)*—a daily nutrient level estimated to meet the needs of 50% of the healthy population in a particular life cycle and gender
- *recommended daily intake (RDI)*—a daily nutrient intake estimated to meet the needs of up to 98% of healthy people in a particular life cycle and gender
- *adequate intake (AI) when RDI cannot be determined*—based on observed or experimentally derived estimates of daily nutrient intake to meet the needs of healthy individuals; produced when the available evidence is insufficient or conflicting
- *upper level (UL) of intake*—the highest daily nutrient intake estimated to pose no risk to almost all people in the general community.

In some instances, the new RDI values for specific nutrients have increased substantially since the previous guidelines (e.g. for iron and folate), whereas others have increased marginally (e.g. for calcium) or decreased (e.g. zinc requirements for adult females).

PITFALLS OF THIS SYSTEM

Setting nutrient reference values presents many challenges. Russell,[2] from the Human Nutrition Research Center on Aging at Tufts University in the USA has outlined eight obstacles.

- Many of the databases used when determining reference values provided information from studies that only evaluated dietary intakes and ignored supplemental intakes.
- Most studies fail to consider the differences in bioavailability of nutrients depending on the food matrixes they are in.
- Few long-term studies are available, so information is extrapolated from short-term studies (e.g. 1–2 weeks).
- There is a paucity of information about children, adolescents and the elderly from which to establish reference values with any degree of certainty.
- Most experiments fail to consider the interaction between nutrients.
- There is a lack of information about individual variability in response to the indicators in question.
- There is a lack of dose–response information—that is, responses to multiple levels of the same nutrient in the same individual.
- There are doubts about the purported action of the nutrient on the indicator being considered—e.g. multiple factors affect an outcome, so a cause and effect relationship can be uncertain and only speculative.

Overall, for many nutrients and food components there is no adequate database to confidently set an RDI or UL, and the scientific basis for many of the reference values is weak. Clearly the reference values we now use can only be a general approximation and loosely relevant to the general healthy population, with even less relevance to the individual with comorbidities or special needs.

To create a set of reference values with greater accuracy and relevance, substantial research funding is required. Even then, some values such as ULs may never be entirely accurate, as ethical considerations would prevent such research from ever being conducted.

MOVING BEYOND RDIs: OPTIMAL NUTRITION

There is now strong international awareness that nutritional intakes at levels beyond RDI have a role in the prevention of many degenerative diseases such as cancer, cardiovascular disease, macular degeneration and cataract, cognitive decline and Alzheimer's dementia, and developmental conditions such as neural tube defects.[1] The new NHMRC guidelines for the adequate intake of vitamins and minerals recognise this fact and state that 'there is some evidence that a range of nutrients could have benefits in chronic disease aetiology at levels above the RDI or AI'.[3]

This has given rise to a new concept, of 'suboptimal nutrition'. A major systematic review of the international literature conducted by Fairfield and Fletcher describes suboptimal nutrition as a state in which nutritional intake is sufficient to prevent the classical symptoms and signs of deficiency, yet insufficient to significantly reduce the risk of developmental or degenerative diseases.[4]

As such, avoiding a state of suboptimal nutrition requires adequate dietary intakes of all key food groups, and possibly the use of additional nutritional supplements. Nutrients associated with a reduced risk of chronic disease when consumed in quantities higher than the RDI are many and include the antioxidant vitamins C, E and A, the mineral selenium and nutrients such as folate, omega-3 fatty acids and dietary fibre.[3] It is also becoming clear that the balance between nutrients or macronutrients is important for optimal health and disease prevention—examples are the ratio of omega-3 to omega-6 fatty acids and high to low glycaemic carbohydrates.

MULTIVITAMINS FOR PREVENTATIVE HEALTH?

In 2003, the Lewin Report quantified the preventative health benefits of multivitamin supplementation using the US health insurance model.[5] It was established that multivitamin use by older adults could lead to more than US $1.6 billion in Medicare cost savings over the next 5 years in the United States. The significant cost savings were based on improved immune function and a reduction in relative risk of coronary artery disease achievable with daily multivitamin supplementation in people over 65 years old. Furthermore, the authors state that this is a conservative estimate that does not take into account cost savings from decreased ambulatory care and assumes that only one-third of adults will experience benefits. Reductions in the incidence of other diseases such as cancer were not considered in this review but may also be reduced.

An extension of this work was carried out by Huang and colleagues, who conducted another comprehensive review of the published literature to determine whether evidence supported the use of multivitamin/mineral supplements and certain single-nutrient supplements in the primary prevention of chronic disease in the general adult population.[6] Their review concluded that multivitamin/mineral supplement use may prevent cancer in individuals with poor or suboptimal nutritional status.

Given their relative safety and general health benefits, the evidence suggests that multivitamins may extend the benefits afforded by healthy eating. Accordingly, it would be prudent for all adults to take multivitamins regularly to prevent chronic disease.[4,7] In particular, they should be recommended for people with barely adequate diets, older adults, alcohol-dependent individuals, fussy eaters and those with malabsorption syndromes and intolerances.

WHAT DEFINES AN ESSENTIAL NUTRIENT TODAY?

Clearly, the line between essential and non-essential nutrients has blurred as a result of modern scientific enquiry and experimentation.[8] In the first half of the twentieth century, nutrients were termed 'essential' when their removal from the diet caused severe organ dysfunction or death. Since then, modern scientific techniques have enabled us to detect finer gradations of inadequacy well before severe organ failure sets in, such as a decline in health status or ability to function optimally. This raises the question of whether nutrients and food components that are vital for optimal function and disease prevention should also be termed 'essential'. This would assume that the traditional aim of clinical nutrition has broadened beyond preventing deficiency to include the promotion of wellness and optimal health.

Many nutrients currently classified as non-essential may in future prove to be essential, if a longer-term view is taken than has been previously. For example, it is feasible that organ failure and death may result from years of inadequate intake and not be apparent in the short term or only manifest after a long latency period. While identifying which non-essential nutrients and food components may turn out to be essential is a difficult task, evidence suggests that some specific diets consisting of multiple food components have substantial health-promoting effects. In particular, evidence to support the Mediterranean diet stands out—this may be the 'essential diet'.

FOOD AS MEDICINE

Food provides us with physical and emotional nourishment. Most obviously, it provides macronutrients (carbohydrates, protein, fat) and micronutrients (vitamins, minerals) that help to sustain health. Many foods also contain a variety of active phytochemicals that exert pharmacological effects, giving those foods health benefits beyond their nutritional content. These non-nutrient constituents are sometimes known as *functional components*. Identification of functional components in everyday foods has led to a greater understanding of their health-giving properties. Table 10.3 provides examples of functional components found in everyday foods.

FUNCTIONAL FOODS AND FOOD SUPPLEMENTS

The term 'functional food' is widely used to describe foods that provide more health benefits than mere nutritional content alone. In many cases, functional attributes are being discovered for everyday fruits and vegetables, causing the mainstream media to call them 'superfoods'. Food technology has allowed the development of food products that may provide even greater health benefits than nature has provided, such as fortified foods. Nutraceutical companies take this one step further and manufacture concentrated food

TABLE 10.3. Examples of functional food components

Food component	Source	Potential benefit
Carotenoids		
Beta carotene	Carrots, various fruits and vegetables	Boosts cellular antioxidant protection; may reduce risk of CHD and contribute to healthy vision
Zeaxanthin/lutein	Collards, spinach, corn, egg yolk, orange peppers	May contribute to healthy vision and reduce incidence of several cancers
Dietary fibre		
Beta glucan	Oat bran, rolled oats	May reduce risk of CHD and aid metabolic control in diabetes
Soluble fibre	*Psyllium* seed husk	May reduce risk of CHD and aid metabolic control in diabetes
Fatty acids		
Omega-3 fatty acids	Deep sea oily fish (e.g. mackerel, salmon, tuna)	May reduce risk of CHD; reduces all-cause mortality; numerous other health benefits
Flavonoids		
Anthocyanidins	Red berries, red grapes	Boosts cellular antioxidant protection; numerous health benefits
Proanthocyanidins	Apples, pears, cranberries, cocoa, wine (esp. red), grapes, peanuts	Boosts cellular antioxidant protection; numerous health benefits
Isothyocyanates		
Indole-3-carbinol and sulphorafane	Cauliflower, broccoli, cabbage, kale, brussels sprouts	Boosts cellular antioxidant protection and influences detoxification pathways; may reduce incidence of various cancers
Phenols		
Caffeic acid, ferulic acid	Coffee, apple, brown rice, citrus fruits, pears and some vegetables	Boosts cellular antioxidant protection; may contribute to healthy vision and heart and reduce incidence of various cancers
Stanols and sterols		
Stanols/sterol esters	Fortified table spreads	May reduce risk of CHD
Prebiotics/probiotics		
Inulin	Whole grains, some fruit, onions	May improve gastrointestinal health and immune function
Bifidobacteria and lactobacilli	Fermented milk products (e.g. yoghurt)	May improve gastrointestinal health and immune function
Phyto-oestrogens		
Isoflavones	Soy-based foods	May reduce risk of CHD
Sulfides/thiols		
Diallyl sulfinate (allicin)/ allyl methyltrisulfide	Garlic, onion, leek (found in allium vegetables)	Boosts cellular antioxidant protection and influences detoxification pathways; may maintain healthy heart and immune function

Source: adapted from the International Food Information Council Foundation[9]

supplements, such as fish oil products with predefined levels of eicosapentaenoic acid (EPA) and docosahexaenoic acid (DHA), and concentrated probiotic supplements containing specific bacterial strains. In many cases, the supplemental forms contain a higher concentration of the functional component than is naturally found in food. There may be other advantages to food supplements, such as more stringent quality control (e.g. fish oil products being tested for heavy metal contamination, whereas fish in the local market are not), consistency in concentration of key active ingredients using standardisation techniques, and palatability, for fussy eaters.

FOUR POPULAR FOOD SUPPLEMENTS

Fish oils

Fish oils, also known as marine oils, contain several types of vitamin B, fat-soluble vitamins, calcium, magnesium and potassium. Importantly, they contain the essential fatty acids EPA and DHA, which exert a myriad effects on the heart and vessels that have been demonstrated in both experimental models and human studies.[1] Clinical trials generally support the use of fish oils in a range of inflammatory and autoimmune diseases, such as rheumatoid arthritis and atopic dermatitis, elevated triglycerides, hypertension and other cardiovascular conditions, poor cognitive function, diabetes and possibly depression.[1]

Although eating fish regularly is the ideal, this is not always practical or even palatable for some people. Fish oil supplements provide one solution and are extremely popular. They contain standardised levels of DHA and EPA, must meet quality control standards and are available in different administration forms (liquids, tablets and capsules). Products containing different EPA:DHA ratios are also available, which enables more specific prescribing.

Ginger

Ginger is a spice that is widely recognised as a food with medicinal qualities. The main pharmacological actions of ginger and its isolated compounds include immunomodulatory, anti-tumorigenic, anti-inflammatory, anti-apoptotic, antihyperglycaemic, antilipidaemic and antiemetic.[10] In Australia, commercially produced ginger tablets are most commonly used to prevent travel sickness and to relieve the symptoms of morning sickness, dyspepsia, nausea and inflammatory joint diseases such as osteoarthritis.

Probiotics

Probiotic-containing foods such as yoghurt are widely recognised as health-promoting foods. Immune system modulation and the prevention of gastrointestinal tract colonisation by a variety of pathogens are perhaps the most important actions of probiotics.[1] Probiotic supplements containing different bacterial strains in concentrated levels have been investigated in numerous clinical trials. For example, a Cochrane review of 23 RCTs found that probiotic supplementation was a useful adjunct to rehydration therapy in treating acute infectious diarrhoea in adults and children.[11] Two trials in the review used the yeast *Saccharomyces boulardii*, whereas the other trials used supplements of lactic acid bacilli. Some clinical studies have also found a protective effect against traveller's diarrhoea, but no single probiotic strain has demonstrated clinically relevant protection worldwide.

Many different probiotic supplements are available. They usually contain a standardised number of living organisms per unit of volume, and dosages range from 1 billion to 450 billion colonies daily. This is in excess of concentrations typically found in yoghurt. Some products contain a single bacterial strain, and others contain multiple strains.

Cranberries

Cranberries are small, dark red, acidic berries. They are available from grocery stores in punnets and are widely consumed as juice or sauce. Besides being an excellent source of vitamin C, a Cochrane systematic review concluded that cranberry products significantly reduce the incidence of urinary tract infections (UTIs) compared with placebo/controls in women. There was no significant difference in the incidence of UTIs between cranberry juice and cranberry capsules.[12] Capsules containing cranberry extract are popular among older women and are used in many nursing homes because of their ease of use.

THE HEALTHIEST DIET: MEDITERRANEAN?

Defining what constitutes a healthy diet is difficult and open to debate. Nutritional pyramids developed by government agencies provide a general guide; however, every few years another dietary approach emerges (e.g. Pritikin, Atkins, vegan) that challenges accepted thought and reminds us how little we truly know about nutrition.

The substantial health benefits afforded to people who adhere to the Mediterranean diet in the long term is a consistent finding in the peer-reviewed literature, making it a strong candidate for the healthiest diet. In 2002, Panagiotakos and colleagues found that a combination of Mediterranean diet and healthy lifestyle (non-smoking, physically active, moderate drinking) was associated with a greater than 50% lower rate of all-causes and cause-specific mortality (e.g. from coronary heart disease, cardiovascular diseases and cancer).[13] The cohort study involved 1507 apparently healthy men and 832 women, aged 70 to 90 years, in 11 European countries. A year later, Trichopoulou also reported a positive association between longevity and the Mediterranean diet that was significant in people aged 55 years or older.[14] More recently, a 2004 review of five cohort studies confirmed these findings and

TABLE 10.4 Summary of foods typically included in the Mediterranean diet and modification generally required to the Western diet

Food	Recommendations for a Mediterranean style of eating
Fish	Increase intake to at least three times a week
Olives, olive oil	Replace current oils and spreads with olive oil
Nuts	Eat regularly, especially walnuts
Vegetables	Eat regularly, especially dark-green leafy types and coloured vegetables (e.g. cooked tomatoes)
Fruit	Eat regularly, especially fresh fruit grown locally in season
Garlic	Eat regularly
Red wine	Moderate amounts taken with meals (1 glass daily)
Red meat—eaten only on occasion	Decrease consumption
Dairy products—eaten only on occasion	Decrease consumption (especially trans fatty acids)
Processed foods—eaten only on occasion	Decrease consumption (especially high glycaemic index foods)

concluded that there is now sufficient evidence to show that diet does indeed influence longevity.[15]

Table 10.4 lists the main foods typically included in the Mediterranean diet. Not surprisingly, many contain functional components discussed in this chapter.

NUTRITIONAL SUPPLEMENTS

Nutritional supplements can never replace a balanced diet or provide all the health benefits of a whole food, but they can provide nutritional assistance and therapeutic effects in three different ways, as discussed below.

Supplementation to correct a gross deficiency

A patient presenting with signs and symptoms of nutritional deficiency will require nutritional counselling and possibly nutritional supplementation to quickly address the situation.

Supplementation to address a subclinical deficiency

A nutritional substance can be used to promote optimal health and/or prevent future disease.

Example: folic acid and gestational health and development

Folate plays an important role in the genomic stability of human cells. Numerous studies have identified a beneficial effect of folate supplementation during the periconceptional period.

A Cochrane systematic review concluded that periconceptional folate supplementation has a strong protective effect against neural tube defects and that information about folate should be made more widely available throughout the health and education systems. Women whose fetuses or babies have neural tube defects should be advised of the risk of recurrence in a subsequent pregnancy and offered continuing folate supplementation. There is also emerging evidence that folate supplementation around the time of conception has the potential to reduce the frequency of Down syndrome.[16] Additionally, a large European study has identified that higher folate levels prior to conception and during pregnancy are linked to the prevention of miscarriages and increased birth weight in the offspring of smoking mothers.[17]

High-dose supplementation as a therapeutic medicine

Nutritional supplements can be used in pharmacological doses to achieve a specific health-related purpose, much like a therapeutic drug. The intended purpose appears to bear no relation to the nutrient's deficiency signs or symptoms.

Example: riboflavin and migraine prophylaxis

The RDI of riboflavin for adults is 1.1–1.6 mg, depending on gender and age. In developed nations, gross deficiency is rare, as most individuals consume dietary amounts greater than the RDI. Riboflavin in much larger doses has been investigated as a prophylactic treatment for migraine headache and found to be effective in some individuals. In three clinical studies of various designs, a daily dose of 400 mg was administered, and a reduction in migraine headache frequency was observed.[18–20] Additionally, one clinical study compared the effects of high-dose riboflavin to those of standard beta-adrenergic antagonists and found that both treatments significantly improved the clinical symptoms of migraine headache.[21] It is suspected that riboflavin activity in mitochondrial metabolism is responsible for its benefits in migraine.

Example: coenzyme Q10 and hypertension

Coenzyme Q10 (CoQ10) is a vitamin-like substance with antioxidant activity. It is found in every cell in

BOX 10.1 Steps in prescribing food and nutritional supplements

1 *Know the benefits and risks.*
Know the benefits and risks associated with popular and evidence-based nutritional and food supplements, including potential drug interactions. If in doubt, refer to a credible resource or trained expert, e.g. a dietician for predominantly food-based solutions or a naturopath for both food-based and supplement-based approaches.
2 *Choose quality products.*
If the product comes from Australia, ensure that the product label includes an AUST L or AUST R number and expiry date. If the product comes from a country other than Australia, make sure it is manufactured according to the Code of Good Manufacturing Practice.
3 *Choose the correct dose.*
Choose the correct dose for the intended outcome—e.g. is it being used to address a deficiency or as a therapeutic agent to treat a disease? Use information from clinical trials, reference texts and manufacturer information for guidance.
4 *Provide instructions.*
Supply the patient with instructions on where the product can be bought—e.g. supermarket, pharmacy, health-food store, other.
5 *Identify a time frame.*
Select a sensible time frame for treatment—some nutritional deficiencies can be effectively treated within a few days, whereas the health benefits of some food supplements may take several months to manifest.

the body. It is essential for adenosine triphosphate synthesis in the mitochondrial inner membrane, and it stabilises cell membranes, preserving cellular integrity and function. It also reconstitutes vitamin E back into its antioxidant form[22] and affects the expression of genes involved in human cell signalling, metabolism and transport.[23] This mechanism may account for some of the pharmacological effects observed with supplementation.

No RDI levels have been established but there has been some speculation as to possible deficiency signs and symptoms. These include fatigue, muscle aches and pains and chronic gum disease.[1] Numerous studies show that supplementation with CoQ10 has beneficial effects on various diseases.

For example, in 2007 a meta-analysis of 12 clinical trials ($n = 362$), comprising three RCTs, one crossover study and eight open-label studies, concluded that supplementation with CoQ10 in hypertensive patients has the potential to lower systolic blood pressure by up to 17 mmHg and diastolic blood pressure by up to 10 mmHg without significant side effects.[24]

PRESCRIBING NUTRITIONAL AND FOOD SUPPLEMENTS

Nutritional and food supplements can play an important role in general practice and provide practitioners with many additional therapeutic tools. While the fully fledged practice of dietetics and clinical nutrition requires several years of specialised training, general practitioners can successfully integrate some simple, pre-prepared treatments into their practice (Box 10.1).

A practitioner who lacks confidence or knowledge about nutrition and food concentrates should consider referring the patient to an accredited dietician for food-based solutions, or a naturopath for both food-based and supplement-based approaches. Some pharmacists have undergone additional training and can provide general information about popular over-the-counter products. For general practitioners who are keen to learn more about this expanding area, several GP-specific short courses are provided by accredited course providers such as the Australasian College of Nutritional and Environmental Medicine (ACNEM).

RESOURCES

American Society for Nutrition, http://www.nutrition.org/
Arbor Nutrition Guide, http://www.arborcom.com/frame/arb_nutr.htm
Braun L, Cohen M. Herbs and natural supplements: an evidence-based guide. 3rd edn. Sydney: Elsevier; 2010 (provides comprehensive, evidence-based information about 130 complementary medicines popular in Australia and New Zealand and detailed drug–nutrient interaction charts)
Jamison J. Clinical guide to nutritional and dietary supplements. Sydney: Elsevier; 2003.
MedlinePlus, http://www.nlm.nih.gov/medlineplus/druginformation.html

REFERENCES

1 Braun L, Cohen M. Introduction to clinical nutrition. In: Herbs and natural supplements: an evidence-based guide. 3rd edn. Sydney: Elsevier; 2010:23–35.
2 Russell R. Setting dietary intake levels: problems and pitfalls. Dietary supplements and health. Chichester: Wiley; 2007:29–45.
3 National Health and Medical Research Council (NHMRC). Nutrient reference values for Australia and New Zealand; 2006. Online. Available: http://www.nhmrc.gov.au/publications/synopses/n35syn.htm 4 Nov 2007.
4 Fairfield KM, Fletcher RH. Vitamins for chronic disease prevention in adults: scientific review. JAMA 2002; 287(23):3116–3126.

5 The Lewin Group. A study of the cost effects of multivitamins in selected populations. 2003. Online. Available: http://www.highbeam.com/doc/1G1-113138553.html
6 Huang HY, Caballero B, Chang S et al. Multivitamin/mineral supplements and prevention of chronic disease. Evid Rep Technol Assess (Full Rep) 2006; 139:1–117.
7 Fletcher RH, Fairfield KM. Vitamins for chronic disease prevention in adults: clinical applications. JAMA 2002; 287(23):3127–3129.
8 Yates AA. Nutrient requirements, international perspectives. In: Benjamin C, ed. Encyclopedia of human nutrition. Oxford: Elsevier; 2005:282–292.
9 International Food Information Council Foundation. Report February 2004. Online. Available: http://www.ific.org/ 4 November 2007.
10 Ali BH, Blunden G, Tanira MO et al. Some phytochemical, pharmacological and toxicological properties of ginger (*Zingiber officinale* Roscoe): a review of recent research. Food Chem Toxicol 2008; 46(2):409–420.
11 Allen SJ, Okoko B, Martinez E et al. Probiotics for treating infectious diarrhoea. Cochrane Database Syst Rev 2004; (2):CD003048.
12 Jepson RG, Mihaljevic L, Craig J. Cranberries for preventing urinary tract infections. Cochrane Database Syst Rev 2004; 2:CD001321.
13 Knoops KT, de Groot LC, Kromhout D et al. Mediterranean diet, lifestyle factors, and 10-year mortality in elderly European men and women: the HALE project. JAMA 2004; 292(12):1433–1439.
14 Trichopoulou A. Traditional Mediterranean diet and longevity in the elderly: a review. Public Health Nutr 2004; 7(7):943–947.
15 Trichopoulou A, Critselis E. Mediterranean diet and longevity. Eur J Cancer Prev 2004; 13(5):453–456.
16 Eskes TK. Abnormal folate metabolism in mothers with Down syndrome offspring: review of the literature. Eur J Obstet Gynecol Reprod Biol 2006; 124(2):130–133.
17 Sram RJ, Binkova B, Lnenickova Z et al. The impact of plasma folate levels of mothers and newborns on intrauterine growth retardation and birth weight. Mutat Res 2005; 591(1/2):302–310.
18 Schoenen J, Lenaerts M, Bastings E. High-dose riboflavin as a prophylactic treatment of migraine: results of an open pilot study. Cephalalgia 1994; 14(5):328–329.
19 Schoenen J, Jacquy J, Lenaerts M. Effectiveness of high-dose riboflavin in migraine prophylaxis. A randomized controlled trial. Neurology 1998; 50(2):466–470.
20 Boehnke C, Reuter U, Flach U et al. High-dose riboflavin treatment is efficacious in migraine prophylaxis: an open study in a tertiary care centre. Eur J Neurol 2004; 11(7):475–477.
21 Sandor PS, Afra J, Ambrosini A et al. Prophylactic treatment of migraine with beta-blockers and riboflavin: differential effects on the intensity dependence of auditory evoked cortical potentials. Headache 2000; 40(1):30–35.
22 Kaikkonen J, Tuomainen TP, Nyyssonen K et al. Coenzyme Q10: absorption, antioxidative properties, determinants, and plasma levels. Free Radic Res 2002; 36(4):389–397.
23 Groneberg DA, Kindermann B, Althammer M. Coenzyme Q10 affects expression of genes involved in cell signalling, metabolism and transport in human CaCo-2 cells. Int J Biochem Cell Biol 2005; 37(6):1208–1218.
24 Rosenfeldt FL, Haas SJ, Krum H et al. Coenzyme Q10 in the treatment of hypertension: a meta-analysis of the clinical trials. J Hum Hypertens 2007; 21(4): 297–306.

chapter 11

Connectedness: the role of social support

INTRODUCTION AND OVERVIEW

'Connectedness' is a term denoting the level of social support experienced in one's life, or the connection we feel to the people, society and social institutions around us. The most important areas of connectedness vary with one's age, and include family, friends, school, workplace and workmates, and one's local community. The opposite of connectedness is social isolation.

Human beings by nature are social creatures. Original hunter-gatherer communities have steadily grown into the urban environments we now know. As a species our survival and continued productivity depend upon our ability to live and work as functioning groups, and so connectedness is deeply etched into our natures genetically, psychologically, socially and behaviourally. An indication of the importance of connectedness is the fact that social isolation is a significant risk factor for mental and physical illness, even independent of other lifestyle factors.

Social isolation is not the same as solitude. Solitude can be healthy, such as when we need time to reflect, or to enjoy peace and space. We can feel 'connected' and be in solitude at the same time. Conversely, we can be among many people and feel 'socially isolated' at the same time, if we do not feel at ease in the environment or are not relating to people in the way we wish to. Therefore, social isolation is more related to our internal state than our external state.

Connectedness can be expressed and fostered in many ways. This chapter looks at the impact of connectedness on health at different stages in the life cycle. This chapter also examines the use of 'social support' in healthcare settings.

TAKING A SOCIAL HISTORY

Doctors learn to take a 'social history' in medical school as a part of a full history, although the importance of a social history has not always been appreciated. A full social history includes questions such as the following:

- Who are you living with at home?
- What type of work do you do?
- What is your family situation and structure?
- What social activities do you engage in?
- What interests and hobbies do you have?
- What is your financial situation like?
- What is your cultural background?
- Have you had any family or social stressors lately?

More important and telling can be open-ended questions such as:

- How would you describe the quality of your family/work/personal relationships?
- Who do you rely on in a challenging situation or under stress?
- Do you feel connected to the people you interact with on a day-to-day basis?
- Do you find it easy to discuss your feelings or important decisions with the people in your life?
- What impact have family and social stressors had on you and your life?
- What part does your cultural heritage play in your life?
- What part does religion or spirituality play in your life?

If we wait to listen and follow up on cues, such questions can reveal a lot more than just information about the practicalities of family, social and work structures. Rather than just describing our external circumstances, they can be windows into the inner world of our social interactions.

SOCIAL ISOLATION AND STRESS

Social isolation is painful, so much so that it figures prominently among the top 10 stressors in the Holmes and Rahe scale.[1] Top among stressors is the grief associated with the loss of a family member. Next come a range of issues related to marriage and workplace stress. Conflict at work is also among the most stressful events in most people's lives. Most of us will wish, at various times, to shun social connection, but the pain associated with feeling socially isolated indicates that the need for connection is part of human nature. As such, it is expressed in many ways, including physical illness, anxiety, depression, low productivity, substance abuse and domestic violence.

SOCIAL ISOLATION AND ILLNESS

Until recent times, the importance of connectedness—or the lack thereof—as a causal factor in illness has been under-recognised. It is important to remember that although social isolation is a precipitator or aggravating factor for many illnesses, social support is equally protective. Further, social support does not just determine whether we become ill but also significantly contributes to our lifestyle and how we cope with illness.

Social isolation, being a considerable stressor, has a significant impact upon our emotional state and therefore on our physical state. The chapter on mind–body medicine (Ch 8) gives a more detailed account of this. Some of the illnesses and problems associated with social isolation include:

- mental illness and suicide
- alcoholism and other forms of substance abuse
- violence
- heart disease
- infectious disease
- inflammatory and autoimmune diseases
- unhealthy lifestyle
- loss of social skills
- cognitive decline and dementia.

Although social isolation can contribute to various illnesses, it should equally be noted that these illnesses can contribute to people becoming socially isolated. As risk factors, social isolation and socioeconomic factors make a major contribution to many common illnesses.[2,3] They are as important as smoking, being overweight or hypercholesterolaemia. Equally, connectedness is protective against the same illnesses. Some examples:

- Sociability is associated with a decreased probability of developing a cold if exposed to the virus, independent of other health factors.[4]
- Social and productive activities such as games, work and social outings are protective against death and cognitive decline in the elderly.[5]
- Social support is a major prognostic factor for those with cardiovascular disease.[6]
- Following a heart attack, men were three times more likely to die from their heart disease in the following 6 months if they were socially isolated.[7]

Some factors that are particularly important include being married, having contact with family and friends, group affiliation and church membership. Even if someone has a chronic illness such as heart disease, the progression of the illness is significantly slowed or accelerated depending on the level of connectedness. The effects are especially significant for the elderly, with the risk of death among those who were isolated being increased fourfold in the months after a heart attack.[8] Such findings are largely independent of access to medical care.

THE SOCIAL GRADIENT

Research, conducted largely through the work of Michael Marmot and colleagues, has consistently demonstrated that one's social position or class has a significant effect on health outcomes.[9] This is not explainable simply in terms of access or lack of access to health resources, particularly in countries with a good standard of universal health cover. It is also not just related to occupational exposure and unhealthier lifestyle, which are more common in lower socioeconomic groups. Other explanations for the findings include:

- lower levels of education
- learned helplessness and disempowerment
- diminished autonomy
- less community engagement
- less-developed capacity for assimilating information and problem solving.

If social isolation contributes significantly to illness, then the solutions to these problems lie in social structures, attitudes and community values. If, for example, relationships are not valued, or if working conditions do not make it easy for parents to spend time with their families, or if an increasing number of parents have to bring up children as a sole parent, then problems are being bred not just for the current generation but also for those coming after.

CONNECTEDNESS AND MENTAL HEALTH

Study findings have suggested that, of young people who present to a general practitioner for any reason, over 20% will have had suicidal ideation in the preceding fortnight.[10] In addressing issues such as youth suicide, much attention has been given to identifying risk factors and intervening with at-risk individuals. Risk factors for suicide include:

- depression and hopelessness
- guilt
- substance abuse
- concurrent physical illness
- bereavement

- recent abortion
- previous attempted suicide
- living alone
- unemployment
- custody and marital problems
- family history
- absence of religion and meaning
- being male.

Such statistics, along with the almost ubiquitous presence of risk factors, can contribute to the creation of a sense of fear and a tendency to overreact to the ordinary vicissitudes of adolescence. Risk factors generally come in multiples and when they do, they have a synergistic effect, making the risk of suicide much greater. Equally important in a positive sense are protective factors. Protective factors, such as employment or connectedness at home, help to neutralise the effects of risk factors. Always thinking of risk rather than protection is not only symbolic of our community's concentration on illness rather than wellness, but also leads to an atmosphere of negativity. A major study of the effect of connectedness on adolescents showed it to be tremendously protective not just against youth suicide and emotional distress but also against substance use and violence.[11] The protective effect was significant regardless of ethnic or socioeconomic background. Connectedness at home and at school were the two most important factors. The effect of multiple risk factors in the absence of protective factors is enormous, but the effect of multiple protective factors, even in the presence of multiple risk factors, is to reduce risk to near normal. The most protective aspect of family connectedness was having a parental presence in the house at important times in the day, such as on waking, after school, at dinner and at bedtime. Having shared activities between parents and their children was also very important. A lack of parental presence, especially where the child had access to drugs and guns at home, was associated with a range of risk-taking behaviours.

Promoting protective factors will require the co-operation of a great many individuals and groups in society. Policy makers, politicians and funds providers need to create conditions that are conducive to community building and strong family structures. Researchers need to provide evidence that community building is a major health priority and also to help guide policy. Schools need to recognise connectedness as a core educational objective. Parents need to acknowledge the importance of connectedness and be supported in the community and workplace to make family and community a priority. Healthcare professionals need to identify those at risk and provide therapy or referral as appropriate. General practitioners can also play a number of other roles, such as:

- raising awareness about the links between social factors and health
- providing encouragement and support to people wishing to improve their 'social health'
- counselling to help people with communication, conflict and relationship issues
- being aware of local resources and support services
- providing support groups within the practice.

POVERTY

Studies examining the impact of income on health status have found that poverty is associated with a significantly increased risk for mortality over a given period compared with high-income groups,[12] and that this is not explainable by other risk factors. As a risk factor for illness, poverty is at least as significant as smoking, drinking, being overweight and being inactive. The reasons are complex but include the fact that those from less affluent backgrounds:

- are more often exposed to occupational hazards
- have poor access to healthcare
- have higher work stress
- are subject to racism and classism
- have less sense of control and self-mastery.

RELATIONSHIPS AND EMOTIONAL EXPRESSION

People have a basic need to belong to families and communities and also to get along well with others. Relating poorly to others is both a risk factor for mental health problems and an indication of them. Bullying, for example, is common at all ages. In children it tends to be more open and transparent; in adults, consciously or unconsciously, it tends to be more concealed. Although bullying is common, it is not 'normal' behaviour or a sign of healthy psychology. Studies of children suggest that bullies are as depressed as their victims.[13] Depression among bullies is four times as common as in the general population and they are far more likely to have suicidal ideation and psychosomatic symptoms. Bullying, whether perpetrated by individuals, groups or countries, rather than being an expression of strength is really an expression of aggression masking emotional weakness and vulnerability.

Developmentally, how we learn to deal with difficult emotions like anger during our upbringing has major implications for the rest of our lives. Two particularly important periods for the development of emotional health are early childhood and adolescence. A lack of warmth and nurture as a child means that important pathways from the prefrontal lobes that govern reasoning and emotional regulation will not be laid down adequately. Even in a normal adolescent these pathways are not well developed, in part explaining why adolescents have difficulty controlling impulses and empathising with others at this age.

There are healthy and unhealthy ways of dealing with anger. Among the unhealthy ways are suppression and aggression; and even 'catharsis' can engender more anger in the longer term.[14] These will tend to be destructive to oneself or others. Healthy ways of dealing with anger include education, improving one's communication skills, cognitive behaviour therapy, mindfulness-based therapies, assertiveness training and many other approaches. There are also useful and regulated outlets for pent-up emotions, such as sport, provided the expression is within the laws of the game.

Anger and hostility have detrimental effects on health. Apart from being pro-inflammatory and immunosuppressive, they also accelerate the progression of cardiovascular disease. For example, a study of young adults (18–30 years) followed up for 10 years clearly showed that hostility was associated with a significantly higher rate of coronary calcification independent of other lifestyle factors.[15] Hostility is defined as a personality trait associated with an attitude of cynicism and mistrust, high levels of anger, and behaviour such as overt or repressed aggression.

MARRIAGE AND LONG-TERM PARTNERSHIPS

In the adult years, the marital or long-term partner relationship is probably the most important relationship with regard to physical and mental health. The fact that virtually every culture fosters the family unit based upon the marital relationship suggests that it is written deeply into human biology and psyche.

It has long been acknowledged that marriage is associated with positive health outcomes even if it is only moderately happy.[16] Most studies have focused on heterosexual relationships, but similar findings are likely for other long-term and cohabiting relationships. For example, a growing number of countries have introduced a form of marriage or civil partnership registration for same-sex couples. It is argued that legal and social recognition of same-sex relationships may reduce discrimination, increase the stability of same-sex relationships and lead to better physical and mental health for gay and lesbian people.[17]

Marriage is protective for both sexes, although in male–female partnerships it may be relatively more protective for men than for women.[18–20] Roles within a relationship also have a different effect for men and women. Greater companionship and equality in decision-making have a strong positive influence on women, but less so on men. A significant part of the positive effect of marriage on the health of men is related to the role that marriage has in improving men's lifestyle, hygiene and health behaviours. Although a significant life transition in itself, marriage largely acts as a buffer for stress and is protective for depression and other mental health problems.[21,22] Obviously, chronically unhappy marriages do not exert a positive health influence and in such a situation an unmarried person is likely to be happier and healthier than an unhappily married one.[23] A patient's response to the question, 'How critical is your spouse of you?'[24] is a very strong predictor of depression relapse. Living with a partner who is constantly undermining one's self-esteem is not conducive to self-development and empowerment. The level of confidence in a relationship is also predictive of the development of mental health problems.[25] The recalling of marital conflict, particularly for women, has a significantly negative effect on blood pressure, and induces many of the effects of the fight-or-flight response, as would be expected.[26] An unhappy marriage is therefore a significant contributor to high allostatic load if prolonged.

Stable long-term relationships are associated with lower all-cause mortality and cause-specific mortality from cancer and heart disease.[27] Recent bereavement or a chronically unhappy cohabiting relationship, on the other hand, is a significant risk factor for death from a whole range of causes.[28] This is illustrated by the fact that women with heart disease had a three times higher chance of further relapse and death over the following 5 years if they had a stressful marital or other cohabiting relationship.[29] Marriage also has effects upon immunity. For example, recent bereavement is associated with poor immunity and response to immunisation, whereas happy and stable relationships are associated with better immune function.[30] Recent separation or divorce is associated with a significant increase in the risk of infectious disease, such as a six-fold increase in the chance of death due to pneumonia.[31] There is even more significant immunosuppression during marital separation.[32,33] In summary, the stress of negative relationships and hostility in marriage produces a clinically significant compromise of immunity.[34] Marriage can also, for better or for worse, affect the progression of chronic fatigue syndrome,[35] the experience of acute and chronic pain[36] and the progression of cancer. Social support in the form of marriage or a committed long-term relationship, or frequent daily contact with others, and the presence of a close confidant, seem to have a protective effect against cancer progression.[37]

Relationship counselling needs to be sensitive to the differing needs and approaches of men and women. This is one of the main reasons that some men will avoid marriage counselling. Women, for example, may feel more comfortable in speaking about emotions than men, and men may wish to take a more pragmatic or cognitive approach. Considering the varying ways in which men and women tend to respond to stress (see the section on the 'fight-or-flight' and 'tend-and-befriend' responses in Ch 8), there may be biological as well as socially conditioned reasons for this. This does not preclude the fact that it is likely that communication skills and emotional sensitivity will need to be enhanced, particularly in men.

Relationship counselling will also need to take into account the religious and cultural background of the individual, couple or family. These factors can have an enormous impact on attitudes to roles, sexuality, family structures and divorce. The counsellor and patient(s) may be unaware of the other's perspective or have widely divergent views on a range of matters. This can make unbiased and patient-centred counselling difficult and may mean that it is sometimes appropriate to refer a patient or couple to a culturally appropriate counsellor.

Important adjuncts to relationship counselling will also include building social and psychological skills and capacities, including emotional intelligence, mindfulness, positive psychology and communication skills.

SOCIAL SUPPORT IN HEALTHCARE

Social support can be provided in healthcare settings in a number of ways. First, many people find visiting the doctor an important source of emotional support, as the doctor plays the role of a close confidant. The medical consultation in itself provides perspective, a sympathetic ear, reassurance and comfort.

In a more formal sense, social support is built into healthcare through the use of support groups, group therapy and group-based education. These are important vehicles for healthcare that have been far under-recognised by practitioners and the healthcare system alike. There are formal and informal support groups related to just about any condition. Support groups are generally built on a few basic principles.

- Participants have a common bond, whether it is having the same medical condition or confronting the same life issue.
- Formal programs are most often run by trained health carers and counsellors. Some successful groups can be run by the participants themselves.
- Support programs can provide participants with access to information, skills and services.
- They provide a safe place for participants to share concerns as well as insights, motivation and the celebration of breakthroughs.
- Support programs can be confronting for some people and so one-on-one support may be more appropriate in these circumstances.

Doctors interested in running support programs or group-based activities would be advised to receive further training in these approaches as they require different skills in facilitation and communication than those required for individually delivered interventions.

Accessing information is one of the most important reasons for accessing support. Studies suggest that the most important information sources are doctors, but family members, nurses, friends, the internet, other medical personnel and other patients are also very important sources.[38] Information technology is becoming an increasingly important means of accessing support and information, although it has its risks and is no substitute for people connecting personally. In spite of this limitation, the internet may play an important and beneficial role, particularly for young people who are reluctant to speak to healthcare professionals.[39] It can also be a cost-efficient way of delivering services to an audience who would otherwise not access them.

Incidental social support is provided in an informal way through one's daily social interactions, employment, being a member of an organisation or club and by being a member of a family. An approach to dealing with any health issue should include an examination of the extent and quality of the person's social interactions and an exploration of how to improve their quality and possibly their quantity.

RESOURCES

Goleman D. Emotional intelligence. New York: Bantam Books; 2006.

Peterson C. A primer in positive psychology. New York: Oxford University Press; 2006.

Psychology Today, http://www.psychologytoday.com/topics/relationships

Relationships Australia, http://www.relationships.com.au/

Relationships Help Online, http://www.relationshiphelponline.com.au/

REFERENCES

1 Miller M, Rahe R. Life changes scaling for the 1990s. J Psychosom Res 1997; 43(3):279–292.

2 House JS, Landis KR, Umberson D. Social relationships and health. Science 1988; 241:540–545.

3 Lantz PM, House JS, Lepkowski JM et al. Socioeconomic factors, health behaviours, and mortality: results from a nationally representative prospective study of US adults. JAMA 1998; 279(21):1703–1708.

4 Cohen S, Doyle WJ, Turner R et al. Sociability and susceptibility to the common cold. Psychol Sci 2003; 14(5):389–395.

5 Glass TA, de Leon CM, Marottoli RA et al. Population-based study of social and productive activities as

predictors of survival among elderly Americans. BMJ 1999; 319:478–483.
6 Hemingway H, Marmot M. Evidence-based cardiology: psychosocial factors in the aetiology and prognosis of coronary heart disease. Systematic review of prospective cohort studies. BMJ 1999; 318(7196):1460–1467.
7 Berkman L, Leo-Summers L, Horwitz R. Emotional support and survival after AMI: a prospective population-based study of the elderly. Ann Int Med 1992; 117:1003–1009.
8 Ruberman W, Weinblatt E. Goldberg JD et al. Psychosocial influences on mortality after AMI. N Engl J Med 1984; 311:552–559.
9 Hemingway H, Marmot M. Evidence-based cardiology: psychosocial factors in the aetiology and prognosis of coronary heart disease. Systematic review of prospective cohort studies. BMJ 1999; 318(7196):1460–1467.
10 McKelvey R, Davies L, Pfaff J et al. Psychological distress and suicidal ideation among 15–24 year olds presenting to a general practice: a pilot study. ANZ J Psychiatry 1998; 32(3):344–348.
11 Resnick MD, Bearman P, Blum R et al. Protecting adolescents from harm; findings from the National Longitudinal Study on Adolescent Health. JAMA 1997; 278(10):823–832.
12 Lantz PM, House JS, Lepkowski JM et al. Socioeconomic factors, health behaviours, and mortality: results from a nationally representative prospective study of US adults. JAMA 1998; 279:1703–1708.
13 Forero R, McLellan L, Rissel C et al. Bullying behaviour and psychosocial health among school students in New South Wales, Australia: cross-sectional survey. BMJ 1999; 319:344–351.
14 Bushman BJ, Baumeister RF, Stack AD. Catharsis, aggression and persuasive influence: self-fulfilling or self-defeating prophecies? J Pers Soc Psychol 1999; 76:367–376.
15 Iribarren C, Sidney S, Bild DE et al. Association of hostility with coronary artery calcification in young adults: the CARDIA study. Coronary artery risk development in young adults. JAMA 2000; 283(19):2546–2551.
16 Kiecolt-Glaser J, Newton T. Marriage and health: his and hers. Psychol Bull 2001; 127(4):472–503.
17 King M, Bartlett A. What same sex civil partnerships may mean for health. J Epidemiol Community Health 2006; 60(3):188–191.
18 Litwak E, Messeri P. Organizational theory, social supports, and mortality rates: a theoretical convergence. Am Sociological Rev 1989; 54:49–66.
19 Ross C, Mirowsky J, Goldsteen K. The impact of the family on health: the decade in review. J Marriage Fam 1990; 52:1059–1078.
20 Hibbard JH, Pope CR. The quality of social roles as predictors of morbidity and mortality. Soc Sci Med 1993; 36:217–225.
21 Beach SRH, Fincham FD, Katz J. Marital therapy in the treatment of depression: toward a third generation of therapy and research. Clin Psychol Rev 1998; 18:635–661.
22 Lee C, Gramotnev H. Life transitions and mental health in a national cohort of young Australian women. Dev Psychol 2007; 43(4):877–888.
23 Glenn ND, Weaver CN. The contribution of marital happiness to global happiness. J Marriage Fam 1981; 43:161–168.
24 Hooley JM, Teasdale JD. Predictors of relapse in unipolar depressives: expressed emotion, marital distress, and perceived criticism. J Abnormal Psychol 1989; 98:229–235.
25 Whitton SW, Olmos-Gallo PA, Stanley SM et al. Depressive symptoms in early marriage: predictions from relationship confidence and negative marital interaction. J Fam Psychol 2007; 21(2):297–306.
26 Carels RA, Sherwood A, Blumenthal JA. Psychosocial influences on blood pressure during daily life. Int J Psychophysiol 1998; 28:117–129.
27 Jaffe DH, Manor O, Eisenbach Z et al. The protective effect of marriage on mortality in a dynamic society. Ann Epidemiol 2007; 17(7):540–547.
28 Hart CL, Hole DJ, Lawlor DA et al. Effect of conjugal bereavement on mortality of the bereaved spouse in participants of the Renfrew/Paisley Study. J Epidemiol Comm Health 2007; 61(5):455–460.
29 Orth-Gomér K, Wamala SP, Horsten M et al. Marital stress worsens prognosis in women with coronary heart disease: the Stockholm Female Coronary Risk Study. JAMA 2000; 284:3008–3014.
30 Phillips AC, Carroll D, Burns VE et al. Bereavement and marriage are associated with antibody response to influenza vaccination in the elderly. Brain Behav Immun 2006; 20(3):279–289.
31 Verbrugge L. Sex differentials in health. Public Health Rep 1982; 97:417–437.
32 Kiecolt-Glaser JK, Fisher LK, Oqricki P et al. Marital quality, marital disruption and immune function. Psychosom Med 1987; 50:213–229.
33 Kiecolt-Glaser JK, Kennedy S, Malkoff S et al. Marital discord and immunity in males. Psychosom Med 1988; 50:213–229.
34 Kiecolt-Glaser JK. Stress, personal relationships, and immune function: health implications. Brain Behav Immun 1999; 13:61–72.
35 Goodwin S. The marital relationship and health in women with chronic fatigue and immune dysfunction syndrome: views of wives and husbands. Nurs Res 1997; 46:138–146.

36 Flor H, Breitenstein C, Birbaumer N et al. A psychophysiological analysis of spouse solicitousness towards pain behaviors, spouse interaction, and pain perception. Behav Ther 1995; 26:255–272.
37 Spiegel D, Sephton SE, Terr AI et al. Effects of psychosocial treatment in prolonging cancer survival may be mediated by neuroimmune pathways. Ann NY Acad Sci 1998; 840:674–683.
38 Pecchioni LL, Sparks L. Health information sources of individuals with cancer and their family members. Health Comm 2007; 21(2):143–151.
39 Heinicke BE, Paxton SJ, McLean SA et al. Internet-delivered targeted group intervention for body dissatisfaction and disordered eating in adolescent girls: a randomized controlled trial. J Abnorm Child Psychol 2007; 35(3):379–391.

chapter 12

Spirituality

INTRODUCTION AND OVERVIEW

'Spirituality' means different things to different individuals and there is no one way of exploring or expressing it. The search for meaning is ubiquitous to humankind, and being able to make meaning of life, and especially adversity, can have an enormously protective effect on people's mental health when coping with major life events. Most commonly, people take spirituality and religion to be synonymous, but there are many other ways, aside from religious practice, of exploring and expressing spirituality—through philosophical enquiry, the pursuit of science, creativity, relationships, environmentalism, altruism and social justice, to name a few.

Spirituality, in the broad sense described above, is relevant to healthcare because it has a direct impact on a range of health determinants, mental health, lifestyle choices, relationships and coping. This chapter explores the relationships between spirituality, meaning and health.

SPIRITUALITY, RELIGION AND MEANING

Most people who call themselves 'spiritual' do so within a religious context. Although religion and spirituality overlap, they are not the same thing. Because of the religious connotations, many people avoid the word 'spirituality' altogether and instead use a term such as 'meaning', as in the following quote by Jung:

> The lack of meaning in life is a soul-sickness whose full extent and full import our age has not yet begun to comprehend.
>
> Carl Jung[1]

The terms most commonly used in the medical and psychological literature examining these phenomena are 'religious commitment' or 'religiosity', which refer to the 'participation in or endorsement of practices, beliefs, attitudes, or sentiments that are associated with an organised community of faith'.[2] One can be 'extrinsically religious' by adopting the trappings of religious behaviours and attitudes, but holding a strong commitment to a religious ideology or core values is associated with being 'intrinsically religious'. Intrinsic religiosity is more protective for mental health than extrinsic religiosity. 'Spirituality' overlaps with intrinsic religiosity and refers to things that are hard to define and measure, such as 'personal views and behaviours that express a sense of relatedness to the transcendental dimension or to something greater than the self'.[3] It can encompass things such as a belief in a higher being, meaning, purpose and connectedness.

It is important that patients, and doctors for that matter, define, explore and express 'spirituality' or 'meaning' in a way that is relevant to one's own views, culture and background. Whatever our background, an active search for meaning is an integral part of what makes us human and able to cope with adversity. Everybody looks for meaning in one way or another—through, for example:

- meaningful relationships and how we respect others around us
- contributing to the world through our work
- a sense of connectedness with others in the community
- science and the pursuit of knowledge in all its forms
- respect for social justice, morality and human rights.

The search for meaning helps to keep individuals and communities healthy.[4] It is the lens through which we look at the world.

In the following discussion, the terms 'religious commitment', 'religiosity' and 'churchgoers' are used because they are the terms used in the research. The findings should be taken in the context of the above discussion about religion, spirituality and meaning.

SPIRITUALITY, MENTAL HEALTH AND SUICIDE

In view of predictions that depression will soon be the leading burden of disease[5] and the escalating trends in youth suicide rates,[6] there may be too little attention being given to the protective factors against mental illness. One important protective factor for mental health is a sense of meaning, spirituality or religion. It has become increasingly clear in reviews of the literature that spirituality has a positive impact on social, mental and emotional health.[7,8] Therefore, a possible contributing factor to the widespread decline in mental health in developed and materially wealthy societies is a lack of meaning and spiritual fulfillment. Whether it is the cause or a marker for other phenomena is hard to say. This is seen among doctors as well as in the general public. Doctors who rate themselves as having lower levels of spiritual wellbeing are more prone to depression and poor health.[9]

Studies suggest that most doctors believe religion and spirituality (R/S) has a significant influence on health[10] and that R/S:

- often helps patients to cope
- gives patients a positive state of mind
- provides emotional and practical support via the religious community.

Doctors with high religiosity are substantially more likely to:

- report that patients often mention R/S issues
- believe that R/S strongly influences health
- interpret the influence of R/S in positive rather than negative ways.

Among doctors, the least likely to have religious beliefs are psychiatrists. Psychiatrists are also more likely to call themselves spiritual but not religious. Doctors with strong religious beliefs are less likely to refer patients to psychiatrists and more likely to refer patients to clergy or religious counsellors for mental health problems.[11] The ignoring of issues related to religion, meaning and spirituality is reflected in medical and psychological education and practice, where religious issues are often marginalised or pathologised.[12] This has been entrenched for some time. Freud, for example, described religion as 'a universal obsessional neurosis' and the 'mystical experience of unity' as a 'regression to primary narcissism'.[13] Jung, one of the early pioneers of a more modern approach to psychotherapy, saw the search for meaning as the central human motivation. Some people undoubtedly have significantly negative experiences in their religious life and upbringing, and religious content is not uncommonly a part of psychosis. Furthermore, although most mainstream religious groups, and the individuals who are a part of them, tend to be moderate and tolerant in their practices and integration into multicultural societies, some religious groups and individuals do tend towards aggressive and intolerant forms of fundamentalism.[14] Such an expression of religiosity appeals to some of the more alienated members of the community and has produced some of the most aggressive and difficult to understand crimes in modern times. Despite this, there is gathering evidence confirming the overall protective effect of 'religiosity' on mental and physical health, and it will be a significant aspect of many patients' ability to cope with and recover from illness. According to large population studies of adolescents, among the most important of protective factors are 'connectedness' and 'spirituality'.[15]

Unfortunately, the negative attitude in many quarters of contemporary medicine and psychiatry is out of keeping with the weight of evidence, which clearly shows that having a healthy spiritual life is beneficial for mental and physical health. The findings are consistent, whether the studies are prospective (following people forward over time) or retrospective (looking back at the past). The relationship seems to hold whether the studies control for other lifestyle and socioeconomic factors or not. It seems to hold whether the studies examine the prevention of, coping with or recovery from illness. Causal relationships between religiosity and good health are sometimes hard to be sure about, but it is certain that something is going on. However, it must be acknowledged that, in cases where a religion or member of the clergy has been responsible for negative experiences, alternative expressions of spirituality that do not include organised religion are likely to be of greater value to that individual.

A number of studies link a lack of religiosity to depression. Religious commitment is associated with a reduced incidence of[16] and significantly faster recovery from depression for the elderly.[17] Those with high levels of 'religious involvement', 'religious salience' and 'intrinsic religious motivation' are at reduced risk of depression.[18] Furthermore, religious commitment is inversely related to suicide risk,[19,20] including risk in those with a comorbidity such as childhood abuse[21] and psychosis.[22] There is a fourfold increased risk for adolescent suicide for 'non-churchgoers' compared to regular attendees.[23] No study has shown an increased risk for people with a regular spiritual or religious dimension to their lives. Despite the overall positive associations between spirituality and mental health, some questions still remain to be resolved. For example, Sorri and colleagues[24] found a high incidence of intense religious activity in 18% of suicide victims, as well as a greater severity of mental illness in either deeply religious or completely non-religious suicide victims. This contrasts with the findings of Krause,[25] which suggest that self-esteem was highest in highly religious and non-religious groups, but was lowest in those of intermediate religious devotion. The explanation for some of this might lie in how things like 'intense religious activity' (e.g. obsessive and anxiety-driven adherence to strict religious doctrines and practices) and 'highly religious' (e.g. religion is a deep and integrated part of a person's life) are defined. The issue of the role of religious commitment to mental health is consequently far from being settled.[26]

SPIRITUALITY AND SUBSTANCE ABUSE

Studies suggest that religiosity protects against drug and alcohol abuse,[27] one of the most commonly used and maladaptive ways of dealing with mental health problems. The risk of substance abuse is probably increased two- to threefold for those without a religious dimension to their lives. One study showed that 89% of alcoholics had lost interest in religious issues in their teenage years, whereas among those without an alcohol problem only 20% had lost interest.[28] Doctors are also a high-risk group for substance abuse. Religious commitment while in medical school has been found to be protective against the development of an alcohol problem in later life.[29]

Religious affiliation, even where alcohol abuse has become a problem, protects against extremely heavy use with all its associated extreme health and social consequences. For those recovering from substance abuse, greater spiritual or religious involvement, interest or practice can have a positive effect on recovery. Programs based on such principles as Alcoholics Anonymous and the 12-Step Program can be beneficial for appropriately motivated patients,[30,31] although such programs will not be of benefit to all.[32] Adolescents can also benefit from programs that include meaning or spiritually focused content.[33]

PHYSICAL HEALTH

The significant role that a spiritual life plays in fostering good mental health, healthy lifestyle and the ability to cope with adversity goes part of the way to explaining why it is also associated with reduced risk for physical illnesses such as hypertension, heart disease and cancer,[34–37] and with a longer life expectancy (Box 12.1). A population study over 9 years showed that death from all causes was significantly reduced and life expectancy increased (75 years versus 82 years) for those who attended church regularly. Again, these findings were not entirely explainable by accepted lifestyle and social variables.[38,39] Although most of this research has been carried out in Western countries, if studies were done in other countries with other religious or spiritual traditions they would probably produce similar findings.

BOX 12.1 Summary of currently studied relationships between spirituality and health

- Mental and social health
- Reduced incidence of depression
- Faster recovery from depression
- Recovery from major surgery with less depression
- Improved coping with disability,[40] illness and stress[41]
- Reduced substance abuse, including alcohol and illicit drugs
- Facilitation of psychotherapy
- Improved palliative care outcomes
- Greater social support
- Physical health
- Reduced all-cause mortality and greater longevity
- Reduced incidence of heart disease and hypertension
- Improved recovery from cardiac surgery[42]
- Reduced incidence of and longer survival with cancer (e.g. bowel cancer)
- Modification of physical risk factors with associated reductions in lifestyle-related illnesses such as emphysema and cirrhosis

BRAIN SCIENCES AND SPIRITUALITY

Some say that spiritual experiences can simply be explained as chemical and electrical changes in the brain. Biological and neural correlates of spiritual experiences have been identified through functional MRI and, to an extent, can be artificially induced through drugs or electrical stimulation. During religious recitation, religious subjects activate areas of the prefrontal and parietal cortex.[43] Activity in the temporal lobes of the brain is also associated with a number of religious and psychological phenomena, including blurring of interpersonal or ego boundaries.[44,45] Whether the neurological changes are the cause of psychological or spiritual phenomena or the effect of them is a source of ongoing debate.

WHY MIGHT SPIRITUALITY BE PROTECTIVE?

Having an active spiritual life can protect people against various problems by:

- providing a high level of social connectedness and support through a religious group

- making the person more likely to receive positive messages about healthy living
- reducing exposure to violence or drug-taking behaviour
- disposing towards more supportive parenting styles
- helping the person to deal more effectively with mental health and relationship issues
- providing a buffer against stressful life events
- enabling the person to find meaning in adverse life events
- providing explanations for problems and events (although metaphysical explanations are harder to validate scientifically).

Religious experience is among the hardest fields of psychology and sociology to study because it is not easily defined, isolated and measured.

RELEVANCE TO CLINICAL MEDICINE

Spirituality has tended to sit uneasily alongside medical science and practice. Valid concerns and questions arise as to the appropriate level and manner of spiritual content in medical consultations. Overall, spiritual issues tend not to be discussed between doctors and patients, perhaps because doctors believe that these issues have little impact upon physical and mental health, that it would be unscientific to discuss them, or that having such discussions is the role of someone more specifically trained to deal with them. However, evidence suggests that most patients wish to discuss spiritual issues with their doctors in particular situations, such as when dealing with major and life-threatening illness. Over four out of five people:

> wanted physicians to ask about spiritual beliefs in at least some circumstances. The most acceptable scenarios for spiritual discussion were life-threatening illnesses (77%), serious medical conditions (74%) and loss of loved ones (70%). Among those who wanted to discuss spirituality, the most important reason for discussion was desire for physician–patient understanding (87%). Patients believed that information concerning their spiritual beliefs would affect physicians' ability to encourage realistic hope (67%), give medical advice (66%), and change medical treatment (62%).[46]

This suggests that, from a patient's perspective at least, spiritual issues are very relevant to the doctor–patient relationship.

Some of the key points about the interaction between spiritual issues and medicine are identified by D'Souza as follows:[47]

- There is a need to incorporate the spiritual and religious dimension of patients into their management.
- By keeping patients' beliefs, spiritual/religious needs and supports separate from their care, we are potentially ignoring an important element that may be at the core of patients' coping and support systems and may be integral to their wellbeing and recovery.
- Doctors and clinicians should not 'prescribe' religious beliefs or activities or impose their religious or spiritual beliefs on patients. The task of in-depth religious counselling of patients is best done by trained clergy.
- In considering the spiritual dimension of the patient, the clinician is sending an important message that he or she is concerned with the whole person. This enhances the patient–physician relationship and is likely to increase the therapeutic impact of interventions.
- Doctors, health care professionals and mental health clinicians should be required to learn about the ways in which religion and culture can influence patients' needs and recovery.

Unfortunately, a perceived lack of holism is a central reason that many patients look outside the biomedical model for their healthcare.[48] Gauging a patient's spiritual interests and involvement, or exploring the ways in which they search for meaning, should form an important part of a thorough medical history, especially when dealing with mental health issues and major illness. One cannot really be said to know another person well without considering such questions. Approaching the management of conditions like depression or terminal illness will take place without an understanding of a person's deepest motivations, fears and hopes.

A consensus panel of the American College of Physicians suggested four simple questions that physicians could ask patients:[49]

- Is faith (religion and spirituality) important to you?
- Has faith been important to you at other times in your life?
- Do you have someone to talk to about religious matters?
- Would you like to explore religious and spiritual matters with someone?

Four basic considerations should be kept in mind when taking a spiritual history:[50]

- Does the patient use religion or spirituality to help cope with illness or is it a source of stress, and how?
- Is the patient a member of a supportive spiritual community?
- Does the patient have any troubling spiritual questions or concerns?
- Does the patient have any spiritual beliefs that might influence their medical care?

Broaching philosophical and spiritual issues within the medical consultation obviously requires skill and sensitivity on the part of the doctor. It also requires courage, trust and openness on the part of the patient. It cannot take place meaningfully and successfully without cultural tolerance and the ability to be non-dogmatic. When done effectively it facilitates counselling and psychotherapy.[51] Each patient needs to explore spiritual issues in their own way.

If a doctor is not religious, it does not relieve them of the responsibility to respectfully enquire about such issues. It is then up to the patient as to how far they take the conversation. Part of inviting discussion in a respectful way is the doctor taking care not to push a line of thought, whether it be religious or secular. Religious, spiritual or philosophical sensitivities and biases can make discussion divisive and difficult. If significant spiritual or religious issues are uncovered then the doctor may be able to direct the patient to the best avenue for follow-up. More in-depth questions about spirituality and religion should be referred to culturally appropriate 'non-medical experts'.

THE SEARCH FOR MEANING

Science without religion is lame, religion without science is blind.

Albert Einstein

For many, especially the young, the search for meaning is becoming a rarer commodity, in the hustle and bustle of modern life with its increasing focus on material concerns. There is an obvious need for balance between material concerns and those related to meaning and values.

The search for meaning is a basic human need, and a prerequisite for growth and understanding. It is the firm foundation upon which we build resilience and gives life its richness, direction and fulfillment. There are many ways of searching for meaning, but it is up to each of us to search for it in a way that is meaningful to us. We all make meaning out of what happens to us, whether we are aware of it or not. Even the vigorous questioning of religious assumptions or dogma is an active search for meaning. It simply means that it is being sought through enquiry, reason and the search for knowledge.

RESOURCES

Cox R, Ervin-Cox B, Hoffman L. (eds) Spirituality and psychological health. Colorado Springs: Colorado School of Professional Psychology Press; 2005.

Duke University Center for Spirituality, Theology and Health,. http://www.spiritualityandhealth.duke.edu/

Journal of Religion and Health, http://www.springer.com/public+health/journal/10943

Koenig H, McCullough M, Larson D. Handbook of religion and health. New York: Oxford University Press; 2001.

Psychology Today. 'Spirituality', http://www.psychologytoday.com/articles/199909/spirituality

REFERENCES

1 Jung C. Jung on synchronicity and the paranormal. London: Routledge; 1997:145.

2 Matthews D, McCullough M, Larson D et al. Religious commitment and health status: a review of the research and implications for family medicine. Arch Fam Med 1998; 7(2):118–124.

3 Reed P. Spirituality and wellbeing in terminally ill hospitalised patients. Res Nurs Health 1987; 9:35–41.

4 Hassed C. Depression: dispirited or spiritually deprived? Med J Aust 2000; 173(10):545–547.

5 Murray C, Lopez A. The global burden of disease. World Health Organization; 1996.

6 Cantor C, Neulinger K, De Leo D. Australian suicide trends 1964–1997: youth and beyond? Med J Aust 1999; 171:137–141.

7 Matthews D, McCullough M, Larson D et al. Religious commitment and health status: a review of the research and implications for family medicine. Arch Fam Med 1998; 7(2):118–124.

8 Moreira-Almeida A, Neto FL, Koenig HG. Religiousness and mental health: a review. Rev Bras Psiquiatr 2006; 28(3):242–250.

9 Yi MS, Mrus JM, Mueller CV et al. Self-rated health of primary care house officers and its relationship to psychological and spiritual well-being. BMC Med Educ 2007; 7:9.

10 Curlin FA, Sellergren SA, Lantos JD et al. Physicians' observations and interpretations of the influence of religion and spirituality on health. Arch Intern Med 2007; 167(7):649–654.

11 Curlin FA, Odell SV, Lawrence RE et al. The relationship between psychiatry and religion among US physicians. Psychiatr Serv 2007; 58(9):1193–1198.

12 Lukoff D, Fu F, Turner R. Cultural considerations in the assessment and treatment of religious and spiritual problems. Psychiatr Clin North Am 1995; 18(3):467–484.

13 Freud S. Obsessive actions and religious practices. In: Sigmund Freud: the standard edition, vol. 9. Trans JA Strachey. London: Hogarth Press; 1959.

14 Hartz G, Everett H. Fundamentalist religion and its effect on mental health. J Relig Health 1989; 28(3):207–217.

15 Resnick M, Bearman P, Blum R et al. Protecting adolescents from harm; findings from the National Longitudinal Study on Adolescent Health. JAMA 1997; 278(10):823–832.

16 Gartner J, Larson D, Allen G. Religious commitment and mental health: a review of the empirical literature. J Psychol Theol 1991; 19:6–25.

17 Koenig H, George L, Perterson B. Religiosity and remission of depression in medically ill older patients. Am J Psychiatry 1998; 155:536–542.

18 McCullough M, Larson D. Religion and depression: a review of the literature. Twin Research 1999; 2(2): 126–136.

19 Gartner J, Larson D, Allen G. Religious commitment and mental health: a review of the empirical literature. J Psychol Theol 1991; 19:6–25.

20 Gonda X, Fountoulakis KN, Kaprinis G et al. Prediction and prevention of suicide in patients with unipolar depression and anxiety. Ann Gen Psychiatry 2007; 6(1):23.

21 Dervic K, Grunebaum MF, Burke AK et al. Protective factors against suicidal behavior in depressed adults reporting childhood abuse. J Nerv Ment Dis 2006; 194(12):971–974.

22 Huguelet P, Mohr S, Jung V et al. Effect of religion on suicide attempts in outpatients with schizophrenia or schizo-affective disorders compared with inpatients with non-psychotic disorders. Eur Psychiatry 2007; 22(3):188–194.

23 Comstock G, Partridge K. Church attendance and health. J Chronic Dis 1972; 25:665–672.

24 Sorri H, Henriksson M, Lionnqvist J. Religiosity and suicide: findings from a nationwide psychological autopsy study. Crisis 1996; 17(3):123–127.

25 Krause N. Religiosity and self-esteem among older adults. J Gerontol B Psychol Sci Soc Sci 1995; 50(5):236–246.

26 Glenn C. Relationship of mental health to religiosity. McGill J Med 1997; 3(2):86–92. Online. Available: http://www.medicine.mcgill.ca/mjm/v03n02/v03p086/v03p086main.htm

27 Koenig HG, McCullough M, Larson DB. Handbook of religion and health: a century of research reviewed. New York: Oxford University Press; 2001.

28 Larson D, Wilson W. The religious life of alcoholics. South Med J 1980; 73:723–727.

29 Moore R, Mead L, Pearson T. Youthful precursors of alcohol abuse in physicians. Am J Med 1990; 88: 332–336.

30 Brown AE, Pavlik VN, Shegog R et al. Association of spirituality and sobriety during a behavioral spirituality intervention for Twelve Step (TS) recovery. Am J Drug Alcohol Abuse 2007; 33(4):611–617.

31 Piderman KM, Schneekloth TD, Pankratz VS et al. Spirituality in alcoholics during treatment. Am J Addict 2007; 16(3):232–237.

32 Galanter M. Spirituality and addiction: a research and clinical perspective. Am J Addict 2006; 15(4):286–292.

33 Hopkins GL, McBride D, Marshak HH et al. Developing healthy kids in healthy communities: eight evidence-based strategies for preventing high-risk behaviour. Med J Aust 2007; 186(Suppl 10):S70–S73.

34 Fraser G, Sharlik D. Risk factors for all-cause and coronary heart disease mortality in the oldest old: the Adventist's Health Study. Arch Intern Med 1997; 157(19):2249–2258.

35 Levin J, Vanderpool H. Is frequent religious attendance really conducive to better health? Toward an epidemiology of religion. Soc Sci Med 1987; 24: 589–600.

36 Kune G, Kune S, Watson L. Perceived religiousness is protective for colorectal cancer: data from the Melbourne Colorectal Cancer Study. J R Soc Med 1993; 86:645–647.

37 Craigie F, Larson D, Liu I. References to religion in the Journal of Family Practice: dimensions and valency of spirituality. J Fam Pract 1990; 30:477–480.

38 Hummer R, Rogers R, Nam C. et al. Religious involvement and US adult mortality. Demography 1999; 36(2):273–285.

39 Clark K, Friedman H, Martin L. A longitudinal study of religiosity and mortality risk. J Health Psychol 1999; 4(3):381–391.

40 Koenig H, Cohen H, Blazer D et al. Religious coping and depression in elderly, hospitalised medically-ill men. Am J Psychiatry 1992; 149:1693–1700.

41 Williams D, Larson D, Buckler R et al. Religion and psychological distress in a community sample. Soc Sci Med 1991; 32:1257–1262.

42 Oxman T, Freeman D, Manheimer E. Lack of social participation or religious strength and comfort as risk factors for death after cardiac surgery in the elderly. Psychosom Med 1995; 57:5–15.

43 Azari NP, Nickel J, Wunderlich G et al. Neural correlates of religious experience. Eur J Neurosci 2001; 13(8):1649–1652.

44 Persinger MA. Preadolescent religious experience enhances temporal lobe signs in normal young adults. Percept Mot Skills 1991; 72(2):453–454.

45 Beauregard M, Paquette V. Neural correlates of a mystical experience in Carmelite nuns. Neurosci Lett 2006; 405(3):186–190.

46 McCord G, Gilchrist VJ, Grossman SD et al. Discussing spirituality with patients: a rational and ethical approach. Ann Fam Med 2004; 2(4):356–361.

47 D'Souza R. The importance of spirituality in medicine and its application to clinical practice. Med J Aust 2007; 186(Suppl 10):S57–S59.

48 Astin J. Why patients use alternative medicine: results of a national study. JAMA 1998; 279(19): 1548–1553.

49 Lo B, Quill T, Tulsky J. Discussing palliative care with patients. Ann Intern Med 1999; 130:744–749.

50 Koenig HG. Espiritualidade no Cuidado com o Paciente. São Paulo: Editora FE; 2005.

51 Hassed C. Western psychology meets Eastern philosophy. Aust Fam Physician 1999; 28(10): 1057–1058.

chapter 13

Screening and prevention

INTRODUCTION AND OVERVIEW

Although the healthcare system still tends to undervalue and under-fund preventive medicine and health promotion, there has nevertheless been a growing recognition of the need to undertake preventive activities and screening within primary healthcare. General practitioners are well placed to be at the forefront of these activities because of their long-term and regular contact with patients and families, providing avenues for both opportunistic and structured approaches.

Preventive and screening activities require informed, disciplined and motivated patients as well as doctors. It also requires the support of reliable systems for recording data and sending reminders. Respective colleges in Australia through the RACGP,[1] and in the United Kingdom, United States and many other countries, along with the World Health Organization,[2] have actively reviewed evidence and made recommendations for best practice in screening and preventive activities. This chapter attempts to distill some of the key points raised by these recommendations.

PREVENTION

There are three main levels of prevention.

- *Primary*—the aim is to prevent an illness before it has got under way, such as through the promotion of healthy lifestyle and nutrition to prevent bowel cancer. Here the cost/benefit ratio tends to be most favourable but it can be difficult to motivate patients who are still 'well' to make the changes required to prevent an illness many years hence. Here the side effects of lifestyle change are beneficial.
- *Secondary*—the aim is to identify an illness early in its development before it has caused significant symptoms and while it is still reversible, such as the early detection of bowel cancer with faecal occult blood measurement or colonoscopy. This is where most funding for prevention and screening is directed within the healthcare system.
- *Tertiary*—here the condition is well under way and causing symptoms. Now the aim is to prevent further recurrence and complications through more radical treatments, such as for advanced bowel cancer. Here the cost/benefit ratio is least favourable and the side effects of treatment can be considerable.

PATIENT EDUCATION

Helping patients to make healthy change in their lives is one aspect of clinical medicine that requires as much art as science. Factors that enhance this process include:[3]

- *health literacy* and making sure the message is appropriate to the patient's education level, language skills and cultural background
- the *doctor–patient relationship*, which is based on trust and mutual agreement
- provision of *enabling strategies* such as stress management, goal setting, the cycle of change and behavioural strategies (see Ch 7, Behaviour change, for more details)
- *communication* skills and methods such as a face-to-face delivery, providing the opportunity to ask questions, reinforcing key messages, using motivational interviewing skills and clarifying concerns and misconceptions
- consideration of the *costs and benefits* for changing or not changing the given behaviour
- *individualising advice* to better manage the behavioural enhancers and barriers
- *managing relapse* and reframing it as a learning opportunity rather than a failure
- the use of *decision aids* and reading materials such as *patient education* sheets.

SCREENING

Screening, whether through physical examination (e.g. blood pressure, random blood glucose) or special tests (e.g. mammography, colonoscopy), is the mainstay of preventive activities within general practice. Which tests to order, how often to perform them and for whom—and whether to order them at all—are far from clear-cut. Guidelines often shift with each new study that comes out, making decisions difficult for clinicians and patients.

Research must determine whether there are significant gains to be made that outweigh the costs to the patient and community in terms of time, emotional and physical discomfort, side effects and monetary expense, before a test can be widely recommended and funded. These issues may also need to be addressed with an individual patient in order for them to have a positive attitude to screening activities. In other words, the case for screening needs to be made—it should not be assumed that a patient will wish to follow guidelines just because they are there.

The WHO recommends that for a screening activity to be widely taken up, it should be identifying important health *conditions* (i.e. common, disabling and/or life-threatening) where there is a window of opportunity between latency and clinical manifestation. The *test* should be simple, as uninvasive as possible, safe, accurate and supported by evidence. *Treatment* for the health condition should be available and have been demonstrated to have a beneficial outcome. The *outcomes* should be of benefit in terms of morbidity or mortality, the benefits should outweigh the side effects and it should be cost-effective.

There are many shades of grey in answering these questions and in deciding who, where and when people are screened. Ultimately, it is the patient who will make their own informed choice as to whether to accept the guidelines or their doctor's advice, and so although guidelines are useful, they will need to be individualised for each patient. A very anxious patient, for example, may be a candidate for screening at an earlier age than someone less anxious. Furthermore, guidelines may vary between various groups in the community (e.g. taking into account the relevance of ethnic background or socioeconomic status) as to who may be at greater or lesser risk.

Specific recommendations on screening for various conditions in children and adults are given in the charts in *Guidelines for Preventive Activities Over the Lifecycle*, which can be downloaded and/or printed for use in the patient records (see the Resources list at the end of this chapter). The charts provide an excellent summary that can be used to help to keep track of which examinations and tests have been done and what the key findings were. Further details regarding each of these activities can also be explored on the RACGP *Red Book* (page numbers are given on the charts), which can also be downloaded and/or printed.

ISSUES IN PREVENTION AND SCREENING

This section comments on some specific issues in relation to particular conditions or patient groups. Other chapters also have content on this topic—see, for example, the chapters on sexual health (Ch 61), cardiovascular disease (Ch 25), diabetes (Ch 26), cancer (Ch 24) and psychiatry and psychology (Ch 40).

PREGNANCY

Apart from the usual medical care and attention to gynaecological history, a number of factors need attention prior to and during pregnancy. These include:

- history of previous pregnancies, past medical history, blood pressure, blood glucose level, BMI, periodontal disease, thyroid function, family history of genetic illnesses
- vaccinations (e.g. varicella, hepatitis B, diphtheria/tetanus/pertussis, rubella, measles, mumps); other immunisation screening
- folic acid—an adequate intake from diet and supplementation (0.5 mg daily) at least a month before planned pregnancy
- healthy weight—achieve and maintain a healthy weight range prior to conception
- healthy diet—a nutritionally rich diet based on whole foods and including sources of omega-3 fatty acids, iron and essential vitamins and minerals; a discussion about a pre-conception multivitamin and mineral supplement is advisable
- regular, moderate, aerobic physical exercise, and specific exercises aimed at flexibility and relaxation
- adequate vitamin D—regular, moderate sunlight, and vitamin D supplements if vitamin D deficient
- good mental health—poor mental health and chronic stress can both affect fetal development as well as maternal wellbeing
- social and emotional support, and an exploration of parenting philosophies
- avoiding cigarettes and alcohol altogether during pregnancy
- avoiding environmental exposure to infections such as toxoplasmosis (sources include garden soil, uncooked meat, unpasteurised milk), cytomegalovirus (CMV sources include dirty hands, soiled nappies; risk for healthcare workers) and listeriosis (sources include pâté, soft cheeses, delicatessen meats, chilled seafood)

- (consider) taking a regular supplement of omega-3 fatty acids, especially so for women choosing to avoid seafood during pregnancy
- avoiding unnecessary medications and over-the-counter preparations; if any are taken, ensure they are safe during pregnancy.

CHILDREN

The health and development of children is exquisitely affected by the family as well as the educational, cultural and environmental milieu within which the child is raised. The prevention or management of illnesses in children should therefore never be in isolation from these factors, particularly parenting and schooling. If parents, particularly mothers, are at risk, then children are at risk. Preventive issues therefore involve:

- parental education and support, including:
  - screening mothers for postnatal depression, and both parents for substance abuse
  - screening for neglect or mistreatment—the presence or absence of local laws on the mandatory reporting of such problems need to be considered
  - provision of advice, particularly for first-time mothers, on accident and injury prevention, especially for young children (e.g. stair guards, fire alarms, electric socket protectors, fire guards, safe storage of poisons and medications, water safety and monitoring, car safety and appropriate car restraints, bike helmets and safety in the kitchen)
- keeping up to date with immunisations
- according to the skin type, time of year and environment, following guidelines on safe sun exposure, taking care to avoid inadequate sun exposure as well as sunburn or excessive sun exposure
- weight and nutritional management:
  - educating the parents as well as the children, especially when parents are overweight
  - promoting breastfeeding
  - promoting daily physical activity and recommending limiting 'screen time' (television and computer) during leisure time to 2 hours per day
  - promoting a nutritious whole-food diet (everyday foods) and limiting empty calories, fast food and processed food (sometimes foods)
  - preferring water to sweet soft-drinks
  - following growth charts, BMI and pattern of fat distribution
- promoting spending meal times with the family as a very important part of enhancing connectedness
- encouraging good dental care
- regular vision and hearing assessments, especially in early childhood and school years
- being on the lookout for emerging behavioural problems—attention deficit disorder is also often used as a coverall for behavioural and family problems
- as a child gets older, providing education about avoidance of substance abuse or considering harm minimisation where necessary
- encouraging healthy 'food for the mind' as much as healthy food for the body
- developing coping and stress management skills from an early age
- developing regular and healthy sleep patterns.

GENETIC COUNSELLING AND TESTING

Current recommendations largely focus on targeted screening of at-risk individuals based on a detailed family history, association with the early onset of chronic illnesses, or illnesses within a family when they are at a far higher rate than would be expected (e.g. breast or colon cancer) in the general community. Other indications include birth-related health problems, intellectual disability, multiple stillbirths or congenital abnormalities. Genetic conditions common enough to be seen on a semi-regular basis in the primary care setting include cystic fibrosis, Down syndrome, haemachromotosis, thalassaemia and fragile-X syndrome. Where these conditions are suspected, reliable sources of information and specialist opinion should be consulted in order to confirm the diagnosis and direct treatment.

MIDDLE AGE AND OLD AGE

The preventive and screening issues for these age groups are well covered in the RACGP lifecycle chart for adults (see Resources list). The aim should be to add not just years to life, but also quality to those years. In order for people to take the time to engage in preventive activities during young adulthood and middle age—which is often the busiest time in a person's life because of work and family commitments—it is important for regular encouragement and reminders to be given, particularly for men, who are far more likely to avoid self-care and health maintenance. Particular issues for men and women are covered in the chapters on men's health (chs 48–50), and women's health (chs 51–53).

For the elderly, isolation and lack of mobility can be significant impediments to taking up preventive opportunities. Polypharmacy is also a major source of iatrogenic illness, and so review and rationalisation of medications should be a regular practice. Attitudes to ageing can also affect quality of life and the progression of chronic illnesses, and so positive attitudes to ageing should be cultivated from an early age.

INFECTIOUS DISEASES

Patterns of infectious and communicable disease vary from country to country, and laws on the notification of these diseases will also vary. Immunisation is obviously the most important preventive strategy available, although concerns arise for an increasing number of people as to which immunisations to have and how often they are really necessary. People with an interest in complementary medicine (CM) are more likely to have an anti-immunisation stance, although the great majority of people with an interest in CM do not have a negative attitude towards immunisation. This issue needs to be negotiated with each patient or parent. The most common reasons for failure of completion of immunisation schedules are system failure and patient/parent apathy or fear of adverse effects.

Doctors should be well-prepared with detailed information to address patients' concerns, as many of them will have investigated the issue extensively for themselves. Local immunisation schedules should be consulted and a reliable system of patient reminders and recall put in place. In parallel with immunisation is the behavioural and lifestyle prevention of infectious diseases. For example, good mental health is also associated with a reduced risk of infections, as are regular physical exercise, healthy nutrition and being an optimal weight.

Vector avoidance is essential along with appropriate immunisation, in prevention of travel-associated infectious diseases.

CHRONIC DISEASE PREVENTION AND SELF-MANAGEMENT

The SNAP (smoking, nutrition, alcohol and physical activity) guidelines[4] are a good starting point for the prevention and management of chronic illnesses. In this book, the ESSENCE Model (education, stress management, spirituality, exercise, nutrition, connectedness, environment) has been used and is more comprehensive because it includes environment, and psychological and social factors.[5]

The '5A's approach'[6] has been used in order to help streamline and systematise the assessment of various risk and protective factors.

- *Ask*—all patients about smoking, nutrition, alcohol or physical activity.
- *Assess*—the patient's readiness to change, and dependence (smoking and alcohol).
- *Advise*—provide brief, non-judgmental advice with patient education materials (e.g. life scripts) and motivational interviewing.
- *Assist*—by providing motivational counselling and a prescription (life script or pharmacotherapy if indicated for nicotine or alcohol dependence).
- *Arrange*—referral to telephone support services, group lifestyle programs or an individual provider (e.g. dietician or exercise physiologist) and a regular follow-up visit.

In considering the prevention or management of any particular chronic condition, the relevant chapters of this book should be consulted.

RESOURCES

American Academy of Family Physicians, guidelines on prevention, http://www.aafp.org/online/en/home/clinical/exam.html

Royal Australia College of General Practitioners (RACGP, Melbourne), guidelines for preventive activities in general practice, http://www.racgp.org.au/guidelines/redbook

UK National Health Services, UK National Screening Committee, http://www.nsc.nhs.uk/index.htm

World Health Organization. Screening for various cancers, http://www.who.int/cancer/detection/variouscancer/en/

REFERENCES

1 Royal Australian College of General Practitioners. Guidelines for preventive activities in general practice. Melbourne: RACGP; 2009. Online. Available: http://www.racgp.org.au/guidelines/redbook

2 World Health Organization. Screening for various cancers. Geneva: WHO; 2005. Online. Available: http://www.who.int/cancer/detection/various cancer/en/

3 Mullen P, Simons-Morton DG, Ramirez G et al. A meta-analysis of trials evaluating patient education and counselling for three groups of preventive health behaviours. Patient Educ Couns 1997; 32(3):159–173.

4 Royal Australian College of General Practitioners. Smoking, nutrition, alcohol and physical activity: a population health guide to behavioural risk factors for general practices. Melbourne: RACGP; 2004.

5 Hassed C. The Essence of health: the seven pillars of wellbeing. Sydney: Random House; 2008.

6 Cited in the RACGP 'Red book' (see reference 1): Dolan M, Mullen P, Simons-Morton DG et al. A meta-analysis of trials evaluating patient education and counselling for three groups of preventive health behaviours. Cochrane Database Syst Rev 1997.

chapter 14

Detoxification

INTRODUCTION AND OVERVIEW

Toxins are ubiquitous in modern life, from the air we breathe to the food we eat. Today's lifestyles and the increase in environmental pollutants have significantly increased the average person's exposure to toxins,[1] and this is placing new demands on natural detoxification mechanisms and causing an accumulation of toxins in our bodies.[2]

Detoxification is garnering more public recognition and many critics have dismissed 'detox' as a popular buzz term, promising a cure-all for better health and vitality but failing to deliver.[3] It is true that many detoxification treatments lack efficacy, and certain protocols such as water fasting are rightfully criticised as detrimental to human health.[2,3]

However, as we become increasingly aware of the effects of pollution and globalisation on human health, it is important to consider the full spectrum of possible causes of illness and the damaging role toxins play in disease. While more clinical-based research is needed in this area, there is growing evidence that toxicity plays a major role in disease and must be addressed. Healthcare professionals are considering the importance of supporting the body's natural detoxification mechanisms and identifying effective techniques to achieve this.[4]

In this chapter we examine what toxins are, where they are found and how they can affect body systems to cause illness. We also examine the underlying principles of detoxification protocols. While these are commonly used by doctors with training in environmental medicine and complementary therapies, it is important to remember that the concept of detoxification will continue to be subject to rigorous debate in the field of medicine.

WHAT ARE TOXINS?

The US Environmental Protection Agency recognises the existence of over 4 million toxic compounds,[5] which can be categorised as follows:

- *exotoxins*—exposure from the modern environment:
  - industrial chemicals, (e.g. polychlorinated biphenyls (PCBs), furans and dioxins)
  - pesticides (e.g. DDT)
  - plasticisers (e.g. phthalates and bisphenol-A)
  - lifestyle toxins (e.g. cigarettes, alcohol, recreational drugs, caffeine, sugar)
  - heavy metals (e.g. mercury, aluminium, cadmium, lead)
  - many artificial food additives
  - pharmaceutical drugs
  - bacterial endotoxins
- *endotoxins*—produced in the body:
  - oxidative stress and free radical production from daily cellular functions
  - hormones (e.g. oestradiol, C16, C4 oestrogens)
  - emotional stress and negative memories, which can produce biochemical and physiological changes that some would classify as 'toxins'.[6]

Most toxins concentrate in adipose tissue and accumulate during a lifetime, leading to increasing toxic loads with age.[7] Often, toxins are also transferred through the umbilical cord, paternal DNA and breast milk, and may even affect gene expression in the unborn child, passing the burden on to future generations.[8–10]

THE EFFECTS OF TOXINS

Toxins contribute to a wide range of diseases and pathological conditions. The effects of toxins are wide-reaching, and studies have identified direct relationships between toxic compounds and disorders of the nervous, endocrine and immune systems.[1,11–13] This may help to explain the aetiology and increasing prevalence of diseases such as ADHD, asthma and allergies, systemic lupus erythematosus (SLE), chronic fatigue syndrome, depression, reproductive disorders, diabetes and cancer.

NEUROLOGICAL

Neurological illnesses including Parkinson's disease, ADHD and Alzheimer's disease have been linked to toxins,[1,14,15] possibly due to the omnipresence of major neurotoxic pesticides that are readily available—from the local grocery produce to commonly used backyard herbicides.[1]

Interestingly, farmed Atlantic salmon, once considered 'brain-health food', has been found to contain high levels of methylmercury and PCBs, which can lead to neuronal decline, necrosis and demyelination if consumed over many years.[16] Additionally, chemotherapeutic drugs such as doxorubicin and cisplatin have also been shown to cause direct damage to the nervous system.[1]

Recent studies have found additives in processed and convenience foods that can trigger mild thyrotoxicosis and dopamine deficiency, and this may play a role in explaining why so many of today's children are affected by attention deficits and other mental disorders.[15,17]

IMMUNE

Some toxic compounds can lower the body's immunity and increase the likelihood of infection and cancer. Others are known to promote inflammation and are strongly linked to common allergic reactions.[13,18,19]

The World Health Organization (WHO) reports that there is growing evidence that a vast number of environmental agents and therapeutics cause auto-immune-like diseases. For example, while the underlying aetiology of SLE is unknown, research points towards possible adverse reactions to toxic chemicals including pharmaceutical drugs such as hydralazine, isoniazid and minocycline.[1,20,21]

ENDOCRINE

Many environmental chemicals are xeno-oestrogens or endocrine disruptors that can affect the endocrine system. Known hormone disruptors, such as the plasticisers (phthalates and bisphenol-A), are readily found in the environment and common goods such as children's toys and baby bottles, plastic food wrap, cosmetics and tinned food cans. This may help explain the rise in premature puberty among girls.[22] These common plasticisers and other environmental chemicals have been shown to lower progesterone, which may contribute to PMS symptoms, breast cysts, miscarriages and even breast cancer.[6,23–25] Additionally, atrazine, the most commonly used herbicide in America's agriculture industry, is also a xeno-oestrogen and is strongly linked to breast, uterine and ovarian cancers.[26,27] Many harsh toxic chemicals can also cross the placenta and are passed on to children in utero and through breast milk.[6,8]

Male fertility has also not escaped the effects of environmental toxins. Since the 1940s, there has been a drop in sperm count, with an overall reduction of 50%.[28,29] Toxins such as PCBs have also had 'gender-bender' effects, reversing the sex of male turtle eggs.[30]

In addition to affecting reproductive tissues, toxins take their toll on the hypothalamus–pituitary–adrenal axis, influencing sleep patterns, mood, libido and energy levels.[1] Solvents found in petrol, glue and fabric cleansers cause destruction of the adrenal glands and disrupt cortisol production.[16,31]

If liver or gut function is compromised due to a nutrient deficiency, toxic stress or imbalances in gut flora, endogenous hormones such as oestradiol and its metabolites may accumulate in the body, causing oestrogen dominance and increasing the risk of breast and ovarian cancer.[6]

BODY WEIGHT

Toxins accumulate in adipose tissue and lead to difficulties in losing weight. Studies have shown that the heavy metals and industrial chemicals such as those found in car exhaust fumes concentrate in cellular mitochondria.[32] These toxins infiltrate the mitochondria and alter the cells' normal biochemistry and energy production, resulting in reduced lipolysis, thermogenesis and ATP production. Thus, toxic exposure will reduce fat breakdown, basal metabolic rate and energy production.[32]

It is not uncommon to have a patient who, after calorie restriction and increased exercise, is still unable to lose weight. It is important to consider toxins as a potential contributor to this difficult clinical scenario.

DIABETES

Based on current research, a new school of thought is emerging on the aetiology of diabetes. As scientific research in this field evolves, scientists are beginning to see a link between diabetes and the level of toxins stored in the body. For example, people with the highest level of stored toxins (such as those found in dry cleaning and lindane shampoo) are almost 40 times more likely to have diabetes.[33] *The Lancet* has gone as far as to say that obesity is a major contributor to type 2 diabetes primarily because fat is a vehicle for persistent organic pollutants.[34]

CANCER

There is increasing evidence to suggest that toxicity is a major contributor to cancer incidence. The *Journal of the American Medical Association* holds that even once smoking is factored out, the rates of cancer are higher for those born after 1940 and can partly be attributed to an increased exposure to environmental carcinogens.[35] The *British Medical Journal* further vindicates this theory in saying that, 'Environmental and lifestyle factors are key determinants of human disease—accounting for perhaps 75 per cent of most cancers'.[36]

The mechanisms of action to explain the carcinogenic effects of toxins of course include potential direct mutagenic effects on cells. Other indirect mechanisms have been postulated. Heavy metals, pesticides and drugs such as cimetidine are known disruptors of mitochondrial function, increasing the production of reactive oxygen species (ROS).[37] In turn, the ROS activate inflammatory transcription factors and cause oxidative damage to nuclear DNA, leading to mutations and carcinogenesis.[38,39]

Breast adipose tissue is found to concentrate organochlorine compounds (OCCs) more than other bodily adipose cells and has been found in higher concentrations in women with breast cancer.[40–42] Another study found a fourfold increased risk of breast cancer associated with raised serum PCB and DDE.[43] However, other studies have failed to observe an increased risk.[44,45]

Exposure to environmental toxins is also implicated in the development of other adult and childhood cancers, particularly haematological and brain.[46–50]

CARDIORESPIRATORY

The APHENA (Air Pollution And Health: A Combined European And North American Approach) study combines health data and air pollution monitoring from cities across Europe, the United States and Canada. The results confirm earlier findings of an increased all-cause mortality associated with air pollution, especially particulate matter with a diameter less than 10 nm. Elderly and unemployed people were more at risk, as were Canadians.[51]

Other epidemiological studies have also found an association with daily fluctuations in particulate matter as well as sulfur- and nitrogen-based air pollutants. Air pollution is positively associated with school absenteeism, reduced peak flow rates in normal children and acute cardio and respiratory admissions to hospital, and mortality.[52] Long-term exposures of over 3 years may even increase these risks.[53] Furthermore, there appears to be no safe lower limit where the rates of illness plateau. The levels set for public health pollution alerts are therefore arbitrary.

Increased rates of asthma and chronic bronchitis, especially in children, have been observed with higher indoor air levels of solvents and formaldehyde.[54]

DETOXIFICATION: HOW THE BODY PROCESSES TOXINS

GASTROINTESTINAL TRACT

Over the course of a lifetime, the gastrointestinal tract processes more than 25 tons of food, which represents the largest load of antigens and xenobiotics confronting the human body.[55]

Toxins are expelled through the body via the intestines. Hence it is vital to have optimal gastrointestinal functioning to ensure adequate elimination of toxins and maximum nutrient absorption.

As many toxins are stored in adipose tissue, the best way to eliminate toxic load is to increase the amount of fat excreted in the stool.[32] In the small intestine, toxins from food and bile are mixed with pancreatic enzymes that emulsify fat for absorption. Importantly, this leads to an increase in the absorption of toxins.

Gastrointestinal flora are important for the proper elimination of toxins, especially hormone metabolites. For example, after being metabolised by the liver, conjugated oestrogens are eliminated through the bowels. Gut dysbiosis with pathogenic bacteria can produce deconjugating enzymes such as beta-glucuronidase that cleave oestrogen metabolites from their neutralising conjugates. The metabolites are reabsorbed via the enterohepatic circulation.[56]

LIVER

The liver is the main organ for detoxifying lipophilic chemicals, filtering about one litre of blood per minute.[6] The rate of detoxification is a function of hepatic blood flow and liver enzyme activity. The detoxification pathways can be divided into two main phases. Most chemicals are first activated through phase 1 before being conjugated in phase 2. However, some chemicals bypass phase 1 and are simply conjugated for renal or biliary excretion.

Phase 1 detoxification

Phase 1 pathways include the flavine-containing monooxygenases (FMO) (NADPH-dependent oxidation), alcohol dehydrogenase and the famous cytochrome P-450 superfamily of enzymes, which metabolise thousands of exogenous and endogenous compounds and are responsible for the activation and detoxification of over 90% of pharmaceuticals. The majority of *phase 1* metabolites are reactive, highly volatile substances and require *phase 2* for neutralisation. These reactive intermediates are up to 60 times more toxic than their parent molecules and can act as free radicals in the body, capable of causing significant oxidative damage, inflammation, DNA mutations and cancer.[57] For example, paracetomol-associated hepatotoxicity does not result from the drug itself but from depleted hepatic glutathione stores (an important hepatic antioxidant) and accumulation of a hepatotoxic *phase 1* metabolite N-acetyl-p-benzoquinoneimine.[58]

Alcohol, nicotine, caffeine, drugs such as HRT, exposure to stress and large amounts of protein have all been shown to increase the speed of *phase 1* detoxification pathways, while benzodiazepines, antihistamines and H_2 blockers will slow phase 1. Genetic polymorphism in cytochrome P-450 may further contribute to variations in *phase 1* detoxification. Under- or over-activity of *phase 1* enzymes may result in a build-up of unprocessed toxins and reactive metabolites.

Phase 2 detoxification

Phase 2 detoxification generally follows *phase 1*, and is a crucial step in the liver detoxification process. It works to neutralise the reactive products from *phase 1*, allowing them to be eliminated from the body.

During phase 2, a number of conjugation reactions occur to bind metabolites to cofactors like glycine, taurine, glutathione, sulfur and methylation co-factors. From here neutralised toxins can be expelled through the blood serum and kidneys and the intestines via the gallbladder.

KIDNEYS

The kidneys are the primary organs for excretion of water-soluble endogenous and exogenous toxins. Smaller-sized toxins unbound to plasma proteins filter through the glomeruli, which act like a sieve. Other toxins, including metals and drugs, urea and uric acid, are passively and actively excreted via tubule secretion. The ionisation of weak organic acids and bases in the tubules is also used to excrete many toxins, especially drugs.[59] As well as increasing the reabsorption of water, antidiuretic hormone (ADH) increases the reabsorption of urea and reduces urine flow and thus the clearance of toxins.[59]

OTHER PATHWAYS OF DETOXIFICATION

Toxins are mobilised from tissues via the body's circulatory systems. Stimulating these systems will boost lymphatic and blood flow, potentially increasing toxin elimination from stored tissues.

As the largest organ in the body, the skin can eliminate heavy metals and chemical xenobiotics through perspiration.[60] Furthermore, when other organs of elimination such as the kidneys are failing, the skin aids in the elimination process, as is seen in uraemic frost.

Toxins may also be eliminated through breast milk and exhaled air.

ASSESSMENT OF TOXICITY AND DETOXIFICATION

AIMS OF DETOXIFICATION

The goal of detoxification programs is to support and enhance the body's natural detoxification mechanisms. This is achieved by reducing exposure to and absorption of toxins and increasing elimination of stored toxins. Through easing the toxic burden, cellular function can improve, restoring health and vitality.

ASSESSMENT FOR A DETOXIFICATION PROGRAM

The assessment of the patient should begin with a thorough case history to evaluate exposure to toxins (Box 14.1) and the potential impact on the patient's health (Boxes 14.2 and 14.3). For each exposure, the patient should be asked about any health complaints experienced at the time or shortly after exposure as well as any potential sequelae. It is also important to appreciate that due to genetic variability, some patients are more affected by toxic chemicals than others. It is

BOX 14.1 History to assess exposure to toxins

- Use of pharmaceutical drugs
- Use of recreational drugs, alcohol and cigarettes
- Past exposure to toxic chemicals
- Occupational history (painter, construction worker, hairdresser, artist etc)
- Pesticide use
- Non-organic meat and dairy consumption
- Fish consumption, particularly farmed fish
- Convenience food consumption
- Use of household cleaners and disinfectants
- Residing in areas of high pollution
- Residing in homes with attached garages
- Digestive function and frequency of elimination
- Family history, including parents' exposure to toxins before conception

BOX 14.2 Diseases associated with increased toxicity[1]

- Parkinson's disease
- Multiple sclerosis
- Alzheimer's disease
- Attention deficit disorder
- Systemic lupus erythematosus and other autoimmune disorders
- Allergies and asthma
- Chronic fatigue syndrome and fibromyalgia
- Endocrine disorders and non-insulin-dependent diabetes
- Cancer
- Dermatological conditions (acne and dermatitis)

BOX 14.3 Other conditions associated with toxicity[4,32]

- Headaches and migraines
- Irritable bowel syndrome or irritable bowel disease
- Fatigue and low energy
- Infertility
- Musculoskeletal pain
- Inflammatory conditions
- Idiopathic undiagnosed chronic conditions

therefore vital to assess each patient on an individual basis and to not discount even small amounts of exposure.

Examination of the patient is guided by the history and clinical presentation to confirm or exclude pathology.

LABORATORY TESTING

Laboratory tests can be used to measure the levels of some toxins, assess physiological detoxification pathways and identify or exclude pathology. Given that many accumulated toxins are stored in adipose tissue, serum, urinary and hair measurements will only provide a proxy measurement for the true levels of toxicity.

Examples of testing methods:

- *Hair mineral analysis*—can be used as a screening tool to test for heavy metal exposure (e.g. mercury, aluminium, arsenic, cadmium) and nutrient deficiency (calcium, magnesium, selenium, zinc, boron). The test requires a 0.5 g hair sample. The results reflect the body's exposure to common toxins and nutrients for the past 2–3 months. Chemicals in hair products can interfere with the results. Depending on the results, further tests from blood and urine may be warranted.
- *Serum, urine and faecal heavy metal tests*—for measuring aluminium, arsenic, cadmium, chromium, lead and mercury. Interpreting these tests requires a thorough understanding of the excretion and storage of each metal.
- *Functional liver tests—phase 1* and *phase 2* (glutathionation, sulfation, glucoronidation and glycination) liver detoxification pathways can be assessed by exposing the patient to metered doses of three toxins (caffeine, paracetamol and aspirin) and measuring the levels of their metabolites in serum, urine and/or saliva over the next 24 hours. The results can help pinpoint imbalances in liver detoxification to help tailor a treatment plan.
- *Gut dysbiosis tests*—both urine and faeces may be tested for evidence of dysbiosis. As well as identifying pathogenic bacteria, parasites and yeasts, stool tests can also measure the levels of healthy bacterial flora in the faeces. Faecal metabolic markers such as beta-glucuronidase can also be measured. The presence of organic compounds such as p-hydroxybenzoate, p-hydroxyphenylacetate and tricarballylate in the urine may also point towards significant dysbiosis.[61,62]

While laboratory tests can be helpful in assessing patients, they are costly and many are only performed by a small number of laboratories. Patients may also find that the tests are not refundable through government or private health insurance. As is the case with any further investigations in clinical medicine, testing should be used judiciously to confirm or exclude pathology and guide management.

DETOXIFICATION PROTOCOLS

Today's practitioners administer a wide variety of detoxification protocols. It is worth noting, however, that few are evidence-based and that they are supported by limited clinical research. A recent clinical trial that used traditional ayurvedic methods had promising results, with its ability to reduce PCBs and beta-HCH levels.[63] Consequently, rather than presenting a protocol, we will present the main elements often prescribed in detoxification therapy.

The first step in a detoxification program is to reduce environmental exposure to toxins. Following this, specific interventions using lifestyle modification, diet, supplements, herbs and topical treatments may help reduce the toxic load. This is usually achieved by focusing on the gastrointestinal tract, liver, kidneys, skin and circulation. If you are untrained in this area, it may be better to refer your patient to an experienced practitioner.

TIMELINE

A detoxification regimen should be individualised and can be administered for any period of time but usually from 2 weeks to 3 months.

GUIDELINES FOR REDUCING TOXIN EXPOSURE

While it is difficult to escape environmental toxins, it is important to take measures to avoid exposure to toxic substances as much as possible. The following guidelines are helpful in reducing toxin exposure:

- Eat organic food.
- Avoiding storing or heating food and drinks in plastic.
- If there is no alternative, choose higher food grade plastics with a number greater than or equal to 5; 7 is ideal. Many plastic containers are marked with a triangle with this number in the centre.
- Use natural alternatives to lindane shampoo to treat lice.

- Avoid dry-cleaning as much as possible—use natural dry-cleaning.
- Practise good dental hygiene—choose non-mercury amalgams and avoid those containing bisphenol-A. However, removal of mercury amalgams should be done with caution due to the risk to both the patient and dental staff of significant exposure to elemental mercury levels from inhaling mercury vapours during the extraction.[64]
- Choose cosmetics containing natural products—avoid those containing parabens.

DIET PLAN AND SUPPLEMENTS TO SUPPORT DETOXIFICATION

First-line therapy with any detoxification protocol is dietary. Dietary changes should be made at the beginning of a detox program and maintained throughout.

A detox diet should include:

- certified organic food sources wherever possible
- a variety of fruits and vegetables, with plenty of leafy green and brassica vegetables, and dark red/purple fruits and vegetables such as beetroot and berries
- whole grains including brown rice, quinoa and amaranth
- legumes and beans
- raw nuts and seeds
- avoidance of peanuts—they may contain aflatoxin
- certified organic sources of lean protein, such as chicken and turkey breast and fish; amino acids are essential for detoxification; the diet must provide adequate daily protein intake
- avoidance of fish or fish oil supplements high in heavy metals. Eat more small oily fish such as sardines and mackerel (note: fish oil supplements are tested for mercury and other environmental toxins; however, those sourced from smaller fish may still be safer to consume)
- fresh leeks, onion, garlic, ginger, turmeric, rosemary in cooking
- drinking 2–3 litres of filtered water daily with squeezed lemon or lime
- drinking green or oolong tea
- complete elimination of all red meat and pork
- complete elimination of dairy products
- complete elimination of all wheat and flour (from any source)
- nothing processed, refined, preserved or canned
- no refined sugar or hydrogenated oils.

Methods to support gastrointestinal elimination of toxins include:

- *Probiotics*—inoculating the bowels with healthy bacteria will reduce dysbiosis and improve elimination of toxins such as oestrogen.[65] This can be achieved through supplementing with probiotic capsules or powder and through the consumption of fermented foods.
- *Fibre*—rice bran fibre has been shown to be a very effective toxic binder.[66,67] In addition, rice is also a pancreatic lipase inhibitor that helps decrease lipid absorption.[32] The same applies for brown rice. *Psyllium* husk is also a mucilaginous fibre that binds lipids and fat-soluble toxins and increases stool bulk. Given the high prevalence of gluten sensitivities, choosing a gluten-free fibre will help reduce the risk of inflammation in these patients. It is important to couple adequate amounts of water with the addition of any supplemental fibre to prevent constipation.
- Methods such as *natural pancreatic lipase inhibition* increase fat in the stool, and have been proved to be safe and effective in decreasing toxic load (not resulting in diarrhoea or fat-soluble vitamin deficiency).[32] Botanical pancreatic-lipase inhibitors increase lipid excretion, augmenting elimination of fat-soluble toxins.[32] Research has found that botanicals such as *Panax* ginseng, green and oolong tea, wild yam, horse chestnut, ginger and hops (beer not included) when mixed with a high-fat diet prevented weight gain, increased faecal fat and increased cholesterol excretion.[68,69] If used correctly it will not cause diarrhoea or fat-soluble vitamin deficiency.[32] One small study found that people given 750 mL of oolong tea three times a day for 10 days had a two-fold increase in faecal fat and increased faecal cholesterol excretion.[70] These results could lead to cutting PCB content by 50%.[32] Simple dietary interventions such as including more green tea and ginger in the diet are easy ways to support ongoing detoxification in patients.
- *Chlorophyll or chlorella*—increases the excretion of fat-soluble toxins. A Japanese study showed that women who took chlorella during pregnancy had a 40% decrease in dioxin levels in their breast milk.[71] It can be supplemented or found in high amounts in green, leafy vegetables and algae.
- *Seaweed*—in a recent study, rats were given dioxin and nori seaweed, which prevented the absorption of toxins, increased overall excretion and reduced body stores of dioxin.[72]
- *Iodine*—is abundant in seaweeds and some algae. It is a vital nutrient that is depleted in most Western diets.[73] In addition to immuno-protective properties, iodine increases the elimination of toxins such as fluorides, bromides and even certain heavy metals.[73]

LIVER DETOXIFICATION

Many studies suggest that a lack of balance between the two liver detoxification phases can increase the risks of drug reactions and oxidative stress, as well as contributing to the aetiology of chronic diseases such as cancer, Parkinson's disease and systemic lupus erythematosus.[74–78] As such, practitioners aim to achieve a balance between the two phases, to reduce the accumulation of both unprocessed toxins and reactive intermediate metabolites.[65,79]

Liver detoxification is influenced by herbal and nutritional supplements, along with diet. These can be used to help create optimal liver detoxification (Table 14.1). It is important to ensure adequate intake of antioxidants to protect the body from any free-radical formation caused by the accumulation of the reactive intermediates formed by *phase 1*.

KIDNEY DETOX

Increasing hydration is the simplest method of enhancing the kidneys' elimination of toxins. As well as increasing glomerular filtration and urine flow, a high water intake reduces ADH secretion and its consequent reabsorption of urea[92] and other water-soluble toxins.[59]

TABLE 14.1 Supplements to support liver detoxification

Phase 1	
Vitamins	Riboflavin (B_2), niacin (B_3), pyridoxine (B_6), B_{12}
Herbs	Schizandra, St John's wort, rosemary, green tea, curcumin • Up-regulate phase 1 activity • Avoid with certain pharmaceuticals and chemotherapeutics[6] • Milk thistle • Down-regulate phase 1 activity[6] • It is common to need to down-regulate phase 1 secondary to high consumption of caffeine, charbroiled meats and alcohol[6] • In vivo studies have shown no interference with the pharmacokinetics of drug metabolism[80]
Other	Glutathione, branched chain amino acids, flavonoids, phospholipids
Antioxidant vitamins & minerals	Carotenes (vitamin A), ascorbic acid (vitamin C), tocopherols (vitamin E), selenium, copper, zinc, manganese, coenzyme Q10, bioflavonoids
Phase 2	
Amino acids	Cysteine, glutathione, L-glycine, L-glutamine, taurine, methylation cofactors • Essential nutrients for phase 2 which constantly need to be replenished through the diet • Glutathione, although extremely important, is not effectively absorbed when supplemented orally. It is therefore crucial to supplement its precursors: cysteine, N-acetyl cysteine and glycine.[32]
Vitamins	Thiamin (B_1), riboflavin (B_2), niacin (B_3), pyridoxine (B_6), B_{12}, folic acid
Herbs	Milk thistle • Contains liver-protective flavonoids[81] • Significantly increases glutathione levels and bile flow[81,82] Dandelion root • Increases bile output and has been shown to reduce oestrogen levels[6] Curcumin • Active ingredient in turmeric • Up-regulates phase 2 while slowing down phase 1 • Elevates levels of glutathione S-transferase, an enzyme responsible for conjugating glutathione[83] • Potent antioxidant, inactivating toxic intermediates[6]
Other micronutrients	Indole-3-carbinol, found in *Brassica* vegetables • Important for proper oestrogen metabolism[84] Calcium D-glucuronate • Needed for oestrogen elimination from the bowel[85] Alpha lipoic acid, flavonoids, zinc, selenium
Food shown to induce phase 2 enzyme activity	• *Brassica* vegetables: broccoli, brussel sprouts, cabbage, kale[86] • Sources of amino acids: lean meats, legumes, beans, whey, whole grains, soy[87] • Fruits containing ellagic acid: raspberries and red grapes[88] • Spices: garlic, onions, rosemary, fennel, turmeric[89–91]

The consumption of 2–3 litres per day of filtered water for an average-sized adult is recommended during a detoxification program. Herbs and foods traditionally used for their diuretic properties, such as dandelion, nettle, parsley, watermelon and asparagus, may also be used.[6]

SKIN, LYMPHATIC AND CIRCULATORY STIMULANTS

The following can be used to increase lymphatic and blood flow, in order to improve circulation and waste removal.

- *Dry skin brushing*—traditionally used to increase lymphatic circulation, dispelling toxins through the skin. Using a loofah or dry body brush, gently brush the skin from the bottom of the feet and the palms towards the heart. Follow with a hot and cold shower.
- *Rotating hot and cold showers*—traditionally used to improve blood circulation, flushing out toxins and improving immunity. Shower for two minutes on hot, thirty seconds on cold, and repeat three times, finishing with cold.
- *Castor oil*—applied topically, penetrates as deep as 10 centimetres into tissue, improving lymphatic circulation, enhancing elimination and drawing out toxins.[52]
    - Rub castor oil onto the liver or the entire abdomen, cover with a towel and plastic wrap to contain any mess.
    - Cover with a dry towel and place a non-electric heating pad or hot water bottle on top.
    - Leave it on the abdomen for 45 minutes to one hour.
    - Should be avoided during menstruation, as it can interfere with uterine blood flow.
- *Saunas*—can help mobilise toxins stored in fat and increase the excretion of toxins through perspiration. Clinical trials have demonstrated the efficacy of saunas in reducing levels of PCBs and pesticides.[93,94] In order to eliminate stored xenobiotics and heavy metals, sauna treatments need to be longer than 15 minutes.[60] Saunas are not advised for pregnant or nursing mothers, or for patients with severe cardiovascular conditions. Doctors should assess patients on an individual basis to determine whether this is a safe treatment.

OTHER INTERVENTIONS TO AUGMENT DETOXIFICATION

- *Exercise*—this is an important component of any detoxification protocol. In addition to mobilising stored fat and thus fat-soluble toxins, exercise stimulates the circulatory and lymphatic systems, to help remove toxins stored in body tissues and organs. Saunas post exercise will help eliminate toxins that have been released from fat cells.
- *Sleep*—this is the body's time for cellular repair and regeneration.[95] An emphasis on adequate sleep supports detoxification and general wellbeing. Advise 8 hours of sleep, because the last 1–2 hours appear to be the most restorative.[96]
- *Emotional and stress detox*—when we experience negative emotions and stress, this physicallyaffects the body through changes in neurotransmitters, the autonomic nervous system, hormones and immunity. A detoxification protocol needs to be holistic and include treatments that support the mental–emotional–spiritual level. To reduce the impact of stress and negative emotional states, a detoxification regimen can include simple breathing exercises, meditation, t'ai chi or yoga, as well as counselling or support groups when necessary. Chapter 8 (mind–body medicine) deals with these issues in more detail.

HEAVY METALS DETOXIFICATION

Environmental exposure to heavy metals, in particular mercury and lead, continues to receive significant attention in the mainstream media. For most individuals, low levels of heavy metals are tolerable because cells have a variety of mechanisms to help defend against injury. Detoxification methods for heavy metals involve either the active chelation and removal of heavy metals, or supportive measures to help reduce their toxic effects on cells and enhance excretion.

Chelation therapy is used for treating acute heavy metal poisoning. Common chelating agents include 2,3-dimercapto-1-propane sulfonic acid (DMPS), meso-2,3-dimercaptosuccinic acid isomer (DMSA), D-penicillamine, British antilewisite (BAL) and ethylene diamine tetra-acetic acid (EDTA). However, the use of chelating agents for the removal of stored heavy metals from low-level chronic exposure is controversial. Advocates for the wider use of chelation therapy use chelators such as EDTA for a range of conditions from metal toxicity to cardiovascular disease, macular degeneration and cancer.[97–99] While chelation therapy may be an effective method for treating heavy metal poisoning such as mercury, lead, iron or copper, the compounds used are potentially toxic and they chelate other essential minerals such as calcium and zinc. As such, the risks and benefits must be weighed up before proceeding and it should only be administered by an experienced practitioner.

Metallothioneins (MTs) are a group of endogenously produced proteins and have been shown to provide protection against heavy metals.[100,101] MTs have been shown to bind to toxic metals such as cadmium, lead, aluminum and inorganic mercury.[100,102,103] In order to form their structures, MTs require zinc, copper, histidine and cysteine.[104] Therefore it is wise to consider supplementing with these nutrients if there is heavy metal exposure.

Other promising supportive therapies have included the use of selenium,[105] coline[106] and glutathione[101] to treat the ill health allegedly arising from mercury cytotoxicity and/or to reduce mercury levels.[103] A combination of vitamin B complex, vitamin C, vitamin E and sodium selenite showed promising results on a range of biochemical and haematological parameters when used as adjuvant therapy during the removal of mercury amalgams.[107]

CONTRAINDICATIONS

Detoxification is a safe and effective form of treatment when administered by an experienced practitioner, but it may not be without side effects. Many are caused as a result of toxins and waste products being mobilised and metabolised. Others can be explained by withdrawal symptoms from drugs such as caffeine and alcohol. Most of these symptoms will subside within a week of treatment. Common side effects include headaches, nausea, irregular bowel function, dizziness, irritability, anxiety and fatigue.

It is important to remember that detoxification needs to be tailored to the individual and that there are no set contraindications. Medical practitioners need to use clinical discretion when prescribing detoxification programs and must not devise programs for pregnant women, or for underweight or cachexic patients.

CONCLUSION

Every day we are exposed to toxins from our environment, from the air we breathe to polluted waterways and industrial and agricultural toxins in our homes. Detoxification programs can enhance the body's natural healing abilities and provide a means to achieve a better state of health. If a patient is suffering from the effects of an unhealthy diet and years of toxic exposure, a good detoxification program that eliminates toxins from the body may be a part of the answer.

REFERENCES

1 Crinnion WJ. Environmental medicine, part 1: the human burden of environmental toxins and their common health effects. Altern Med Rev 2000; 5(1): 52–63.

2 Liska DJ, Bland JS. Emerging clinical science of bifunctional support for detoxification. Townsend Letter 2002; 231:42–43.

3 The dubious practice of detox. Internal cleansing may empty your wallet, but is it good for your health? Harvard Women's Health Watch 2008; 15(9):1–3. [no authors listed]

4 Rogers S. Detoxify or die. Syracuse: Prestige Publishers; 2002.

5 William JR. Chemical sensitivity, volume 1. Boca Raton: Lewis Publishers; 1992.

6 Kaur SD. The complete natural medicine guide to breast cancer: a practical manual for understanding, prevention and care. Toronto: Robert Rose; 2003.

7 US Environmental Protection Agency. Breaking the cycle: 2001–2002 PBT Program Accomplishments. 2002. Online. Available: http://www.epa.gov/pbt/pubs/pbtreport2002.htm.

8 Landrigan PJ, Sonawane B, Mattison D et al. Chemical contaminants in breast milk and their impacts on children's health: an overview. Environ Health Persp 2002; 110:A313–A315.

9 Crinnion WJ. Environmental medicine, Part 4. Pesticides—biologically persistent and ubiquitous toxins. Altern Med Rev 2000; 5(5):432–447.

10 Young E. Rewriting Darwin: The new non-genetic inheritance. New Scientist 2008; 2664. Online. Available: http://www.newscientist.com/article/mg19926641.500-rewriting-darwin-the-new-nongenetic-inheritance.html 26 March 2009.

11 Sotom AM, Vandenberg LN, Maffini MV et al. Does breast cancer start in the womb? Basic Clin Pharmacol Toxicol 2008; 102(2):125–133.

12 Luster MI, Rosenthal GJ. Chemical agents and the immune response. Environ Health Persp 1993; 100: 219–226.

13 Hueser G. Diagnostic markers in clinical immunotoxicology and neurotoxicology. J Occup Med Toxicol 1992; 1:5–9.

14 Synder SH, D'Amato RJ. Predicting Parkinson's disease. Nature 1985; 317:198–199.

15 Hungerford C. Good health in the 21st century: a family doctor's unconventional guide. Melbourne: Scribe; 2006.

16 Haschek WM, Rousseaux CG. Handbook of toxicologic pathology. San Diego: Academic Press; 1991.

17 Buist R. Food chemical sensitivity. North Ryde: Collins/Angus and Robertson; 1990.

18 Kuhnlein HV, Receveur O, Muir DC et al. Arctic indigenous women consume greater than acceptable levels of organochlorines. J Nutr 1995; 125:2501–2510.

19 Vial T, Nicolas B, Descotes J. Clinical immunotoxicity of pesticides. J Toxicol 1996; 48:215–229.

20 World Health Organization. Principles and methods for assessing autoimmunity associated with exposure to chemicals. Environmental Health Criteria Series no. 236. Geneva: WHO; 2006.

21 D'Cruz D. Testing for autoimmunity in humans. Toxicol Lett 2002; 127(1–3):93–100.
22 Massart F, Parrino R, Seppia P et al. How do environmental estrogen disruptors induce precocious puberty? Minerva Pediatr 2006; 58(3):247–254.
23 Lee JR. What your doctor may not tell you about menopause. New York: Time Warner; 1996.
24 Boulakoud MS, Mosbah R, Abdennour C et al. The toxicological effects of the herbicide 2,4-DCPA on progesterone levels and mortality in Wistar female rats. Meded Rijksuniv Gent Fak Landbourwkd Toegep Biol Wet 2001; 66(2b):891–895.
25 Foster WG, McMahon A, Villeneuve DC et al. Hexachlorobenzene (HCB) suppresses circulating progesterone concentrations during the luteal phase in the cynomolgus monkey. J App Toxicol 1992; 12:13–17.
26 Epstein SS. The politics of cancer. Hankins, NY: East Ridge Press; 1998.
27 Bradlow HL, Davis DL, Lin G et al. Effects of pesticides on the ratio of 16 alpha/2-hydroxyestrone: a biologic marker of breast cancer risk. Environ Health Persp 1995; 103(7):147–150.
28 Sharpe R, Shakkeback N. Are oestrogens involved in falling male sperm counts and disorders of the male reproductive tract? Lancet 1993; 41:1392–1395.
29 Carlsen E, Givercman A, Skakkebaek NE. Evidence for decreasing quality of semen during past 50 years. BMJ 1992; 305:609–613.
30 Colborn T, Dumanoski D, Peterson Myers J. Our stolen future. New York: Penguin; 1996.
31 Lund B, Bergman A, Brandt I. Metabolic activation and toxicity of a DDT-metabolite, 3-methylsulphonyl-DDE, in the adrenal zona fasciculata in mice. Chem Biol Interact 1988; 65:25–40.
32 Crinnion WJ. The effective use of botanicals, dietary agents and food additives to enhance the clearance of lipophilic xenobiotics from the body. Lecture given at American Association of Naturopathic Physicians Annual Convention, Phoenix, Arizona; 2008.
33 Ryan A. Inflammation linked to postmenopausal glucose metabolism. Diabetes Care 2004; 27:1699–1705.
34 Porta M. Persistent organic pollutants and the burden of diabetes. Lancet 2006; 9535:558–559.
35 Davis DL, Dinse GE, Hoel DG. Decreasing cardiovascular disease and increasing cancer among whites in the United States from 1973 through 1987. JAMA 1994; 271:431–437.
36 Sharpe RM, Irvine SD. How strong is the evidence of a link between environmental chemicals and adverse effects on human reproductive health? BMJ 2004; 328:447–451.
37 Plaza S, Lamson D. How does it happen? An origin of mutations for malignancy. American College of Advancement in Medicine National Meeting; 2003.
38 Toyokuni S, Okamoto K, Yodoi J et al. Persistent oxidative stress in cancer. FEBS Lett 1995; 358(1): 1–3.
39 Davidson JF, Schiestl RH. Mitochondrial respiratory electron carriers are involved in oxidative stress during heat stress in *Saccharomyces cerevisiae.* Mol Cell Biol 2001; 21(24):8483–8489.
40 Wasserman M, Nogueira DP, Tomatis L et al. Organochlorine compounds in neoplastic and adjacent apparently normal breast tissue. Bull Environ Contam Toxicol 1976; 15:478–484.
41 Mussalo-Rauhamaa H. Occurrence of betahexachlorocyclohexane in breast cancer patients. Cancer 1990; 66:2124–2128.
42 Falck F. Pesticides and polychlorinated biphenyl residues in human breast lipids and their relation to breast cancer. Arch Environ Health 1992; 47:143–146.
43 Wolff MS, Toniolo PG, Lee EW et al. Blood levels of organochlorine residues and risk of breast cancer. J Natl Cancer Inst 1993; 85:648–652.
44 Hunter DJ, Hankinson SE, Laden F et al. Plasma organochlorine levels and the risk of breast cancer. N Engl J Med 1997; 337:1253–1258.
45 Krieger N, Wolff M, Hiatt RA et al. Breast cancer and serum organochlorines: a prospective study among white, black, and Asian women. J Natl Cancer Inst 1994; 86:589–599.
46 Davis JR, Brownson RC, Garcia R et al. Family pesticide use and childhood brain cancer. Arch Environ Contam Toxicol 1993; 24:87–92.
47 Leiss J, Savitz D. Home pesticide use and childhood cancer: a case control study. Am J Pub Health 1995; 85:249–252.
48 Claggett S. 2,4-D Information packet. Northwest Coalition for Alternatives to Pesticides; 1990.
49 Eriksson M, Karlsson M. Occupational and other environmental factors and multiple myeloma: a population based case-control study. Br J Ind Med 1992; 49:95–103.
50 Anttila A, Pukkala E, Sallman M et al. Cancer incidence among Finnish workers exposed to halogenated hydrocarbons, J Occup Environ Med 1995; 37:797–806.
51 Samoli E, Peng R, Ramsay T et al. Acute effects of ambient particulate matter on mortality in Europe and North America: results from the APHENA study. Environ Health Perspect 2008; 116(11):1480–1486.
52 Committee of the Environmental and Occupational Health Assembly of the American Thoracic Society. Health effects of outdoor air pollution. Am J Respir Crit Care Med 1996; 153(1):3–50.
53 Lee D, Ferguson C, Mitchell R. Air pollution and health in Scotland: a multicity study. Biostatistics 2009; 10(3):409–423.

54 Krzyzanowski M, Quackenboss JJ, Lebowitz MD. Chronic respiratory effects of indoor formaldehyde exposure. Environ Res 1990; 52:117–1125.
55 Liska DJ. The detoxification enzyme systems. Altern Med Rev 1998; 3(3):187–198.
56 Fujisawa T, Mori M. Influence of bile salts on beta-glucuronidase activity of intestinal bacteria. Lett Appl Microbiol 1996; 22(4):271–274.
57 Meyer UA, Zanger UM, Skoda RC et al. Genetic polymorphisms of drug metabolism. Prog Liver Dis 1990; 9:307–323.
58 Ioannides C. Cytochromes P450: metabolic and toxicological aspects. Boca Raton, Florida: CRC Press; 1996.
59 Golan DE, Tashjian AH, Armstrong EJ et al. Principles of pharmacology: the pathophysiologic basis of drug therapy. 2nd edn. Philadelphia: Lippincott Williams & Wilkins; 2007.
60 Crinnion WJ. Components of practical clinical detox programs—sauna as a therapeutic tool. Altern Ther Health Med 2007; 13(2):154–156.
61 Chalmers RA, Valman HB, Liberman MM. Measurement of 4-hydroxyphenylacetic aciduria as a screening test for small bowel disease. Clin Chem 1979; 25:1791–1794.
62 Lindblad BS, Alm J, Lundsjo A et al. Absorption of biological amines of bacterial origin in normal and sick infants. Ciba Found Symp 1979; 70:281–291.
63 Herron RE, Fagan JB. Lipophil-mediated reduction of toxicants in humans: an evaluation of an ayurvedic detoxification procedure. Altern Ther Health Med 2002; 8(5):40–51.
64 Molin M, Bergman B, Marklund SL et al. Mercury, selenium, and glutathione peroxidase before and after amalgam removal in man. Acta Odontol Scand 1990; 48(3):189–202.
65 Hall DC. Nutritional influences on estrogen metabolism. Applied Nutritional Science Reports 2001; 1–8. Nutrition Publications Inc.
66 Harris PJ, Sasidharan VK, Robertson AM et al. Adsorption of a hydrophobic mutagen to cereal brans and cereal bran and dietary fibres. Mutation Res 1998; 412:323–331.
67 Sera N, Morita K, Nagasoe M et al. Binding effect of polychlorinated compounds and environmental carcinogens on rice bran fiber. J Nutr Biochem 2005; 16(1):50–58.
68 Han LK, Nose R, Li W et al. Reduction in fat storage in mice fed a high-fat diet long term by treatment with saponins prepared from Kochia scoparia fruit. Phytother Res 2006; 20(10):877–882.
69 Kimura H, Ogawa S, Katsube T et al. Antiobese effects of novel saponins from edible seeds of Japanese horse chestnut (*Aesculus turbinate* BLUME) after treatment with wood ashes. J Agric Food Chem 2008; 56(12):4783–4788.
70 Hsu TF, Kusumoto A, Abe K et al. Polyphenol-enriched oolong tea increases fecal lipid excretion. Eur J Clin Nutr 2006; 20(11):1330–1336.
71 Nakano S, Takekoshi H, Nakano MJ. Chlorella (*Chlorella pyrenoidosa*) supplementation decreases dioxin and increases immunoglobulin A concentrations in breast milk. J Med Food 2007; 10(1):134–142.
72 Morita K, Nakano T. Seaweed accelerates the excretion of dioxin stored in rats. J Agric Food Chem 2002; 50(4):910–917.
73 Abraham GE. The safe and effective implementation of orthoiodosupplementation in medical practice. The Original Internist 2004; 11(1):17–36.
74 Daly AK, Cholerton S, Gregory W et al. Metabolic polymorphisms. Pharmac Ther 1993; 57:129–160.
75 Kawajiri K, Nakachi K, Imai K et al. Identification of genetically high risk individuals to lung cancer by DNA polymorphisms of the cytochrome P4501A1 gene. FEBS Lett 1990; 263:131–133.
76 Nebert DW, Petersen DD, Puga A et al. Locus polymorphism and cancer: inducibility of CYP1A1 and other genes by combustion products and dioxin. Pharmacogenetic 1991; 1:68–78.
77 Bandmann O, Vaughan J, Holmans P et al. Association of slow acetylator genotype for N-acetyltransferase 2 with familial Parkinson's disease. Lancet 1997; 350:1136–1139.
78 Meyer UA, Zanger UM, Skoda RC et al. Genetic polymorphisms of drug metabolism. Prog Liver Dis 1990; 9:307–323.
79 Liska DJ. The detoxification enzyme systems. Alt Med Rev 1998; 3(3):187–198.
80 Wu JW, Lin LC, Tsai TH. Drug-drug interactions of silymarin on the perspective of pharmacokinetics. J Ethnopharmacol 2009; 121(2):185–193.
81 Hoffman D. Medical herbalism: the science and practice of herbal medicine. Rochester: Healing Arts Press; 2003.
82 Das SK, Vasudevan DM. Protective effects of silymarin, a milk thistle (*Silybum marianum*) derivative on ethanol-induced oxidative stress in liver. Indian J Biochem Biophys 2006; 43(5): 306–311.
83 Goud VK, Polasa K, Krishnaswarmy K. Effect of turmeric on xenobiotic metabolising. Plant Foods Hum Nutr 1993; 44(1):87–92.
84 Weng JR, Tsai CH, Kulp SK. Indole-3-carbinol as a chemopreventative and anti-cancer agent. Cancer Lett 2008; 262(2):153–163.
85 Minton JP, Walaszek Z, Schooley W. Beta-glucuronidase levels in patients with fibrocystic breast disease. Breast Cancer Res Treat 1986; 8:217–222.

86 Pantuck EJ, Pantuck CB, Garland WA et al. Stimulatory effect of brussels sprouts and cabbage on human drug metabolism. Clin Pharm Ther 1979; 25:88–95.

87 Appelt LC, Reicks MM. Soy feeding induces phase II enzymes in rat tissues. Nutr Cancer 1997; 28:270–275.

88 Barch DH, Rundhaugen LM. Ellagic acid induces NAD(P)H:quinone reductase through activation of the antioxidant responsive element of the rat NAD(P)H:quinone reductase gene. Carcinogenesis 1994; 15:2065–2068.

89 Singh B, Kale RK. Chemomodulatory action of *Foeniculum vulgare* (Fennel) on skin and forestomach papillomagenesis, enzymes associated with xenobiotic metabolism and antioxidant status in murine model system. Food Chem Toxicol 2008; 46(12):3842–3850.

90 Offord EA, Mace K, Ruffieux C et al. Rosemary components inhibit benzo[a]pyrene-induced genotoxicity in human bronchial cells. Carcinogenesis 1995; 16:2057–2062.

91 Lisk DJ. Modulation of Phase I and Phase II xenobiotic-metabolizing enzymes by selenium-enriched garlic in rats. Nutr Cancer 1997; 28:184–188.

92 Sircar S. Principles of medical physiology. New York: Thieme; 2009.

93 Tretzak Z, Shields M, Beckmann SL. PCB reduction and clinical improvement by detoxification: an unexploited approach? Hum Exp Toxicol 1990; 9:235–244.

94 Schnare DW, Ben M, Shields MG. Body burden reduction of PCBs, PBBs and chlorinated pesticides in human subjects. Ambio 1984; 13(5/6):378–380.

95 Seigel JM. Why we sleep. Sci Am 2003; 89(5):92–97.

96 Dickson Thom. Health of business, business of health. Seminar, Toronto, Ontario; May 2008.

97 Kondrot ED. Healing the eye the natural way. Carson City, NV: Nutritional Research Press; 2000.

98 Godfrey ME. EDTA chelation as a treatment of arterioscleros. NZ Med J 1990; 93:100.

99 Gordon GF. EDTA and chelation therapy: history and mechanisms of action, an update. Payson, AZ: Gordon Research Institute. Online. Available: http://www.gordonresearch.com/articles_oral_chelation/edtachel.html 21 March 2009.

100 Szitanyi Z, Nemes C, Rozlosnik N. Metallothionein and heavy metal concentration in blood. Microchemical Journal 1996; 54(3):246–251.

101 Satoh M, Nishimura N, Kanayama Y et al. Enhanced renal toxicity by inorganic mercury in metallothionein-null mice. J Pharmacol Exp Ther 1997; 283: 1529–1533.

102 Ikemoto T, Kunito T, Anan Y et al. Association of heavy metals with metallothionein and other proteins in hepatic cytosol of marine mammals and seabirds. Environ Toxicol Chem 2004; 23(8): 2008–2016.

103 Guzzi G, La Porta CA. Molecular mechanisms triggered by mercury. Toxicology 2008; 244(1):1–12.

104 Wikipedia. Metallothionein. Wiki article; 2008. Online. Available: http://en.wikipedia.org/wiki/Metallothionein 16 March 2009.

105 Rooney JP. The role of thiols, dithiols, nutritional factors and interacting ligands in the toxicology of mercury. Toxicology 2007; 234:145–156.

106 Clarkson TW, Strain JJ. Nutritional factor may modify the toxic action of methyl mercury in fish-eating populations. J Nutr 2003; 133:1539S–1542S.

107 Frisk P, Danersund A, Hudecek R. Changed clinical chemistry pattern in blood after removal of dental amalgam and other metal alloys supported by antioxidant therapy. Biol Trace Elem Res 2007; 120 (1–3):163–170.

part TWO

Principles of general practice

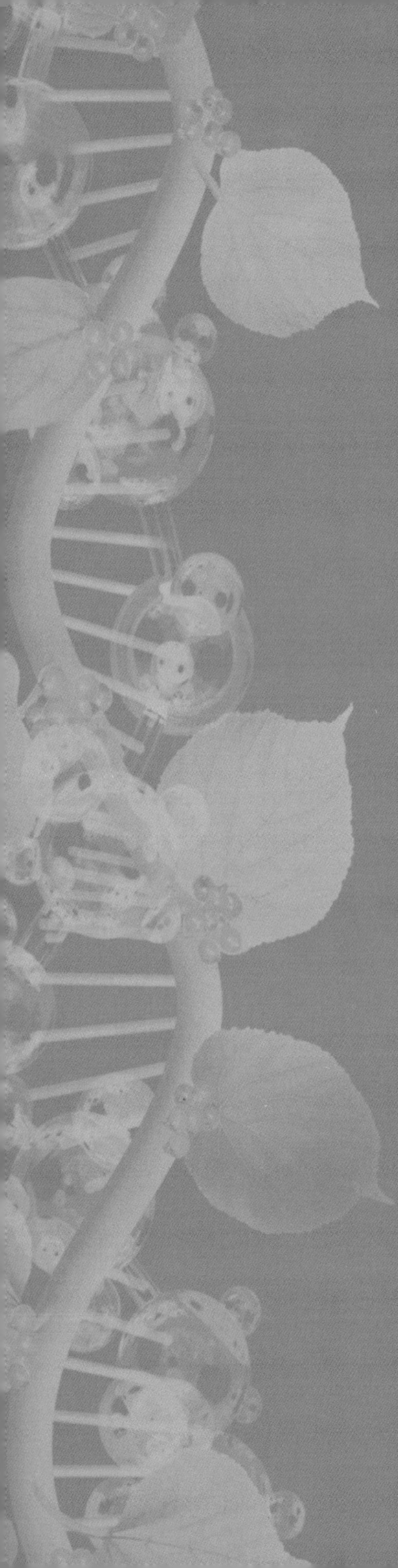

chapter 15

The consulting room

INTRODUCTION

A consulting room should be comfortable, functional, efficient and able to meet your patients' healthcare needs. Your working environment also makes a statement about your personality, professionalism and attitude towards your patients. When designing the layout and planning the equipment for your consulting room, you need to consider the therapeutic modalities you will be using, as well as your style of practice. For example, a practitioner who teaches yoga techniques or provides remedial massage or manipulative therapies will require particular types of beds and sufficient floor space to move around. Acupuncture may require a number of adjoining rooms where patients can be left to relax while their treatment proceeds and the practitioner commences face-to-face consultations with other patients.

SEATING

In general, the layout of a consulting room should provide sufficient space to accommodate all equipment as well as several chairs for patients, as there will be times when three or more members of a family attend a session. If space allows, you may want to provide your patients with the choice of sitting opposite you or at the side of the desk. Some patients prefer physical proximity to the doctor without a barrier, whereas others like to know there is a desk between them.

SPACE

You should be able to move freely around the room and have space at the head end of the bed (about 60 cm) to examine the patient and conduct procedural work around the head and face with the patient lying down. There should be sufficient room at the foot of the bed (about 60 cm) to allow you to stand and bend to examine the feet, even with tall patients.

COMPUTER

The computer should be situated so that it does not obstruct your view of the patient's face, but also so that you do not have to turn your back to the patient to make notes. The workstation (adjustable chair, seat height, level of keyboard and monitor) should be ergonomically designed to accommodate many hours of sitting, as well as unimpeded access to the other side of the desk and to the examination bed.

FLOOR

The flooring should be made of a washable material, preferably hospital-grade welded vinyl or its equivalent.

LIGHTING

Lighting should provide 'white light' and be portable so that it can be used to examine patients either on the examination bed or in their chair.

SINK

The sink should be supplied with hot and cold water and have a handle that can be operated without touching it with the hands. Antiseptic hand wash in a pump pack should be on the sink. A dispenser for disposable hand towels should be mounted on the wall adjacent to the sink.

PRIVACY

The door should be sound-proofed for privacy and there should be a privacy latch on the inside, to prevent unwanted entry. A privacy curtain should surround the bed, allowing enough space for the patient to stand behind it in order to dress and undress and ensuring that the bed cannot be viewed from outside the room if the door is opened.

BOX 15.1 Consulting room equipment

Office furniture & supplies

- Computer with clinical and practice management software with fast broadband access
- Ergonomically sound adjustable office chair
- Examination light
- Examination/treatment bed with a padded washable surface
- Office desk
- Patient chairs
- Prescription and OTC stationery
- Stationery
- Wastepaper bin

Medical equipment & supplies

Storage/disposal:

- Drug safe and log book
- Instrument trays
- Medical waste receptacle
- Sharps bin
- Specimen jars
- Trolley with drawer and work surface (on wheels)
- Vaccine fridge stocked with supply of vaccines

Measuring devices/monitors:

- Baby length measuring device
- Baby scales (digital)
- Blood glucose monitor
- Electrocardiograph compatible with practice software
- Fetal heart Doppler
- Sphygmomanometer
- Spirometer with disposable mouthpieces
- Tape measure
- Thermometer and disposable covers
- Wall-mounted height meter
- Weight scales

Procedural equipment:

- Alcohol wipes
- Antiseptic lotion, hydrogen peroxide, normal saline
- Auriscope with disposable covers
- Biopsy punches
- Blood and specimen collection equipment
- Dermatoscope
- Diathermy
- Disposable proctoscopes (small and large)
- Disposable tongue depressors
- Dressing packs
- Dressings and bandages
- Ear syringe
- Gauze swabs, cotton wool
- Guedel's airway
- Hand mirror
- Liquid nitrogen and cryotherapy gun
- Local anaesthetic, with and without adrenaline
- Magnifiers
- Needle holders, forceps, scissors
- Needles: 18 G, 21 G, 23 G, 25 G (long and short)
- Ophthalmoscope
- Pap smear equipment:
  - disposable speculums (small and large)
  - glass slides and slide holders
  - Pap smear brushes
  - spray fixative
  - swabs for viral and bacterial culture and PCR for chlamydia and HPV testing
- Patella hammer
- Spacer and bronchodilator
- Stethoscope
- Suture material
- Syringes: 50 mL, 20 mL, 10 mL, 5 mL, 3 mL, 1 mL
- Tourniquets
- Tuning fork
- Zinc solution for zinc taste test

Charts:

- Ishihara charts
- Snellen chart

Other equipment:

- Autoclave
- Blood and body fluids spill kit, containing:
  - 1 small bucket to contain all equipment
  - 1 pair heavy duty rubber gloves
  - 1 pair safety glasses or face shield
  - 1 preferably disposable impermeable/plastic apron
  - 1 pair forceps
  - 1 roll paper towelling or paper towels
  - 2 pieces firm cardboard to be used as scrapers or 1 scoop or small dustpan
  - 2 plastic waste bags
  - body fluid clean-up absorbent powder or granules (kitty litter, polymerising beads or other absorbent material)
  - detergent to be made up when needed
  - hazard sign when needed to quarantine an area
- Disposable paper sheets
- Emergency drugs
- Face masks
- Other disposable gloves
- Oxygen cylinder with masks
- Pillow, pillow cases
- Sheets
- Sterile gloves, correctly sized for practitioners using the room
- Torch

It is useful to keep a vomit bowl/bags at reception and another within reach in your office.

Source: QIP/AGPAL

BOX 15.2 Doctor's bag: suggested contents

Emergency equipment

- Airway 110 mm (orange)
- Airway 50 mm (blue)
- Airway 60 mm (black)
- Airway 90 mm (yellow)
- Alcohol swabs
- Ambu bag (resuscitator bag) and mask (single use)
- Auriscope/ophthalmoscope with spare batteries
- Crepe bandage roll
- Disposable gloves
- Dwellcath (12 g × 2)
- Emergency guidelines manual
- Gauze squares
- Giving set
- Hartmann's solution (500 mL)
- IV cannulae
- Micropore tape
- Needles (variety)
- Normal saline ampoules
- Schedule 8 drug record book
- Sharps container
- Single-use scalpel
- Sphygmomanometer
- Syringes (variety)
- Thermometer
- Tongue depressor
- Tourniquet
- Tracheal tube adaptor 3.5 mm
- Tracheal tube adaptor 8 mm
- Tracheal tube uncuffed 3.5 mm
- Volumatic spacer with bronchodilator aerosol
- Winged infusion set

Emergency bag drugs[1] (depending on your clinical circumstances)

- Storage and safekeeping should be considered in selecting appropriate drugs.
- Adrenaline
- Antibiotics—range of samples
- Atropine (600 mcg/mL), lignocaine (100 mg/5 mL) and verapamil (5 mg/2 mL) for management of arrhythmias
- Benzotropine mesylate (Cogentin®)
- Bronchodilator (salbutamol)
- Buscopan
- Diazepam (10 mg/2 mL)
- Frusemide
- Glucose (50%)
- Glyceryl trinitrate sublingual spray or tablets
- Hydrocortisone sodium succinate
- Indomethacin suppositories (for renal colic)
- Maxolon® (metoclopramide hydrochloride)
- Morphine sulfate (15 mg/mL)
- Naloxone hydrochloride (2 mg/5 mL) (for opioid respiratory depression)
- Oral analgesics (a range of)
- Parenteral penicillin and ceftriaxone
- Pethidine (100 mg/2 mL)
- Phenergan® (promethazine hydrochloride)
- Soluble aspirin (300 mg)
- Stemetil® (prochlorperazine)
- Sumatriptan

STORAGE

You will need sufficient storage space for consumables. This improves efficiency by cutting down on time wasted going to a common storage area. Staff members should be assigned to check and replenish supplies daily, and check expiry dates regularly.

UNIFORMITY

If several practitioners are sharing space or working in different consulting rooms, uniformity of layout and equipment will be important for efficiency.

EQUIPMENT

An efficient general practice requires baseline equipment to facilitate emergency and procedural treatments. Specialised equipment will be determined by the individual practitioner's style of practice. Box 15.1 gives a list of basic equipment.

EMERGENCY AND RESUSCITATION TROLLEY

This should be located centrally in the practice so it can be accessed at any time by any doctor and/or the practice's registered nurse. Your choice of emergency trolley drugs and equipment will depend on the types of clinical conditions you are likely to encounter and your proximity to tertiary emergency services, so it is important that you customise it according to your practice's needs.

DOCTOR'S BAG

The contents of your doctor's bag (Box 15.2) should allow you to perform a basic patient examination outside the consulting room setting. Clearly, it will not be possible to carry everything you might need in one carrying case, so the bag needs to be planned and maintained to take into account the most likely clinical situations in which you might be called upon to do a house call or out-of-rooms visit.

The bag should be lightweight and waterproof, and contain layered shelves for easy access.

You should check the contents of your bag routinely. It should be restocked after each use, and all use-by dates checked about once a month.

REFERENCE

1 Murtagh J. Drugs for the doctor's bag. Australian Prescriber 1996; 19:89–92. Online. Available: http:www.australianprescriber.com/magazine/19/4/89/92/

chapter 16

Communicating with patients

INTRODUCTION

Listen to the patient, he is telling you the diagnosis.

Sir William Osler, 1904

THE PATIENT-CENTRED APPROACH

At around the same time that 'The Progress of Medicine' (see overleaf) was created, a number of clinicians began expressing similar concerns about the increasing disease-focus of modern medicine, and the corresponding decrease in attention to the patient as an individual. They began to articulate a different approach, one that did not ignore the great gains made in the scientific understanding, diagnosis and management of disease, but advocated an integration of all these advances with the individual patient's experiences, beliefs, feelings, fears and expectations.[1–3] They differentiated between disease and illness, disease being the 'biological processes physicians use as an explanatory model for illness',[2] and illness being the patient's experience of that physical or psychological disturbance.[3,4] The disease describes the common features between patients with a particular disorder, and is therefore invaluable in establishing the pattern recognition required for effective diagnosis, prognostic predictions and treatment. However, the illness experience of each patient is unique, and encompasses the 'real life' complexity of the disorder, which often does not fit neatly into textbook descriptions or investigation results. Disregarding the illness can lead to the depersonalisation of medicine, and a disconnection between doctor and patient, with no shared understanding of the very nature of the problem, and the intent and aim of treatment.[5] Medical historian Brian Hodges identifies a paradox: that by the middle of the twentieth century, when doctors were more able to offer hope of effective treatment, and even cure, than at any other time in history, patients were losing confidence in 'traditional medicine'.[6] This is not necessarily contradictory, if one considers that these scientific advances and the resultant increasing ability of doctors to effectively intervene shifted the focus to disease, with a gradual, inadvertent lessening in attention on and even respect for the illness experience. This is not to say that these doctors were uncaring, just that there was a mismatch between what patients were seeking and what doctors understood they were being asked to provide.

As general practitioners, we are often witness to the discordance between a patient's complaint that a doctor did not listen or seemed uninterested and the comprehensive history and differential diagnoses detailed in the correspondence back to us. Usually this discordance represents a disease-focused consultation—the doctor has heard the parts of the story that fit the disease model, but has had selective deafness to the patient's experiences that lie outside this construct or, at least, has not reflected back to the patient that they have heard and understood. Often these are the aspects of the story that are of most importance to the patient—the effect of the illness on their life, their fears, their struggles to make sense of the illness, its causation and prognosis. Of course, GPs are also susceptible to this 'selective deafness'. The integration of both the disease and the illness experience improves our understanding of the disorder, and the patient, and subsequently our management options (see Fig 16.1). Hippocrates himself stressed the importance of considering both 'what is common to every and particular to each case'.[2]

Initially described as the disease–illness model, the clinical approach outlined in Figure 16.1 became the foundation of patient-centredness, to contrast with a disease-centred approach. It grew out of real clinical experience in general practice / family medicine, rather

PROGRESS OF MEDICINE

The artwork, 'Progress of Medicine', by E. Fries, which graces the entrance to the medical building at the University of Melbourne, has always held a special significance for me, although the personal meaning has changed over the years. When I first entered the building as a newly accepted medical student, it represented the long tradition of healers, stretching back millennia, whose ranks I was about to join. This was both humbling and awe-inspiring.

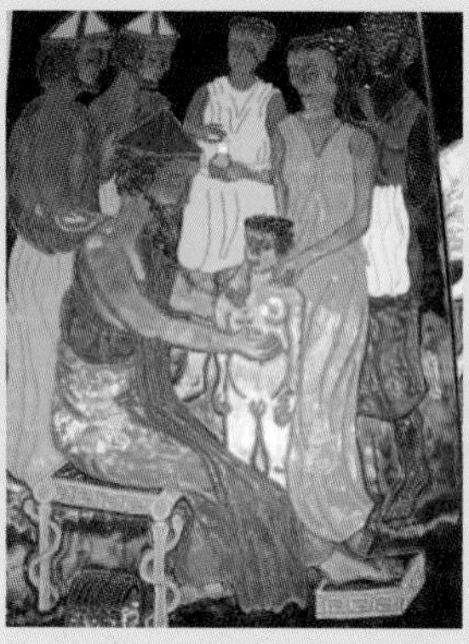

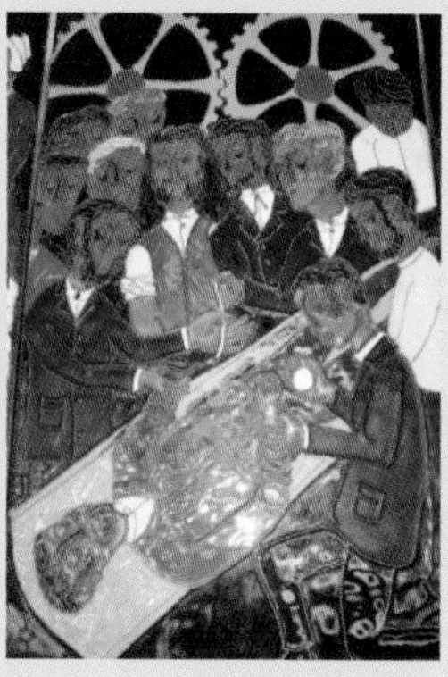

In my middle student years, chock-full of education in the medical sciences such as biochemistry, microbiology, physiology and pharmacology, I gazed at the panels and wondered how my medical forebears had been able to practise without such detailed knowledge. The depiction of the Caesarean without anaesthetic, the surgery conducted in street clothes, were horribly fascinating. How many patients had died as a result of their medical care? How did patients survive despite it? Of course, the doctors and nurses were well-intentioned, and providing the best care they could within the limitations of the current knowledge, but how very limited that seemed. It also prompted me to wonder which of the knowledge I was accepting as part of my study would be regarded askance at some future time, much as 'bleeding the patient' is regarded today.

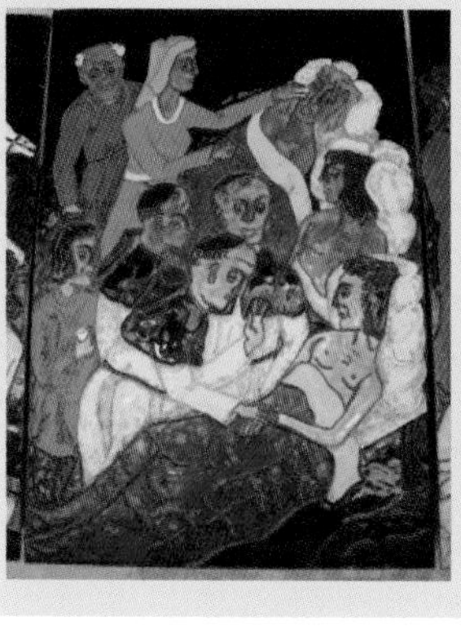

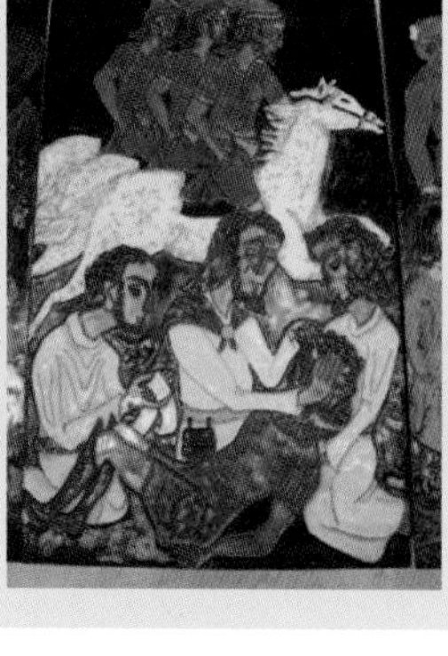

Later, I returned to the university as a senior lecturer, primarily to coordinate the teaching of communication and consulting skills. I was now a practising clinician. I stood again before the artwork which had formed the backdrop of my professional life. But now my eye was drawn to the last of the panels—depicting the modern era.

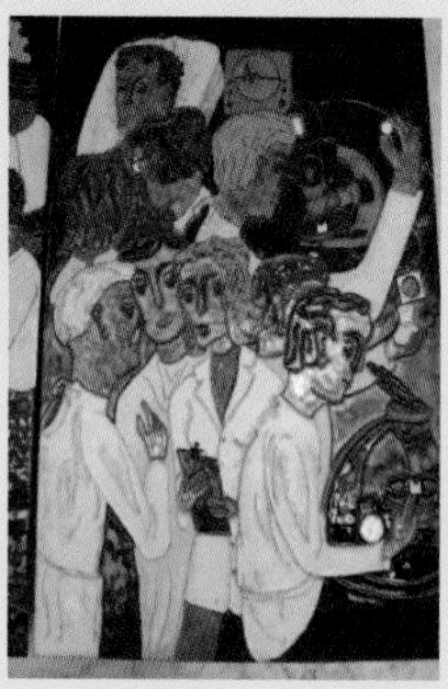

I had previously regarded this as a proper celebration and acknowledgement of the scientific advances which underpinned the current practice of medicine, many of which had been discovered and developed within the corridors around me. But now something else struck me, so forcibly that I wonder still at the intentions of the artist and the faculty fathers who had selected this piece as their prominent statement about healthcare at the building's entrance. Were they, in fact, issuing a silent challenge to all who passed? For where was the patient? They have been pushed into the background by all the technology. Whereas in the previous panels, the patient was at the centre of everyone's attention, the focus had now fundamentally shifted. And in their scientific white coats, the doctors appeared less as individuals, more depersonalised than in the earlier panels. Did this truly reflect the evolution of medicine?

Kathryn Robertson

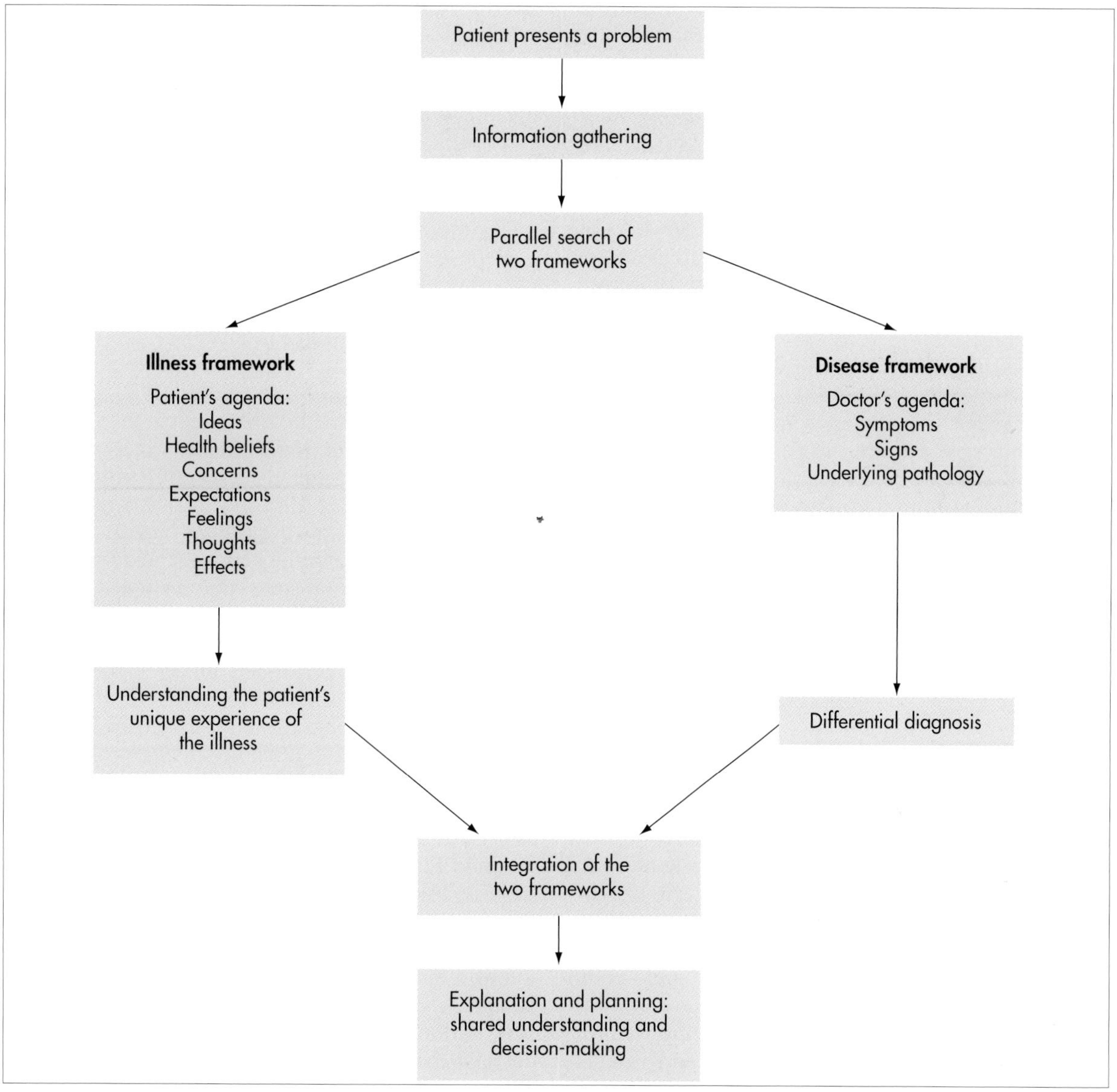

FIGURE 16.1 The disease–illness model

than being developed in theoretical and academic circles and, as such, resonated with GPs and their clinical experiences. It now has a broader currency within other medical specialties, although some find the term 'patient-centredness' quite threatening, as it is wrongly assumed that its opposite is 'doctor-centredness', with the inference that a choice has to made between the doctor's and the patient's agendas, therefore implying that patient-centredness is akin to consumerist medicine rather than a relationship based on mutuality[8] and a collaborative partnership.[7] Patient-centredness does not mean 'giving in' to the patient: an overt exploration of the patient's agenda allows an open discussion of their expectations, and a clear explanation for refusal, if required.

A key component of patient-centredness is to negotiate a balance between physician authority and patient autonomy, to achieve an optimal outcome for all involved. In some consultations, such as those involving health promotion or motivational interviewing, the scales will tip more towards patient autonomy. In other consultations the doctor may need to take on more of the decision-making responsibility. An extreme example of this would be in an emergency situation, or when the patient's decision-making capacity is impaired. Recognising patient autonomy does not mean handing over all responsibility for decision-making to the patient, but using both doctor and patient expertise to inform the process. While the doctor brings their medical expertise to the consultation, patients are experts on themselves, with invaluable insights and knowledge of their own health status. In fact, patients' self-assessments of their health have been shown to be a more accurate predictor of their survival, in both the short term and the long term, than more 'objective' measures from physical examination or a wide range of investigations.[8]

Most doctors have a preferred position on the spectrum between total patient autonomy and total physician authority, and tend to attract patients, where there is choice, who match this position. Although not all patients want to be actively involved in decision-making, most want to understand the options and the reasoning behind decisions.[9] This interplay of roles potentially fluctuates with every consultation, not just with individual patient characteristics, but also with the same patient, depending on the nature and stage of the illness and the available management options acceptable to both parties. The truly patient-centred practitioner needs to be flexible enough to modify their approach accordingly.

McWhinney thus described two of the major tasks of the consultation to be to understand both the disease and the illness, and to integrate both the doctor's and the patient's agendas.[2] The patient's beliefs, concerns, expectations and preferences are actively sought and openly addressed, and the doctor's reasoning in considering these made clear. Discordance between the doctor's and the patient's explanatory understandings of illness leads to misunderstanding and poor outcomes.[2] One only has to consider three common examples to recognise the potential for dissonance: the cultural differences in health beliefs and health-seeking behaviours; the increased general acceptance of alternative and complementary therapies, many of which have significantly different underlying explanatory models; and the use by patients of information of variable quality accessed from the internet. A patient-centred approach leads to a greater understanding of the patient's reasons for seeking help, and addressing of the patient's specific concerns.[7] This approach is associated with higher patient satisfaction and compliance than if their agenda was never explored, and with a significant improvement in clinical outcomes.[4,5,7,8,10–13] Clinical competence also, not surprisingly, leads to patient satisfaction, although some studies have suggested that patients are unable to objectively assess technical competence except in glaring examples, and tend to infer it from the doctor's interpersonal skills. Paling suggests that patient trust is a function of perceived competence and caring.[14]

Incorporating the patient's agenda also has positive outcomes for doctors, such as more accurate, effective and efficient consultations, increased doctor satisfaction and decreased frustration.[5,7,13] A patient-centred approach has been shown to positively correlate with such clinical measures as taking a reliable history, prescribing the correct medications and giving appropriate information.[8]

The concern of many doctors is that a patient-centred approach will mean longer consultations. Numerous studies have demonstrated little or no increase in the length of consultations,[4,5,7,8,11] especially once practitioners have become adept in the skills. This is attributed to the improved efficiency of ascertaining, and therefore addressing, the patient's agenda early in the consultation, and realistically establishing what can be achieved in the time available, which may include negotiating what would be better left to a future consultation. Levinson suggests that patients may feel subjectively that they have had enough time if there has been effective communication, rather than the consultation actually running longer.[12] McWhinney proposed that even a longer consultation may be an effective investment of time in the long term, if it more accurately establishes the nature of the problem and mutually acceptable action plans, compared with a series of consultations where both doctor and patient struggle to establish shared understanding and common ground.[2] Effective communication has been shown to decrease the need for follow-up appointments, as well as leading to fewer investigations and fewer referrals.[7]

An overt discussion of the two agendas, including the reasoning that underlies them, can help overcome an apparent conundrum in modern medicine. A solid body of research and literature supports a collaborative decision-making approach that respects patient autonomy. However, many doctors feel very exposed by the medico-legal implications of a patient taking a decision that subsequently leads to a negative outcome, for example by not following through a referral or investigation request. Identification of the patient's agenda helps the doctor identify any discordance, and enables them to frame the consultation around the patient's needs. Sharing the doctor's thoughts involves the patient in problem solving, helps patients understand why the doctor is asking a particular question, performing a particular test or examination, or making a referral, and provides an opportunity for elaboration and clarification. When the doctor's hypothesis forming and testing occurs internally, patients may not be able to distinguish between a suggestion, which they may choose to follow or not, and an imperative, or appreciate the intended urgency.

Poor doctor–patient communication is a leading factor in 70% of litigation, particularly when patients feel deserted, that their views are devalued or not understood, or that the information they receive is delivered poorly.[12,15] Doctors who explicitly negotiate the structure and expectations of the consultation with their patients are less likely to be sued.[7]

The process of negotiating an integration of both agendas can help develop a stronger doctor–patient relationship, which can be therapeutic in itself.[8] It conveys the doctor's interest and respect for the individual patient, and enables the patient to 'tell their story', which is a fundamental human need, particularly at a time of anxiety and uncertainty such as when confronting illness.[8] As well as being cathartic, in finding the words to describe their situation to the doctor, the patient can make more sense of it themselves, and perhaps develop insights and new awareness.[8] Stories change in the telling, greatly influenced by the responses of the audience, and in this way we help shape—consciously or unconsciously, for better or worse—the patient's understanding of their illness experience.

McWhinney stated that the greatest single problem in clinical interviewing is the failure to let the patient tell their story.[2] In a frequently cited 1984 study, Beckman and Frankel demonstrated that in only 23% of consultations was the patient able to complete their response to the opening question, and that most doctors interrupted after 15–18 seconds.[16] The longest any patient took to complete their story uninterrupted was 2½ minutes, with most completed by 45 seconds. Of particular note was the observation that the patients' most clinically significant concerns were often raised later in their story—they 'built up' to them, often establishing the context initially. Directing the consultation to the earliest issues will mean that these other, more significant concerns will either not be raised at all, or raised much later in a consultation that has already been spent on less important or urgent issues. This leads to poor time management and both patient and doctor frustration.[8] Of course, trying to establish all the patient's agenda at the outset is not fail-safe, and many patients need time to develop the relationship, trust and confidence through the consultation to raise their most significant concerns, particularly if they are embarrassed or fearful.

Thus, the tasks of the consultation go beyond making an accurate and comprehensive diagnosis/diagnoses, and formulating an appropriate management plan. They include understanding the patient and their illness and agenda, establishing and maintaining a collaborative relationship based on mutual trust and respect, appropriately shared decision-making, patient education and managing time and resources effectively. Communication skills are the tools that allow these tasks to be met.

COMMUNICATION SKILLS

Silverman and colleagues assert that the four essential components of clinical competence are knowledge, skills in communication, physical examination and problem solving.[5,7] Communication skills are important not just for the interpersonal aspects of our work, but equally for the 'technical' tasks.[8] Medical knowledge, physical examination and problem-solving skills are only useful if we can apply them, and for this we need to be able to take a relevant history, explain the reasons for examinations and investigations and ensure that the patient is giving informed consent, elucidate our diagnoses and management, and share our conclusions. This includes communication with our colleagues and other members of the healthcare team.

Effective communication is a clinical skill that can be learned.[2,4,5,7,8,17] Communication skills do not depend on personality traits, and are not just about being 'nice' to patients. Certainly, they can be misused if the intent is not in the patient's best interest and based on respect and positive regard. Although with practice they will become almost second nature, their use is still deliberate, and their selection based on the desired outcome. Until the doctor is practised and adept, they might feel forced, and sometimes their use will not be smooth; however, patients will usually still respond to the underlying intent, and forgive the occasional rough spot or backtracking.

Different skills are usually required at different stages of the consultation, and this provides a useful structure for discussing them. Silverman and colleagues[7] provide a detailed description of the structure of a typical medical consultation that incorporates a patient-centred approach, and identify the main tasks of each stage. Box 16.1 provides a summary of their framework.

In reality, these stages merge, and some may not even be necessary in every consultation. If this is a repeat consultation with a patient, there will already be some existing rapport developed in earlier consultations, and instead there will be a reconnection—often through brief social conversation. Sometimes the reason for attendance is obvious—an acute injury, for example—or it may have been initiated by the doctor as a follow-up. Nevertheless, even if the reason is apparent, it is worth checking whether there are other concerns as well. An explanation may not be necessary in every consultation for a chronic illness, but it is still important to check that both the patient and the doctor have a shared understanding, especially as the illness changes over time, or complications arise. Building the relationship

BOX 16.1 Silverman et al's expanded framework of the consultation

1. Initiating the session
   - Establish the initial rapport
   - Identify the reason(s) for the consultation
2. Gathering information
   - Explore the problems
   - Understand the patient's perspective
   - Provide structure to the consultation
3. Building the relationship
   - Develop rapport
   - Involve the patient
4. Explanation and planning
   - Provide the correct amount and type of information
   - Aid accurate recall and understanding
   - Achieve a shared understanding: incorporate the patient's perspective
   - Plan: share decision-making
   - Options in explanation and planning:
     - if discussing opinion and significance of problems
     - if negotiating mutual plan of action
     - if discussing investigations and procedures
5. Closing the session

Source: Silverman et al. 1998[7]

takes place throughout the consultation, and the skills used for maximal effectiveness in the other stages also foster a positive doctor–patient relationship.

INITIATING THE SESSION AND GATHERING INFORMATION

Traditionally, when trained to take a history, medical students are taught about questioning. They memorise a checklist of questions for each body system to provide structure to the patient's symptoms. However, in the patient-centred approach, the focus is more on listening to the patient's story and using a range of responding skills to draw out their experience. Questioning still has a place, even closed questions, as in the traditional checklist as a means to 'fill in the gaps' in the patient's narrative.

Clinical studies consistently show that the patient's history contributes 60–80% of the information needed to make a diagnosis, even with all the technological advances in investigations. We have already discussed the importance of gathering information about the patient's experience and agenda and establishing the doctor–patient relationship. Information is also gathered by physical examination and investigations, of course, and communication skills are vital here to explain to the patient what is intended, and why, to obtain informed consent, to ease anxiety, and to ensure patient engagement.[14] This is an area where misunderstandings are too frequent and often lead to complaints against the doctor.

Listening

... we listen not only with our ears but with our eyes, mind, heart and imagination as well. We listen to what is going on within ourselves, as well as to what is taking place in the person we are hearing.

Carl Rogers (cited in McWhinney 1989, p 100[2])

Effective listening includes paying attention to the non-verbal communication and the emotional content as well as the verbal content. Patient satisfaction is linked to the doctor's skills in accurately interpreting emotions conveyed by body language.[8] Yet body language can be culturally specific. Culture is not just related to ethnicity, but also includes sub-cultural characteristics such as those based on age, sex, education, socioeconomic status and occupation. The medical profession itself is a sub-cultural group with its own shared beliefs and assumptions.

Responding

Listening is not a passive activity. The patient will be guided by our response as to whether to continue and will often need encouragement. Our responses will direct the focus to particular aspects of their story. Which aspects we focus on will be determined by a range of factors: cues as to their apparent significance to the patient, relevance to our diagnostic hypotheses, and our own particular biases and interests. Self-knowledge is therefore important, as the doctor subtly but very definitely influences the patient's story. This should be based on the value of further exploration either to the doctor in understanding the problems for the patient, or to the patient in telling their story. Responding skills can be thought of as falling into five categories:

- attending skills
- following skills
- questioning skills
- reflecting skills
- advanced responding skills.

Attending skills

Attending skills are the non-verbal behaviours that demonstrate our interest and attention. Attending skills are usually unconscious indications of an attentive listener—the speaker will respond to the interest. Although they can be adopted consciously, there is the danger that the listener's attention will then be shifted away from the patient to themselves. The behaviours can become overly studied, and the attention lost. Rather than consciously trying to adopt these behaviours, it is more useful to note their absence, as a clue that perhaps we are not fully attentive, and to direct our attention back to the patient and their story.

Attending skills include:

- *an open posture*, facing or slightly side-on to the patient. When a listener is fully engaged, they will often mirror the posture of the speaker. Looking at the notes or computer is distracting and conveys a lack of attention. Even though the doctor may be able to repeat the content of what has been said, they will have missed important body language, and the patient's story will often have petered out, in the face of perceived lack of interest.
- *appropriate body movement and distance* from the patient
- *appropriate eye contact*—this can be very culturally specific, including different comfort levels across genders and ages
- *an open facial expression*, appropriately responsive to the patient's story
- *consideration of the environmental cues*, such as noise, privacy and patient comfort.

Following skills

Using following skills affords the patient the opportunity to tell their story in their own way, without the doctor overtly providing direction, but still seeking clarification where necessary.

Following skills include:

- *Interpreting and following non-verbal cues*—cues signal the significance of a particular issue. They may be verbal or non-verbal, but non-verbal cues are often an accurate indication of the meaning. Identifying possible cues requires an alert doctor. They may acknowledge the cue (e.g. '*You seem worried about your daughter ...*'), provide an opportunity to elaborate ('*Would you like to talk about it?*') and then provide the silent space for the patient to respond if they would like, with the doctor demonstrating appropriate attending skills. The doctor must remain open to the possibility that they have misinterpreted the cue—they are gently raising a possibility, rather than playing detective in looking for a 'dead give-away'. It is important to verify the interpretation with the patient.
- *Clarifying responses*—this is an attempt to more clearly define the patient's perspective. Often this clarification is as useful for the patient as it is for the doctor. Helping the doctor to understand the issues for the patient can make them more defined for the patient as well. Sometimes this also makes them less overwhelming and more manageable (e.g. '*Can I check that I've understood you correctly? ...*').
- *Confirmation*—this can demonstrate support or agreement (e.g. '*I'm glad you came in today. These symptoms have obviously been worrying you.*').

  Confirmation involves accepting non-judgmentally what the patient has to say, acknowledging the legitimacy of the patient to hold their own views and emotions (even if these differ from those of the doctor) and valuing their contributions.[7] Doctors are highly skilled in continuously evaluating the information presented to them, and they can often inadvertently inhibit the patient's story-telling by agreeing or disagreeing, or offering premature reassurance.
- *Minimal verbal and non-verbal encouragers*—these are the way we indicate our interest and attention. They include head nods, facial expressions in response to what the patient is conveying, and verbal prompts such as '*aha, hmm, I see, aah*'. Beckman and Frankel demonstrated that the more doctors used non- and sub-verbal encouragers in the first 90 seconds, the more likely the patient's main concerns and reasons for the visit are to be elicited.[16] By using these encouragers, the doctor enables the patient to complete their opening statements rather than interrupting and cutting the story off.
- *Probes*—a probe is an open-ended request for more elaboration on a particular issue. Examples are: '*Tell me more about your abdominal pain*', '*You mentioned your husband. How are things at home?*'
- *Attentive silence*—silence can be very powerful but very difficult to master. Silence provides the space for the patient and their internal experiences—their thoughts and their emotions. It gives them time to reflect and consider where and how to continue. It may enable them to regain their composure. It can convey support and comfort, particularly when accompanied by empathic attending skills.

Questioning skills

Open-ended questions give the patient a broad scope in the area they wish to cover in their reply, and encourage elaboration. Examples are: '*What can I do for you today?*', '*Can you tell me more about yourself?*' Patients' responses to open-ended questions reveal significantly more relevant information than their responses to closed questions.[8]

In using focused questions, the doctor starts to narrow down the area of enquiry. For example: '*Can you tell me more about the pain?*', '*Tell me about your diet—can you describe a typical day for you?*'

Closed questions invite a one-word answer—usually 'yes' or 'no' or a numerical answer. Because they tend to shut down elaboration by the patient and convey high control by the questioner, they can feel interrogatory unless 'signposted' or introduced. For example: '*There are a few symptoms I need to check out specifically to help me work out the likely cause of your pain. Does the pain move into your neck? … Your arm? … Do you have any nausea? … Any shortness of breath or feeling puffed out? …'*

There are two further question styles that are not usually helpful, and are better avoided.

- *Leading questions* imply the desired answer, and are difficult for the patient to disagree with. For example: *'The pain doesn't move down your arm, does it?', 'And you haven't had any change in vision?'*
- *Compound questions* often lead to confusion, for doctor and/or patient. For example: *'Have you had any nausea, vomiting, diarrhoea or constipation?'*. The patient usually responds to the first or last item on the list, and so other symptoms may be overlooked. Or the patient might answer 'Yes', and the list will then need to be broken down into its individual items to clarify the symptoms anyway. Compound questions are often used when the doctor is in a hurry, in an attempt to speed up the consultation, but often they actually slow everything as the information has to be checked and clarified.

Traditional teaching in history-taking trains doctors to ask a series of closed questions. (Paper-based checklists tend to follow the same model.) However, these can make hard work of the consultation for the doctor, as the onus is on them to think of all possible symptoms or issues, rather than allowing the patient to raise them themselves. The doctor is often distracted from listening to the patient's response, because they are thinking so hard about the next question. If they listen to the patient, the next question will usually be obvious. If the doctor does not think of a particular issue to raise, it is difficult for the patient to interrupt and introduce it themselves, so the issue or symptoms may remain unidentified.

When a patient tells their story in their own way, and the doctor fills in the gaps, there is usually a richness, internal logic and 'flow' to the story—one issue leads logically onto the next, and the significance of each is more apparent in its context. The story is therefore easier to process and remember than the 'shotgun' approach of a checklist of closed questions. Being able to recall the story in this way makes it possible to defer note taking, and focus completely on the patient.

To counteract traditional training there has been a move to encourage the greater use of open-ended questions. This is not to imply, however, that open-ended questions are intrinsically 'better' than closed or focused questions. Open, focused and closed questions all have their place, depending on the outcome one is seeking. For example, very talkative or disorganised patients can benefit from the structure provided to the consultation by focused or closed questions. Silverman and colleagues conceptualise the typical medical consultation as an 'open-to-closed cone',[7] describing the progression of the questioning style, as the doctor enables the patient to tell their story initially, then 'fills in the gaps' with increasingly focused questions. Question styles are part of a continuum rather than discrete, different categories.

Reflecting skills

In using reflecting skills the doctor conveys that they are not just listening, but understand the patient's perspective. Understanding is different from agreeing with that view. Reflection is particularly useful for conveying empathy, which is concerned with the patient's experience, rather than the doctor's own response to or interpretation of that experience.

- *Empathy* is a powerful communication skill that deepens the relationship and can be therapeutic in itself. Empathy involves both listening to the patient and reflecting back their experience, particularly their emotions. The empathic doctor needs to be open to the patient's perspective and actively put aside their own response, projections or assumptions about how the patient might feel.

  Useful starting phrases include: *'It sounds as though you felt …'* or *'I can see/sense how sad/angry/frightened … you have been …'*

  Empathy is also conveyed non-verbally, by expression, posture, tone of voice or touch, and sometimes does not need words at all.
- *Paraphrasing* is repeating back to the patient what has just been said in slightly different words. It provides an opportunity to check that the doctor has accurately understood the issue(s), indicates empathy and prompts and guides further elaboration. For example:

  Patient: *'I just feel my body is falling apart since I turned 50! I have put on weight, my blood pressure has gone up and now you are telling me my cholesterol is too high!'*

  Doctor: *'It sounds like your health has become a real concern now that you're over 50.'*
- *Restatement* is an echo of the key point in the patient's statement, usually with a vocal inflection turning the statement into a question, in effect asking for elaboration on that point. It demonstrates that the doctor is listening, but also enables the doctor to gently steer the interaction in a particular direction. For example:

  Patient: *'I'm finding it hard to cope with all this pain.'*

  The doctor can choose to restate: *'All this pain?'* or *'Hard to cope?'* The choice will guide the patient in which direction to elaborate (and may therefore affect the course of the rest of the consultation).

- *Summarising*, like empathy, can be a very powerful and useful communication skill. Depending on when and how it is used, it can actually express empathy. When the patient's story has been lengthy, or disorganised, a summary can also be a check that the doctor has understood the key points. It can be useful to feed back to the patient that the doctor has listened and understood, and can signal a change in focus in the consultation.

Advanced responding skills

- *Interpretation* extrapolates beyond what the patient presents verbally and non-verbally, to aid further insights. Both content and emotion can be interpreted to deepen understanding for both doctor and patient. For example:

  Patient: *'My cousin had to have surgery for breast cancer, and it all happened so quickly that she couldn't really get her head around it until months later, when it was all over.'*

  Doctor: *'Do you feel you are being rushed into making a decision? … It must be really difficult to have to make choices at a time like this.'*

  The second part of the doctor's statement is an empathic response, which can be particularly useful when using the advanced responding skills.
- *Reflection of discordance*—gently pointing out discordance between, for example, a patient's verbal and non-verbal messages, or between their stated aspirations and their behaviour, or between their understanding and reality can powerfully focus the consultation. For example:

  'You say you really don't mind having to work late, and yet you sound quite angry about it.'

  'On the one hand you are quite worried about the possible complications of your diabetes, but on the other hand you continue to smoke. That's quite a dilemma …'

  Sometimes called confrontation, reflecting discordance can appear aggressive, unless it is delivered empathically and non-judgmentally.
- *Active listening* is giving one's complete attention to another person and requires the listener to put aside any personal concerns, distractions and preconceptions, to make their total awareness available to the speaker. It is a profound validation of the speaker and their thought processes (although again not necessarily of the views being expressed).[18] This is an act of generosity and courage,[19] especially as it is difficult and tiring to do well. It is an extension of all the communication skills outlined above, but is done for the intrinsic benefit of the listening rather than to gather information to make a diagnosis or develop solutions, which are the very skills for which doctors have been trained.

> You can learn to be a better listener, but learning it is not like learning a skill that is added to what we know. It is a peeling away of things which interfere with listening, our preoccupations, our fear, of how we might respond to what we hear.
>
> Ian McWhinney (cited by Kelly, p 168)[20]

EXPLANATION AND PLANNING

This phase of the consultation typically refers to the task of explaining the doctor's assessment and negotiating a mutually acceptable management plan, and therefore usually occurs in the second half of the consultation. However, it is important to remember the importance of planning the consultation itself, and explaining the rationale, which occurs much earlier. Doctors might see 30 or more patients a day in familiar surroundings, and it is easy for them to underestimate the uncertainty and anxiety about the consultation itself that many patients experience. Simple assumptions such as which aspects of the history are relevant, which examinations are indicated and the details of what the examinations involve can lead to misunderstandings. There are a number of specific techniques that are useful:[7]

- *Sharing the doctor's thoughts* makes the doctor's reasoning, hypothesis forming and testing open, and thereby helps the patient understand why the doctor is asking a particular question or performing a particular test or examination. It involves the patient in problem solving.
- Similarly, *providing a rationale* for the doctor's questioning and examination can prevent misunderstanding. For example, a patient may see no obvious reason for the doctor to examine their axillae and inguinal regions for lymph nodes, suggesting glandular fever when their presenting complaint was a sore throat, unless the connection is made clear.
- *Signposting* also makes the underlying rationale clear and smoothes the transition between topics. It indicates the direction of the consultation, and is often used in conjunction with summarising to check with the patient before progressing. For example:

  'Let me check that I have understood you correctly—the pain came on while you were resting after dinner last night. It was in the centre of your chest and felt like something was stuck in your gullet. It settled after you had a drink of milk. Is that right? … There are a few other specific questions I would like to ask you, to check out the possible causes of the pain [signpost]. Did it move anywhere else? …'

The management phase

The management phase is built on the earlier stages of the consultation, and difficulties at this point have usually originated earlier, such as failure to identify or explore the patient agenda, or develop an effective relationship.

Studies have repeatedly shown that patients want more information from their doctors,[6–8] and that the information they do receive does not match their needs. Doctors generally overestimate the amount of time they spend on explanation and information giving, and they tend to focus on treatment, especially drug treatment, whereas patients want information on diagnosis, causation and prognosis.[6–8] Patients perceive doctors who provide clear, relevant and useful information as more personally caring, sincere and dedicated,[8] but too often the information is incomprehensible to patients, being incomplete or full of technical terms, which adversely affects the patient's understanding of their condition and its appropriate management.[7]

The doctor–patient relationship will affect how comfortable the patient feels in asking questions and seeking clarification. Patients are often concerned that the doctor will think badly of them if they ask too many questions—that they haven't understood or are pushy, that they are questioning the doctor's judgment or that they are taking too much of the busy doctor's time.[8] Perhaps not surprisingly, patients who ask questions receive more information[7]; ironically, however, those patients who have been involved throughout the consultation and shared in the doctor's thoughts and rationale are likely to feel most comfortable and have the least need to seek clarification at this stage.

The following skills can be particularly useful in structuring the management phase of the consultation.

- *Check the patient's information need.* In the patient-centred approach, the patient's prior knowledge, experience, fears, beliefs and expectations will have been ascertained during the information-gathering phase, and this will form the basis for determining what information is needed and how the information should be best presented. It can be helpful to check this with the patient, as well as providing encouragement or explicit permission to the patient to interrupt, question or clarify any of the information.
- *Having ascertained what information needs to be conveyed, deliver it in 'chunks and checks'.* This can aid patient understanding, recall and compliance.[7] It can sometimes be helpful to think about delivering information as similar to reading a newspaper article. Newspaper articles are laid out in paragraphs with headings and subheadings to direct the reader's attention to the key messages and to facilitate comprehension. Verbal information can be delivered in the same manner, in 'chunks', punctuated with checks of the patient's understanding and the opportunity for questions and concerns to be addressed. Repetition, and the skills discussed earlier of signposting, summarising and attending to the patient's verbal and non-verbal cues, can also assist patient's comprehension and subsequent adherence to the plan.[7]

It is important that, at the end of the consultation, the doctor and patient have a clear and shared understanding of what is expected to happen from then on. For example, the patient should have an appreciation of the expected course of the illness, and what action to take if it varies from this course, including specific developments that would raise concern and what to do if they occur. This is sometimes called *safety-netting*. For example, a provisional diagnosis of gastroenteritis may have been made, but the patient might be advised about symptoms and signs that could indicate the development of appendicitis.

Similarly the patient should have a clear plan for any follow-up, or any further action such as investigations or referrals, including intended urgency.

CLOSING THE CONSULTATION

Problems in closing the consultation most often relate to the patient raising a totally new symptom or concern, often in response to the doctor asking an open question such as: 'Is there anything else?'. This is a very useful question to ask when establishing the patient's agenda early in the consultation, but is almost certain to lead to mutual frustration if left until the very end. But if both agendas were integrated earlier, if patients have been able to ask questions throughout, and if their understanding and commitment have been checked, closure will usually follow naturally. Signposting that the consultation is drawing to a close, summarising the diagnosis and management plan and doing a final check that this concurs with the patient's understanding are usually all that is required. It is usually considered polite to accompany the patient to the door, perhaps with a farewell handshake, and this is an additional non-verbal signal that the consultation has concluded.

SUMMARY

In the medical consultation, effective communication:

- fosters a relationship based on mutuality and a partnership between doctor and patient
- is patient-centred—both the patient's and doctor's agendas are explored and integrated
- explores both illness and disease frameworks
- is framed around the individual patient's needs, including using language and concepts that are comprehensible to the patient

- is flexible—responsive to the individual patient, the individual situation and the individual doctor
- is empathic
- is reflective—the doctor is consciously concerned with the communication processes and their outcomes
- facilitates the process of negotiating disagreements and establishing boundaries
- is interactive—that is, a two-way communication; the doctor checks throughout the consultation that the patient understands and is in agreement with both the process and the content of the interaction. The doctor shares their thought processes and rationale with the patient.

Finally, it seems appropriate to give Ian McWhinney the last word.

> If we could all just learn to listen, everything else would fall into place. Listening is the key to being patient centered.
>
> Ian McWhinney (cited in Kelly, p 168[20])

Acknowledgments

Kathryn Robertson would like to acknowledge the invaluable contributions of her colleagues Heather MacCormack, Ruth McNair and Professor Doris Young to the various incarnations of communication skills training at the University of Melbourne.

The specific communication skills that form the body of this chapter have been adapted and modified from numerous sources over the years, but the most influential texts have been *A Textbook of Family Medicine* by Ian R. McWhinney, *Skills for Communicating with Patients* by Silverman, Kurtz and Draper, and Robert Bolton's generic text on communication: *People Skills.*

Especial thanks go to Mr E. Fries for his kind permission in allowing reproduction of his artwork: 'Progress of Medicine'.

RESOURCES

Bolton R. People skills. How to assert yourself, listen to others and resolve conflicts. Sydney: Prentice Hall; 1986.

McWhinney IR. A textbook of family medicine. 2nd edn. New York: Oxford University Press; 1997.

Silverman J, Kurtz S, Draper J. Skills for communicating with patients. Oxford: Radcliffe Medical Press; 1998.

REFERENCES

1 Levenstein JH, McCracken EC, McWhinney IR et al. The patient-centred clinical method. 1. A model for the doctor-patient interaction in family medicine. Fam Pract 1986; 3(1):24–30.

2 McWhinney IR. A textbook of family medicine. New York: Oxford University Press; 1989.

3 Weston WW, Brown JB, Stewart MA. Patient-centred interviewing. Part I: Understanding patients' experiences. Can Fam Physician 1989; 35:147–151.

4 Stewart M, Brown BB, Weston WW et al. Patient-centred medicine. Transforming the clinical method. Thousand Oaks, CA: Sage; 1995.

5 Kurtz S, Silverman J, Draper J. Teaching and learning communication skills in medicine. Oxford: Radcliffe Medical Press; 1998.

6 Hodges B. The many and conflicting histories of medical education in Canada and the USA: an introduction to the paradigm wars. Med Educ 2005; 39:613–621.

7 Silverman J, Kurtz S, Draper J. Skills for communicating with patients. Oxford: Radcliffe Medical Press; 1998.

8 Roter DL, Hall JA. Doctors talking with patients. Patients talking with doctors. Improving communication in medical visits. Westport, CN: Auburn House; 1992.

9 Levinson W, Kao A, Kuby A et al. Shared decision-making not for all patients. J Gen Intern Med 2005; 54(12):531–535.

10 Horder J, Moore GT. The consultation and health outcomes. Br J Gen Prac 1990; 40(340):442–443.

11 Simpson M, Buckman R, Stewart M. Doctor–patient communication: the Toronto consensus. Br Med J 1991; 303:1385–1387.

12 Levinson W. Physician–patient communication: a key to malpractice prevention. JAMA 1994; 272(20): 1619–1620.

13 Thiedke CC. What do we really know about patient satisfaction? Fam Pract Manage 2007; 14(1):33–36.

14 Paling J. Strategies to help patients understand risks. Br Med J 2003; 327:745–748.

15 Beckman HB, Markakis KM, Suchman AL et al. The doctor–patient relationship and malpractice. Arch Intern Med 1994; 154:1365–1370.

16 Beckman HB, Frankel RM. The effect of physician behaviour on the collection of data. Ann Intern Med 1984; 101:692–696.

17 Bolton R. People skills. How to assert yourself, listen to others and resolve conflicts. Sydney: Prentice Hall; 1986.

18 Robertson K. Active listening. More than just paying attention. Aust Fam Physician 2005; 34(12): 1053–1055.

19 Mackay H. The good listener. Better relationships through better communication. Sydney: Pan Macmillan; 1994.

20 Kelly L. Listening to patients: a lifetime perspective from Ian McWhinney. Can J Rural Med 1998; 3:168–169.

chapter 17

The general check-up

More is missed by not looking than by not knowing.

INTRODUCTION AND OVERVIEW

Many patients will present without a specific symptom or disease, instead requesting a 'general check-up'. Other patients, presenting with undifferentiated symptoms and signs, will need a more thorough history and examination than would normally be the case for most presentations. For your schedule to run smoothly, you will need to ensure that reception staff allow adequate time for new patients and for those who request a general check-up. This should average about 45 minutes to an hour and will usually require a follow-up appointment for discussion of results and health advice.

MOTIVATORS

It is worth ascertaining the patient's motivation for their appointment, to ensure that you address the underlying reason for their presentation on this occasion. Some possible reasons:

- Their partner or a family member is concerned about an aspect of their health.
- They require a medical report for insurance or employment purposes.
- They are approaching a milestone birthday or event and want to assess their state of health.
- They feel non-specifically unwell and want to exclude disease.
- They have a friend or family member recently diagnosed with a health problem such as a cancer, diabetes or a cardiac event.
- They have become aware of a family history of disease for which they want to be screened.
- They have seen or heard a public health message and have decided to act on it.
- They have a health concern such as depression or sexual dysfunction, but they feel uncomfortable talking about it and are 'checking you out' to see if they trust you enough to discuss it with you.

HOW OFTEN?

How often a person should have a medical check-up depends on their age and general health status.

- *Babies*—should be opportunistically examined at the first encounter with a GP. This is often at the time of the first immunisation at 2 months, then again at 4 months, 6 months, 12 months and 18 months.
- *Children and adolescents*—preschoolers should have a comprehensive check-up every 6–12 months; older children and adolescents, once a year.
- *Adults*—if there are no specific health problems, annually.

HISTORY

As in all areas of medical care, a comprehensive history is the foundation of quality practice. Questions that probe the patient's physical, emotional and spiritual wellbeing will be required, to form a picture of their overall health.

New patients should be encouraged to collate and bring with them any previous documentation, including specialists' or allied health professionals' reports, investigation results, X-rays, CT scans, MRIs and hospital discharge summaries. They should also be asked to bring any bottles or packets of prescribed or over-the-counter (OTC) medications, supplements or herbal medicines they are taking. This will enable you to check ingredients and doses of combination preparations.

ELEMENTS OF THE HISTORY

Elements of the history are as follows:

- *establish patient's reason for appointment*
- *current symptoms* and health concerns
- *past medical history*—including any hospitalisations and significant diagnoses
- *obstetric* (female)—date of last normal menstrual period; frequency and duration of periods; obstetric history: number of pregnancies, deliveries (vaginal and caesarean), premature births, neonatal deaths, ectopic pregnancies, miscarriages, terminations, infertility, continence
- *occupation(s)*—present and past, including any occupational exposures to toxins, chemicals or pollutants
- *family medical history*—including age and cause of death of first- and second-degree relatives. Ask particularly about heart disease, asthma, diabetes, cancers and depression
- *medication*—prescription, OTC remedies and supplements and self-medication including dosage, frequency and route of administration. Women often need to be prompted about the oral contraceptive pill, many not viewing it as 'medication'
- *past and current use of recreational drugs*—type, route of administration and frequency of use
- *lifestyle*—type of work, working hours, how they spend their leisure time, recent travel
- *emotional health*—moods; sleep pattern; relationships; attitude to work; signs of depression; level of satisfaction with job; family; friends; anxiety; use of alcohol, caffeine, tobacco or other drugs to alter mood
- *sleep pattern*—sleep latency, time of retiring to bed and waking, and total hours of sleep. Is it interrupted? Snoring or breathing pattern while sleeping, daytime sleeping and tiredness
- *exercise routine*—type, time, intensity, preferences for types of activity
- *diet, nutrition*—appetite, digestion, breakfast, snacks, lunch, dinner, fluid intake. For accuracy, this may require a food diary to be kept for several days to a week to indicate types and amounts of foods eaten
- *for babies*—feeding patterns and difficulties. Is the child breastfed? What formula if they are bottle-fed? Solids?
- *smoking*—past or current tobacco use. Did they ever smoke? How much and for how long? When did they quit? If still smoking, are they considering quitting?
- *alcohol*—frequency, type, amount (recorded as standard drinks per day and number of days per week or month)
- *sexual history*—current partner(s), new partner(s), previous sexual partner(s), previous testing for sexually transmissible infections, unprotected intercourse, sexual functioning, contraception
- *immunisation*—routine and travel vaccinations, with dosages and dates according to the relevant standard vaccination schedule
- *previous check-ups and investigations*—dates and results of previous Pap smears, prostate-specific antigen (PSA) tests, blood glucose, lipids, ECGs, chest X-rays etc.

GENERAL PHYSICAL EXAMINATION

Despite some medical debate about its value, the comprehensive physical examination is a core clinical skill essential to the integrative approach to healthcare, described in the *Medical Journal of Australia* as 'the doctor's best kept secret—powerful, portable, fast, cheap, durable, reproducible and fun'.[1] It is about confirming the normal and looking for the abnormal. It will interact with and complement the medical history, which will have revealed areas that may require special attention and is an absolute prerequisite to further investigation of symptoms and signs.

Before you commence:

- Observe the patient's demeanour, body habitus, facial expressions, mobility and gait as they enter the room, take a seat and transfer from chair to examination couch.
- Check that you have everything you need, so you do not have to interrupt the consultation to go hunting for an essential piece of equipment.
- Ensure that you have the patient's (or, for children, their parent's) permission to proceed with the examination.
- Allow the patient to remove their own clothes without your assistance, unless they request that you assist.

It is also important to explain to the patient what you are doing throughout the examination. The sequence in which you conduct the examination will depend on your training and on any particular issues raised by the history.

BABIES

- Measurements—length, weight, head circumference. Check against percentile chart for age.
- Head—shape, fontanelles.
- Ears—external canals, eardrums. Does the baby startle to noise?
- Eyes—fix and follow? Strabismus? Check lenses for signs of cataract.
- Mouth—tongue tie, thrush, teething.

- Skin—jaundice, rashes, birthmarks.
- Heart—check for murmurs.
- Lungs—breath sounds, respiratory rate and effort.
- Abdomen—liver, spleen, umbilicus.
- Hips and legs—check for congenital dislocation of the hips.
- Genitalia—check for inguinal hernia. In boys, check both testes in the scrotum, look for hydrocele.
- Developmental assessment checked against appropriate age milestones.
- Moro reflex (normal if bilateral and present from birth to 4 months).
- Immunisation status.

CHILDREN

- Height and weight, chart percentiles.
- Blood pressure and heart rate. Check for murmurs.
- Teeth, gums, tongue and throat.
- Reflexes.
- Eyes, ears, nose.
- Skin.
- Lungs.
- Abdomen.
- Fine motor development, e.g. ability to pick up small objects, write or tie shoes.
- Gross motor development, e.g. ability to walk, climb stairs, skip or jump.
- Spinal alignment—for signs of curvature (scoliosis).
- Genitalia, confirming a normal level of maturation, and checking for hernia or other possible problems.
- Check immunisation status.

ADOLESCENTS

(see Ch 56, Adolescent health and development.)

- Physical examination—as for adults.
- Check stage of sexual maturation.

ADULTS

- General demeanour, body shape, facial expression, vocal tone, gait, tremor.
- Colour—pallor, florid, peripheral or central cyanosis.
- Weight (kg).
- Height (cm).
- Waist and hip measurements (cm).
- BMI and waist–hip ratio (< 1.0 for women and 0.9 for men).
- Blood pressure (sitting and standing). If elevated on first reading, ask the patient to take a deep breath in and out and allow themselves to relax back in their chair. Then repeat. The blood pressure will often settle once the initial performance anxiety passes.
- Temperature.
- Pulse—rate, character and rhythm.
- Auscultation—heart sounds, murmurs.
- Jugular venous pressure.
- Precordial movement.
- Arterial pulses.
- Lungs—air entry, chest expansion, rhonchi, rales.
- Genitalia—male: urethra, testes, STI check; female: gynaecological examination including speculum, Pap smear if required and swabs for STI including *Chlamydia* if indicated.
- Breast examination (female).
- Abdomen—liver, spleen, masses, tenderness or guarding, rebound, distension, digital rectal examination (DRE), inguinal nodes, axillary nodes.
- Hernias—check with patient standing, lying and straining with head lifted off the pillow.
- Eyes—acuity, pupils, fundi, eye movements, colour perception (Ishihara chart).
- Ears, nose and throat:
  - ears—hearing, screening, ear canals, tympanic membranes
  - nose—airway
  - tongue—mouth, throat, teeth
  - thyroid—check for goitre or thyroid nodule
  - cervical, axillary and inguinal lymph nodes
  - cranial nerve examination.
- Neurological examination:
  - deep tendon reflexes (upper limb and lower limb)
  - cranial nerves
  - gait
  - muscle strength
  - coordination
  - sensory perception.
- Spinal movement—scoliosis, forward flexion, extension, rotation, neck range of motion.
- Joints—signs of joint swelling, inflammation or limitation of movement; single or multiple joint involvement.
- Skin—lesions, rashes, birthmarks, naevi (dermatoscope for greater detail of suspicious lesions), nails, hair, scalp.
- Urinalysis—collect midstream at the time of examination and observe macroscopically for blood, sediment and clarity.
- Dipstick test for white cells, red cells, nitrites, glucose and microalbuminuria.
- Resting ECG.
- Mental state examination:
  - appearance
  - attitude
  - behaviour
  - mood and affect
  - speech

    - thought process
    - thought content
    - perceptions
    - cognition
    - insight
    - judgment.
- Mini mental state examination (MMSE) if screening for dementia/memory:
    - time and place of the test
    - remembering a list of words
    - arithmetic (e.g. serial sevens)
    - language use
    - language comprehension
    - basic motor skills.

INVESTIGATIONS

Investigations will depend on the patient's age, gender, personal and family medical history, health behaviours and any relevant findings on history and examination. Guidelines also change and evolve as evidence emerges of the costs and benefits of individual case-finding or population screening.

A comprehensive medical check-up may require referral for:

- electrocardiogram (exercise)
- intraocular pressure (tonometry) and retinal examination
- laboratory tests—full blood examination
- iron studies—iron, ferritin
- liver function tests—bilirubin, albumin, total protein, alkaline phosphatase, alanine transferase (ALT), aspartate aminotransferase (AST), gamma glutamyl transferase (GGT)
- kidney function tests—blood urea, creatinine, calcium, sodium, potassium, glomerular filtration rate (GFR), microalbuminuria
- diabetes screening (fasting blood glucose)
- HIV and hepatitis B and C serology
- prostate-specific antigen (PSA) testing for males
- lipid profile—total cholesterol, HDL, LDL, triglycerides
- thyroid function tests T4, TSH (thyroid-stimulating hormone)
- stool for occult blood (or colonoscopy, depending on age and family history of bowel cancer)
- chest X-ray
- 24-hour ambulatory blood pressure monitoring if resting BP is elevated on successive readings
- osteoporosis screening—peripheral bone densitometry (DEXA); vitamin D
- female—mammogram, pelvic ultrasound, CA-125
- audiometry
- mini mental state assessment—if signs of short-term memory loss
- biopsy or referral for suspicious skin lesions.

PREVENTIVE INTERVENTIONS

Armed with the results of your history, examination and investigations, the follow-up consultation is the opportunity to formulate a health management plan or to provide advice on preventive health measures. Any features of concern need to be addressed and interventions discussed.

Preventive strategies will depend on the patient's age and state of health (see chapters on babies and children (Ch 55), adolescents (Ch 56), pregnancy and antenatal care (Ch 54) and the elderly (Ch 57)) and can have a powerful effect on reducing the future risk of chronic disease.

Interventions might include:

- smoking cessation advice
- discussion of safe alcohol drinking limits
- physical activity plan (see Ch 9)
- healthy weight and waist measurement, and weight management plan
- nutrition advice, including appropriate diet and supplements
- medication review, including potential side effects and interactions
- immunisation update
- sexual safety counselling where appropriate
- advice on sun protection, skin self-examination and adequate sun exposure
- advice on oral hygiene and referral for dental check.

RESOURCES

Talley NJ, O'Connor S. Clinical examination: a systematic guide to physical diagnosis. 6th edn. Sydney: Elsevier; 2010.

REFERENCE

1 Reilly BM, Smith CA, Lucas BP. Physical examination: bewitched, bothered and bewildered. (Editorial) Med J Aust 2005; 182(8):375–376.

chapter 18

Practice management principles

INTRODUCTION

This chapter provides a checklist of the important factors to consider in establishing and operating an integrative health clinic. It is not a definitive practice management manual. Most of the principles described here are the same as for other medical clinics, but there are some distinctive features.

When considering establishing or changing your practice to an integrative model, you will have a range of options to consider. Your practice might consist of:

- general practitioners (GPs) only, without special CM training, who refer actively to a 'virtual team' of CM practitioners outside the clinic
- GPs only, who have an understanding of or special training in one or more CM modalities, which they incorporate into their therapeutics advice to patients
- GPs with or without in-depth knowledge of one or more CM modalities working in a co-located integrated team with CM practitioners, with an in-house inter-referral pattern.

MISSION STATEMENT

An important first step is to know who and what you are, and to be able to articulate this. Writing a mission statement may sound like a simple task, but it can take a significant amount of thought and negotiation to make sure everyone, from the front desk staff to the most senior practitioners, shares the belief described in the mission statement.

Your practice management style will reflect the type of practice, your underpinning philosophy and the mix of practitioners working in your team. Adopting an integrative model of practice should also begin with the practitioners as role models themselves, by incorporating health principles into their own personal beliefs and health habits.

BUSINESS PLAN

Whatever your mission and philosophy, for your practice to survive and thrive, its business fundamentals must be sound. A business strategy needs to be based on the most likely scenario, but it also has to consider the potential 'worst case' financial scenarios.

An initial scoping exercise will assess the existing services in your local area and whether there is a demand for the services you are planning to provide. If you provide a largely locally based service then you will need to assess the likely patient demographic and the patients' special health needs. If your practice is likely to draw from a wider area because it provides more specialised services for which patients are prepared to travel, then that demographic will be different and may only become evident with time as the clinic and its practitioners develop a reputation for expertise in particular areas.

All potential costs need to be factored in, as well as realistic projections of turnover and growth trajectory, including buying or leasing costs of furniture, phone systems, IT, medical equipment, leasing or holding costs of premises, insurances, cleaning, utilities, consumables and staffing.

Material resources need to be planned and discussed with team members and administration staff. Decisions on big-ticket items like computer systems and software need to be made very carefully, with a view to future capacity, not just current need. You also need to decide whether to buy, lease or hire-purchase major equipment.

Staffing levels for administration need to be appropriate to the required skill set and demand due to current and anticipated patient traffic. Staff levels will need to be adjusted as required. The selection of practice manager will be central to your success and your own mental health. This person will need to have the skills to set up and operate the office systems, deal with staff and suppliers, and ensure the smooth running of the business. A mixture of full-time and part-time staff can provide the continuity and flexibility required in a small to medium-sized practice.

Employment contracts that comply with relevant legislation need to be created. It is important to have an occupational health and safety policy and an equal opportunity and anti-discrimination policy in place as an appendix to employment contracts.

Establishing a service-oriented culture from the front desk that pervades your organisation will not only help deliver efficient patient care but also increase the likelihood of profit.

REVOLUTION OR EVOLUTION

Becoming an integrative practice can be a revolution or an evolution. Existing general practices might begin the process by maximising the health promotion opportunities and chronic disease management options offered to patients, as well as encouraging self-care strategies adopted by practitioners and staff.

An existing general practice might also survey its local area for qualified CM practitioners, arrange meetings to discuss practitioners' areas of expertise and broaden the practice's referral base beyond the existing list of allied health professionals. For example, an osteopath, an acupuncturist and a chiropractor might be added to the existing referral list where more appropriate than a physiotherapist in some clinical circumstances. The most 'integrated' approach is to incorporate CM practices or CM practitioners into an existing GP-only practice, or to establish a planned integrated team de novo.

Your strategic plan ideally will include a statement of goals, objectives, opportunities and potential barriers.

AUDIT THE PRESENT

If you have an existing practice and are planning to move towards an integrative model, you can begin with an audit of the practice's current performance in this area.

- What does your practice (or practitioners) already offer or provide referrals for in areas such as stress management, dietary advice, exercise advice, risk reduction interventions, community education programs and support groups?
- What are the needs and beliefs of your patients? Rather than taking a wild guess, consider using a carefully constructed patient questionnaire.
- Update your existing referral base to include practitioners who can offer care in a form that your patients would find useful. This would include such things as yoga or Pilates teachers/classes, meditation, t'ai chi, aquafitness, qualified personal trainers, massage therapists, nutrition education classes, counselling services, help lines and so on.

SET UP THE INFRASTRUCTURE

Once you have decided which practices or practitioners you intend to include in your integrative model, you need to adjust your infrastructure to accommodate any changes.

- Are your consulting rooms the appropriate size for the planned activity?
- What is the appropriate duration of consultations?
- Does your practice software have the capacity to accommodate different types of practitioners?
- What equipment is needed? (e.g. massage tables, acupuncture needles)
- Is your communication network (phones, faxes, email) appropriate for your purposes or does it need to be upgraded?
- Staff members need to be educated about the treatments offered by the clinic and the appropriate responses to enquiries from patients and potential patients.
- A website is a useful tool that patients can access for practice details, practitioner profiles and health news and information.

IS YOUR CLINIC AS 'GREEN' AS IT COULD BE?

According to the Australian Conservation Foundation,[1] saving just one ream of paper will save 20 kg of greenhouse gases and reduce your stationery bill.

- Print on both sides of paper, and use the back of used paper for intra-office memos.
- Aim for a 'paper-free' office by moving to computerised records, and arrange for results to be sent online. Ask drug reps to leave only one copy of promotional material, which can then be circulated to all doctors.
- Have a paper shredder to shred privacy-sensitive documents before recycling.
- Buy recycled paper and toilet paper.
- A single incandescent globe switched over to a compact fluorescent globe will save 0.5 tonnes of greenhouse gas and save you $70 in energy costs in its lifetime.
- Installing a $4 tap aerator in the bathroom or kitchen can cut water use there by half. Fix any dripping taps.
- Buy green power for your clinic.
- Turn off computers and appliances when they are not in use, and make sure all lights are switched off out of hours.
- Check that refrigerators are working efficiently and with seals intact.
- Check the cleaning products in your clinic and ensure they are non-toxic.
- Ventilate your clinic with natural air and minimise the use of air conditioning.

REGULATORY CONSIDERATIONS

Specific regulatory requirements will vary from one jurisdiction to another, but practice management requires detailed attention to:

- insurances—professional indemnity, building and contents, public liability, workers' compensation, key personnel etc
- financial record-keeping and accounting
- staff superannuation
- taxation, including employees' PAYG withholding
- goods and services tax or other consumption taxes.

OUTSOURCING

Referral to CM practitioners requires some knowledge of the evidence base regarding the safety, efficacy and cost-effectiveness of various modalities for different conditions. It is important to be able to identify the most appropriate therapies for given conditions based on the evidence, and the patient's needs, previous experiences and personal preferences. For example, there is little point in referring a patient for acupuncture if they have a phobia about needles.

A referral base takes some time and effort to build and will come from a variety of sources including professional recommendations, local networks and patient recommendations.

Practitioners outside the practice could be invited to submit their credentials and references prior to referrals. You will need to know details of the practitioners' academic qualifications, clinical experience and areas of expertise, registration (if the modality has a register), fee structure, insurance rebates available to patients and professional liability insurance.

IN-HOUSE

If you decide to integrate CM practitioners into an existing general practice, there needs to be consensus on the types of modalities that would be most suitable for inclusion. The type of financial or business arrangement also needs to be considered. This might be in the form of:

- room rental with or without administration services
- contractor on a commission basis
- employee
- associateship
- partnership.

Legal advice should be sought to determine the exact nature of the arrangement and this should be codified and agreed on prior to the commencement of that practitioner. You will need documentation confirming practitioners' qualifications, references, registration and professional indemnity insurance.

REFERRAL PATTERNS

A general practitioner-centred model of integrative practice has the GP as the initial contact within the practice. The doctor would carry out an assessment of the patient's health status and their healthcare needs, and then discuss and coordinate the most appropriate strategies to reduce health risk, prevent disease or manage illness.

Referral to practitioners with the appropriate knowledge and skills occurs in the same way as referral to medical specialists, with a requirement for monitoring clinical progress either through an integrated record system or through progress reports being communicated back to the referring doctor. There should also be an agreed time frame for medical re-evaluation of the patient's progress.

An integrative practice where there is a variety of primary care providers may have either a GP, an allied healthcare or CM practitioner outside the clinic, or another practitioner within the clinic (such as a naturopath, a physiotherapist or a psychologist) as the initial contact. In these cases the non-medical practitioners need to be very clear on when it is appropriate to refer for medical assessment, or to refer back to the referring GP once treatment is concluded or if medical review is required.

Communication protocols between practitioners need to be carefully established and followed.

COMMUNICATION

Communication is an important feature of efficient practice management and team development.

FROM THE PRACTICE TO PATIENTS AND POTENTIAL PATIENTS

A practice brochure in hard copy and on your website should contain, as a minimum, information on your mission statement, practitioners, location, contact details, public transport, directions and parking, how to make appointments, what your after-hours and emergency arrangements are, your billing rates for various practitioners, and forms of payment.

Prior to your launch or relaunch you will need to organise a graphic designer to design a logo and colours for your brochure, letterhead, business cards and other stationery. Patients could be offered the opportunity for email newsletters.

Appointments, particularly for booked long consultations, can be confirmed via bulk email or SMS messaging through practice software.

Patients also need to be informed of the practice's privacy policy and what happens to their confidential information, and agree to clinically relevant information being transmitted between practitioners involved in their care.

BETWEEN PRACTITIONERS

As in any group practice, group meetings are an essential form of communication for the purpose of exchanging information on practice management matters and improving efficiency. Meetings should be held regularly by agreement at a time suitable for most practitioners and staff. Minutes should be kept and circulated with a note of actions taken or planned, as soon as practicable after the meeting. Practitioners may wish to hold separate clinical meetings to discuss difficult or complex cases, with appropriate measures taken to protect patient confidentiality.

An integrative practice provides the opportunity for joint consultations. For example, a patient wanting to combine medical, herbal and/or acupuncture treatments might benefit from a part of the consultation being conducted with two or more practitioners from different disciplines involved in their care present to discuss their management plan.

Where the integrative practice operates as a 'virtual' team, clinical feedback about patient progress ideally needs to be done in writing. Or, if feedback is provided by phone, a contemporaneous record of conversation must be kept in the patient's records. Significant changes in treatment or the patient's condition should be communicated with all practitioners involved in the patient's care.

PATIENT RECORD KEEPING

Medical practitioners are generally well aware of their responsibility to keep contemporaneous and legible records of patient encounters. Confidential patient information must be protected and patients informed if there is a shared record system accessible to other practitioners. These principles must be emphasised for all healthcare practitioners in an integrative clinic.

Some practitioners, such as psychologists, may prefer to maintain their own separate records and communicate patients' progress back to the referring practitioner by letter rather than shared records.

The clinical record must:

- identify the patient
- be comprehensible to another practitioner
- contain details of the history and examination, clinical opinion and management plan, including medication or supplements prescribed, procedures, counselling and advice.

Records must be kept for at least seven years from the date of the last entry. If the patient is a minor, the record must be kept until the patient turns 25. Within reason, records must be stored so that confidentially is maintained and so that they are not lost, stolen or damaged.

ONGOING EVALUATION

Successful practice management requires an ongoing system of performance assessment. This will include clinical and financial aspects of the practice as well as less tangible outcomes like practitioner and staff satisfaction.

Patient satisfaction can be gauged by surveys designed to assess how happy patients are with the current service and what they would like to see done to improve their experience of the clinic.

RESOURCES

American Medical Association, Solutions for Managing Your Practice, http://www.ama-assn.org/ama/pub/physician-resources/solutions-managing-your-practice.shtml

Australian Medical Association Guidelines on Service Contracts between Doctors and Medical Practice Principals, http://www.ama.com.au/node/3760

The Drs Reference Site, Practice Management, http://www.drsref.com.au/business.html

REFERENCE

1 The Australian Conservation Foundation's GreenClinic Guide can be downloaded from the ACF website at http://www.acfonline.org.au/uploads/res/res_greenclinicguide.pdf

chapter 19

Integrative medicine and the law*

INTRODUCTION

Integrative medicine is a major development within the healthcare systems of the Western world, including the United States, the United Kingdom, Canada and Europe. All doctors need to understand the legal implications of the practice of integrative medicine. Doctors need to be aware, for example, of the requirements for informed decision-making, and know how complementary medicines (CMs) and complementary practitioners (CPs) are regulated. While this chapter focuses on the Australian legal context, doctors in other jurisdictions will find the general discussion helpful.

Integrative medicine involves the blending of conventional and complementary and alternative medicine (CAM) 'with the aim of using the most appropriate of either or both modalities to care for the patient as a whole'.[1] There have been many attempts at defining CAM and a frequently cited definition is:

> a broad domain of healing resources that encompasses all health systems, modalities, and practices and their accompanying theories and beliefs, other than those intrinsic to the politically dominant health system of a particular society or culture in a given historical period.[i]

CAM includes a diverse group of healing practices such as traditional Chinese medicine, ayurvedic medicine, Western herbal medicine and naturopathy. Different taxonomies of CAM have been proposed and one frequently cited is that of the National Center for Complementary and Alternative Medicine.[2] This taxonomy divides CAM into five categories:

- alternative medical systems, such as traditional Chinese medicine and Ayurveda
- mind–body interventions, such as meditation
- biologically based therapies, such as herbs
- manipulative and body-based methods, such as osteopathy
- energy therapies—modalities that involve the use of energy fields.

The term 'CAM' has traditionally described the 'relationship between unconventional healthcare disciplines and conventional care' but is now more of 'a collective label for the disciplines themselves'.[3a] CAM brings different approaches to diagnosis and treatment, and a central focus is prevention and wellness, which complements biomedicine.[4]

While historically CAM has been on the margins of healthcare, developments in the past decade that have accorded it greater legitimacy within mainstream healthcare include a massive investment in CAM research, particularly in the United States, increasing evidence of its safety and efficacy, acknowledgement of a role for evidence-based CAM in mainstream healthcare by professional medical bodies, and a number of high-level government and institutional inquiries around the world into the role of CAM.[ii] These inquiries have focused on the regulatory interventions necessary for a planned and systematic integration of CAM into mainstream healthcare. Although a wide-ranging inquiry has not been held in Australia, there have been three recent inquiries with a narrower focus on CMs, CPs and health services.[iii] The implementation of recommendations from these inquiries is assisting, or when implemented will assist, with the promotion of integration in Australia.

Significantly, it is the ad hoc integration occurring at the level of the consumer and the health practitioner, including the general practitioner (GP), that has been driving these developments at the state and national policy level. The most recent and comprehensive data show that nearly 70% of Australians use CAM.[5] It means that Australians have one of the highest rates of CAM

* As at 28 February 2009.

usage among Western nations.[5] In the 12 months prior to the 2005 survey by Xue and colleagues, more than 44% had consulted a CP, resulting in an estimated 69.2 million visits to CPs.[5] This figure approximates the number of visits to medical practitioners during the same period.[5]

There is evidence that consumers use CAM because of a desire for holistic and natural treatment, to fill gaps in medical care, such as the management of chronic illness, and the perceived effectiveness of CAM.[6–8] It is also clear from prevalence studies that consumers use CAM as part of self-care, and in combination with biomedicine, to achieve their own type of integration. CAM users like to pragmatically pick and mix biomedical and CAM options to address their healthcare needs.[5,9,10] One difficulty with this trend is that a high proportion of patients use CAM and biomedicine concurrently, and do not inform their doctor about the CAM use and, in addition, many doctors fail to ask patients about CAM use.[5,10–16]

Doctors, and particularly GPs, have been responding to consumer demand and integrating CAM treatments into treatment plans. In 2000, 20% of GPs in Victoria and 38% of GPs in Perth, Western Australia, had practised one or more CAM modalities. Eighty-two per cent of the Victorian GPs had referred patients for a complementary therapy, and nearly 68% of Perth GPs were in favour of referring patients to CPs as part of their medical care.[17,18] A national survey of Australian GPs in 2000 (published in 2005) found that CAM, non-medicinal therapies, such as acupuncture, massage, meditation, yoga, hypnosis and chiropractic, 'are widely accepted and can be considered mainstream in Australian general practice'.[13a] At the same time, the Victorian study showed that herbal medicine, naturopathy, vitamin and mineral therapy, osteopathy and homeopathy were 'accepted by a sizable minority of doctors'.[17a] In a 2008 survey of Australian GPs, one-third reported practising integrative medicine and about 90% had recommended at least one CM in the past 12 months.[16]

Doctors may be motivated by a number of factors to integrate CAM, including the desire to address consumer preferences in healthcare, an interest in working with safer remedies, and the need to contain costs. It is also reasonable to assume that integrative doctors believe that CAM complements biomedical care, and can also be the primary treatment for patients suffering from chronic conditions who are unresponsive to conventional treatment.[3,13,19]

LEGAL OBLIGATIONS IN THE PRACTICE OF INTEGRATIVE MEDICINE

It is not possible to outline all the legal obligations that may be relevant to this context, or how those obligations impinge on integrative medical practice. The ethical and legal obligations relevant to medical practice are, of course, also relevant to the practice of integrative medicine, including professional codes of conduct, the criminal law, and obligations related to confidentiality and privacy. There are texts providing information about these obligations that are written specifically for medical practice.[iv] It is a matter of applying the relevant laws to the integrative context.

Because doctors who practise integrative medicine are firstly biomedical practitioners, obligations stemming from statutory registration are of particular importance. The doctor's duty to exercise reasonable care and skill in the care of the patient is also central, as it affects every area of practice including the provision of information and advice to the patient to enable the patient to make an informed decision. There are also laws that are particularly important in the integrative context, and these include the regulation of CMs and CPs.

There is little legal authority relevant to integrative medicine, as the medico-legal issues are, for the most part, yet to be tested in the courts in Australia, the United Kingdom and the United States. This chapter therefore addresses general legal considerations and refers to tools that may assist doctors to manage the risks and generally navigate this new terrain. The chapter focuses primarily on the doctor's duty of care, and the regulation of CMs, CPs and healthcare services.

THE DOCTOR'S DUTY OF CARE TO THE PATIENT

Through the law of negligence, the law imposes on a doctor an obligation to exercise reasonable care and skill in examination, diagnosis, treatment, and provision of information and advice, that duty being a 'single comprehensive duty'.[v] The relevant law has been affected by reforms arising from the Review of the Law of Negligence (Ipp Review) initiated by the Australian Government in 2002 in response to an insurance crisis.[20] Although it was originally intended that a model statute be developed to implement the reforms recommended by the Ipp Review in all Australian states and territories, this did not eventuate. As a result, there are a number of differences in the legislative provisions enacted in the states and territories.

There is currently little guidance from the courts on the meaning of the new statutory provisions and how they affect the common law, which applied across Australia prior to the Ipp Review reforms. What follows therefore is a discussion of elements of the law that doctors need to bear in mind in their daily practice. It is, of necessity, a broad brush approach, as it is not possible to provide specific guidance in relation to each state or territory.

A doctor owes a duty of care to each patient to take reasonable care to avoid acts and omissions that a reasonable doctor would foresee as likely to cause harm. It is an obligation to take reasonable steps to avoid foreseeable risks of harm that are 'not insignificant'. In ascertaining what, if any, precautions a reasonable doctor would take in response to a foreseeable risk, consideration needs to be given to:

- the probability of the harm occurring
- the likely seriousness of the harm
- the expense, difficulty and inconvenience of taking precautionary action
- any other conflicting responsibilities you may have, and
- the social utility of the activity.[vi]

The greater the probability of a risk and the greater the magnitude of the harm, the greater the need to take steps to minimise that risk, particularly where the cost of doing so is reasonable.

Although CAM therapies are not without their risks, generally speaking CAM as a whole does have a lower risk profile than biomedicine. Adverse events do occur in CAM but are much less common than in biomedicine.[vii] And there are fewer complaints and claims against CPs. A US study found that claims against complementary practitioners 'occurred less frequently and typically involved less severe injury than did those against conventional practitioners in the same period'.[21a]

Doctors need to become familiar with the risks of integrative practice. The major risks include harm stemming from:

- the failure to provide safe and efficacious biomedical treatment
- a missed or delayed diagnosis of a biomedical condition, and
- complications arising from the combined use of pharmaceuticals and CMs.

Reasonable responses to these risks would generally include:

- undertaking a biomedical differential diagnosis before embarking on a treatment plan
- ensuring that patients are offered safe and efficacious biomedical treatment, and
- asking patients about CM use and taking this into account when prescribing pharmaceuticals.

These matters are all considered further below.

THE SCOPE OF THE DOCTOR'S DUTY

At this time the scope of a doctor's duty of care extends to the provision of biomedicine only. However, according to the Australian Medical Association's (AMA) position statement on CM, a doctor appears to have an ethical obligation to at least ask a patient about CAM use in medical consultations.[22] Although the ethical obligation to engage with patients about CAM is unlikely to be enforced by the AMA, it may increasingly be recognised and enforced in other forums, such as professional disciplinary hearings and in medical litigation, because of the risks stemming from patients combining CAM and biomedicine. A doctor may also have a legal obligation to provide information and advice to some patients about evidence-based CAM treatment options, and this is discussed below (see 'Informed decision-making in integrative practice').

At present, a doctor has no positive duty, ethically or legally, to integrate CAM therapies into medical practice. At the same time, it is ethical and lawful for a doctor to provide evidence-based CAM treatments to a patient, or to refer a patient to receive such healthcare.[viii] However, once a doctor chooses to integrate CAM into conventional medical practice, the scope of the doctor's duty of care expands to include integrative practice.

MEETING THE REQUIRED STANDARD OF CARE

The standard of reasonable care and skill required of a medical practitioner under the common law is 'that of the ordinary skilled person exercising and professing to have that special skill'.[ix] In the case of a GP, the standard of reasonable care and skill is that of a doctor who specialises in general practice.

Following the 1992 High Court decision of *Rogers v Whitaker*, the court became the final arbiter of whether or not the standard of care had been met (although medical evidence has always been influential in the view formed by the court), but this has now been modified in most jurisdictions as a result of recommendations arising from the Ipp Review. The means by which any liability in negligence will ultimately be determined is now set out in most jurisdictions in statutory provisions, such as s. 59 of the *Wrongs Act 1958* (Vic). Under s. 59 a doctor will not be negligent if he or she acts in a way that at the time is 'widely accepted in Australia by a significant number of respected practitioners in the field (the peer professional opinion) as competent professional practice in the circumstances' (*the peer professional opinion test*). The fact that there are differing opinions that are widely accepted 'does not prevent any one or more (or all) of those opinions being relied on'. Further, the peer professional opinion does not have to be universally accepted in order to be widely accepted. However, where the court determines that the peer professional opinion is unreasonable, it cannot be relied on.

The peer professional opinion test appears to create a type of defence in medical litigation.[x] This means that if a doctor is able to provide probative evidence that his or her conduct or opinion is widely accepted as competent professional practice in the circumstances, he or she will not be negligent (provided the court considers that the opinion is reasonable).

The peer professional opinion test is similar in other states, although the widely accepted practices and opinions are not limited to Australian ones, in Queensland and Western Australia.[xi] In those states a doctor could draw on widely accepted practices in integrative medicine outside Australia, to establish that he or she had acted within the standard of care.

There is little authority on the meaning of the peer professional opinion test, but it has been suggested that:

- 'widely accepted' may require that the practice be accepted by various groups across the nation, rather than limited, for example, to a group within one region
- 'a significant number of practitioners' may mean that a large portion of those practising the medical speciality accept the conduct, although not necessarily 50% or more as there is clearly room for different schools of thought
- expert medical evidence in medical litigation should come from respected practitioners and must support the conduct of the doctor as competent.[23]

There have been no decisions where the courts have determined that peer professional opinion is irrational or unreasonable, and it is likely that this will occur only in very exceptional circumstances.[20]

PROFESSIONAL STANDARDS AND THE PEER DEFENCE

The need to meet the standard of reasonable care and skill, and the availability of the peer defence, point to the importance of professional standards and guidelines on the practice of integrative medicine, integrative medical texts, peer-reviewed journals on evidence-based CAM, and educational programs. These professional resources will provide important guidance on what is expected.

Medical boards are the primary regulator of doctors and have ultimate responsibility for those who are integrating CAM into conventional practice.[22] Guidance on professional standards is found in the codes and guidelines published by the medical boards.[xii] Although the codes and guidelines are recommendations of the medical boards and are not legally binding, they are authoritative and an important guide to professional standards and what is expected of medical practice and performance. They are potentially enforceable through disciplinary processes in relation to allegations of unprofessional conduct and unsatisfactory professional performance. The codes and guidelines need to be applied to the integrative context. They are not comprehensive and do not cover every possibility, and it is expected that doctors will apply general principles to different circumstances as they arise.

Most medical boards have a specific policy statement on CAM and doctors should be familiar with the relevant policy and its application to practice.[xiii] However, there are a number of differences in the policies, raising questions about what the appropriate professional standards are in this area. The establishment of the National Registration and Accreditation Scheme for the health professions, including medical practitioners, in 2010 will provide the opportunity for the development of a national integrative medicine policy.[xiv]

A number of jurisdictions in the United States have passed legislation intended to protect doctors from being inappropriately targeted and disciplined for the practice of CAM.[24] Inappropriate targeting would involve findings related to the use of CAM as substandard, on the basis that a CAM treatment is different from a biomedical treatment.[25] The Medical Council of New Zealand has made provision for a similar protective clause within its policy statement on CAM.[26]

There are no similar legislative or policy provisions within Australia, but the process for dealing with CAM-related complaints by medical boards may have a similar effect. The Western Australia Medical Board, for example, makes it clear that any investigation into a complaint will involve an assessment of the overall competence of the practitioner, some assurance that integrating CAM will not in itself result in a finding of unprofessional conduct.[27] However, where CAM use forms a part of the complaint, there will be specific inquiries into matters such as the risk/benefit ratio of the treatment and whether it is greater or less than that of other treatments.[27] It is likely that this will be the approach across all Australian jurisdictions. Doctors should therefore be prepared to produce evidence of the reasoning process that led to the decision-making, as well as the informed decision-making of the patient.

There is a need for consistent guidelines in relation to CAM, and national and integrative medicine bodies, such as the Royal Australian College of General Practitioners (RACGP) and the Australian Integrative Medicine Association (AIMA), are taking a lead in this respect.

AIMA, established in 1992, is the peak body for integrative medicine in Australia. The members of AIMA are doctors who are interested or involved in integrating natural and holistic approaches into conventional care. AIMA provides a vehicle for peer support for integrative doctors, provides educational programs and resources (including a journal) and acts as an advocate of integrative medicine with government and professional bodies.[28]

The RACGP sets standards for general practice in Australia. The RACGP seeks to ensure that the general practice training curriculum reflects 'both the fundamental nature of Australian general practice and the evolution of … [the] discipline in response to community needs and advances in science and technology'.[29a] The RACGP has a major role to play in standard setting in integrative medicine, as most doctors integrating CAM are GPs. Hence the college collaborates with AIMA through a joint working party to provide guidance to practitioners on good medical practice in the evolving field of integrative medicine.

The RACGP/AIMA Joint Working Party (JWP) was established in 2005 and the terms of reference include establishing how complementary medicine can be incorporated into high-quality clinical practice.[xv] A *Joint Position Statement on Complementary Medicine* was released in 2005 and the primary position of the JWP is that 'evidence based aspects of complementary medicine are part of the repertoire of patient care in mainstream medical practice'.[30a]

More recently the RACGP has established a Chapter of Integrative Medicine within the college and there are plans to introduce a Fellowship of Integrative Medicine and standards for integrative practice.[xvi] An integrative medicine curriculum was published in 2007.[xvii] This incorporates the skills and knowledge needed by GPs in integrative medicine across five domains of general practice. The curriculum, Chapter and proposed Fellowship are key developments, as they direct, or will direct, doctors to the skills that they need to acquire to achieve competent practice in this area. It is clear that the RACGP is committed to addressing the integrative medicine educational needs of GPs and providing guidance in relation to the standard of care expected. When fully implemented these developments will play a highly significant role in carving out what amounts to widely accepted, competent professional practice for integrative medicine in Australia, particularly in general practice.

Other integrative medical bodies, such as the Australian Medical Acupuncture College, and the Australian College of Nutritional and Environmental Medicine, are currently playing, and will continue to play, a role in defining standards in these more specific aspects of integrative medicine—that is, acupuncture, and nutritional and environmental medicine.

Membership in the RACGP and integrative medical bodies will assist doctors to keep in touch with relevant standards and widely accepted practice in this rapidly developing area of medical practice. Such membership will also provide access to resources and peer networks for resolving the integrative medicine and medico-legal issues that will inevitably arise.

The remainder of this section considers the doctor's duty in the therapeutic encounter, with particular reference to examination, diagnosis, treatment, referral, and the provision of information and advice.

EXAMINATION, DIAGNOSIS AND TREATMENT IN INTEGRATIVE PRACTICE

For doctors, integrative medicine involves integrating CAM into conventional medical practice. This is clear from the entire legal context. It is also apparent from guidelines, such as the Western Australia policy statement on complementary, alternative and unconventional medicine, which refers to the doctor's obligation to undertake a proper assessment, arrive at a diagnosis according to biomedical principles, devise a treatment plan, and provide information in relation to any conventional treatment, and its risks and benefits.[28]

As is illustrated in a number of chapters in this integrative medicine text, the doctor will need to make a differential biomedical diagnosis according to the usual methods of history taking, examination and diagnostic testing. And, as is standard practice within general practice, it will be necessary to exclude particular diseases, such as cancer, as a cause of symptoms (see, for example, Ch 51, Breast disease). CAM diagnostic testing may be appropriate if it will provide further information to assist in the care of the patient (see, for example, alternative testing methods in Ch 21, Allergies).

In the treatment phase, it is a matter of ascertaining treatments for the patient's condition, including any appropriate CAM options, and working with the patient to devise a treatment plan. An integrative approach may be appropriate for some conditions but not others (see, for example, Ch 42, Skin).

It is clear from existing professional guidelines that evidence-based CAM is relevant to the practice of integrative medicine.[22,30] The RACGP-AIMA position statement on complementary medicine states that:

> evidence based medicine should be the basis of evaluating complementary medicine and/or therapies and their use by the medical profession. It should also be the basis of any collaborative relationship between general practitioners and complementary therapists.[30b]

The RACGP-AIMA statement adopts the Sackett et al definition of evidence-based medicine as:

> the conscientious, explicit, and judicious use of current best evidence in making decisions about the care of individual patients. The practice of evidence based medicine means integrating individual clinical expertise with the best available external clinical evidence from systematic research. By individual clinical expertise we mean the proficiency and judgment that individual clinicians acquire through clinical experience and clinical practice.[30c,31]

The RACGP policy on evidence-based medicine is also relevant to decision-making about CAM treatments. This policy refers to the evidence-based approach incorporating three components: the best evidence available, the biopsychosocial circumstances of the patient, and the clinical skills and judgment of the doctor.[32] Evidence-based medicine therefore involves more than the highest levels of scientific validation. It is an assessment that considers all treatments, conventional and complementary, across a multidimensional spectrum that takes into account safety and efficacy, and 'practicality, availability, utility and cost effectiveness as well as other dimensions'.[33a] And adopting an evidence-based approach to CAM is not so much about having specific knowledge as it is about acquiring evidence-based medicine problem-solving skills, and having access to texts, databases, peer networks and CAM prescribing software.[34a]

Bearing in mind the legal obligation to act reasonably and take reasonable steps to avoid foreseeable risks that are 'not insignificant', the level of evidence required will depend on the circumstances. Where treatments are potentially toxic, or where the treatment is being proposed as an alternative to biomedicine, higher levels of evidence will be necessary. With low-risk therapies, or where there is no biomedical treatment available for the condition and the CAM treatment is known to be safe, lower levels of evidence are more likely to be acceptable. Of course, doctors should ensure that the patient has realistic expectations about what can be achieved by the CAM therapy, particularly where the evidence available is equivocal.[35a]

Cohen and Eisenberg have devised a decision-making grid based on an analysis of the evidence available for safety and efficacy.[36] The grid is a useful risk management tool and provides guidelines on when CAM could be recommended, when it should be avoided, and when it could be implemented with close monitoring.

REFERRAL IN INTEGRATIVE PRACTICE

In referral, as with the other aspects of the doctor's duty, reliance must be placed on the general principles of the law of negligence and relevant professional guidelines.

Doctors may be concerned about the potential for legal liability, such as vicarious liability (liability for the negligent conduct of another), arising from referral to CPs. Whether a referral from a doctor to a CP gives rise to the potential for vicarious liability will depend on the nature of the relationship. Where the CP is someone with whom the doctor has a pre-existing legal relationship—employee, independent contractor, business partner or licensee—there may be the potential for such liability. Doctors making referrals to such CPs should seek legal advice.

Where there is no pre-existing legal relationship, it is unlikely that the doctor will be found responsible for any negligent conduct of the CP to whom a patient is referred. However, the doctor may be liable for making a negligent referral because, for example, the CAM modality was inappropriate for the patient's condition, or the CP was not appropriately qualified to provide the healthcare. The 2002 decision of the New South Wales Court of Appeal, *McGroder v Maguire,* illustrates the difference well, because in that case the doctor was liable for a negligent referral to a chiropractor, but not for the negligence of the chiropractor to whom the referral had been made.[xviii]

To avoid a negligent referral, there appear to be two primary considerations—choosing a modality that is appropriate for the patient's condition, and referring the patient to a suitably qualified health practitioner, whether that be another doctor or a CP. Other considerations relate to the need to establish reasonable communication with the health practitioner, and an appropriate level of biomedical review of the patient's condition.

The RACGP-AIMA joint position statement refers to the need for referral to be based on evidence-based medicine. This means that the evidence-based considerations outlined above in relation to treatment also apply to decision-making about referral.[30b]

The referral from a doctor to a CP may be viewed as similar to a referral to an allied health practitioner, such as a physiotherapist, particularly where the CP is regulated by statute—that is, osteopaths and chiropractors in all Australian jurisdictions, and traditional Chinese medicine practitioners in Victoria. Where a CP is regulated by statute, the task of referral is simplified, as it is reasonable for a doctor to rely on statutory registration as indicating an acceptable level of knowledge and competence, in the absence of evidence to the contrary. However, there are many CPs within Australia who are not regulated by statute. Instead, most CPs are self-regulated through professional associations, although there may be some CPs who are not regulated at all, as membership of professional associations is voluntary.

The La Trobe University School of Public Health review of the regulation of naturopathy and Western herbal medicine severely criticised the self-regulation of these two CAM modalities.[6] Among the factors criticised were: the proliferation of education providers in the CAM field, which had resulted in a lack of appropriately qualified teaching staff (most are sessional); a limited research environment; inconsistent arrangements for clinical training; and lack of standardisation of educational requirements or significant movement to align curricula so that practitioners using the same title, such as 'naturopath', have the same knowledge base.[6] Given this recent evidence, a CP's membership in one or more of the numerous self-regulating professional associations may not be a sufficient basis for decisions in relation to referral. The reasonable doctor may need to take further steps to ensure that the CP is qualified to provide the necessary healthcare to the patient.

General practitioners surveyed in 2000 were noted to be more concerned about CPs (such as practitioners of chiropractic, Chinese herbal medicine, herbal medicine, naturopathy and homeopathy) acting as primary carers, including in relation to serious illness, without recourse to GPs, and the potential for delayed and missed diagnosis, than the risk posed by the actual CAM therapies.[13] Therefore, setting aside formal considerations, such as qualifications, there are other matters that a doctor may also want to be reasonably confident about when making a referral. For example, does the CP regularly assess the progress of a patient and cease treatment when the condition is alleviated or the treatment is shown to be ineffective? Does the CP know when and how to refer the patient on for medical management?[35,37]

It may also be prudent to provide a written referral to the CP. A written referral provides contemporaneous documentary evidence of the nature of the referral and the expectations of the doctor. This will become relevant in the event of an adverse outcome and any subsequent legal or complaints processes. Relevant referral information may include the medical history, the clinical examination and findings, the biomedical diagnosis and treatments, and the goals of treatment.[35] It is reasonable to suggest that the more serious the condition, the greater the need for comprehensive information. In some circumstances it may also be appropriate for the doctor to ask the CP to assess the patient and provide advice about whether the practitioner and the CAM modality could assist in the care of the patient's medical condition.

There is a great deal that needs to occur at the state and national policy level to facilitate appropriate referrals between doctors and CPs, including the regulation of CPs. Traditional Chinese medicine practitioners will be regulated under the National Registration and Accreditation Scheme for the healthcare professions from 1 July 2012.[xix] There are no current plans for naturopaths and Western herbal medicine practitioners to be included in the national scheme although there have been recommendations that these healthcare professions be regulated by statute.[6,38]

There is a need for detailed guidelines and protocols for doctors in relation to referral, and no doubt these will be forthcoming from bodies such as the RACGP and AIMA in the near future. In the meantime, enquiries to professional bodies will assist in establishing relevant standards and widely accepted practice in the area of referral. For example, do GPs interview CPs and seek reference checks from peers who have worked with a CP before making a referral?[35]

INFORMED DECISION-MAKING IN INTEGRATIVE PRACTICE

A doctor has an ethical and legal obligation to provide information and advice to enable a patient to make an informed decision, and increasingly this includes evidence-based CAM options for healthcare.

The doctor's *ethical* obligation to provide information and advice is set out in the *General Guidelines for Medical Practitioners on Providing Information to Patients*.[39,xx] The guidelines are not mandatory standards but they reflect good medical practice and may be relevant evidence in disciplinary proceedings or medical litigation. The professional obligation includes not only information about risks, such as the possibility and probability of complications and side effects, but also the benefits and likely outcomes of treatment, and alternative treatment options.

In the 1992 decision of *Rogers v Whitaker*, the Australian High Court held that a doctor has a duty to provide information and advice about the material risks of any planned procedure. A risk is material:

> if, in the circumstances of the particular case, a reasonable person in the patient's position, if warned of the risk, would be likely to attach significance to it [the proactive limb of the test] or if the medical practitioner is or should be reasonably aware that the particular patient, if warned of the risk, would be likely to attach significance to it [the reactive limb of the test] *(the test of materiality)*.[xxi]

While in *Rogers v Whitaker* the court was focused on material risks (the case was concerned with the risks of eye surgery), the doctor's legal obligation to provide information and advice also includes other types of information, such as benefits and alternative treatment options, to enable a patient to make a meaningful decision.

If the proactive limb of the test of materiality is operating, a doctor has to turn his or her mind to what the reasonable person in the position of the patient would want to know. On the other hand, if the patient asks questions, the reactive limb of the test is engaged and the specific concerns of the patient must be addressed, no matter how unreasonable those concerns may be.[xxii] And the reactive limb will operate not only where the doctor knows of the specific concerns of the patient, but also where the doctor should have known of those concerns. If, for example, the patient does not expressly ask about CAM options but the doctor is aware from the patient's history that the patient regularly uses CAM, then it is likely that the doctor should have known that the patient would find information about CAM options material.

The peer professional opinion test pertaining to the doctor's duty in relation to examination, diagnosis, treatment and referral is not applicable to the provision of information and advice. Instead of medical opinion, it is the court that is the final arbiter as to whether the doctor acted reasonably in providing information and advice, given the application of the patient-centred test of materiality outlined above.

While the AMA left it to the individual doctor to decide whether to adopt direct use of CAM therapies, it clearly saw the need for doctors to have at least a basic understanding of CAM, to enable advice to be provided to patients about CAM.[22] The RACGP-AIMA position statement on complementary medicine also notes that GPs 'should be sufficiently well informed about complementary medicines and/or therapies to be able to provide advice to patients when appropriate'.[30d]

I have argued elsewhere that a doctor may have a legal obligation to advise a patient about evidence-based CAM treatment options where those options are reasonably available, and where that information would be significant to the particular patient or the reasonable person in the position of the patient.[40] Since the publication of that argument there have been a number of changes that put the argument on a stronger footing. Not changes in the law but, rather, the increasing evidence of safe and efficacious CAM, and evidence that nearly 70% of the population now have an interest in CAM healthcare options (it was previously thought that 52% of the population were CAM users).[5,12]

Of course, in the integrative context it is important to remember that patients should also be advised about standard biomedical treatments. And if a patient refuses to accept biomedical treatment after being informed and advised, trying to persuade the patient to submit to biomedical treatment may not be helpful or necessary from a legal point of view. Instead, through discussion and negotiation, a 'wise agreement' can be developed in relation to a treatment plan which may include the trialling of CAM options with an appropriate level of monitoring.[41a] A doctor can also enhance, rather than jeopardise, the therapeutic relationship by engaging in a dialogue with the patient. It is necessary for the doctor to remain open to the patient's use of CAM and explore the patient's concerns, health goals and reasons for using CAM.[7,42] It is also important from a professional and a legal point of view that the treatment plan and the patient's informed decision be documented. This documentation will assist in the event of an adverse outcome, if the matter becomes the subject of disciplinary proceedings, a coronial inquiry or medical litigation.

REGULATION OF COMPLEMENTARY MEDICINES

It is essential for doctors to have a good working knowledge of how CMs are regulated. Without this information, practitioners are not in a position to advise consumers and prescribe such treatments competently.

Complementary medicines include vitamins, minerals, herbs and nutritional supplements, homeopathic medicines and some aromatherapy products. Complementary medicines are given different labels in other countries. In Canada, for example, they are referred to as 'natural health products'. The regulation of CMs also varies greatly internationally. There is minimal regulation in some countries, such as New Zealand, where there is no pre-market scrutiny of safety and quality.[43] In other jurisdictions, CMs are heavily regulated. In Germany and France, for example, herbal medicines at least are regulated like pharmaceuticals, with pre-market approval of safety, quality and efficacy.[44] Australia's regulatory scheme for CMs is robust but the regulatory approach is based on the low-risk profile of CMs. A brief introduction to the regulatory scheme is provided here. For more details, you are referred to other resources.[xxiii]

Complementary medicines are regulated under the Therapeutic Goods Act 1989 (Cth) (TG Act) and Therapeutic Goods Regulations 1990 (Cth) (TG Regs).[xxiv] The regulatory scheme is administered by the Therapeutic Goods Administration (TGA). The Office of Complementary Medicines (OCM) is a discrete, administrative group within the TGA established to focus exclusively on the regulation of CMs. The Complementary Medicines Evaluation Committee (CMEC) is an expert committee that evaluates CMs and provides scientific and policy advice to the TGA.

All therapeutic goods (including CMs) must be registered with the Australian Register of Therapeutic Goods (ARTG) established under the TG Act. Most CMs are 'listed' goods and prescription medicines are 'registered' goods under the ARTG. The distinction is important, as registered goods are subject to efficacy requirements prior to marketing, but listed goods are not.[xxv]

The Australian regulatory approach aims to achieve a balance between the four regulatory objectives (safety, efficacy, quality and timely availability) through the licensing of manufacturers, good manufacturing requirements, a pre-market safety evaluation of therapeutic substances to be included in CMs, and post-market surveillance, including a system for reporting adverse events.[xxvi]

Pharmaceuticals have a narrow therapeutic window, and apart from over-the-counter medication, access is restricted via prescription according to requirements under drugs and poisons legislation.[xxvii] Many complementary medicines, on the other hand, have a wide therapeutic window, and are widely available without prescription through outlets such as pharmacies, health food stores and supermarkets.

Listed CMs are not evaluated for safety, although the therapeutic ingredients that are incorporated into listed CMs are evaluated. Listed CMs are also not evaluated for efficacy in the same way as prescription medicines, and this enables the products to be marketed fairly quickly. At the same time, the claims that can be made for listed CMs are limited to general and medium-level claims. For example, a medium-level claim based on traditional use of the medicine could state that: 'this traditional Chinese medicine has been used for the relief of the symptoms of eczema. If symptoms persist, consult your healthcare practitioner'.[45a] Sponsors of the CM must hold evidence related to the level of the claim that is made prior to marketing.[xxviii]

The Australian regulatory scheme was evaluated in 2003 and considered appropriate for CMs, but doctors should be aware of current gaps in the regulation of CMs. First, there are risks that arise as a result of the lack of regulation of raw herbs, including misidentification, heavy metal and toxin contamination, inadvertent or deliberate substitution, and adulteration with Western pharmaceutical products.[6] While these matters are being addressed by the regulator it may be necessary to inform a patient about such risks. Second, there is no regulation requiring the standardisation of herbal ingredients in CMs. Without regulation to define the standardisation of herbal ingredients, and what is necessary to meet that definition, there is no consistent approach between manufacturers. This can lead to potential variations in dosages within and between brands, even resulting in sub-potent and super-potent dosages, compromising herbal treatment.[6] These matters may need to be considered when informing a patient about the risks of some treatments and when prescribing CMs.

The regulatory scheme for CMs includes a voluntary scheme for reporting adverse events. It would be prudent to be aware of reports of adverse reactions as well as alerts and advisories provided by the TGA in relation to complementary medicines, and to take these into consideration when prescribing treatment and advising patients. Information can be received regularly via email through the *Australian Adverse Drug Reactions Bulletin*.[46]

Australia's National Medicines Policy (NMP) complements the regulation of pharmaceuticals and CMs by the TGA. It focuses on the appropriate use of medicines once they are in the market. Central to this policy is the National Strategy for Quality Use of Medicines (QUM) authored by G Moses.[47] Moses, a pharmacist, has developed guidelines based on the QUM principles—called 'complementary medicine protocols'—to assist pharmacists and other integrative health practitioners to advise consumers about CMs. The guidelines assist a practitioner to make decisions about CM use through a six-step analysis. For example, in the case of heart failure, is it appropriate to use the herb hawthorn 'before, with or after digoxin?'.[47] The protocols may be a useful tool to assist with integrating CMs into the care of a patient.

REGULATION OF HEALTH SERVICES UNDER MEDICARE

Integrative medicine involves more than substituting CMs for pharmaceuticals. Integrative medicine also:

> aims to shift some of the basic orientations of medicine: toward healing rather than symptomatic treatment, toward a closer relationship with nature, toward a strengthened doctor–patient relationship and an emphasis on mind and spirit in addition to body.[48a]

And this broad vision is incorporated into the RACGP definition of integrative medicine.[1] The RACGP acknowledges that the integration of complementary medicines is a central aspect of integrative medicine, but also emphasises that, like general practice, integrative medicine 'embraces and encourages a holistic approach to practice incorporating patient involvement in self health care, prevention and lifestyle interventions'.[1a]

The holistic approach to the patient and relationship in integrative practice may diminish the potential for legal liability, as it is well documented that lack of good communication and failure to include the patient's perspective is responsible for most formal complaints and litigation.[49] However, working with the patient to strengthen the relationship and empower the patient to take greater responsibility for the healthcare takes time, and longer patient consultations tend to be a feature of integrative practice. As integrative practitioners often work with those with chronic and complex conditions, this care also takes time and may require greater pathology testing.[50] It is important therefore that doctors practising integrative medicine meet regulatory requirements when providing services funded by Medicare Australia.

Patient consultations, and other services such as pathology requests, provided by doctors and other health practitioners under Medicare are monitored and, where considered necessary, investigated. The regulatory task is shared by three entities: Medicare Australia, the Professional Services Review Scheme (PSRS) and the Determining Authority.[xxix]

The object of the regulation is to protect patients from the risks, and the public purse from the cost, of inappropriate practice. The regulator is concerned with conduct, such as a high volume of rendered services, a high average number of services per patient and high levels of prescribing under the Pharmaceutical Benefits Scheme (PBS). The services of practitioners are monitored by Medicare Australia through a review process that includes the use of statistics, and in particular the use of a normal distribution or bell curve.[xxx] The focus of the monitoring is usually the outer right of the bell curve within the third standard deviation from the mean, where 2.5% of occurrences sit. For example, GPs who are the highest users of a particular Medical Benefits Schedule (MBS) item under Medicare, such as long consultations and pathology testing, have the potential to come under the scrutiny of the regulator, because their pattern of consultations will lie outside that of most GPs.

The CEO of Medicare Australia can request that the director of the PSRS review the provision of services of a practitioner. This review may result in the director taking no further action or entering into an agreement with the practitioner about future conduct. Alternatively, the director may make a referral to the Professional Services Review Committee (PSRC), who investigate and make findings about whether the practitioner has engaged in 'inappropriate practice' in connection with the rendering or initiation of services for which a Medicare benefit was payable. A GP would be engaging in inappropriate practice if his or her conduct in rendering or initiating a service was such that it could reasonably be concluded that the conduct would be unacceptable to the general body of GPs. A service provided must be clinically relevant—that is, generally accepted by the medical profession as necessary for the appropriate treatment of the patient. And the PSRC must have regard (in addition to other relevant matters) as to whether or not the practitioner kept adequate and contemporaneous records in the rendering of the services.[xxxi]

In the event of a finding of inappropriate practice, the Determining Authority decides what sanctions to impose. This will include one or more sanctions such as a reprimand, counselling or cessation of Medicare payments.

Under Medicare, eligibility for rebates is limited by strict criteria, as set out under the MBS item. When billing for long consultations (or other MBS items) it is recommended that GPs consider two questions: does the service rendered comply with the time and content requirements of the MBS item descriptor; and would the majority of my peers accept that the treatment provided during the service is clinically appropriate for this patient? If the answer is a confident yes to both questions and the GP has adequate, contemporaneous documentation of the consultation, this should place the GP in good stead in the event of an audit by the regulator.[xxxii] Where a doctor is also engaged in 'integrative medicine' tasks, they need to be accommodated in addition to the MBS criteria for the specific consultation claimed.

Doctors should ensure that pathology testing is clinically appropriate for the treatment of the patient. Sometimes it is necessary to educate patients who are anxious to have regular pathology tests that clinical outcomes are often more important than pathology tests. And there may be circumstances where it is appropriate to pass on the costs of some pathology tests to patients.[xxxiii]

A recent review of the PSRS has recommended a number of changes to the scheme. The review acknowledges the growing number of special-interest practices, such as integrative medicine, and the difficulty of identifying inappropriate practice in these areas, due to different work practices.[51] This acknowledgement provides an opening for bodies such as the RACGP and AIMA to raise concerns about Medicare and integrative practice, including the role and significance of long consultations, with the aim of bringing about appropriate regulatory change to facilitate the practice of integrative medicine. Some initial discussions have taken place between the AIMA and the PSRS.[xxxiv] In 2008 the Minister for Health, Nicola Roxon, also indicated that the Department of Health and Ageing will examine whether current general practice requires changes to Medicare items, including items for long consultations.[xxxv]

CONCLUSION

Integrative medicine is evolving rapidly and there is an increasing obligation on the part of doctors to become familiar with evidence-based CAM and to provide information and advice to patients about CAM options, to enable patients to make informed decisions. It is critical that doctors acquire the necessary knowledge and skills and become familiar with guidelines that are indicative of the standard of care and widely accepted practice before embarking on an integrative approach. The law does not make allowances for the inexperienced.[xxxvi]

It would be prudent to check with your medical indemnity insurer to establish that the particular practices you plan to adopt are covered by the insurer. And always consult with professional and regulatory bodies, and seek legal advice about particular circumstances where necessary.

RESOURCES

Australian Integrative Medicine Association (AIMA). Position statement on sale of complementary medicines by medical practitioners; 2006. Online. Available: http://www.aima.net.au 24 March 2009.

Brophy E. In the surgery: informed consent and CM. J Complement Med 2003; 2(4):23–28.

Brophy E. Medico-legal implications of complementary medicine. In: Cohen M, ed. Holistic healthcare in practice. Melbourne: AIMA; 2003:24–38.
Brophy E. Referral to complementary therapists. J Complement Med 2003; 2(6):42–48.
Brophy E. The GP's duty of care. J Complement Med 2009; 8(2):20–24.
Federation of State Medical Boards. Model guidelines for the use of complementary and alternative therapies in medical practice; 2005. Online. Available: http://www.fsmb.org/pdf/2002_grpol_Complementary_Alternative_Therapies.pdf 24 March 2009.
National Health and Medical Research Council. Communicating with patients: advice for medical practitioners; 2004. Online. Available: http://www.nhmrc.gov.au/publications/synopses/e58syn.htm 24 March 2009.
National Health and Medical Research Council. Making decisions about tests and treatments: principles for better communication between healthcare consumers and healthcare professionals; 2006. Online. Available: http://www.nhmrc.gov.au/publications/synopses/_files/hpr25.pdf 24 March 2009.
Weir M. Complementary medicine: ethics and law. 3rd edn. Brisbane: Prometheus; 2007.

REFERENCES

1 Royal Australian College of General Practitioners. RACGP Curriculum for Australian General Practice. Curriculum statement: integrative medicine; 2007. Online. Available: http://www.racgp.org.au/scriptcontent/curriculum/pdf/integrativemedicine.pdf 24 March 2009. a p 2.
2 National Center for Complementary and Alternative Medicine. What is complementary and alternative medicine? 2003. Online. Available: http://www.nccam.nih.gov/health/whatiscam/index.htm 24 March 2009.
3 Peters D, Chaitow L, Harris G et al. Integrating complementary therapies in primary care—a practical guide for health professionals. London: Churchill Livingstone; 2002. a p 5.
4 Select Committee on Science and Technology. Complementary and alternative medicine. HL Paper 123. House of Lords; 2000.
5 Xue CC, Zhang L, Lin V et al. Complementary and alternative medicine use in Australia: a national population-based survey. J Alt Complement Med 2007; 13(6):643–650.
6 La Trobe University School of Public Health. The practice and regulatory requirements of naturopathy and western herbal medicine. Final Report; 2006. Online. Available: http://www.health.vic.gov.au/pracreg/naturopathy 24 March 2009.
7 Sanderson CR, Koczwara B, Currow DC. The therapeutic footprint of medical, complementary and alternative therapies and a doctor's duty of care. Med J Aust 2006; 185(7):373–376.
8 Smallwood C. The role of complementary and alternative medicine in the NHS; 2005. Online. Available: http://research.freshminds.co.uk/files/u1/freshminds_report_complimentarymedicine.pdf 24 March 2009.
9 Adams J, Sibritt DW, Easthope G. The profile of women who consult alternative health practitioners in Australia. Med J Aust 2003; 179:297–300.
10 American Association of Retired Persons and National Center for Complementary and Alternative Medicine. Complementary and alternative medicine: what people 50 and older are using and discussing with their physicians; 2007. Online. Available: http://www.aarp.org/research/health/prevention/cam_2007.html 24 March 2009.
11 MacLennan AH, Wilson DH, Taylor AW. The escalating cost and prevalence of alternative medicine. Prev Med 2002; 35:166–173.
12 MacLennan AH, Myers S, Taylor A. The continuing use of complementary and alternative medicine in South Australia: costs and beliefs in 2004. Med J Aust 2006; 184(1):27–31.
13 Cohen M, Penman S, Pirotta M. The integration of complementary therapies in Australian medical practice: results of a national survey. J Altern Complement Med 2005; 11(6):995–1004. a p 1003.
14 Robinson A, McGrail MR. Disclosure of CAM use to medical practitioners: a review of qualitative and quantitative studies. Complement Ther Med 2004; 12(2/3):90–98.
15 Williamson M, Tudball J, Toms M et al. Information use and needs of complementary medicines users. Sydney: National Prescribing Service; October 2008.
16 Brown J, Morgan T, Adams J et al. Complementary medicines information use and needs of health professionals: general practitioners and pharmacists. Sydney: National Prescribing Service; December 2008.
17 Pirotta, MV, Cohen M, Kotsirilos V. Complementary therapies: have they become accepted in general practice? Med J Aust 2000;172:105–109. a p 109.
18 Hall K, Giles-Corti B. Complementary therapies and the general practitioner: a survey of Perth GPs. Aust Fam Physician 2000; 29(6):602–606.
19 Eastwood HL. Complementary therapies: the appeal to general practitioners. Med J Aust 2000; 173(2):95–98.
20 Commonwealth of Australia, Department of the Treasury. Review of the law of negligence. Final report; 2002. Online. Available: http://revofneg.treasury.gov.au/content/review2.asp 24 March 2009.
21 Studdert DM, Eisenberg DM, Miller FH et al. Medical malpractice implications of alternative medicine. JAMA 1998; 280(18):1610–1615. a p 1612.

22 Australian Medical Association. AMA position statement: complementary medicine; 2002. Online. Available: http://www.ama.com.au/node/2214 24 March 2009.
23 Douglas R, Mullins G, Grant S. The annotated Civil Liability Act 2003 (Qld). 2nd edn. Sydney: LexisNexis Butterworths; 2008.
24 Dumoff A. Protecting ACM physicians from undeserved discipline. Altern Complement Ther 2002; 8(2):120–126.
25 Dumoff A. Federation of State Medical Boards' new guidelines for ACM: improvements and concerns. Altern Complement Ther 2002; 8(5):305–309.
26 Medical Council of New Zealand. Statement on complementary and alternative medicine; 2005. Online. Available: http://www.mcnz.org.nz/portals/0/guidance/comp_alternative.pdf 24 March 2009.
27 Medical Board of Western Australia. Complementary, alternative and unconventional medicine; 2004. Online. Available: http://www.medicalboard.com.au/pdfs/Alternative%20Medicine%20Draft%20-%20March%202002.pdf 24 March 2009.
28 Australian Integrative Medicine Association. AIMA information. J Aust Integ Med Assoc 2004; 22.
29 Royal Australian College of General Practitioners. Application to the Australian Medical Council for reaccreditation of its general practice education standards and processes; 2006. Online. Available: http://www.racgp.org.au/amc 24 March 2009. a p 22.
30 Royal Australian College of General Practitioners RACGP-AIMA joint position statement on complementary medicine; 2005. Online. Available: http://www.racgp.org.au/policy/complementary_medicine.pdf 24 March 2009. a p 3, b p 2.3, c p 2.4, d p 4.4.
31 Sackett DL, Rosenberg WMC, Gray JAM et al. Evidence-based medicine: what it is and what it isn't. BMJ 1996; 312(7023):71–72.
32 Royal Australian College of General Practitioners (RACGP). Position statement: evidence based medicine; 2001. Online. Available: http://www.racgp.org.au/policy/Evidence_Based_Medicine.pdf 19 March 2009.
33 Cohen M. From complementary to integrative and holistic medicine. In: Cohen M, ed. Perspectives on holistic health. Melbourne: AIMA; 2000:38. a p 38.
34 Jonas WB, Linde K, Walach H. How to practice evidence-based complementary and alternative medicine. In: Jonas WB, Levin JS, eds. Essentials of complementary and alternative medicine. Maryland: Lippincott, William & Wilkins; 1999:72–87. a p 73.
35 Novey DW. Integration. In: Novey DW, ed. Clinician's complete reference to complementary and alternative medicine. Missouri: Mosby; 2000:13–16. a p 16.
36 Cohen MH, Eisenberg DM. Potential physician malpractice liability associated with complementary and integrative medical therapies. Ann Intern Med 2002; 136(8):596–603.
37 Zollman C, Vickers A. ABC of complementary medicine. London: BMJ Books; 2000.
38 Australian Government, Therapeutic Goods Administration. Implementation of the government response to the recommendations of the Expert Committee on Complementary Medicines in the Health System: Progress Report; October 2006. Online. Available: http://www.tga.gov.au/cm/cmreport3.pdf 24 March 2009.
39 National Health and Medical Research Council. General guidelines for medical practitioners on providing information to patients; 2004. Canberra: NHMRC.
40 Brophy E. Does a doctor have a duty to provide information and advice about complementary and alternative medicine? J Law Med 2003; 10:271–284.
41 Cohen MH. Negotiating integrative medicine: a framework for provider–patient conversations. Negotiation J 2004; 30(3):409–433. a p 424.
42 Kerridge IH, McPhee JR. Ethical and legal issues at the interface of complementary and conventional medicine. MJA 2004; 181(3):164–166.
43 Australia New Zealand Products Authority. The proposed Joint Regulatory Scheme for Complementary Medicines; 2007. Online. Available http://www.anztpa.org/cm/fs-cm.htm#why 6 November 2009.
44 Institute of Medicine. Complementary and Alternative Medicine in the United States. Washington DC: National Academies Press; 2005.
45 Australian Government, Therapeutic Goods Administration. Guidelines for levels and kinds of evidence to support indications and claims: for non-registrable medicines, including complementary medicines and other listable medicines; 2001. Online. Available: http://www.tga.gov.au/docs/pdf/tgaccevi.pdf 24 March 2009. a p 15.
46 Australian Government, Therapeutic Good Administration. Australian Adverse Drug Reactions Bulletin. Online. Available: http://www.tga.gov.au/adr/aadrb.htm 9 November 2009.
47 Moses G. In the pharmacy: pharmacy protocols and professionalism. J Complement Med 2002; 1(1):36–39.
48 Cohen MH, Ruggie M, Micozzi MS. The practice of integrative medicine: a legal and operational guide. New York: Springer; 2007. a p 47.
49 Coulter A. The autonomous patient: ending paternalism in medical care. London: Stationery Office; 2002.
50 Australasian Integrative Medicine Association (AIMA). Long consultations. J Australasian Integrative Medicine Association 2002; 19:19–22.
51 Australian Government Department of Health and Ageing. Review of the Professional Services Review

Scheme; 2007. Online. Available: http://www.psr.gov.au/docs/publications/PSRReview-FindJuly2007.pdf 24 March 2009.

Cases

Dobler v Kenneth Halverson (2007) 70 NSWLR 151
Imbree v McNeilly [2008] Aust Torts Reps 81-966
Jones v Manchester Corporation (1952) 2 QB 852
McGroder v Maguire [2002] NSWCA 261 (unreported Handley, Sheller and Beazley JJA, 13 August 2002)
Rogers v Whitaker (1992) 175 CLR 479, 487
Rosenberg v Percival (2001) 205 CLR 434
Wyong Shire Council v Shirt (1980) 146 CLR 40.

Legislation

Civil Law (Wrongs) Act 2002 (ACT)
Civil Liability Act 1936 (SA)
Civil Liability Act 2002 (NSW)
Civil Liability Act 2002 (Tas)
Civil Liability Act 2002 (WA)
Civil Liability Act 2003 (Qld)
Drugs, Poisons and Controlled Substances Act 1981 (Vic)
Drugs, Poisons and Controlled Substances Regulations 2006 (Vic)
Health Insurance Act 1973 (Cth)
Therapeutic Goods Act 1989 (Cth)
Therapeutic Goods Regulations 1990 (Cth)
Wrongs Act 1958 (Vic)

NOTES

i This definition appears frequently in the literature. It is variously attributed to the Office of Alternative Medicine (now the National Center for Complementary and Alternative Medicine) and the Cochrane Collaboration, but does not appear on either website. The definition appears to be in general usage.

ii See, for example: Select Committee on Science and Technology, 'Complementary and Alternative Medicine', HL paper 123, House of Lords, 2000; White House Commission, 'White House Commission on Complementary and Alternative Medicine Policy: Final Report', 2002, http://whccamp.hhs.gov/pdfs/fr2002_document.pdf 24 March 2009.

iii See: Commonwealth of Australia, 'Expert Committee on Complementary Medicines in the Health System—Report to the Parliamentary Secretary to the Minister for Health and Ageing', 2003, http://www.tga.gov.au/docs/html/cmreport1.htm 24 March 2009; LaTrobe University School of Public Health, 'The Practice and Regulatory Requirements of Naturopathy and Western Herbal Medicine Final Report', 2006; Department of Human Services, http://www.health.vic.gov.au/pracreg/naturopathy 24 March 2009; The Senate Community Affairs References Committee, 'The Cancer Journey: Informing Choice', 2005, Commonwealth of Australia, http://www.aph.gov.au/Senate/committee/clac_ctte/cancer/report/index.htm 24 March 2009.

iv See, for example: Stewart C, Kerridge I, Parker M. The Australian medico-legal handbook. Sydney, Elsevier 2008; Loane S. Law and medical practice: rights, duties, claims and defences. 2nd edn. Sydney: Lexis Nexis, 2004.

v *Rogers v Whitaker* (1992) 175 CLR 479, 483 (Mason CJ, Brennan, Dawson, Toohey and McHugh JJ).

vi See: *Wyong Shire Council v Shirt* (1980) 146 CLR 40, 47-8 (Mason J); Wrongs Act 1958 (Vic) s. 48; Civil Liability Act 2003 (Qld) s. 9; Civil Liability Act 2002 (NSW) s. 5B; Civil Liability Act 2002 (Tas) s. 11; Civil Law (Wrongs) Act 2002 (ACT) s. 43; Civil Liability Act 2002 (WA) s. 5B(1); and Civil Liability Act 1936 (SA) s. 32.

vii Australian data for adverse events arising from the use of listed CMs in 2008, for example, show that there were a total of 109 reports where a CM was the sole suspected possible, probable or certain cause of an adverse patient reaction. There were no deaths where a CM was suspected. During the same period there were 7372 cases where a medicine (prescription, over-the-counter medication and other products registered on the ARTG including registered rather than listed CMs) was the sole suspected possible, probable or certain cause of an adverse patient reaction. In the same period the Therapeutic Goods Administration received 157 reports of a fatality where the reporter suspected that the medicine contributed to the death. In many cases the contribution of the suspected medicine to the death is uncertain; however, based on the information reported it is not possible to entirely exclude the possibility that the suspected medicine contributed to the fatal outcome. (Statistics provided by the Office of Medicines Safety Monitoring at the Therapeutic Goods Administration, 25 March 2009.) The reporting of adverse events is voluntary and the data are mostly provided by doctors, dentists and pharmacists. There may be under-reporting of adverse events related to CMs for a number of reasons, including patients not informing their doctors about adverse events. It is also pertinent to note that patients using prescription medicines can be very ill. For a review of the medical literature documenting the potential side effects of CAM see Markman M. Safety issues in using complementary and alternative medicine. J Clin Oncol 2002; 20(Suppl 18):39S–41S.

viii But note that the Queensland Medical Board advises doctors to avoid referral of patients to 'unconventional' health practitioners: Queensland,

Medical Board of. Unconventional medical practice; 2006. http://www.medicalboard.qld.gov.au/pdfs/unconventional-medical-practice.pdf 24 March 2009.

ix *Rogers v Whitaker* (1992) 175 CLR 479, 487. This common law test has been restated as a part of recent tort reforms arising from the Review of the Law of Negligence (the Ipp Review) in Victoria, South Australia and the Australian Capital Territory, and is similar in effect. See Wrongs Act 2003 (Vic) s. 58, Civil Liability Act 1936 (SA) s. 40; Civil Law (Wrongs) Act 2002 (ACT) s. 42.

x See *Dobler v Kenneth Halverson* (2007) 70 NSWLR 151 (Giles, Ipp and Basten JJA).

xi See Civil Liability Act 2003 (Qld) s. 22 (not limited to Australian opinion); Civil Liability Act 2002 (NSW) s. 50 (limited to Australian opinion); Civil Liability Act 2002 (Tas) s. 22 (limited to Australian opinion); Civil Liability Act 1936 (SA) s. 41 (limited to Australian opinion); Civil Liability Act 2002 (WA) s. 5PB (not limited to Australian opinion). In these jurisdictions if the court determines that the peer professional opinion is irrational (rather than unreasonable, as in Victoria) it cannot be relied on. Ipp-related statutory reforms in the Northern Territory and the Australian Capital Territory do not include the peer professional opinion test and so the common law remains applicable. See *Rogers v Whitaker* (1992) 175 CLR 479.

xii See, for example: NSW Medical Board. Code of professional conduct: good medical practice http://www.nswmb.org.au/index.pl?page=44&search_key=code%20of%20professional%20conduct 23 March 2009.

xiii See: New South Wales Medical Board, Complementary health care, 2004, http://www.nswmb.org.au/index.pl?page=58&search_key=complementary 23 March 2009; Medical Board of Queensland, Unconventional medical practice, 2006, http://www.medicalboard.qld.gov.au/pdfs/unconventional-medical-practice.pdf 23 March 2009; Medical Practitioners Board of Victoria, Alternative or complementary medicines, 2005, http://medicalboardvic.org.au/content.php?sec=35 23 March 2009; Medical Board of Western Australia, Complementary, alternative and unconventional medicine, 2004, http://www.medicalboard.com.au/pdfs/Alternative%20Medicine%20Draft%20-%20March%202002.pdf 23 March 2009; Medical Board of the Northern Territory, Guidelines for the practice of alternative and experimental treatments, 2007, http://www.health.nt.gov.au/library/scripts/objectifyMedia.aspx?file=pdf/13/05.pdf&siteID=1&str_title=Guidelines%20Practice%20of%20Alternative%20Medicine%20and%20Experiment.pdf 23 March 2009.

xiv See National Health Workforce Taskforce, http://www.nhwt.gov.au/nhwt.asp 20 March 2009.

xv Joint RACGP/AIMA Working Party Terms of Reference. Online. Available: http://www.racgp.org.au/racgpaimajwp 24 March 2009.

xvi Communication with Dr Vicki Kotsirilos, Chair, RACGP/AIMA Joint Working Party, 5 February 2009.

xvii RACGP. Integrative medicine. 2007. The RACGP curriculum for Australian general practice. Online. Available: http://www.racgp.org.au/scriptcontent/curriculum/pdf/integrativemedicine/pdf 24 March 2009.

xviii *McGroder v Maguire* (2002) NSWCA 261 (unreported, Handley, Sheller and Beazley JJA, 13 August 2002).

xix Joint RACGP/AIMA Working Party Terms of Reference. Online. Available: http://www.racgp.org.au/racgpaimajwp 24 March 2009

xx See also guidelines on informed decision-making provided by Medical Boards and the RACGP.

xxi *Rogers v Whitaker* (1992) 175 CLR 479, 490 (Mason CJ, Brennan J, Dawson J, Toohey J, McHugh J).

xxii *Rosenberg v Percival* (2001) 205 CLR 434, 500 (Callinan J).

xxiii See: Therapeutic Goods Administration website at http://tga.com.au; Commonwealth of Australia, *Expert Committee on Complementary Medicines in the Health System—Report to the Parliamentary Secretary to the Minister for Health and Ageing* (2003) http://www.tga.gov.au/docs/html/cmreport1.htm 24 March 2009; Hall J. Recent developments in complementary medicines regulation. In: Cohen M, ed. The art and science of holistic health; 2005:120.

xxiv Because of the Commonwealth's limited ability to regulate the entire field of therapeutic goods, and the failure of most other jurisdictions to pass complementary legislation, some 'therapeutic goods' may not be regulated. Commonwealth of Australia, Expert Committee on Complementary Medicines in the Health System – Report to the Parliamentary Secretary to the Minister for Health and Ageing, 2003, http://www.tga.gov.au/docs/html/cmreport1.htm 24 March 2009.

xxv It is possible for CMs to be registered goods provided they meet all the requirements of registration. As it is a lengthy and costly process and is not mandatory for CMs, few are actually registered goods: Commonwealth of Australia, Expert Committee on Complementary Medicines in the Health System—Report to the Parliamentary Secretary to the Minister for Health and Ageing, 2003, http://www.tga.gov.au/docs/html/cmreport1.htm 24 March 2009.

xxvi There are also labelling and advertising requirements under the TG Act, TG Regs and the Therapeutic Goods Advertising Code 2007.

xxvii See, for example, Drugs, Poisons and Controlled Substances Act 1986 (Vic) and Drugs, Poisons and Controlled Substances Regulations 2006.

xxviii The evidence can be traditional use, including evidence set out in a TGA-approved monograph, or it may be scientific evidence, including evidence such as case studies: Australian Government Therapeutic Goods Administration, Guidelines for levels and kinds of evidence to support indications and claims: for non-registrable medicines, including complementary medicines and other listable medicines, 2001, http://www.tga.gov.au/docs/pdf/tgaccevi.pdf 24 March 2009.

xxix See Health Insurance Act 1973 (Cth) Part VAA.

xxx See Bell R. Medicare regulation through professional services review—lessons learned. In: Freckleton I, ed. Regulating health practitioners; 2006:113.

xxxi Health Insurance Act 1973 (Cth) s. 82, s. 10, s. 3.

xxxii Department of Health and Ageing. Fact sheet: Correct claiming of Medicare Group A1- level C and D items, http://www.health.gov.au/internet/mbsonline/publishing.nsf/Content/AD01CA668C5E4588CA2574E40017C10D/$File/Fact_Sheet-Level_C_and_D_items.pdf 24 March 2009.

xxxiii See Woolhouse M. Feeling safe under the Medicare system. JAIMA 2009; 14(1):6–7.

xxxiv See Woolhouse M. Feeling safe under the Medicare system. JAIMA 2009; 14(1):6–7.

xxxv Department of Health and Ageing. Fact sheet: Correct claiming of Medicare Group A1- level C and D items, http://www.health.gov.au/internet/mbsonline/publishing.nsf/Content/AD01CA668C5E4588CA2574E40017C10D/$File/Fact_Sheet-Level_C_and_D_items.pdf 24 March 2009.

xxxvi *Jones v Manchester Corporation* (1952) 2 QB 852; *Imbree v McNeilly* [2008] Aust Torts Reports 81-966.

chapter 20

Medical ethics

INTRODUCTION

Ethics: 'Relating to morals, treating of moral questions. Set of principles of morals, science of morals, moral principles, rules of conduct.'

Oxford Dictionary

'Ethics' is a word derived from the Greek *ethikos*, which means 'habit' or 'custom'. Put simply, in modern usage it is the study of how we ought to live or act in response to the situations confronting us in daily life. Medical ethics in particular is a branch of bioethics and is the study of how we ought to live or act as doctors. Ethics, being a branch of philosophy, relates to things such as 'right', 'wrong', 'duty' and 'morality'. Making decisions of an ethical nature in medical practice is often difficult and demanding, and the clinician has to balance medical considerations with legal and moral ones.

Taking the time to reflect upon ethical issues, and having a structured approach to doing this, can help clinicians to navigate through many potentially challenging situations. Not taking time for this can compound ethical and moral concerns. This has effects upon our wellbeing and can also have medico-legal implications. As with many medico-legal dilemmas, ethical problems are often compounded by poor communication.

This chapter does not present a detailed analysis of particular and complex bioethical issues such as euthanasia, stem cell research or abortion. Nor does it make concrete pronouncements about the 'correct' view on given topics or course of action in given situations. It does, however, give an overview of generic ethical terms, concepts and methods that can be applied by the clinician to particular situations. We are interested here in 'applied ethics' and not simply 'theoretical ethics' or 'meta-ethics'.

DEFINITIONS, TERMS AND MEANING

Many ethical conflicts lie in our understanding and interpretation of words. It is therefore useful before considering principles and concepts in more detail that some remarks are made about the language of ethics and the meaning of words commonly used in ethical discourse. It is easy to assume that different people mean the same thing by a word when they use it. This assumption gives rise to many misunderstandings. For example, one person might interpret 'freedom' as having all external restraints removed from their behaviour, whereas another might equate freedom with an internal state of self-awareness, balance and self-control. One person might equate happiness with pleasure or wealth, whereas another might equate it with spiritual enlightenment. One of the first points is that we should reflect on the meaning of the words we often take for granted.

As was mentioned, there is a distinction between meta-ethics and applied ethics. *Meta-ethics* is the 'philosophical inquiry into the concepts, theories, language and intellectual foundations of ethics—as opposed to practical ethical questions'.[1] So when a moral philosopher seeks to say what it means to say that something (a value or action) is 'right' or 'wrong', they are seeking to clarify the language or concepts of moral judgments rather than to say what one ought or ought not to do.[2] It is like standing beside (meta) ethical actions and seeking to provide conceptual clarity to the usage of moral language.

Normative ethics is 'concerned with establishing basic ethical principles or standards ("norms"—from the Greek for builder's rule or square). Examples include normative theories (e.g. deontology or teleological), normative principles (e.g. the principles of bioethics), and declarations or statements whether on the core values of medicine or on specific duties of doctors and nurses in particular circumstances'.[1] The following definitions of terms commonly used in ethical discourse are from the *Oxford Dictionary*.

- *autonomy* 'right of self-government; personal freedom'. Sometimes seen as a principle opposed to paternalism, it relates to the patient's right to make decisions about their healthcare on their own behalf
- *beneficence* 'doing good; active kindness'. It is derived from the word 'benefit' and also carries the sense of providing advantage
- *competence* 'ability to do a task'. In the medical context it usually relates to a person's mental state, ability to understand information, and to make decisions.
- *confidential* 'spoken or written in confidence; entrusted with secrets'
- *consent* 'voluntary agreement, compliance'
- *deontology* 'the science of duty'
- *duty* 'moral or legal obligation; binding force of what is right'
- *due* 'person's right; what is owed him'
- *inform* 'tell a person of or about a thing or subject'
- *informed consent* giving that consent having been previously informed in an appropriate way of all relevant background and facts
- *justice* 'fairness; exercise of authority in maintenance of right. Due allocation of reward of virtue and punishment of vice'. In its most general sense it relates to the lawfulness (natural or human-made) of actions, but in the context of medical ethics justice is most often associated with fairness in relation to the distribution of resources
- *non-maleficence* to be maleficent is to be 'hurtful, criminal', so non-maleficence means to do nothing hurtful or unlawful
- *paternalism* 'of or like a father; government limiting the subject by well meant regulations'. In the medical context it relates to the doctor being granted a position of authority on the basis of their knowledge, skills and care for the patient.
- *right* 'just, required by morality or duty, proper, true, correct. What is just or fair treatment of a person'
- *rights* carries the meaning as above; also taken as a complementary principle to duties in that rights don't exist in the absence of a corresponding duty and vice versa
- *trust* 'firm belief in reliability, honesty, veracity, justice, strength'
- *utilitarianism* 'doctrine that actions are right because they are useful'
- *virtue* 'moral excellence, uprightness, goodness'.

ETHICAL APPROACHES

MICRO-ETHICS AND MACRO-ETHICS

In ethical discourse, community debate and media coverage, most attention is given to *macro-ethical* issues such as euthanasia, abortion, stem cell research and genetic engineering. These issues, as important as they are, are nevertheless far removed from the vast majority of clinical encounters between doctors and patients. All clinical encounters contain ethical issues but they are generally not obvious. These *micro-ethical* issues include everyday ethical concerns relating to such things as the doctor–patient relationship, communication, information giving, certificate writing, the management of common problems, and physical examination. As every clinical encounter contains ethical content and is ethically relevant, it is deserving of consideration, whether it be:

- the way the doctor does or does not inform the patient about what treatment is being offered,
- whether the doctor does or does not include the patient in the decision-making process,
- the level of care and compassion shown by the doctor towards the patient,
- the way in which a patient's medical records are stored, or
- how much care the doctor takes to avoid drug interactions.

It is therefore important to be reflective about all aspects of clinical medicine and not just those aspects that are more prominent in the media. When considering the factors that affect patient satisfaction or have potential medico-legal implications, it is far more common for these to involve the micro-ethical rather than the macro-ethical.

MEDICAL ETHICS AND THE LAW

It is beyond the scope of this chapter to give a detailed discussion of the laws pertaining to medical practice. In any case, laws vary so widely between and within countries that any such overview would be of little relevance. The best source of information relating to medical law is likely to be one's medical defence association. The broader issue relevant to ethicists regarding the relationship between law and ethics is: are they the same and do they lead to the same course of action?

The case could be made that they reflect each other in that laws reflect ethical principles and morality, and ethical and moral precepts are enshrined in law. Indeed, some would argue, as Plato did, that ethics is the bedrock of the law. If you offend one you offend them both, if the laws of the land are just.

Another case could be made that ethics and law are different. They may overlap but they are not the same, in that what is considered legal is generally, but not always, ethical. For example, a law could be made that some might consider unethical, such as apartheid being written into law. Equally, a thing that some people might consider ethical could be illegal, such as abortion.

In an endeavour to resolve the potential conflict, some might argue that if ethics and law appear to conflict then we may be confused about what is ethical, or an unjust law has been enacted. Either:

- what is considered ethical but illegal at one time or by one group of people is not truly ethical, or
- what has been written into law but is considered unethical is not a wise and just law, or
- law and ethics only fit in relation to natural law rather than human-made law, and they do not fit if human-made laws do not reflect natural law.

From a clinician's perspective, when there is concern about a course of conduct that seems ethical but conflicts with the law, it is pertinent to seek advice from a legally qualified person or organisation. If there is no way of following what seems to be legal and ethical at the same time then it might be useful to reflect more deeply on our assumptions about what is truly ethical. Sometimes, in an attempt to preserve both, a difficult decision remains that depends upon a clinician weighing up how important the ethical principle is versus how severe the legal consequences are for not following the law.

PRINCIPLES-BASED ETHICS[3]

The meaning of the word 'principle', in the broadest sense, comes from the Latin *principium* meaning 'beginning or source'. It also carries the meaning of a fundamental truth, law or motive force. It is also a starting assumption as the basis for further reasoning or the foundation upon which many other things are based. The principle 'Do no harm', for example, spawns a vast array of other societal morals, manners, customs, precepts, rules and laws. Whether we accept the validity of traditional principles or not, principles of one sort or other, consciously or unconsciously, form the basis of our actions. We may govern our actions with one overriding principle, a number of complementary ones, or even a number of conflicting principles. We could be consciously aware of those principles we live by or completely oblivious to them; nevertheless they govern our conduct.

Principles-based ethics has been the most widely adopted and taught paradigm in contemporary medical ethics. Some of these, such as autonomy and paternalism, and beneficence and non-maleficence, are complementary, like two sides of the same coin. In medical ethics discourse, the most commonly cited principles are:

- autonomy
- paternalism
- consent
- justice
- confidentiality
- beneficence
- non-maleficence.

A common argument against principles-based ethics, or a potential weakness in it, is that principles don't necessarily provide us with consistent, unambiguous conclusions and therefore we have to trade one principle off against another. Put another way, some would say that no principle is ever found to be absolute—that is, operating under all cases—and so in order to maintain autonomy, for example, you might sometimes have to sacrifice beneficence. Such might be the case if a doctor recommends a course of management that appears to be beneficial to the patient but the patient chooses to decline the treatment. Even more problematic is when a patient requests a course of management that appears to be detrimental. Here the ethicist may say that the doctor needs to prioritise their principles and also to remember that, at the end of the day, the doctor is an autonomous agent as well. Regardless of what a patient chooses, the doctor is largely concerned with determining what they will do rather than what the patient will do.

It is often assumed that the various considerations affecting decisions necessarily conflict or compete. They need not, but it is often difficult to transcend apparent contradictions in competing principles and values as well as to balance medical, legal, social and moral 'goods'. Reflecting upon values is often considered a luxury that busy clinicians do not have time for, but many ethical conflicts arise as the result of an unreflective and inflexible approach to understanding values and principles. Conflicts are often resolved as a result of taking the time for a broader or deeper view of the issues involved.

Autonomy and paternalism

The balance between autonomy (personal freedom to choose) and paternalism (respect for the advice of an authority figure) is a hotly contested ethical issue. The boundaries of personal freedom and liberties are being pushed ever further, often at the expense of traditional values and authority figures such as parents, governments, teachers and, of course, doctors. The traditional role of the doctor has been that of a 'paternal' or parental figure who, like a parent, has knowledge, skills, objectivity, experience, integrity, self-sacrifice and strength that the patient—child—needs but may not have. Like a parent, a paternalistic doctor is obliged to care wholeheartedly for the wellbeing of the patient, who may be unwell and vulnerable.

Being paternalistic can also encompass the fostering of the eventual independence or autonomy of the patient, although conventional use of the word in ethical discourse tends to ignore this aspect of paternalism. Paternalism has therefore come in for considerable criticism in recent times, and perhaps rightly so, if it is missing one or more of the abovementioned pillars upon which a reasonable application of paternalism rests (that is, knowledge, skills, objectivity, experience, integrity, self-sacrifice and strength). For example, a doctor may be deficient in knowledge or skills about technical or human matters. The doctor may lack objectivity, care, integrity or strength, or may seek to gain some personal benefit by fostering the dependence of the patient. These examples of how paternalism breaks down are not an argument against the need for authority altogether but, rather, against its misuse. A more enlightened view of paternalism may encompass the practice of a beneficent, compassionate, moderate and reasonable style of paternalistic medicine, also aimed at educating the patient towards independence and informed decision-making. That form of paternalism which is associated with the dependency and negation of a rightful use of self-determination is rightly coming under close scrutiny.

To say that autonomy or self-government is inherently and always good is as questionable as asserting that paternalism is always bad. Reflecting on the rightful use of autonomy also raises the question, 'Which part of the "self" should one be governed by?'. What is the natural order of the elements in human nature for sound self-government and ethical behaviour? Are there some aspects of ourselves that we would do well not to be governed by? It would seem obvious that many impulses, emotions and unreflective reactions are not a sound basis for autonomy and can lead to much harm for oneself and others. For true autonomy we need competence that is associated with internal qualities such as awareness, reason, emotional regulation and impulse control as well as the more commonly recognised requirements such as having and understanding information (informed consent) and freedom from coercion. Therefore, a simple and more enlightened conception of autonomy can coexist with and support a more enlightened view of paternalism. When the rightful use of either breaks down, ethical complexity and conflicts tend to follow.

Consent

Consent is a principle that links closely with autonomy and relates to our innate right to self-determination. For someone to have a treatment or any limitation of their freedom against their consent would have to be underpinned by very powerful arguments for such strong use of paternalism. Such arguments could include that the person was a significant danger to themselves or others or that their competence was so severely affected that they were unable to make a reasonable decision.

When ethicists speak about consent it is nearly always linked with the word 'informed'. When a patient gives consent we assume that they have been informed of all the relevant information in a way that they can understand. Being aware of and responsive to the amount of information that an individual patient requires and wants is an important micro-ethical aspect of the doctor–patient relationship.

Patients who are considered incompetent—such as children, the unconscious, the demented, the intoxicated and those with a major mental illness or brain syndrome—would not generally be considered able to give informed consent. Although such a person (a child, for example) may not be able to give informed consent because of their inability to understand information, this does not mean that a treatment should be given to them without trying to enlist their trust, willingness and cooperation. When a person is unable to give informed consent, the duty for making decisions may move to another party such as a parent, the doctor, someone who has been granted power of attorney or a guardian determined by the courts. It is not that the decision-making principle has changed—the decision should still be ruled by reason and compassion, but the reason and compassion will be delivered from another source until the person is able to give consent themselves.

Justice

In most ethical discourse, justice is generally interpreted as being related to the fair and equitable distribution of resources—distributive justice. To consider justice in such a narrow way is to do an injustice to its full meaning and importance. Distributive justice is just one way of expressing justice, but there are many more. The more important question relates to what justice is in a more universal sense.

Plato's conception of justice related to a harmony and order of the psyche from which flowed the actions of a just person or community, whether in relation to money or anything else. Others relate justice to observing basic rights, obedience to natural law or the laws and conventions of society as dictated by the law makers and interpreters. The fact that many have received justice according to the laws of the land but still feel that they have been treated unjustly suggests that community laws do not always reflect justice. Reflecting upon the relationship between law and justice raises a number of questions, including the following:

- Are there different levels of laws? Are the universal laws of nature confined to physics and chemistry, or is there also a natural order in the workings of the mind, and the conduct of society?

- Who ultimately makes the law? Is the individual a law unto themselves? Does the community make the laws, or is it God?
- Is law universal or is it relative to place, culture and time? Has every society recognised and legislated for a universal quality called 'justice', but expressed it in a different form?

Humankind could see itself as the master of the law or the servant of the law. For example, an assertion that all laws of morality and human conduct are human-made, and that there is no higher authority, has many implications. It will be likely to lead to a law-making process based on the opinions and fashions of the time. We have the freedom to make them as we choose. On the other hand, an assertion that laws are absolute and made by some higher authority, although expressed in different ways by different societies, makes it imperative to delineate and obey these laws. In this view, anything but obedience is futile, as true laws are non-negotiable. By one means or another, nature will enforce its own laws and will teach us the principles of morality.

Our answers to questions such as those posed above also lead to quite different interpretations of the origin of natural phenomena such as illness. One interpretation might say that illness is a chance event, and another might call it the working of natural justice.

Confidentiality

From the time of Hippocrates, confidentiality has been one of the most fiercely protected ethical principles. Patients confide information to doctors that they may never have told another human being, and they have a right to determine what happens to that information. This information should not be given to others without the patient's consent unless under the most extenuating circumstances. Even when there is a need to pass on information to third parties that would otherwise be considered confidential, the doctor is advised to make the most strenuous efforts to inform the patient of their reasons and to gain their consent.

Circumstances in which confidentiality might need to be breached include where the law requires it (e.g. illegal activities), where there are public safety issues (e.g. notifiable diseases) and in emergency situations. The doctor is very unlikely to be at risk of litigation in such situations, particularly where the reasons for breaching confidentiality are compelling and attempts were made to pass on information with the patient's consent first. To not breach confidentiality when one is legally, medically or morally obliged to would be more contentious and dangerous than breaching confidentiality.

Beneficence and non-maleficence

Two of the most fundamental ethical principles since the time of Hippocrates have been beneficence (do good) and non-maleficence (do no harm). They would seem to be self-evident and simple ethical principles against which no reasonable ethicist would argue, and about which there should be no contention. They are not, however, as simple as they appear. One reason is that we all value different things and what we value has a direct effect upon what we believe are ethical and unethical actions. What one person thinks is a good another thinks is a harm, and vice versa. For example, say one person values personal integrity and another values material wealth or status. In both cases each person is pursuing what they value as they perceive it, and interpretations of benefits and harms will be interpreted through the filter of such perceptions. Secondly, we can value physical, psychological, social, economic and spiritual goods and will prioritise them differently. Good on one level might also be associated with harm on another. So, for example, a person might benefit physically from receiving an organ transplant but perceive a moral harm if that organ was attained in an unethical way.

Other questions that could be asked include:

- Do we sometimes value things that are harmful to us and avoid things that are good for us? (Changing such perceptions is the premise upon which motivational interviewing is based.)
- Are some things superficially pleasant but ultimately unsatisfying, and can other things be superficially unpleasant but ultimately satisfying?
- Are some goods short-term and others long-term?
- Is there such a thing as the 'absolute good' which is larger, more valuable and permanent than that of individual preferences for the various forms of good?

The more usual usage of beneficence and non-maleficence implies that it is the doctor's duty at all times to benefit their patients—physically, psychologically and socially—and not to harm them in any way unless the harm (e.g. performing a painful procedure) is an unavoidable result of attaining a greater benefit (e.g. curing an illness). Harms occur in clinical medicine even with the best intentions in the world, but it is incumbent upon the doctor to take all reasonable steps to prevent such harms and to intervene if they occur. Indeed, with the rise of technology, the increasing tendency towards intervention and the increasing use of pharmaceuticals, the potential for harm has escalated enormously in modern medicine. Harms as a result of an unforeseen side effect of a medication, however, would be seen as far less an ethical concern than the same harms as a result of medical negligence.

VIRTUE ETHICS

Virtues have been written about and exhorted in myth and fable in every culture since the dawn of human history. Cultures often vary widely on particular customs but they tend to agree on the core virtues, although they may give slightly different emphasis or precedence to one or another.

Virtues were previously defined as moral excellence, uprightness and goodness. Although they may bear a resemblance to the principles previously described, they are not the same thing. Virtues are qualities of our nature that are reflected in our words and conduct. We may feel unfamiliar with an overarching definition of virtue or find it less than instructive, but we will all be familiar with the common virtues. The four cardinal virtues (the original meaning of *cardinal* is 'hinge') spoken of by Plato are wisdom, justice, temperance (moderation) and courage. In Christian theology were added the other three virtues of faith, hope and charity. The list, however, could be extensive: patience, kindness, compassion, honesty, determination, magnanimity and so on. Although we might agree about the importance of virtues, we often disagree about them in practice. In viewing events, individuals often vary in their interpretation of virtue or its absence. For example, what one may interpret as patience and meekness another may interpret as weakness.

Some philosophers and ethicists, like Plato, exhorted people to observe a purity and kind of transcendent quality in their pursuit of virtue. Plato said that they are the expression of an enlightened, happy and refined soul or psyche. Aristotle, on the other hand, exhorted the middle ground between virtues and vices, or the 'mean' between the two as being the more practical path.

To use virtues as a moral guide for decision-making means that one would have to reflect on them sufficiently to be able to recognise them and then to practise them over a considerable period of time until they became natural to us. Thus, upbringing and education are the first and most important training grounds for the development of virtue.

CONSEQUENTIALISM AND DEONTOLOGY

In ethical debate there are two popular ways of deciding the rightness or wrongness of an action. These can be broadly categorised as conseqentialism and deontology.

Deontology (*deon* is a Greek word meaning 'duty') is the oldest and most widely used approach to ethics. It says that actions are right or wrong depending upon whether or not they accord with duty. In this view, consequences are not irrelevant, but are of secondary importance compared to what one is duty-bound to do. The eighteenth-century philosopher Immanuel Kant is the most often quoted deontologist in the study of ethics, and ethical formulations such as the Ten Commandments and the Hippocratic Oath would be considered well-known deontological frameworks. Most deontological codes contain broad and concrete statements about what should or should not be done, and such codes are a common part of daily life. Codes of conduct and practice guidelines could also be considered examples. Common arguments against deontological approaches are that it is a simplistic approach but not reflective or perhaps reasoned. Further, although they may help to guide conduct in the majority of cases, they are not flexible enough to accommodate all situations. It would not be difficult to come up with circumstances where one deontological precept conflicted with another. In such a situation one would either need to sacrifice a duty, prioritise duties, or have a more flexible interpretation of them.

Consequentialism is an approach which says that actions are right or wrong not because of anything inherently right or wrong in them but because of the consequences that those actions are expected to produce. Utilitarianism, originally described by Jeremy Bentham and John Stuart Mill, two eighteenth-century English philosophers, is the most popular form of consequentialism and has three main tenets. First, consequences are the mark of the ethical rightness of actions; second, the best consequence is to maximise happiness (that is, the greatest happiness for the greatest number); and third, happiness largely equates with pleasure (that is, what pleases the greatest number). Some would say that the approach could be summed up by the statement, 'The end justifies the means'. There are some difficulties with this approach despite the fact that it is attractive at first glance. Although it sounds simple in theory, in practice it is very difficult to predict the outcomes of actions, especially in complex moral, political or social situations. Furthermore, it is not difficult to justify actions that would otherwise seem unjust, on the basis that the injustice affects a smaller segment of the community and if one appeals to some future desirable outcome. It would not be difficult to make a utilitarian argument to support many things that might otherwise be considered morally repugnant.

RIGHTS AND DUTIES

Another way of considering ethical decisions is by appeal to basic rights. Most would agree that we have, for example, a right to food, water, education, shelter, safety and basic medical care. To have these things is right and to be denied them is wrong. Hence there are an increasing number of bills of rights with their spheres of influence, all the way from international politics to family conduct.

Unfortunately, much discussion about rights tends to revolve around the things that people expect to be provided with, but tends to ignore the fact that a right to anything is only meaningful in relation to the duty required to provide that right. If, for example, we have a right to healthcare then that implies that someone has a duty to provide it, such as government, community, doctors or other health workers. Rights without duties are largely meaningless. Therefore, if one wishes to promote human rights then one really needs to promote human duties.

Another problem with the rights-based approach is that although most would agree about basic rights like the ones mentioned above, many would argue about rights in relation to more contentious issues. For example, some would say that the right to freedom of speech only goes so far and that at some point speech has to be censored if it is harmful to individuals or communities in some way. A socially liberal view might support the right to gay marriage, but a more conservative or religious view might deny that there is any such right when it is counter to their definition of 'natural' laws. People also argue about who is or is not a morally relevant entity with regard to rights. For example, some argue for animal rights and against the rights of the unborn fetus. If one is deemed to be morally irrelevant and therefore not protected by rights, then, as a natural consequence, a range of actions become valid which would have otherwise have been considered wrong, such as animal abuse or abortion.

THEOLOGICAL APPROACHES AND NATURAL LAW

A small number of major religions give moral guidance to the majority of people on the planet. This should make ethical decision-making a simple process, but it does not. There are enormous variations within those religions through the various denominations and sects, and there are a large number of minor religions. Further, cultural influences on religious precepts and interpretations are enormous and blur the distinctions between what is spiritually right and what is culturally expected. Added to this is the fact that, rightly or wrongly, groups and individuals interpret those religious precepts in many different ways.

Despite this, the similarities between different religions' ethical instructions are probably greater than the differences, although the differences are often what attracts the most attention. Although religions might differ in emphasis and expression, they largely condone virtues such as compassion, truthfulness, justice and wisdom, and denounce such things as stealing, taking life and adultery.

The main underpinning of religious-based ethical approaches is through the appeal to natural law. In this view, nature—whether it be the nature of the physical universe, society or human psychology—is governed by natural laws given by a higher being. Human-made laws exist only to reflect these laws and uphold them. Disobedience of these laws, no matter whether it seemed expedient at the time, will inevitably lead to greater problems later on.

Problems with this approach obviously relate to disagreement about what these natural laws are, even among people from the same religious group. The other issue is that we live in an age where an increasing proportion of the community hold secular views and do not recognise that such laws exist. As a result there is an increasing move towards the separation of religion and the judiciary and parliament in most countries around the world.

OTHER THEORIES

Cultural relativism

According to this view, what is right or wrong is arbitrary and determined by the prevailing views of a culture rather than any universal or transcendent principles. A practice considered appropriate in one culture, such as polygamy or female circumcision, might be considered inappropriate in another. Generally speaking, within most democratic societies there is a wide tolerance of cultural practices and variations except when such practices have the potential for significant harm and/or conflict with the law.

Ethical egoism

Some ethicists say that all decisions are, at their core, decided by what is best for ourselves, even decisions that seem to be altruistic on the surface. In such situations we might, for example, anticipate something good in return, such as praise, favours or feeling good about ourselves. They might argue that any ethical conduct directed at the good of others is really only an expression of enlightened self-interest.

Intuitionism

Intuitionism refers to an approach where intuition is taken as the best yardstick of what is right or wrong. Conscience (from the Latin *con*—to connect with, and *science*—knowledge) carries the meaning of connecting with an inner knowledge of what is right or wrong. Such a view implies that humans have moral or ethical precepts written into the very fabric of their nature but they are only clearly seen in a higher state of awareness. Thus, unless there is something significantly wrong with our genes, level of awareness or upbringing, it feels innately wrong to lie, take life or steal. Indeed, the lie detector test is merely a stress test. Other ethicists discount the possibility of such intuition and see appealing to it as an easy escape from more strenuous ethical reflection. To them, intuition is little more than an automatic, unconscious or conditioned response to a given stimulus.

RESOURCES

American Medical Association, 'Medical ethics', http://www.ama-assn.org/ama/no-index/physician-resources/2416.shtml

Beauchamp TL, Childress JF. Principles of biomedical ethics. 5th edn. New York: Oxford University Press; 2001.

BMC Medical Ethics, http://www.biomedcentral.com/bmcmedethics/

Journal of Medical Ethics, http://jme.bmj.com/

Veatch R. Medical ethics. Boston, MA: Jones & Bartlett; 1989.

REFERENCES

1 Boyd K, Higgs R, Pinching A. The new dictionary of medical ethics. London: BMJ Publishing; 1997.

2 Billimoria P. Course notes, MFM1017, Graduate Diploma in Family Medicine, Department of General Practice, Monash University, Melbourne; 2007.

3 Hassed C. Course notes, MFM1017, Graduate Diploma in Family Medicine, Department of General Practice, Monash University, Melbourne; 2008.

part THREE

Systems

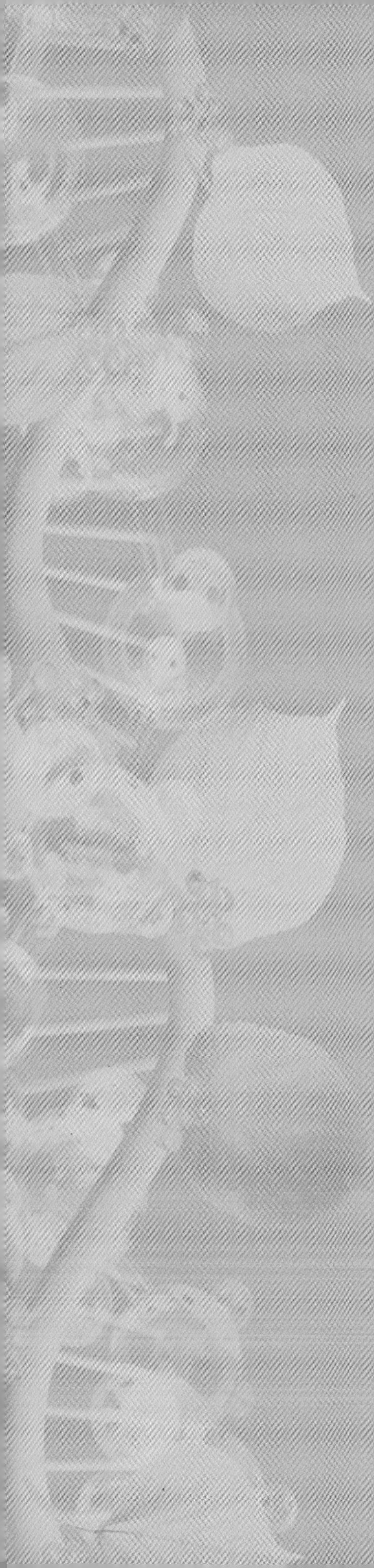

chapter 21

Allergies

INTRODUCTION AND OVERVIEW

The purpose of this chapter is to introduce you to the basics of allergy, what the practitioner should know in order to plan an effective integrative treatment strategy, and to provide an overview of some therapies that have been used successfully to treat different aspects of allergy. For the patient, an integrative approach usually means making lifestyle changes and being more attentive to what they allow inside their body and their home. For the practitioner, it means becoming more informed about allergy and treatment options in order to make better treatment decisions for each patient.

Millions of people worldwide endure the misery of allergies and suffer from their effects, seeking relief through conventional pharmacological remedies. However, most conventional remedies only treat the symptoms of allergies with antihistamines, decongestants or immunosuppressive medications, which, while offering welcome relief or even saving lives, do not treat the allergy itself. Untreated allergies can spread, worsen or cause other health problems. Also, reliance on drugs is always problematic, as most drugs have undesirable side effects.

One problem that has so far limited our ability to successfully treat allergy is what Dr Merv Garrett of the Australasian College of Nutritional and Environmental Medicine refers to as 'labelling disease'.[1] Allergy is a multifactorial problem, attributable to so many causal factors and appearing in so many different ways that labelling all its manifestations as allergy can mislead the practitioner into a narrow pattern of diagnosis and treatment. Any diagnosis of allergy should include a thorough investigation of the influences on that particular case, and investigation into the likely effectiveness and appropriateness of different possible treatments.

DEFINITION OF TERMS

Most natural or complementary healthcare practitioners use the term 'allergy' to refer to situations in which the immune system overreacts to a normally harmless substance, causing an exaggerated sensitivity (hypersensitivity) to that substance. However, medical doctors and scientists often recognise only reactions that result from the activation of immunoglobulin E (IgE) antibodies as allergies—that is, the 'classic' allergy. People who experience allergic symptoms without the antibody reaction are said to have an intolerance or a hypersensitivity to a particular substance.

Some people, however, may have many of the symptoms of classical allergy, but reactions, which may occur hours or days after the exposure, involving little or no IgE. While these people may experience delayed skin reactions, their immediate skin reactions and blood tests for allergens may be negative or weak. More than a decade later, there is much wider recognition of the diversity of allergic responses, and of the fact that IgE-mediated responses do not account for all allergies, especially food allergies.[2–4]

Because medical terminology must be precise in order to facilitate proper diagnosis and treatment, the following distinctions are made between allergy, sensitivity and intolerance.

- *Allergy* refers to the immune system's hypersensitivity upon re-exposure to a sensitising agent, an allergen, which results in the release of inflammatory chemicals and development of various symptoms. Although the presence of IgE has traditionally been the marker of an allergy, the correct term applies to elevation of specific antibodies due to antigen stimulus.
- *Sensitivity* refers to adverse reactions in the body upon exposure to a sensitising agent in the environment. It does not involve antibodies,

although it may involve other immunological processes. Most food and chemical reactions are sensitivities.
- *Intolerance* refers to the absence of a particular chemical (e.g. the enzyme lactase) or physiological process needed to digest a food substance, and the reaction is the result of non-immunological response of the body. Food intolerance is responsible for most adverse reactions to food, but it is not a true allergy; correcting the defect ends the symptoms.

BACKGROUND AND PREVALENCE

It is difficult to obtain solid, consistent, up-to-date statistics on allergy, but throughout the Western world, a significant rise in the incidence of allergy has been reported since the 1950s. A report released by the House of Lords Select Committee on Science and Technology in July 2007 stated that, 'Allergy in the United Kingdom has now reached epidemic proportions, with new, more complex and potentially life threatening allergies'.[5] Allergies are also on the rise in Australia, which has one of the highest rates in the world.

A study by the Australian Centre for Asthma Monitoring revealed that, 'the number of Australians hospitalised for severe life-threatening allergic reactions has more than doubled in the past 15 years', particularly among young children.[6] In a lecture at the Onassis Foundation in Greece, Dr Daphne Tsitoura said that if something is not done to stem this growth, one in two Europeans will have allergies or allergy-related conditions by 2015.[7]

Food allergies, many of which do not fit the IgE-mediated reaction pattern, are on the rise globally. In 2001, the US Food and Drug Administration reported that 'Only about 1.5 percent of adults and up to 6 percent of children younger than 3 years in the United States—about 4 million people—have a true food allergy, according to researchers who have examined the prevalence of food allergies', but those statistics only included 'classic' allergies involving IgE. After surveying 14,948 people about seafood allergies, Sicherer and colleagues concluded that 2.3% of the general population had credible seafood allergy, suggesting that food allergies are much more prevalent than generally allowed for in US government statistics.[8]

The House of Lords report on allergy noted the adverse effects of allergy on quality of life, especially for children, and on school and workplace performance.[5] In addition to this, allergy places an enormous economic burden on society. For these reasons alone, it is not to be taken lightly, even when the allergies are mild. Even more insidious are the less obvious and 'hidden' health effects of allergy. It makes life miserable for many sufferers, and has been implicated in a large number of diseases and disorders, including degenerative disease.

AETIOLOGY

Allergy means that the person's body, for one reason or another, has lost the normal ability to cope appropriately with one or more substances. While heredity makes some people more susceptible to allergy than others, the causes of allergy and sensitivity are multifactorial. Specifically, genetic susceptibility and some dietary, environmental and lifestyle factors that break down or disrupt the individual's immune system and barrier defences are in varying degrees responsible for the development and progress of allergy and sensitivity.

GENETIC INFLUENCES ON ALLERGY

An allergic predisposition or tendency is inherited, so allergy often runs in families. The age of onset of an allergic condition depends on the degree of inheritance: the stronger the genetic factor, the earlier in life is the probable onset. Genes do increase children's risk of allergies, from 50–58% if one parent has allergies to 60–80% if both are affected. This risk seems to be higher if the mother has allergies. Even with a family history of allergy, however, a child may not develop allergies until later in life, or may never develop the condition, because allergy results from a combination of other factors that determine whether a person's genetic susceptibility will be realised.

OTHER PARENTAL INFLUENCES ON INFANT ALLERGY

The development of allergy in people with or without a family history of allergies is usually triggered by pre-existing environmental influences that can affect a person even before birth. A mother with allergies can transmit them, and the antibodies against them, to her unborn child through the placenta, or after birth in the breast milk. A mother without allergies can transmit toxins, biochemicals resulting from chronic stress or trauma, or pathogens to the unborn child or infant in the same ways: via the placenta or through breastfeeding. This can set the stage within that child's body for allergies. Some early influences on allergy are:

- serious parental disease or condition prior to conception or birth
- maternal exposure to harmful substances during pregnancy
- parental exposure to toxins prior to conception
- toxins in the child's body resulting from disease (e.g. streptococcal infection as in strep throat, measles or chicken pox)
- maternal emotional or physiological trauma during pregnancy

- in utero and postnatal stress. Maternal stress, including parenting stresses and maternal depression, has been identified as a factor in early onset of asthma in children by age 3 years, and research suggests that the in utero environment, including maternal stress, affects atopy[9–11]
- weakness of the child's immune system due to infection, drugs, malnutrition etc.

ENVIRONMENTAL AND LIFESTYLE FACTORS

External factors can cause allergy in children and adults. In 1998, Dr Stephen Holgate wrote, in the *Quarterly Journal of Medicine*, 'While ~40% of the clinical expression of an allergic disorder can be accounted for by genetic factors, for these to be manifest there is an absolute requirement for interactions with environmental factors'.[12] The World Health Organization reported that, 'convincing evidence demonstrates that a number of environmental factors—environmental tobacco smoke, poor indoor/outdoor climate and some allergens—contribute to the onset of allergic disease. Once the disease is established, these factors may also trigger symptoms'.[13]

Additional factors linked to the development of allergies include:

- diet—lack of variety, too much of one food, overeating or binge eating
- lack of breastfeeding
- early introduction of cow's milk
- early introduction of solid food
- dysbiosis
- toxins
- other factors such as hormonal imbalances, infections, metabolic diseases, seasons, altitude, nutritional imbalances, heredity and race.

In an article on preventing allergies, AB Becker of the University of Manitoba, Canada, wrote: 'It is increasingly clear that gene-directed environmental manipulation of allergy in a multifaceted manner during a "window of opportunity" is critical in the primary prevention of allergy and allergic diseases like asthma'.[14] The 'window of opportunity' for most people is in the first year of life, when a multifaceted preventive strategy can help develop the child's resistance to allergies. Research suggests that in the first year of life, allergies may be prevented by:

- breastfeeding
- delayed introduction of cow's milk
- delayed introduction of solid foods
- providing a wide variety of balanced dietary elements
- maternal and infant supplementation with probiotics.

(For more details, see below, under 'Prevention'.)

THE TWO PATHWAYS TO ALLERGY

In general, some or all of the above-mentioned influences lead to allergies through one or both of two pathways:

- immune system hypersensitivity
- damage to the mucous membranes in the body's natural defence barriers (gut, airways and skin).

Immune overreactivity

An immune system stressed by infection, stress or toxins can become hypersensitive and overreact to an otherwise safe substance. The first time this occurs, antibodies are produced that attach to basophils and mast cells embedded in the mucous membranes, creating sensitivity to that substance, but no allergic reaction. On the next exposure to that allergen, the antibodies 'remember' the substance, and stimulate release of chemicals, including histamines. Together with other cells also rushed to the affected site, these cause inflammation and the typical symptoms of allergy: coughing, sneezing, runny nose, swelling, itching and so on.

Failure of the mucous membranes

The cells of the mucous membranes lining the intestines, respiratory passages and skin are held together with 'tight junctions'. When the membranes become irritated and inflamed, the tight junctions weaken, allowing food particles, bacteria or toxins to pass through the walls prematurely, which once again can lead to allergy.

One very important example of this is 'leaky gut syndrome', which researchers have shown to contribute to the development of allergies.[15–18] The mucous membrane lining of the gut wall can be compromised by:

- dysbiosis and/or faulty digestion
- infestation by bacteria, parasites, fungus, yeasts or protozoa
- chemical irritants or toxins
- poor diet
- inflammatory bowel conditions such as colitis, Crohn's disease, coeliac disease (which may in turn be associated with hidden food allergies)
- chronic stress (leading to the over-release of certain chemicals and hormones)
- genetic or acquired enzyme deficiencies (e.g. lactose deficiency and coeliac disease).

DIAGNOSIS

The practitioner taking an integrative approach to allergies must be willing to look beyond the expected parameters of diagnosis, as allergies have a varied and complex pathology due to the interactions of so many different elements: physiology, psychology, genetic make-up, situation, family and environment. Not only do different people manifest the same kinds of allergies in different ways, and not only are they multifactorial in cause, but one must consider the possibility of cross-reactions, where sensitivity to one substance causes a person to be sensitive to ingredients in several other substances. For example, a person with an allergy to melons may also be allergic to other fruits or even to pollen because of certain similar ingredients. Assessment of cross-reactive food allergens requires careful history, testing and perhaps oral food challenges.[19]

Below is a simple but practical model for diagnosing allergies. Note the central role of the history in determining what might be causing the allergic symptoms.

HISTORY

The clinical pattern of allergies and food intolerances is often exposed in the history taken from the patient. The practitioner needs to identify childhood problems such as intolerance to milk feeding, frequent diagnosis of upper respiratory tract infections, ear infections, tonsillitis and sinusitis, which could all be due to dairy intolerance in particular. The history should include any history of eczema, information about dairy and wheat reactions, frequency and duration of reactions, possible or likely triggers, seasonal or other influences on reactions, such as presence of animals or certain locations, family history of any reactions or allergy disorders, age of onset of reactions or condition, and changes over time.

Through an examination of an infant's dietary history, for instance, it is easy to establish a relationship between severe colic and cow's milk, from which the practitioner can surmise that the colic is associated with cow's milk intolerance (as reported by Iacono and colleagues[20] and Hill & Hosking[21]) without resorting to distressing skin tests, and recommend dietary treatment.

Also ask about the emotional environment and the emotional context of reactions, as this can play a role in the onset and worsening of allergies.

History and other investigations are critical, even when the symptoms seem to indicate one kind of allergy. Food allergies or sensitivities, for instance, can lead to lung disease, asthma, eczema, and rhinitis, wheezing and other respiratory symptoms. Asthma can show up as food allergies and gastrointestinal symptoms. Food allergy or sensitivity is, in fact, often overlooked as a cause of asthma, especially because food allergies do not always show up in standard skin tests. Multiple chemical sensitivity with its complex combination of factors can also be missed by standard tests, and is usually diagnosed by history.[22]

Dietary and environmental history

The purpose of taking a dietary and environmental history is to get an idea of which foods and toxins may be causing reactions. A week-long food diary can be adequate, showing where the food was bought, prepared and eaten, and any effects from eating the food. Include snacks, takeaway food, beverages and meals out.

Some reactions to food will be almost immediate, within an hour or two of consumption or even of contact with the food. These are usually obvious reactions such as stomach cramps, itching, vomiting or anaphylaxis, a severe and potentially fatal reaction which can involve light-headedness, swollen tongue or throat, difficulty breathing, fainting or facial swelling. Anaphylaxis usually occurs immediately or within 2 hours of food ingestion, and requires immediate emergency care. Other reactions may be 'hidden', occurring from 24 hours to days after ingestion, and this can make it difficult to relate them to particular foods. This is why a food diary is so important, as it can reveal otherwise hidden patterns of reaction. An elimination diet can be a useful diagnostic tool in this case (see below, under 'Investigations'). Hidden reactions can include physiological reactions such as swollen lymph nodes or unexplained body aches, or they can be psychological, showing up as clusters of cognitive or behavioural problems.

Exposure to toxins

Clues to environmental factors are also to be found in the patterns of presentation of symptoms, and also in chemical testing, such as hair or urinary testing to identify environmental pollutants such as arsenic or mercury.[22] Because a person can be allergic to just about anything, everything with which the person comes into contact should be considered, including common household chemicals such as:

- fluoride in toothpaste
- chlorine and/or fluoride in water (which can enter through the skin when bathing)
- chemical solvents and toxic fumes in building materials
- aluminium in deodorants
- nickel in jewellery
- latex in dish-washing gloves
- petrochemicals in many personal care products and cleaning products
- food additives and colours
- electromagnetic frequencies from computers, microwaves and mobile phones
- dust, which contains allergens such as mould, dust mites, pollen, debris from cockroaches, and household and animal dander
- toxins in sprays and treatments against cockroaches and ants

- formaldehyde in carpets, polyester clothing, spray starch and paper products
- Scotchgard™ on furniture
- poisons in fire retardants in clothing and upholstery.

SIGNS AND SYMPTOMS

How do you recognise an allergy? You look for signs, though you will only be able to see some for yourself, if any, so history is your primary diagnostic tool and can lead you to a correct diagnosis even when tests indicate to the contrary. Below are some signs and symptoms that can indicate allergy. You can include them in your consultation interviews or checklists.

First, suspect allergy whenever inflammation is present. If the allergic reaction is near the skin, you will often see all four cardinal signs of inflammation: pain, swelling, heat and redness. For example, hives will show up as a red, warm, painful and swollen rash. In the gut, allergies will cause inflammation in the gut lining, compromising nutrient absorption and digestion. Depending on where the reaction takes place, you will have different symptoms. Allergy can occur anywhere in the body, even in the brain.

There are two categories of allergy sufferers: those with obvious allergy symptoms and signs, and those with 'hidden' signs that may be easily overlooked. Signs of allergy include:

- nasal congestion, drippy nose, itchy teary eyes
- tender sinuses
- swelling of face, tongue or limbs
- skin rashes, eczema or hives
- coughing or wheezing
- dark, blue or black eye circles (sometimes called 'allergic shiners')
- crease at the bridge of the nose.
- wrinkles or abnormally puffy bags under the eyes
- a 'spaced-out' look
- bright red cheeks, nose tip or earlobes
- 'wiggly' or restless legs
- frequent nose rubbing
- frequent throat clearing or coughing
- a puffy look to face, hands and knuckles, ankles and lower leg
- eye problems—red, itching, burning, running, heavy puffy eyelids
- acne, acne rosacea, hives, eczema, dermatitis, boils, psoriasis
- sleep disturbances
- frequent colds and flu
- mental and behavioural—depression, irritability, agitation, mood swings, anxiety, anger, panic attacks, delusions, epilepsy, insomnia, restlessness, falling asleep at inappropriate times, or manifesting unusual behaviour
- persistent throat clearing, coughing
- burning or numbness of the face, arms, legs or feet, or a creepy crawly feeling under the skin.

INVESTIGATIONS

Most information will come from the history, and tests may also be administered, to identify or confirm major allergies and allow strategies to be precisely targeted. Various diagnostic procedures are available to test allergies and IgE-mediated allergies. Allopathic medicine uses various testing modalities to identify allergens and allergic reactions in sensitive individuals. Other diagnostic approaches include allergy symptom-rating questionnaire, food avoidance test, food challenge test, scratch test, elimination and challenge diet, rotation diet,[23] pulse difference test,[24,25] patch test, skin prick test (SPT), radioallergosorbent test (RAST), provocative neutralisation testing, immunoglobulin studies (IgE, IgA, IgM, IgG) and IgE-specific antigen studies.

The most commonly performed allergy tests are the SPT, the RAST and the enzyme-linked immunosorbent assay (ELISA). They evaluate whether a person is producing specific IgE to ingested or inhaled allergens.

Scratch or prick test

A drop of concentrated antigen is placed on the skin, usually on the inner forearm, which is then pricked or scratched so that a minute amount of antigen is absorbed. The size of a wheal surrounded by erythema compared with the control indicates a response to a problem substance. Generally, a wheal diameter of 3 mm × 3 mm is considered positive. However, there are several complexities and pitfalls in interpreting SPTs. If a sensitive person has high IgE levels, the scratch or

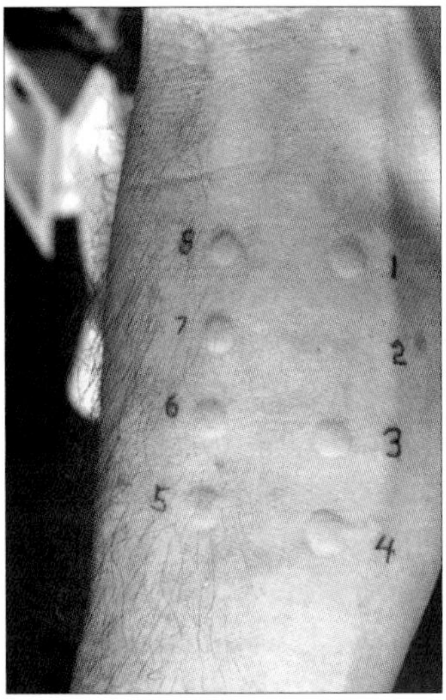

FIGURE 21.1 Positive prick test

prick test can accurately determine allergy to pollens, moulds, dust, dust mite and animal dander. However, if IgE levels are low, a wheal may not develop even if the person tested is sensitive to these inhalants. There is no standard battery of allergens tested—the history guides which allergen extracts are used.

When the scratch test is used for food testing, only food allergies for which the person has an extremely high IgE level will be uncovered. Because over 85% of food allergy is non-IgE mediated, this type of testing cannot give an accurate picture of a person's food problems. The scratch test also cannot be used for testing chemicals, because most chemical reactions are not IgE mediated.

The test will not be effective if the person is taking antihistamines or antidepressants, as these will inhibit the skin reaction. The person must not take the test if on beta-blockers, as these will intensify the skin reaction, possibly leading to a severe reaction.

Patch test

The patch test is used to diagnose contact allergies. A patch with an antigen on it is applied to the skin and is left in place for 24–48 hours. Lesions, a rash, erythema or hardness of the skin under the patch indicate sensitivity to the test substance.

Blood tests

Several allergy testing methods use the person's blood. The radioallergosorbent test (RAST) is a blood test in which IgE and IgG antibodies are labelled with a radioactive substance. The amount of antibody found in the blood in response to a given food, pollen, mould, dust and so on can be measured with a Geiger-counter type of instrument. RASTs are useful when SPTs cannot be performed. The RAST can test for sensitivities to a large number of substances in a short period of time. It works only with immunological antibodies; it cannot identify problem substances for which there is no antigen–antibody response, but it does have the advantage of measuring IgG antibodies, confirming an IgG-mediated immune response to milk in milk-intolerant individuals.[26]

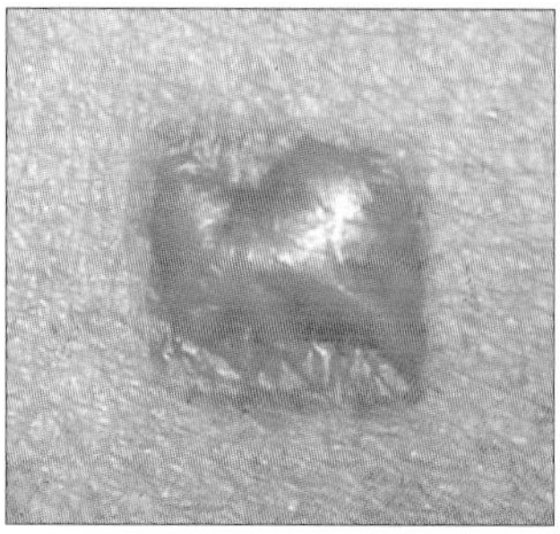

FIGURE 21.2 Positive patch test

Different laboratories use different panels of allergens for RASTs. The CAP RAST (ImmunoCAP® specific IgE blood test) system, which gives a quantified result for the IgE level, is superior to the traditional + to +++ system. Laboratories will do RASTs against specific foods if requested, and these results are much more helpful than the completely non-specific 'food-mix positive' result.

The enzyme-linked immunosorbent assay (ELISA) can detect IgE antibodies in serum. A variation of this test, called the ELISA/ACT, can diagnose all delayed immune reactions that involve other types of antibodies. This technique uses the antigen-binding properties of antibodies to detect specific antigens or antibodies in the serum of the patient.

Dietary elimination and challenge test

In the dietary elimination and challenge test, the body is cleared of possible food allergens, then foods are reintroduced one at a time, and any resulting symptoms noted. Semi-fasting detoxifies the body, unmasks sensitivities and makes it easier to identify an offending food, but because of the detoxification, any reaction may be exaggerated.

Elimination diet

This very reliable and effective test for food allergies was first developed by Californian Dr Albert Rowe and expounded in his book, *Elimination Diets and the Patient's Allergies* (1941), and later enabled Australian researchers to establish the role played by dietary factors in certain allergies.[27] Dr Rowe, formerly of the University of California School of Medicine in San Francisco, California, is considered the father of the concept of food allergy. He realised that foods can cause a problem even though the reaction is not IgE mediated. He is best known for his elimination diet, which is still important in identifying and treating food allergy.

The procedure involves two steps: elimination and reintroduction of foods.

Step 1: Elimination phase

Eliminate all suspect foods for 4–7 days, to clear the body of any delayed reactions to the food. This may require a semi-fast of mainly vegetables, which has the added benefit of giving the person's system a break from unhealthy or allergenic foods. Eliminating suspect foods one at a time is not recommended, as a person often has multiple food allergies. If a semi-fast is not feasible, begin by eliminating:

- those foods that are suspect (any foods that appear to affect the person physically or mentally)
- common allergenic foods—dairy, wheat, eggs, nuts, fish and seafood, citrus, food additives, sugar

- foods that are craved or eaten a lot, as food cravings and addictions can result from allergies.

If the person continues to show any signs of allergy, continue eliminating foods, starting with chocolate, pork and beef, tomatoes and kiwifruit. The person may experience withdrawal symptoms—irritability, emotionality, headaches or lethargy—which may also show that the body is detoxifying, but these will pass quickly.

Step 2: Challenge phase

It may take 4–5 days to completely clear the body of food allergens and eliminate allergy symptoms, and to notice the positive effects on health and behaviour. Then you can begin to reintroduce the eliminated foods in the following way, to allow more accurate identification of food allergens.

- At first, reintroduce organic, whole foods where possible, as the person may be reacting to pesticides or additives in a food or during food processing, not to the food itself.
- Add only one food each day, to be eaten alone as a meal, not in combination with other foods.
- Portions should be moderate, not large.
- Note any symptoms—such as pain, bloating, gas, fatigue, difficulty concentrating, gloominess, overexcitability, stuffy nose—that occur after that food is eaten. If symptoms are noted, this indicates a food allergy, sensitivity or intolerance, and the food should be avoided. Some symptoms may surface a few days later, and foods reintroduced over that time may need to be re-tested for.
- Sugary, fatty and stimulant foods should be avoided, as they can interfere with the results.
- The foods used in the test meals must be free of chemical contaminants and seasonings, to avoid confusing the results.

When done properly, the food challenge gives very accurate results. Although the test can be done at home, it is not safe for everyone. Also, because of the allergy/addiction phenomenon, withdrawal symptoms from foods can be severe. For those with strong or severe allergic reactions, multiple symptoms or other medical conditions, the challenge phase is best done under medical supervision. There is a risk of a severe reaction associated with the challenge, but given its diagnostic benefit, it might be considered worthwhile if carried out under the guidance of an experienced practitioner who is also equipped for emergencies.

Rotation diet

If the elimination/challenge test is not successful or is too difficult, a rotation diet can be used to reduce symptoms and reduce the likelihood that the patient will develop further food sensitivities. This is because food from each food category is only eaten once every 4 days, which is about the time it takes most allergens to clear the body. Therefore, the allergen does not build up in the body, so food allergens can be identified with little risk of an allergic reaction.

Alternative testing methods

Alternative medicine practitioners also employ a variety of other tests for detecting allergies, sensitivities and food intolerances. Some of the commonly used non-traditional medical screening tests include: electrodermal screening test (also known as electroacupuncture by Voll (EAV)), muscle response testing, cytotoxic test, prime test, applied kinesiological screening, pulse test, saliva test, meridian scanning test, computerised organ scanners, Kirlian photography, electromagnetic force measurements and serial end-point titration, which is also used therapeutically (see below, under 'Complementary or alternative therapies for allergy').

FINAL THOUGHTS ON DIAGNOSING ALLERGIES

Food allergies and intolerances are suggested by: early age of onset of symptoms (before 12 months old); past history of atopic dermatitis; infective pattern to asthma, sinusitis, recurrent ear infections, repeated grommets, recurrent croup; and associated symptoms such as migraines, undue fatigue, irritable bowel syndrome, behaviour problems in children, obstructive nasal or pharyngeal symptoms, poor response to prophylactic drug therapy, and negative skin tests to inhalants. A family history of atopy needs to be identified, as food sensitivities often run right through families.

Inhalant allergies are often suggested by: age of onset after 18 months; anterior nasal symptoms such as itching, sneezing, clear rhinorrhoea; ticklish cough; history of asthma; and skin prick tests. They usually respond well to prophylactic drug therapy. Parents often have similar allergies. Also consider that around 20% of people with inhalant allergies also have food allergies or sensitivities. There are many cross-reactions between foods and pollens, probably because of the underlying phenolics and the homologous conserved proteins in these foods and non-food proteins.[28]

MANAGEMENT

PREVENTION

The first major challenge in treating allergies is to change the emphasis from drug treatment to prevention. Prevention is rarely funded, but it is the best approach to ward off the development of allergies, chronic disease and morbidity. The most effective preventive strategies are those targeting the newborn and small child, but the

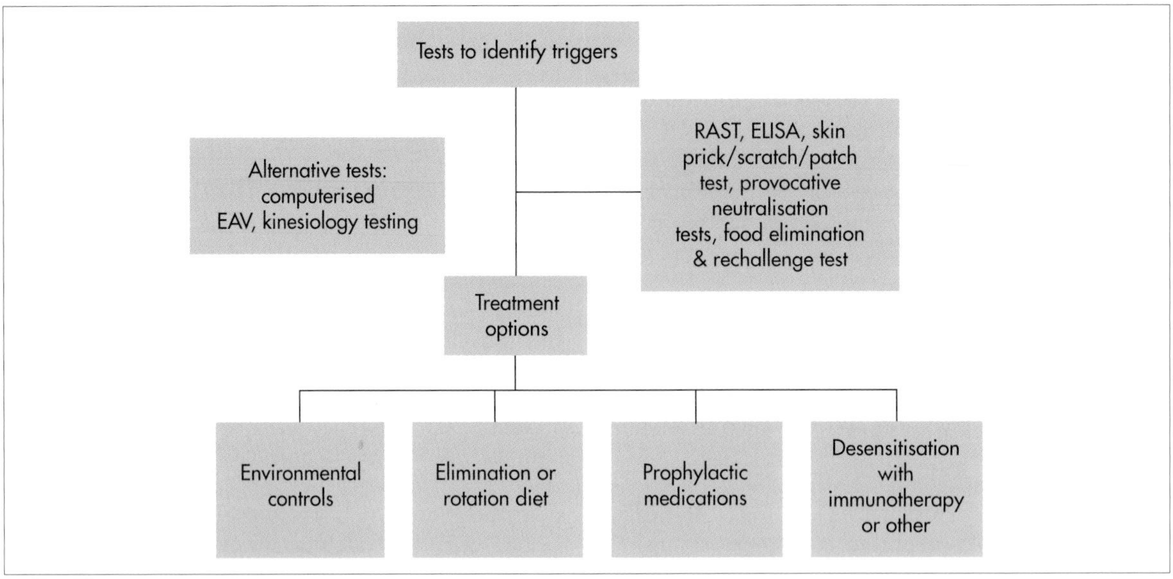

FIGURE 21.3 Testing and treatment options

onset of allergies can occur at any time of life. Therefore, the preventive strategies below include some that are also relevant to adults.

Exclusive breastfeeding

If continued for at least the first 4 months, breastfeeding helps protect against allergies, strengthens the immune system and ensures good use of nutrients to build a strong barrier system. Exclusive breastfeeding means no additional liquids or foods. If breastfeeding isn't possible, a hydrolysed (hypoallergenic) formula rather than one based on cow's milk is recommended for the first 12 months. Because allergies and allergens can be transmitted by an allergic mother to her infant via breastfeeding, preventive measures should begin with identification and avoidance of all allergens that affect the mother before pregnancy and during breastfeeding.

Delayed introduction of cow's milk

Cow's milk is best avoided for the first 12 months of life. It is higher in fat and protein than breast milk, and contains substances that the infant's digestive tract is not normally able to handle. The infant's immature digestive system must therefore work much harder to digest cow's milk. This probably explains why it is one of the most common allergens for children. Also, cow's milk and milk-based formulas lack the enzymes found in breast milk that help break it down. This means that partially digested protein may be absorbed by the infant's more permeable digestive system, resulting in an allergy to cow's milk. Allergy to milk will cause colic in infants, and can result in gastrointestinal bleeding, anaemia, chronic diarrhoea, fibrosis and coeliac disease.

Later introduction of solid foods

With the rapid rise in food allergies over the past decades, dietary strategies are especially crucial. Solid foods put an unnecessary burden on the infant's immature digestive system, and may not be properly digested; therefore, it is advisable to delay solids until at least 6 months, when the child's digestive tract has been able to develop healthy colonies of microflora, and is more mature. This also helps minimise the child's exposure to toxins, such as those found in many foods, including baby foods, and to potentially allergic foods, until the child's system is better able to handle them.

Foods should be introduced one at a time, beginning with mostly vegetables and some fruits (many fruits are quite allergenic). Rice and oatmeal can be added later, but common allergenic foods—wheat, eggs, nuts, corn, fish, beef, kiwifruit and citrus—should only be added after 12–18 months, and withdrawn if they seem to bring on symptoms such as rash, hyperactivity, ear infection, red cheeks, diarrhoea, runny or stuffy nose, pain, itchiness or unusual irritability.

Modified maternal diet during pregnancy and breastfeeding

An allergic mother should eliminate common allergenic foods and foods to which she is allergic from her diet before (if possible) and during pregnancy, to eliminate common allergens. The Allergy Unit of the Royal Prince Alfred Hospital in Sydney reported that children whose mothers eliminated allergenic foods from their diet had at least 50% fewer allergies than children whose mothers did not modify their diet, and that 'there were fewer problems with egg, milk, and peanut allergies'.[29] Citrus, kiwifruit, large fish, soy, legumes and wheat should also be avoided.

Delayed vaccinations

Some researchers have raised concerns about possible effects of early vaccinations on the child's immature immune system.[30,31] The general consensus, however, is that the protective benefits of vaccines outweigh the possible risks. Vaccination induces a predominately Th2-mediated immune response and probiotics may be beneficial during routine vaccinations, to manage the effects of vaccinations in children.

Promotion of beneficial intestinal microflora

Beneficial intestinal microflora help protect against damage to the digestive tract, reverse intestinal permeability and reduce antigen load in the gut by degrading and modifying potentially harmful macromolecules. A maternal probiotic supplement is suggested during pregnancy and breastfeeding, and also for the baby from birth, and in the event of antibiotic treatment. Antibiotics can disrupt the balance of intestinal bacteria, allowing pathogens to proliferate, which has been shown to cause allergies.[32,33] Research into the effects of intestinal microflora on allergy indicated that infants with greater diversity of microbial colonisation by 1 month of age were less likely to develop allergies.[33]

A wide variety of balanced dietary elements

Good nutrition can help prevent allergies in both children and adults. Allergies can result from eating too much of one kind of food, perhaps because the enzymes for that food are depleted or due to biochemical changes. A balanced, varied diet also ensures adequate nutrition, a key factor in allergy prevention and treatment, and can help reduce allergy symptoms, as particular foods are less likely to accumulate in the body.

Stress management

Stress is increasingly recognised as a factor in the onset of allergies, possibly even a major factor. Effective stress management can prevent the development of some allergies, and can significantly reduce the severity of reactions.

Reduced exposure to toxins

Toxic chemicals, pesticides, heavy metals and fumes are ubiquitous in the modern environment, found in our soil, water, air, food, medications, homes, workplaces and personal care products. Toxins are a major culprit in the onset of allergies and many other diseases. While the body can usually cope with a certain level of toxins, when the body is overloaded with toxins, its normal detoxification processes are overwhelmed, and key organs can be affected. Toxic overload severely disrupts body processes and stresses the immune system, leading to allergies. In our increasingly toxic world, the best protection one can have against allergies is reduced exposure to toxins, which in most situations requires conscious lifestyle choices.

PLANNING THE INTEGRATIVE STRATEGY

You have investigated the situation for your client who has allergies. Some preventive measures can already be put into place to prevent the development of further or worse allergies, but you are ready to consider treatment options. The next step is to work out what the triggers are and what causes the allergy symptoms in the first place. For example, we have to stop regarding asthma, glue ears, migraines, hay fever, irritable bowel syndrome and sinusitis as the end of the story. They should all qualify for a thorough diagnostic work-up to establish the underlying causes and triggers. For example, a 5-year-old with a recurring wheezy bronchitis since birth could be suffering from classic cow milk intolerance, and a 5-year-old with a 2-year history of recurring nocturnal asthmatic symptoms could be suffering from dust mite sensitivity. Both children have similar symptom presentations, but a closer look at the history reveals different aetiologies that require different management strategies.

To understand the clinical patterns of allergies, you need to ask some critical questions:

1. Could the patient's symptoms be related to underlying allergies? Chemical sensitivities? Food intolerance?
2. What additional tests would be useful to identify triggers or causes?
3. What are the treatment options? Is antigen desensitisation with immunotherapy an option?
4. Are changes to the environment necessary? Are dietary modifications required?
5. What prophylactic pharmacology is likely to be effective?
6. What is the overall toxic load on the patient's immune system?
7. What is the nutritional status of the patient and can it be improved?

The answers to these questions will assist in planning treatment strategies. While different doctors may respond to this information by selecting different methods and resources, a multi-track strategy is the only way to address the complexity of factors associated with allergy, and to provide a holistic healing framework for each patient. Some of the many possible treatment options that different practitioners and patients have reported to be effective are described in the following sections.

A six-step approach to allergy

Once the contributing factors and nature of the allergy have been defined, the first line of action is to address the person's lifestyle, diet and environment, in order to reduce or remove those elements that caused the development of allergy and contribute to allergic symptoms. The second line of action is to rebuild the person's health and capacity to heal, thereby building lasting resistance to allergies.

A basic program for treating and even preventing nearly all allergies and sensitivities is as follows:

1. Avoid/eliminate and/or desensitise the person to the identified allergens in their environment.
2. Alleviate the chronic inflammatory action.
3. Detoxify and reduce the total toxic load (in the body and the environment).
4. Stabilise the barrier systems, whether gut, skin or respiratory system.
5. Correct nutritional deficiencies and rebuild the immune system.
6. Reduce and manage stress.

KEY ELEMENTS OF AN INTEGRATIVE APPROACH TO TREATING ALLERGIES

The processes discussed below are the backbone of the six-step program outlined above, because they address the major contributing factors of allergy and allergy-related disorders. These processes are: detoxification, reduced exposure to toxins and allergen, identification of the allergens causing reactions, and desensitisation to those allergens, repair of the body's natural defence barriers, recolonisation of the gut with beneficial microflora, correction of digestive processes, nutritional therapy, and stress reduction and management.

The overall aim of these processes is to restore health to the whole patient, rather than simply providing superficial allergy symptom relief, and to also help the person achieve a balance between the physical, mental–emotional and even spiritual aspects of life. Many healthcare practitioners have successfully and effectively integrated these processes into holistic programs of treatment for allergies and other disorders.

Reducing toxic load

Studies by environmental scientists and physicians indicate that pollutants play a role in the creation of all allergies, as well as arthritis and autoimmune illnesses. Reducing the toxic load on a person's body involves reducing exposure to environmental toxins in the home, workplace or outdoors as well as detoxifying the body. Enzyme therapy is also very helpful, as some enzymes help break down toxins and irritants that would otherwise accumulate and aggravate or cause allergies. The broken-down toxins can then be more easily eliminated.

Nutritional support

Nutrition should be part of any comprehensive allergy treatment program, firstly because good nutrition helps to build a strong immune system and flush allergens and toxins from the body, and secondly because it is needed to correct existing nutritional imbalances and to protect against allergy. Essential foods include essential fatty acids, probiotic and prebiotic foods, fruits and vegetables, greens and lots of water.

Essential fatty acids (EFAs) can inhibit the inflammation that leads to many allergic reactions and help strengthen the body's mucous membranes, reducing the risk and severity of allergic reaction, including eczema and bronchial symptoms. EFAs also reduce inflammation in the nerves and brain that can cause behavioural symptoms such as autism, which has been also associated with EFA deficiencies. EFAs include omega-3, found in fish oil, and omega-6, found in evening primrose oil, blackcurrant seed oil and borage oil. Foods high in EFAs include sardines, mackerel, salmon, tuna, sunflower and pumpkin seeds, nuts, olives, soybeans, pumpkin, walnuts, eggs, soybeans, avocados and certain oils, such as olive, flaxseed, sunflower and borage oil.

Prebiotics are indigestible ingredients found in some foods whose role is to nourish probiotics: they *feed* the probiotics in the gut. They are found in fruits and vegetables, and some whole grains. Recommended foods include whole oats and barley (and whole wheat if the person is not allergic to it), legumes, artichokes, asparagus, onions, leeks, garlic, chicory, burdock, bananas, raw honey and maple syrup.

Probiotics are supplements or foods containing beneficial bacteria that help maintain digestive and gut health, preventing leaky gut and other causes of allergy. Clinical studies suggest that they help reduce inflammatory bowel conditions, improve milk intolerance and reduce atopic eczema in children. They may also reduce the symptoms of food allergies, and are associated with increased overall health. Probiotic foods include unsweetened, live culture yoghurt, buttermilk, sauerkraut, lightly cooked and raw cabbage, blueberries and miso.

Supplements—because allergies often deplete the body of certain nutrients, supplements may also be required, including vitamin C to reduce atopy in infants,[34] essential fatty acids, minerals and vitamin E. Consumption of sugar and unhealthy fats should be reduced, as they impair immunity.

Avoidance of allergens

Exposure to allergens has been shown to set off allergies,[35] and some people with multiple chemical sensitivities (acute hypersensitivity to low levels of everyday chemicals) can begin reacting to more and more specific environmental chemicals found in the workplace, school or home as their allergies spread.[36] Avoidance and clearing the home of known contact and inhalant allergens is especially recommended for high-risk children or adults, and for those with a weakened immune system. Avoidance is an essential component of treatment as it allows the person's system to become clear of allergens and recover from the effects of reactions, many of which do not show up as symptoms. Pay particular attention to substances that are known to commonly cause allergies, such as dust mites, pesticides and household chemicals.

Promotion of intestinal microflora

We have already seen that beneficial microflora have a protective effect against allergy. Healthy populations of beneficial microflora also prevent infection from harmful microbes such as *Escherichia coli*, chlamydia, candida, clostridia and so on. Epidemiological and clinical studies conducted over the past decade indicate that probiotics in the gut might be a major factor essential for the maturation of the immune system. Probiotics provide a non-pathogenic challenge to the Th1 immune system, which has an inhibitory effect on atopy. Administering probiotics during pregnancy and breastfeeding has been found to offer a safe and effective mode of promoting the immunoprotective potential of breastfeeding and provides protection against atopic eczema during the first 2 years of life. The best therapeutic strains recommended for allergies include:

- *Lactobacillus rhamnosus* HN001—a highly bioactive strain of probiotic that enhances cellular immune response by increasing natural killer cell activity and polymorphonuclear phagocytic activity, making it extremely useful in managing infectious diarrhoea and allergies and in supporting healthy immunity in adults
- *Bifidobacterium lactis* HN019—a special strain of *Bifidobacterium* that has been proved to assist immune function. This specific strain may help normalise T-helper cell responses in allergies and autoimmunity, thereby assisting in the maintenance of healthy immune responses. It has been shown to be useful for allergic conditions including atopic eczema, particularly in children.

Stress management

Stress is widely acknowledged as a critical element of most disease and allergy. It adds to the toxic load, disrupts communication between cells, and puts considerable strain on the immune system. Reducing and managing stress can remove a significant factor in both the development of allergy and the worsening of allergic responses. The practitioner should be prepared to address emotional issues, refer a patient to a counsellor or encourage regular de-stressing strategies.

TREATMENT

Most standard allergy therapies are pharmacological, and are predominantly aimed at preventing, relieving or reducing the severity of symptoms. The allergy is usually not addressed, and there is a widespread belief among practitioners that there is no remedy for allergy, just for its symptoms. However, therapies that were once considered alternative, and therefore questionable, are now gaining respect as viable treatment options. Others are still controversial, although many doctors have used some of them with good results, while some seem to be of little value; the latter have not been included in this chapter.

PHARMACOLOGICAL TREATMENTS

Prophylactic (preventive) drug therapy for allergies or allergy-related conditions can only be interpreted if there is an understanding of the aetiological factors and mechanisms involved. However, as a profession we seem to be in a pattern of acceptance of the allergic state, with management devoted almost entirely to pharmacological control rather than to working out why the patient has become sick in the first place. Treatment is not investigative, simply pharmacological, and focuses on treating the effect rather than the cause. Large improvements in our management of these conditions have concentrated on reducing allergic inflammation and the mediators involved using appropriate medications.

Drugs do have a place, even in a natural healing context, in improving quality of life for some patients and allowing them to physically and mentally recharge and prepare for healing. Pharmacological treatments can be used to alleviate symptoms or to lessen their severity. There are two types of medical treatments for allergies: drugs and immunotherapy. Appropriate drugs include antihistamines, decongestants, antihistamine–decongestant combinations, anti-inflammatory drugs and adrenaline (epinephrine) (for life-threatening or serious reactions). People with allergic asthma may also require other medications—specifically bronchodilators and mucokinetic drugs.

Antihistamines work by blocking histamine from H_1 receptors, and are used for relief and to prevent symptoms when exposure to allergens is unavoidable.

They are delivered as nasal sprays, eye drops, oral tablets and topical creams and sprays. *Decongestants* work by reducing swelling of mucous membranes and blood vessels. It is recommended that topical decongestants, if used at all, not be used for more than 3–5 days, to avoid a rebound nasal reaction. Systemic decongestants can be used for longer periods of time. However, stimulant side effects require care for people with high blood pressure or heart disease.

Anti-inflammatory drugs include mast cell stabilisers and the corticosteroids. Mast cell stabilisers have a prophylactic action and can be used regularly or as needed to reduce symptoms from exposure to specific, known allergens, or before an allergy hay fever season. The oldest and best known mast cell stabiliser is cromolyn sodium. Anti-inflammatories can be delivered as a nasal spray, eye drops (to treat allergic conjunctivitis) or a metered-dose inhaler, nebulised liquid or powder-filled capsule for the management of asthma (Intal® (cromolyn sodium)).

Corticosteroids are powerful anti-inflammatory drugs. They are more potent than antihistamines, decongestants and mast cell stabilisers. They have a greater side-effect profile, and so should be used with caution in the long term, especially with systemic corticosteroids (which can suppress the body's normal production of adrenal hormones). The form in which they are used varies according to the allergy they are used to treat: nasal sprays and inhalers for respiratory allergies, creams and ointments for skin allergies, oral tablets for more serious conditions.

Adrenaline is the primary treatment for anaphylaxis or in cases of emergency. It constricts blood vessels, increases lowered blood pressure, increases the heart rate and relaxes smooth muscles in the airways. It often comes in prescribed kits under the brand names EpiPen® and EpiPen Jr®, with pre-measured doses of adrenaline.

Immunotherapy

The goal of immunotherapy is to desensitise a person to an allergen to which they are sensitised. When immunotherapy is successful, a person's sensitivity to an allergen decreases and, in some cases, disappears. Thus, it decreases both the frequency and the severity of allergy symptoms. It can also reduce a person's need for medication. Immunotherapy is generally used mostly in the management of allergic rhinitis and allergic asthma. Food allergies or sensitivities, which often cause hives and other symptoms, do not generally respond well to immunotherapy. Immunotherapy is usually continued for 3–5 years.

This treatment uses serums containing extracts of allergens to stimulate the immune system with gradually increasing doses of the substances to which a patient is allergic, with the aim of weakening or ending the allergic response. It has been found most effective for IgE-mediated inhalant sensitivities such as persistent allergic rhinitis, which puts patients at risk of developing asthma,[37] especially for allergies to dust mites, pollens, animal dander and insect bites. Immunotherapy can take 6–12 months to become effective, with injections required every few years thereafter. Immunotherapy may be suggested for those whose response to drugs has been poor, and when the allergen cannot be avoided. Contraindications are beta-blockers, autoimmune disease, other serious conditions, pregnancy, multiple allergies and lymphoproliferative disorders.[1]

There are two forms of immunotherapy available: injections and sublingual drops. Some people obtain greater relief when the extracts are administered by injections. However, most people get significant relief from and prefer sublingual use of extracts, and it has the advantage of being easier to take.

Management of anaphylaxis

Every physician should be prepared for the most serious of allergic reactions. If a patient presents with strong allergy symptoms, or has multiple allergies or sensitivities, you should discuss the possibility of anaphylaxis, and devise an emergency strategy.

Signs of a severe allergic reaction

- Difficulty breathing
- Swollen tongue or throat
- Swollen joints
- Facial swelling
- Sneezing and coughing
- Light headedness, dizziness or fainting
- Severe hives
- Heart palpitations.

If any of these signs occurs immediately or within 2 hours of eating or coming into contact with food, an insect bite or any allergen, treat it as an emergency.

Prepare for an emergency

For every patient presenting with allergies, consider the possibility that a serious reaction may occur, even if it has not occurred before. It is strongly recommended that you put emergency strategies in place, whether this means providing emergency phone numbers, telling the patient how to contact you in case of emergency, or prescribing emergency medication.

A comprehensive emergency strategy might include the following steps:

- *Decide whether the patient's symptoms warrant prescribing medicine for anaphylaxis.* It is usually given by injection administered by an EpiPen®.

Adrenaline is the most frequently prescribed drug. Steroids or antihistamines may also be used.
- *Teach the patient or the patient's care provider how to safely administer the medication.* An EpiPen® is quite easy to use. Teach the patient or care provider how and when to give antihistamines as well, in an emergency.
- *Teach the care provider how to do mouth-to-mouth resuscitation, in case the patient stops breathing.* Encourage the person to teach other family members, teachers and work colleagues also.
- *Instruct the patient to keep the medication on hand at all times,* even when away from home.
- *Advise the patient to go to hospital emergency or a medical facility immediately after administering the injection.* Additional treatment may be needed. Up to one-third of anaphylactic reactions are followed by other reactions within hours of the initial attack. The patient should be under close supervision by a medical practitioner for 4–8 hours after an attack.
- *Ensure that staff at your medical facility know the correct emergency procedure* and can quickly direct a patient or family member to emergency care.

If the patient is not carrying self-administered adrenaline for anaphylaxis

- Teach the patient or a relevant family member to recognise the signs of anaphylaxis.
- Discuss emergency options with your patient and the patient's care provider.
- Ensure that the patient knows exactly how to get to immediate emergency care, and has emergency phone numbers.

Emergency protocol in general practice

- Assess for life-threatening features (stridor, bronchospasm, hypotension).
- Assess associated features (urticaria, pruritis, nausea, vomiting, diarrhoea, abdominal cramps).
- Dial emergency number for ambulance support.
- Administer adrenaline:
  - *Dose*:
    - 0.01 mg/kg of 1/1000 or 0.1 mg/kg of 1/10,000 SC or IM for children
    - 0.3–0.5 mL of 1/1000 SC or IM for adults.
  - Repeat 5-minutely if necessary.
- Apply oxygen by mask at 6 L/min.
- Salbutamol inhalation if significant bronchospasm present after adrenaline.
- Prepare to intubate if obstruction worsens.
- IV access with large-bore cannula.
- Run IV normal saline if hypotensive.
- *TRANSFER TO HOSPITAL*. Condition may deteriorate again 12 hours after initial episode.
- Methylprednisolone, 1 mg/kg IVI
- Promethazine, 1 mg/kg/dose to maximum of 10 mg IM or 25 mg orally, for relief of urticaria.

COMPLEMENTARY OR ALTERNATIVE THERAPIES FOR ALLERGY

Many complementary therapies aim at preparing the body for healing, reducing toxic load and desensitising or eliminating identified allergens, and some patients have reported that their allergies have been completely healed, although that could be a result of increased awareness, better intervention, and self- and environmental management. Nevertheless, there is good evidence that desensitisation can be achieved and can alter the clinical course of the disease.

If the immune system is constantly stressed by adverse reactions to foods, chemicals or inhalants, its efficiency decreases over time, and target organ damage can occur. Also, if the immune cascade is allowed to proceed unchecked, tissue damage will follow. Therapies that stop the process, or stop further reactions from happening, give the immune system a rest and a chance to repair and heal. These therapies offer protection and relief from unwanted symptoms, although, for lasting results, other factors such as diet and lifestyle will usually need to be addressed.

Serial endpoint titration

Used as both a diagnostic tool and a desensitisation therapy, serial endpoint titration (SET) is immunotherapy tailored to each particular patient's tolerance of the allergen. In a series of steps, the patient's skin on the upper arm is exposed to progressively more diluted amounts of the extract-containing serum until no wheal results from the exposure. The process is repeated for each allergen known to affect that person. The endpoint dilution of the allergen extracts represents the maximum tolerance for those allergens, and it is the amount of extract that is then administered intradermally or sublingually. The patient may not see positive results for a few months. Although complete desensitisation might not be achieved, SET greatly increases the patient's tolerance to allergens.

Enzyme-potentiated desensitisation

Developed in the 1960s by British immunologist Dr Leonard McEwen, enzyme-potentiated desensitisation (EPD) is used to train the patient's immune system to not react to allergens. Like other forms of immunotherapy, it uses extracts of allergens, but with three significant differences: the dilutions are even weaker than is usually used; extracts of multiple related allergens are used in each serum; and the serum also contains an enzyme called beta-glucuronidase. This enzyme, which is used at a similar strength to that at which it occurs in the body, makes the vaccine more potent. The serum is believed to activate suppressor T-cells. Once these are activated, injections are spaced weeks or months apart.

RESOURCES

Websites

Allergy information sheets, Royal Prince Alfred Hospital, Sydney, http://www.sswahs.nsw.gov.au/rpa/allergy/default.htm

Auckland Allergy Clinic, food cross-reactions, http://www.allergyclinic.co.nz/guides/42.html

Food Intolerance Network, http://www.fedupwithfoodadditives.info/

Health Professional Information, Australasian Society Clinical Immunology and Allergy, ASCIA Education Resources, http://www.allergy.org.au/content/view/139/114/

National Asthma Council Australia, http://www.nationalasthma.org.au/content/view/176/25/

Victorian Department of Health, Better Health Channel. Food allergy and intolerance, http://www.betterhealth.vic.gov.au/bhcv2/bhcarticles.nsf/pages/Food_allergy_and_intolerance/

Books, articles

Debarry J, Garn H, Hanuszkiewicz A et al. *Acinetobacter lwoffii* and *Lactococcus lactis* strains isolated from farm cowsheds possess strong allergy-protective properties. J Allergy Clin Immunol 2007; 119(6):1514–1521.

Eaton KK, Howard M, Howard JM, Princess Margaret Hospital, Windsor, Berkshire, UK. Gut permeability measured by polyethylene glycol absorption in abnormal gut fermentation as compared with food intolerance. J R Soc Med 1995; 88(2):63–66.

Formanek Jr R. Food allergies: when food becomes the enemy. FDA Consumer magazine 2001; July/August:10–16. Pub No. FDA 04-1312C

Kemp AS, Mullins RJ, Weiner JM. The allergy epidemic: what is the Australian response? Med J Aust 2006; 185(4):226–227.

Law M, Morris J, Wald N et al. Changes in atopy over a quarter of a century, based on cross-sectional data at three time periods. Br Med J 2005; 330:1187–1188.

Mrazek DA, Schuman WB, Klinnert M. Early asthma onset: risk of emotional and behavioral difficulties. J Child Psychol Psychiatry 1998; 39:247–254.

Nsouli TM, Nsouli SM, Linde RE et al. Role of food allergy in serous otitis media. Ann Allergy 1994; 73(3):215–219.

Ouwehand A, Kirjavainen P, Laiho K et al. From hypoallergenic foods to anti-allergenic foods. Food Science & Technology Bulletin: Functional Foods 2003; 1(5):1–12.

Pelto L, Isolauri E, Lilius E-M et al. Probiotic bacteria down-regulate the milk-induced inflammatory response in milk-hypersensitive subjects but have an immunostimulatory effect in healthy subjects. Clin Exp Allergy 1998; 28:1474–1479.

Prescott SL, Tang M. ASCIA Position Statement: Summary of Allergy Prevention in Children, as published in the Medical Journal of Australia 2005; 182(9):464–467. Online. Available: http://www.mja.com.au/public/issues/182_09_020505/pre10874_fm.html

Rapp DJ. Allergies and your family. New York: Sterling; 1984.

Randolph T. Environmental medicine: beginnings and biographies of clinical ecology. Fort Collins, CO: Clinical Ecology Publications; 1987.

Rea WJ. Chemical sensitivity, Vols 1–4. Boca Raton, FL: Lewis; 1992–97.

Reynolds G. Food allergies rise 12-fold in Australian children. AP-FoodTechnology.com; 2007. Online. Available: http://www.ap-foodtechnology.com/news/ng.asp?id=77467 19 October 2007.

Sampson HA. Food allergy. JAMA 1997; 278(22):1888–1894.

Sampson H, Muñoz-Furlong A, Campbell R et al. Second symposium on the definition and management of anaphylaxis: summary report—second National Institute of Allergy and Infectious Disease/Food Allergy and Anaphylaxis Network symposium. J Aller Clin Immunol 2005; 117(2):391–397.

Simpson A, Custovic A. Pets and the development of allergic sensitization. Curr Allergy Asthma Rep 2005; 5(3):212–220.

Tamburlini G, von Ehrenstein O, Bertolini R, eds. Children's health and environment: a review of evidence: a joint report from the European Environment Agency and the WHO Regional Office for Europe, Copenhagen. European Environment Agency. 2002:48–49. Environmental Issue Report No. 29.

Taylor F, Krohn J. Allergy relief and prevention. A practical encyclopedia. A doctor's complete guide to treatment and self care. 3rd edn. Vancouver: Hartley & Marks; 2000.

Wright RJ. Stress and atopic disorders. J Allergy Clin Immunol 2006; 116(6):1301–1306.

REFERENCES

1 Garrett M. Allergy in general practice. Paper presented at the Gold Coast Allergy and Sensitivity Specialist Training Program, Gold Coast, Queensland, Australia, 16–17 July 2005.

2 Schmid-Grendelmeier P, Simon D, Simon H et al. Epidemiology, clinical features, and immunology of the 'intrinsic' (non-IgE-mediated) type of atopic dermatitis (constitutional dermatitis). Allergy 2001; 56(9):841–849.

3 Sabra A, Bellanti J, Rais JM et al. IgE and non-IgE food allergy. Ann Allergy, Asthma Immunol 2003; 90(6 Suppl 1):71–76.

4 Sampson HA. Food allergy. J Allergy Clin Immunol 2003; 111(2):540–547.
5 House of Lords Science and Technology Committee. Allergy, Volume 1: Report. 26 September 2007. London: House of Lords; 2007: 6.
6 The Age, 12 October 2007. Severe allergic reactions on the rise. Online. Available: http://www.theage.com.au/news/NATIONAL/Severe-allergic-reactions-on-the-rise/2007/10/12/1191696150293.html
7 Tsitoura D. Allergy: a novel epidemic in the developed world of 21st century. AΩ International Online Magazine 2007; March (5). Online. Available: http://www.onassis.gr/enim_deltio/foreign/05/story_04.php
8 Sicherer SH, Munoz-Furlong A, Sampson HA. Prevalence of seafood allergy in the United States determined by a random telephone survey. J Allergy Clin Immunol 2004; 114(1):159–165.
9 Klinnert MD, Nelson HS, Price MR et al. Onset and persistence of childhood asthma: predictors from infancy. Pediatrics 2001; 108(4):69.
10 American Thoracic Society. Mother's prenatal stress predisposes their babies to asthma and allergy, study shows. Science Daily 19 May 2008. Online. Available: http://www.sciencedaily.com/releases/2008/05/080518122143.htm
11 Wright RJ. Stress and atopic disorders. J Allergy Clin Immunol 2006; 116(6):1301–1306.
12 Holgate ST. Asthma and allergy—disorders of civilization? Q J Med 1998; 91:171–184.
13 World Health Organization, Environmental hazards trigger childhood allergic disorders. 1 Fact sheet EURO/01/03 Copenhagen, Bonn, Brussels, Moscow, Oslo, Rome, Stockholm, 4 April 2003, p. 2. Online. Available: http://www.euro.who.int/document/mediacentre/fswhde.pdf
14 Becker AB. Primary prevention of allergy and asthma is possible. Clin Rev Allergy Immunol 2005: 28(1):5–16.
15 Cereijido M, Contreras RG, Flores-Benitez D et al. New diseases derived or associated with the tight junction. Arch Med Res 2007; 38(5):465–478.
16 Kirjavainen PV, Apostolou E, Arvola T et al. Characterizing the composition of intestinal microflora as a prospective treatment target in infant allergic disease. FEMS Immunol Med Microbiol 2001; 32(1): 1–7.
17 Liu Z, Li N, Neu J. Tight junctions, leaky intestines, and pediatric diseases. Acta Paediatr 2005; 94(4):386–393.
18 Taylor L, Hale J, Wiltschut J et al. Effects of probiotic supplementation for the first 6 months of life on allergen- and vaccine-specific immune responses. Clin Exp Allergy 2006; 36(10):1227–1235.
19 Auckland Allergy Clinic. Oral (provocation) challenges; 2005. Online. Available: http://www.allergyclinic.co.nz/guides/68.html
20 Iacono G, Carroccio A, Montalto G et al. Severe infantile colic and food intolerance: a long-term prospective study. J Pediatr Gastroenterol Nutr 1991; 12:332–335.
21 Hill DJ, Hosking CS. Infantile colic and food hypersensitivity. J Pediatr Gastroenterol Nutr 2000; 30(1 Suppl):67–76.
22 Hromek K. Taking a dietary/environmental history. Paper presented at the Gold Coast Allergy and Sensitivity Specialist Training Program, Gold Coast, Queensland, Australia, 16–17 July 2005.
23 Randolph TG, Rinkel H, Zeller M. Food allergy. Springfield, IL: Charles C Thomas; 1951.
24 Coca A. Familial nonreagenic food allergy. Springfield; 1942.
25 Coca A. The pulse test. New York: Lyle Stewart; 1956.
26 Little, CH, Georgiou GM, Shelton MJ et al. Production of serum immunoglobulins and T-cell antigen binding molecules specific for cow's milk antigens in adults intolerant to cow's milk. Clin Immunol Immunopathol 1998; 89(2):160–170.
27 Gibson A, Clancy R. Management of chronic idiopathic urticaria by the identification and exclusion of dietary factors. Clin Allergy 1980;10(6):699–704.
28 Garrett M. Inhalent allergy. Paper presented at the Gold Coast Allergy and Sensitivity Specialist Training Program, Gold Coast, Queensland, Australia, 16–17 July 2005.
29 Soutter V, Swain A, Loblay R. Food allergy prevention. Royal Prince Alfred Hospital, Sydney, 2002. Online. Available: http://www.cs.nsw.gov.au/rpa/allergy/resources/allergy/prevention.pdf
30 Hurwitz E, Morgenstern H. Effects of diphtheria-tetanus-pertussis or tetanus vaccination on allergies and allergy-related respiratory symptoms among children and adolescents in the United States. J Manipulative Physiol Ther 2000; 23:81–90. Abstract available online: http://www.ncbi.nlm.nih.gov/pubmed/10714532
31 Sakaguchi M, Inouye S. IgE sensitization to gelatin: the probable role of gelatin-containing diphtheria–tetanus–acellular pertussis (DTaP) vaccines. Vaccine 2000; 18(19):2055–2058.
32 Noverr M, Noggle RM, Toews GB et al. Role of antibiotics and fungal microbiota in driving pulmonary allergic responses. Infect Immun 2004; 72(9):4996–5003. Abstract. Online. Available: http://iai.asm.org/cgi/content/abstract/70/1/400
33 Wold A, Strachan D, Matricardi P et al. Impact of intestinal microflora on allergy development (Allergyflora); 2005. Online. Available: http://ec.europa.eu/research/quality-of-life/ka4/pdf/report_allergyflora_en.pdf 20 October 2007.

34 Hoppu U, Rinne M, Salo-Väänänen P et al. Vitamin C in breast milk may reduce the risk of atopy in the infant. Abstract. Eur J Clin Nutr 2005; 59(1):123–128.

35 Sporik R, Holgate ST, Platts-Mills TAE et al. Exposure to house dust mite allergen (DerP1) and the development of asthma in childhood. N Engl J Med 1990; 323: 502–507.

36 Beresford P. Report on Environmental Hypersensitivity in response to the Report of the Advisory Committee to the Minister of Health, Province of Nova Scotia; 5 January 1998. Online. Available: http://www.environmentalhealth.ca/Jan98report.html

37 Marogna M, Falagiani P, Bruno M et al. The allergic march in pollinosis: natural history and therapeutic implications. Int Arch Allergy Immunol 2004; 135(4):336–342. Abstract. Online. Available: http://www.ncbi.nlm.nih.gov/pubmed/15564776

chapter 22

Blood

INTRODUCTION AND OVERVIEW

This chapter examines the management of patients with haematological disorders likely to be encountered in general practice.

Haematology in general practice involves the care and monitoring of a very broad and disparate group of medical conditions and syndromes, ranging from investigation of anaemia and iron disorders, bleeding diatheses, venous thromboembolism and thrombophilias, to blood-product administration, and the initial diagnosis and comanagement of patients with haematological malignancy.

In recent years, patients with haematological conditions may have been treated with new therapies, including immunotherapy (e.g. rituximab for non-Hodgkin's lymphomas) or molecularly targeted therapies ('designer drugs' or 'magic bullets' such as imatinib mesylate for chronic myeloid leukaemia (CML)).[1] The impact of these new therapies and the rapidly changing treatment of blood cancers is discussed.

ANAEMIA AND HAEMATINIC DEFICIENCY STATES

The patient with anaemia or haematinic deficiency may be asymptomatic, with anaemia having been identified on blood tests performed for other reasons.

Symptoms that are often present, and may alert you to the presence of anaemia, include:

- fatigue and reduced exercise tolerance
- muscle weakness
- headache
- lack of concentration
- dizziness
- palpitations
- dyspnoea
- angina of effort.

Signs may include pallor, tachycardia and systolic flow murmur. You should also check for signs of cardiac failure, including peripheral oedema, jaundice and koilonychias.

The history, in a simplified clinical approach, should focus on:

- possible dietary causes (iron, folate, vitamin B_{12} deficiency, vegetarian)
- blood loss (ingestion of non-steroidal anti-inflammatory drugs (NSAIDs)), menorrhagia, gut symptoms)
- underlying infection
- previous gut surgery
- symptoms suggesting coeliac disease or inflammatory bowel disease
- inflammation (diabetes, renal insufficiency especially)
- possibility of pregnancy, in women of childbearing age
- malignancy
- lead exposure in children.

In the patient without obvious cause, anaemia itself is best regarded as a symptom, not a diagnosis.

The full blood count (FBC), mean red cell volume (MCV) and examination of the blood film remain the cornerstones of investigation. Anaemia types are classified according to red cell size:

- microcytic
- macrocytic
- normocytic.

Microcytic anaemia results mostly from iron deficiency, anaemia of chronic disease or thalassaemia/haemoglobinopathy. The most common causes of *macrocytic anaemia* are alcohol, pregnancy, and vitamin B_{12} and folate deficiency (Table 22.1).

When the bone marrow responds to an insult such as haemorrhage or haemolysis with a brisk increase

TABLE 22.1 Red cell size as a pointer to the likely cause of anaemia

Microcytic	Normocytic	Macrocytic
Iron deficiency	Chronic disease*	Pregnancy
Chronic disease*	Combined haematinic deficiencies	Reticulocytosis
Thalassaemias & haemoglobinopathies	Renal failure	Megaloblastosis Vitamin B_{12}/folate deficiency
Sideroblastic anaemia	Liver disease	Myeloma
		Alcohol
		Drugs (chemotherapy)
		Hypothyroidism

*Anaemia of chronic disease can cause normocytic or microcytic anaemia.

in reticulocytes (immature red cell forms), they can increase the MCV. For example, a reticulocytosis of over 10% may bring the MCV up to 105 fL (normal range: approx. 80–100). Rarer causes include hypothyroidism, myeloma and many chemotherapy drugs.

The diagnosis may be more difficult in those with a *normocytic anaemia*; in this situation, review of the blood film can be diagnostic. Such red cell changes include:

- increased numbers of spherocytes (small, rounded red cells without central pallor), which indicate immune-mediated haemolytic anaemia
- fragmented red cells with so-called 'helmet cells' (think of an American GI's helmet), seen in syndromes such as glomerulonephritis, malignant hypertension, disseminated intravascular coagulation and the rare thrombotic thrombocytopenic purpura
- nucleated red cells, coupled with markedly left-shifted granulocytes, which define leuco-erythroblastic change that implies marrow invasion (metastatic cancer) or compromise (extreme sepsis). A leuco-erythroblastic blood film without a known cause warrants immediate referral to a haematologist and consideration of marrow biopsy for occult cancer.

Where the cause of anaemia is still obscure, it may be appropriate to proceed to referral for further investigation, including a bone marrow biopsy; generally, if this is contemplated, the focus has shifted to the possibility of intrinsic marrow disorders such as myelodysplastic syndrome. The biopsy is taken from the posterior iliac crest and includes: an aspirate, to look at cellular morphology; a bone marrow core or trephine biopsy, which gives a better indication of the overall cellularity and the presence of the occult malignancy; and cytogenetic examination, which often gives the best yield for diagnosing early myelodysplastic syndrome. A sample is also frequently collected for flow cytometry to quantify blast cells (acute leukaemia), plasma cells (myeloma) or lymphoid cells (lymphoma). Bone marrow biopsy is best performed at a specialised centre, to allow optimum specimen collection and handling.

ANAEMIA OF CHRONIC DISEASE

The onset can be within 2 weeks of acute illness. The pathophysiology results in part from suboptimal erythropoietin activity, due to inhibition of gene expression by the inflammatory cytokines interleukin-1 and tumour necrosis factor. However, we now know that the principal mediator is hepcidin, which is synthesised in the liver, and this is upregulated by (other) inflammatory cytokines. High levels of hepcidin reduce iron absorption from the gut and inhibit iron release from macrophages. The net effect is that iron is unavailable for erythropoiesis.[2] The resulting anaemia can be normocytic or microcytic (25% of cases). In renal failure, lack of erythropoietin probably plays a larger part, and the anaemia can be profound, even with relatively mild renal insufficiency.

IRON DEFICIENCY ANAEMIA

In iron deficiency anaemia (Fig 22.1), the usual aetiology is negative iron balance, either from inadequate dietary intake or from gastrointestinal loss, menorrhagia or, more rarely, haemolysis. Iron deficiency is often symp-

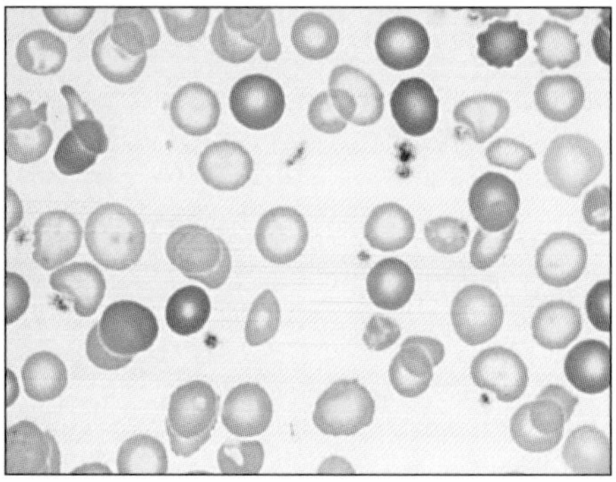

FIGURE 22.1 Iron deficiency anaemia

tomatic in the absence of anaemia. It can be associated with impaired mentation ('thinking through a cloud of cotton wool'), excessive fatigue, restless legs, a mild subjective peripheral neuritis and the rare pica syndrome (the urge to eat bizarre foods such as plaster or ice in excessive amounts). The history should include careful assessment of dietary iron, blood loss with menses, and asking about possible melaena, and haematuria or haemoglobinuria with dark urine. Physical examination may reveal classic stigmata, including glossitis, angular cheilosis and koilonychia, but these may not be present even with severe deficiency.

The serum iron value gives no guide to bodily iron stores; it reflects only the state of iron transport in the body. The diagnosis is made if the ferritin is below the lower limit of the normal reference range in a given laboratory. This is a pathognomonic result. However, ferritin is also an acute phase reactant, and so, in the iron-deficient individual with an inflammatory process, it may be inappropriately normal. Ferritin is also raised by infection, iron overload and malignancy.

In the asymptomatic patient, test for faecal blood loss and consider panendoscopy. In men and postmenopausal women, iron deficiency usually signifies gastrointestinal blood loss.[3]

Absorption of dietary iron is best (around 20%) as haem iron from animal sources such as red meat, white meat and fish. Iron in the non-haem form is less well absorbed (< 5%), and is found in cereals, legumes, vegetables and nuts. Iron enhancers can improve non-haem iron absorption two- to three-fold, and include vitamin C (citrus, tomato and broccoli), animal protein and vitamin A (spreads, oils, dairy products). Oxalates in spinach, tannin in tea and phytates in certain foods are iron inhibitors; so, for example, spinach eaten with tomato or broccoli improves iron bio-availability.

Occasional patients are seen in whom dietary intake of iron is adequate and no ongoing source of blood or iron loss is identified. Recently described mutations of the TMPRSS6 gene leading to impaired iron absorption may explain why some patients are refractory to oral iron replacement therapy. However, it appears that patients with these mutations are rare.[4,5]

Oral iron supplements are effective and well tolerated in about 80% of patients.[6] Slow-release ferrous sulfate preparations are better tolerated than the iron salt, but rates of discontinuation in randomised trials are the same. Patients should be warned of possible constipation, and increased bloating, wind or flatulence, probably attributable to rapid bacterial overgrowth in the presence of increased available iron. Co-prescribing live culture yoghurts or probiotics may minimise this. Bowel motions will turn black (it is, however, a greenish-black, rather than the reddish-black of melaena). Oral iron should never be taken with tea (because of its tannin content), but rather with orange juice for its vitamin C content. Indeed, some iron formulations incorporate vitamin C. One tablet a day is usually enough; some patients tolerate two tablets daily without problems, but others find even one a day difficult. For these patients, taking the supplement with food may still provide enough iron to raise body stores. You will need to check the elemental iron equivalent in different supplements.

Some 20% of patients are genuinely intolerant of oral iron.[6] It can lead to pseudo bowel obstruction and even surgical abdominal crises. For these patients, intravenous iron infusions are greatly preferable to intramuscular iron. The latter is poorly bio-available, and persists under the skin, leaving scarring and pigmentation. Whereas earlier IV preparations (iron dextran) were associated with cardiac arrhythmias, modern preparations (e.g. iron polymaltose, iron sucrose) have a far lower incidence of anaphylaxis and can be given rapidly without requiring electrocardiographic monitoring. This is best done in a specialised unit. Medical supervision should be on hand for the rare instance of anaphylaxis. Some patients experience arthralgia for 48 hours and this may require paracetamol. The response in many is gratifying, although it can take 2–6 weeks to become maximal. Thereafter, patients can be monitored with iron studies every 3 months, as many, but not all, will need further infusions in the future.

MEGALOBLASTIC ANAEMIA

A megaloblast is a morphologically abnormal red cell precursor with features of delayed nuclear maturation (Fig 22.2). The common causes are dietary vitamin B_{12} or folate deficiency, some antimetabolite drugs and, infrequently, myelodysplasia with 'megaloblastoid' changes. In the history, check diet, drugs and past history of abdominal surgery or autoimmune disease. The physical examination may reveal evidence of dementia or loss of ankle reflexes and proprioception in the lower limbs. Vitamin B_{12} deficiency anaemia can occur without the neurological deficits (subacute combined degeneration of the spinal cord, dementia) and vice versa.

Animal products (meat and dairy) are the only sources of vitamin B_{12}. Adequate absorption requires intact gastric mucosa, liberation of intrinsic factor and R binders, and small intestinal integrity. The modern diagnosis of pernicious anaemia has dispensed with the Schilling test and now relies upon direct measurement of intrinsic factor and gastric parietal cell auto-antibodies.

Folate deficiency is mostly seen with poor diet and alcoholism.

The combination of folate and iron deficiency is highly suggestive of coeliac disease.

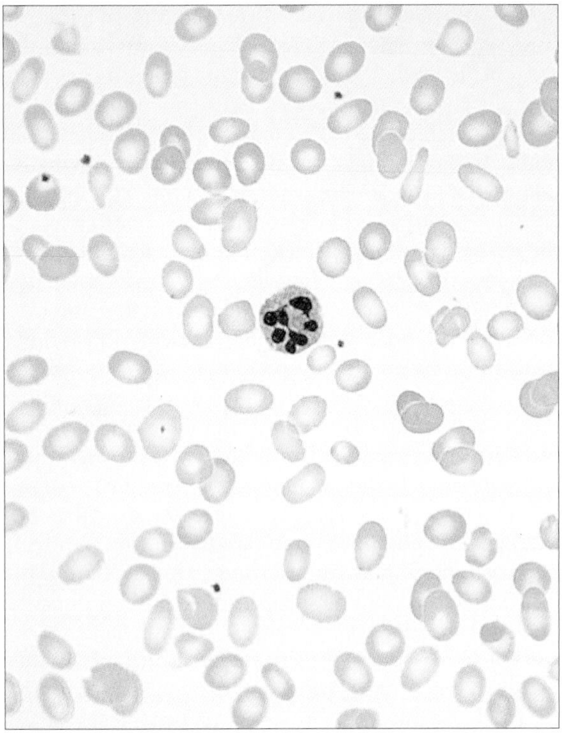

FIGURE 22.2 Megaloblastic anaemia

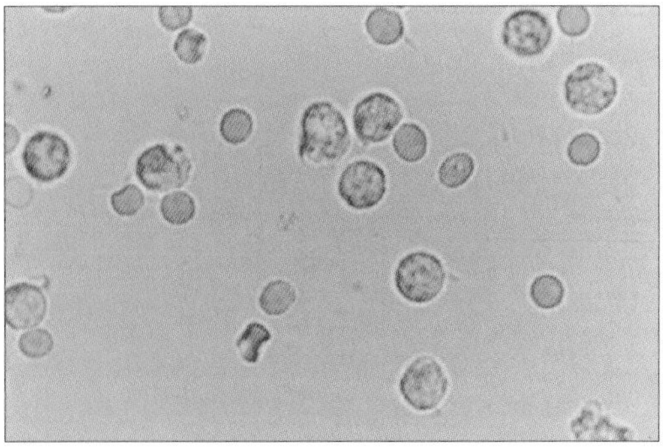

FIGURE 22.3 White blood cells of a healthy person

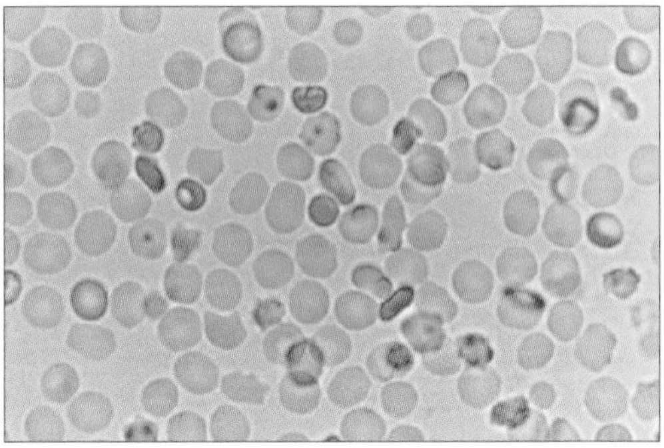

FIGURE 22.4 Red blood cells of a healthy person

Some medications inhibit dihydrofolate reductase and antagonise folate metabolism. Examples are trimethoprim, primethamine, phenytoin and methotrexate. Because both vitamin B_{12} and folate are not injurious, therapeutic trials are a reasonable manoeuvre in cases where megaloblastic anaemia has been identified.

IMMUNE-MEDIATED CYTOPENIA

Whereas white cells (Fig 22.3) mostly leave the circulation to perform their various functions, red blood cells (Fig 22.4) and platelets are recycled. This recycling is one of the two functions of the spleen. The other function of the spleen is to act as a lymph gland for the bloodstream. Splenectomised patients are therefore at increased risk of septicaemia, with well-known encapsulated organisms including *Neisseria meningitidis*, *Streptococcus pneumoniae* and *Haemophilus influenzae*. Galen believed that the spleen was the 'seat of the soul'. In evolutionary terms, the spleen was also the site of haematopoiesis, so it made sense to recycle blood cell components there.

As red blood cells and platelets age, they accumulate molecules, mostly immunoglobulins, on their surface, with the antibody molecule stem (the Fc portion) protruding. In normal transit through the spleen, blood cells pass from the venous circulation into the splenic sinusoids, lined with macrophages. If the antibody density on the cell surface of the cell is high enough, the cell binds to the Fc receptors of macrophages, is removed from the circulation and its components recycled. In this way, normally senescent red cells and platelets are removed from circulation. However, in the presence of an anomalous autoimmune process, where an antibody (often post-infectious) cross-reacts with red cell or platelet cell surface antigens, younger cells rapidly acquire a density of antibodies that leads to premature removal. If the marrow response is overwhelmed, the resulting cytopenia is referred to as immune-mediated thrombocytopenia (ITP) or autoimmune haemolytic anaemia (AIHA). Red cell production can increase six-fold, which will compensate for red cell survival reduced from the normal 120 days to about 16, but not shorter.

It follows that treatment of ITP and AIHA is aimed at:

- reducing antibody production with immune suppression, such as corticosteroids or rituximab (a more elegant way of inhibiting antibody production without systemic steroid side effects)
- 'mopping up' circulating antibody, which is thought to be one mechanism of efficacy of intravenous immunoglobulin or intragam, as well as saturation of the Fc receptors of the macrophages lining the splenic sinusoids, or
- removing the location of cellular removal (i.e. splenectomy).

IMMUNE-MEDIATED THROMBOCYTOPENIA

Immune-mediated thrombocytopenia may present after recent viral illness or be apparently unprovoked. A range of drugs can cause ITP, including quinine, chemotherapy agents and methotrexate, valproic acid and interferon. The prognosis in children is good, with a self-limiting course being typical. Steroids can be given to hasten platelet count recovery. In adults, the natural history is unpredictable, and up to 40% may pursue a multiplying–relapsing course. Adult-onset ITP may be associated with chronic viral infections such as HIV, hepatitis B or hepatitis C, and also with autoimmune diseases such as systemic lupus erythematosus (SLE). Patients with bleeding, or platelet counts of less than 20 $\times 10^9$/L, should be referred urgently to a haematology centre.

Therapeutics

Steroids (e.g. prednisolone 1 mg/kg/day) remain the first line of therapy in all patients. Intragam (IVIg) can be given if the response is inadequate, partly to shorten the length of time spent in hospital. Once a response is achieved, steroids can be weaned. Should relapse occur, options now include further steroids, rituximab and/or splenectomy. Thrombopoietin receptor agonists, including romiplostim (a platelet lineage equivalent of erythropoietin), show promising results and may eventually reduce the need for splenectomy.

Splenectomy is effective in about 50–75% of cases of chronic refractory ITP or AIHA. Other indications include diagnostic splenectomy (rare, for suspected primary splenic lymphoma), symptomatic hereditary spherocytosis, Gaucher's disease, Felty's syndrome, and after traumatic or spontaneous splenic rupture. Electively, it can be done laparoscopically, which is far less invasive and traumatic for the patient, who can often go home by the second postoperative day. (Much smaller incisions are made; the splenic pedicle is clamped and the spleen enclosed in a plastic bag; the organ is then mulched to a deformable state and passed out through one of the small incisions.) Recent guidelines for the management of splenectomised patients are provided in Box 22.1.[7]

INTEGRATIVE MEDICINE IN GENERAL HAEMATOLOGY

Simply put, there are no dietary ways to raise the white cell or platelet counts. Nor is there evidence to support the 'blood group' diet. (A Google search in May 2010 produced over 4 million hits!)

COAGULATION DISORDERS

The modern understanding of haemostasis describes a primary phase and a secondary phase. The actions of blood vessels and platelets constitute the primary phase. In response to injury, blood vessels constrict.

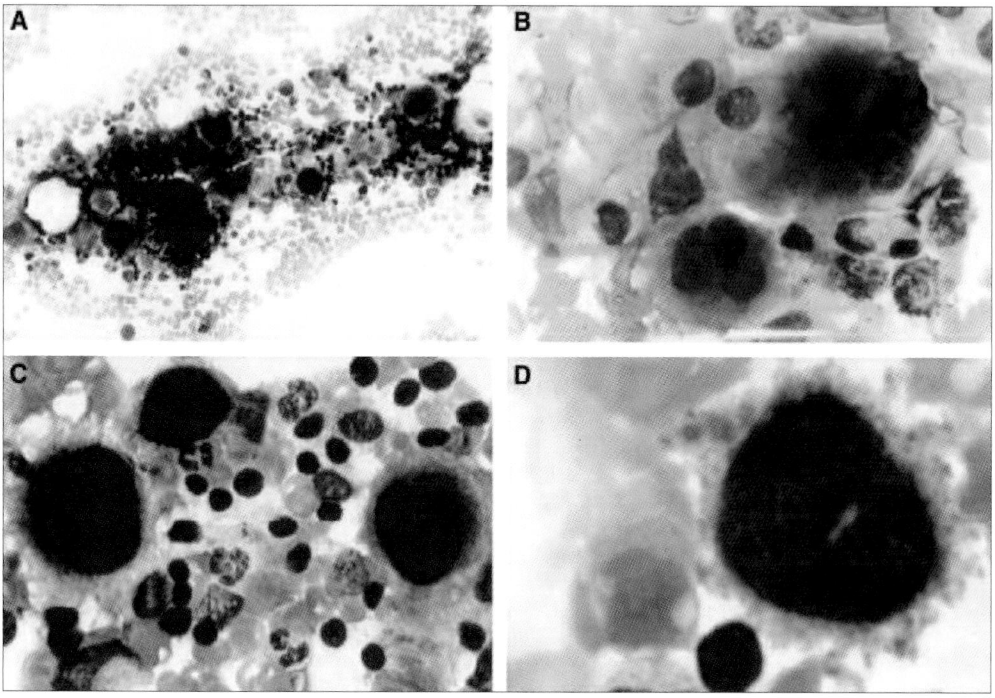

FIGURE 22.5 Immune thrombocytopenia: **A** ×250; **B** ×1000; **C** ×200; **D** ×1600

BOX 22.1 Guidelines for the management of asplenic patients

1. Educate about the risk and need for prompt antibiotics.
2. Preoperative vaccination:
   - *Pneumococcus*: 23vPPv
   - *Meningococcus*: MenCCV, then 4vMenPV 4 weeks later
   - *Haemophilus influenzae*: Hib vax
3. Revaccination:
   - 23vPPv at 5 years; 4vMenPV at 3–5 years, annual influenza vaccination
4. Consider antibiotic prophylaxis:
   - 1–2 years, then re-evaluate need
   - standby antibiotics with instructions
   - include probiotics

Source: Spelman et al. 2008[7]

Platelets, in response to newly exposed collagen, ADP and adrenaline, undergo the shape change reaction, rather like inflating an inverted rubber glove. Thus, previously hidden, or cryptic, molecules are exposed on the platelet surface, allowing interaction principally with von Willebrand factor (vWf). Platelets can now bind to injured endothelium (adhesion) and each other (aggregation), leading to a 'stacks on the mill' aggregation of platelets, and thrombus formation.

The coagulation protein reactions constitute the second phase of haemostasis. This generates fibrin in high local concentration at the site of injury or thrombosis, in effect 'throwing a net' over the platelet aggregate, anchoring it in place. These protein reactions occur as a sequence of macromolecular aggregates (not a 'cascade', Fig 22.6), mediated on the platelet surface, at the site of injury. In the current view, tissue factor has a crucial role as the initiator of haemostasis, down both the intrinsic and the extrinsic pathways (see below). The last step involves the conversion of fibrinogen to fibrin (factors I and Ia respectively) by thrombin (also called factor IIa). Fibrinogen's shape becomes linear and it spontaneously polymerises (side-to-side and end-to-end, making D-dimers) to create the fibrin net. Finally, this fibrin mesh is stabilised by cross-linkage with factor XIII.

The endothelial cell has a key role in locally regulating pro-coagulant and anti-coagulant proteins,

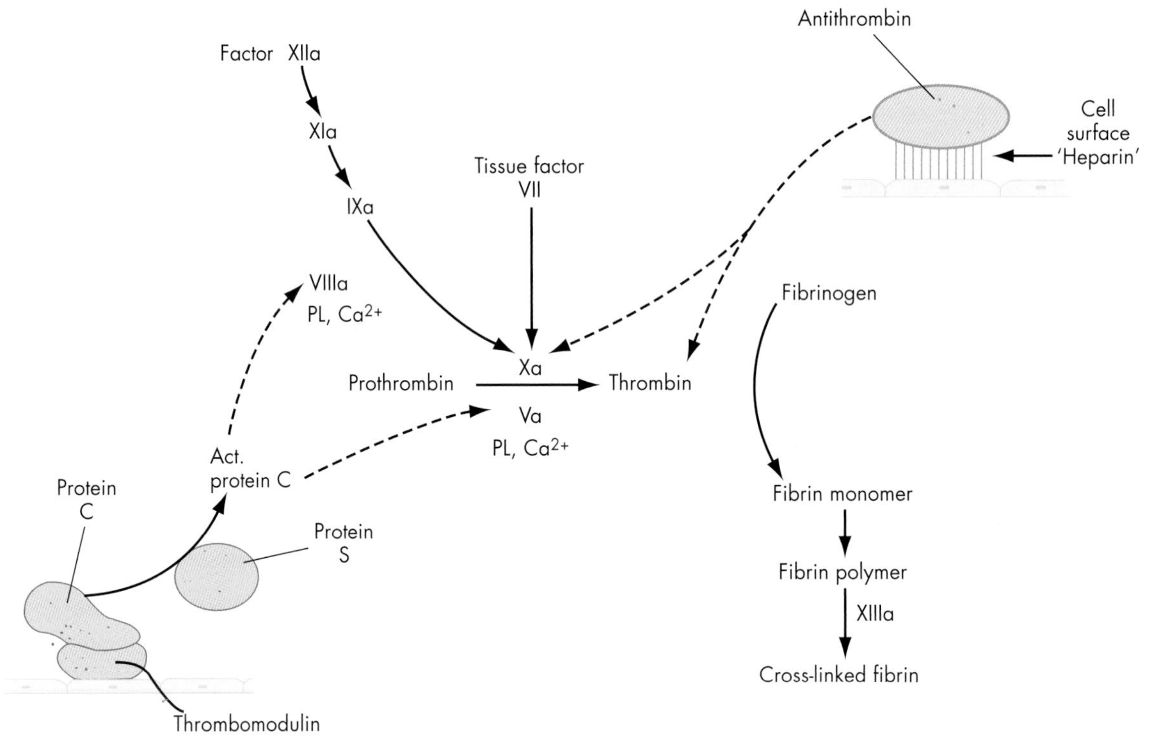

Note: Dashed lines indicate inhibited clotting and thrombolytic factor

FIGURE 22.6 Coagulation cascade; a denotes activated factor. Ca: calcium; PL: phospholipid to allow a thrombus to form where needed, but inhibit propagation too widely. There are complex local mechanisms controlling levels of required proteins, cofactors and substrates in these reactions. Ex vivo testing of plasma cannot accurately reflect these events in the body.

Defects in the primary phase usually manifest with mucosal-style bleeding, such as epistaxis, menorrhagia, petechial rashes, haematuria and blood blisters in the oral mucosa. Mild von Willebrand's disease is the classic example. Defects in the secondary phase of haemostasis, including haemophilia, mostly lead to deep tissue bleeding with haematomas and haemarthroses.

Causes of a bleeding diathesis (referring here to mild or asymptomatic) are listed in Table 22.2. Congenital causes include mild phenotypes of the classic bleeding disorders, haemophilia A (factor VIII deficiency), haemophilia B (factor IX deficiency) and von Willebrand's disease, and rarer deficiencies of other clotting factors.

Liver disease, warfarin overdose and vitamin K deficiency (secondary to antibiotic use) are the more common acquired causes. Haemophilia can be acquired; this is an acquired antibody that binds to factor VIII or IX, resulting in plasma clearance and functional deficiency. Antibodies to other plasma proteins are called *inhibitors of coagulation*; the lupus anticoagulant is one example. Low-grade disseminated intravascular coagulation (DIC) occurs in some cancers, mostly adenocarcinomas. Purpura simplex is a diagnosis of exclusion in women with increased bruising linked to their menstrual cycle. In the absence of abnormal coagulation times, it is not clinically significant.

INVESTIGATING THE PATIENT WITH EASY BRUISING

Congenital disorders can manifest in adulthood, and acquired causes can appear in the elderly. Moreover, phenotypically mild bleeding problems may be very significant in the face of a major haemostatic challenge such as trauma or surgery. Patients who develop easy bruising or recurrent bleeding at any age should not be dismissed. Preoperative assessment may be another indication for investigation.

From the history, determine whether bleeding or bruising is longstanding or recent, and if it has been in pathological amounts. Endeavour to ascertain whether it has a mucosal (primary haemostasis defect, i.e. thrombocytopenia or platelet dysfunction) or deep-tissue pattern (defect implied in secondary haemostasis). Trauma, surgery, dental extractions and childbirth are all good in vivo tests of haemostasis. So, while many report heavy bleeding after dental extractions or childbirth, in only a few does this persist for more than a day and/or require transfusion.

Transfusion history, menses, family history and comorbidities such as liver disease or renal failure are all relevant.

Current drugs and complementary medicine use must be ascertained, including particularly aspirin, antiplatelet drugs (clopidogrel), NSAIDs and herbal supplements, notably gingko, garlic, ginger and ginseng. These all reduce platelet function. Commencing such medicines can be enough to unmask a hitherto hidden bleeding diathesis, especially mild von Willebrand's disease. Drugs that cause thrombocytopenia are discussed below.

TABLE 22.2 A guide to bleeding diagnoses and typical coagulation test results

	Bleeding time	PT	APTT	TCT	Notes
Primary phase					
Vasculopathies etc	Long	Normal	Normal	Normal	e.g. steroid purpura
Thrombocytopenia	Long	Normal	Normal	Normal	See text for causes; the APTT is long in HITTS
Platelet dysfunction syndromes	Long	Normal	Normal	Normal	Perform platelet function testing to confirm
Secondary phase					
Haemophilia A, B (fVIII, IX deficiency)	Normal	Normal	Long	Normal	Perform specific factor assays
von Willebrand's disease	Long	Normal	Long	Normal	The APTT may be normal in those with vWf > 30%
Inhibitors of coagulation	Normal	Normal	Long	Normal	APTT fails to normalise with pooled 50:50 normal plasma
Lupus anticoagulant	Normal	Normal	Long	Normal	Further special testing required

APTT: activated partial thromboplastin time; HITTS: heparin-induced thrombocytopenia-thrombosis syndrome; PT: prothrombin time; TCT: thrombin clotting time.

In the examination, the findings may point to a platelet-type bleeding defect or to a coagulation pathway problem with deep tissue bleeding. Look for bruises of differing ages, gum bleeding, haematuria and, possibly, fundoscopy for retinal haemorrhages. Tall stature, cardiac murmurs or loose skin could point to a collagen disorder, such as Marfan's syndrome.

If the history and examination are worrying enough to warrant referral to a haematologist, it is appropriate to perform an initial FBC, Urea and electrolys (U&E), liver function tests, PT, APTT and TCT, as well as von Willebrand factor (vWf) assays and ABO blood typing.

Individuals with blood group O have 30% less vWf, although the clinical significance of this is doubtful. The results of these may help the haematologist proceed, after clinical review, to a subsequent round of tests if needed (discussed below).

DISORDERS OF PLATELET NUMBER AND FUNCTION

In the absence of any cause for platelet dysfunction, the risk of spontaneous bleeding corresponds to a platelet count of 20×10^9/L or less. Patients with platelets $< 50 \times 10^9$/L should be referred urgently. Thrombocytopenia can be spurious, as in up to 1% of some populations, individuals form platelet clumps with EDTA, the most common sample tube anticoagulant. (The laboratory will request a citrate sample if this is suspected.) Partially clotted samples may also give a low platelet count.

Isolated thrombocytopenia is only rarely due to under-production (called 'amegakaryocytic thrombocytopenia'), and far more commonly to platelet peripheral destruction from idiopathic immune mechanisms (ITP) or drug-associated. (Treatment of ITP is discussed under the cytopenias.)

Heparin and low molecular weight heparin (LMWH) are the most common drug cause of thrombocytopenia, referred to as the heparin-induced thrombocytopenia-thrombosis syndrome (HITTS). Classically, the platelet count starts halving daily 5–10 days after regular heparin or LMWH is commenced. The incidence is 1.5% and 1.2% of exposed individuals respectively in heparin-naive individuals.

Aggregates form that consist of drug, antibody (to complexes of heparin and platelet factor 4) and platelets; these can be life-, organ- and limb-threatening.

Referral to a haematologist is urgent, for accurate diagnosis and prompt treatment. This includes stopping heparin and, often, finding an alternative anticoagulant such as lepirudin or danaparoid.[8] Re-exposure to heparin may induce an anamnestic response and a much more rapid fall in platelet count. This rapid-onset HITTS occurs mostly when the prior exposure was within the previous 3 months or, more typically, 30 days.

Other drugs causing thrombocytopenia include quinine (or quinidine), even in trace amounts in tonic water or angostura bitters; ranitidine, rifampicin, cotrimoxazole and others are rarer culprits.[9] The full list is daunting, and any drug should be suspected.

Platelet function is affected in rare congenital syndromes including intrinsic platelet disorders, and collagen abnormalities like Ehlers-Danlos and Marfan's syndromes, in some marrow disorders (e.g. myeloproliferative disease), in chronic liver and renal disease, and by many drugs as above.

COAGULATION PROFILE TESTS AND ASSOCIATED DISORDERS

The coagulation profile includes the prothrombin time (PT), the activated partial thromboplastin time (APTT), and sometimes the thrombin clotting time (TCT). The principle in all these tests is that factor levels of 30% or more give normal clotting times. Mild bleeding disorders (factor levels 30–50%) may give normal results, but a careful history may point to the need for factor assays when these are suspected.

The PT provides a measure of the extrinsic pathway. It measures functional tissue factor, factors VII, X, II (prothrombin) and fibrinogen. As factor VII has the shortest half-life of the plasma proteins targeted by warfarin, the PT is the best test to monitor warfarin. Causes of a long PT include warfarin, liver disease, vitamin K deficiency and factor VII deficiency.

The APTT measures the intrinsic pathway involving factors XII, XI, VIII, IX, X, prothrombin and fibrinogen. Causes of a long APTT include heparin, haemophilias, lupus anticoagulant and other inhibitors.

The PT and APTT are both long in liver disease, severe warfarin overdose, disseminated intravascular coagulopathy (DIC) and deficiencies of fibrinogen, thrombin and factors V and X.

The TCT is performed by measuring excess bovine thrombin to the sample, and the time taken to clot is proportional to the amount of functional fibrinogen present. Prolongation of the TCT is seen in afibrinogenaemia, hypofibrinogenaemia (e.g. DIC) and dysfibrinogenaemia (congenital, liver disease). Heparin, paraproteins and clot breakdown products can interfere with the TCT. As this is the final step in both pathways, if the TCT is prolonged, the other tests usually are as well.

There are recognised haemostatic defects that may be clinically significant, even if the coagulation profile is normal:

- mild deficiency states
- mild von Willebrand's disease
- platelet dysfunction syndromes
- acquired inhibitors to anticoagulant proteins; factor XIII deficiency

- rare fibrinolytic disorders
- vasculopathies
- corticosteroids, like old age (and scurvy!), lead to small vessel fragility, and secondary purpura and ecchymoses.

More-specific tests may be performed. The bleeding time is the only in vivo measure of primary haemostasis. Individual factor assays may be warranted by the clinical scenario, particularly to exclude mild bleeding disorders such as von Willebrand's disease or similar. Tests of platelet function include platelet aggregometry.

Mild von Willebrand's disease requires specifically assaying vWf. Various subtypes are recognised. Bleeding may manifest only after an antiplatelet agent is started, including some herbs as above. A distinction is increasingly being drawn between those with low vWf (30–50%) and those with mild von Willebrand's disease (levels usually 10–30%).[10,11]

Acquired inhibitors may manifest as a sudden onset of a bleeding diathesis in adults. Their detection relies upon demonstrating a prolonged APTT that fails to ameliorate after 50 : 50 pooling with normal plasma, which should normalise all clotting times (as all factor levels should be at least 50% or more). Repeating the test after a 2-hour incubation increases the sensitivity.

Diagnosing the lupus anticoagulant requires a battery of specialised tests, which should be positive on at least two occasions 3 months apart. If found, related autoantibodies should be checked, such as antiphospholipid and beta-2-glycoprotein I antibodies, plus tests for SLE.

In summary, a good history is the key to guide appropriate testing. When a mild bleeding diathesis is found, the implications of the diagnosis need to be explained, as well as any lifestyle and medication implications. A family study may be considered.

INTEGRATIVE MEDICINE IN BLEEDING DISORDERS

Aspirin, antiplatelet drugs (clopidogrel), NSAIDs and herbal supplements, notably gingko, garlic, ginger and ginseng, all reduce platelet function.

VENOUS THROMBOEMBOLIC DISEASE

Venous thromboembolism (VTE) remains the most common preventable cause of hospital death, and the management of newly diagnosed cases has shifted to the GP in recent years.

CAUSES AND DIAGNOSIS

Thrombosis occurs with perturbations of Virchoff's triad of intrinsic properties of the blood favouring thrombosis, vascular injury and stasis. The thrombophilias are a group of inherited and acquired measurable abnormalities of the blood associated with increased VTE risk. These can be distinguished from the hypercoagulable states (discussed below). Examples of vascular injury include trauma and venous cannulation. Immobility, left ventricular dysfunction, atrial fibrillation and venous insufficiency may all contribute to stasis.

Hypercoagulable states (Fig 22.7) refer to clinical settings associated with increased thrombosis risk:

- pregnancy
- malignancy
- sepsis
- oestrogen therapy
- postoperative status
- prolonged immobility during travel ('economy class syndrome').

The diagnosis of VTE is notoriously prone to false-negative clinical examination. Tests should be used and interpreted in the light of clinical suspicion. Undue credence is given by many clinicians to the D-dimer test. A positive result is not helpful: there are many things that can cause it to be elevated, and in a hospital ward or emergency room population, specificity is very low. However, a negative result (normal titre) in an outpatient with a low possibility of thrombosis helps to exclude recent VTE. Ultrasound examination results are operator-dependent; venography is still the gold standard in clinical trials. CT pulmonary angiogram (CTPA) and/or ventilation-perfusion (VQ) scanning remain important in diagnosing pulmonary embolism (PE).

TREATMENT

Treatment is usually with heparin in some form, and warfarin. The two can often be started together. Unfractionated heparin (MW 15,000 Dalton), first isolated from ox liver in 1916, has marked variation in effect, partly due to its high negative charge and non-specific binding to a variety of plasma proteins, and to unpredictable antiplatelet effects. It is fully and rapidly reversible with protamine and is best reserved for patients who must be anticoagulated but who are at high risk of bleeding. Heparin is also preferred over LMWH in the treatment of major or life-threatening pulmonary embolism (PE), but lesser PE can be safely treated with LMWH.

If heparin is used, a baseline APTT should be raised two-fold over baseline within 8–24 hours, to reduce the chance of VTE progression.[12,13] Monitoring of the APTT is required.

Low molecular weight heparins have a molecular weight of 4000–7000 Dalton, greater predictability in effect, longer half-life, greater specificity of action

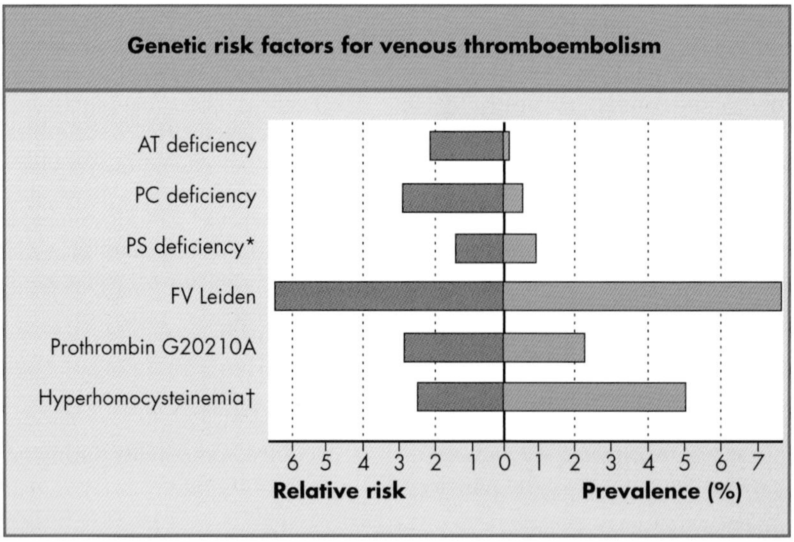

FIGURE 22.7 Hypercoagulable states and thrombosis risk. * Prevalence unknown. † includes acquired defects. AT: antithrombin III; FV: factor V; PC: protein C; PS: protein S

(inhibition of activated factor Xa and IIa, i.e. thrombin), and better correlation of effect with body weight. A Cochrane review concluded that once-daily treatment for deep vein thrombosis (DVT) and sub-massive PE at home with LMWH is safer than with heparin.[14] Levels may accumulate in renal failure or be low in the very obese. Reversibility with protamine is incomplete. Monitoring is not usually needed, but can be achieved by measuring anti-factor Xa activity in, for example, those with renal insufficiency or the very obese.

Warfarin was discovered in rotten hay when a herd of cattle bled to death at the Wisconsin Agricultural Research Facility (WARF) in 1936—hence its name. There is marked inter-individual variation in dose (doses vary between 1 and 15 mg daily) and the effect of any dose is maximal 36 hours later—so be aware that, when adjusting the dose, it is in response to today's blood test and the day before yesterday's dose. Many patients are tested too frequently and dose-adjusted too often for the pharmacokinetics of the drug. It is still often poorly prescribed, especivally initially and later, when over-confidence can occur in either patient or physician.

The international normalised ratio (INR) is a mathematical manipulation of the prothrombin time to equalise different laboratories and reagents, such that the patient can be advised that, 'An INR of 2.0 means your blood is taking twice as long to clot as someone not taking warfarin; and any laboratory the world over would get a similar result'. The INR has been a meaningful advance for those who travel while taking warfarin.

Five milligrams daily will achieve therapeutic levels in 80% within 4 days.[15]

When starting a patient on warfarin, be satisfied that they will be able to comply, and check other drugs and supplements, noting any that may be likely to affect the INR and/or be stopped (e.g. antibiotics). Ensure that the patient has a monitoring book; explain the meaning of the INR result and the risks of over-dosage. Explain the role of diet (capsicum and alfalfa have high doses of the antagonist vitamin K, but the dose can be adjusted according to usual diet) and alcohol (maximum two standard drinks in any one sitting; some say none at all). Many patients ultimately require a dose between discrete daily doses, and patients should have a monitoring book with allocated spaces for each day of the week so that, in long-term patients, the weekly rather than the daily dose can be changed.

Antiplatelet agents should be used with great caution with warfarin, especially aspirin and clopidogrel, with a half-life of 10 days (in terms of antiplatelet effects) compared with 2 days for NSAIDs.

The duration of anticoagulation for a DVT should be at least 3 months.[16] A meta-analysis found that recurrence is 40% less with 12–24 weeks of anti-coagulation after unprovoked DVT, than with 3–6 weeks, without increased risk of major bleeding.[17] For 'provoked' (e.g. associated with a venous catheter, or injury) and calf vein DVT, some say a shorter course can be given. With the latter, a repeat ultrasound at 10 days to exclude more proximal extension and higher risk of PE may be worthwhile.[18] For superficial vein thrombosis and thrombophlebitis, topical hyaluronidase and aspirin are more appropriate therapy. For a PE, anticoagulation is usually for 6–12 months.

TABLE 22.3 Anticoagulation recommendations after VTE

	Intensity (target INR)
All patients, except ...	2.0–3.0
Mechanical heart valves (caged ball, caged disc)	3.0–4.5
	Duration (risk stratification)
First episode	3 months
First episode, provoked (e.g. venous catheter) or calf vein DVT	6–12 weeks
First episode, permanent risk factors	3–6 months, consider indefinite
Two episodes	Indefinite

TABLE 22.4 High-risk groups

Indication	Medication	Duration
Orthopaedic surgery (total hip, total knee, hip fracture)	LMWH + GCS/IPC	35 days
Major abdominal surgery and age > 40	LMWH + GCS/IPC	Until discharge or 28 days if high risk
Acute medical illness requiring immobility, with other risk factors	LMWH	Until ambulant
Pregnancy and postpartum with other risk factor	LMWH	During pregnancy and 4–6 weeks post-partum
Travel over 8 hours	LMWH Compression stockings, adequate hydration, movement, avoid alcohol, no restrictive clothing	24 hours before flight, again just before flying and 24 hours later

GCS: graduated compression stockings; IPC: intermittent pneumatic compression; LMWH: low molecular weight heparin.

For a second confirmed episode of VTE, lifelong anticoagulation should be strongly considered.[19] The intensity of anticoagulation with warfarin (target INR) is 2.0–3.0 in all circumstances, save one: mechanical left-sided cardiac valves require anticoagulation to an intensity of INR 3.0–4.5. See Table 22.3 for guidelines on target and duration of therapy, based on published Australian recommendations.[20]

There has been much interest in warfarin pharmacogenomics. CYPC29 polymorphisms are seen in 1% of the population, in whom a lower dose of warfarin may be needed and there is higher risk of bleeding. Conversely, VKORC1 refers to genetic variations of the vitamin K epoxide reductase subunit 1 gene; they are rare and associated with clotting factor deficiencies and warfarin resistance. The value of screening the population is debated.[21]

Ultimately, the decision to anticoagulate must be a clinical one, weighing up the potential benefits and risks in any one case. The decision should be re-evaluated periodically; the risk of major bleeding with warfarin rises to over 5% in the over-75 years age bracket and, for example, this may swing the cost-benefit equation against continuing warfarin in an elderly patient with atrial fibrillation and declining ability to comply.

Warfarin reversal can be achieved with vitamin K, fresh frozen plasma or Prothrombinex®, depending upon urgency (see Baker et al 2004[22] for guidelines). Prothrombinex® contains concentrates of factors II, VII and IX; although it is recommended that cryoprecipitate or fresh frozen plasma (FFP) be given as well, to supply factor X, it might not be needed.[23]

PREVENTION OF VTE

Primary prevention, using either low-dose heparin or LMWH, is recommended by most authorities perioperatively in all patients for some forms of surgery (such as orthopaedics) and in hospitalised or critically ill patients (Table 22.4).

Secondary prevention measures should be applied equally to those with a prior episode of VTE, a thrombophilic state (see below) or both.[22,24] Long-haul travel (in planes, cars and trains for longer than 8 hours) is associated with a small absolute increase in thrombosis, possibly as little as one per two million arriving passengers over the subsequent 30 days.[25] Recommended measures include wearing loose clothing, drinking plenty of fluids, frequent calf muscle contraction and, for those at higher risk (past VTE, thrombophilia), fitted compression stockings and LMWH

TABLE 22.5 Frequency and effect (increased thrombosis risk) of selected thrombophilias[27]

Syndrome	Frequency in Caucasian population	Prothrombotic effect
Congenital		
Factor V Leiden	3–5%	× 3–7*
Anti-thrombin III deficiency	< 1%	× 10
Protein C deficiency	< 1%	× 10
Protein S deficiency	< 1%	× 10
Prothrombin 20210A mutation	3%	× 3
Hyperhomocysteinaemia	5% have level > 18 μmol/L	mild
Acquired		
Lupus anticoagulant	Rare	× 10

*Homozygotes, however, have a 30-fold increased risk.

immediately pre-travel (repeating the dose 24 hours later).

Aspirin is not an effective thromboprophylactic in this setting.[24] Travel within 3 weeks of a VTE or high-risk event (e.g. surgery) is best avoided, even for those on warfarin. In cancer patients, VTE is best treated indefinitely with LMWH, not warfarin, as recurrence is halved.[26]

HYPERCOAGULABLE STATES AND THROMBOPHILIA

Hypercoagulable states refer to clinical settings associated with increased thrombosis risk: pregnancy, malignancy, sepsis, oestrogen therapy, postoperative status and prolonged immobility during travel ('economy class syndrome'). *Thrombophilia* is a growing list of measurable inherited and acquired disorders that predispose an individual to thrombosis to varying degrees (Table 22.5). There is much debate over who to screen, but probably the indications include younger VTE patients (< 40 years); those with unprovoked 'atypical' VTE; those with VTE in an unusual site such as cerebral, renal, hepatic or mesenteric veins; those with a strong family history; and perhaps those in whom elective pro-thrombotic therapy is contemplated. Patients should be assessed individually, as the familial predispositions tend to 'run true' in kindreds, and family history is important.

Inherited thrombophilias include:

- factor V Leiden mutation
- antithrombin
- protein C and protein S deficiency
- prothrombin gene mutation.

The most common inherited thrombophilia in Caucasians is factor V Leiden, with an incidence of around 3–5%, associated with a three- to seven-fold increased risk.

However, the diagnosis of thrombophilia has little impact on the management of the individual patient. Asymptomatic thrombophilic patients should be advised to avoid oestrogens and consider prophylactic measures for long-haul plane travel or surgery.

Thrombophilic individuals after one episode of VTE are at only a modestly increased risk of a second DVT, compared with others who have had a VTE episode.[28,29] Anticoagulation should be at the usual level and duration. Exceptions include homozygosity for factor V Leiden and those with two thrombophilic states, which confer a much higher thrombosis risk. Such individuals should be reviewed by a haematologist, and lifelong therapy offered.

EXOGENOUS OESTROGEN

Oestrogen is pro-thrombotic in a dose-dependent way, mostly through lowering proteins C and S. Advising women with a history of DVT, or those found to have a thrombophilia state, and who want to take oestrogen for contraception or as hormone replacement therapy (HRT), is particularly difficult. All alternative forms of contraception or menopause management should be discussed. Once again, individual assessment of risk, including assessment of provoked or unprovoked VTE, and family history, are important.

Screening all women contemplating HRT for a thrombophilic state is not feasible, and this raises a dilemma. A meta-analysis of 81 studies concluded that screening of all women is impractical and not cost-effective, whereas screening of higher-risk groups based on individual assessment of risk is.[30]

For thrombophilic or post-VTE women, other forms of contraception should be encouraged. There is no evidence that progesterone alone is pro-thrombotic. Some women find menopausal symptoms so bad that they will take HRT against haematological advice. Some find symptom relief with phyto-oestrogens and other

TABLE 22.6 Overview of myeloid pathology

Pathological process	Aplasia	Hypoplasia	Normal	Hyperplasia	Neoplasia
Haematological term	Aplastic anaemia	Myelodysplasia	Normal	Myeloproliferative disorders	Acute leukaemia
Blood counts	Very low	Low		High: • raised Hb in PRV • raised platelets in ET • raised WCC in CML	Low (WCC low, normal or high)
Bone marrow	Empty	Abnormal morphology Blasts 5–20%	Blasts < 5%	Normal morphology or increased megakaryocytes or fibrosis	> 20% blasts
Notes	Immune-mediated; treat with immune suppression or marrow transplant	Risk of progression to AML: 20–60%		JAK2 mutation: 95% PRV 50% ET Risk of progression to AML: 5–15%	

AML: acute myeloid leukaemia; CML: chronic myeloid leukaemia; ET: essential thrombocythaemia; Hb: haemoglobin; PRV: polycythaemia rubra vera; WCC: white cell count.

treatments (see Ch 53, Menopause). Transcutaneous oestrogen patches, due to first-pass metabolism, are less thrombogenic.[31,32] The French ESTHER study performed a multi-centre case-control study of 271 consecutive cases of VTE among postmenopausal women aged 45–70 years and 610 controls (426 hospital controls, 184 community controls) matched for centre, age and admission date. After adjustment for potential confounding factors, the odds ratios (ORs) for VTE in current users of oral and transdermal oestrogen compared with non-users were 4.2 (95% CI 1.5–11.6) and 0.9 (95% CI 0.4–2.1), respectively.[31] These findings suggest that transdermal oestrogen may not be thrombogenic at all.

MALIGNANT HAEMATOLOGY

After an infection, the white cell count rises, sometimes with the platelet count, and then falls to the same premorbid level. Thus, marrow haemopoietic tissue, some 5 kg scattered around the long and flat bones of the body, behaves in a coordinated way, as a single organ. Moreover, it is subject to the same pathological processes as other organs. For historical reasons, the terminology is different. Table 22.6 shows how haematological terms correspond conceptually to the more familiar terms *aplasia*, *dysplasia*, *hyperplasia* and *neoplasia* in the spectrum of primary bone marrow pathologies. On the deficit side, complete loss of marrow or marrow function is called *aplastic anaemia* (a better term would be *aplastic pancytopenia*). Hypoplasia of the marrow usually maps to the myelodysplastic syndromes. In contrast, hyperplastic disorders of the marrow are referred to as the *myeloproliferative syndromes*. Neoplasia of the marrow stem cell is *acute leukaemia*.

Symptoms in patients with haematological malignancies can be considered negative or positive.

Negative symptoms arise from marrow hypofunction, manifesting with:

- symptomatic anaemia
- infection—for example, a common presentation of acute leukaemia is recurrent sore throat
- bleeding—due to lack of red cells, white cells or platelets respectively.

Positive symptoms are a characteristic complex arising from increased levels of cytokines liberated by white blood and immune cells, such as tumour necrosis factor, interleukin-1, IL-3 and IL-6. These cause the classic 'B' symptoms of:

- unintentional weight loss (> 10%)
- fevers (> 38.5°C on two occasions without cause) and drenching night sweats
- fatigue, and spontaneous cigarette, alcohol or meat intolerance—may occur, as with any malignancy
- itch—common in Hodgkin's lymphoma, T-cell non-Hodgkin's lymphomas and some of the myeloproliferative disorders; it may be provoked by exercise or hot water
- bone pain—can mimic acute back pain; is often felt in the back, pelvis and thighs
- very high white cell counts—may cause leucostasis, manifesting as pseudo-strokes, dyspnoea, angina and even priapism.

Physical examination should include assessment of all peripheral lymph node stations, including visualising the tonsils and palpating the epitrochlear and popliteal lymph nodes; plus a careful check for splenomegaly; and gently testing for bone tenderness over the sternum.

Often the first indication is, of course, the blood count. The more of the three blood cell lineages that are numerically abnormal, the more likely there is to be primary marrow pathology, such as myelodysplasia or acute leukaemia. For example, isolated thrombocytopenia of 3×10^9/L in a young adult is probably ITP; but if the Hb is 90 g/L and the neutrophils 1.1×10^9/L, then more-sinister pathology is likely.

In those with suspected haematological malignancy, referral should be made urgently for haematological assessment. It is very helpful to perform FBC, U&E, liver function tests, serum LDH, blood film, uric acid, serum calcium and possibly flow cytometry of peripheral blood lymphocytes; chest X-ray and CT scans of thorax and abdomen are always appropriate in those with suspected lymphoma.

A brief summary of the main haematological cancers now follows.

CHRONIC MYELOID LEUKAEMIA

Chronic myeloid leukaemia (CML) (Fig 22.8) is a misnomer, as it is really a myeloproliferative pre-leukaemia, albeit one that had a 100% risk of progression to acute leukaemia before effective therapies were available. It has a unique triphasic natural history, from chronic phase, to accelerated and, finally, transformed CML. Patients may present late in the chronic phase, with a white cell count as high as $600{,}000 \times 10^{12}$/L. Fatigue, moderate or massive splenomegaly, early satiety, night sweats and weight loss are classic symptoms. Increasingly the diagnosis is made in asymptomatic patients as an incidental finding—at a health or insurance check, for example.

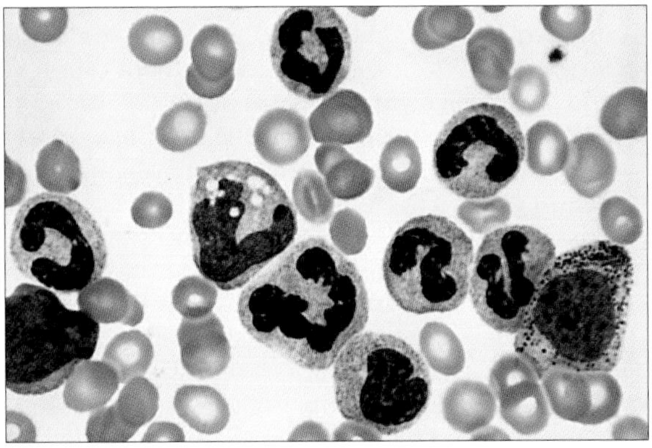

FIGURE 22.8 Chronic myeloid leukaemia

Treatment has changed from busulphan in the 1970s, to interferon in the 1980s, to the astonishing success of imatinib mesylate in the early 2000s. This has provided proof-of-concept that the molecular biology revolution can deliver to the clinic. Imatinib is the first widely used drug targeted at a pathological molecule—that is, BCR-ABL, a tyrosine kinase, generated by the famous Philadelphia chromosome (translocation 9;22). The full story has been told recently elsewhere.[1] For many with CML, lifelong disease control with tyrosine kinase inhibitors, such as imatinib and its successors, appears probable, after our first 10 years' experience at least; bone marrow transplantation, although still the only cure, is reserved for those with accelerated or transformed disease, which remains much feared.

CHRONIC LYMPHOCYTIC LEUKAEMIA

Rather than abnormal cell growth, chronic lymphocytic leukaemia (CLL) (Fig 22.9) is characterised by the accumulation over time of lymphocytes in the bloodstream, lymph glands and/or bone marrow, or combinations thereof. Again, increasingly the diagnosis is made incidentally. The diagnostic test is no longer the bone marrow biopsy. Peripheral blood flow cytometry is easier and gives a pathognomic result, although the marrow often shows unexpectedly high numbers of CLL cells, and this may influence clinical decision-making. Treatment is indicated for symptomatic disease, bulky or disfiguring lymphadenopathy, or cytopenia. Most haematologists recommend treatment when the lymphocyte count hits 100×10^{12}/L, for at this level, the other triggers for treatment usually soon follow.

The treatment paradigm has shifted from oral chlorambucil to more aggressive combination chemotherapy, with good evidence that this confers better survival and longer remissions.[33]

For many newly diagnosed patients, treatment is not immediately indicated. Nevertheless, all patients

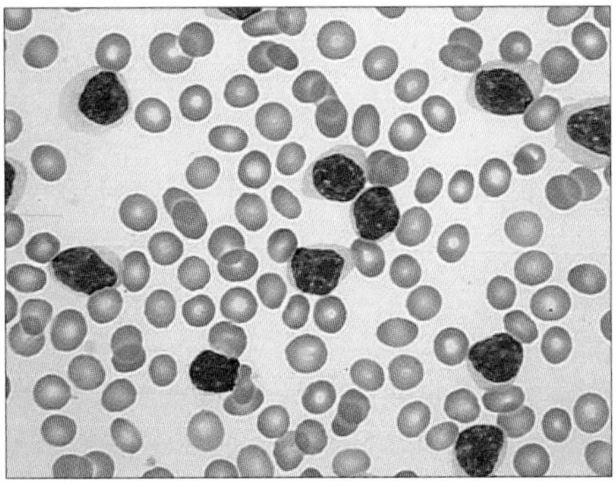

FIGURE 22.9 Chronic lymphocytic leukaemia

should be referred for haematological review, even if asymptomatic, as the immediate implications for health include advice to start antibiotics promptly for suspected bacterial infection, to take measures to reduce solar skin damage and to assess for complications. As with any B-cell tumour, hypogammaglobulinaemia may occur (IgG < 2 g/L). Other complications include increased second cancers including skin and other cancers, autoimmune haemolytic anaemia in up to 20% of cases, and Richter's transformation, a rare progression to aggressive non-Hodgkin's lymphoma.

ACUTE LEUKAEMIA

When the term *leukaemia* was coined, in the nineteenth century, it referred to an excess of white cells in the bloodstream. Those with normal-appearing white cells lived longer (hence *chronic leukaemia*), whereas those with abnormal, or blast, cells, died rapidly, and so this was called *acute leukaemia*. We now recognise acute leukaemia (Fig 22.10) as a cancer of the bone marrow stem cell. The modern definition is: more than 20% blast cells in the marrow. (Less than 2% blast cells is normal; 5–20% blast cells characterises myelodysplasia.) *Acute lymphoblastic leukaemia* (ALL) is seven times more common than *acute myeloid leukaemia* (AML) in children; the ratio is reversed in adults.

The history is typically of two or more infections in the previous 3 months, or increasing bone pain; rarer presentations include DIC, priapism and meningism. Usually there is pancytopenia (i.e. neutropenia, anaemia, thrombocytopenia), in which the neutropenia may or may not be masked by a high blast cell count. Thus, the white cell count in acute leukaemia can be high, normal or low, depending upon the readiness of the blast cells to leave the marrow compartment for the bloodstream. Bone marrow biopsy remains essential for medico-legal and prognostic reasons, even if the diagnosis is evident in the blood film.

It is good practice to refrain from giving the diagnosis to the patient until the bone marrow biopsy is done. Obviously, patients will need to be told 'there is concern over a possible bone marrow disorder' to explain the prompt contact and recommendation to attend hospital.

The diagnosis of acute leukaemia is a medical emergency. In some forms, notably *acute promyelocytic leukaemia* (APML), prompt institution of appropriate therapy can be life-saving. Patients should be managed at a centre with expertise.

Therapeutics

Curative management of acute leukaemia requires 3 or 4 months of intensive chemotherapy in or near hospital. In ALL, the central nervous system is recognised as a possible sanctuary site for future relapse, and chemotherapy or adjunctive radiotherapy is given accordingly. Some 80% of patients achieve an initial response or remission; the problem then is keeping it. Paediatric ALL has cure rates approaching 90%, a great success story. Present cure rates in adults rest at 40%

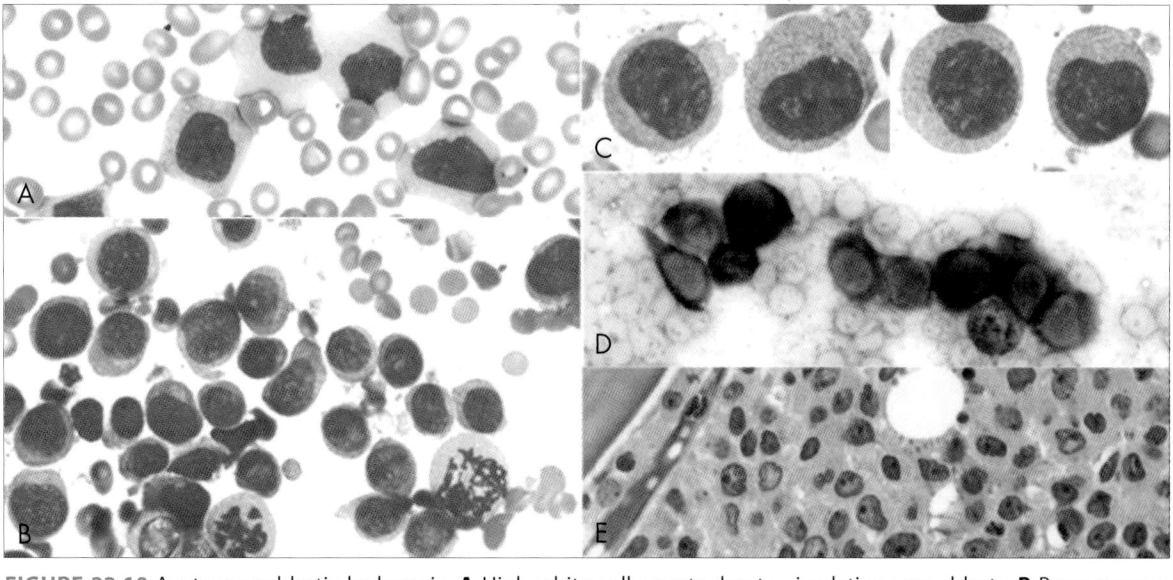

FIGURE 22.10 Acute monoblastic leukaemia. **A** High white cell counts due to circulating monoblasts; **B** Bone marrow aspirate packed with monoblasts (**C**) and showing few granulocytic elements; **D** Rare granulocytes show the blue reaction product from the combined esterase reaction while the rest show orange-brown; **E** Biopsy sample is unusually packed with sheets of monoblasts with fine nuclear chromatin and abundant pink cytoplasm

for AML and 25% for ALL. There are better results with some subtypes, including AML with certain karyotypic abnormalities and APML. Bone marrow transplantation is offered to selected patients in first remission as the best chance of cure, and has become less dangerous with improvements in tissue typing, viral and fungal antibiotics and supportive care for graft versus host disease. For the very elderly, a palliative chemotherapy approach may give surprising longevity (over a year) with good quality of life.

MYELODYSPLASIA

The myelodysplastic syndromes occur mostly in the elderly. Causes include prior chemotherapy and/or radiotherapy. Characteristically there are low peripheral blood counts, leading to negative symptoms of marrow failure. The cells look abnormal in the bone marrow biopsy (Fig 22.11). It is a morphogical diagnosis. Abnormal marrow cytogenetics are found in up 60% of cases, and there is a 20–80% risk of progression to acute leukaemia.

Therapeutics

Treatment is supportive, with blood and platelet transfusions, and growth factor injections; some will respond to erythropoietin. New therapies are in clinical trials worldwide. Quality of life is usually poor once transfusion dependence reaches every 3 weeks or less. Iron overload can occur rapidly.

MYELOPROLIFERATIVE DISORDERS

Symptoms common to all these diseases include:

- fatigue
- weight loss
- itch
- headache.

Very high platelet counts can lead to burning pain of the extremities (often in individual digits)—that is, erythromelalgia.

High haemoglobin levels may cause facial plethora, conjunctival injection and gritty eyes. A patient with an elevated haemoglobin may have plasma volume contraction (Gaisbock's syndrome, associated with diuretic and tobacco use), secondary polycythaemia (to chronic

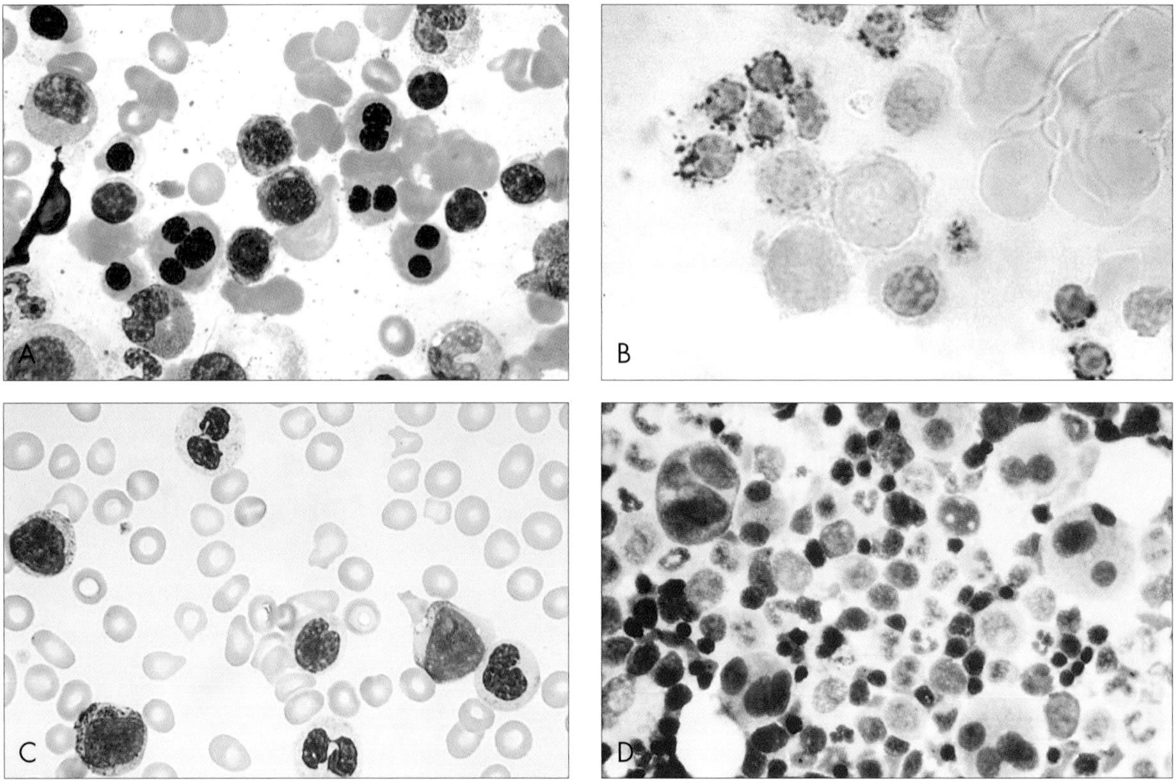

FIGURE 22.11 Characteristic forms of myelodysplasia: **A** Nucleated red cell progenitors with multi-lobed or multiple nuclei; **B** Ringed sideroblasts—erythroid progenitors with iron-laden mitochondria seen stained with Prussian blue; **C** Pseudo-Pelger-Hüet cells (top and bottom)—neutrophils with only two nuclear lobes instead of the normal three or four; **D** Megakaryocytes with multiple nucleii instead of normal single, multi-lobed nucleus

hypoxia from cardiorespiratory disease) or true polycythaemia rubra vera (PRV). Rarer causes of secondary polycythaemia include various erythropoietin-secreting tumours.

The clinical approach should therefore cover prescribed and other drug history, exercise tolerance, and careful physical examination of the cardiac and respiratory systems. Two-thirds of PRV patients have splenomegaly.

Cellular morphology in the blood film is generally normal, with a raised peripheral blood cell count along one or other cell lineage: the red cells in PRV, the platelets in essential thrombocythaemia (ET), and the granulocytes in CML. In myelofibrosis, the peripheral blood is often leuco-erythroblastic and there are increased marrow stromal cells and collagen deposition in the marrow. Very high haemoglobin levels (e.g. > 20 g/L) are a haematological emergency due to high risk of stroke, and urgent referral for therapeutic venesection is recommended. The risk of progression to acute leukaemia in these myeloproliferative disorders (except CML) is 5–15%.

The recent description of an acquired mutation of the JAK2 kinase gene in the MPS has revolutionised the diagnosis.[34] It is positive in 95% of those with PRV and 50% of those with ET. Previously, nuclear medicine scans and bone marrow biopsy were needed to diagnose PRV and ET respectively. Now, screening for the JAK2 kinase mutation is diagnostic in most cases (now readily available in many countries) and it is an appropriate step for the GP to perform prior to referral.

Therapeutics

Although the lifespan for most is near normal, management of these patients is complex, and options include hydroxyurea, interferon, anagrelide and venesection (PRV only). Low-dose aspirin is also given to many patients, to reduce the risk of thrombosis. New drugs targeting the JAK2 kinase mutation are in clinical trials in the United States and elsewhere, with encouraging early results.

LYMPHOMA

Lymphoma (Fig 22.12) is cancer of the immune system, and this in part explains the difficulty in classification over many years. Modern understanding of the immune system only began with the identification of B- and T-lymphocytes around 1970. Seeing lymphomas in this way also explains their heterogeneity, as there are many types of lymphocytes, with specialised roles and organ sites. Nevertheless, some broad generalisations can be made.

- Lymphoma can occur anywhere in the body. Rarer locations for lymphomas include the skin, central nervous system and testes.
- Generally, there is a lump. This is because lymphoma is a cancer of a committed lymphopoietic progenitor, and these are cells programmed to grow in lumps—unlike marrow stem cells in leukaemia. Lymphadenopathy from lymphoma is rarely painful and may fluctuate in size.
- In Hodgkin's lymphoma, 90% of cases arise in lymph glands ('nodal disease'); in non-Hodgkin's lymphoma (NHL), 40% of cases are extra-nodal and sites include mucosal associated lymphoid tissue (MALT) lymphomas of the stomach, and cutaneous mycosis fungoides.
- Eighty per cent of lymphomas are of B-cell origin. T-cell lymphomas tend to be slower growing but more resistant to therapy.
- Fine needle aspiration (FNA) biopsy is inadequate for accurate lymphoma diagnosis. Core or open biopsy is mandatory.
- Surgery is never curative. Lymphoma is not a surgical disease. Patients presenting with imminent or completed bowel obstruction are an exception.
- Some 10–20% of lymphoma cases have marrow involvement, and marrow biopsy should be included in staging tests, as well as serum lactate dehydrogenase (LDH), uric acid, flow cytometry, FBC, urea and electrolytes, CT and PET scanning.
- In NHL, smaller tumour cells and follicular (once called 'nodular') growth patterns are mostly associated with a better prognosis. There are exceptions (e.g. mantle cell lymphoma, where the cells are small, but the prognosis is poor).

Therapeutics

Lymphoma management is complex and changing.[35] Multidisciplinary care, as for many solid tumours, is increasingly used, principally with consolidative radiotherapy. In aggressive NHL, cure rates are high

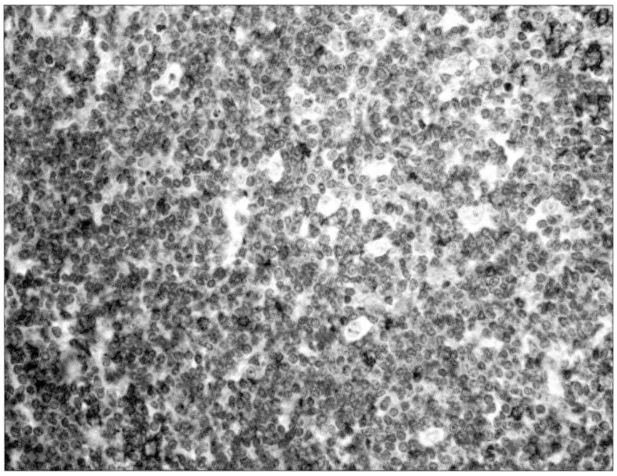

FIGURE 22.12 Lymphoma

(around 70%). Randomised, controlled clinical trials have generally shown no benefit for more intensive regimens or for up-front bone marrow transplantation for aggressive NHL. Instead, cure rates improved in B-cell lymphomas with the addition of rituximab to the familiar CHOP regimen (R-CHOP). This is a humanised antibody to CD20, a pan-B-cell antigen found on most B-lymphoma cell types; it seems to work essentially by 'lighting up' the B-cells for the patient's own T-cells to kill. Rituximab has rewritten the NHL landscape and represents an advance that proved elusive with intensified chemotherapy. Very high-grade lymphomas are treated essentially as for acute leukaemia.

Cases of follicular, or low-grade, NHL often present beyond stage II and are rarely curable with radiotherapy. Worldwide, with evidence that the addition of rituximab improves survival, the treatment paradigm has shifted to a more aggressive approach, also using R-CHOP, followed by maintenance rituximab, after which fully 80% can expect a remission lasting 4 years.[36]

Hodgkin's lymphoma, now recognised as a B-cell tumour although lacking the usual B-cell surface antigens, has a cure rate of around 85–90%, mostly with the relatively non-toxic regimen of ABVD. Nevertheless, using a prognostic scoring system,[37] cases at high risk of relapse can be identified and should be treated with a more intensive approach, such as BEACOPP or variants.

Relapses of many kinds of lymphomas are best managed with an autologous stem cell transplant in suitable patients, and this may require planning in the initial phases of treatment, to collect marrow stem cells before they are depleted by chemotherapy.

INVESTIGATION OF A PATIENT WITH LYMPHADENOPATHY

Lymph nodal enlargement of greater than 1 cm persisting for more than 4 weeks in an adult may warrant further investigation. Referral to a haematologist prior to surgical referral is recommended. It is reasonable for the GP also to organise FBC, U&E, serum LDH, chest X-ray and FNA. If the last suggests a lymphoma, CT scanning of the chest and abdomen are helpful.

However, open biopsy will still be necessary to provide tissue for the large battery of tests in modern histopathology to grade a lymphoma. There are often up to 12 different immuno-histochemical stains, plus fluorescence in situ hybridisation, flow cytometry of cell suspensions and molecular work-up of tumour cell DNA. Lymphoma work-up in a larger pathology laboratory with an interest in lymphoma diagnosis will reclassify about 1 in 20 cases, leading to possible changes in treatment.[38–40]

MULTIPLE MYELOMA

Multiple myeloma (Fig 22.13) is not a tumour of bone, as the name suggests. Rather, it is a tumour of antibody-secreting (into the plasma, hence 'plasma cells') immune cells that reside in the marrow. It is an insidious process of unknown cause, and the diagnosis may easily be missed for several years. These cells can erode bone, and crowd out the normal production of blood cells, and the protein they secrete can induce renal failure. Classic presentations are covered by the CRAB acronym: hyper**c**alcaemia, **r**enal failure, **a**naemia and **b**one pain or fractures. It may mimic osteoporotic spinal fractures. Rarer presentations include neutropenia or other cytopenia, hyperviscosity syndrome (headaches, blurred vision, dyspnoea and organ dysfunction), pyrexia of unknown origin and splenomegaly. Physical examination has little diagnostic value.

Screening is best done with a full blood count and film (background protein staining may be noticed in the haematology laboratory), a serum QEPP and serum free light chain (SFLC) assay. Until recently, a urinary QEPP was also required to exclude myeloma, because in some 20% of cases, the plasma cells secrete light chains only. These are small molecules that spill over from the bloodstream into the urine, leading to a negative serum QEPP, and positive urinary light chain (Bence-Jones) proteins. Light chains do not give a positive result on dipstick protein analysis. Most laboratories now perform, or have access to, the SFLC, which will detect light chains in serum at low levels (mg/L rather than g/L), and urine collection is no longer needed. A skeletal survey is more sensitive than a nucleotide bone scan for lytic lesions.

Therapeutics

Treatment is indicated for those with symptoms, high tumour burden or evidence of end-organ damage, such as lytic lesions or fractures, anaemia or renal failure. Components of treatment include chemotherapy, radiotherapy and bisphosphonates. Management of myeloma

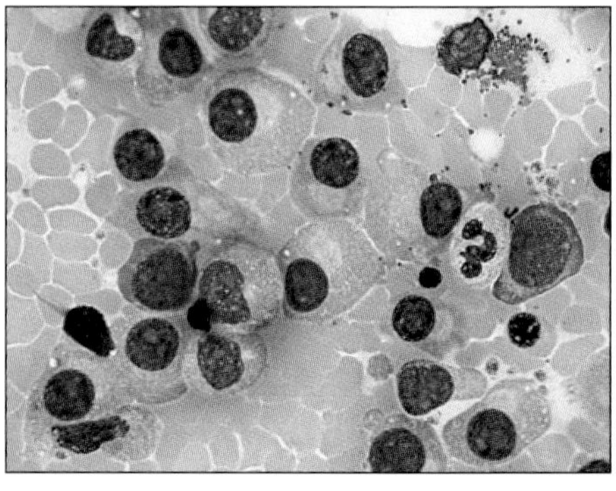

FIGURE 22.13 Myeloma

is also complex and rapidly changing—the past 15 years or so have seen the introduction of autologous stem cell transplantation, thalidomide, bortezomib and lenalidomide, all effective and capable of improving survival.[41] Thus, for many, myeloma can be brought into remission for periods lasting several years at a time between lines of therapy and a more optimistic message can and should be given to myeloma patients. Oral or IV bisphosphonate therapy reduces bony adverse events by some 40%; recently, a rare complication, osteonecrosis of the jaw, has been recognised.[42]

INTEGRATIVE MANAGEMENT OF BLOOD CANCERS

The GP has a responsibility to be well informed about the adjunctive treatments that may be of benefit to patients in alleviating side effects of cancer treatments and enhancing the patient's ability to cope with the disease and its treatment. There is also a valuable role for adjunctive therapies in rehabilitation after treatment with surgery, chemotherapy or radiotherapy (see Ch 24, Cancer).

Surveys in all developed countries consistently report that around 80% of cancer patients turn to complementary and alternative medicine (CAM). Ignoring this is dangerous (the risk of herb–drug interactions) and, at worst, humiliating for patients, who are, after all, trying to be proactive about their health.

Cancer patients have traditionally been advised by medical experts to stay away from the many self-cures, unproven remedies, fad diets and dietary supplements, sometimes but not always for good reason. These are a vulnerable patient group, and unfounded, frequently expensive, promises of cure are all too seductive. Moreover, many cancer patients will be deluged with well-meaning advice, and need help to react appropriately.

Encouraging the patient to develop a personal approach to their illness can be very empowering for them, and can improve compliance with mainstream treatment.[43] The patient must be involved in treatment and have the chance to buy into the therapeutic decisions, rather than having assumptions made and choice removed. There is good (level 2) evidence that lifestyle interventions can alleviate or reduce cancer symptoms and treatment side effects. This has recently been reviewed.[44] A number of these interventions are now discussed here.

Lifestyle

Exercise

Perhaps the best single lifestyle intervention before, during and after cancer is exercise. It has been shown to have primary cancer preventive effect in the Californian teachers' study, in which women who exercised (very hard, it must be said) reduced their breast cancer risk by 20%.[45] Secondary cancer preventive benefit has been suggested in the setting of colorectal cancer,[46,47] breast cancer and prostate cancer. Exercise promotes immune cell function and changes circulating white cell and lymphocyte subsets. Chemotherapy causes muscle catabolism and widespread loss of muscle mass; this may be potentiated by steroid myopathy. Resistance training in various muscle groups is more likely to help retain muscle mass, and reduce fatigue, than is mild aerobic exercise such as walking.[48] High-intensity exercise is inappropriate, if not impossible, during chemotherapy, and a rough rule of thumb is: never exercise so hard that you can't complete a sentence.

Diet

Diet is a focus for many cancer patients. Patients are encouraged to include all the food groups and specifically vitamin B_{12}, folate and iron, in their diet, to aid haemopoietic recovery after each cycle of chemotherapy. (This is specious, as no dietary manipulation has been demonstrated to improve white cell or platelet counts, save that 10% of iron-deficient individuals manifest thrombocytopenia.) The dangers of mono-food and fad diets should be expressly mentioned. Weight gain above the healthy BMI range increases mortality after cancer.[43]

Antioxidants

Antioxidants clearly have some anti-cancer effects in vitro, and their proponents argue that they may confer cytoprotective effects upon normal cells exposed to chemo-radiotherapy as well. However, human clinical trials have been disappointing. Indeed, a 2008 review cast a shadow over supplemental antioxidants during chemotherapy, raising the possibility of worse outcomes.[49] Furthermore, a Cochrane non-cancer-related review that included 67 randomised trials with 232,550 participants found that although vitamin C and selenium appeared safe, vitamin A, beta-carotene and vitamin E may be associated with increased mortality.[50] Long-term selenium use has been linked to increased risk of type II diabetes,[51] but appeared to reduce radiation-associated diarrhoea seen with treatment of gynaecological cancer.[52]

High-dose vitamin C may potentiate the activity of some chemotherapy regimens. Higher serum levels are achievable with IV than with oral preparations, and only recently has this been investigated in a more open way.[53] Evidence of benefit remains scanty. Although it appears safe, it may precipitate haemolysis in G6PD-deficient individuals and promote urinary stone formation.

These are cautionary notes and, for these reasons, a blended fruit/vegetable drink is recommended as a healthier source of antioxidants, and possibly a multivitamin three times a week, as B-group vitamins may aid neurological recovery after insult (e.g. peripheral neuropathy after vinca alkaloids).

Other good sources of antioxidants include green tea and red wine. A molecule in green tea is under study at the Mayo Clinic for its powerful anti-CLL effect. Many other supplements and herbal preparations are generally discouraged by oncologists during chemotherapy; rather, they should be reserved until after chemotherapy, to reduce the risk of interactions. However, some, such as *Astragalus*, have been found to reduce the incidence of leukopenia, and nausea and vomiting related to chemotherapy.

Asking patients what they are taking, and checking with a desktop reference of alternative and herbal preparations,[54] shows a preparedness to discuss CAM use, and can help prevent dangerous herb–drug interactions.

Acupuncture

There is Cochrane meta-analysis evidence from 11 trials that acupuncture reduces acute post-chemotherapy vomiting (less so nausea or late vomiting).[55]

Music therapy

Music therapy can be passive (listening) or active (playing in any form, singing, etc). In an RCT of patients undergoing autologous stem cell transplantation, subjects receiving an individualised program of live music therapy had a significant total improvement in mood.[56]

Massage

There are many forms of massage, such as therapeutic massage, aromatherapy and reflexology. There is no single report in the literature that massage promotes cancer spread, although it seems prudent not to massage known sites of disease. Massage seems mostly to have an anti-anxiety effect. A recent well-conducted multicentre RCT of aromatherapy massage showed short-term benefit (6 weeks, but not 10 weeks).[57,58]

Homeopathy

Recent meta-analyses from the United Kingdom, where homeopathy enjoys more mainstream support, have found no evidence of efficacy.

Overseas cures

Patients or carers may ask for advice about travelling to either reputed centres of excellence (e.g. the MD Anderson Cancer Center in Houston), or to more clearly 'left-field' therapies including certain remedies in Mexico. With the former, care should be taken to ascertain whether there is access to a tumour-specific agent not available in their country of residence—that is, there should be a particular reason to go. In the latter, the lack of published evidence may fail to dissuade, in which case an 'open-door' policy should be offered. In either case, the very real cost, disruption, lack of local supports, and potential for distress caused to others, should be mentioned. Often the disruption and subsequent stress may outweigh any small incremental benefit in prolonging survival.

This discussion can be very difficult, because it often arises after a failure of local treatment, and advising against travel may seem to be removing hope—and hope is part of the human condition. However, it may also be an opportunity to change expectations from immortality, to a period of good life before a good death. Leading such a discussion can be courageous, but a key point at which the latter becomes possible.

Stress

There is some evidence that major life stresses predispose to cancer, but the small number of papers reporting a positive association are outweighed by many more finding no such link. A study in Sydney failed to show increased breast cancer rates in 239 women with breast carcinoma and 275 women with benign breast disease, after multiple regression analyses of carefully measured psychosocial factors.[59]

Positive mental attitude: 'fighting the cancer'

Cancer patients are often encouraged and expected to show the much-quoted 'positive mental attitude'. Many don't feel they can achieve this, and feel guilty as a result of not meeting the expectations of those around them. A meta-analysis failed to show any survival benefit of any particular coping style.[60] Admittedly, the point here is not survival, but making treatment more tolerable.

Instead, patients should be encouraged to reach a state of calmness about their cancer. How to do this will vary from person to person. Learning about the cancer may vary from acceptance of medical advice for some, to long hours on the internet to others. Patients should satisfy themselves that their mainstream advice is good, and decide how to face their illness in their own way. GPs can have a key role in providing some support to this process. There is growing evidence that some complementary therapies can reduce anxiety, ameliorate pain and fatigue and empower cancer patients.[43,61] Positive self-imagery—an image of lying on a beach in Bali after treatment, for example—helps some.

Carers

Carers are part of the equation, and their attitude and capacity to assist a loved one through illness is clearly important. They should be encouraged to touch the patient—touch is a powerful form of human communication. They must respect the patient's approach to their illness, which may be difficult, and keep aside some time and energy for self-care. Appointing a spokesperson for updates outside the cancer-afflicted household can save much energy, distress and time. Friends can help by providing ready-made meals, transport assistance and acceptance of the path chosen by the patient.

HAEMATOLOGICAL CANCER SURVIVORSHIP

Often after very intensive periods of therapy, requiring much time at or in the hospital, survivors of blood cancers arrive at a point of apparently suddenly being 'cut adrift' from their haematological team. This can be a profound shock, and can bring to the surface issues of avoidance of psychological reconciliation with the diagnosis, as well as uncertainty about returning home and to the workplace and current or future relationships. Such stressors may be magnified in patients who have had to move to a major centre for care that may have involved more than 6 months away from home, in the case of a bone marrow transplant.

Identified unmet needs in haematological cancer survivors include advice on financial and employment implications, the surveillance plan and information on lifestyle changes and long-term side effects, including infertility and second cancer risk; but the major unmet need by far is the fear of relapse.[62]

Strategies to help cope with fear of relapse can include pointing out that many cancer relapses occur in a similar way or place to the original presentation, and that vague symptoms can often be appropriately dismissed. It may help to make explicit to the patient which markers (symptoms, physical signs, blood tests and scans) are being monitored as well. Having the GP available as a first contact point is of comfort to some; others will insist upon unplanned review by their specialist, which will become increasingly impractical as pressure on tertiary care grows.

Even if cured, this cannot be ascertained for 3–5 years, and the patient must live with the sword of Damocles over their head for this time. All cancers, curable or not, should be viewed as a chronic illness.

Strategies for resuming life after cancer therapy include practical advice on late side effects and information on the surveillance plan; and encouragement to improve lifestyle and make health changes as above. Cancer should never be regarded as some kind of bonus, but planting the seed of positive life changes—resolving long-term stresses, good diet, exercise and plentiful sleep—may allow personal affirmation from the experience. There is increasing research and interest in survivorship, and the likelihood is that GPs will have more opportunity to be part of post-cancer surveillance and the supportive framework for the cancer survivor in the near future.

RESOURCES

Haematology Education Resource, http://www.haematology.org/

Haematology Society of Australia and New Zealand, http://www.hsanz.org.au/

Hoffbrand AV, Moss PAH, Pettit JE. Essential haematology. 5th edn. Oxford:Blackwell; 2006.

Rosenthal DS, Dean-Clower E. Integrative medicine in hematology/oncology: benefits, ethical considerations, and controversies. Hematology 2005; 1:491–497. Online. Available: http://asheducationbook.hematologylibrary.org/cgi/content/full/2005/1/491

REFERENCES

1 Joske DJ. Chronic myeloid leukemia: the evolution of gene-targeted therapy. Med J Aust 2008; 189(5):277–282.

2 Argawal N, Prchal J. Anemia of chronic disease (anaemia of inflammation). Acta Haematologica 2009: 122:103–108.

3 Ioannou GN, Rockey DC, Bryson CL et al. Iron deficiency and gastrointestinal malignancy: a population cohort study. Am J Med 2002: 113:276–280.

4 Finberg K, Heeney MM, Campagna DR et al. Mutations in TMPRSS6 cause iron-refractory iron deficiency anemia (IRIDA). Nat Genet 2008; 40(5):569–571.

5 Beutler E, van Geet C, te Loo DM et al. Polymorphisms and mutations of human TMPRSS6 in iron deficiency anemia. Blood Cell Molec Dis 2010; 44:16–21.

6 McDiarmid T, Johnson ED. Clinical inquiries. Are any oral iron formulations better tolerated than ferrous sulphate? J Fam Prac 2002: 51(6):576.

7 Spelman D, Buttery J, Daley A et al. Guidelines for the prevention of sepsis in asplenic and hyposplenic patients. Australasian Society for Infectious Diseases. Intern Med J 2008; 38(5):349–356.

8 Ortel T. Heparin-induced thrombocytopenia: when a low platelet count is a mandate for anticoagulation. Hematology 2009; 1:225–232.

9 George J, Aster R. Drug-induced thrombocytopenia: pathogenesis, evaluation and management. Hematology 2009; 153–158.

10 Hayward C. Diagnosis and management of mild bleeding disorders. Hematology 2005; 1:423–428.

11 Leung L. Perioperative evaluation of a bleeding diathesis. Hematology 2006; 1:457–461.

12 Hull RD, Raskob GE, Rosenbloom D et al. Optimal therapeutic level of heparin therapy in patients with venous thrombosis. Arch Intern Med 1992; 152:1589–1595.

13 Raschke RA, Reilly BM, Guidry JR et al. The weight-based heparin dosing nomogram compared with a 'standard care' nomogram: a randomised controlled trial. Ann Intern Med 1993; 119: 874–881.

14 Othieno R, Abu Affan M, Okpo E. Home versus in-patient treatment for deep vein thrombosis. Cochrane Database Syst Rev 2007; 3:CD003076.

15 Crowther MA, Ginsberg JB, Kearon C et al. A randomized trial comparing 5 mg and 10 mg warfarin loading doses. Arch Intern Med 1999; 159:46–48.

16 Schulman S, Rhedin AS, Lindmaker P et al; Duration of Anticoagulation Study Group. A comparison of six weeks with six months of oral anticoagulant therapy after a first episode of venous thrombo-embolism. N Eng J Med 1995; 332:1661–1665.

17 Pinede L, Duhaut P, Cucherat M et al. Comparison of long versus short duration of anticoagulant therapy after a first episode of venous thromboembolism a meta-analysis of randomised controlled trials. J Intern Med 2000; 247(5):553–562.

18 Prandoni P, Prins MH, Lensing AW et al. AESOPUS Investigators. Residual thrombosis on ultrasonography to guide the duration of anticoagulation in patients with deep vein thrombosis: a randomized trial. Ann Int Med 2009; 150(9):577–585.

19 Schulman S, Granqvist S, Holmstrom M et al. The duration of oral anticoagulant therapy after a second episode of venous thromboembolism. N Engl J Med 1997; 336(6):393–398.

20 Gallus A, Baker R, Chong B et al. Consensus guidelines for warfarin therapy. Recommendations from the Australasian Society of Thrombosis and Haemostasis. Med J Aust 2000; 172:600–605.

21 Rosove MH, Grody WW. Should we be applying warfarin pharmacogenetics to clinical practice? No, not now. Ann Intern Med 2009; 151:270–273.

22 Baker R, Coughlin PB, Gallus AS et al. Warfarin reversal: consensus guidelines, on behalf of the Australasian Society of Thrombosis and Haemostasis. Med J Aust 2004; 181:492–497.

23 Crawford JH, Augustson BM. Prothrombinex use for the reversal of warfarin: is fresh frozen plasma needed? Med J Aust 2006; 184:365–366.

24 Geerts WD, Berqvist D, Pineo GF et al. Prevention of venous thromboembolism: American College of Chest Physicians, evidence-based clinical practice guidelines, 8th edn. Chest, 2008; 133(6 Suppl):381S–453S.

25 Kelman CW, Kortt MA, Becker NG et al. Deep vein thrombosis and air travel: record linkage study. BMJ 2003; 327:1072–1075.

26 Lee AY, Levine MN, Baker RI et al. Low-molecular-weight heparin versus coumarin for the prevention of recurrent venous thromboembolism in patients with cancer. N Engl J Med 2003; 349(2):146–153.

27 De Stefano V, Finazzi G, Mannucci PM. Inherited thrombophilia: pathogenesis, clinical syndromes, and management. Blood 1996; 87:3531–3544.

28 De Stefano V, Martinelli I, Mannuci PM et al. The risk of recurrent deep vein thrombosis among heterozygous carriers of both factor V Leiden and the G20210 A prothrombin mutation. N Engl J Med 1999; 341(11):801–806.

29 Ho WK, Hankey GJ, Quinlan DJ et al. Risk of recurrent venous thromboembolism in patients with common thrombophilia: a systematic review. Arch Intern Med 2006; 166:729–736.

30 Wu O, Robertson L, Twaddle S et al. Screening for thrombophilia in high-risk situations: systematic review and cost-effectiveness analysis. The Thrombosis; Risk and Economic Assessment of Thrombophilia Screening (TREATS) study. Health Technol Assess 2006; 1–110.

31 Canonico M, Oger E, Plu-Bureau G et al; Estrogen and Thromboembolism Risk (ESTHER) Study Group. Hormone therapy and venous thromboembolism among postmenopausal women: impact of the route of estrogen administration and progestogens: the ESTHER study. Circulation; 2007; 115(7):840–845.

32 Canonico M, Plu-Bureau G, Lowe GD et al. Hormone replacement therapy and risk of venous thromboembolism in postmenopausal women: systematic review and meta-analysis. BMJ 2008; 36(7655):1227–1231.

33 Carney DA, Mulligan SP. Chronic lymphocytic leukemia: current first-line therapy. Intern Med J 2009: 39(1):44–48.

34 Levine RL, Gilliland DG. Myeloproliferative disorders. Blood 2008; 112(6):2190–2198. Review.

35 Young GA, Iland HJ. Clinical perspectives in lymphoma. Intern Med J 2007; 37(7):478–484.

36 van Oers MH, Klasa R, Marcus RE et al. Rituximab maintenance improves clinical outcomes of relapsed/resistant follicular non-Hodgkin lymphoma in patients both with and without rituximab during induction: results of a prospective randomised phase 3 intergroup trial. Blood 2006: 108(10):3295–3301.

37 Hasenclever D, Diehl V. A prognostic score for advanced Hodgkin's disease. International Prognostic Factors Project on Advanced Hodgkin's Disease. N Engl J Med 1998; 339(21):1506–1514.

38 Clarke CA, Undurraga DM, Harasty PJ et al. Changes in cancer registry coding for lymphoma subtypes: reliability over time and relevance for surveillance and study. Cancer Epidemiology Biomarkers Prev 2006; 15(4):630–638.

39 LaCasce A, Kho M, Friedberg J et al. Comparison of referring and final pathology for patients with non-Hodgkin's lymphoma in the National Comprehensive Cancer Network. J Clin Oncol 2008; 26(31):5107–5112.

40 Prescott R, Wells S, Bisset DL et al. Audit of tumour histopathology reviewed by a regional oncology centre. J Clin Path 1995; 48:245–249.
41 Raab MS, Podar K, Breitkreutz I et al. Multiple myeloma. Lancet 2009; 374(9686):324–339. Review.
42 Dickinson M, Prince HM, Kirsa S et al. Osteonecrosis of the jaw complicating bisphosphonate treatment for bone disease in multiple myeloma: an overview with recommendations for prevention and treatment. Intern Med J 2009: 39(5):304–316.
43 Jones LW, Demark-Wahnefried W. Diet, exercise and complementary therapies after primary treatment for cancer. Lancet Oncol 2006; 7:1017–1026.
44 Joske DJ, Rao A, Kristjanson L. Critical review of complementary therapies in haemato-oncology. Intern Med J 2006; 36(9):579–586.
45 Dallal CM, Sullivan-Halley J, Ross RK et al. Long-term recreational physical activity and risk of invasive in situ breast cancer: the California teachers' study. Arch Intern Med 2007; 167(4):408–415.
46 Meyerhardt JA, Giovannucci EL, Holmes MD et al. Physical activity and survival after colorectal cancer diagnosis. J Clin Oncol 2006; 24(22):3527–3534.
47 Meyerhardt JA, Giovannucci EL, Ogino S et al. Physical activity and male colorectal cancer survival. Arch Intern Med 2009; 169(22):2102–2108.
48 Galvao DA, Newton RU. Review of exercise intervention studies in cancer patients. J Clin Oncol 2005; 23(4):899–909.
49 Lawenda BD, Kelly KM, Ladas EJ et al. Should supplemental antioxidant administration be avoided during chemotherapy and radiation therapy? J Natl Cancer Inst 2008; 100(11):773–783.
50 Bjelakovic G, Nikolova D, Gluud LL et al. Antioxidant supplements for prevention of mortality in healthy participants and patients with various diseases. Cochrane Database Syst Rev 2008; 2:CD007176.
51 Stranges S, Marshall JR, Natarajan R et al. Effects of long-term selenium supplementation on the incidence of type 2 diabetes: a randomised trial. Ann Intern Med 2007; 147(4):217–223.
52 Muecke R, Schomburg L, Glatzel M et al. Multicentre, phase 3 trial comparing selenium supplementation with observation in gynecologic radiation oncology. Int J Radiat Oncol Biol Phys 2010; 2 Feb [Epub ahead of print].
53 Verrax J, Buc Calderon P. The controversial place of vitamin C in cancer treatment. Biochem Pharmacol 2008; 76(12):1644–1652.
54 Ernst E, ed. The desktop guide to complementary and alternative medicine. An evidence-based approach. Edinburgh:Mosby; 2001.
55 Ezzo JM, Richardson MA, Vickers A et al. Acupuncture point stimulation for chemotherapy induced nausea or vomiting. Cochrane Database Syst Rev 2006; 2:CD002285.
56 Casileth BR, Vickers AJ, Magill LA. Music therapy for mood disturbance during hospitalisation for autologous stem cell transplantation: a randomised controlled trial. Cancer 2003; 98(12):2723–2729.
57 Post-White J, Kinney ME, Savik K et al. Therapeutic massage and healing touch improve symptoms in cancer. Integr Cancer Ther 2003; 2(4):332–334.
58 Wilkinson SM, Love SB, Westcombe AM et al. Effectiveness of aromatherapy massage in the management of anxiety and depression in patients with cancer: a multicentre randomised controlled trial. J Clin Oncol 2007: 25(5):532–539.
59 Price MA, Tennant CC, Butow PN et al. The role of psychosocial factors in the development of breast carcinoma, Part II. Life event stressors, social support, defense style emotional control and their interactions. Cancer 2001: 91(4):686–697.
60 Petticrew M, Bell R, Hunter D. Influence of psychological coping on survival and recurrence in people with cancer: systematic review. BMJ 2002: 325(7372):1066. Review.
61 Diehl V. The bridge between patient and doctor: the shift from CAM to integrative medicine. Hematology 2009; 1:320–325. Review.
62 Lobb E, Joske D, Butow P et al. When the safety net of treatment has been removed: patients' unmet needs at the completion of treatment for haematological malignancies. Patient Educ Couns 2009; 77(1):103–108.

chapter 23

Bones

INTRODUCTION AND OVERVIEW

Bones are complex organs with many important functions, the most obvious being structural. They provide support for the body and the means by which muscles can insert into fixed structures in order to allow movement. They are also important in hearing, through the transduction of sound via the ear's ossicles, and they protect other soft organs that are easily damaged, such as the brain, eyes, kidneys, lungs and spleen. Bone marrow, which is largely within the medulla of the long bones, is the centre for production of blood cells (haematopoesis) and an important site for storage of fatty acids. Bones also have important metabolic functions, including:

- mineral storage and regulation—in particular calcium and phosphorus
- acid–base balance—through storing and releasing salts
- storage of heavy metals—important for detoxifying the body
- releasing hormones—helps the kidneys to regulate phosphate absorption.

Bone strength depends not only on the hardness of the minerals within bone, but also the structure and organisation of the connective tissue—largely collagen. Despite the brittleness of bone, the network of collagen fibres gives it some flexibility. It is the movement of bone and the action of forces through the harder layer of compact or cortical bone as it grows and repairs that tells bone how to lay down and organise its structure. Weight-bearing exercise, particularly for the long bones, is vital for maintenance of bone strength and structure, whereas physical inactivity and immobilisation of bones will lead to weakening of those bones. The interior of bone—the medulla or trabecular bone—is far more porous and provides an environment for the bone marrow.

Bone is in a continual process of rebuilding itself through the action of osteoblasts and osteocytes, which lay down and maintain new bone, and osteoclasts, which resorb bone. The balance between these cells gives bone the capacity to repair itself and to remodel itself over time. Imbalances between the activity of these cells can predispose to development of bone pathology, such as osteoporosis. Maintenance of healthy bones requires vitamin D (dietary and from sunlight), a balanced diet with adequate fruit, vegetables, protein, calcium and other minerals, growth hormone, and thyroid and sex hormones. The resorption of bone by osteoclasts is inhibited by calcitonin secreted by the parafollicular cells in the thyroid gland.

Bones develop from cartilage, and by the time of birth only the metaphyses of the long bones are visible on X-ray. Bone growth throughout childhood takes place at the epiphyses or the growth plate of the long bones, which slowly narrow. By the time they fuse, at the end of adolescence, no further growth is possible and the person will have attained their adult height. The eventual height of a person depends on many factors including genetics, nutrition, hormonal status and injuries. Injuries such as fractures (e.g. involving the epiphysis) can lead to premature fusion and reduced growth of that bone. Height can also be reduced when there is inherited short stature, significant malnutrition, inadequate sex hormones, growth hormone deficiency or hypothyroidism.

This chapter describes the following conditions affecting bones:

- osteoporosis
- rickets
- osteomalacia
- Paget's disease
- bone cancer.

OSTEOPOROSIS

DEFINITION

In 1991, *osteoporosis* was defined as a metabolic bone disease characterised by 'low bone mass, microarchitectural deterioration of bone tissue leading to enhanced bone fragility and a consequent increase in fracture risk'.[1] However, the current conception of osteoporosis is as a disease of compromised bone strength that predisposes an individual to an increased risk of fracture.[2] In this new definition, osteoporosis is a dynamic, rather than an anatomical, condition. The *disease* is thus low bone mass and deteriorated bone quality, and *fracture* is the clinical consequence of the disease.

The 'bone strength' component of the definition refers to the integration of bone mass and bone quality. 'Bone quality' primarily refers to bone architecture, metabolic turnover, damage accumulation (e.g. micro-fractures) and demineralisation. At present, the most clinically relevant indicator of bone quality is a history of personal fracture. The current definition of osteoporosis represents it as both a disease and a risk factor, and this has important implications for the pathogenesis, prevention and treatment of the disease.

Osteoporosis is highly prevalent in the general population. Using the operational definition of osteoporosis (based on measurement of bone mineral density (BMD)), the prevalence of osteoporosis in Australian men and women aged 60 years and above was estimated to be 11% and 27% respectively.[3] As expected, the prevalence of osteoporosis increases with advancing age, from approximately 5% (men) and 13% (women) at 60 years of age to over 28% (men) and 63% (women) at age 80 or above.[4] With a rapidly ageing population, it is expected that osteoporosis will be an even greater problem in the next 20 years or so.

The outcome of osteoporosis is *fragility fracture.* Fractures are a major public health problem because of their high incidence rate in the population, and because individuals with fracture are at increased risk of mortality and morbidity and reduced quality of life, and incur significant healthcare costs. In several population-based epidemiological studies, all major fractures were associated with increased mortality, especially in men.[5] Even in healthy older women, clinical vertebral fractures, commonly manifested as asymptomatic fracture, and hip fractures, are substantially associated with increased mortality.[6,7] A more recent study demonstrated that asymptomatic vertebral deformity is a major risk factor for subsequent fracture and mortality.[8]

The increase in fracture cases will result in a significant increase in healthcare costs. The annual cost of treatment of fractures and associated sequelae has been estimated at $10–20 billion in the United States and £3 billion in England and Wales. Within the next 50 years the cost of hip fracture alone in the United States may exceed $240 billion.[9] In Canada, the annual cost of hip fracture is estimated at $650 million and is expected to rise to $2.4 billion by 2041.[10] In Australia, the direct and indirect costs of fracture have been estimated at $7.5 billion.[11]

EPIDEMIOLOGY OF FRACTURES

Theoretically, any fracture related to low bone density may be considered an *osteoporotic fracture.* Fractures of the spine (vertebrae), hip and wrist (distal forearm) have long been regarded as typical osteoporotic fractures.[12–16] Most types of fracture occur more often in patients with low BMD,[17,18] and therefore most types of age-related fractures are osteoporotic in nature. According to this definition, the following fracture types are considered osteoporotic:

- in women—vertebrae, hip and other femoral, wrist–forearm, humeral, rib, pelvic, clavicle, scapula, sternum, tibia and fibula
- in men—similar to women, except that tibia and fibular fractures are not considered osteoporotic.

In both women and men, fractures occurring at the skull and face, hands and fingers, feet and toes, ankle and patella are classified as not due to osteoporosis.[19]

Because fragility or osteoporotic fracture is defined as fracture-related with minimal trauma (i.e. a fall from standing height or less),[20,21] in the research setting, fractures clearly due to major trauma (such as motor vehicle accidents) or due to underlying diseases (such as cancer or bone-related diseases) were excluded from analysis.[5,16,18,22–26]

Overall, the incidence of any fracture in women and men increases with advancing age, and is greater in women than in men. The incidence of fracture also varies according to geographic variations between and within countries. Fracture rates in women aged 60 or older are six times higher than those in women aged 35–59 years; in men aged 60 or older the rate is 1.4-fold greater than in men less than 60 years of age.[27]

Overall fracture rates are greater in urban than in rural areas.[28,29] The difference is more pronounced in those aged 60 years or over, suggesting that environmental factors have an impact on bone health.

The magnitude of osteoporosis-related fracture can be quantified by the lifetime risk of fracture. In developed countries it is estimated that the residual lifetime risk of any fracture for men and women from age 60 is approximately a quarter and just under a half respectively.[16] For individuals with osteoporosis, the mortality-adjusted lifetime risk of any fracture is probably over 40% for men and 65% for women.[3] The three most common sites are hip, vertebral and Colles' fracture.

TYPES OF FRACTURE

Hip fracture

Hip fractures include femoral neck, intertrochanteric or subtrochanteric fractures. Hip fracture is the most serious consequence of osteoporosis because it incurs many subsequent complications, including pain and disability.[30]

It is estimated that, from the age of 60 years, 11 out of 100 women will sustain a hip fracture during their remaining lifetime. This risk is higher than the risk of being diagnosed with breast cancer (around 10%). Approximately 17% of women and 30% of men who have sustained a fracture will die within 12 months after the event.[31] However, the exact causes of death among these individuals are not clear. Among women who survive the fracture, over 20% require long-term care and over a third are unable to return to their prior work,[32] and have a significantly reduced quality of life.[33]

Vertebral fracture

Osteoporosis has sometimes been referred to as a 'silent disease' because individuals often do not have apparent symptoms and pain until a fracture occurs. Asymptomatic vertebral fracture can be considered a silent disease, because patients do not realise that they have a fracture and do not seek medical attention. Currently, there is no 'gold standard' for the identification of vertebral fracture[34,35]; estimates of its overall prevalence and incidence rate in elderly women and men depends in part on the definition used.[36]

Asymptomatic vertebral fracture can be detected by conventional radiology, but it is not an attractive means of large-scale screening, because of cost and radiation exposure. In a large-scale study,[37] vertebral fracture was present in 12% of women and men. As expected, the prevalence of vertebral fracture increases with age, more sharply in women.[38] The use of corticosteroid therapy doubles the risk.[39] Studies have found that about 33% of vertebral fractures or deformities are symptomatic[40] and that only 23% of vertebral deformities in women were diagnosed clinically.[41] In other words, there are many 'silent' vertebral fractures that produce no obvious symptoms. Vertebral deformities, whether clinically recognised or not, are related to an increase in chronic back pain and disability,[42,43] and to low health-related quality of life[44] and an increase in mortality.[8,45]

Distal forearm fracture

A fracture of the distal forearm is one that occurs through the distal third of the radius and/or ulna. It is frequently and typically seen in women.[46,47] Although its consequence is less serious than that of a hip fracture, it is associated with significant pain and may be associated with severe and long-term complications.[48,49] The incidence increases rapidly with advancing age in women (but less so with men), for up to 10 years following menopause, and tends to slow thereafter.[50]

CLINICAL ASSESSMENT OF OSTEOPOROSIS

The clinical assessment of osteoporosis and fracture risk is based on assessment of:

- clinical risk factors, including the possibility of secondary causes of osteoporosis or bone loss
- bone strength.

Risk factors

Risk factors can be broadly classified into modifiable and non-modifiable risk factors (listed in Box 23.1). Of these, the four key risk factors are:

- advancing age
- personal history of a fragility fracture
- family history of fracture
- low BMD (or osteoporosis).

A prior fragility fracture substantially elevates an individual's risk of future fracture.[5,8,51,52] The elevated risk is 1.5- to 9.5-fold depending on age at assessment, number of prior fractures and the site of the incident fracture. A pre-existing asymptomatic vertebral fracture increases the risk of a second vertebral fracture and non-vertebral fracture at least four-fold.[8] A study of a placebo group showed that 20% of those who experienced a vertebral fracture during the period of observation had a second vertebral fracture within 1 year. Patients with a

BOX 23.1 Risk factors for osteoporosis

Non-modifiable risk factors

- Personal history of fracture as an adult
- History of fracture in first-degree relative
- Advanced age (> 65 years)
- Female
- Genetic factors

Potentially modifiable risk factors

- Current cigarette smoking
- Low body weight
- Oestrogen deficiency, early menopause or hypogonadism (in men)
- Long-term exposure to anticonvulsant drugs or SSRIs
- Lifelong low vitamin D and calcium intake
- Alcoholism
- Inadequate physical activity
- Poor health/frailty (e.g. rheumatoid arthritis, hyperthyroidism, dementia, impaired eyesight)
- History of falls or recurrent falls
- Chronic stress and depression (due to high cortisol levels leaching calcium out of the bones)
- Hyperparathyroidism

hip fracture are at increased risk of a second hip fracture. The risk of subsequent fracture among those with a prior fracture at any site is 2.2 times that of people without a prior fragility fracture.[52] A family history of osteoporotic fracture is also a major risk factor for fracture.

Although most studies have focused on the index person's mother or other female family members, the genetic influence on risk of osteoporosis is multifactorial, and one should not ignore a history of osteoporotic fracture in first- or second-degree male relatives. Therefore, other family members should be included during assessment of genetic contribution to osteoporosis risk.

Bone strength

At present there is no direct method for reliably measuring bone strength. However, BMD, measured by dual-energy X-ray absorptiometry (DXA), provides a benchmark for bone strength. BMD measurement could account for up to 70–75% of variance in bone strength.[53] BMD is often standardised by expressing it as a T-score, i.e. the number of standard deviations (SD) from the young normal mean, taken as aged between 20 and 30 years.

There is a strong, continuous and consistent relationship between BMD and fracture risk, such that each SD lowering in BMD is associated with a 1.6-fold increase in fracture risk in both men and women.[54] In Chinese women, the relative risk of fracture for each SD lowering in femoral neck BMD was two-fold.[55] There is evidence that the magnitude of association between BMD and hip fracture risk (with relative risk being 2.2[56] to 3.6[57]) is equivalent to or even stronger than the association between serum cholesterol and cardiovascular disease. Measurement of BMD is therefore considered the gold standard for diagnosis of osteoporosis in elderly men and postmenopausal women.

An operational definition of osteoporosis, by which a postmenopausal woman is considered to have osteoporosis, is if her femoral neck BMD (which is more reliable than lumbar spine measurements) is decreased by at least 2.5 SD compared with the mean value in young adults.[58] The WHO classification also includes definitions of osteopenia and normal BMD (Table 23.1). The operational criteria of osteoporosis for women has also been adopted for men.[59] These classifications do not apply to children.

Who should have a BMD measurement?

Mass screening using DXA scanning is not recommended or feasible without some selection of the target population. One important and difficult question is how to decide which women should undergo BMD measurement and further evaluation based on the results of BMD scan. It is suggested that a case-finding strategy be adopted, to identify individuals ideally eligible for a BMD scan[61]—that is:

- women aged > 65 years, or men aged > 70 years
- women aged < 65 years, or men aged < 70 years, with risk factors for fracture (as in Box 23.1).

In the absence of BMD measurement, a number of clinical prediction rules, including the Osteoporosis Self-assessment Tool for Asians (OSTA), have been developed,[62,63] to identify 'candidates' for a BMD scan. Most of these scores, based only on age and body weight, are a simple prediction rule that can potentially be useful in identifying women at high risk of osteoporosis. These scoring systems[64,65] can be useful in ruling out osteoporosis.

Quantitative ultrasonography (QUS) is a portable, less expensive, less time-consuming and radiation-free technology, although there is limited evidence of its clinical usefulness.

TABLE 23.1 WHO diagnostic categories for BMD in postmenopausal women

Category	Projected proportion of population*
Normal	BMD not more than 1 SD below peak BMD in young adult mean (T-score > −1)
Osteopenia	BMD 1–2.5 SD below young adult mean (T-score −1 to −2.5)
Osteoporosis	BMD 2.5 SD or more below young adult mean (T-score at or below −2.5)
Established osteoporosis	BMD 2.5 SD or more below young adult mean, and the presence of one or more fragility fractures

*Urban, 2020 (%). SD: standard deviation. BMD: bone mineral density.

Source: Nolla et al. 2002[60]

Bone turnover markers

Bone is a net result of two counteracting processes of *bone resorption* and *bone formation*, often referred to as *bone remodelling*.

- *Bone remodelling* is a normal, natural process that maintains skeletal strength, enables repair of microfractures and is essential for calcium homeostasis. During the remodelling process, osteoblasts produce a number of cytokines, peptides and growth factors that are released into the circulation. Their concentration thus reflects the rate of bone formation.
- *Bone formation* markers include serum osteocalcin, bone-specific alkaline phosphatase and procollagen I carboxyterminal propeptide (PICP).

- Most biochemical indices of *bone resorption* are related to collagen breakdown products such as hydroxyproline or the various collagen cross-links and telopeptides. Bone resorption markers include urinary hydroxyproline, urinary pyridinoline (PYR), urinary deoxypyridinoline (D-PYR) as well as collagen type I cross-linked N telopeptide (NTX) and collagen Type I cross-linked C telopeptide (CTX).

Bone turnover rate in postmenopausal women correlates negatively with BMD, and markers of bone resorption are associated with fracture risk.[66] A reduction in biochemical markers appears to be correlated with a decrease in vertebral fracture incidence[67] in some studies, but is not necessarily always predictive of response to therapies. Nevertheless, the predictive value of biomarkers in assessing an individual patient can be limited by their high variability within individuals.[68]

Assessment of absolute fracture risk

At any given level of BMD, fracture risk varies widely in relation to the burden of other risk factors[56] (some modifiable), such as:

- advancing age
- low dietary calcium intake
- low vitamin D levels and inadequate sunlight
- family history of fracture
- steroid use
- low BMI
- increased propensity to fall
- smoking
- chronic stress and poor mental health
- excessive alcohol ingestion.

Thus, for any one individual, the likelihood of fracture depends onavv a combination of risk factors. This means that two individuals, both with osteoporosis, can have different risks of fracture because they have different non-BMD risk profiles. Likewise, an osteoporotic

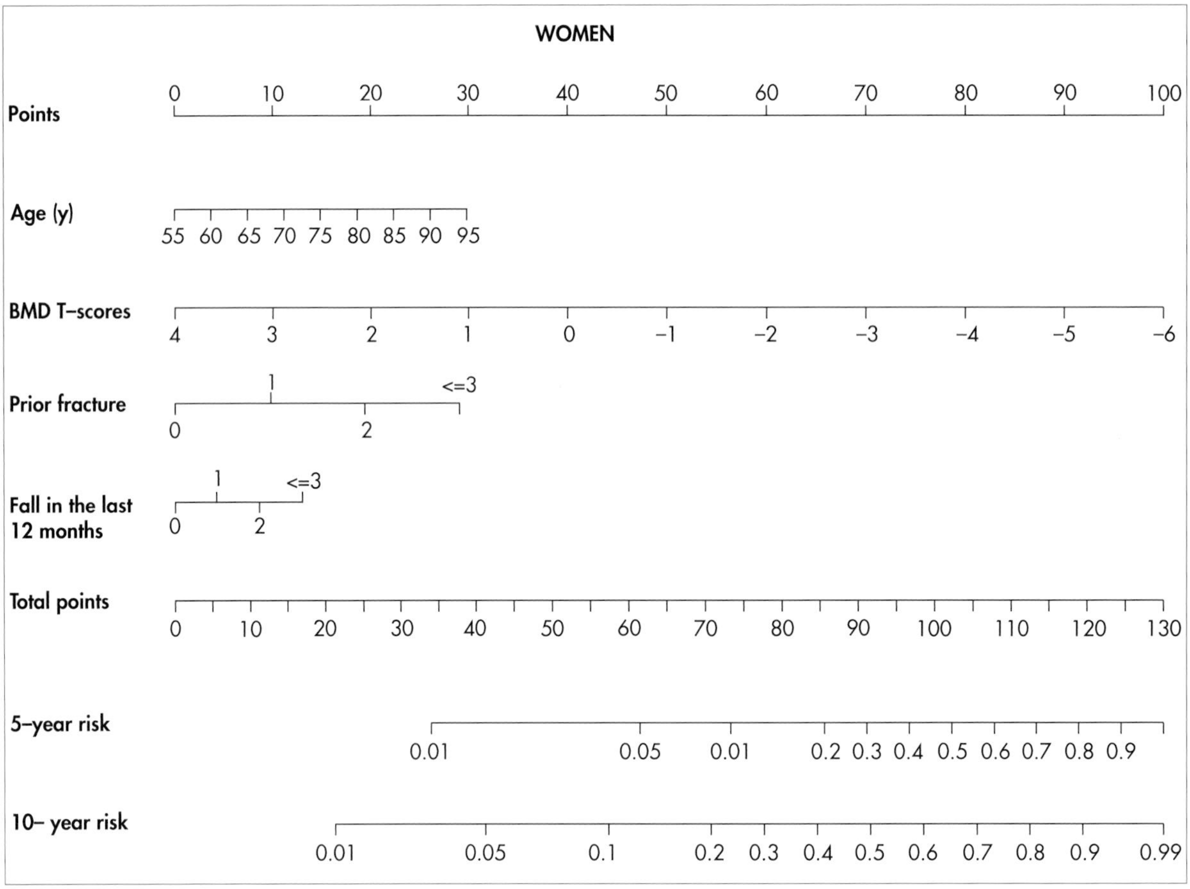

FIGURE 23.1 Nomogram for predicting 5-year and 10-year probability of hip fracture.[69] To use, mark the age of an individual on the 'Age' axis and take a vertical line up to the 'Points' axis. Repeat this process for each additional risk factor, then sum the points. Locate the final sum on the 'Total points' axis and take a vertical line down to the 5-year and 10-year risk lines to determine the individual's probability of sustaining a hip fracture within these timeframes

individual can have the same risk of fracture as a non-osteoporotic individual. A logical and appropriate assessment of fracture risk for an individual should therefore take into account the individual's risk profile, including BMD and a history of fracture. A multivariable-based nomogram such as the one developed by Nguyen and colleagues[69,70] and the WHO's FRAX model[71] can be used to estimate an individual's absolute risk of fracture, and help select patients suitable for intervention.

The critical question of who should be treated can only be answered by a complete evaluation of an individual's risk profile. Treatment is cost-effective if an individual's 10-year risk of hip fracture is between 1.2% and 9.0%, depending on age.[72] To facilitate the estimation of this threshold, a nomogram (Figure 23.1) is used to estimate the probability of fracture based on age, BMD and history of fractures and falls.

TREATMENT

Lifestyle advice

- Exercise—childhood and adolescence are particularly important life stages for laying down bone mass through exercise. Physical activity is an essential part of maintenance of bone mass in adulthood. It is also an essential part of rehabilitation, falls prevention and treatment of established osteoporosis.
- Resistance training.
- Eliminate avoidable risk factors—such as smoking, excessive alcohol.
- Ensure adequate nutrition.
- Safe exposure to sunlight.
- Eliminate or substitute, where possible, drugs likely to cause or contribute to osteoporosis (e.g. steroids, SSRIs, anticonvulsant drugs).
- Stress management.
- Control of any underlying chronic medical conditions.

Nutrition and supplements

Nutrition

Preventive nutrition begins in early childhood. Adequate levels of calcium intake can maximise the positive effect of physical activity on bone health during the growth period of children. Adequate dietary magnesium and calcium intake throughout life is essential to bone health.

Higher dietary protein intake is associated with a lower rate of age-related bone loss,[73] and fruit and vegetable intake is positively associated with bone density in men and women.[74]

Salt intake should be reduced.

Calcium and vitamin D

A combination of calcium and vitamin D reduces the incidence of hip and non-vertebral fractures.[75–77] Elderly women (aged 69+ years) taking calcium (1200 mg/day) and vitamin D (800 IU) for 18 months had their risk of hip fracture reduced by 43% and non-vertebral fracture by 32%, although in a recent meta-analysis it was shown that the use of calcium or calcium plus vitamin D reduced fracture risk by 12%.[55] In summary, calcium and vitamin D appear to be efficacious in reducing the risk of hip fracture and non-vertebral fractures. There is some evidence, however, that calcium supplements can lead to a moderately increased risk of myocardial infarction. Regular moderate sun exposure should also be remembered as a valuable way of maintaining adequate vitamin D levels. If vitamin D levels are very low (< 50 nmol/L[2]), a large loading dose of vitamin D of up to 50,000 IU per month until the level is at least > 75 nmol/L[2] and then a maintenance dose of 2000 IU daily with 3-monthly monitoring.[78] Some advocate a larger loading dose of 100,000 IU as being helpful in bringing up the levels more quickly, followed by a supplement of 1000–5000 IU daily, monitored at 3-monthly intervals until normal range is achieved. Then maintenance of 1000 IU daily if sun exposure has not increased.

Pharmacological

During the past two decades, several major advances in the treatment of osteoporosis have been made. There are now more therapeutic options available than at any time before. Anti-fracture therapies can be broadly divided into two groups: *anti-resorptive* and *bone-forming* (anabolic) agents. The former reduces bone turnover, while the latter increases bone formation. Both agents have been shown to reduce fracture risk for some, although not necessarily all, fragility fractures. It is difficult to assess the relative anti-fracture efficacy of the various therapies, as there have not been any head-to-head comparative trials.

Hormone therapy

Hormone therapy (HT) has been used in treating osteoporosis for some time, despite there having been no randomised controlled trial or large-scale prospective studies of the efficacy of HT in postmenopausal women with osteoporosis or a pre-existing fracture. The Women's Health Initiatives (WHI) study found that HT reduced the risk of hip fracture by an average of 34%, vertebral fracture by 34% and all fractures by 24%.[79–81] However, women on HT in the HERS study (designed to evaluate the effect of oestrogen plus progestin on the risk of coronary heart disease) found no significant reduction in hip fracture risk and any fracture.[80] Still, a recent meta-analysis of women who had been treated with HT for 12–120 months showed that HT could reduce non-vertebral fracture risk by 28% and vertebral fracture risk.[82] Although these data collectively suggest that HT may reduce fracture risk with a modest efficacy, its anti-fracture benefit must be weighed against other adverse effects such as increased risk of breast cancer, thromboembolic disease and stroke.

Selective oestrogen receptor modulators

In postmenopausal women suffering from osteoporosis, raloxifene (at the dose of 60 mg/day) has been shown to significantly reduce the risk of vertebral fracture by as much as 50%.[83,84] However, its effects on hip and non-vertebral fractures have not been consistent. Raloxifene could also reduce the risk of non-vertebral fractures in women with severe osteoporosis. The drug is mostly used in younger postmenopausal women who have bone loss predominantly at the spine, not the hip.

Calcitonin

Calcitonin (generally given as a nasal spray), due to its antiresorptive properties, has been used in the treatment of osteoporosis for many years, with significant beneficial effects in reducing bone loss and fracture risk, possibly up to 33% when combined with calcium (1000 mg/day) and vitamin D (400 IU per day).[85] Similar risk reduction was also observed in those with a pre-existing vertebral fracture.[85] A meta-analysis including four studies conducted between 1966 and 2000 found that calcitonin reduced vertebral fracture risk by 54%. However, its effect on non-vertebral fractures has not been shown. Calcitonin is also associated with pain relief in patients following acute osteoporotic vertebral fractures.

Bisphosphonates

Bisphosphonates are currently a mainstay of pharmacological therapy for the treatment of osteoporosis in both postmenopausal women and elderly men. Bisphosphonates inhibit bone resorption through their effects on osteoclasts, and other complex cellular mechanisms that are not well understood. Their potential benefits need to be weighed against the risk of side effects, including jaw necrosis in long-term use.

There are a number of agents in this class, and based on their mode of action they can be classified into two main groups: those that closely resemble pyrophosphate (clodronate and etidronate), and nitrogen-containing bisphosphonates (alendronate, risedronate and ibandronate). Currently, alendronate (Fosamax®), risedronate (Actonel®) and ibandronate (Boniva®) are FDA-approved for osteoporosis treatment.

- *Alendronate*—has been extensively studied in the treatment and prevention of fracture. In a three-year study of postmenopausal women[86] it significantly reduced the incidence of new fractures, possibly by up to 47% over three years.[87] In this group of patients it also reduced the risk of hip fracture and wrist fracture. It is effective in the treatment of glucocorticoid-induced osteoporosis, increases BMD[88,89] and decreases the incidence of vertebral fractures at 2 years (6.8% *vs* 0.7%) in glucocorticoid-treated men and women.[89] It also has beneficial effects in men.[90]
- *Risedronate*—in women with osteoporosis, treatment with risedronate (5 mg/day) for 3 years reduced the incidence of vertebral fractures by 41–49% and non-vertebral fractures by 39–33%.[91–93] Among those with a prior vertebral fracture, it reduced hip fracture by 60%, although no significant reduction of hip fracture may be seen in elderly women who were selected on the basis of clinical risk factors other than low BMD.
- *Other bisphosphonates*—*etidronate* is not FDA-approved for the prevention or treatment of osteoporosis, but it may reduce the risk of vertebral fracture by up to 37%.[94] Nevertheless, concerns about its efficacy and safety have limited its use. *Ibandronate* is FDA-approved for the prevention and treatment of postmenopausal osteoporosis at a dose of 2.5 mg/day, and may reduce vertebral fracture and increase BMD.[95]
- *Zoledronic acid* is more potent than other bisphosphonates such as alendronate and risedronate, and has been approved by the FDA for the treatment of hypercalcaemia of malignancy, multiple myeloma, and bone metastases from solid tumours. It has been found to reduce the incidence of vertebral fractures by 70%, clinical vertebral fracture by 77%, and hip fracture by 41%.[96]

Parathyroid hormone

Parathyroid hormone (PTH) is an anabolic agent[97] and is FDA-approved for the treatment of postmenopausal osteoporosis. Although it has been found to reduce the incidence of fractures in men and women,[98] there is concern regarding osteosarcomas in long-term use. PTH also has a beneficial effect on bone health in men[99,100] and in women with glucocorticoid-induced osteoporosis.[101,102]

Strontium ranelate

Strontium ranelate (SR) is a trace element that stimulates bone formation and suppresses bone resorption.[103,104] Two grams per day has been shown to reduce the incidence of vertebral fractures by 41% over 3 years.

Fluoride

Sodium fluoride is a potent stimulator of bone formation[105] and gained popularity in the 1970s and 1980s.[106] There was, however, concern about the high incidence of side effects, particularly with some formulations, and sodium fluoride therapy has not been shown to be effective in preventing fractures in postmenopausal osteoporosis. There have been no studies in premenopausal women.

Combined therapies

Combining anti-resorptive agents is not recommended, because there is no documented additive benefit or cost consideration. Current data discourage the concomitant use of alendronate and PTH because the bisphosphonate appears to inhibit the anabolic action of PTH. Whether this also applies to other bisphosphonates or inhibitors of resorption remains unknown.

BMD and drug-induced fracture risk reduction

There is no strong (or linear) relationship between increases in BMD or decreases in bone turnover markers and fracture risk reduction. A modest change in BMD may not be an indicator of anti-fracture efficacy.

Who should be treated?

This is a complex issue because it depends on the patient's preference and economic consideration. Experts suggest that pharmacological intervention should be considered for women with:

- a pre-existing fragility fracture and
- a BMD T-score less than –2.5 without a fracture.[107]

Women with BMD in the osteopenic range may require treatment, depending on the number and severity of clinical risk factors.

Duration of treatment

The best duration of treatment is not known yet. Most randomised clinical trials followed patients for 3 years, with the longest study running for 7 years.[102] Therefore, from the principle of evidence-based medicine, it seems that 3-year duration is the logical answer. However, stopping treatment could result in increased bone remodelling, bone loss, structural damage and increased fracture risk. It has been suggested that if treatment restores BMD to the normal range, it may be reasonable to consider stopping treatment and monitoring bone turnover markers and rates of bone loss.[108]

Monitoring response to drug therapy

Testing may be recommended, to monitor a patient's response to osteoporosis therapy. This may include measurement of BMD, or laboratory tests that indicate bone turnover (i.e. rate of new bone formation and breakdown). Testing is typically done before treatment begins, to get a baseline measurement. Laboratory testing may be repeated 3 months after treatment begins, while bone density testing may be repeated after 2 years.

Side effects of bisphosphonates

Most individuals who take bisphosphonates for prevention or treatment of osteoporosis do not have any serious side effects related to the medication. However, there has been concern about a risk from bisphosphonates in patients who require invasive dental work. A problem known as avascular necrosis or osteonecrosis of the jaw has rarely developed in a small number of people who used bisphosphonates in cancer therapy. The risk of this problem is small in patients who take bisphosphonates for osteoporosis prevention and treatment. However, there is a slightly higher risk of this problem when higher doses of bisphosphonates are given intravenously during cancer treatment. Bisphosphonates are not recommended for premenopausal women who could become pregnant, because of the unknown effects on a developing fetus.

Alternative or adjunct therapies

Vitamin K and ipriflavone (a synthetic phyto-oestrogen) are the only alternative therapies for which sufficient data on BMD and fracture outcomes are available for evaluation. Phyto-oestrogens are weak oestrogen-like chemicals produced by plants, which have been shown to have oestrogen agonist and antagonist properties. There are three major groups of naturally occurring phyto-oestrogens: isoflavones (found principally in soybeans and other legumes), lignans (found principally in flax seed, fruits and vegetables) and coumestans (found in bean sprouts and fodder crops). Ecological studies have shown that communities with a high phyto-oestrogen intake (such as Asians living in Asia) have lower rates of hip fracture than North Americans.[109] However, direct epidemiological and clinical evidence for a protective effect of natural phyto-oestrogens in humans is not yet conclusive. Although vitamin K may be efficacious in slowing bone loss in postmenopausal women with osteoporosis, it has not been shown to be superior to calcium and vitamin D. It is not efficacious in preventing bone loss associated with medication-induced ovarian failure.[110] In summary, the data available to date suggest that vitamin K may be efficacious in the treatment of postmenopausal women with severe osteoporosis, but has not been shown to be superior to calcium and vitamin D.[111]

DHEA

Low dehydroepiandrosterone (DHEA) levels have been associated with decreased bone mineral density[112] and an increased risk of fracture. DHEA supplementation is indicated where there is demonstrated to be a low serum DHEA level. Dose begins at 10 mg orally per day, reviewed monthly. The aim is to achieve normal serum level. Excessive levels should be avoided because of potential for androgenic side effects.

OSTEOPOROSIS IN MEN

Because of its oestrogen-related mechanism, osteoporosis has been commonly perceived as a disease of postmenopausal women. However, emerging evidence in recent years suggests that this perception is an oversight, because men are also susceptible to osteoporosis. Indeed, approximately one-third of all fracture cases in the general population occur in men.[113] Furthermore, the lifetime risk of fracture in men is 1 in 4.[3,114] Outcomes of fracture in men are often worse than in women. For instance, men who have sustained a fracture have an increased risk of mortality compared to women.[5] Men are twice as likely as women to die in hospital after a hip fracture.[115] However, most studies of osteoporosis have largely been conducted in women and, as a result, osteoporosis in men has not been well documented.

Men have, on average, higher BMD and lower rate of bone loss than women[4,116] and they tend have a lower risk of fracture at a later age than women.[117] Major risk factors for osteoporosis in men include:

- a history of atraumatic fracture
- osteopenia on radiograph
- glucocorticosteroid use > 5 mg/day
- hypogonadism
- hyperparathyroidism[24,118,119]
- use of anticonvulsant drugs
- excessive alcohol consumption
- tobacco use
- rheumatoid or other inflammatory arthritis
- multiple myeloma or lymphoma
- family history of osteoporosis
- concomitant diseases (e.g. Cushing's disease, chronic liver or kidney disease, pernicious anaemia, gastric resection)
- nutritional calcium, magnesium and/or vitamin D deficiency

Although reduced testosterone is a risk factor for fracture in men,[70] lower level of oestrogen is also a risk factor for low bone mass and fracture.[120–122] Low BMD is a major risk factor for fracture;[18,56,123] therefore, evaluation of BMD by DEXA and radiograph can be used to make a diagnosis of osteoporosis in men. It has been estimated that approximately 10% of men aged 60 years or above have osteoporosis.[4] Prognostic models that take into account various simple risk factors can be used to estimate the risk of fracture for a man.[69] In randomised controlled clinical trials, bisphosphonates[89,124] (alendronate and risedronate) and PTH[125] (teriparatide, recombinant parathyhroid hormone) have been shown to be effective in reducing fracture risk in men. Calcium and vitamin D supplementation can also be useful in preventing osteoporosis and fracture in men.[118]

PREVENTION

Calcium

Calcium is an important component of fracture prevention. Although calcium alone may not prevent osteoporosis, having adequate calcium, whether through food or supplementation, is an important and practical way to maintain bone health. Low dietary calcium intake is associated with lower BMD and increased fracture risk.[4] Up to 75% of women may have a calcium intake (including supplemental calcium) less than the recommended daily intake.[126] Although a lower calcium intake is associated with greater risk of hip fracture,[127] calcium supplementation appears to improve BMD.[128,129] Despite this limited evidence, the public health message is that people should have adequate dietary calcium intake throughout life (Table 23.2). More recently, concerns have arisen regarding a potentially increased risk of myocardial infarction among people taking calcium supplements over the long term.

Vitamin D

Although most calcium is deposited in bone, bone is not just calcium, and calcium does not function in isolation but in interaction with vitamin D—adequate vitamin D is important for bone health, as it regulates the efficiency of calcium absorption. Vitamin D here includes cholecalciferol (vitamin D_3) and ergocalciferol (vitamin D_2). Despite the common perception of Australia as 'sunshine country', there is a high prevalence

TABLE 23.2 Recommended daily calcium intakes*

Age/gender	Recommended daily calcium intake (mg)
< 6 months	300
6 months – 1 year	500
1–3 years	700
4–7 years	900
Girls:	
8–11 years	900
12–15 years	1000
16–18 years	800
Women:	
19–54 years	800
> 54 years	1000
pregnant	1100–1200
Boys:	
8–11 years	800
12–15 years	1200
16–18 years	1000
Men:	
19–64 years	800
> 64 years	800

*Australia, National Health and Medical Research Council

Source: NHMRC 1991[130]

of vitamin D deficiency among elderly people. For example, a study of institutionalised or housebound individuals found that up to 80% of women and 70% of men were deficient in vitamin D and, of these, 97% had a blood level of vitamin D below the median value of the healthy reference range.[131,132]

People with vitamin D deficiency may need a loading dose, depending on the vitamin D levels, and supplementation with 3000–5000 IU vitamin D_3 per day for 12 weeks, before repeating the test o fvitamin D levels and reviewing.[133]

Lifestyle and dietary factors

Lifestyle and dietary factors, including caffeine, alcohol, smoking and salt intake, have been shown to be associated with fracture risk.[134–138] In Caucasian populations, heavy caffeine ingestion (> 4 cups coffee/day) has been shown to be associated with hip fracture in men and women.[139,140] The effect of sodium on bone health remains unclear; however, studies have shown a significant negative effect[141] when daily intake exceeds 2100 mg (90 mmol). Cigarette smoking is a significant risk factor for hip fracture.[134] Modification of lifestyle, including reducing or stopping smoking, and reducing alcohol, caffeine and salt intake, is recommended as a practical way to slow the progression of osteoporosis or to reduce the risk of fracture. Other factors such as dietary magnesium and protein are also important.

Physical activity

Adequate physical activity is an important factor in reducing the risk of fracture and falls[142]; however, excessive physical activity can be harmful to bone health.[143] It is recommended that older adults maintain regular physical activity such as jogging, field and racquet sports and swimming to reduce bone loss and fracture risk. Weight-bearing exercise is the most useful in osteoporosis prevention and management. Appropriate resistance exercise is also recommended.

Fall prevention

In the elderly, approximately one-third of women and 20% of men fall each year.[144] About half of falls occur indoors, mainly in the living room (30%), bathroom/toilet (23%), dining room (14.4%) and bedroom (12.3%). Falls are an important risk factor for fracture.[56] Over 90% of hip fractures are a result of a fall[145] but only 1–2% of all falls of the elderly lead to a hip fracture.[146,147] Therefore, fall prevention is an important approach, to reduce the risk of fracture in the elderly.

Practical strategies of fall prevention include:

- modifying the home to remove slippery surfaces and dangerous furniture
- correcting poor vision
- installing appropriate aids in the bathroom
- modifying medications such as sedatives.

Physical therapies aimed at improving strength and balance, including resistance training and t'ai chi, have been found to be beneficial in reducing falls in the elderly.

POST-FRACTURE MANAGEMENT

An existing fracture increases the risk of subsequent fractures.[8,148,149] Individuals with a personal history fracture—with or without osteoporosis—should be considered for treatment. However, several studies have suggested a very low uptake of treatment. In a study of 502 hip-fracture patients in a hospital setting, only 14% underwent BMD scan, 13% received calcium/vitamin D, and only 18% received HRT, calcitonin or bisphosphonates.[150] Other studies have reported that only 5% of patients with recent hip fractures left the hospital with a new medication prescribed to reduce the risk of subsequent fractures.[151–153] Most women attending primary care physicians who reported a fracture after menopause are not on any specific anti-osteoporotic therapy.[153] Thus, despite both the magnitude of the problem and the introduction of osteoporosis treatment guidelines, most high-risk individuals (possibly 80%) are still not identified, and therefore not treated. An information-based intervention could increase the uptake of anti-fracture treatment among high-risk patients.[154] Other strategies for improving treatment uptake include fracture discharge pathways, increased nurse contact and patient education.

There was a concern that anti-resorptive therapies may interfere with the bone healing process; however, there is no consistent evidence that the use of anti-resorptive agents soon after fracture impairs fracture healing. There is a view that older patients with a pre-existing fracture may not benefit from treatment. However, evidence from clinical trials clearly indicates that older patients with fracture benefit from anti-osteoporosis therapy, similarly to younger individuals.

RICKETS

Rickets is a condition associated with softening of bones, leaving them vulnerable to deformity and fracture. The main cause is vitamin D deficiency, although a significant and prolonged poor intake or malabsorption of calcium can also cause it.

Rickets was a once common bone disease of children and it is still common in poorer countries where nutrition is inadequate. Although far less common until recently in developed countries, it is now making a comeback in many places around the world, probably due to inadequate sun exposure leading to inadequate vitamin D levels. This rise in the incidence of rickets can be contributed to by a predominance of indoor activities, physical inactivity and an over-aggressive approach to sun protection. The breastfeeding children of mothers with inadequate vitamin D levels are also more likely to develop rickets. Dark-skinned children, especially those living in countries with relatively low levels of sunlight, are at greater risk, as are children who are not consuming milk. Vitamin D deficiency can also result in hypocalcaemia and hyperexcitability of muscles.

SYMPTOMS

The symptoms associated with rickets include:

- bone deformities:
  - most obvious in the legs, with bowlegs (genu varum) in young children developing into knock-knees (genu valgum) in older children
  - soft skull and square-headed appearance
  - dental problems
  - costochondral swelling (rickety rosary)
  - widening of the wrist
- poor growth
- bone pain
- neuromuscular problems—including muscle weakness and tetany due to hypocalcaemia
- fractures—due to bone softening, all fractures, particularly greenstick, are more common.

DIAGNOSIS

Rickets is classically diagnosed on the clinical picture in association with the following tests.

- X-rays—revealing classic deformities listed above
- low serum calcium and serum phosphorus
- high serum alkaline phosphatase (ALP)
- low vitamin D.

MANAGEMENT

If diagnosed and managed in childhood, the problems associated with rickets respond well without long-term disability or deformity. If not managed, however, the deformities can become permanent.

Clinically evident rickets requires co-management with a paediatric endocrinologist.

Neonates and infants under 3 months:

- vitamin D level 25–50 nmol/L—400 IU vitamin D_3 (cholecalciferol daily)
- vitamin D level < 25 nmol/L—1000 IU daily for 3 months.

Infants 4–12 months:

- vitamin D level 25–50 nmol/L—50,000 IU stat or 400 IU daily for 3 months, then maintenance 400 IU daily
- vitamin D level < 25 nmol/L—100,000 IU stat or 1000 IU daily for 3 months, then maintenance 400 IU daily.

Children and adolescents 1–18 years:

- vitamin D level 25–50 nmol/L—150,000 IU stat or 1000–2000 IU daily for 3 months
- vitamin D level < 25 nmol/L—150,000 IU stat repeated at 6 weeks, or 1000–2000 IU daily for 6 months plus regular moderate safe sun exposure (ultraviolet B).

For all ages, re-check vitamin D, calcium, phosphate and ALP at 3 months, then vitamin D and ALP annually.

Cod liver oil is also a good source of vitamin D but should not be considered for high-dose vitamin D, because of concerns about vitamin A toxicity. Generally speaking, 10–20 minutes per day is sufficient exposure on a regular basis, with the amount of sun exposure with skin unprotected by sunscreen and/or glass varying according to the season, colour of the skin and latitude. Avoiding sunburn is of course advisable, to avoid the risk of melanoma; and if a child is going to be out in the sun for a more prolonged period of time, particularly in the summer months of the year, then all the usual measures for sun protection should be undertaken. Increasing the dietary intake of calcium is also advisable.

OSTEOMALACIA

Osteomalacia is a milder form of rickets seen in adults. It is also a softening of the bone due to vitamin D deficiency causing poor bone mineralisation. It is associated with diffuse bone pain, weakness and a tendency to fracture. Adults at particular risk of osteomalacia are those who have inadequate ultraviolet B exposure, such as those with dark skin who are living in countries with low levels of sunlight, those who cover their skin for cultural reasons and institutionalised elderly perople who rarely go outdoors. It can also be found in people with a poor diet or who are unable to absorb vitamin D from their food due to malabsorption or coeliac disease. Patients with chronic renal failure and renal tubular acidosis can also suffer from osteomalacia.

The symptoms of and laboratory tests for osteomalacia are similar to those for rickets and osteoporosis. A technetium bone scan will indicate increased bone activity, and X-rays may also show pseudofractures (Looser's zones).

Management of osteomalacia is by administration of vitamin D_3. A very low vitamin D level can be an indication for a larger stat dose of vitamin D, for example 100,000 IU IM or orally as drops, followed by a maintenance dose of 10,000–20,000 IU per week until the vitamin D levels are again adequate. A lower maintenance dose may then be required, particularly if the cause of vitamin D deficiency cannot be resolved. Malabsorption syndromes may require vitamin D injections rather than oral administration.

PAGET'S DISEASE

Paget's disease (osteitis deformans) is a condition of bone that tends to affect the elderly. About 10% of 90-year-olds have it, although a great proportion of these will be asymptomatic. Paget's disease is of uncertain origin, although a viral aetiology is suspected. A genetic predisposition may also play a role, and men are more commonly affected than women.

The pathological process in Paget's disease involves bone resorption by osteoclasts, followed by new, softer bone being laid down by osteoblasts—that is, there is an increase in bone turnover. The new bone being laid down tends to be more disorganised—the so-called 'mosaic' pattern—and is hypervascular, which can cause problems during surgery.

SYMPTOMS

Some patients with Paget's disease will be diagnosed based on tests taken for other reasons, such as X-ray findings or serum ALP levels. For patients who are symptomatic, the following are common symptoms:

- bone pain—in affected bones, most commonly the spine; it is like a deep aching feeling, often worse at night, causing disturbed sleep.
- joint pain and osteoarthritis—particularly of the hip or knee
- headaches—can be associated with Paget's disease of the skull
- sometimes growth of the bones of the skull can also cause hearing loss or pressure on other cranial or spinal nerves
- bone deformity—such as enlargement of the skull, spreading of the teeth or bowing of the tibia
- gait problems
- cardiovascular complications—including calcification of the aortic valve and cardiac failure, in severe Paget's disease
- kidney stones—more common in people with Paget's disease.

DIAGNOSIS

Diagnosis can be made clinically and confirmed by the following tests where indicated:

- X-ray or skeletal survey showing areas of dense and thickened bone
- raised ALP—can also be useful in monitoring the level of disease activity
- normal calcium and phosphate levels
- radioisotope bone scans—can help to gauge the level of disease activity.

Although an uncommon presentation, bony metastases from prostate cancer can mimic X-ray lesions suggestive or Paget's disease, and so it will be helpful to exclude this before confirming a new diagnosis of Paget's disease in an elderly male. Osteogenic sarcoma is also a rare complication of Paget's disease.

MANAGEMENT

If treated early, the outcome for Paget's disease patients is good, in terms of slowing the progression of the condition and associated symptoms. The disease process, however, and the secondary impact of it, will not go away.

General measures as outlined in the chapter on pain management (Ch 38) will be useful for those with more severe and chronic pain. The mainstays of medical management are aimed at reducing pain and minimising deformities that can lead to complications such as hearing loss. Drugs commonly used for Paget's disease (see the section above on osteoporosis) are:

- bisphosphonates—generally considered first-line therapy
- calcitonin.

Surgery can sometimes be necessary for those who have severely involved joints, after fractures or when bone deformity is causing significant problems.

Lifestyle measures such as adequate vitamin D_3 intake (a supplement of 1000 IU daily may be beneficial), regular moderate sun exposure and calcium intake are recommended. Regular exercise is important for maintaining healthy weight, mobility and bone integrity. Patients should discuss the appropriate level and form of exercise with a healthcare professional.

BONE CANCER

As with tumours of other parts of the body, primary bone tumours can be benign or malignant. Bone is a common site for metastases from other parts of the body, such as breast and prostate, and can be involved in haematological malignancies involving the bone marrow, such as multiple myeloma and leukaemia.

Benign bone tumours include osteoma, bone cysts and osteochondroma. Malignant tumours of the bone include osteogenic sarcoma, chondrosarcoma and Ewing's tumour. Although bone tumours are not one of the more common tumours, they tend to be aggressive and need to be diagnosed and treated early.

The most common presentation of bone tumours is worsening bone pain (characteristically worst at night) and pathological fractures, particularly of the long bones. They are diagnosed by X-ray and biopsy.

As with other tumours, the management approaches for bone cancer are primarily:

- surgical—amputation of the affected bone/limb
- chemotherapy
- radiotherapy
- symptomatic management—e.g. managing pain, phantom pain, nausea, treatment-related side effects

- lifestyle management as outlined in the cancer chapter
- complementary therapies—many will be helpful with symptomatic control.

The chapter on cancer (Ch 24) outlines these various therapies in more detail.

RESOURCES

Dubbo Osteoporosis Epidemiology Study, fracture risk calculator, http://www.fractureriskcalculator.com

World Health Organization, Prevention and management of osteoporosis (report, 2003), http://whqlibdoc.who.int/trs/WHO_TRS_921.pdf

REFERENCES

1 Anonymous. Consensus development conference: prophylaxis and treatment of osteoporosis. Am J Med 1991; 90(1):107–110.

2 NIH Consensus Development Panel on Osteoporosis. Osteoporosis prevention, diagnosis and therapy. JAMA 2001; 285:785–795.

3 Nguyen ND, Ahlborg HG, Center JR et al. Residual lifetime risk of fractures in women and men. J Bone Miner Res 2007; 22(6):781–788.

4 Nguyen TV, Center JR, Eisman JA. Osteoporosis in elderly men and women: effects of dietary calcium, physical activity, and body mass index. J Bone Miner Res 2000; 15(2):322–331.

5 Center JR, Nguyen TV, Schneider D et al. Mortality after all major types of osteoporotic fracture in men and women: an observational study. Lancet 1999; 353(9156):878–882.

6 Cauley JA, Thompson DE, Ensrud KC et al. Risk of mortality following clinical fractures. Osteoporos Int 2000; 11(7):556–561.

7 Cooper C, Atkinson EJ, Jacobsen SJ et al. Population-based study of survival after osteoporotic fractures. Am J Epidemiol 1993; 137(9):1001–1005.

8 Pongchaiyakul C, Nguyen ND, Jones G et al. Asymptomatic vertebral deformity as a major risk factor for subsequent fractures and mortality: a long-term prospective study. J Bone Miner Res 2005; 20(8):1349–1355.

9 Lindsay R. The burden of osteoporosis: cost. Am J Med 1995; 98(2A):9S–11S.

10 Wiktorowicz ME, Goeree R, Papaioannou A et al. Economic implications of hip fracture: health service use, institutional care and cost in Canada. Osteoporos Int 2001; 12(4):271–278.

11 Access Economics Pty Ltd. The burden of brittle bones: costing osteoporosis in Australia. Canberra, ACT: Access Economics Pty Ltd; 2001.

12 Cooper C, Shah S, Hand DJ et al. Screening for vertebral osteoporosis using individual risk factors. The Multicentre Vertebral Fracture Study Group. Osteoporos Int 1991; 2(1):48–53.

13 Cooper C. Bone mass, muscle function and fracture of the proximal femur. Br J Hosp Med 1989; 42(4):277–280.

14 Cumming RG, Klineberg RJ. Epidemiological study of the relation between arthritis of the hip and hip fractures. Ann Rheum Dis 1993; 52(10):707–710.

15 Cummings SR, Kelsey JL, Nevitt MC et al. Epidemiology of osteoporosis and osteoporotic fractures. Epidemiol Rev 1985; 7:178–208.

16 Nguyen T, Sambrook P, Kelly P et al. Prediction of osteoporotic fractures by postural instability and bone density. BMJ 1993; 307(6912):1111–1115.

17 Seeley DG, Kelsey J, Jergas M et al. Predictors of ankle and foot fractures in older women. The Study of Osteoporotic Fractures Research Group. J Bone Miner Res 1996; 11(9):1347–1355.

18 Nguyen TV, Center JR, Sambrook PN et al. Risk factors for proximal humerus, forearm, and wrist fractures in elderly men and women: the Dubbo Osteoporosis Epidemiology Study. Am J Epidemiol 2001; 153(6): 587–595.

19 Kanis JA, Oden A, Johnell O et al. The burden of osteoporotic fractures: a method for setting intervention thresholds. Osteoporos Int 2001; 12(5):417–427.

20 Compston JE, Cooper C, Kanis JA. Bone densitometry in clinical practice. BMJ 1995; 310(6993):1507–1510.

21 Kanis JA, Devogelaer JP, Gennari C. Practical guide for the use of bone mineral measurements in the assessment of treatment of osteoporosis: a position paper of the European foundation for osteoporosis and bone disease. The Scientific Advisory Board and the Board of National Societies. Osteoporos Int 1996; 6(3):256–261.

22 LeBoff MS, Bermas B, Ginsburg E et al. Osteoporosis. Guide to prevention, diagnosis, and treatment. Boston, MA: Brigham and Women's Hospital; 2001.

23 Melton LJ III, Atkinson EJ, O'Connor MK et al. Fracture prediction by BMD in men versus women. J Bone Miner Res 1997; 12(Suppl 1):S362.

24 Nguyen TV, Eisman JA, Kelly PJ et al. Risk factors for osteoporotic fractures in elderly men. Am J Epidemiol 1996; 144(3):255–263.

25 Keen RW, Hart DJ, Arden NK et al. Family history of appendicular fracture and risk of osteoporosis: a population-based study. Osteoporos Int 1999; 10(2):161–166.

26 Hu R, Mustard CA, Burns C. Epidemiology of incident spinal fracture in a complete population. Spine 1996; 21(4):492–499.

27 Sanders KM, Seeman E, Ugoni AM et al. Age- and gender-specific rate of fractures in Australia: a population-based study. Osteoporos Int 1999; 10(3):240–247.

28 Johnell O, Melton LJ III, Nilsson JA. Are annual fluctuations in hip fracture incidence dependent upon the underlying mortality rate? Osteoporos Int 1998; 8(2):192–195.
29 Melton LJ III, Crowson CS, O'Fallon WM. Fracture incidence in Olmsted County, Minnesota: comparison of urban with rural rates and changes in urban rates over time. Osteoporos Int 1999; 9(1):29–37.
30 Keene GS, Parker MJ, Pryor GA. Mortality and morbidity after hip fractures. BMJ 1993; 307(6914):1248–1250.
31 Wehren LE, Orwig DL, Hebel JR et al. Gender differences in mortality after hip fracture: the role of infection. J Bone Miner Res 2003; 18(12): 2231–2237.
32 Goeree R, O'Brien B, Pettit D et al. An assessment of the burden of illness due to osteoporosis in Canada. J Soc Obstet Gynaecol Can 1996; 18:15–24.
33 Randell AG, Nguyen TV, Bhalerao N et al. Deterioration in quality of life following hip fracture: a prospective study. Osteoporos Int 2000; 11(5):460–466.
34 Delmas PD, van de Langerijt L, Watts NB et al. Underdiagnosis of vertebral fractures is a worldwide problem: the IMPACT study. J Bone Miner Res 2005; 20(4):557–563.
35 Genant HK, Jergas M. Assessment of prevalent and incident vertebral fractures in osteoporosis research. Osteoporos Int 2003; 14(Suppl 3):S43–S55.
36 Black DM, Cummings SR, Stone K et al. A new approach to defining normal vertebral dimensions. J Bone Miner Res 1991; 6(8):883–892.
37 McCloskey EV, Spector TD, Eyres KS et al. The assessment of vertebral deformity: a method for use in population studies and clinical trials. Osteoporos Int 1993; 3(3):138–147.
38 O'Neill TW, Felsenberg D, Varlow J et al. The prevalence of vertebral deformity in european men and women: the European Vertebral Osteoporosis Study. J Bone Miner Res 1996; 11(7):1010–1018.
39 de Nijs RN, Bijlsma JW, Lems WF et al. Osteoporosis Working Group, Dutch Society for Rheumatology. Prevalence of vertebral deformities and symptomatic vertebral fractures in corticosteroid treated patients with rheumatoid arthritis. Rheumatology (Oxford) 2001; 40(12):1375–1385.
40 Jones G, White C, Nguyen T et al. Prevalent vertebral deformities: relationship to bone mineral density and spinal osteophytosis in elderly men and women. Osteoporos Int 1996; 6(3):233–239.
41 Kanis JA, Johnell O, Oden A et al. The risk and burden of vertebral fractures in Sweden. Osteoporos Int 2004; 15(1):20–26.
42 Nevitt MC, Ettinger B, Black DM et al. The association of radiographically detected vertebral fractures with back pain and function: a prospective study. Ann Intern Med 1998; 128(10):793–800.
43 O'Neill TW, Cockerill W, Matthis C et al. Back pain, disability, and radiographic vertebral fracture in European women: a prospective study. Osteoporos Int 2004; 15(9):760–765.
44 Cockerill W, Lunt M, Silman AJ et al. Health-related quality of life and radiographic vertebral fracture. Osteoporos Int 2004; 15(2):113–119.
45 Kado DM, Duong T, Stone KL et al. Incident vertebral fractures and mortality in older women: a prospective study. Osteoporos Int 2003; 14(7):589–594.
46 Eastell R. Forearm fracture. Bone 1996; 18(Suppl 3):203S–207S.
47 Cuddihy MT, Gabriel SE, Crowson CS et al. Forearm fractures as predictors of subsequent osteoporotic fractures. Osteoporos Int 1999; 9(6):469–475.
48 de Bruijn HP. The Colles' fracture, review and literature. Acta Orthop Scand 1987; 58(Suppl 23):7–25.
49 Cooney WP III, Dobyns JH, Linscheid RL. Complications of Colles' fractures. J Bone Joint Surg Am 1980; 62(4):613–619.
50 Melton LJ III, Amadio PC, Crowson CS et al. Long-term trends in the incidence of distal forearm fractures. Osteoporos Int 1998; 8(4):341–348.
51 Ismail AA, Cockerill W, Cooper C et al. Prevalent vertebral deformity predicts incident hip though not distal forearm fracture: results from the European Prospective Osteoporosis Study. Osteoporos Int 2001; 12(2):85–90.
52 Klotzbuecher CM, Ross PD, Landsman PB et al. Patients with prior fractures have an increased risk of future fractures: a summary of the literature and statistical synthesis. J Bone Miner Res 2000; 15(4): 721–739.
53 Ammann P, Rizzoli R. Bone strength and its determinants. Osteoporos Int 2003; 14(Suppl 3):S13–S18.
54 Johnell O, Kanis JA, Oden A et al. Predictive value of BMD for hip and other fractures. J Bone Miner Res 2005; 20(7):1185–1194.
55 Kung AW, Lee KK, Ho AK et al. Ten-year risk of osteoporotic fractures in postmenopausal Chinese women according to clinical risk factors and BMD T-scores: a prospective study. J Bone Miner Res 2007; 22(7):1080–1087.
56 Nguyen ND, Pongchaiyakul C, Center JR et al. Identification of high-risk individuals for hip fracture: a 14-year prospective study. J Bone Miner Res 2005; 20(11):1921–1928.
57 Marshall D, Johnell O, Wedel H. Meta-analysis of how well measures of bone mineral density predict occurrence of osteoporotic fractures. BMJ 1996; 312(7041):1254–1259.

58 Kanis JA, Melton LJ III, Christiansen C et al. The diagnosis of osteoporosis. J Bone Miner Res 1994; 9(8):1137–1141.
59 Writing Group for the ISCD Position Development Conference. Diagnosis of osteoporosis in men, premenopausal women, and children. J Clin Densitom 2004; 7(1):17–26.
60 Nolla JM, Gómez-Vaquero C, Fiter J et al. Usefulness of bone densitometry in postmenopausal women with clinically diagnosed vertebral fractures. Ann Rheum Dis 2002; 61:73–75.
61 Delmas PD, Rizzoli R, Cooper C et al. Treatment of patients with postmenopausal osteoporosis is worthwhile. The position of the International Osteoporosis Foundation. Osteoporos Int 2005; 16(1):1–5.
62 Koh LK, Sedrine WB, Torralba TP et al. A simple tool to identify Asian women at increased risk of osteoporosis. Osteoporos Int 2001; 12(8):699–705.
63 Pongchaiyakul C, Nguyen ND, Nguyen TV. Development and validation of a new clinical risk index for prediction of osteoporosis in Thai women. J Med Assoc Thai 2004; 87(8):910–916.
64 Nguyen TV. Individualization of osteoporosis risk. Osteoporos Int 2007; 18(9):1153–1156.
65 Hillier TA, Stone KL, Bauer DC et al. Evaluating the value of repeat bone mineral density measurement and prediction of fractures in older women: the study of osteoporotic fractures. Arch Intern Med 2007; 167(2):155–160.
66 van Daele PL, Seibel MJ, Burger H et al. Case-control analysis of bone resorption markers, disability, and hip fracture risk: the Rotterdam study. BMJ 1996; 312(7029):482–483.
67 Eastell R, Barton I, Hannon RA et al. Relationship of early changes in bone resorption to the reduction in fracture risk with risedronate. J Bone Miner Res 2003; 18(6):1051–1056.
68 Nguyen TV, Meier C, Center JR et al. Bone turnover in elderly men: relationships to change in bone mineral density. BMC Musculoskelet Disord 2007; 8(1):13.
69 Nguyen ND, Frost SA, Center JR et al. Development of prognostic nomograms for individualizing 5-year and 10-year fracture risks. Osteoporos Int 2008; 19(10):1431–1444.
70 Meier C, Nguyen TV, Handelsman DJ et al. Endogenous sex hormones and incident fracture risk in older men: the Dubbo Osteoporosis Epidemiology Study. Arch Intern Med 2008; 168(1):47–54.
71 Kanis JA, Johnell O, Oden A et al. FRAX and the assessment of fracture probability in men and women from the UK. Osteoporos Int 2008; 19(4):385–397.
72 Kanis JA, Borgstrom F, Zethraeus N et al. Intervention thresholds for osteoporosis in the UK. Bone 2005; 36(1):22–32.
73 Hannan MT, Tucker KL, Dawson-Hughes B et al. Effect of dietary protein on bone loss in elderly men and women: the Framingham Osteoporosis Study. J Bone Miner Res 2000; 15:2504.
74 Tucker KL, Hannan MT, Chen H et al. Potassium, magnesium, and fruit and vegetable intakes are associated with greater bone mineral density in elderly men and women. Am J Clin Nutr 1999; 69:727.
75 Chapuy MC, Arlot ME, Duboeuf F et al. Vitamin D_3 and calcium to prevent hip fractures in the elderly woman. N Engl J Med 1992; 327(23):1637–1642.
76 Chapuy MC, Pamphile R, Paris E et al. Combined calcium and vitamin D_3 supplementation in elderly women: confirmation of reversal of secondary hyperparathyroidism and hip fracture risk: the Decalyos II study. Osteoporos Int 2002; 13(3):257–264.
77 Dawson-Hughes B, Harris SS, Krall EA et al. Effect of calcium and vitamin D supplementation on bone density in men and women 65 years of age or older. N Engl J Med 1997; 337(10):670–676.
78 Victorian Government (Australia), Department of Health. Low vitamin D in Victoria: key health promotion messages for community health workers; December 2009. Online. Available: http://www.health.vic.gov.au/chiefhealthofficer/downloads/vitamin_d_comm.pdf
79 Anderson GL, Limacher M, Assaf AR et al. Effects of conjugated equine estrogen in postmenopausal women with hysterectomy: the Women's Health Initiative randomized controlled trial. JAMA 2004; 291(14):1701–1712.
80 Wedick NM, Barrett-Connor E, Knoke JD et al. The relationship between weight loss and all-cause mortality in older men and women with and without diabetes mellitus: the Rancho Bernardo Study. J Am Geriatr Soc 2002; 50(11):1810–1815.
81 Rossouw JE, Anderson GL, Prentice RL et al. Risks and benefits of estrogen plus progestin in healthy postmenopausal women: principal results From the Women's Health Initiative randomized controlled trial. JAMA 2002; 288(3):321–333.
82 Torgerson DJ, Bell-Syer SE. Hormone replacement therapy and prevention of nonvertebral fractures: a meta-analysis of randomized trials. JAMA 2001; 285(22):2891–2897.
83 Ettinger B, Black DM, Mitlak BH et al. Reduction of vertebral fracture risk in postmenopausal women with osteoporosis treated with raloxifene: results from a 3-year randomized clinical trial. Multiple Outcomes of Raloxifene Evaluation (MORE) Investigators. JAMA 1999; 282(7):637–645.
84 Delmas PD, Ensrud KE, Adachi JD et al. Efficacy of raloxifene on vertebral fracture risk reduction in postmenopausal women with osteoporosis: four-year

results from a randomized clinical trial. J Clin Endocrinol Metab 2002; 87(8):3609–3617.
85 Chesnut CH III, Silverman S, Andriano K et al. A randomized trial of nasal spray salmon calcitonin in postmenopausal women with established osteoporosis: the prevent recurrence of osteoporotic fractures study. PROOF Study Group. Am J Med 2000; 109(4):267–276.
86 Liberman UA, Weiss SR, Broll J et al. Effect of oral alendronate on bone mineral density and the incidence of fractures in postmenopausal osteoporosis. The Alendronate Phase III Osteoporosis Treatment Study Group. N Engl J Med 1995; 333(22):1437–1443.
87 Black DM, Cummings SR, Karpf DB et al. Randomised trial of effect of alendronate on risk of fracture in women with existing vertebral fractures. Fracture Intervention Trial Research Group. Lancet 1996; 348(9041):1535–1541.
88 Saag KG, Emkey R, Schnitzer TJ et al. Alendronate for the prevention and treatment of glucocorticoid-induced osteoporosis. Glucocorticoid-Induced Osteoporosis Intervention Study Group. N Engl J Med 1998; 339(5):292–299.
89 Adachi JD, Saag KG, Delmas PD et al. Two-year effects of alendronate on bone mineral density and vertebral fracture in patients receiving glucocorticoids: a randomized, double-blind, placebo-controlled extension trial. Arthritis Rheum 2001; 44(1):202–211.
90 Orwoll E, Ettinger M, Weiss S et al. Alendronate for the treatment of osteoporosis in men. N Engl J Med 2000; 343(9):604–610.
91 Harris ST, Watts NB, Genant HK et al. Effects of risedronate treatment on vertebral and nonvertebral fractures in women with postmenopausal osteoporosis: a randomized controlled trial. Vertebral Efficacy With Risedronate Therapy (VERT) Study Group. JAMA 1999; 282(14):1344–1352.
92 Reginster J, Minne HW, Sorensen OH et al. Randomized trial of the effects of risedronate on vertebral fractures in women with established postmenopausal osteoporosis. Vertebral Efficacy with Risedronate Therapy (VERT) Study Group. Osteoporos Int 2000; 11(1):83–91.
93 McClung MR, Geusens P, Miller PD et al. Effect of risedronate on the risk of hip fracture in elderly women. Hip Intervention Program Study Group. N Engl J Med 2001; 344(5):333–340.
94 Cranney A, Guyatt G, Krolicki N et al. A meta-analysis of etidronate for the treatment of postmenopausal osteoporosis. Osteoporos Int 2001; 12(2):140–151.
95 Chesnut IC, Skag A, Christiansen C et al. Effects of oral ibandronate administered daily or intermittently on fracture risk in postmenopausal osteoporosis. J Bone Miner Res 2004; 19(8):1241–1249.
96 Black DM, Delmas PD, Eastell R et al. Once–yearly zoledronic acid for treatment of postmenopausal osteoporosis. N Engl J Med 2007; 356(18):1809–1822.
97 Reeve J, Meunier PJ, Parsons JA et al. Anabolic effect of human parathyroid hormone fragment on trabecular bone in involutional osteoporosis: a multicentre trial. BMJ 1980; 280(6228):1340–1344.
98 Neer RM, Arnaud CD, Zanchetta JR et al. Effect of parathyroid hormone (1–34) on fractures and bone mineral density in postmenopausal women with osteoporosis. N Engl J Med 2001; 344(19):1434–1441.
99 Slovik DM, Adams JS, Neer RM et al. Deficient production of 1,25–dihydroxyvitamin D in elderly osteoporotic patients. N Engl J Med 1981; 305(7): 372–374.
100 Kurland ES, Cosman F, McMahon DJ et al. Parathyroid hormone as a therapy for idiopathic osteoporosis in men: effects on bone mineral density and bone markers. J Clin Endocrinol Metab 2000; 85(9):3069–3076.
101 Lane JM, Russell L, Khan SN. Osteoporosis. Clin Orthop 2000; 372:139–150.
102 Lane NE, Sanchez S, Modin GW et al. Parathyroid hormone treatment can reverse corticosteroid-induced osteoporosis. Results of a randomized controlled clinical trial. J Clin Invest 1998; 102(8):1627–1633.
103 Delmas PD. Clinical effects of strontium ranelate in women with postmenopausal osteoporosis. Osteoporos Int 2005; 16(Suppl 1):S16–S19.
104 Meunier PJ, Roux C, Seeman E et al. The effects of strontium ranelate on the risk of vertebral fracture in women with postmenopausal osteoporosis. N Engl J Med 2004; 350(5):459–468.
105 Rich C, Ensinck J, Ivanovich P. The effects of sodium floride on calcium metabolism of subjects with metabolic bone diseases. J Clin Invest 1964; 43: 545–555.
106 Riggs BL, Arnaud CD, Jowsey J et al. Parathyroid function in primary osteoporosis. J Clin Invest 1973; 52(1):181–184.
107 Sambrook PN, Seeman E, Phillips SR et al. Preventing osteoporosis: outcomes of the Australian Fracture Prevention Summit. Med J Aust 2002; 176(Suppl):S1–S16.
108 Tonino RP, Meunier PJ, Emkey R et al. Skeletal benefits of alendronate: 7-year treatment of postmenopausal osteoporotic women. Phase III Osteoporosis Treatment Study Group. J Clin Endocrinol Metab 2000; 85(9):3109–3115.
109 Scheiber MD, Rebar RW. Isoflavones and postmenopausal bone health: a viable alternative to estrogen therapy? Menopause 1999; 6(3):233–241.
110 Somekawa Y, Chigughi M, Harada M et al. Use of vitamin K_2 (menatetrenone) and 1,25-dihydroxyvitamin D_3 in the prevention of bone

loss induced by leuprolide. J Clin Endocrinol Metab 1999; 84(8):2700–2704.

111 Shiraki M, Shiraki Y, Aoki C et al. Vitamin K_2 (menatetrenone) effectively prevents fractures and sustains lumbar bone mineral density in osteoporosis. J Bone Miner Res 2000; 15(3):515–521.

112 Osmanagaoglu MA, Okumus B, Osmanagaoglu T et al. The relationship between serum dehydroepiandrosterone sulfate concentration and bone mineral density, lipids, and hormone replacement therapy in premenopausal and postmenopausal women. J Womens Health (Larchmt) 2004; 13(9):993–999.

113 Jones G, Nguyen T, Sambrook PN et al. Symptomatic fracture incidence in elderly men and women: the Dubbo Osteoporosis Epidemiology Study (DOES). Osteoporos Int 1994; 4(5):277–282.

114 Narayan KM, Boyle JP, Thompson TJ et al. Lifetime risk for diabetes mellitus in the United States. JAMA 2003; 290(14):1884–1890.

115 Myers AH, Robinson EG, van Natta ML et al. Hip fractures among the elderly: factors associated with in-hospital mortality. Am J Epidemiol 1991; 134(10): 1128–1137.

116 Nguyen ND, Center JR, Eisman JA et al. Bone loss, weight loss, and weight fluctuation predict mortality risk in elderly men and women. J Bone Miner Res 2007; 22(8):1147–1154.

117 Nguyen TV, Eisman JA. Risk factors for low bone mass in men. In: Orwoll ES, ed. Osteoporosis in men. San Diego, Ca: Academic Press; 1999:335–361.

118 Amin S, Felson DT. Osteoporosis in men. Rheum Dis Clin North Am 2001; 27(1):19–47.

119 Orwoll ES. Osteoporosis in men. Endocrinol Metab Clin North Am 1998; 27(2):349–367.

120 Khosla S, Melton LJ III, Robb RA et al. Relationship of volumetric BMD and structural parameters at different skeletal sites to sex steroid levels in men. J Bone Miner Res 2005; 20(5):730–740.

121 Gennari L, Merlotti D, Martini G et al. Longitudinal association between sex hormone levels, bone loss, and bone turnover in elderly men. J Clin Endocrinol Metab 2003; 88(11):5327–5333.

122 Khosla S, Melton LJ III, Atkinson EJ et al. Relationship of serum sex steroid levels to longitudinal changes in bone density in young versus elderly men. J Clin Endocrinol Metab 2001; 86(8):3555–3561.

123 Nguyen ND, Eisman JA, Center JR et al. Risk factors for fracture in nonosteoporotic men and women. J Clin Endocrinol Metab 2007; 92(3):955–962.

124 Wallach S, Cohen S, Reid DM et al. Effects of risedronate treatment on bone density and vertebral fracture in patients on corticosteroid therapy. Calcif Tissue Int 2000; 67(4):277–285.

125 Orwoll ES, Scheele WH, Paul S et al. The effect of teriparatide [human parathyroid hormone (1–34)] therapy on bone density in men with osteoporosis. J Bone Miner Res 2003; 18(1):9–17.

126 Pasco JA, Sanders KM, Henry MJ et al. Calcium intakes among Australian women: Geelong Osteoporosis Study. Aust NZ J Med 2000; 30(1):21–27.

127 Lau E, Donnan S, Barker DJ et al. Physical activity and calcium intake in fracture of the proximal femur in Hong Kong. BMJ 1988; 297(6661):1441–1443.

128 Lau EM, Woo J, Leung PC et al. The effects of calcium supplementation and exercise on bone density in elderly Chinese women. Osteoporos Int 1992; 2(4):168–173.

129 Shea B, Wells G, Cranney A et al. Meta-analyses of therapies for postmenopausal osteoporosis. VII. Meta-analysis of calcium supplementation for the prevention of postmenopausal osteoporosis. Endocr Rev 2002; 23(4):552–559.

130 National Health and Medical Research Council. Recommended dietary intakes for use in Australia. Canberra: AGPS; 1991. Online. Available: http://www.nhmrc.gov.au/publications/synopses/n6syn.htm

131 Flicker L, Mead K, MacInnis RJ et al. Serum vitamin D and falls in older women in residential care in Australia. J Am Geriatr Soc 2003; 51(11):1533–1538.

132 Sambrook PN, Cameron ID, Cumming RG et al. Vitamin D deficiency is common in frail institutionalised older people in northern Sydney. Med J Aust 2002; 176(11):560.

133 Working Group of the Australian and New Zealand Bone and Mineral Society. Vitamin D and adult bone health in Australia and New Zealand: a position statement. Med J Aust 2005; 182(6):281–285.

134 Kanis JA, Johnell O, Oden A et al. Smoking and fracture risk: a meta-analysis. Osteoporos Int 2005; 16(2):155–162.

135 Hallstrom H, Wolk A, Glynn A et al. Coffee, tea and caffeine consumption in relation to osteoporotic fracture risk in a cohort of Swedish women. Osteoporos Int 2006; 17(7):1055–1064.

136 Heaney RP. Role of dietary sodium in osteoporosis. J Am Coll Nutr 2006; 25(Suppl 3):271S–276S.

137 Morris RC Jr, Schmidlin O, Frassetto LA et al. Relationship and interaction between sodium and potassium. J Am Coll Nutr 2006; 25(Suppl 3):262S–270S.

138 Kanis JA, Johansson H, Johnell O et al. Alcohol intake as a risk factor for fracture. Osteoporos Int 2005; 16(7):737–742.

139 Kiel DP, Felson DT, Hannan MT et al. Caffeine and the risk of hip fracture: the Framingham Study. Am J Epidemiol 1990; 132(4):675–684.

140 Prince R, Devine A, Dick I et al. The effects of calcium supplementation (milk powder or tablets) and exercise

on bone density in postmenopausal women. J Bone Miner Res 1995; 10(7):1068–1075.

141 Yano K, Heilbrun LK, Wasnich RD et al. The relationship between diet and bone mineral content of multiple skeletal sites in elderly Japanese-American men and women living in Hawaii. Am J Clin Nutr 1985; 42(5):877–888.

142 Sinaki M. The role of physical activity in bone health: a new hypothesis to reduce risk of vertebral fracture. Phys Med Rehabil Clin N Am 2007; 18(3):593–608, xi–xii.

143 National Osteoporosis Foundation. Physician's guide to prevention and treatment of osteoporosis. Washington DC: National Osteoporosis Foundation; 2003.

144 Lord SR, Sambrook PN, Gilbert C et al. Postural stability, falls and fractures in the elderly: results from the Dubbo Osteoporosis Epidemiology Study. Med J Aust 1994; 160(11):684–685, 688–691.

145 Grisso JA, Kelsey JL, Strom BL et al. Risk factors for falls as a cause of hip fracture in women. The Northeast Hip Fracture Study Group. N Engl J Med 1991; 324(19):1326–1331.

146 Nevitt MC, Cummings SR, Kidd S et al. Risk factors for recurrent nonsyncopal falls. A prospective study. JAMA 1989; 261(18):2663–2668.

147 Tinetti ME, Speechley M, Ginter SF. Risk factors for falls among elderly persons living in the community. N Engl J Med 1988; 319(26):1701–1707.

148 Center JR, Bliuc D, Nguyen TV et al. Risk of subsequent fracture after low-trauma fracture in men and women. JAMA 2007; 297(4):387–394.

149 Kanis JA, Johansson H, Oden A et al. A family history of fracture and fracture risk: a meta-analysis. Bone 2004; 35(5):1029–1037.

150 Harrington JT, Broy SB, Derosa AM et al. Hip fracture patients are not treated for osteoporosis: a call to action. Arthritis Rheum 2002; 47(6):651–654.

151 Kamel HK, Hussain MS, Tariq S et al. Failure to diagnose and treat osteoporosis in elderly patients hospitalized with hip fracture. Am J Med 2000; 109(4):326–328.

152 Bauer DC. Osteoporotic fractures: ignorance is bliss? Am J Med 2000; 109(4):338–339.

153 Eisman J, Clapham S, Kehoe L. Osteoporosis prevalence and levels of treatment in primary care: the Australian Bone Care Study. J Bone Miner Res 2004; 19(12):1969–1975.

154 Bliuc D, Eisman JA, Center JR. A randomized study of two different information-based interventions on the management of osteoporosis in minimal and moderate trauma fractures. Osteoporos Int 2006; 17(9):1309–1317.

Acknowledgments

The Dubbo Osteoporosis Epidemiology Study, from where several key data are used in this chapter, has been supported by the National Health and Medical Research Council, and untied educational grants from GE-Lunar, Merck Australia, Eli Lilly International and Aventis Australia. One author (Tuan V. Nguyen) is supported by a Senior Research Fellowship from the National Health and Medical Research Council.

chapter 24

Cancer

INTRODUCTION AND OVERVIEW

Integrative cancer care requires a comprehensive and well-coordinated team or virtual team approach. The general practitioner with an integrative philosophy is well placed to coordinate appropriate screening, prevention, case finding and treatment services for patients at all stages of their journey. The cancer journey begins with awareness of risk factors and preventive strategies, and continues through diagnosis of the type and stage of cancer, decisions about conventional treatment and adjunctive therapies.

It is estimated that up to 80% of patients with cancer seek complementary and alternative therapies, almost entirely as adjunctive treatment. A study published in the *Journal of Clinical Oncology* reported that 88% of 102 people with cancer who were enrolled in phase I clinical trials (research studies in people) at the Mayo Comprehensive Cancer Center had used at least one CAM therapy.[1] Of those, 93% had used supplements (such as vitamins or minerals), 53% had used non-supplement forms of CAM (such as prayer/spiritual practices or chiropractic care), and almost 47% had used both.

The choice of integrative therapy depends on the type and stage of the cancer, the gender and age of the patient, their preferences and previous experience of CAM, the conventional treatment being undertaken for the particular stage of the cancer, and what you and the patient are seeking to achieve through their treatment plan.

Patients diagnosed with cancer are often in a particularly vulnerable situation and are looking for guidance, which needs to be provided with a clear description of what is known about the efficacy and safety of each treatment modality. The role of each practitioner is to guide patients to decisions about treatments that are likely to enhance longevity and quality of life, to be aware of and avoid harmful interactions, and to guide them away from treatments that are potentially harmful or have little evidence or likelihood of improving outcomes for them.

Ideally, the integrative approach to cancer management improves a patient's sense of self-control, reduces anxiety and aims to maximise the body's potential to heal.

CANCER AND THE ESSENCE MODEL

Cancer is a very real risk, with one person in three being affected before the age of 75. As the major cause of death in developed countries it is closing in on heart disease. Cancer is also an entirely different disease than cardiovascular disease. First, it is not one disease but many, all with differing causes and treatments. Secondly, cancers vary enormously in how aggressive or life-threatening they are. Although there tends to be dread of receiving a cancer diagnosis, many cancers are not life-threatening, and even for those that are, early diagnosis and treatment can have a significant impact upon outcome. Thirdly, because cancer includes such a wide variety of conditions, some have been extensively researched and others have not. Despite all we do know, cancer largely remains something of a mystery.

Although it has just been said that cancer is different from other diseases, the ESSENCE principles of cancer prevention and management[2] (see Ch 6) are very similar whatever the cancer type. The important thing is to understand the principles, which are largely the same whatever the cancer, and not get concerned because there might be less information on one particular type of cancer. Although most research data is drawn from the more common cancers, the same rules apply for others.

PATIENT EDUCATION

In the most general sense, cancer is a disease in which a cell changes in such a way that it:

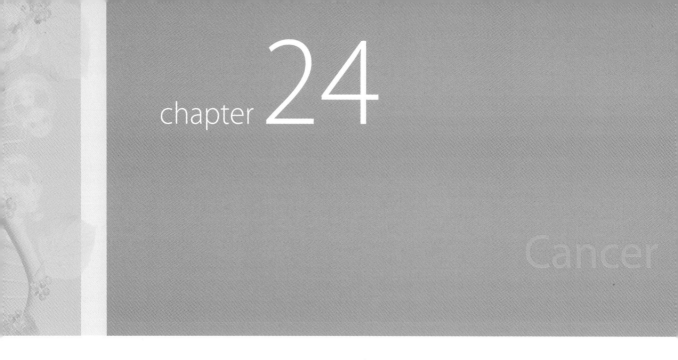

- *divides at a rapid rate*—cells normally obey hormonal and other messages from the body about when to divide and how fast. They can multiply faster in response to demand. Cancer cells multiply far beyond what they should and do not respond to the body's messages about stopping their multiplication
- *lives far longer than it should*—all cells have a regulated lifespan through 'inbuilt obsolescence'. It can vary from a relatively short time (days for the cells lining the gut) to many years (brain cells). Because of their genetic changes, cancer cells often don't seem to know when to die
- *doesn't obey the normal boundaries*—cells in the body tend to stay within well-demarcated boundaries and don't spread into other tissues. Cancer cells will press on or invade surrounding organs, causing loss of function and destruction of healthy tissues. Cancer can spread through the body to distant sites via the bloodstream and lymph vessels, and can spread directly to local tissues. Cells that have spread to distant parts of the body are called 'secondary cancer' or metastases, whereas the original site of the cancer is called the 'primary'
- *consumes considerable resources but has no useful function in the body*—cancer cells are hungry cells but they produce nothing useful. This consumption of energy/food can leave the rest of the body depleted (cachectic) when it is advanced. Interestingly, a nutritionally rich but calorie-restricted diet is associated with a reduced risk of cancer and slower cancer progression
- *is no longer part of the 'self'*—as cancer cells change and further mutate over time, they resemble less and less the original tissue from which they came. As they do this they are no longer recognised by the body as part of the self. If the immune system can recognise cells as cancerous it will attack them as if they were foreign tissue.

Causes

The causes of cancer are many and varied, like the disease itself. There is an ongoing battle between cancer cells being produced within the body on a regular basis, and the body's defences. Whatever increases the risk of cancer cells being made, or reduces the body's defences against cancer, will increase the chances that cancerous cells will evade the body's defences and cause a cancer that poses a risk to life. There is no one factor by itself that can be implicated; it tends to be the interplay of a range of factors such as genetics (e.g. family history), chemical exposure (e.g. smoking), lifestyle (e.g. diet and exercise), mental health (e.g. chronic stress and depression), social circumstances, environment (e.g. radiation exposure), chronic inflammation (e.g. chronic hepatitis or inflammatory bowel disease), poor immunity (e.g. AIDS) and many others. There are undoubtedly many potential risk factors that we don't know about. Whether known or unknown, these factors affect risk. Whatever the interplay of causes, it is generally thought that one way or another, a range of genetic mutations and switches are activated, which starts the disease. It is also now understood that the body makes cancer cells on a regular basis but, through a range of defences, stops the cancerous cells before they cause any noticeable illness. This is called 'tumour surveillance'. Things that lower our bodily defences (such as stress or an unhealthy lifestyle) or increase the number of cancer cells that the body is making (such as smoking) can push the balance in favour of the cancer cells and thus allow a cancer to slip through the safety net. A cancer will often have been growing for a number of years before it is obvious as a lump or causes symptoms that bring it to the attention of the patient or doctor.

Staging

Cancers can be largely divided into two groups: solid and blood-borne malignancies.

Cancers are generally staged according to their level of spread and how aggressive or mutated they are. The TNM system is one of the most commonly used staging systems.[3] This system has been accepted by the International Union Against Cancer (UICC) and the American Joint Committee on Cancer (AJCC). Most medical facilities use the TNM system as their main method of cancer reporting.

The TNM system is based on the extent of the tumour (T), the extent of spread to the lymph nodes (N) and the presence of metastasis (M). A number is added to each letter to indicate the size or extent of the tumour and the extent of spread (Box 24.1).

Cancers of the brain and spinal cord are not given a TNM designation but rather are classified according to their cell type and grade. Different staging systems are also used for haematological cancers and lymphomas.

Staging is important because the treatment and prognosis will vary accordingly. Obviously, if a cancer is treated in the early stages, the outcome will tend to be far more optimistic.

Hence, it is not just the primary prevention of cancer through healthy lifestyle that is important, but also secondary prevention through early detection and screening. There are many forms of screening for particular cancers, such as breast self-examination and mammography for breast cancer, faecal occult blood or colonoscopy for bowel cancer, digital rectal examination and prostate-specific antigen (PSA) for prostate cancer

BOX 24.1 TNM staging system

Primary tumour (T)	
TX	Primary tumour cannot be evaluated
T0	No evidence of primary tumour
Tis	Carcinoma in situ (early cancer that has not spread to neighbouring tissue)
T1, T2, T3, T4	Size and/or extent of the primary tumour
Regional lymph nodes (N)	
NX	Regional lymph nodes cannot be evaluated
N0	No regional lymph node involvement (no cancer found in the lymph nodes)
N1, N2, N3	Involvement of regional lymph nodes (number and/or extent of spread)
Distant metastasis (M)	
MX	Distant metastasis cannot be evaluated
M0	No distant metastasis (cancer has not spread to other parts of the body)
M1	Distant metastasis (cancer has spread to distant parts of the body)

Source: National Cancer Institute 2004[3]

and chest X-ray for lung cancer. Cancers picked up on routine screening are more likely to be in an earlier stage of growth and of a lower level of malignancy than cancers detected because they have produced symptoms.

Treatment

The most widely used conventional cancer treatments tend to fall into three categories, sometimes unflatteringly referred to as:

- *slash (surgery)*—cut out the tumour and/or try to minimise its impact upon the body by, for example, debulking, taking pressure off the brain or unblocking the bowel
- *burn (radiotherapy)*—X-rays are concentrated on and kill tumour cells, even those deep in the body. The more accurately this can be done, the less damage to and inflammation of surrounding healthy tissues there will be.
- *poison (chemotherapy)*—substances are administered that are poisonous to dividing cells. The dose is measured so that it most affects rapidly dividing cells—the cancer—but does not overly damage healthy cells that also divide at a fast pace (e.g. blood, gut, hair follicles). It is in these tissues that many of the side effects of chemotherapy are felt. There are also longer-term effects of chemotherapy such as memory loss and, strangely, an increased risk of other cancers.

Other forms of therapy are being developed, such as hormonal treatments, adjuvant therapy, vaccines and immunotherapy. Some promising treatments derived from plant-based products are also being researched. Some therapies are aimed at prolonging survival and others are aimed at palliation of symptoms, whether caused by the disease itself or by the treatments being administered.

Many complementary therapies have also been found to be useful for symptom control and improving quality of life. Cancer treatment can have a major impact on quality of life—for the better when it kills the tumour, and for the worse when it attacks the rest of the body, causing side effects. It is beyond the scope of this book to describe all the potential cancer therapies in detail. Suffice it to say that it is important to have full and open conversations with the team members who are helping to manage the cancer. Such a team could include oncologists, surgeons, general practitioners, counsellors, social workers, nursing, allied healthcare and complementary medicine practitioners. Other important sources of information include the community cancer agencies and support groups, medical databases such as PubMed and other respectable websites.

It is important that patients are given the opportunity to ask questions and to have them answered to their satisfaction. If they do not find the answers and resources they need, then it is important to offer them a second opinion. It is also vital that patients feel as empowered and involved as they wish to be in decisions about their cancer management. The therapeutic team plays an important role in helping patients make responsible decisions regarding their cancer care. A poor decision could be to decline a clearly beneficial conventional treatment, or to undertake a line of therapy with considerable side effects and little prospect of cure. A problem arises from the fact that cancer patients and their families are often vulnerable and can be taken advantage of through unrealistic expectations in relation to exotic and sometimes harmful or very expensive treatments that have no reasonable prospect of benefit. There are examples of both complementary and conventional treatments in this category.

This having been said, if a patient feels obstructed, undermined or disempowered in their cancer management, if they are told there is nothing they can do for themselves, if they are told that lifestyle doesn't matter or that there is nothing outside the medical model that can help them, then they need to think seriously about finding another practitioner. Quality information and respectful and open lines of communication are much needed for both practitioner and patient, so that neither is making uninformed decisions and so that outcomes can be optimised. The Australian Senate Inquiry into the management of cancer made a number of findings and clearly indicated that the 'cancer establishment' should be doing a far better job in this regard.[4]

MIND–BODY THERAPIES

There has been much debate over the years, some of it heated, about the role of psychosocial factors in cancer. There is little debate that better mental and social health is associated with better coping and quality of life for cancer patients, but their role in the causation and progression of cancer remains controversial in conventional cancer circles. Many studies have suggested a link between psychosocial factors and cancer causes, but others have not. Some studies have looked at outcomes and others at the possible mechanisms whereby patients' mental and emotional health changes outcomes. Because there are so many factors potentially affecting cancer, doubt often exists as to how much of a contribution psychological factors make.

In an authoritative review, Professor David Spiegel concluded that chronic and severe depression is probably associated with an increased risk of cancer, but that there is 'stronger evidence that depression predicts cancer progression and mortality'.[5a] Of all the emotional factors, depression is probably the most important.[6] Further, providing psychosocial support, through a support group for example, 'reduces depression, anxiety, and pain, and may increase survival time with cancer'.[5a] The longer the depression has existed, say for longer than 6 years, the greater the risk factor it is. The risk is nearly doubled, independent of other lifestyle variables, and is not related to any particular cancer.[7,8] The most recent review of the effect of depression on survival for patients who already have cancer concluded that clinical depression played a causal role in cancer mortality and was associated with a 39% increased mortality rate.[9]

Poor coping, distress and depression have been linked to poor survival for various cancers, including cancer of liver and bile duct (hepatobiliary),[10] lung cancer,[11] breast cancer[12], malignant melanoma[13] and bowel cancer. Some studies have not confirmed a link.[14] Having a good global quality of life is associated with better survival for a variety of cancers.[15–18] Other factors, including the perceived aim of treatment, minimisation, quality of life and anger, all influence survival.[19] *Minimisation* refers to a person minimising the importance or impact of the cancer. It is not denial, but reflects an ability to adapt or to see the illness in a larger perspective.

If psychological and social factors do play a role in the cause and prognosis of cancer, the important question is whether psychosocial interventions such as group support, relaxation and meditation and CBT produce better survival chances. That they can improve quality of life for cancer patients is clear, but unfortunately there are very few completed controlled trials examining the survival outcomes of such interventions. A number of studies have shown a significant improvement in both quality of life and survival time, but others have not.[20]

The most noted and first study of its type was done by David Spiegel, who studied women with metastatic breast cancer. His results showed a doubling of average survival time from 18.9 months to 36.6 months for the women who received the support program, compared with those who didn't. The intervention included group support focused on improving emotional expression, some simple relaxation and self-hypnosis techniques, plus the usual medical management.[21] Ten years after the study, three women in the intervention group were still alive but none in the group that had had the usual medical management alone were.

Another well-performed study by Fawzy and colleagues looked at outcomes for 68 patients with early-stage malignant melanoma.[22] The patients were divided into two groups and followed for 6 years, at which time those who had had the usual surgical care and monitoring plus stress management showed a halving of the recurrence rate (7/34 *vs* 13/34) and much lower death rate (3/34 *vs* 10/34) than the group who had had the usual surgical management and monitoring alone. The intervention on this occasion was only 6 weeks of stress management. In this study, immune function was also followed. Originally the two groups were comparable but the stress management group had significantly better immune function 6 months into the study. We know that melanoma is one of the cancers that is aggressively attacked by natural killer (NK) cells and this probably contributed to the major difference in survival rates—that is, the immune system, monitoring for any cancer spread, was able to deal with it before the cancer had a chance to grow. Ten-year follow-up on the Fawzy program still shows a positive survival effect, although this has weakened a little over time,[23] so it may be that people lose motivation over time, and 'boosters' may be required to maintain the therapeutic effect.

Other studies have also yielded promising results in terms of survival, for cancer of the liver,[24] gastrointestinal tract[25] and lymphoma.[26] A number of trials have shown equivocal or negative results from a psychosocial support program, in terms of improved survival.[27–31] One of these trials was an attempt to replicate the Spiegel study but the results showed that, despite some improvements in mental health and quality of life, there was no significant effect on survival. An even more recent study of group support for breast cancer survival showed that the intervention did not statistically significantly prolong survival, although the average survival time in the support group was 24.0 months, compared with 18.3 months in the control group. The support program did, however, help to treat and prevented new depressive disorders, reduced hopeless-helplessness and trauma symptoms, and improved social functioning.[32] Another recent study on psychotherapeutic support for gastrointestinal malignancies like stomach and bowel cancer showed a clinically and statistically significant survival benefit. This hospital-based psychosocial support program was delivered to individuals rather than in a group format. Over twice the number of gastrointestinal cancer patients were alive at 10 years if they had a psychotherapeutic intervention.[33] The work by the Ornish group on support programs and cancer is probably the best researched and has shown excellent results, but this included a range of other lifestyle factors apart from psychosocial support.

Therefore, in summary, of the six trials not showing longer survival, three have shown a positive effect on mental health and the other three have not. Of the trials that showed a positive effect on survival, all showed improved mental health as a result of the intervention. So the trend seems to be that where the psychosocial intervention has marginal or no long-term benefit on mood or quality of life, it tends not to translate into longer survival. If the support program produces a significant and enduring improvement in mental health and quality of life, then it tends to have a 'side effect' of improving survival. Nine out of 12 studies have followed this rule so far.

Support programs vary enormously in content, duration and delivery, thus many questions in the area of psychosocial support and cancer survival will need to be answered in future research.[34] For example: What kinds of programs work best? Who should they be run by? How long is the optimal duration for such a program? What are the essential ingredients? What advice should a doctor give to a patient regarding whether or not to attend a support group? To what extent does compliance affect the outcome? Does having a residential component improve outcomes?

It is likely that it is not just being in a program that is protective but also the level to which a person participates in it and lives by it. This was demonstrated by one of the studies referred to above, showing that high involvement in the program was associated with better survival, and that there was no benefit from just 'going through the motions'.[35] One paper suggested that programs of 12 weeks or longer duration were more likely to be effective.[36] Those that use validated forms of meditation and also foster positive emotional responses including humour and hope are more likely to be successful. Although programs attempting to deal with psychological factors need to take into account the fact that personality traits and coping styles can affect quality of survival, there are mixed results from research on whether things such as 'helplessness',[37,38] 'fighting spirit' and 'optimism'[39] affect survival. Despite the fact that a number of studies suggest that they do, other studies throw this into doubt.[40]

If improving mental health does indeed have survival benefits, the potential mechanisms explaining that longer survival are worth considering.[41] Below is a summary of key points, followed by a more extensive discussion of each.

Direct physiological and metabolic effects

- *The stress response*—when stressed or depressed, the body produces high levels of cortisol and other stress and inflammatory hormones, such as interleukins. These not only affect the body's defences but also accelerate cancer cell replication. High and 'flattened' cortisol levels associated with high allostatic load have been found to be a poor prognostic finding for cancer patients,[42–44] whereas cancer patients who apply strategies such as mindfulness-based stress management show significant improvement in these parameters.[45]
- *Genetic mutation and expression*—stress increases the likelihood of expressing genetic tendencies towards illness, increases genetic mutations and impairs the body's ability to repair them. Again, psychological strategies that reduce stress have the effect of reducing genetic damage and improving genetic repair.[46]
- *Immunosuppression*—stress causes suppression of immune cells, in particular NK cells. This leads to reduced defences and poor cancer surveillance for some cancers.[47]
- *Effects of 'anti-cancer' hormones such as melatonin*—melatonin has a number of beneficial effects on genes and immunity that have important implications for cancer.[48] Poor mental health is associated with low levels of melatonin, whereas healthy lifestyle and stress reduction increase melatonin. Melatonin supplements have been associated with 34% lower recurrence rates and better cancer survival,[49,50] although if taking it as a supplement it is important not to take excess doses and to monitor for side effects. The most commonly used dosages administered in these cancer trials was 20 mg taken orally in the evening.
- *Angiogenesis*—this is the ability of tissues to make new blood vessels. Solid cancers thrive on many of the stress hormones such as interleukins, which increase angiogenesis and therefore the cancer's ability to spread. It is known that cancer patients with depression have high levels of the hormones that stimulate angiogenesis compared with cancer patients who are not depressed. These elevations in interleukin (IL-4, IL-6 and IL-10) levels are reversible with mind–body therapies.[51]

- *Metabolic syndrome*—metabolic syndrome has been linked as a risk factor with a range of cancers[52,53]; and poor mental health is associated with high allostatic load and an increased risk of metabolic syndrome. The relationship goes a significant way to explaining why a range of healthy lifestyle changes have such positive effects on cancer outcome.
- *Oxidative damage*—stress is pro-oxidative and this has been linked to cancer risk and progression. Other markers of DNA repair are commonly suppressed in cancer patients and are potential markers of cancer susceptibility.[54] Thus oxidative stress due to psychological stress coupled with a low intake of dietary antioxidants may be crucial factors in the evolution and progression of cancer. There is even evidence from animal studies that oxidative DNA damage can be classically conditioned.[55] The implications of all these findings are significant but as yet barely explored. Reducing stress and having an adequate dietary intake of antioxidants are therefore important.

Indirect effects

- *Better compliance with treatment*—it may be that those with better mental health comply better with treatment and use more avenues of therapy.
- *Improved lifestyle*—it is known that those who feel better psychologically also find it easier to make healthy changes in other parts of their lives. This has secondary effects on improving survival.

The original belief in psycho-oncology circles was that immune cells were the main explanation for why the mind has effects on cancer outcomes, but there is much more to it than that. Immunity may explain some of the beneficial effects of stress management for some tumours, but not all. In some cancers, such as malignant melanoma or those where viral infections are an important cause, the immune system may be the main defence, but it is probably less important for cancers that are primarily caused by chemical injury, such as lung cancer. Many cancers do not wear their mutated antigens on their surface and therefore the immune system cannot recognise and attack them.[56]

Some hormones can also suppress cancer growth and even induce cancer cell apoptosis. The ability to change the activity of such chemical mediators may in part explain why various activities prolong a healthy lifespan in humans, such as cognitive behaviour therapy, meditation-based therapies, stress reduction, anti-inflammatory techniques, dietary (calorie) restriction and aerobic exercise. These all affect molecular mediators including dehydroepiandrosterone (DHEA), interleukins and especially melatonin.[57]

Chronic inflammation is not a good combination with cancer. Even the inflammation associated with major surgery has been shown to increase the growth of tumour metastases at distant sites via these hormones,[58] so it is important for patients with disseminated cancer only to have surgery if it is really necessary. Reducing stress hormones[59] and inducing hormones associated with wellbeing and relaxation, such as melatonin, may be part of the reason that stress reduction and psychosocial interventions help cancer survival.[60]

Some immune mediators (e.g. TNF-alpha) can kill tumour cells and have anti-tumour effects. We now know that many tumours are 'dormant' through a balance between cell division, cell death and the body's defences.[61] Upsetting this balance may explain why the occurrence and recurrence of cancer often follow recent traumatic events that were not well dealt with.[62] In such a case it may be more accurate to say that emotional disturbance is a contributing or precipitating factor accelerating the cancer's growth, rather than it being the cause of the cancer.

Apart from having significant effects on immunity[63] and ageing,[64] melatonin also has anti-tumour effects. It slows cancer cell replication, helps to switch off cancer genes, and inhibits the release and activity of cancer growth factors, promotes better sleep and helps to enhance the immune response.[65,66] Because of the biological activity of melatonin, this has a number of implications for cancer therapy.[67,68] Helping the body to stimulate its own melatonin production has many beneficial effects. Among the things which stimulate melatonin endogenously are many of the interventions that are part of holistic cancer support programs (Box 24.2).

Melatonin regulates our body clock, and therefore sleep is intimately linked with melatonin levels and thereby with cancer progression.[75] This may partly explain why things that affect melatonin (e.g. doing shift work or working in the airline industry) may also be risk factors for cancer.[76] Body-clock alterations commonly occur in cancer patients, with greater disruption seen in more advanced cases. Emotional and social factors as well as many symptoms associated with cancer can have a significantly negative effect on sleep rhythms. From a therapeutic perspective, using behavioural interventions to enhance sleep is a vital part of coping with cancer but it also helps to improve cancer defences and prognosis. The chapter on sleep strategies (see Ch 43) would be useful to read if sleep is a problem.

Psychological states affect genetics. We can have a genetic disposition to cancer but, equally, DNA has protective genes such as 'cancer suppressor genes'. It has been shown that stress impairs repair of genetic mutations[77] and causes oxidative damage to DNA. In

BOX 24.2 Mediation of melatonin[69,70,71,72]

Enhanced by:
- meditation[73,74]
- subdued lighting after sunset
- calorie restriction
- exercise
- diet: foods rich in Ca, Mg, B_6, tryptophan-rich foods (e.g. milk, spirulina seaweed)
- relaxing music

Inhibited by:
- stress
- drugs, especially before bed (e.g. caffeine, beta-blockers, alcohol, sedatives)
- inactivity
- electromagnetic radiation
- working night shift
- jet lag
- excessive calories

experiments on workers, perceived workload, perceived stress and the 'impossibility of alleviating stress' were all associated with high levels of DNA damage.[78,79] Personality factors were also linked to oxidative DNA damage, with high 'tension-anxiety', particularly for males, or 'depression-rejection', particularly for females, correlating with the level of DNA damage.[80] A low level of closeness to parents during childhood, or bereavement in the previous 3 years, were also associated with greater DNA damage. Psychological stress reduces the ability of immune cells to initiate genetically programmed cancer cell suicide.[81]

Angiogenesis, which is the process of new blood vessel formation, is vital for tissue repair but also for the growth of tumours. Solid tumours can only grow into other tissues because they are able to lay down new blood vessels. Blood vessel growth is also mediated via various cytokines. One particularly important one is vascular endothelial growth factor (VEGF), and in cancer patients high levels of this cytokine are associated with poor prognosis. Sympathetic nervous system activation, a vital part of the stress response, increases the level of VEGF, and cancer patients who report higher levels of social wellbeing have lower levels of VEGF, a good prognostic sign. 'Helplessness' and 'worthlessness' are also associated with higher levels of VEGF.[82] Other studies emphasising the importance of angiogenesis in tumour progression have found links with depression.[83] Tumours in stressed animals showed markedly increased vascularisation (angiogenesis) and increased levels of the hormones that produce these effects.[84]

As ever, we are more interested in the therapeutic potential of strategies for improving psychological wellbeing. Support groups have already been discussed but other research with bearing on this topic is also of interest. A study has been performed on the effects of mindfulness-based stress reduction (MBSR) on quality of life, stress, mood, hormonal and immune function in early-stage breast and prostate cancer patients.[85] The 8-week MBSR program included relaxation, meditation, gentle yoga and daily home practice, and followed patients for 12 months. The participants showed and maintained significant improvements in symptoms of stress, their cortisol levels decreased (a good prognostic sign) and physiological markers of stress reduced, as did pro-inflammatory cytokines: 'MBSR program participation was associated with enhanced quality of life and decreased stress symptoms, altered cortisol and immune patterns consistent with less stress and mood disturbance, and decreased blood pressure'.[85a]

Much more work needs to be done, but the signs are looking increasingly positive and are confirming what many patients intuitively sense and have found in their own experience—that taking an active role in enhancing mental health has positive effects on coping and quality of life, and also on outcomes.

SPIRITUALITY

Cancer, more than most illnesses, raises the prospect of one's own mortality. As such it is a common catalyst for looking at one's life and reconsidering what is important. Cancer can therefore be a powerful stimulus for personal growth, but for many it will lead to an emotional implosion unless motivation is positive and adequate support is given. Much has already been said in the chapter on spirituality (Ch 12) about how having an active search for meaning or a spiritual dimension in one's life:

- enhances mental health and reduces stress
- improves one's ability to cope with adversity and symptoms
- helps to support healthy lifestyle change
- is associated with greater life expectancy.

These are all reasons in themselves to consider 'spirituality', however one relates to it, as an important part of the management of cancer. Indeed, it has already been mentioned in the chapter on spirituality (Ch 12) that approximately 80% of patients dealing with major illness wished to discuss spiritual issues with their doctor. Among cancer survivors, the relationship between social functioning and distress was significantly affected by having a sense of meaning in life, whereas the relationship between physical functioning and distress was partially mediated by meaning.[86] There have been precious few studies on whether spirituality or religion is protective against cancer. The only well-performed trial found a significantly lower incidence of bowel cancer among those with a religious dimension to their lives, and this could not be explained by other risk factors.[87] This study also found longer survival in those with bowel cancer.

A related issue is whether various forms of 'distant healing' can assist in healing or in symptom control. A review showed that there was some evidence, albeit a little sparse and inconsistent, to suggest that forms of healing including therapeutic touch, faith healing and reiki may be helpful.[88] Most of the results demonstrated so far, however, are reduction in pain and anxiety, and improvement in function. Grander claims, such as effects on tumour regression through prayer, therapeutic touch and faith healing, are mainly anecdotal and have not been rigorously investigated or proved.

CONNECTEDNESS

Connectedness can be important for different reasons at different times throughout the progression of cancer. There is the initial adjustment to a cancer diagnosis and what it potentially entails. There is the support needed in coping with cancer treatment. There is the support required in the time after treatment as one returns to work and family life, and thereafter lives with the diagnosis of being a 'cancer patient'. It is often a lonely place to be, as many people will avoid contact with a friend or family member with cancer because they may find it confronting or not know how to deal with the potentially emotionally sensitive situation. A person with cancer may crave solitude or, conversely, feel isolated. We will not know unless we ask. Finally, if the cancer becomes advanced then there is the important phase of palliative care and dealing with the prospect of death. Support will significantly affect how this is dealt with. There is potentially no more lonely time in a person's life and yet, with care and encouragement, it can be the most uplifting and inspiring. Ultimately, death is not optional for any of us, but how we confront death is. For those caring for a dying loved one it is important to help the loved one find their way and not to project our assumptions and fears onto them.

As has been discussed, social isolation predisposes a person to a whole range of illnesses including cancer and is associated with a higher mortality rate.[89] Population studies of adults demonstrated that socially isolated males were 2 to 3 times more likely to die over the following 9 to 12 years and that socially isolated women were 1.5 times as likely to die.[90] This is not explained by other lifestyle factors, although our social context has a significant influence on our lifestyle. This influence can be positive or negative. Having support to give up smoking, for example, makes it much easier, whereas a lack of support can make it all but impossible.

The most common sources of social support are family and friends. It has been shown that cancer patients who are married or have a stable relationship survive for longer than would otherwise be expected. Reviews of the studies have shown an 'association between at least one psychosocial variable and disease outcome. Parameters associated with better breast cancer prognosis are social support, marriage, and minimising and denial, while depression and constraint of emotions are associated with decreased breast cancer survival'.[91]

In cancer management, social support can be provided or enhanced in a number of ways. These include the informal support provided by helpful and nurturing health-carers and the formal provision of cancer support programs. The effects of such programs have been discussed above and providing them should be part of standard cancer care.

EXERCISE THERAPY

Evidence for the role of exercise in the prevention and management of cancer is significant and growing. Regular moderate exercise helps to prevent a range of cancers, including cancers of the bowel, prostate and breast, and prolongs survival for those who already have cancer.

Reviewing the vast body of evidence, the World Cancer Research Fund has declared that physical inactivity is clearly a risk factor for cancer.[92] This can be illustrated by examining some of the studies reviewed.

Over 30 studies have shown a protective relationship between physical activity and colon cancer mortality.[93,94] This protective effect also extends to precancerous bowel polyps. The reduction of bowel cancer risk is around 50%.

Large-scale Norwegian studies show a 37% reduction in the risk of breast cancer in all women who exercise regularly, particularly in those less than 45 years of age, for whom the risk was 62% lower. In those who were lean, exercised approximately 4 hours per week and were premenopausal, the risk was reduced by 72%.[95] Similar findings have been found for lung cancer.[95] This is confirmed in an analysis of the Nurses' Health Study.[96] In postmenopausal women, brisk walking has been shown to reduce breast cancer risk. Another study looked at 75,000 postmenopausal women aged between 50 and 79 years, and showed that those who exercised at a level equivalent to brisk walking for 1¼ to 2½ hours per week had a significant breast cancer risk reduction of 18%.[97] This increased to 22% in those who exercised up to 10 hours per week. A past history of strenuous exercise at age 35 or 50 was associated with a breast cancer risk reduction. Independent of smoking and nutritional status, the Norwegian study mentioned above also showed a reduced risk of lung cancer in those who exercised. Aerobic exercise seems to be the best protection against cancer, and the suggested reasons as to why exercise protects against cancer include:

- changes to prostaglandins and other modulators of inflammation
- antioxidant effects
- maintaining a regular bowel habit and reducing bowel transit time
- protecting against obesity and metabolic syndrome by contributing to better overall energy balance
- facilitating other healthy lifestyle changes, such as better diet
- improvements in mental health and depression
- improvements in immune function
- stimulation of melatonin production.

Even more interesting are studies of the effect of exercise after a cancer diagnosis. The following studies illustrate this.

- A study of 2987 women with stage 1–3 breast cancer followed for up to 18 years found that the risk of death for those women who engaged in 9–15 MET-hr/week (approximately equivalent to walking 3–5 hr/week) was 0.50—that is, they had half the chance of dying during that time.[98] This was confirmed in another study over a 9-year follow-up on women with breast cancer, where regular exercise was associated with a 44% reduction in death rates.[99]
- A study of 47,620 men who were followed for over 14 years found that approximately 3000 had developed prostate cancer during that time. Many prostate cancers are very slow growing and not life threatening, but some become aggressive and can advance rapidly. In men older than 65, the risk of getting advanced prostate cancer was one-third as great if they exercised regularly.[100]
- A study followed 526 patients with bowel (colorectal) cancer for over 5 years and found that the risk of death was halved in those with stage II and III bowel cancer if they exercised regularly.[101]

The above findings could be contrasted with the 'success' of chemotherapy for adult malignancies, which has tended to be much oversold to cancer patients.

It is very clear that cytotoxic chemotherapy only makes a minor contribution (2%) to (5-year) cancer survival. To justify the continued funding and availability of drugs used in cytotoxic chemotherapy, a rigorous evaluation of the cost-effectiveness and impact on quality of life is urgently required.[102]

Hopefully, if cancer patients understand the benefits of exercise for cancer, they will be motivated to do it.

Exercise must be a part of your management plan for preventing or treating any type of cancer. When initiating an exercise program, working the body regularly through exercise is useful, provided you carefully consider the patient's age, previous exercise history and current level of fitness.

Exercise not only helps with preventing and managing cancer, it also helps with many symptoms common among cancer patients. It is associated with reduced fatigue, greater quality of life, reduced emotional distress, improved immunological parameters, and improved aerobic capacity and muscle strength.[103] It can also help with other symptoms common in cancer, such as chronic pain.[104] The reduction in pain is largely due to the fact that exercise induces endorphins but is also because of its positive effects on mood, muscle relaxation and its anti-inflammatory effect, which is important for those whose pain is secondary to an inflammatory process.

NUTRITION

It is clear that what we eat contributes to our risk of developing cancer. Research is seeking to establish which foods protect and which increase risk, and how much is optimal. Overall, a poor diet increases cancer risk, probably by 30%.[105,106] One point to emphasise in the information given below is that although most studies look at just one food group or one type of cancer, the same principle is likely to hold for other cancers. Although there may be some individual foods that have a particularly important role for individual cancers, as a general rule, if a food has been found to be good for one cancer it is likely to be good for other cancers as well.

Oxidation is part of the ageing process and is largely mediated by 'free radicals'. Antioxidants help to 'mop up' excess free radicals and slow the ageing process. Principally, dietary antioxidants reduce cancer risk, and a healthy diet with nutritious whole food prepared in a way that preserves its nutritional value is most protective. 'Protective elements in a cancer-preventive diet include selenium, folic acid, vitamin B_{12}, vitamin D, chlorophyll and antioxidants such as carotenoids (alpha-carotene, beta-carotene, lycopene, lutein, cryptoxanthin).'[107]

Although there is evidence that some antioxidant supplements, such as selenium, can have a protective effect, the best protection is gained through a healthy diet rather than taking supplements, particularly in the presence of a deficient diet. This point is illustrated by a study on breast cancer, which concluded: 'Vegetable and, particularly, fruit consumption contributed to the decreased risk ... These results indicate the importance of diet, rather than supplement use ... in the reduction of breast cancer risk.'[108] Antioxidant supplementation may be more helpful, particularly in helping to reduce the negative impact of radiotherapy for cancer patients.[109] The chapter on genetics (Ch 31) will also provide some useful information about nutrition, genetics, antioxidants and cancer.

Lowering total calorie intake, otherwise known as calorie restriction, helps to reduce the risk not only of cancer but also of a range of other illnesses, and significantly increases longevity. According to the World Cancer Research Fund International (WCRF):

> Sweet drinks such as colas and fruit squashes can also contribute to weight gain. Fruit juices, even without added sugar, are likely to have a similar effect. Try to eat lower energy-dense foods such as vegetables, fruits and whole-grains. Opt for water or unsweetened tea or coffee in place of sugary drinks.[110]

The WCRF also advocates a diet low in saturated fats. A trial on nearly 2500 women with breast cancer found that a low-fat diet was associated with a 24% reduction in recurrence and 19% improvement in survival after 5 years.[111]

The WCRF recommendation is that there is no amount of processed meat (bacon, ham, salami, corned beef and some sausages) that can be confidently shown not to increase cancer risk, particularly for bowel cancer. One should limit total intake of red meat to < 500 g cooked weight, which is equivalent to about 700–750 g raw weight, per week. Red meat probably increases the risk for a range of cancers other than bowel cancers,[112] although other white meats or fish are probably less problematic. If eating meat, where possible, certified organic and free range are preferred. There are a range of hormones, antibiotics and chemicals used by many commercial meat producers that may be more problematic than is currently known.

To date, evidence does not support a 'miracle' food to cure cancer, but many foods have been identified that significantly contribute to cancer prevention and treatment. Below are some of the most important foods, remembering that it is the consistent intake of a balanced, varied and healthy diet that is best.

- The American Institute of Cancer Research estimates that if the only dietary change made was to increase the daily intake of *fruits and vegetables* to five servings per day, cancer rates could decline significantly.
- Cabbage, broccoli, brussel sprouts, kale, watercress, bok choy, turnip and cauliflower are part of the *cabbage or cruciferous family*. Although not the most popular vegetables for many people they are very prominent when it comes to cancer management, especially slowing the spread of cancer.[113,114] In a study involving 47,909 people over a 10-year period, eating five or more weekly servings of cruciferous vegetables, especially broccoli and cabbage, was associated with half the risk of developing cancer compared with people consuming one or no servings per week. Other studies confirm their protective effect—for example: 'strong evidence for a substantial protective effect (approximately 35% reduced risk) of cruciferous vegetable consumption on lung cancer.'[115] The cancer-protective effects of broccoli are significantly diminished when it is over-cooked.[116] Women with breast cancer are significantly less likely to have recurrences if they eat five or more *vegetable* servings per day.[117] These findings are similar to those of another study, which found that women with breast cancer who had a high intake of fruit and vegetables—as indicated by a high blood carotenoid concentration—had a 43% reduced risk for breast cancer recurrence.[118]
- Eating *certified organic fruits and vegetables* is probably advisable, because of their much higher concentrations of important vitamins, minerals and antioxidants.
- Current information suggests that garlic may play an important part in the prevention of prostate, stomach, colon and oesophageal cancers[119] and possibly breast cancer. Freshly crushed garlic is the best nutritionally.
- *Citrus fruits* such as oranges, grapefruits, mandarins and lemons are essential foods in cancer prevention.
- *Red grapes* (and wine) contain a compound in their skins called resveratrol, which has anti-cancer activity, so moderate consumption of resveratrol supplements, red grapes (or wine) may be useful.
- *Tomatoes* have high levels of lycopene, a pigment that gives tomatoes their bright red colour and their anti-cancer potential. Lycopene's anti-cancer effect is increased by cooking tomatoes in the presence of vegetable fats such as olive oil.
- *Soy*—there are great differences in the rates of hormone-dependent cancers (breast and prostate) between Eastern and Western countries.[120] This may be related to the consumption of soy-based foods in Asian countries, especially when consumption begins before puberty. Soy foods include soybeans, soy flour, miso, tofu and soy milk. Studies have shown that, for a person to benefit from the anti-cancer effects of soy, they need to consume about 50 g per day of soy-based food. Only whole soy foods are considered cancer protective. Supplements containing isoflavones are not considered useful. Soy foods have also been found to be protective against colorectal cancer.[121] For people with existing hormone-dependent cancers there is some concern regarding the safety of soy products, although at the moment it is difficult to delineate the extent to which the risk is anticipated or real. Some studies have even suggested a protective role of genistein, a form of phyto-oestrogen, in reducing the risk of breast cancer recurrence.

- Green tea contains large amounts of catechins, which are compounds that may have many anti-cancer properties.[122]
- *Strawberries, raspberries, blueberries, goji berries and cranberries*[123] have high levels of antioxidants and anti-cancer phytochemicals.[124]
- *Omega-3 fatty acids*, found in sardines, mackerel, salmon, flax seed, soy and nuts, especially walnuts, can help to prevent cancer.[125] Studies have shown that consuming fish rich in omega-3 decreases the risk of developing breast, prostate or colon cancer.
- *Insoluble fibre* helps to prevent bowel cancer. Studies suggest that people in the top 20% for fibre intake, who ate an average of 35 g of fibre daily, had the risk of colorectal cancer reduced by 40%, compared to those eating 15 g of fibre daily.[126]

  Insoluble fibre is not absorbed from the gut and therefore bulks and loosens stools, which helps to reduce the transit time.
- Seasonings and herbs such as *turmeric, parsley, thyme, mint* or *capers*[127,128] have been found to have inhibitory activity on the growth of cancer cells, as well as preventing the development of tumours.
- Good-quality *dark chocolate*[129] that contains 70% cocoa mass (plenty of cocoa but not too much fat or sugar) contains polyphenols, which can help with cancer management. Eating two 20 g squares a day is enough.

The diet that is part of the Ornish program used for cancer is described in more detail later in this chapter.

ENVIRONMENT

Many patients who have been diagnosed with cancer will be interested in ways of altering their environment to reduce future risk for themselves and their families. There are various ways in which one's environment can increase the risk of cancer. For example, there are five major household and environmental cancer hazards.[130]

- *Pollution and passive smoking*:
  - Heavy air pollution makes a contribution to cancer risk, mostly lung cancer, but nowhere near as great as smoking. Diesel is more problematic than other pollutants.
  - Regular and long-standing exposure to passive smoking increases the risk of some forms of lung and throat cancer. For those with heavy exposure, the risk is nearly doubled.[131] Avoiding regular contact with passive smoking is advised, and legislation on smoking in public places has made this much easier.
- *Asbestos fibre*:
  - Asbestos was a common building and insulation material used last century. When asbestos materials become damaged and crumble, the tiny fibres can be breathed in and cause cell damage leading to lung (mesothelioma) and throat cancer.
  - Asbestos was commonly used in older homes built before the 1960s, and it is important to have it removed by persons qualified to do this work. There are a range of procedures required to do this safely.
- *Pesticides, insecticides and weed-killers*:
  - People who are exposed to a range of agricultural chemicals are at a higher risk of a variety of cancers, including lymphoma, leukaemia and prostate, skin and lung cancers. Farmers are at particular risk.
  - Correct use and storage of these chemicals is important. Only use them if necessary. If possible, to minimise the need to use them, use natural methods such as companion planting and mulching.
  - Use as little as possible, follow safety precautions, wear protective clothes, wash after use and keep poisons away from children.
- *Household cleaners, solvents and chemicals*:
  - There is not nearly enough research into the potentially harmful effects of many household products. Products containing benzene and methylene chloride (present in some paint strippers and paints) can cause cancer.
  - Use these products sparingly and use environmentally friendly products wherever possible. Take appropriate precautions, ventilate the area adequately, avoid contact with skin, wash after use, and store safely.
- *Electromagnetic fields (EMF)*:
  - Radiation and magnetic fields are a normal part of our environment and all exposure is not necessarily bad. Low-level exposure from sources such as household exposure, mobile phones or computers probably does not increase cancer risk, according to the current balance of evidence.[132]
  - Higher-level exposure, such as living in close proximity (within 200–300 metres) of high-voltage power lines or radio towers, probably does increase cancer risk, particularly for children.[133] Part of the reason may be because such fields disrupt melatonin secretion.
  - Having a simple procedure like a chest X-ray has been assumed to be safe, and this may be so for those with a low cancer risk, but the story may not be the same for those with a strong genetic predisposition to cancer. For example, women with breast cancer genes (BRCA1/2) had double the risk of getting breast cancer if they had had a chest X-ray, and if they had had the chest X-ray

before the age of 20 then the risk was increased four-fold.[134] This may be because it takes relatively less radiation exposure to cause DNA damage in genetically predisposed individuals. This should be taken into account before having radiological tests.
- Sunburn increases the risk of malignant melanoma and high-level sun exposure increases the risk of less dangerous skin cancers. Regular and moderate sun exposure, however, reduces the risk of a whole range of cancers, probably because of beneficial effects on vitamin D, melatonin, immunity, mood and lifestyle.

THE ORNISH PROGRAM

To date, the Ornish program is the only comprehensive lifestyle program to have been trialled on any form of cancer.

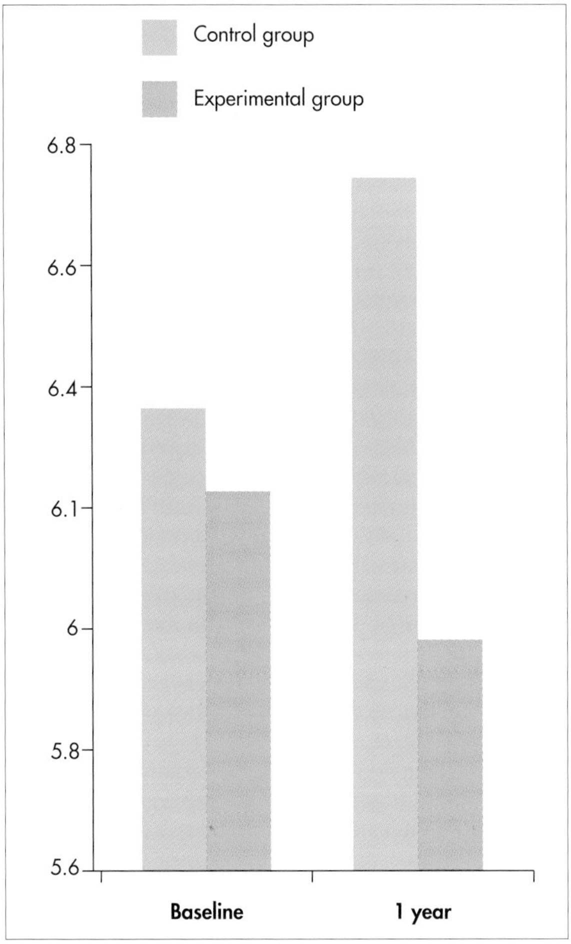

FIGURE 24.1 Change in PSA levels for controls and Ornish (experimental) group

A study of men with early prostate cancer evaluated the effects, after 1 year of comprehensive lifestyle changes, on PSA and LNCaP (a marker of the body's defences against prostate cancer).[135] Eighty men with early, biopsy-proven prostate cancer who had chosen active surveillance were chosen for the study.

The men who had chosen to watch and wait were randomly assigned to the experimental (Ornish lifestyle program) group or the control (usual lifestyle) group. The Ornish program chosen for men with prostate cancer included:

- vegan diet:
  - fruits, vegetables, whole grains, legumes and soy
  - low fat (10% calories from fat), particularly saturated/animal product fats
  - supplemented by soy (tofu), fish oil (3 g daily), vitamin E (400 IU daily), selenium (200 mcg daily), vitamin C (2 g daily)
- exercise:
  - walking for 30 minutes, six times weekly
- stress management:
  - gentle yoga, meditation, breathing and progressive muscle relaxation
- support group (1 hour weekly).

What the researchers found was very interesting. Over the following year, no men in the experimental (Ornish) group went on to develop aggressive cancer, but 6 of the 40 men in the control group underwent conventional treatment due to an increase in PSA and/or progression of their disease on MRI.

Figure 24.1 shows the average change in PSA (ng/mL) after 1 year. The average PSA of men in the Ornish group fell, unlike that of the control group. Figures 24.2 and 24.3 show that the changes in PSA and LNCaP cell growth were significantly associated with the degree of lifestyle change, meaning that the more lifestyle change the men adhered to, the greater the improvement in their condition. PSA levels decreased by an average of 4% in the experimental group but increased by an average of 6% in the control group, and growth of LNCaP prostate cancer cells was inhibited eight times more by serum from the experimental group than from the control group.

More recent follow-up of these programs is indicating that the improvements from making these lifestyle changes become more marked with time and is explaining more about the mechanisms whereby the improvements are produced. The lifestyle changes are associated with alterations of cancer gene expression[136] and improved telomerase-based genetic repair[137], both of which indicate good prognosis. This is confirmed with the findings that, at 2-year follow-up, 27% (13/49) of the patients in the control group had gone on to require aggressive cancer treatment because of disease

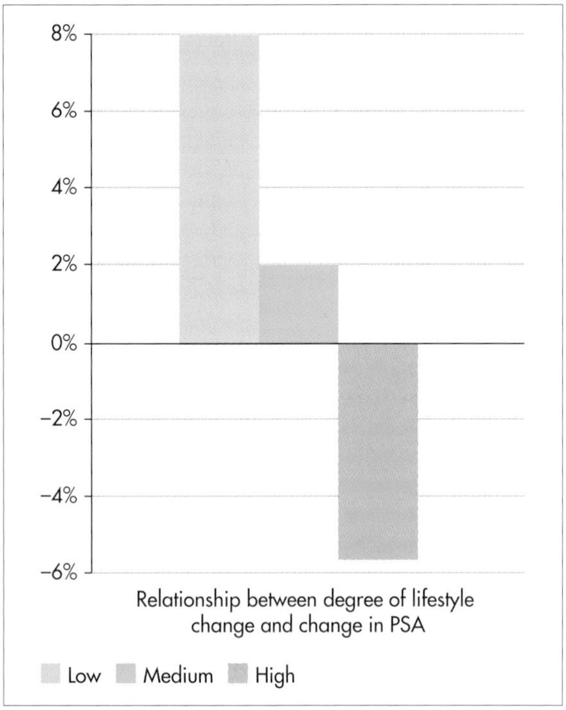

FIGURE 24.2 Relationship between degree of lifestyle change and change in PSA level

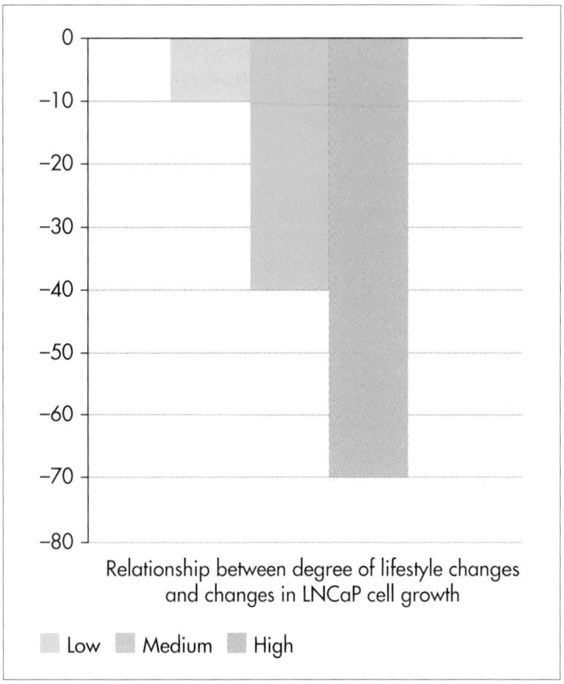

FIGURE 24.3 Relationship between degree of lifestyle change and change in prostate cancer cell growth

progression, whereas only 5% (2/43) of patients in the Ornish lifestyle group had gone on to require cancer treatment because of disease progression.[138]

The belief that cancer, like heart disease, is an inevitably progressive condition may in fact be far from the truth, although more research is desperately needed to see:

- if a similar approach holds for other cancers
- if particular variations on the program are important for certain varieties of cancer
- at what stage and to what extent a lifestyle-based approach can make a difference
- the extent to which such an approach can minimise the need for invasive and expensive cancer treatments
- what the effect of such programs is on cancer treatment and side effects.

It is already well known that such programs improve the quality of life and mental health of participants. If a patentable cancer drug had anywhere near this effect it would be widely publicised as a revolutionary cancer breakthrough and the discoverer would probably have a Nobel Prize for their efforts. Undramatic as it is, it is easy for such an approach to meet with a mentality and system within the healthcare sector that cannot or will not embrace it. It is likely that times will change, and some decades from now we will scratch our heads when we contemplate our current approach to cancer therapy and the slowness to embrace the simplest, safest and most effective strategies.

PREVENTION AND SCREENING

(See also Ch 13, Screening and prevention)

PREVENTION: WCRF RECOMMENDATIONS

A recent statement was issued by the World Cancer Research Fund (WCRF) following a review of decades of research into the prevention of cancer.[139] The WCRF made a series of recommendations for cancer prevention. Box 24.3 is adapted from that list.

CANCER SCREENING ACTIVITIES

Screening activities in general practice with particular relevance to cancer include:

- *taking a comprehensive history of risk factors*—including family history of heritable factors, environmental and occupational risk (e.g. asbestos exposure, sun exposure), nutrition, assessment of activity levels, smoking, alcohol consumption and emotional health
- *evidence-based guidelines*—these change regularly, based on current available evidence, and there will always be a tension between effectiveness and

economics; guidelines for screening should be considered in that context
- *examination and screening tests*—including those described below.

BOX 24.3 WCRF recommendations for cancer prevention[3]

1 **Be as lean as possible without becoming underweight.**
Weight gain and obesity increases the risk of a number of cancers. Maintain a healthy weight through healthy nutrition and regular physical activity to lower cancer risk.

2 **Be physically active for at least 30 minutes every day.**
There is strong evidence that physical activity protects against cancer. Regular physical activity is also vital for maintaining a healthy weight.

3 **Calorie restriction: avoid sweet drinks and limit energy-dense foods, particularly processed foods high in added sugar, low in fibre or high in fat.**
Energy-dense foods are high in fats and/or sugars and generally low in nutrient value (vitamins, antioxidants, minerals etc), and increase the risk of obesity and therefore cancer.

4 **Eat a wide variety of vegetables, fruits, whole grains and pulses such as beans.**
Evidence shows that the above foods containing dietary fibre may protect against a range of cancers and help to protect against weight gain and obesity.

5 **Limit consumption of red meat (e.g. beef, pork and lamb) and avoid processed meat.**
There is strong evidence that red and processed meats are causes of bowel cancer, and probably other cancers.

6 **Limit alcoholic drinks to two for men and one for women a day.**
Any consumption of alcoholic drinks can increase the risk of a number of cancers, although there is evidence to suggest that small amounts of alcohol can help protect against heart disease.

7 **Limit consumption of salty foods and food processed with salt.**
Evidence shows that salt and salt-preserved foods probably cause stomach cancer. Processed foods, including bread and breakfast cereals, can contain large amounts of salt.

8 **Don't use supplements to protect against cancer.**
Research shows that high-dose nutrient supplements can reduce our risk of cancer but it is best to opt for a balanced diet without supplements.

9 **It is best for mothers to breastfeed exclusively for up to 6 months.**
Breastfeeding protects mothers against breast cancer and babies from excess weight gain.

Examination and screening tests

Weight, height and BMI

Body mass index (BMI) is a mathematical formula calculated by measuring weight in kilograms and dividing it by height in metres squared (BMI = kg/m^2). BMI categories are:
- Underweight ≤ 18.5
- Normal weight for young and middle-aged adults = 18.5–24.9
- Overweight = 25–29.9
- Obesity ≥ 30

Waist measurement

Research by the Cancer Council Victoria involving over 40,000 subjects found a direct link between waist measurement and cancer risk.[140] The results showed that being overweight or obese is associated with an increased risk of cancer of the colon, postmenopausal breast cancer and cancers of the endometrium, kidney and oesophagus. Men with a waistline over 100 cm were found to have a 72% greater risk for colon cancer and 43% for prostate cancer. For women with a waistline over 85 cm, the risk was 22% higher for breast cancer and 33% higher for colon cancer. The Cancer Council estimates that in Victoria, Australia, in 2004, 1100 cancer cases and 500 cancer deaths could be attributed to overweight and obesity.

Waist circumference is taken simply by putting a tape measure around the waist at the level of the umbilicus. For men:
- 94 cm or more = increased health risk
- 102 cm or more = substantially increased risk.

For women:
- 80 cm or more = increased health risk
- 88 cm or more = substantially increased risk.

Testicular examination

The peak incidence of testicular cancer is in males aged 15–35 years. It is the most common form of cancer in this age group.

Male babies and infants should be checked opportunistically for maldescent of the testes, a risk factor. Other risk factors are a previous history of testicular cancer, orchidopexy and testicular atrophy.

From puberty, boys should be instructed in testicular self-examination and report any abnormal findings (painless lump, testicular pain, heaviness or swelling). Testicular examination is an important part of regular clinical examination in adolescents and young men.

While to date no studies have been done to determine whether routine screening of asymptomatic patients improves rates of morbidity and mortality, we do know that early detection improves the likelihood of cure.

Abnormal clinical findings are followed up with Doppler ultrasound and tumour markers prior to surgical referral.

Pap smear (women)

A good-quality cell sample from the transformation zone of the cervix for Pap smear testing, ideally with a concurrent ThinPrep sample, should be performed every 2 years for women with no clinical evidence of cervical pathology. Screening should commence at 18–20 years or 1–2 years after first intercourse (whichever is later) until 70 years of age.

Abnormal Pap smears need to be rigorously followed up. There is no international consensus on how women with low-grade abnormalities should be managed, and so the following is based on Australian guidelines.[141]

All women with a first report of a low-grade squamous abnormality, whether possible or definite, should have a repeat Pap smear in 12 months. If this repeat smear shows persistent low-grade abnormalities, the woman should then be referred for a colposcopy. If the second smear is normal, the woman should undergo a repeat Pap test 12 months later.

All women with atypical glandular cell reports should be referred for colposcopy.

If, at any stage, high-grade abnormalities (CIN 2 or above) are detected in any patient, the guidelines recommend automatic referral for a colposcopy.

High-risk HPV testing is used as a test of cure following treatment for CIN 2 and CIN 3.

Ovarian cancer

Current tests used in the diagnosis of ovarian cancer are the CA-125 blood test and transvaginal ultrasound. However, evidence does not support universal screening of asymptomatic women.[142]

Breast cancer

Breast cancer is the most common cancer in women. Women aged 50 or older are encouraged to have a mammogram every 2 years to screen for breast cancer.

Even with a fully implemented mammographic screening program, more than half of all breast cancers in Australia are found by women themselves, or their doctors, as a change in the breast.[143] However, the results of randomised trials do not show that a systematic approach to breast self-examination finds breast cancers early or affects survival.[144] Nevertheless, breast awareness through self-examination is recommended, and women should be encouraged to present to their doctor early with any breast changes that they notice, irrespective of whether they have had recent screening mammography with normal results.[145]

The 'triple test' for breast cancer involves:

- clinical breast examination and taking a personal history
- imaging tests (mammogram, ultrasound and/or MRI)
- if there is a suspicion of breast cancer—a biopsy to remove cells or tissue for examination.

Colorectal cancer

Colonoscopy has the highest level of sensitivity and specificity for detection of colorectal neoplasia and is considered the gold standard for detecting and treating precancerous polyps, but there are no meta-analyses of screening using colonoscopy. Accessibility and affordability are other considerations. Ideally, it should be performed every 5 years from the age of 50 years, starting at 40 years if there is a family history of bowel cancer or polyps, or more often if the patient has previously identified polyps or is at higher risk because of inflammatory bowel disease or coeliac disease.

Faecal occult blood testing (FOBT) trials have shown a link between a favourable shift in staging and mortality reduction in populations aged over 50 years. It fails to detect most polyps and some cancers.

Sigmoidoscopy and FOBT has been found to be cost-effective but will only identify polyps or cancers in the rectum and sigmoid colon.

Digital rectal examination may be performed during a physical examination but only allows examination of the lower part of the rectum.

Skin check

Patients may request a skin check as part of a general health check or present for assessment of a skin lesion they are concerned about. Patients should be encouraged to be alert to any new or changing skin lesions. When a patient presents with concerns about a skin lesion, a whole body skin examination should be conducted.

Prostate cancer

Mass population PSA screening is currently not recommended, does not have international consensus and is the subject of intense debate. The current recommendation is:

- a single PSA test at age 40 years or beyond.[146] If the PSA is above age-specific median levels (higher than 0.6 at age 40, higher than 0.7 at 50), then the intensity of subsequent monitoring of men at higher risk would be individualised according to family history, DRE findings, PSA velocity and PSA derivatives (see Ch 50)
- then annual PSA testing and digital rectal examination from age 50.

Recall and reminder systems

There is a common law duty and a professional standards requirement to have an efficient recall and reminder system for patients, preferably computerised where practical.

TREATMENT

TREATMENT PLAN

Using Figure 24.4 as a decision tool, you can discuss options for what could be included in a treatment plan with the patient and their family. Beginning with the type of cancer, your decision flows to the stage of the cancer journey, and what interventions are appropriate for each stage. Where specific symptom control is required, a decision is made about the combination of treatments and the healthcare professional most appropriate to deliver those treatments.

THE THERAPEUTIC TEAM

Responsible and efficient cancer care requires a team approach, ideally with a central healthcare professional working with the patient and their family to coordinate and facilitate referrals and time treatments on an individualised basis. The team may include but would not be limited to any combination of:

- *GP*—managing all acute and chronic health problems, coordinating referrals and the therapeutic team, and optimising health during the cancer journey
- *surgeon*—advising, planning surgical treatment options, performing surgery and managing the immediate postoperative period
- *oncologist*—staging the cancer and devising and supervising administration of chemotherapy and adjuvant medical therapies

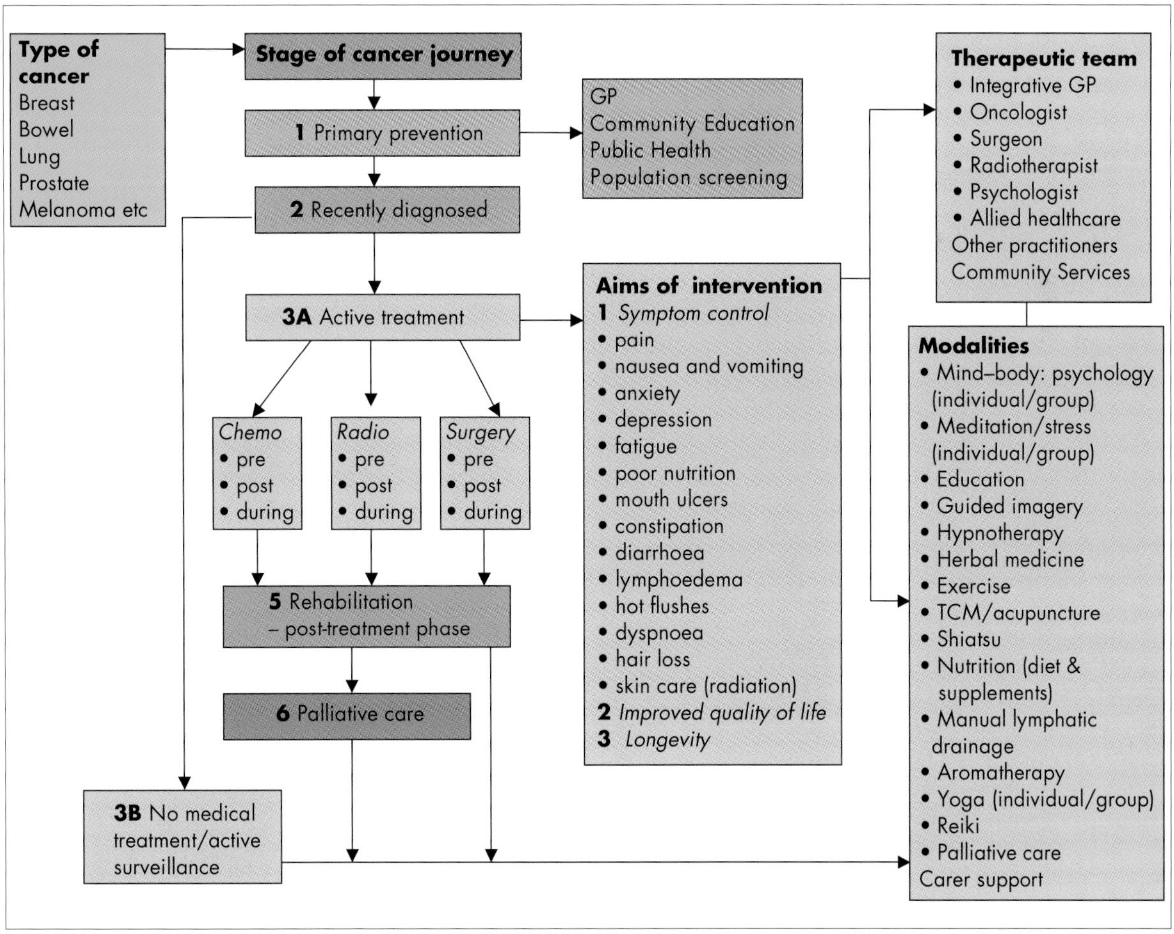

FIGURE 24.4 Decision tool for the cancer treatment plan

- *radiotherapist*—devising and supervising a course of radiotherapy
- *psychologist*—providing individual counselling or group therapy to deal with emotional issues for patients with cancer and their families
- *naturopath*—advising and prescribing lifestyle and natural therapies including diet, herbal treatments and nutritional supplements as an adjunct to medical and surgical treatments, preferably in consultation with the patient's GP and medical specialists
- *cancer nurse*—providing nursing care and support for patients diagnosed with cancer; may be responsible for administering chemotherapy and helping to manage symptoms related to cancer illnesses
- *other allied healthcare personnel*—such as dietician, exercise physiologist, occupational therapist, social worker, massage therapist
- *support groups, family and carer(s)*.

SYMPTOMS AND SIDE EFFECTS

It is important to have a comprehensive discussion with the patient regarding their current symptoms and what to expect. The symptoms may relate to the cancer or to its treatment (surgery, radiotherapy, chemotherapy) and may include:

- pain
- nausea and vomiting
- anxiety
- depression
- fatigue
- poor nutrition
- weight loss
- mouth ulcers
- constipation or diarrhoea
- lymphoedema
- hot flushes
- hair loss
- skin problems (from radiation)
- reduced immune function
- cardiotoxicity.

PAIN

Pain is one of the most common and distressing symptoms experienced by cancer patients. Management of cancer pain needs to consider physiological, psychological, emotional, social, cultural and spiritual factors. For these reasons the integrative approach to cancer pain requires a combination of expertise in medical, surgical, psychological and pharmacological assessment and treatment of the patient. The choice of therapy or combination of therapies depends on the aetiology of the pain, its severity and the availability of skilled practitioners.

Useful modalities include regional anaesthesia techniques, pharmacological analgesia, acupuncture and mind–body techniques (see Ch 38, Pain management).

NAUSEA AND VOMITING

Nausea and vomiting are common adverse effects of chemotherapy. While state-of-the-art antiemetic medications are usually needed, adjunctive therapies can reduce the amount of medication needed, or improve tolerance of chemotherapy.

- *Medication*—patients undergoing chemotherapy are usually provided with antiemetic medication such as metoclopramide or ondansetron (Zofran®) for prophylaxis or symptom relief.

  Dose: metoclopramide 10 mg p.o. or IMI 1–2 hours before chemotherapy administration, then 8-hourly.

  Ondansetron is usually required. It is available in IV, tablet and wafer form.

  Dose: single dose of 8 mg IV prophylactically then 8 mg 6-hourly × 2 doses, plus dexamethasone 8 mg IV 30 minutes before administration of chemotherapy, then 6-hourly.
- *Acupuncture*[147] and acupuncture point stimulation[148] have been shown to relieve nausea associated with chemotherapy. Of all the investigated effects of acupuncture on cancer-related or chemotherapy-related symptoms and disorders, the positive effect of acupuncture on chemotherapy-induced nausea and vomiting is the most convincing.[149]
- Regular sips of *clear, cool drinks* can help to reduce nausea.
- *Cold food* or food at room temperature may be more appealing than hot food, as the smell of cooked food may trigger nausea.
- Nausea can be reduced by eating small amounts of *salty or sour foods* (such as lemon or sour pickles). Sour or mint sweets or chewing gum may also help.
- *Ginger (Zingiber officinale)* has an anti-nausea effect.[150] It can be taken as dried root (1–3 g daily in divided doses or 1–2 g as a single dose) or as a tea infusion (4–6 slices steeped for 30 minutes in boiling water).
- *Baiacal skullcap* has an antiemetic effect, which suggests a role in managing nausea and vomiting.[151]

  Dose: dried herb 6–15 g/day; liquid extract (1:2) 4.5–8.5 mL/day in divided doses.
- *Astragalus*—a Cochrane review of Chinese herbs for chemotherapy side effects in colorectal cancer

patients showed that *Astragalus* can reduce nausea, vomiting and leucopenia.[152]

- *Mind–body techniques* such as hypnosis and mindfulness meditation may help tolerance of nausea.

ANXIETY AND DEPRESSION

Anxiety and depression are frequently associated with the diagnosis of cancer and with its treatment, and health professionals involved in care of cancer patients need to anticipate its possibility and be aware of the signs. Research shows that 20–35% of people with cancer experience ongoing depression, and 15–23% of people with cancer experience anxiety.[153]

Useful interventions include counselling, support groups, hypnotherapy, music therapy, meditation, stress management, acupuncture and yoga. St John's wort may be useful for treatment of depression following treatment but care needs to be taken to check for potential interactions during chemotherapy. Significant interactions include decreased efficacy of cyclosporin, tacrolimus, irinotecan and other chemotherapeutic agents. It has also been shown to have some anti-neoplastic properties.[154]

FATIGUE

Fatigue associated with chemotherapy and radiotherapy is common and often underestimated. Surgery, hormone therapy and immunotherapy can also create fatigue as a side effect. It has biological and psychological causes.

It is important to investigate and treat possible causes such as nutritional deficiency, anaemia, medication side effects, insomnia, underlying infection or depression.

Advice on managing fatigue includes the following:

- Advise patients to anticipate fatigue during treatment and to modify their planned activities in advance.
- Identify and treat any underlying causes.
- Pace activities—include rest periods interspersed with gentle exercise.
- Modify work duties.
- Enlist the help of friends and family for daily chores where possible.
- Avoid alcohol, caffeine and tobacco.
- Nutrition—include plenty of fluids and fresh organic fruit and vegetables, as well as iron-rich foods and complex carbohydrates.
- Cognitive behaviour therapy will help address underlying anxiety and fear.

CONSTIPATION

The most common causes of constipation in patients with cancer are low food intake, low fluid intake, medication side effect, lack of exercise, depression and reluctance to use the bowel because of discomfort or inconvenience.

- Nutritional approach—a diet with adequate amounts of cereals and fibre such as *Psyllium* or oats, and fruit and vegetables, will provide good sources of dietary fibre to prevent constipation.
- Patients should be advised to eat frequent small amounts, chewing thoroughly.
- Drink at least six cups of water, tea, coffee, fruit juices, soup or other liquids every day.
- Attempt some physical activity as tolerated.
- Where codeine or morphine preparations are prescribed, constipation should be anticipated and dietary and laxative measures recommended prophylactically.
- Measures to prevent and manage constipation:
  - bulk-forming laxatives such as *Psyllium* mixed with water or sprinkled into cereal, or Metamucil (processed and flavoured *Psyllium*), flaxseed (*Linum usitatissimum*) powder or seeds, *fenugreek* (*Trigonella foenum-graecum*) or barley[155]
  - stimulant laxatives such as senna (*Cassia acutifolia*, *Cassia angustifolia*, *Cassia senna*) and *Cascara segrada* (300 mg once per day)[155]
  - osmotic laxatives such as lactulose or magnesium citrate
  - stool softeners (Coloxyl®)
  - probiotic supplementation with lactobacillus and *Bifidobacterium*.

POOR NUTRITION

Loss of appetite, nausea and altered taste and smell sensation during chemotherapy can adversely affect a patient's nutritional status. Special attention needs to be paid to nutritional status at times of nausea and vomiting, and diet will need to be adjusted. Advise patients to eat very small, light meals or snacks frequently during the day and to avoid highly seasoned foods, and fried or fatty foods. Fresh organic whole foods are preferred where possible.

Protein, vitamin and mineral supplementation will be required for nutritional support where anorexia prevents adequate intake of food.

MOUTH ULCERS

Cancer-treatment-related mouth ulcers are painful and can make it difficult to talk, breathe, eat and swallow. It might not be possible to prevent mouth ulcers, but there are some measures patients can take prior to treatment, to reduce their severity. A preventive dental check and thorough dental hygiene treatment are recommended prior to chemotherapy or radiotherapy aimed at the head and neck. Patients should be strongly encouraged to stop smoking and to eat a diet rich in fruit and vegetables.Throughout treatment, oral hygiene is essential.

- Rinse mouth with filtered water (with a small amount of salt or bicarbonate of soda added) every 2 hours while awake.
- Low-dose oral glutamine supplementation during and after chemotherapy significantly reduced both the duration and the severity of chemotherapy-associated stomatitis.[156] Swish around the mouth and swallow.
- Use a soft-bristle toothbrush to clean teeth after every meal. If platelet count is adequate, floss with unwaxed floss daily.
- Use an oral lubricant. Avoid mouthwashes containing alcohol.
- Apply lip balm regularly.

Maintain good nutrition focusing on high-protein and high-calorie foods that are soft and/or semi-liquid, and avoid foods that are sharp or brittle, spicy or hot. Avoid acidic food and alcohol (including medication containing alcohol).

Mouth ulcers can also be the result of infection with *Candida* species. Antifungal lozenges, drops or oral tablets may be necessary. Examples: nystatin, clotrimazole, fluconazole. Carafate® (sucralfate) applied to ulcers may provide protection.

Low-energy laser therapy is used in some specialised facilities to heal ulcers.

LYMPHOEDEMA

Lymphoedema can develop as an early or late consequence of disruption of the lymphatic drainage after surgery or radiotherapy. It most commonly affects a limb but can affect more proximal areas of the body, with the affected area becoming swollen, heavy, uncomfortable and less mobile.

Healthcare professionals need to be made aware of the risk and avoid procedures such as blood pressure measurement or venipuncture on the side that has previously been subject to lymphatic damage.

The aim of treatment is to control swelling, prevent infection and maintain function, and is best undertaken by a qualified lymphoedema therapist. A treatment program might need to involve:

- limb exercises
- pressure garments
- skin care
- specialised lymphatic massage
- low-level laser therapy of the whole limb, 2–5 sessions a week for 2–3 weeks.

Horse chestnut standardised extract (HCSE) contains a plant compound (escin) that is well tolerated and has traditional use in strengthening the tissues of the lymph vessels, capillaries and veins.[157] It may be useful in supporting treatment for lymphoedema.

Diuretic medications are not useful for this type of localised oedema.

SKIN INFLAMMATION FROM RADIOTHERAPY

Radiation dermatitis can be distressing for patients. Calendula ointment applied twice daily has been found to be superior to trolamine (a topical non-steroidal anti-inflammatory agent) for the prevention of skin toxicity of grade 2 or higher, and for other end points including allergy, interruption of treatment, patient satisfaction, pain relief and dermatitis.[158]

REDUCED IMMUNE FUNCTION

Stress management through mind–body interventions can help to support the immune system during cancer treatment.

Astragalus (huang-qi) is used in cancer patients to enhance the effectiveness of chemotherapy and reduce associated side effects. It is also used to enhance immune function. It has a wide safety margin. A Cochrane review of Chinese herbs for chemotherapy side effects in colorectal cancer patients showed that *Astragalus* can reduce nausea, vomiting and leucopenia.[159] Increases in the proportion of T-lymphocyte subsets (CD3, CD4 and CD8) were also reported.

Baiacal skullcap may be useful as an adjunctive therapy during cancer treatment to reduce nausea and immune suppression.[160]

There is a potential role for *Withania* as an adjunctive treatment during chemotherapy for the prevention of drug-induced bone marrow suppression.[161]

CARDIOTOXICITY

L-carnitine is an amino acid essential for energy production in mitochondria. Long-term carnitine administration 2 g daily or b.i.d. may reduce cardiotoxic side effects of adriamycin.[162]

Coenzyme Q10 provides some protection against cardiotoxicity caused by some forms of chemotherapy.[163,164]

HEPATOTOXICITY

Milk thistle (*Silybum marianum*)—standardised extract, 80–200 mg 1–3 times daily, has a hepatotoprotective effect in chemotherapy.[165,166]

Coenzyme Q10 provides some protection against hepatotoxicity during cancer treatment.

CHEMOTHERAPY AND RADIOTHERAPY: HERBS AND SUPPLEMENTS

Scientific research into the use of herbal medicine has grown exponentially in recent decades, and the popularity of complementary therapies as adjunctive cancer treatment has stimulated an increase in research into herbal medicines. As with any medicine prescribing, consideration needs to be given to the risks and benefits of any prescribed substance or combination of substances. With herbal medicine prescribing, there is the additional consideration of variability in the original plant material, purity of supply and production methods.

Phytomedicines can play a useful supportive role in cancer treatments. There is evidence to suggest that herbal medicines can reduce multi-drug resistance during chemotherapy as well as reducing the side effects of radiotherapy. Immune-stimulating and antifungal herbs can minimise multi-drug prescriptions.

Some herb–drug interactions are detrimental (see Ch 5, Herb–drug interactions), while others have a beneficial, protective or additive effect in combination with chemotherapy agents. Issues such as combinations, timing in relation to chemotherapy and dosage ranges are important.

Herbs used with radiotherapy are listed in Box 24.4.

In traditional Chinese medicine, cancer is considered a result of long-term accumulation of blood stasis, phlegm and toxins, which are from poor lifestyle factors such as irregular diet, emotional swings, smoking and so on. In Western countries, Chinese herbal treatments are used mainly for the purpose of treating the patient's overall constitution, in order to promote general health and alleviate any discomfort. Western medical practitioners should consult a practitioner trained in herbal medicine to ensure the safety and efficacy of herb–drug combinations.

BOX 24.4 Herbs used with radiotherapy

- Milk thistle (*Silybum marianum*)[166]—standardised extract, 80–200 mg, 1–3 times daily, as an antioxidant and liver protectant
- Green tea (*Camellia sinensis*)[167]—standardised extract, 250–500 mg daily or as a tea, for antioxidant effects
- Panax ginseng (*Panax ginseng*)[168]—standardised extract,100–200 mg twice daily, for symptoms of radiation poisoning
- Reishi mushroom (*Ganoderma lucidum*)[169]—standardised extract, 150–300 mg, 2–3 times daily, for immune effects; also as tincture of this mushroom extract, 30–60 drops, 2–3 times daily
- Holy basil (*Ocimum sanctum*)[170]—standardised extract, 400 mg daily, for radiation protection
- Calendula (*Calendula officinalis*)[171]—topical cream, apply externally to radiation-damaged skin 2–3 times daily

RESOURCES

National Cancer Institute, http://www.cancer.gov

National Cancer Institute, Complementary and alternative medicine in cancer treatment, Questions and answers, http://www.cancer.gov/cancertopics/factsheet/therapy/CAM

National Institutes of Health, National Center for Complementary and Alternative Medicine, Cancer and CAM, http://nccam.nih.gov/health/cancer/camcancer.htm#top

PubMed, http://www.ncbi.nlm.nih.gov/sites/entrez

World Cancer Research Fund International, http://www.wcrf.org

REFERENCES

1 Dy GK, Bekele L, Hanson LJ et al. Complementary and alternative medicine use by patients enrolled onto phase 1 clinical trials. J Clin Oncol 2004; 22(23):4810–4815.

2 Hassed C. The Essence of health: the seven pillars of wellbeing. Sydney: Random House; 2008.

3 National Cancer Institute. Staging: questions and answers; 2004. Online. Available: http://www.cancer.gov/cancertopics/factsheet/detection/staging

4 Commonwealth of Australia, Senate Community Affairs Committee. The cancer journey: informing choice; 2005. Online. Available: http://www.aph.gov.au/SENATE/COMMITTEE/clac_ctte/completed_inquiries/2004-07/cancer/report/index.htm

5 Spiegel D, Giese-Davis J. Depression and cancer: mechanisms and disease progression. Biol Psychiatry 2003; 54(3):269–282. a p 269.

6 Brown KW, Levy AR, Rosberger Z et al. Psychological distress and cancer survival: a follow-up 10 years after diagnosis. Psychosom Med 2003; 65(4): 636–643.

7 Penninx BW, Guralnik JM, Pahor M et al. Chronically depressed mood and cancer risk in older persons. J Natl Cancer Inst 1998; 90(24):1888–1893.

8 Serraino D, Pezzotti P, Fratino L et al. Chronically depressed mood and cancer risk in older persons. J Natl Cancer Inst 1999; 91(12):1080–1081.

9 Satin JR, Linden W, Phillips MJ. Depression as a predictor of disease progression and mortality in cancer patients: a meta-analysis. Cancer 2009; 14 Sep [Epub ahead of print].

10 Steel JL, Geller DA, Gamblin TC et al. Depression, immunity, and survival in patients with hepatobiliary carcinoma. J Clin Oncol 2007; 25(17):2397–2405.

11 Faller H, Bulzebruck H, Drings P et al. Coping, distress, and survival among patients with lung cancer. Arch Gen Psychiatry 1999; 56(8):756–762.
12 Greer S, Morris T, Pettingale KW et al. Psychological response to breast cancer and 15-year outcome. Lancet 1990; 1:49–50.
13 Rogentine GN, van Kammen DP, Fox BH et al. Psychological factors in the prognosis of malignant melanoma: a prospective study. Psychosom Med 1979; 41:647–655.
14 Richardson J, Zarnegar Z, Bisno B et al. Psychosocial status at initiation of cancer treatment and survival. JPsychosom Res 1990; 4(2):189–201.
15 Montazeri A, Gillis CR, McEwen J. Quality of life in patients with lung cancer: a review of literature from 1970 to 1995. Chest 1998; 113:467–481.
16 Coates A, Gebski V, Signorini D et al. for the Australian New Zealand Breast Cancer Trials Group. Prognostic value of quality-of-life scores during chemotherapy for advanced breast cancer. J Clin Oncol 1992;10:1833–1838.
17 Dancey J, Zee B, Osoba D et al. Quality of life scores: an independent prognostic variable in a general population of cancer patients receiving chemotherapy. Qual Life Res 1997; 6:151–158.
18 Coates AS, Hurny C, Peterson HF et al. Quality-of-life scores predict outcome in metastatic but not early breast cancer. International Breast Cancer Study Group. J Clin Oncol 2000; 18(22):3768–3774.
19 Butow P, Coates A, Dunn S. Psychosocial predictors of survival in metastatic melanoma. J Clin Oncol 1999; 17(12):3856–3863.
20 Gottlieb BH, Wachala ED. Cancer support groups: a critical review of empirical studies. Psychooncology 2007; 16(5):379–400.
21 Spiegel D, Bloom JR, Kraemer HC et al. Effect of psychosocial treatment on survival of patients with metastatic breast cancer. Lancet 1989; 2:888–891.
22 Fawzy FI, Fawzy NW, Huyn CS et al. Malignant melanoma: effects of an early structured psychiatric intervention, coping and affective state on recurrence and survival six years later. Arch Gen Psychiatry 1993; 50:681–689.
23 Fawzy FI, Canada AL, Fawzy NW. Malignant melanoma: effects of a brief, structured psychiatric intervention on survival and recurrence at 10-year follow-up. Arch Gen Psychiatry 2003; 60(1):100–103.
24 Richardson JL, Shelton DR, Krailo M et al. The effect of compliance with treatment on survival among patients with hematologic malignancies. J Clin Oncol 1990; 8:356–364.
25 Kuchler T, Henne-Bruns D, Rappat S et al. Impact of psychotherapeutic support on gastrointestinal cancer patients undergoing surgery: survival results of a trial. Hepatogastroenterology 1999; 46(25):322–335.
26 Ratcliffe MA, Dawson AA, Walker LG. Eysenck Personality Inventory L-scores in patients with Hodgkin's disease and non-Hodgkin's lymphoma. Psychooncology 1995; 4:39–45.
27 Cunningham AJ, Edmonds CV, Phillips C et al. A prospective, longitudinal study of the relationship of psychological work to duration of survival in patients with metastatic cancer. Psychooncology 2000; 9(4): 323–339.
28 Edelman S, Lemon J, Bell DR et al. Effects of group CBT on the survival time of patients with metastatic breast cancer. Psychooncology 1999; 8(6):474–481.
29 Ilnyckyj A, Farber J, Cheang MC et al. A randomized controlled trial of psychotherapeutic intervention in cancer patients. Ann R Coll Physicians Surg Can 1994; 27:93–96.
30 Linn MW, Linn BS, Harris R. Effects of counseling for late stage cancer patients. Cancer 1982; 49: 1048–1055.
31 Goodwin PJ, Leszcz M, Ennis M et al. The effect of group psychosocial support on survival in metastatic breast cancer. N Engl J Med 2001; 345:1719–1726.
32 Kissane DW, Grabsch B, Clarke DM et al. Supportive-expressive group therapy for women with metastatic breast cancer: survival and psychosocial outcome from a randomized controlled trial. Psychooncology 2007; 16(4):277–286.
33 Kuchler T, Bestmann B, Rappat S et al. Impact of psychotherapeutic support for patients with gastrointestinal cancer undergoing surgery: 10-year survival results of a randomized trial. J Clin Oncol 2007; 25(19):2702–2708.
34 Fawzy FI. Psychosocial interventions for patients with cancer: what works and what doesn't. Eur J Cancer 1999; 35(11):1559–1564.
35 Cunningham A, Phillips C, Lockwood G et al. Association of involvement in psychological self-regulation with longer survival in patients with metastatic cancer: an exploratory study. Adv Mind Body Med 2000; 16(4):276–287.
36 Rehse B, Pukrop R. Effects of psychosocial interventions on quality of life in adult cancer patients: meta analysis of 37 published controlled outcome studies. Patient Educ Couns 2003; 50(2):179–186.
37 Visintainer MA, Volpicelli JR, Seligman ME. Tumor rejection in rats after inescapable or escapable shock. Science 1982; 216(4544):437–439.
38 Watson M, Homewood J, Haviland J et al. Influence of psychological response on breast cancer survival: 10-year follow-up of a population-based cohort. Eur J Cancer 2005; 41(12):1710–1714.
39 Schulman P, Keith D, Seligman ME. Is optimism heritable? A study of twins. Behav Res Therapy 1993; 31(6):569–574.

40 Petticrew M, Bell R, Hunter D. Influence of psychological coping on survival and recurrence in people with cancer: systematic review. BMJ 2002; 325(7372):1066.
41 Spiegel D, Giese-Davis J. Depression and cancer: mechanisms and disease progression. Biol Psychol 2003; 54(3):269–282.
42 Abercrombie HC, Giese-Davis J, Sephton S et al. Flattened cortisol rhythms in metastatic breast cancer patients. Psychoneuroendocrinology 2004; 29(8):1082–1092.
43 Sephton SE, Sapolsky RM, Kraemer HC et al. Diurnal cortisol rhythm as a predictor of breast cancer survival. J Natl Cancer Inst 2000; 92(12):994–1000.
44 Turner-Cobb JM, Sephton SE, Koopman C et al. Social support and salivary cortisol in women with metastatic breast cancer. Psychosom Med 2000; 62(3):337–345.
45 Pace TW, Negi LT, Adame DD et al. Effect of compassion meditation on neuroendocrine, innate immune and behavioral responses to psychosocial stress. Psychoneuroendocrinology 2009; 34(1):87–98.
46 Epel E, Daubenmier J, Moskowitz JT et al. Can meditation slow rate of cellular aging? Cognitive stress, mindfulness, and telomeres. Ann NY Acad Sci 2009; 1172:34–53.
47 Kiecolt-Glaser JK, Robles TF, Heffner KL et al. Psycho-oncology and cancer: psychoneuroimmunology and cancer. Ann Oncol 2002; 13(Suppl 4):165–169.
48 Miller SC, Pandi-Perumal SR, Esquifino AI et al. The role of melatonin in immuno-enhancement: potential application in cancer. Int J Exp Pathol 2006; 87(2): 81–87.
49 Lissoni P. Biochemotherapy with standard chemotherapies plus the pineal hormone melatonin in the treatment of advanced solid neoplasms. Pathol Biol 2007; 55(3/4):201–204.
50 Mills E, Wu P, Seely D et al. Melatonin in the treatment of cancer: a systematic review of randomized controlled trials and meta-analysis. J Pineal Res 2005; 39(4): 360–366.
51 Witek-Janusek L, Albuquerque K, Chroniak KR et al. Effect of mindfulness-based stress reduction on immune function, quality of life and coping in women newly diagnosed with early stage breast cancer. Brain Behav Immun 2008; 22(6):969–981.
52 Wood PA. Connecting the dots: obesity, fatty acids and cancer. Lab Invest 2009; 89(11):1192–1194.
53 Maiti B, Kundranda MN, Spiro TP et al. The association of metabolic syndrome with triple-negative breast cancer. Breast Cancer Res Treat 2009; 23 Oct [Epub ahead of print].
54 Pero RW, Roush GC, Markowitz MM et al. Oxidative stress, DNA repair, and cancer susceptibility. Cancer Detect Prev 1990; 14(5):555–561.
55 Irie M, Asami S, Nagata S et al. Classical conditioning of oxidative DNA damage in rats. Neurosci Lett 2000; 288(1):13–16.
56 Rabbitts J. Chromosomal translocations in human cancer. Nature 1994; 372:143.
57 Bushell WC. From molecular biology to anti-aging cognitive-behavioral practices: the pioneering research of Walter Pierpaoli on the pineal and bone marrow foreshadows the contemporary revolution in stem cell and regenerative biology. Ann NY Acad Sci 2005; 1057:28–49.
58 Oliver R. Does surgery disseminate or accelerate cancer? Lancet 1995; 346:1506.
59 Chrousos G. The HPA axis and immune mediated inflammation. N Engl J Med 1995; 332:1351.
60 Kearney R. From theory to practice: the implications of the latest psychoneuroimmunology research and how to apply them. MIH Conference Proceedings 1998;171–188.
61 Holmgren L, O'Reilly M, Folkman J et al. Dormancy of micrometastases: balanced proliferation and apoptosis in the presence of angiogenesis suppression. Nat Med 1995; 1:149.
62 Kune S, Kune GA, Watson LF et al. Recent life change and large bowel cancer. J Clin Epidemiol 1991; 44:57–68.
63 Maestroni GJ, Conti A, Pierpaoli W. Role of the pineal gland in immunity. J Neuroimmunol 1986; 13:19–30.
64 Pierpaoli W. Neuroimmunomodulation of aging. A program in the pineal gland. Ann NY Acad Sci 1998; 840:491–497.
65 Reiter R, Robinson J. Melatonin: your body's natural wonder drug. Bantam Books: New York; 1995.
66 Panzer A, Viljoen M. The validity of melatonin as an oncostatic agent. J Pineal Res 1997; 22(4):184–202.
67 Coker KH. Meditation and prostate cancer: integrating a mind/body intervention with traditional therapies. Sem Urol Oncol 1999; 17(2):111–118.
68 Callaghan BD. Does the pineal gland have a role in the psychological mechanisms involved in the progression of cancer? Med Hypotheses 2002; 59(3):302–311.
69 Brzezinski A. Melatonin in humans. N Engl J Med 1997; 336:186.
70 Weindruch R, Walford RL. Dietary restriction in mice beginning at 1 year of age: effect on lifespan and spontaneous cancer incidence. N Engl J Med 1997; 337:986–994.
71 Heuther G. Melatonin synthesis in the GI tract and the impact on nutritional factors on circulating melatonin. Ann NY Acad Sci 1994; 719:146.
72 Cronin A, Keifer J, Davies M et al. Melatonin secretion after surgery. Lancet 2000; 356(9237):1244–1245.
73 Massion AO, Teas J, Hebert JR et al. Meditation, melatonin and breast/prostate cancer: hypothesis and preliminary data. Med Hypotheses 1995; 44(1):39–46.

74 Tooley GA, Armstrong SM, Norman TR et al. Acute increases in night-time plasma melatonin levels following a period of meditation. Biol Psychol 2000; 53(1):69–78.
75 Sephton S, Spiegel D. Circadian disruption in cancer: a neuroendocrine–immune pathway from stress to disease? Brain Behav Immun 2003; 17(5):321–328.
76 Franzese E, Nigri G. Night work as a possible risk factor for breast cancer in nurses. Correlation between the onset of tumors and alterations in blood melatonin levels. Prof Inferm 2007; 60(2):89–93.
77 Kiecolt-Glaser J, Stephens R, Lipetz P et al. Distress and DNA repair in human lymphocytes. J Behav Med 1985; 8(4):311–320.
78 Irie M, Asami S, Nagata S et al. Relationships between perceived workload, stress and oxidative DNA damage. Int Arch Occup Environ Health 2001; 74(2):153–157.
79 Irie M, Asami S, Nagata S et al. Psychological factors as a potential trigger of oxidative DNA damage in human leukocytes. Jpn J Cancer Res 2001; 92(3):367–376.
80 Irie M, Asami S, Nagata S et al. Psychological mediation of a type of oxidative DNA damage, 8-hydroxydeoxyguanosine, in peripheral blood leukocytes of non-smoking and non-drinking workers. Psychother Psychosom 2002; 71(2):90–96.
81 Tomei LD, Kiecolt-Glaser JK, Kennedy S et al. Psychological stress and phorbol ester inhibition of radiation-induced apoptosis in human peripheral blood leukocytes. Psychol Res 1990; 33(1):59–71.
82 Lutgendorf SK, Johnsen EL, Cooper B et al. Vascular endothelial growth factor and social support in patients with ovarian carcinoma. Cancer 2002; 95(4):808–815.
83 Onogawa S, Tanaka S, Oka S et al. Clinical significance of angiogenesis in rectal carcinoid tumors. Oncol Rep 2002; 9(3):489–494.
84 Thaker PH, Han LY, Kamat AA et al. Chronic stress promotes tumor growth and angiogenesis in a mouse model of ovarian carcinoma. Nat Med 2006; 12(8): 939–944.
85 Carlson LE, Speca M, Faris P et al. One year pre-post intervention follow-up of psychological, immune, endocrine and blood pressure outcomes of mindfulness-based stress reduction (MBSR) in breast and prostate cancer outpatients. Brain Behav Immun 2007; 21(8):1038–1049. ap 1038.
86 Jim HS, Andersen BL. Meaning in life mediates the relationship between social and physical functioning and distress in cancer survivors. Br J Health Psychol 2007; 12(3):363–381.
87 Kune G, Kune S, Watson L. Perceived religiousness is protective for colorectal cancer: data from the Melbourne Colorectal Cancer Study. J R Soc Med 1993; 86:645–647.
88 Astin J, Harkness E, Ernst E. The efficacy of 'distant healing': a systematic review of randomised trials. Ann Intern Med 2000; 132(11):903–910.
89 Pelletier K. Mind–body health: research, clinical and policy applications. Am J Health Promot 1992; 6(5):345–358.
90 House J, Landis K, Umberson D. Social relationships and health. Science 1988; 241:540–545.
91 Falagas ME, Zarkadoulia EA, Ioannidou EN et al. The effect of psychosocial factors on breast cancer outcome: a systematic review. Breast Cancer Res 2007; 9(4):R44.
92 World Cancer Research Fund. Online. Available: http://www.wcrf-uk.org/cancer_prevention/index.lasso
93 Slattery M, Potter J, Caan B et al. Energy balance and colon cancer—beyond physical activity. Cancer Res 1997; 57:75–80.
94 Colditz G, Cannuscio C, Grazier A. Physical activity and reduced risk of colon cancer. Cancer Causes Control 1997; 8:649–667.
95 Thune I, Lund E. The influence of physical activity on lung cancer risk. Int J Cancer 1997; 70:57–62.
96 Rockhill B, Willett W, Hunter D et al. A prospective study of recreational activity and breast cancer risk. 1999; 159:2290–2296.
97 McTiernan A, Kooperburg C, White E et al. Recreational physical activity and the risk of breast cancer in post menopausal women: The Women's Health Initiative Cohort Study. JAMA 2003; 290:1331–1336.
98 Holmes MD, Chen WY, Feskanich D et al. Physical activity and survival after breast cancer diagnosis. JAMA 2005; 293(20):2479–2486.
99 Pierce JP, Stefanick ML, Flatt SW et al. Greater survival after breast cancer in physically active women with high vegetable–fruit intake regardless of obesity. J Clin Oncol 2007; 25(17):2345–2351.
100 Giovannucci EL, Liu Y, Leitzmann MF et al. A prospective study of physical activity and incident and fatal prostate cancer. Arch Intern Med 2005; 165(9):1005–1010.
101 Hall NR. Survival in colorectal cancer: impact of body mass and exercise. Gut 2006; 55:62–67.
102 Morgan G, Ward R, Barton M. The contribution of cytotoxic chemotherapy to 5-year survival in adult malignancies. Clin Oncol 2005; 16(8):549–560.
103 Galvao DA, Newton RU. Review of exercise intervention studies in cancer patients. J Clin Oncol 2005; 23(4):899–909.
104 Borjesson M, Karlsson J, Mannheimer C. Relief of pain by exercise! Increased physical activity can be a part of the therapeutic program in both acute and chronic pain. Lakartidningen 2001; 98(15):1786–1791.
105 Doll R, Peto R. The causes of cancer: quantitative estimates of avoidable risks of cancer in the United States today. J Natl Cancer Inst 1981; 66:1196–1265.

106 Key TJ, Allen NE, Spencer EA et al. The effect of diet on risk of cancer. Lancet 2002; 360:861–868.
107 Divisi D, Di Tommaso S, Salvemini S et al. Diet and cancer. Acta Biomed 2006; 77(2):118–123.
108 Ahn J, Gammon MD, Santella RM et al. Associations between breast cancer risk and the catalase genotype, fruit and vegetable consumption, and supplement use. Am J Epidemiol 2005; 162(10):943–952.
109 Moss RW. Do antioxidants interfere with radiation therapy for cancer? Integr Cancer Ther 2007; 6(3): 281–292.
110 World Cancer Research Fund. Expert report recommendations. Online. Available: http://www.wcrf.org/research/expert_report/recommendations.php
111 Chlebowski RT, Blackburn G, Thomson C et al. Dietary fat reduction and breast cancer outcome: interim efficacy results from the Women's Intervention Nutrition Study. J Natl Cancer Inst 2006; 98(24):1767–1776.
112 Bandera EV, Kushi LH, Moore DF et al. Consumption of animal foods and endometrial cancer risk: a systematic literature review and meta-analysis. Cancer Causes Control 2007; 18(9):967–988.
113 Verhoeven DTH, Goldbohm RA, van Poppel G et al. Epidemiological studies on *Brassica* vegetables and cancer risk. Cancer Epidemiol Biomarkers Prev 1996; 5:733–748.
114 Herr I, Büchler MW. Dietary constituents of broccoli and other cruciferous vegetables: implications for prevention and therapy of cancer. Cancer Treat Rev 2010; 19 Feb [Epub ahead of print].
115 Brennan P, Hsu CC, Moullan N et al. Effect of cruciferous vegetables on lung cancer in patients stratified by genetic status: a mendelian randomisation approach. Lancet 2005; 366(9496):1558–1560.
116 Conway C, Getahun S, Liebes L et al. Disposition of glucosinolates and sulforaphane in humans after ingestion of steamed and fresh broccoli. Nutr Cancer 2000; 38(2):168–178.
117 Pierce JP, Stefanick ML, Flatt SW et al. Greater survival after breast cancer in physically active women with high vegetable–fruit intake regardless of obesity. J Clin Oncol 2007; 25(17):2345–2351.
118 Rock CL, Flatt SW, Natarajan L. Plasma carotenoids and recurrence-free survival in women with a history of breast cancer. J Clin Oncol 2005; 23(27):6631–6638.
119 Fleischauer AT, Arab L. Garlic and cancer: a critical review of the epidemoiological literature. J Nutr 2001; 131:1032S–1040S.
120 Madgee PJ, Rowland IR. Phyto-oestrogens, their mechanism of action: current evidence for a role in breast and prostate cancer. Br J Nutr 2004; 91:513–531.
121 Cotterchio M, Boucher BA, Manno M et al. Dietary phytoestrogen intake is associated with reduced colorectal cancer risk 1. J Nutr 2006; 136(12):3046–3053.
122 Shankar S, Ganapathy S, Srivastava RK et al. Green tea polyphenols: biology and therapeutic implications in cancer. Front Biosci 2007; 12:4881–4899.
123 Neto C. Cranberry and blueberry: evidence for protective effects against cancer and vascular diseases. Mol Nutr Food Res 2007; 51(6):652–664.
124 Duthie S. Berry phytochemicals, genomic stability and cancer: evidence for chemoprotection at several stages in the carcinogenic process. Mol Nutr Food Res 2007; 51(6):665–674.
125 Larsson SC, Kumlin M, Ingelman-Sundberg M et al. Dietary long chain ω-3 fatty acids for the prevention of cancer: a review of potential mechanisms. Am J Clin Nutr 2004; 79:935–945.
126 Bingham SA, Day NE, Luben R et al. Dietary fibre in food and protection against colorectal cancer in the European Prospective Investigation into Cancer and Nutrition (EPIC): an observational study. Lancet 2003; 361(9368):1496–1501.
127 Meeran S, Kativar S. Cell cycle control as a basis for cancer chemoprevention through dietary agents. Front Biosci 2008; 13:2191–2202.
128 Krishnaswamy K. Traditional Indian spices and their health significance. Asia Pac J Clin Nutr 2008; 17(Suppl 1):265–268.
129 Maskarinec G. Cancer protective properties of cocoa: a review of the epidemiologic evidence. Nutr Cancer 2009; 61(5):573–579.
130 Kune G. Reducing the odds: a manual for the prevention of cancer. Sydney: Allen & Unwin; 1999.
131 Taylor R, Najafi F, Dobson A. Meta-analysis of studies of passive smoking and lung cancer: effects of study type and continent. Int J Epidemiol 2007; 36(5):1048–1059.
132 Davis S, Mirick DK. Residential magnetic fields, medication use, and the risk of breast cancer. Epidemiology 2007; 18(2):266–269.
133 Henshaw DL, Reiter RJ. Do magnetic fields cause increased risk of childhood leukemia via melatonin disruption? Bioelectromagnetics 2005; 7(Suppl): S86–S97.
134 Epidemiological Study of BRCA1 and BRCA2 Mutation Carriers (EMBRACE); Gene Etude Prospective Sein Ovaire (GENEPSO); Gen en Omgeving studie van de werkgroep Hereditiair Borstkanker Onderzoek Nederland (GEO-HEBON); International BRCA1/2 Carrier Cohort Study (IBCCS) Collaborators' Group, Andrieu N, Easton DF, Chang-Claude J et al. Effect of chest X-rays on the risk of breast cancer among BRCA1/2 mutation carriers in the international BRCA1/2 carrier cohort study: a report from the EMBRACE, GENEPSO, GEO-HEBON, and IBCCS Collaborators' Group. J Clin Oncol 2006; 24(21):3361–3366.

135 Ornish D, Weidner G, Fair WR et al. Intensive lifestyle changes may affect the progression of prostate cancer. J Urol 2005; 174(3):1065–1069.
136 Ornish D, Magbanua MJ, Weidner G et al. Changes in prostate gene expression in men undergoing an intensive nutrition and lifestyle intervention. Proc Natl Acad Sci USA 2008; 105(24):8369–8374.
137 Ornish D, Lin J, Daubenmier J, Weidner G et al. Increased telomerase activity and comprehensive lifestyle changes: a pilot study. Lancet Oncol 2008; 9(11):1048–1057. Erratum in: Lancet Oncol 2008; 9(12):1124.
138 Frattaroli J, Weidner G, Dnistrian AM et al. Clinical events in prostate cancer lifestyle trial: results from two years of follow-up. Urology 2008; 72(6):1319–1323.
139 World Cancer Research Fund. Recommendations for cancer prevention. Online. Available: http://www.wcrf-uk.org/research_science/recommendations.lasso
140 Cancer Council Victoria (Australia). Waistline and cancer risk. Online. Available: http://www.cancervic.org.au/preventing-cancer/weight/calculating_risk
141 National Cervical Screening Program. Online. Available: http://www.health.gov.au/internet/screening/publishing.nsf/Content/cv-guide-article
142 National Breast and Ovarian Cancer Centre. Position Statement on ovarian cancer screening. Aust NZ J Obstet Gynaecol; 5 October 2009.
143 Anti-Cancer Council of Victoria. Surgical management of breast cancer in Australia in 1995. Sydney: NHMRC National Breast Cancer Centre; 1999.
144 Thomas DB, Gao DL, Ray RM et al. Randomized trial of breast self-examination in Shanghai: final results. J Natl Cancer Inst 2002; 94:1445–1457.
145 Zorbas H. Breast cancer screening. Med J Aust 2003; 178(12):651–652.
146 American Urological Association. Prostate-Specific Antigen Best Practice Statement: 2009. Update. Online. Available: http://www.auanet.org/content/guidelines-and-quality-care/clinical-guidelines/main-reports/psa09.pdf
147 Reindl TK, Geilen W, Hartmann R et al. Acupuncture against chemotherapy-induced nausea and vomiting in pediatric oncology. Support Care Cancer 2006; 14(2):172–176.
148 Ezzo J, Vickers A, Richardson MA et al. Acupuncture-point stimulation for chemotherapy-induced nausea and vomiting. J Clin Oncol 2005; 23(28):7188–7198.
149 National Cancer Institute, US National Institutes of Health. Effect of acupuncture on chemotherapy-induced nausea and vomiting. Online. Available: http://www.cancer.gov/cancertopics/pdq/cam/acupuncture/HealthProfessional/page6#Section_58
150 Ryan J L, Heckler C, Dakhil SR et al. Ginger for chemotherapy-related nausea in cancer patients: A URCC CCOP randomized, double-blind, placebo-controlled clinical trial of 644 cancer patients. J Clin Oncol 2009; 27(Suppl abstr 9511):15S.
151 Aung HH, Dey L, Mehendale S et al. *Scutellaria baicalensis* extract decreases cisplatin-induced pica in rats. Cancer Chemother Pharmacol 2003; 52(6): 453–458.
152 Taixiang W, Munro AJ, Guanjian L. Chinese medical herbs for chemotherapy side effects in colorectal cancer patients. Cochrane Database Syst Rev 2005; 1:CD04540.
153 Beyond Blue. Cancer and depression/anxiety. Online. Available: http://www.beyondblue.org.au/index.aspx?link_id=4.1175
154 Medina MA, Martinez-Poveda B, Amores-Sanchez M et al. Hyperforin: more than an antidepressant bioactive compound? Life Sci 2006; 79(2):105–111.
155 Mills S, Bone K. Principles and practice of phytotherapy. Modern herbal medicine. London: Churchill Livingstone; 2000:168–173.
156 Anderson PM, Schroeder G, Skubitz KM. Oral glutamine reduces the duration and severity of stomatitis after cytotoxic cancer chemotherapy. Cancer 19981; 83(7):1433–1439.
157 Pittler M, Ernst E. Horse chestnut seed extract for chronic venous insufficiency. Cochrane Database Syst Rev 2006;25(1):CD003230.
158 Pommier P, Gomez F, Sunyach M et al. Calendula ointment and radiation dermatitis during breast cancer treatment. J Clin Oncol 2004; 22(8):1447–1453.
159 Taixiang W, Munro AJ, Guanjian L. Chinese medical herbs for chemotherapy side effects in colorectal cancer patients. Cochrane Database Syst Rev 2005; 1:CD04540.
160 Sagar S, Yance MN, Wong RK. Natural health products that inhibit angiogenesis: a potential source for investigational new agents to treat cancer Part 1. Curr Oncol 2006; 13(1):14–26.
161 Davis L, Kuttan G. Immunomodulatory activity of *Withania somnifera* extract in mice. J Ethnopharmacol 2000; 71(1/2):193–200.
162 MijaresA, Lopez JR. L carnitine prevents increase in diastolic Ca^{2+} induced by doxorubicin in cardiac cells. Eur J Pharmacol 2001; 425(2):117–120.
163 Bryant J, Picot J, Baxter L et al. Clinical and cost-effectiveness of cardioprotection against the toxic effects of anthracyclines given to children with cancer: a systematic review. Br J Cancer 2007; 96(2):226–230.
164 Roffe L, Schmidt K, Ernst E. Efficacy of coenzyme Q10 for improved tolerability of cancer treatments: a systematic review. J Clin Oncol 2004; 22(21):4418–4424.
165 Ladas EJ, Kroll DJ, Oberlies NH et al. A randomized, controlled, double-blind, pilot study of milk thistle for the treatment of hepatotoxicity in childhood

acute lymphoblastic leukemia (ALL). Cancer 2010; 116(2):506–513.

166 Ramasamy K, Agarwal R. Multitargeted therapy of cancer by silymarin. Cancer Lett 2008; 269(2):352–362.

167 Pajonk F, Reidisser A, Henke M et al. The effects of tea extracts on proinflammatory signaling. BMC Med 2006; 4:28.

168 Kim SH, Cho CK, Yoo SY et al. In vivo radioprotective activity of *Panax* ginseng and diethyl ldithiocarbamate. In Vivo 1993; 7:467–470.

169 Wang D, Weng X. Antitumor activity of extracts of *Ganoderma lucidum* and their protective effects on damaged HL-7702 cells induced by radiotherapy and chemotherapy. Zhongguo Zhong Yao Za Zhi 2006; 31(19):1618–1622.

170 Ganasoundari A, Zare SM, Uma Devi P. Modification of bone marrow radiosensitivity by medicinal plant extracts. Br J Radiol 1997; 70:599–602.

171 Pommier P, Gomez F, Sunyach MP et al. Phase III randomized trial of *Calendula officinalis* compared with trolamine for the prevention of acute dermatitis during irradiation for breast cancer. J Clin Oncol 2004; 22(8):1447–1453.

chapter 25

Cardiology

INTRODUCTION AND OVERVIEW

Cardiovascular disorders are encountered very frequently in the primary care setting. In developed or affluent countries, cardiovascular disease is still the most common cause of mortality, accounting for 38% of all deaths,[1] and a significant cause of disability, particularly due to cerebrovascular disease and congestive cardiac failure. One in five Australians are affected by cardiovascular disease.[2] Cardiovascular disorders are due to pathologies that arise in the:

- coronary circulation (e.g. ischaemic heart disease)
- cardiac musculature (e.g. cardiomyopathies)
- cardiac valves (e.g. aortic stenosis, mitral regurgitation)
- cardiac conduction system (e.g. complete heart block, atrial fibrillation).

The most common presenting complaints associated with cardiac disorders include angina, dyspnoea, palpitations and syncope. Of all cardiac conditions, the most common is coronary heart disease or ischaemic coronary syndrome.

This chapter explores the basic elements of assessing the cardiovascular system and then describes the major cardiovascular conditions presenting in the primary healthcare setting. Lifestyle and complementary therapy recommendations are made, where they can be supported by evidence.

THE INTEGRATIVE APPROACH IN CARDIOLOGY

Integrative cardiology refers to incorporation of what has been termed complementary and alternative medicine (CAM) into orthodox medical practice, including herbs, vitamins and non-herbal dietary supplements as well as therapies conducted around issues such as bioenergetics (e.g. acupuncture and energy fields) and mind–body medicine.

In 2005 the American College of Cardiology published an expert consensus document titled, 'Integrating complementary medicine into cardiovascular medicine'.[3] The authors noted that there was considerable debate regarding the clinical utility of alternative medicine practices, that these practices were widely employed by patients with cardiovascular disease and that there was a need for further research. The authors noted that 'integrating CAM into medicine must be guided by compassion, but enhanced by science and made meaningful through solid doctor/patient relationships. Most importantly CAM involves a commitment from the clinician to the caring of patients on a physical, mental and spiritual level'.[3a]

Treatment of patients with cardiovascular disease follows the usual general principles of management. Lifestyle measures are employed first, then relevant CAMs, followed by drug therapy and, finally, invasive procedures and surgery.

ASSESSMENT OF THE CARDIOVASCULAR SYSTEM

CARDIOVASCULAR HISTORY

A detailed history needs to be obtained on the presenting symptoms. Based on the presenting complaint, further information should be elicited, including the following:

- *Chest pain*—ask about the onset, character, duration, severity (on a scale of 1 to 10, with 10 being the most severe pain the patient has ever experienced), radiation, relieving and exacerbating factors, associated other symptoms (e.g. nausea, vomiting, diaphoresis). If it is effort angina, ask how far the patient can walk before experiencing angina ('angina distance'). Although chest pain of cardiac origin is often of the textbook type

(e.g. severe, central, crushing, radiating to the neck and/or left arm, associated with sweating and nausea), it is also often atypical, especially in women, the elderly and diabetics. Therefore atypical chest pain is often misdiagnosed in these groups and a surprising number of heart attacks are 'silent' or go unrecognised.
- *Dyspnoea*—ask about the onset, duration, progression, relationship to rest or exertion, any associated orthopnoea, paroxysmal nocturnal dyspnoea, level of effort tolerance (how far the patient can walk before feeling breathless—'dyspnoea distance').
- *Palpitations*—ask about the onset, frequency, duration, trigger factors (e.g. caffeine, smoking, anxiety), pattern (ask the patient to tap on a table to demonstrate the rhythm they felt), associated symptoms (presyncope), relieving factors.
- *Syncope*—ask about any premonitions, what the patient was doing at the time of onset, any postural changes, any associated vertigo (a feature that would favour a neurological association), incontinence, any similar previous episodes, post-event drowsiness (may weigh in favour of an ictal episode) and account of a bystander witness.

The above four remain the most common cardiac presentations. Once adequate information has been obtained on the presenting complaint, information about past cardiovascular history should be obtained. Any previous cardiac pathology places the patient at a high risk of recurrent similar events.

- Ask about intercurrent illnesses and past history of other illnesses. Associated kidney disease, endocrine disorders, stroke or peripheral vascular disease has relevance to the cardiovascular system.
- Ask about the risk factors for cardiovascular disease, particularly coronary artery disease (see later section on risk factors). Obtain details about family history of cardiac disease.
- Obtain a detailed medication history, paying particular attention to cardiovascular medications and agents that can affect the cardiovascular system. Always ask about allergies.
- Family history is of significant importance in the cardiac history. Do not forget to probe into the social history, focusing on occupational status, cigarette smoking, alcohol and substance consumption/abuse, dietary habits, recreational physical activity and travels.
- Ask about stress and mental health issues. Ischaemic chest pain is commonly precipitated in response to an acute stressor, and major acute stressors and panic attacks are risk factors for precipitating cardiac events. Poor long-term mental health is also an independent risk factor for cardiovascular disease.

CARDIOVASCULAR EXAMINATION

The cardiovascular examination should be tailored according to the symptoms and other relevant information obtained in the history.

- Ideally the patient should be positioned lying supine with upper body resting at 45 degrees. Establish patient's clinical stability by checking the pulse, blood pressure and pattern of breathing.
- Observe the patient's general appearance and establish the overall level of physical comfort (dyspnoea, malaise, diaphoresis etc.), body habitus (obesity, cachexia etc.) and mental state/alertness. If obese, note where the most adiposity is distributed. Central and abdominal obesity (the so-called 'apple' pattern) is far more strongly associated with cardiovascular risk than obesity in the hips and periphery (the so-called 'pear' pattern).
- Define the rhythm, rate and character of pulse. Exclude a radial–radial or a radial–femoral delay, which can indicate the presence of a coarctation of the aorta or dissection of the aorta.
- Check the upper extremities for any peripheral stigmata of infective endocarditis (not common in contemporary practice) such as clubbing, and splinter haemorrhages. Look for palmar crease pallor indicating anaemia, and capillary return indicating sluggish circulation. Note the shape of the hand and fingers, and do not miss Marfan's syndrome (spindle-shaped, long fingers) and acromegaly (spade-shaped, beefy hands). Exclude finger clubbing, which can be associated with subacute bacterial endocarditis or congenital cyanotic heart disease. Look for tar-stained nails, suggestive of chronic cigarette smoking.
- Look in the elbow for tendon xanthomata, indicating familial hypercholesterolaemia.
- Assess the jugular venous pressure (JVP), its pulse morphology and check the hepatojugular reflex.
- Feel the carotid pulse and listen for any carotid bruits bilaterally.
- Observe the face for any characteristic facies such as the Marfan's face (scaphocephaly, malar hypoplasia, enophthalmos, retrognathies, down-slanting palpebral fissures), acromegalic face (protruding jaw etc.), mitral facies (pink malar discolouration of severe mitral stenosis) and Down syndrome face.
- With regard to the eyes, check for conjunctival pallor and look in the fundus for hypertensive retinal changes, diabetic retinal changes or Roth spots seen in bacterial endocarditis.

- Check the level of dental hygiene and look for the presence of gingivitis, which is associated with a higher risk of cardiovascular disease. Also exclude the presence of a high-arched palate seen in Marfan's syndrome, and macroglossia seen in acromegaly.
- Expose the upper thorax and survey the precordium, looking for obvious apex beat, pectus excavatum or pectus carinatum, sternotomy scar (testimony to previous open heart surgery), thoracotomy scars and implanted devices such as permanent pacemakers and implanted cardiac defibrillators. Feel and locate the apex beat, and feel also for thrills and heaves. Auscultate the precordium to appreciate the heart sounds and murmurs and the radiation of the murmurs. Grade the murmur according to the loudness. Listen under the left clavicle for the machinery murmur of patent ductus arteriosus (PDA). Exclude a pericardial friction rub in the patient presenting with pleuritic precordial pain.
- Seat the patient upright and listen to the back of the thorax, looking for any evidence of pulmonary congestion in the way of mid-course crepitations. If present, define the distribution of the crepitations.
- While examining the chest, also look for pitting sacral oedema, which will be a more reliable indicator of fluid retention or cardiac failure than ankle oedema in a patient who has been supine for some time.
- Lie the patient supine and feel the abdomen in the right upper quadrant for the liver edge. Exclude painful hepatomegaly of right heart failure associated hepatic congestion and pulsatile liver of severe tricuspid regurgitation. Exclude shifting dullness of the abdomen in the patient with signs of heart failure.
- Feel the femoral pulse and check for femoral–femoral delay by feeling the pulse bilaterally. Feel the popliteal and pedal pulse and palpate for ankle oedema. If present, define the extent and severity of the peripheral oedema.

CLINICAL ASSESSMENT OF THE CARDIOVASCULAR SYSTEM IN PATIENTS PRESENTING WITH POTENTIAL CARDIAC EVENTS

This section gives an outline of a structured approach to cardiovascular assessment in patients presenting with signs and symptoms indicating a significant problem of cardiac origin.

In the clinical assessment of the cardiovascular system, the most important first step is to ensure that the patient is not in imminent life-threatening danger due to cardiovascular compromise.

- Check the patient's vital signs:
  - *breathing*—looking for dyspnoea, tachypnoea, hypopnoea and apnoea
  - *blood pressure*—look for hypertension (> 140/90 mmHg), hypotension (< 100/50 mmHg), pulsus paradoxus (weakening of pulse volume and drop in systolic blood pressure of > 10 mmHg with inspiration) or postural drop (any drop in blood pressure with standing up)
  - *pulse*—define the rhythm, rate and character
  - *oxygenation*—ensure adequate oxygen saturation, exclude cyanosis
  - *haemodynamic stability*—ensure that the blood pressure is stable and adequate, and that the peripheral pulse is palpable.
- If possible, an urgent electrocardiogram (ECG) should be performed to ensure that the patient is not having a myocardial infarction or an unstable and abnormal cardiac rhythm. If the patient presents with chest pain and the ECG shows ST segment elevation in at least two contiguous leads or a new left bundle branch block, it should be considered an acute transmural myocardial infarction and as such look at organising urgent reperfusion therapy (discussed later in this chapter). Unstable cardiac rhythms include severe bradycardia, supraventricular tachycardia (SVT), ventricular tachycardia (VT) and ventricular fibrillation.
- If there is any element of clinical instability, such as severe bradycardia (heart rate < 40 beats per minute), severe tachycardia (heart rate > 100 beats per minute) or cardiogenic shock, urgent remedial measures should be put in place and if necessary basic or advanced life support should be initiated immediately, and urgent retrieval to a hospital emergency room should be organised.

Urgent steps to be taken in this setting include the following:

1. Ensure adequate oxygenation—manage airway and breathing.
2. Apply cardiac compression if required, or defibrillation to restore rhythm.
3. Secure vascular access.
4. Administer intravenous agent according to the situation at hand:
   - adrenaline, lignocaine (1.0–1.5 mg/kg IV over 3–5 min, up to a maximum of 3 mg for VT)
   - atropine (0.5 mg IV every 3–5 min up to a maximum total dose of 3 mg for severe bradyarrhythmia)
   - adenosine (6–12 mg as a slow IV push every 1–2 min for SVT).

Once the patient's clinical stability is established, a more thorough assessment can be started.

CARDIOVASCULAR INVESTIGATIONS

Cardiovascular investigations should be guided by the differential diagnoses arrived at based on the history and the physical examination. Most patients require an ECG, a full blood count, electrolyte profile and renal function indices. Those presenting with chest pain should be further investigated for cardiac damage by performing serial serum troponin levels.

Following is a list of common cardiac investigations with indications:

- *ECG*—for patients presenting with syncope, presyncope, palpitations, chest pain, hypertension, high cardiovascular risk (multiple coronary risk factors) or dyspnoea.
- *Exercise stress test / myocardial perfusion scan / exercise stress echocardiogram*—for patients presenting with chest pain on exertion, and those with coronary risk factors commencing on a physical activity program.
- *Transthoracic echocardiogram (TTE)*—for patients with cardiac murmurs, dyspnoea, chronic hypertension, syncope (to exclude severe left ventricular failure, which can lead to malignant ventricular tachyarrhythmias, or critical aortic stenosis, which can cause syncope). Also useful in those with unexplained fevers (to exclude bacterial endocarditis), hypotension with evidence of cardiac tamponade (Kussmaul's sign—rising of JVP with inspiration, pulsus paradoxus), and after a myocardial infarction to define any regional wall motion abnormalities of the ventricles.
- *Transoesophageal echocardiogram (TOE)*—to exclude a patent foramen ovale (PFO) in patients presenting with a cryptogenic stroke, suspected bacterial endocarditis (small vegetations may not be detected in TTE), or to exclude thrombus in the left atrial appendage in patients who have atrial fibrillation (with stroke or prior to direct current cardioversion).

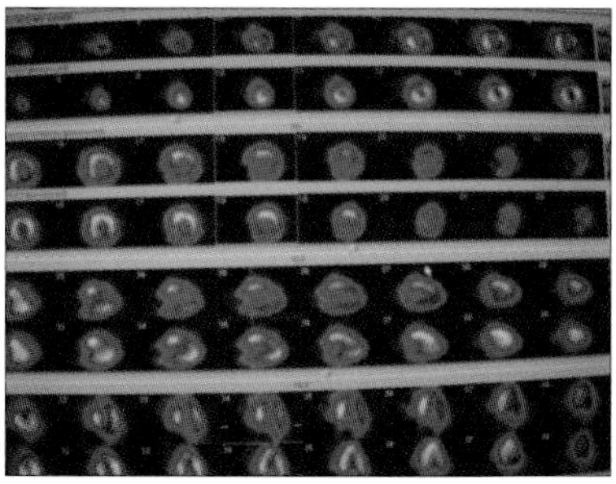

FIGURE 25.1 Nuclear myocardial perfusion scan

- *Holter monitor / event monitor / loop recorder*—for unexplained syncope, palpitations.
- *Coronary angiography*—for patients presenting with acute myocardial infarction, those with post-infarction angina, those with stable angina and a positive exercise stress test or perfusion scan, those presenting with evidence of heart failure possibly due to coronary ischaemia, and those patients who are due to undergo open heart surgery for valvular disorders.
- *Electrophysiological study*—for patients presenting with palpitations or syncope, those with resting ECG evidence of Wolff-Parkinson-White (WPW) syndrome, and those who have documented arrhythmia that can be treated with radiofrequency ablation (RFA).

RISK FACTORS FOR CARDIOVASCULAR DISEASE

Coronary artery disease remains the major cause of morbidity and mortality among the adult population in developed countries around the world. Much progress has been made in preventing and treating coronary artery disease over the past 50 years, but it is still a major health burden. Identifying and addressing coronary risk factors can effectively prevent the development and progression of coronary artery disease and cardiac events.

Non-modifiable coronary risk factors include male gender, postmenopausal state in the female, advancing age and certain ethnicities (such as indigenous groups, Pacific Islanders and African Americans).

Modifiable coronary risk factors include:

- hypertension
- diabetes mellitus
- hypercholesterolaemia
- obesity (especially abdominal adiposity)
- physical inactivity
- smoking
- obstructive sleep apnoea
- chronic kidney disease
- poor mental health (e.g. chronic depression, anxiety and psychological stress).

In hypercholesterolaemia, high low-density lipoprotein (LDL) and triglyceride (TG) levels are associated with heightened risk, while high high-density lipoprotein (HDL) level has a protective effect. Chronic kidney disease, proteinuria and peripheral vascular disease are important coronary risk factors. Familial hypercholesterolaemia and homocysteinuria are associated with coronary artery disease at a young age.

Psychological factors such as chronic stress and depression can contribute significantly to the aetiology and progression of cardiovascular disease, largely due

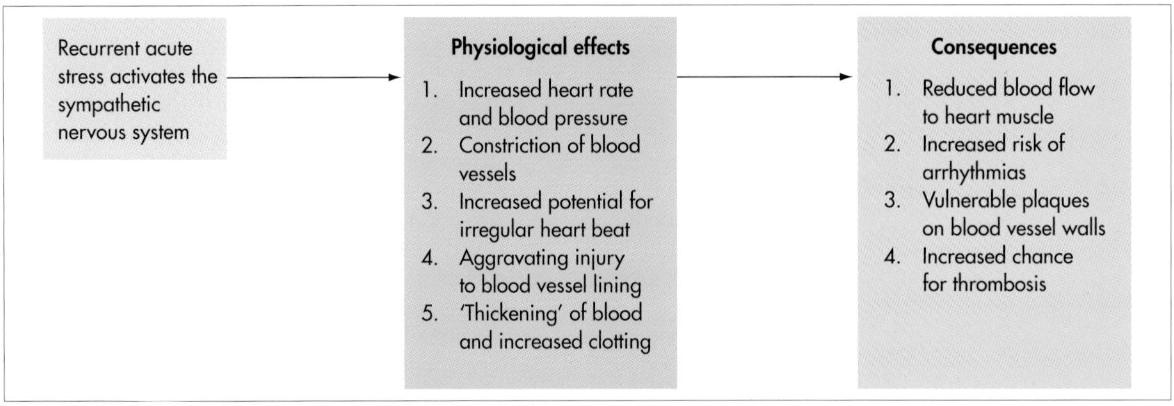

FIGURE 25.2 Effects of psychosocial stress on the heart (adapted from Rozanski et al.[4])

to their association with sympathetic nervous system over-activation and high allostatic load. These effects are summarised in Figure 25.2.

There are also novel risk factors that have been described in the recent past. These include hyperhomocysteinaemia, high-sensitivity C-reactive protein elevation (h-CRP), elevation of lipoprotein(a) (Lpa) and hyperuricaemia. The association of these risk factors to coronary artery disease is variable and the precise means of effectively controlling these, and the absolute benefit from reducing the incidence of coronary events by doing so, are still unclear.

PRIMARY PREVENTION

Primary prevention of acute myocardial infarction requires first and foremost the clear identification of the patient's global risk factor profile. Once this is accomplished, the patient's risk level can be quantified using a coronary risk calculator. The New Zealand risk score and the Framingham risk score are two such practical tools widely used in the primary care setting (Figs 25.3 and 25.4).

DIABETES MELLITUS

- Diabetes increases the cardiovascular risk two- to three-fold. Strict control of blood sugar levels, however, has not shown to be beneficial in the prevention of cardiac events and, in fact, too tight control is associated with a slightly increased risk of mortality.
- However, good blood sugar control helps in the prevention of microvascular complications such as diabetic nephropathy, neuropathy and retinopathy. It is important to aggressively control other cardiovascular risk factors in the diabetic patient.
- Insulin resistance and metabolic syndrome X are associated with increased coronary risk.

HYPERCHOLESTEROLAEMIA

- A high total cholesterol (TC) level, high LDL cholesterol level, low HDL cholesterol level and high TG level are associated with increased coronary risk.
- In the management of high cholesterol levels, lifestyle measures such as dietary discretion, increased physical activity and weight loss should be given first priority. Those who fail lifestyle modification or those at high overall cardiovascular risk can be commenced on lipid-lowering therapy. Although they do not reduce lipid levels as significantly as some pharmaceuticals, omega-3 fatty acids are most effective in reducing cardiac and all-cause mortality. For LDL lowering, statins remain the most potent class of drugs, but they have significant side effects, such as muscle pain and weakness, and reduced cognitive ability. Many patients resist prescription of statins because of concern about side effects. It is important that the patient is offered an alternative plan in addition to lifestyle measures, including:
  - *niacin and fibrates*—useful for raising HDL, although these have less impact on reducing overall mortality; for lowering triglycerides, strict glycaemic control, fish oil supplements and fenofibrate therapy are useful
  - *dietary fibre*—several studies have shown that soluble fibre (found in beans, oats, barley, apples, *Psyllium*[7] and flaxseed) lowers LDL cholesterol and triglycerides
  - *dietary soy*—20 to 50 g/day of dietary soy (tofu, miso, tempeh) can lower total cholesterol, LDL and triglycerides
  - *red yeast rice*—(*Monascus purpureus*, 1200 mg b.i.d.); several studies indicate that a proprietary form of red yeast can lower cholesterol levels

New Zealand cardiovascular risk prediction charts

Risk level: 5-year cardiovascular risk (non-fatal and fatal)		Benefit (1): Cardiovascular events prevented per 100 treated for 5 years*	Benefit (2): Number needed to treat for 5 years to prevent 1 event*
Very high	>30%	>10	<10
	25–30%	9	11
	20–25%	7.5	13
High	15–20%	6	16
Moderate	10–15%	4	25
Mild	5–10%	2.5	40
	2.5–5%	1.25	80
	<2.5%	<0.8	<20

* Based on a 20% reduction in total cholesterol or a reduction in blood pressure of 10–15 mmHg systolic or 5–8 mmHg diastolic, which reduces risk of cardiovascular disease by about one-third over five years

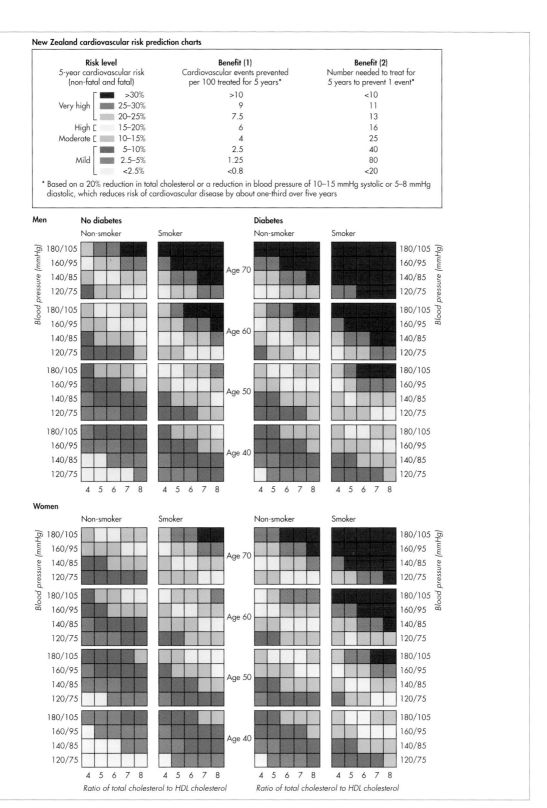

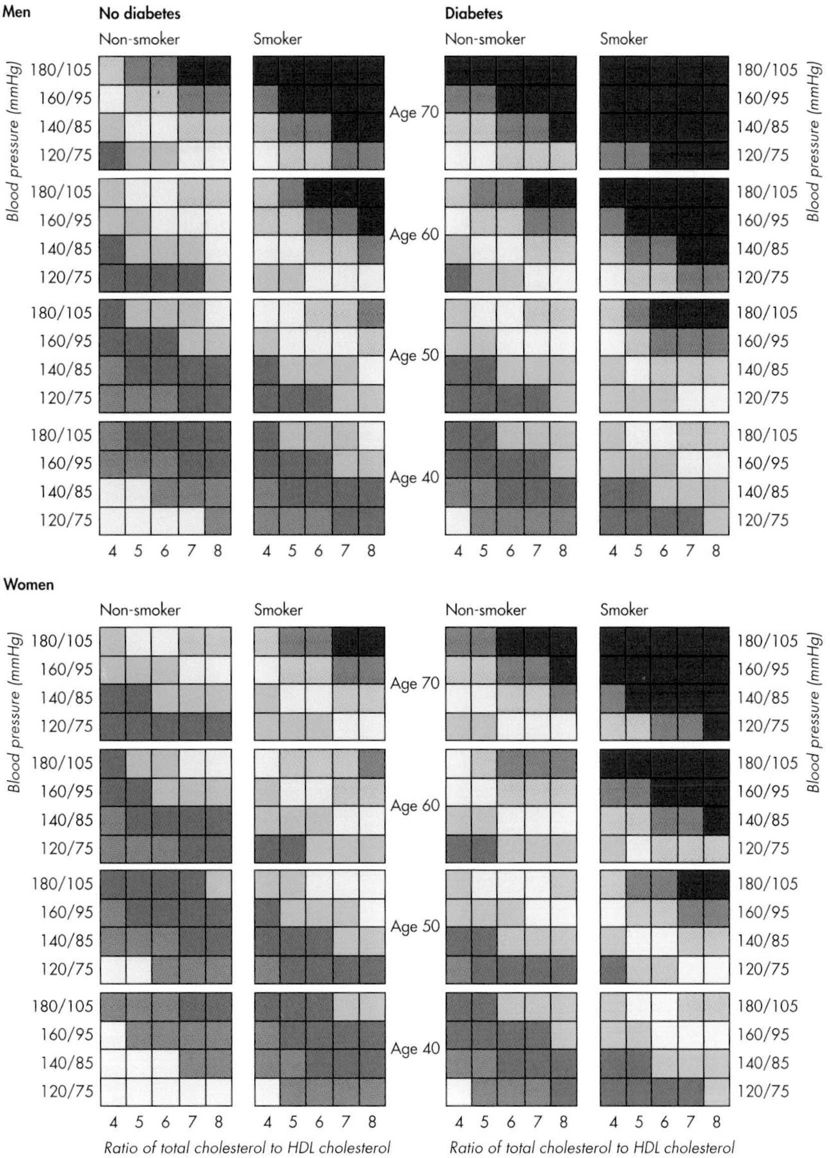

FIGURE 25.3 New Zealand risk score (from Jackson 2000[5])

Step 1

Age		
Years	LDL Pts	Chol Pts
30–34	−9	[−9]
35–39	−4	[−4]
40–44	0	[0]
45–49	3	[3]
50–54	6	[6]
55–59	7	[7]
60–64	8	[8]
65–69	8	[8]
70–74	8	[8]

Step 2

LDL - C		
(mg/dL)	(mmol/L)	LDL Pts
<100	<2.59	−2
100–129	2.60–3.36	0
130–159	3.37–4.14	0
160–190	4.15–4.92	2
≥190	≥4.92	2

Cholesterol		
(mg/dL)	(mmol/L)	Chol Pts
<160	<4.14	[−2]
160–199	4.15–5.17	[0]
200–239	5.18–6.21	[1]
240–279	6.22–7.24	[1]
≥280	≥7.25	[3]

Step 3

HDL-C			
(mg/dL)	(mmol/L)	LDL Pts	Chol Pts
<35	<0.90	5	[5]
35–44	0.91–1.16	2	[2]
45–49	1.17–1.29	1	[1]
50–59	1.30–1.55	0	[0]
≥60	≥1.56	−2	[−3]

Step 4

Blood pressure					
Systolic (mmHg)	Diastolic (mmHg)				
	<80	80–84	85–89	90–99	≥100
<120	−3 [−3] Pts				
120–129		0 [0] Pts			
130–139			0 [0] Pts		
140–159				2 [2] Pts	
≥160					3 [3] Pts

Note: When systolic and diastolic pressures provide different estimates for point scores, use the higher number.

Step 5

Diabetes		
	LDL Pts	Chol Pts
No	0	[0]
Yes	4	[4]

Step 6

Smoker		
	LDL Pts	Chol Pts
No	0	[0]
Yes	2	[2]

Step 7 (sum from steps 1–6)

Adding up the points	
Age	________
LDL-C or Chol	________
HDL-C	________
Blood pressure	________
Diabetes	________
Smoker	________
Point total	________

Step 8 (determine CHD risk from point total)

CHD Risk			
LDL Pts Total	10 yr CHD Risk	Chol Pts Total	10 Yr CHD Risk
≤−2	1%	[≤−2]	[1%]
−1	2%	[−1]	[2%]
0	2%	[0]	[2%]
1	2%	[1]	[2%]
2	3%	[2]	[3%]
3	3%	[3]	[3%]
4	4%	[4]	[4%]
5	5%	[5]	[4%]
6	6%	[6]	[5%]
7	7%	[7]	[6%]
8	8%	[8]	[7%]
9	9%	[9]	[8%]
10	11%	[10]	[10%]
11	13%	[11]	[11%]
12	15%	[13]	[13%]
13	17%	[13]	[15%]
14	20%	[14]	[18%]
15	24%	[15]	[20%]
16	27%	[16]	[24%]
≥17	≥30%	[≥17]	[≥27%]

Step 9 (compare to average person your age)

Comparative Risk			
Age (years)	Average 10 yr CHD risk	Average 10 yr hard* CHD risk	Low** 10 yr CHD risk
30–34	<1%	<1%	<1%
35–39	<1%	<1%	1%
40–44	2%	1%	2%
45–49	5%	2%	3%
50–54	8%	3%	5%
55–59	12%	7%	7%
60–64	12%	8%	8%
65–69	13%	8%	8%
70–74	14%	11%	8%

Key	
Colour	Relative risk
green	very low
white	low
yellow	moderate
rose	high
red	very high

* Hard CHD events exclude angina pectoris.

** Low risk was calculated for a person the same age, optimal blood pressure, LDL-6 100–129 mg/dL or cholesterol 160–199 mg/dL for women, non-smoker, no diabetes.

Risk estimates were derived from the experience of the Framingham Heart Study, a predominantly Caucasian population in Massachusetts, USA

FIGURE 25.4 Framingham risk score (from Wilson et al[6])

- *coenzyme Q10*—may be depleted in patients who take statins; may help reduce the adverse effects of statins
- *hawthorn*—(*Crataegus monogyna*, 900–1800 mg/day in two or three divided doses) has lipid-lowering activity; may potentiate antihypertensive drugs, so monitoring of blood pressure is necessary.

- It is important to note that approximately 40% of patients who are eligible for lipid-lowering therapy do not get treated in the primary care setting and, of those who are treated, approximately 50% fail to reach target levels.[8]
- Current consensus on target lipid levels is as follows:[9]

total cholesterol level	< 4 mmol/L
LDL cholesterol level	< 2.5 mmol/L
HDL cholesterol level	> 1 mmol/L
TG level	< 1.5 mmol/L

HYPERTENSION

- The World Health Organization has defined systolic blood pressure > 140 mmHg and diastolic blood pressure > 90 mmHg as hypertension. In diabetic patients and those who have had a previous myocardial infarction, this cut-off is brought down to 130/85 mmHg.
- Studies of older patients indicate that blood pressure goals that are appropriate for younger patients do not provide added benefits. Treatment regimens to attain such strict blood pressure control can be associated with significant side effects, including drug interactions, postural hypotension and falls. Older patients therefore often do better with more liberal blood pressure targets.
- Over 90% of adult patients with hypertension do not have an underlying cause and therefore have *essential hypertension*. Although it is said that there is no 'underlying cause', a number of factors contribute to the development of essential hypertension, including overweight and obesity, alcohol abuse, excess dietary salt, physical inactivity and psychological factors such as emotional stress, depression and chronic anger. The remainder have *secondary hypertension* due to multiple possible causes such as obstructive sleep apnoea, obesity, alcohol, renal disease, renal artery stenosis, Cushing's syndrome, Conn's syndrome, phaeochromocytoma or acromegaly. A number of medications are also associated with causing or exacerbating hypertension, such as steroids, non-steroidal anti-inflammatories, cocaine, nicotine and licorice (*Glycyrrhiza glabra*).

Left untreated, hypertension can lead to disorders of various organ systems (target organ damage).

- *Heart*—chronic hypertension can cause left ventricular hypertrophy, diastolic heart failure, systolic heart failure, coronary artery disease and myocardial infarction.
- *Brain*—hypertension can lead to ischaemic as well as haemorrhagic stroke.
- *Kidneys*—hypertension can cause hypertensive nephrosclerosis, leading to chronic renal failure.
- *Eyes*—hypertension can lead to retinal changes and bleeding into the retina, eventually leading to papilloedema in its most severe form.
- *Arterial system*—hypertension can lead to arteriosclerosis and aneurysm formation, leading to their rupture.

Investigations

- For the definitive diagnosis of hypertension, high blood pressure reading should be recorded on three occasions separated in time.
- 24-hour ambulatory blood pressure monitoring has become popular and has proved to be a more accurate and comprehensive way of diagnosing hypertension. Usually the systemic pressure should drop by about 5–10 mmHg in the early hours of the night. Absence of this nocturnal dip is associated with increased cardiovascular risk.
- ECG—may show evidence of left ventricular hypertrophy.
- Echocardiography—to demonstrate left ventricular hypertrophy and diastolic impairment.

Management

Initial management of hypertension should involve lifestyle changes and weight loss as the first step. Lifestyle changes that can bring the blood pressure down include reduction in alcohol consumption, reduction in salt consumption, recreational physical activity and mental relaxation. For more severe hypertension, lifestyle changes alone will not be enough to bring the blood pressure into the desirable range and so medications are likely to be required.

A medication review for pro-hypertensive agents (see Boxes 25.1 and 25.2) needs to be performed.

However, any patient at very high overall cardiovascular risk, such as Aboriginals or Torres Strait Islanders, diabetics and those who have suffered end-organ damage, should be commenced on antihypertensive therapy in addition to the institution of positive lifestyle changes.

First-line

If lifestyle modification fails to bring about significant improvement in blood pressure, medical therapy needs to be commenced.

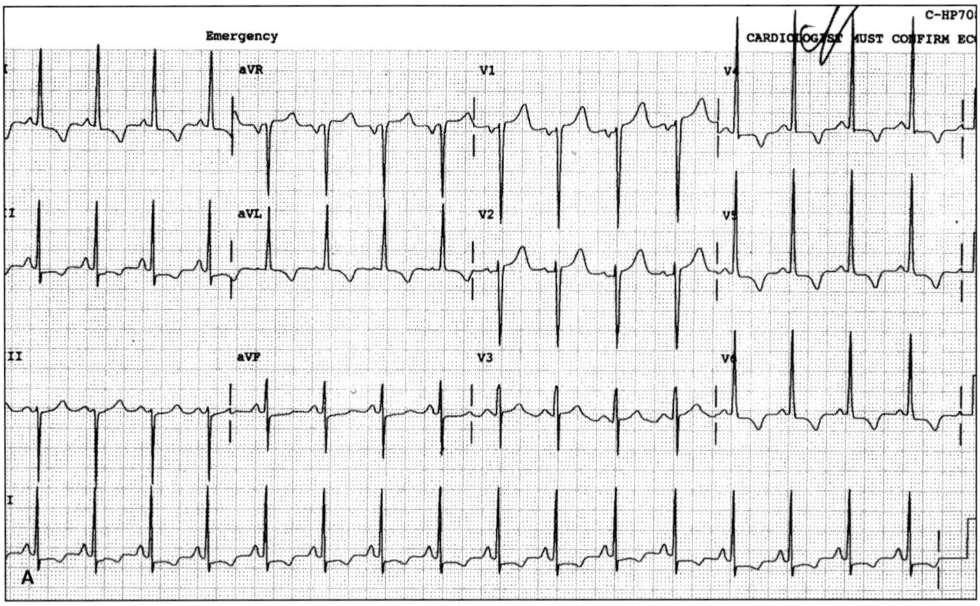

FIGURE 25.5 ECG illustrating hypertension

BOX 25.1 Medications that may have a pro-hypertensive effect[10]

- Corticosteroids
- Non-steroidal anti-inflammatory drugs
- Caffeine
- Cyclosporin
- Hormone replacement therapy
- Oral contraceptive pill
- Pseudoephedrine
- Irreversible MAOIs
- Sibutramine
- Tacrolimus
- Venlafaxine

BOX 25.2 Complementary medicines that may have a pro-hypertensive effect

- American mistletoe
- Angel's trumpet
- Butcher's broom
- Caffeine-containing herbs (green tea, cola nut)
- Dehydroepiandrosterone (DHEA)
- Siberian ginseng
- Guarana
- Hawaiian baby woodrose
- Jimson weed
- Licorice
- Melatonin
- Peyote
- Phenylalanine
- Yohimbine

- *Diet*—ensure adequate fruit and vegetables, nuts and fish (e.g. oily fish such as tuna, salmon and mackerel) at least twice a week and adequate intake of calcium.
- *Fish oil*—reduces all-cause cardiovascular mortality; also reduces incidence of postoperative fibrillation when used prior to cardiac surgery.
- *Coenzyme Q10*—CoQ10 supplements can result in a mean decrease in systolic (16 mmHg) and diastolic (10 mmHg) blood pressure.[11]

  Dose: 100–150 mg daily; well tolerated and no known cardiac interactions.
- *Hawthorn*—has a positive inotropic action, increases coronary blood flow, reduces myocardial oxygen demand and has hypotensive, lipid-lowering and anti-arrhythmic effects; has a low incidence of side effects and is well tolerated. It may potentiate the effect of antihypertensive drugs, so monitor drug dose and modify accordingly.
- *Garlic*—a meta-analysis of clinical trials concluded that garlic is superior to placebo in the treatment of hypercholesterolaemia, but clinical significance is limited by the size of the effect.[12] The small effect on cholesterol is also reflected in the 2007 review by Pittler.[13] Subsequent to Pittler's ambivalence regarding the effect of garlic on blood pressure, two other meta-analyses published in 2008 reported strong evidence for reduction of SBP and DBP in hypertensive patients.[14,15] Lower levels of evidence such as traditional usage, in vitro and animal studies have alluded to other effects, such

as antioxidant, anti-atherosclerosis, antiplatelet, antibacterial, antifungal, antiviral, anti-parasitic, anti-neoplastic, fibrinolytic and immunostimulant, but robust clinical trials to study the mentioned effects are still lacking.

Dose form and dosage:

- Fresh, minced garlic bulb: 2–5 g/day
- Dried powder: 0.4–1.2 g/day
- Aged garlic extracts: 2.4–7.2 g/day
- Oil: 2–5 mg/day
- Fluid extract (1:1): 0.5–2.0 mL three times daily
- Tincture 1:5: 20 mL/day

- *Green tea*—green tea extract has been shown to prevent hypertension and target organ damage induced by a high angotensin II dose, likely by prevention or scavenging of superoxide anion generation.[16] One prospective cohort study reported decreased relative risk of death from CVS disease in participants who consumed more than 10 cups of tea compared with those who consumed fewer than three cups.[17]

  Dose: 3–10 cups green tea per day
- *Magnesium citrate*—360–600 mg daily; magnesium supplementation produces a modest, dose-dependent antihypertensive effect, according to a meta-analysis.[18]
- *L-arginine*—1–2 g t.d.s.; may help blood vessels dilate, lowering blood pressure.
- *Stress management*—see the section below on the Essence of managing CVD.

Pharmaceutical

When selecting antihypertensive drugs, consider potentially favourable and unfavourable effects on coexisting conditions.

Common pharmaceutical agents used in the treatment of hypertension:

- *Thiazide diuretics*—a cheaper agent with moderate potency in lowering blood pressure. Caution should be exercised in diabetic patients, whose blood sugar control may be disrupted. A suitable first-line agent for the elderly patient.
- *Calcium channel blockers (CCBs)*—non-dihydropyridine CCBs are effective antihypertensive agents but can cause bradycardia and worsen heart failure. Dihydropyridine CCBs are useful antihypertensive agents with antianginal properties and do not cause bradycardia. These agents, however, can cause ankle oedema.
- *Angiotensin-converting enzyme (ACE) inhibitors*—very effective and potent antihypertensive agents with beneficial effects in ischaemic heart disease, heart failure and diabetes mellitus. Side effects include dry cough, angio-oedema, hyperkalaemia and postural hypotension.
- Angiotensin II receptor blockers (ARBs)—effective antihypertensive agents with protective effects in heart failure and diabetes.
- Combinations of ACE inhibitors or ARBs with a CCB or a thiazide diuretic in one pill can be used when a single agent fails to control blood pressure effectively. Some evidence suggests superior clinical benefits of the former combination.
- Alpha-blockers, centrally acting agents and vasodilators can be used in resistant hypertension.
- Beta-blockers are also used to treat hypertension, but are less potent than the above agents.
- Aldosterone antagonist spironolactone is also used as an antihypertensive agent; however, worsening of renal function and hyperkalaemia should be watched for.
- According to the National Heart Foundation Guidelines of 2008, ACEs, ARBs and thiazide diuretics are to be considered first-line pharmaceutical agents.[19] In cases of resistant hypertension, further investigations should be carried out to exclude a secondary cause such as renal artery stenosis or hyperaldosteronism.

POOR MENTAL HEALTH

Poor mental health—for example, severe and relapsing depression, chronic anxiety or vital exhaustion—is an independent risk factor for heart disease and should therefore always be assessed and managed accordingly. Furthermore, having heart disease is a significant risk factor for the development of depression.

Psychological strategies that are effective in improving mental health have also been shown to be associated with a reduced incidence of recurrence and cardiac mortality. Including psychological and social support in the management of heart disease produces major reductions in disease progression and the number of deaths.[20] A review of the evidence by Linden and colleagues found that, compared to those who were given psychosocial support, those with no such support were 70% more likely to die from their heart disease and 84% more likely to have a recurrence.[20] Managing depression with antidepressants has not been shown to produce a significant reduction in cardiac risk and, in fact, many of the earlier classes of drugs increased cardiac risk.

CARDIOVASCULAR DISEASES

ISCHAEMIC CHEST PAIN

Chronic stable angina

Ischaemic chest pain that is brought on by exertion, after a meal or emotional stress is known as chronic stable angina. The pathology is usually a stenotic coronary lesion due to stable cholesterol plaque.

History

- Ask about the nature and severity of the chest pain.
- Check whether the pain responds to sublingual nitrate therapy.
- Identify the patient's coronary risk factor profile.
- Define the patient's angina distance and ask whether this has shortened and, if so, over what time frame.
- Remember that the pattern of chest pain and presenting symptoms in women and the elderly can be atypical and sometimes leads to myocardial infarction going unreported or misdiagnosed.

Investigations

Perform a standard cardiovascular examination.

- *Exercise stress test*—has good sensitivity and specificity in the high-risk population. It is not a useful test if the patient's pre-test probability of coronary artery disease is low. Exercise echocardiogram is preferable in women as stress ECG has a higher rate of false positives in women than in men.
- *Exercise or dobutamine stress echocardiogram*—has a higher sensitivity and specificity than the stress test in identifying reversible coronary ischaemia.
- *Myocardial perfusion scan (radionucleoid scan)*—has higher sensitivity and specificity than exercise stress testing in identifying reversible coronary ischaemia. Fixed perfusion defects indicate non-viable myocardium.
- Check the patient's coronary risk factor profile by performing fasting blood sugar levels, fasting cholesterol profile and 24-hour blood pressure monitoring.

Management

- Lifestyle change—patients should be encouraged to make sustained lifestyle changes such as smoking cessation, diet, physical exercise as tolerated within the levels of comfort, and stress management.
- Other aspects of a person's life might need to be looked at, such as mental health, employment, social activities and relationships.
- The patient's coronary risk factor profile should be well controlled.
- Initially the patient could be managed with antianginal therapy: topical or oral nitrates, beta-blockers, calcium channel blockers or ACE inhibitors.
- If the non-invasive test is positive for reversible coronary ischaemia, the patient should be referred for coronary angiography.
- If suitable, the patient should be treated with coronary revascularisation via balloon angioplasty and stent placement, or by referral for coronary artery bypass surgery.
- Patients with left main coronary artery disease or three vessel (left anterior descending, left circumflex and the right coronary) coronary disease benefit from bypass surgery.
- Patients who are not amenable to mechanical coronary revascularisation need optimal medical therapy.
- Recalcitrant angina can be treated with second-line antiangina agents such as nicorandil, perhexiline and ivabradine.
- L-carnitine (2 g daily)—controlled studies have indicated that L-carnitine supplements increase exercise tolerance and reduce frequency of angina attacks, enabling some patients to reduce reliance on nitrates.[21]
- Coenzyme Q10 (150 mg daily)—patients with ischaemic heart disease have a relative deficiency of coenzyme Q10. CoQ10 appears to delay the onset of angina[22] and reduce nitroglycerin consumption.[23]

Acute coronary syndrome: unstable angina and myocardial infarction

Unstable angina is chest pain of ischaemic origin that is increasing in severity and/or frequency or that has an onset at rest.

Acute myocardial infarction (AMI) is a medical emergency. Any patient with high cardiovascular risk presenting with persistent chest pain at rest should be suspected of having an AMI until proved otherwise. It is important to remember that female patients often do not present with the classic retrosternal chest tightness and therefore atypical features in the high-risk female patient should not be ignored.

History

- Take a rapid focused history, first asking about the onset of symptoms and associated symptoms such as diaphoresis and nausea/vomiting. Check the triggers of the pain. Check the details of the pain: severity, location, radiation and relieving factors. Classic angina is retrosternal in location with radiation along the arms unilaterally or bilaterally. It may also radiate up the neck. It is described as a dull ache akin to 'heaviness' or a crushing sensation with no respiratory variation of its severity. Patients may experience diaphoresis and/or nausea. These features should alert to the very high likelihood of a myocardial infarction.
- Ask about coronary risk factors. Enquire about the patient's past history, especially cardiovascular history.

- Check whether the patient has exertional angina. Some people report a change in symptoms in the weeks preceding infarction, including sleep disturbance, dyspnoea and unusual fatigue.

Examination

- First check the vital signs and establish haemodynamic stability. Hypotension, bradycardia, tachyarrhythmia and hypoxia are warning signs of concern. If these signs are present, upon establishing vascular access, antiplatelet therapy and fluid resuscitation (for hypotension) and diuretic therapy (frusemide 40–80 mg IV) (for hypoxia related to pulmonary congestion) should be given. Oxygen (100%) should be made available via (Hudson) mask. Aspirin 150 mg should be given orally, and organise urgent reperfusion therapy if ST segment elevation is observed in the ECG.
- Once the patient is stable, perform a detailed cardiovascular examination. Listen to the heart for additional sounds such as the third and fourth heart sounds. Listen to the lung bases for crepitations associated with congestion.

Investigations

- Perform a 12-lead ECG as soon as possible to confirm the diagnosis and also to define the type of infarction—ST segment elevation myocardial infarction (STEMI) or non-ST segment elevation myocardial infarction (NSTEMI), because the management of the two types is different. In NSTEMI and unstable angina, the ECG shows ST segment depression or T wave inversion
- Perform a standard battery of investigations that include the full blood count, electrolyte profile, renal function indices and cardiac biomarkers such as troponin and CK-MB (creatine kinase-MB) levels.
- Obtain a chest X-ray, looking for pulmonary congestion and the size of the cardiac shadow.

Management of acute myocardial infarction

The primary objective is to restore blood flow to the infarct-related myocardium. If the ECG shows a STEMI:

- Give the patient aspirin and clopidogrel immediately.
- Refer the patient to the nearest hospital for urgent reperfusion therapy: thrombolysis or, if a catheterisation service is available, urgent primary angioplasty.
- If the ECG shows an NSTEMI, the patient should be anticoagulated with fractionated or unfractionated heparin to stabilise the ruptured coronary plaque.
- The patient may benefit from symptomatic therapy with morphine or glyceryl trinitrate (GTN) in tablet or topical form. Ensure that the patient is not significantly hypotensive.
- Patients also benefit from a beta-blocker agent (ensure that the patient does not have bradycardia).
- If the patient has pulmonary crepitation and is not hypotensive, give a low-dose ACE inhibitor.
    - The patient will benefit from HMG-CoA reductase inhibitor (statin) therapy such as simvastatin, atorvastatin or rosuvastatin.
    - Patients with ongoing symptoms and dynamic ECG changes may also benefit from intravenous antiplatelet agents such as glycoprotein IIb/IIIa inhibitors (tirofiban/eptifibatide).

The long-term management plan should be based on a firm partnership between the patient and the primary care doctor.

- Significant lifestyle changes should be advocated, with cessation of smoking, dietary modification and resumption of regular recreational physical activity—at least half an hour a day of brisk walking. Patients will find it far easier to act on lifestyle advice if attention is given to enabling factors such as stress management, behaviour change skills and goal setting.
- The patient should be referred to a cardiac rehabilitation program and should be encouraged to attend the same—without doctor's advice the compliance rate with cardiac rehabilitation is dismal (30% or less).
- Perform an echocardiogram to assess the damage sustained and the residual ejection fraction—if there is impaired systolic function of the left ventricle, the patient may benefit from eprenolone, the new-generation aldosterone antagonist, and third-generation beta-blocker therapy.
- Ongoing angina post AMI is an indication for exercise stress testing and, if positive, for coronary angiography.
- Many patients suffer significant psychological stress with AMI and some develop ongoing subclinical depression. This is associated with a poor prognosis, and therefore it is important to identify and treat the same. Good mental health is also enormously important in helping a person to make and maintain other healthy lifestyle changes.
- Sexual function may also be affected and should be discussed as part of the rehabilitation program.

Preparation for coronary artery bypass surgery

In recent years the increasing incidence of high-risk and elderly patients presenting for major surgery has presented a challenge for surgeons, due to the associated increased mortality and complication rate and costs. Novel ways need to be found to improve the results of surgery in these patients. Over the past 10 years at the Alfred Hospital and the Baker Heart Research Institute in Melbourne, Australia, researchers led by Professor Franklin Rosenfeldt have developed regimens of metabolic therapy with the pyrimidine precursor, orotic acid, and the antioxidant and mitochondrial respiratory chain component, coenzyme Q10.[24] Using test tube studies, animal models and human studies, they have shown that these regimens improve the response of the ageing and failing heart to hypoxia, ischaemia/reperfusion injury and aerobic stress such as occur during cardiac surgery.[24–29] To these original regimens, omega-3 fatty acids (fish oil supplements) and the antioxidant alpha-lipoic acid were added in an attempt to provide better clinical outcomes. The use of coenzyme Q10 supplementation as standalone treatment was validated in a clinical trial, and the entire combination of therapeutic strategies in a 1-year pilot study.[25,26,30] Compared with placebo, treated patients demonstrated improved energy production in the heart muscle, increased resistance to hypoxic stress, one-day shortened hospital stay and improved postoperative quality of life.

A 3-year prospective randomised clinical trial of this integrated 'preoperative rehabilitation' program has been completed at the Alfred Hospital. This study demonstrated that patients experienced reduced length of stay, reduced troponin 1 release, indicating less damage to the myocardium, and, for coronary artery bypass patients, reduced incidence of postoperative atrial fibrillation, and provided a cost saving. In addition, the treatment was well tolerated and patients expressed overwhelming satisfaction with the program (results presented at the Cardiac Society of Australia and New Zealand Annual Meeting, Christchurch 2007 and at the American Heart Association Annual Scientific Sessions, Orlando Florida, November 2007, paper not yet submitted for publication).

It is on this basis that Dr Lesley Braun and Professor Franklin Rosenfeldt developed the Integrative Cardiac Surgery Wellness Program at the Alfred Hospital, which builds research conducted on site and published studies and meta-analyses demonstrating the benefits of such programs.[31–34] It also incorporates research produced by hospital-based integrative cardiology and health promotion units already established in the United States (such as the Mayo Clinic and the Cleveland Clinic).

ARRHYTHMIAS

Paroxysmal supraventricular tachycardia

Paroxysmal supraventricular tachycardia (PSVT) is usually a narrow complex tachycardia, although aberrant conduction may give rise to a wide complex. Based on the site of onset, SVT is classified as atrial, atrioventricular nodal (AVN) or junctional (Fig 25.6).

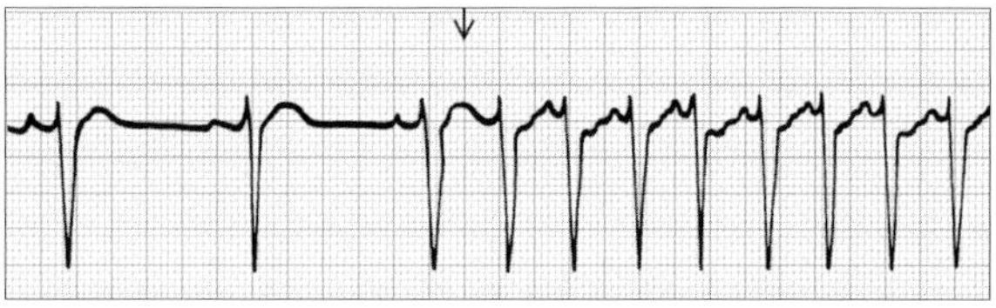

FIGURE 25.6 ECG of supraventricular tachycardia

- *Atrial tachyarrhythmias* include sinus tachycardia, inappropriate sinus tachycardia, atrial tachycardia, sinus node re-entrant tachycardia (SNRT), atrial flutter and atrial fibrillation (atrial fibrillation is discussed separately).
- *Atrioventricular tachycardias* include AV nodal re-entrant tachycardia (AVNRT), AV re-entrant tachycardia (AVRT) and junctional ectopic tachycardia (JET).
- *Sinus tachycardia* is sinus rhythm at a rate over 100 bpm and is usually a response to an identifiable cause such as physical exertion, anxiety, hypovolaemia, hypotension, sepsis, hypoxia, hyperthyroidism or agents that stimulate adrenergic drive and so on.
- *Inappropriate sinus tachycardia* is sinus tachycardia without an identifiable stimulus and is due to hypersensitivity of the sinus node to adrenergic stimuli. This is mostly observed in young females.
- SNRT is due to a re-entrant circuit in or around the sinus node. The rate varies between 100 bpm and 150 bpm. P waves present in the normal manner in the ECG. Episodes are paroxysmal, with spontaneous onset and termination.
- *Atrial tachycardia* arises in the atrial myocardium and its rate varies between 120 bpm and 250 bpm. The P wave morphology is variable.
- *Atrial flutter* arises in the right atrium due to a re-entrant circuit. It has associations with ischaemic heart disease, cardiomyopathy, myocarditis and alcohol. Usual rate is between 250 bpm and 350 bpm, with a ventricular response of 75–150 bpm. Typical flutter waves are seen in leads II, III and aVF. Progression to AF is often observed, and hence the potential risk of thromboembolism.
- *AVNRT* is the most common narrow complex tachycardia with a regular rhythm. It is more commonly seen in young, otherwise healthy females. Rarely it is associated with structural heart disease. This arrhythmia is due to the presence of two conduction pathways in the AV node with different conduction properties (speeds), one slow (alpha) and the other fast (beta), giving rise

to re-entrant circuits. The SVT is triggered by a supraventricular ectopic beat. The common typical AVNRT has the slow pathway conducting antegradely and therefore the PR interval is longer than the RP interval. The P wave is seen embedded in the terminal portion of the QRS complex or after the QRS complex. In the atypical form, where the antegrade conduction is via the fast pathway, the PR interval is shorter than the RP interval. Usually the rate is between 150 bpm and 200 bpm.

- *AVRT* is due to an accessory pathway between the atrial and ventricular myocardium across the mitral or tricuspid valve. It is more common among males and onset is at a younger age. Commonly there is no structural heart abnormality present; however, there is a rare association with Ebstein anomaly. Rate is between 150 bpm and 250 bpm.
  - When the antegrade conduction is via the accessory pathway there is pre-excitation of the ventricle, as in WPW syndrome where there is a short PR interval and slurring of the QRS complex (delta wave).
  - Patients with WPW can develop AF or atrial flutter which, if conducted via the accessory pathway, can lead to VT or ventricular fibrillation (VF). Therefore patients with WPW at risk of AF or atrial flutter should not be given AV nodal blocking agents, due to the risk of sudden death.
  - When the accessory pathway conducts the impulse in a retrograde direction (anterograde conduction via the AV node), it is called *orthodromic AVRT*—this is more commonly seen. This manifests as a narrow complex tachycardia. When the accessory pathway conducts in an anterograde direction it is called *antedromic AVRT* and the ECG shows a bizarre, wide complex tachycardia.
- *JET* is a rare SVT that is associated with underlying cardiac pathology or recent cardiac surgery. ECG shows a narrow complex regular tachycardia with no evidence of P waves.

Presentation

- Patients with SVT present most commonly with palpitations. Other presentations include presyncope, dyspnoea, syncope, angina and diaphoresis.

Investigations

- Investigations in the setting of SVT include (in addition to the ECG) electrolyte profile, full blood count and an echocardiogram to exclude rare but possible structural heart abnormalities. If the arrhythmia was not recorded, an event monitor or a Holter monitor may be useful in capturing future events. Other investigations should be guided by the other symptoms.
- Electrophysiological study is useful in inducing the arrhythmia in order to study the morphology and the mechanism, and also to identify/map the accessory pathways and abnormal circuits.

Management

- Acute management involves vagal manoeuvres such as carotid sinus massage or Valsalva manoeuvre if the patient is haemodynamically stable. Carotid sinus massage should be unilateral and should be done upon excluding a bruit in the older patient. The presence of a bruit is suggestive of an occlusive carotid plaque that can lead to stroke if disrupted and embolised.
- Non-responders to vagal manoeuvres can be treated with intravenous adenosine, which is a very short-acting AV node blocking agent. Other agents that can also be used in this setting include calcium channel blockers such as verapamil or diltiazem, and beta-blockers such as metoprolol.
- Haemodynamically unstable or severely symptomatic (with chest pain or pulmonary oedema) patients require urgent direct current synchronised cardioversion.
- A long-term management strategy should be based on the frequency of episodes, type of arrhythmia, patient's age and other associated cardiac pathology.
- Infrequent episodes in stable and otherwise well patients can be managed with beta-blockers, calcium channel blockers or digoxin.
- Definitive therapy is radiofrequency catheter ablation of the accessory pathway once identified by electrophysiological study.
- Patients with WPW and at risk of sudden death should also be referred for electrophysiological (EP) study and curative radiofrequency ablation (RFA).
- There is a rare risk of complete heart block during the RFA of AVNRT. Other rare (1–3%) risks of EP/RFA include haemorrhage, deep venous thrombosis and cardiac tamponade and death (0.1%).

Atrial fibrillation

Atrial fibrillation (AF) is very common in the primary care setting, with 1% of the adult population estimated to suffer from this arrhythmia. Prevalence increases with age and with structural heart disease. AF can lead to palpitations, angina associated with coronary ischaemia and worsening of heart failure.

- Common aetiologies include hypertension, ischaemic heart disease, valvular disease (especially mitral), cardiomyopathy, thyrotoxicosis and alcohol.

- AF that occurs in patients below the age of 55 with no underlying cause is called *lone AF*.
- AF can increase the risk of thromboembolic stroke five-fold, particularly in older patients (over 65 years), and in those who have other coronary risk factors, a previous history of stroke or structural heart disease.
- The CHADS2 score gives an objective evaluation of the thromboembolic risk and as such helps guide suitable preventative therapy (see Box 25.3). A score of 0 implies a low risk of embolic stroke, 1–2 an intermediate risk, and 3 or above a high risk. A score of 2 in a patient with a prior history of stroke or transient ischaemic attack should be considered high. Therapeutic implications of the score are discussed below.
- Most AF is idiopathic; however, if suggested by the clinical features, investigation for a secondary cause should be carried out. Some secondary causes include hyperthyroidism, mitral valve disease and WPW syndrome.

BOX 25.3 CHADS2 score

Risk factor	Score
Heart failure	1
Hypertension	1
Age 75 or above	1
Diabetes	1
Stroke/TIA	2

(adapted from Gage et al 2001[35])

Investigations

1. A 12-lead ECG to confirm the irregularly irregular rhythm and the absence of 'p' waves.
2. TTE to estimate the size of the left atrium and to look for mitral valve disease.
3. TOE to check for thrombus in the left atrial appendage, especially prior to cardioversion. If a thrombus is present, cardioversion should be postponed by 3 months and the patient should be anticoagulated for 3 weeks.
4. A loop recorder or a Holter monitor may be required for the diagnosis of AF in patients who complain of palpitation but remain in sinus rhythm at presentation (paroxysmal AF).

Management

Management of AF has three immediate objectives: rate control, rhythm control and stroke prevention.

Stroke prevention

- In patients who fail to cardiovert or are in paroxysmal AF, anticoagulation with warfarin is required, to prevent stroke. Warfarin is indicated for high-risk patients (CHADS2 score of 2 or more). The INR (International Normalized Ratio) should be maintained at 2–3. A CHADS2 score of 1 can be treated with aspirin or warfarin, and a

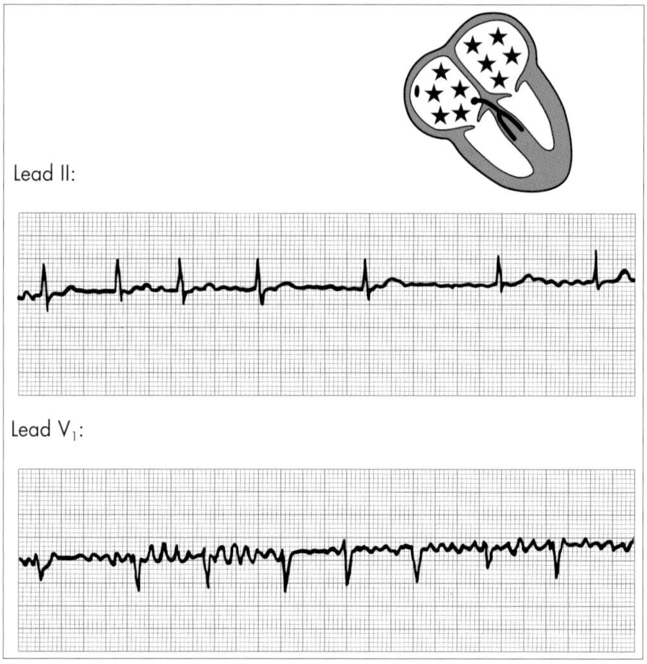

FIGURE 25.7 ECG of atrial fibrillation

score of 0 will benefit from aspirin alone. There is no current role for dual antiplatelet therapy in the prevention of embolic strokes in AF.

- Known precipitants such as alcohol should be avoided.

Rate control

- Rapid rate control is achieved with agents known to block the cardiac conduction system. Common agents used include amiodarone, digoxin, verapamil, diltiazem or a beta-blocker such as atenolol.
- Beta-blocker alone or together with digoxin is the most efficacious at rate control. Often a single agent fails to adequately control the rate and therefore a combination of two agents is required.

Rhythm control

- Rhythm control offers no extra mortality and morbidity benefits over rate control. However, rhythm control precludes the need for anticoagulation and as such may be preferable for the patient's convenience.
- The best means of rhythm control is by DC cardioversion under general anaesthesia (electrical cardioversion).
- Drugs useful in rhythm control include amiodarone, sotalol, flecainide, quinidine and procainamide. Flecainide should not be used in those who have established heart disease or cardiac structural abnormalities.

Those not responding to drug therapy can be helped with radiofrequency ablation of AF by isolation of the pulmonary venous ostea. This procedure has a lower success rate initially and therefore repeat procedures may be required to achieve a lasting effect. Operator and centre experience also affect the success rate and rate of complications.

Surgical maze procedure is another option for resistant cases.

Ventricular tachycardia

Ventricular arrhythmias are often of greater concern because of their association with haemodynamic instability. They need rapid recognition and management. An ECG of VT is shown in Fig 25.8.

- A broad complex (QRS duration of more than 120 ms) regular tachycardia with a rate between 100 bpm and 200 bpm is considered ventricular tachycardia (VT) until proved otherwise. If sustained, the patient can rapidly deteriorate, with haemodynamic compromise and sudden death. The differential diagnosis is supraventricular tachycardia with aberrant ventricular conduction.
- Features of VT include:
  - AV dissociation (P waves occurring with no association to the QRS complexes)
  - capture beats that occur at a shorter RR interval (this is a normal-appearing narrow QRS complex due to ventricular conduction that occurs in the normal AV conduction pathway)
  - fusion beats that morphologically have the appearance of one in between a normal AV conducted beat and a ventricular originated beat. This is due to the simultaneous occurrence of AV conduction and the origin of a ventricular beat. The RR interval will remain stable.
- If the QRS complexes remain in the same morphology it is called *monomorphic VT*, and if it is of varying morphology it is called *polymorphic VT*.
- If the VT lasts less than 30 seconds and does resolve spontaneously, it is called *non-sustained VT*.
- VT is associated with coronary ischaemia, congestive heart failure, cardiomyopathy or QT prolongation and antiarrhythmic agents.

Management

If the patient is haemodynamically stable, a rapid infusion of amiodarone, lignocaine or procainamide may help. This should be carried out in a hospital setting with concurrent ECG monitoring. If the VT is recalcitrant or leads to haemodynamic compromise, cardiopulmonary resuscitation and rapid DC cardioversion are indicated. The initial shock of 200 J is given upon placing the defibrillator pads on the anterior chest wall. Further shocks of 300 J and 360 J should be delivered if required for VT not responding to previous low-energy shocks.

- ECG features of VT–AV dissociation, QRS axis between –90 and ± 180 degrees, positive QRS

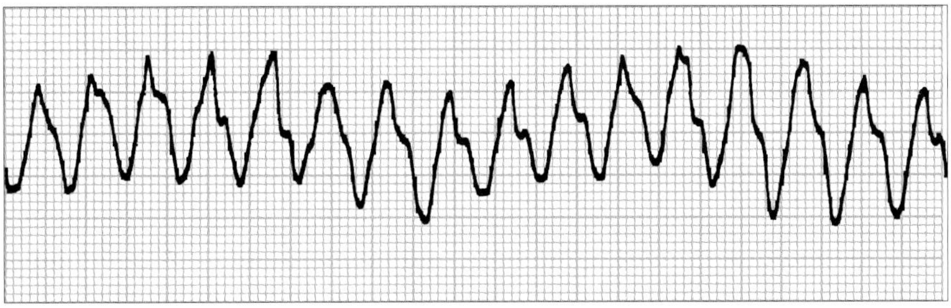

FIGURE 25.8 ECG of ventricular tachycardia

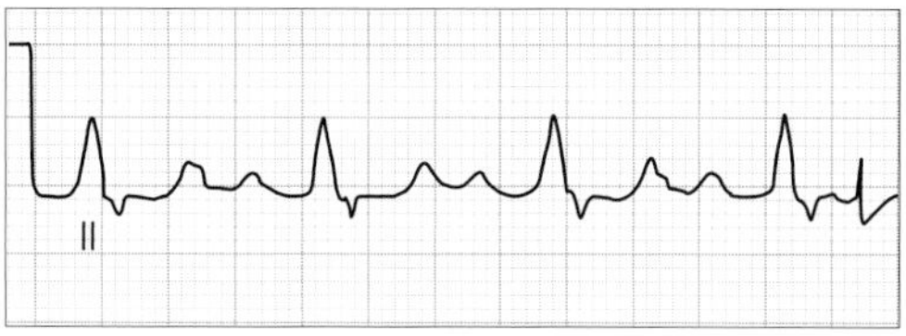

FIGURE 25.9 ECG of AV node block

concordance (positive deflection of QRS in leads V1 to V6), combined left bundle branch block (LBBB) pattern with right axis. If the pattern is that of right bundle branch block (RBBB) the QRS duration is > 140 msec, and with LBBB the QRS duration is > 160 msec.

- A ventricular rhythm at a rate between 75 bpm and 100 bpm is termed *accelerated idioventricular rhythm*. This does not usually cause haemodynamic collapse and often self-terminates or occurs in paroxysms. Associations include myocardial ischaemia and digoxin toxicity.
- Torsades de pointes (polymorphic VT with shifting of axis)—associations include long QT syndrome, drug toxicity (especially antiarrhythmics such as quinidine, procainamide), hypokalaemia, hypomagnesaemia. This rhythm can deteriorate into ventricular fibrillation and cardiac arrest. Management options include DC cardioversion, acceleration of sinus rate with isoprenaline infusion, overdrive pacing or magnesium sulfate infusion. The causative factor should be corrected.

Integrative medicine and arrhythmias

There are a range of options for the integrative management of arrhythmias that may be used as an adjunct to conventional treatments and to reduce complications and relapse.[36] For example, omega-3 fatty acids (fish oils) are useful, and populations with a high fish intake have lower incidence of coronary heart disease and death. Omega-3 fatty acids have anti-arrhythmic effects and have been shown to reduce sudden death from VF. Fish oils have also been shown to reduce the incidence of post-coronary artery bypass AF. Supplementation with coenzyme Q10, L-carnitine and selenium might also be useful. The role of potassium and magnesium is promising. Stress, through raised SNS activity, has also been shown to increase arrhythmic potential and so stress reduction should be considered a core element of the management of any serious arrhythmia.

Sick sinus syndrome

Sick sinus syndrome is a result of a dysfunctional sinus node associated with depressed conduction via the AV node. There may be alternating episodes of SVT (most often AF) and severe bradycardia, which is dubbed tachycardia–bradycardia syndrome). Usually the SA node resumes its activity very slowly after DC cardioversion and sometimes there is no resumption of its activity.

- Symptoms include presyncope, syncope and palpitations. Those with AF are at risk of thromboembolic stroke.
- If the arrhythmias are not recorded or captured during presentation, the patient may require further investigation with a Holter monitor, event monitor or loop recorder.
- Management involves permanent pacemaker implantation and medications for rate or rhythm control for the tachycardia episodes. Those with high-risk features for embolic stroke due to AF require anticoagulation.

CONGESTIVE CARDIAC FAILURE

Heart failure could be due to the impairment of systolic pump function or the diastolic filling function, or both. The patient may have left ventricular failure, right ventricular failure, or both. Heart failure could be due to multiple causes, such as:

- ischaemic cardiomyopathy
- hypertensive heart disease
- idiopathic dilated cardiomyopathy
- cardiomyopathy due to viral illness, cardiotoxins (anthracycline chemotherapeutic agents, alcohol)
- regurgitant valvular disease of the aortic and mitral valves.

The causes of high-output cardiac failure are severe anaemia, beriberi, Paget's disease, thyrotoxicosis and arteriovenous fistulae.

History

- Ask about the patient's exercise tolerance and interpret the severity of heart failure according to the level of effort tolerance (New York Heart Association classification – see Box 25.4).
- Ask about symptoms of orthopnoea (ask how many pillows the patient uses) and paroxysmal nocturnal dyspnoea.
- Check whether the patient has a known history of ischaemic heart disease or hypertension.
- Ask about recent viral illness and alcohol consumption.

Physical examination

- Look for the presence of tachypnoea and tachycardia, and check blood pressure.
- Assess the jugular venous pressure and the character of the arterial pulse. Patients with severe cardiac failure may have Kussmaul's breathing.
- Feel the apex beat, looking for a lateral shift or a heave. Auscultation may reveal an S_3 gallop.

BOX 25.4 NYHA functional classification of patients with heart failure

Class I
No limitation of physical activity. Ordinary physical activity does not cause undue fatigue, palpitation or dyspnoea.
Class II
Slight limitation of physical activity. Comfortable at rest, but ordinary physical activity causes undue fatigue, palpitation or dyspnoea.
Class III
III A Marked limitation of physical activity. Comfortable at rest, but less than ordinary activity causes undue fatigue, palpitations or dyspnoea.
III B Marked limitation of physical activity. Comfortable at rest, but minimal exertion causes undue fatigue, palpitation or dyspnoea.
Class IV
Unable to carry out any physical activity without symptoms or discomfort. Symptoms of cardiac failure present at rest. If any physical activity is undertaken, discomfort is increased.

NYHA: New York Heart Association

Listen for murmurs that would suggest a valvular pathology such as aortic stenosis, aortic regurgitation and/or mitral regurgitation. Left ventricular enlargement may lead to mitral annular dilatation, which may cause functional mitral regurgitation with a pansystolic murmur.

- Listen to the lung fields for crepitations. Examine the abdomen for tender hepatomegaly and ascites. Check for peripheral oedema and define its distribution.
- Check the patient's weight.

Investigations

- Full blood count, electrolyte profile, renal function indices
- ECG and chest X-ray—looking for cardiac enlargement and pulmonary congestion
- Cardiac biomarkers such as troponin, CK-MB
- Echocardiogram—to assess the ventricular systolic and diastolic function and valve function
- BNP (B-type natriuretic peptide) level (see Box 25.5) is useful when the clinical features are not confirmatory of the diagnosis of heart failure in the dyspnoeic patient.

Long-term management of cardiac failure

- Diuretic therapy should be commenced with a loop diuretic such as frusemide. These agents facilitate preload reduction as well as after-load reduction due to their vasodilator effect. The dose may need to be titrated to gain maximum clinical benefit with fewest side effects.
- If a single agent fails to act, combination diuretic therapy can be tried with the addition of a thiazide or spironolactone for the potent effect of sequential diuresis. When patients are on combination diuretic therapy, electrolyte imbalances, particularly hypernatraemia, should be watched for.
- Oral or transdermal GTN therapy for pre-load reduction and relief of cardiac ischaemia.
- Third generation beta-blockers have significant prognostic and survival benefits. Carvedilol is an agent that has alpha- as well as beta-adrenoreceptor blocking qualities. This is indicated in symptomatic cardiac failure with a severity consistent with grade II–III according to the New York Heart Association classification. This drug has to be started at a low dose and the dose gradually increased over a period of a few weeks while observing the level of tolerance and efficacy. It can be commenced in hospital and followed up after discharge. Bisoprolol and long-acting formulation metoprolol also have shown benefit to patients in randomised controlled trials. Bisoprolol has cardiac beta-receptor selectivity and as such can be given to patients with asthma or emphysema. It is better tolerated by patients with low blood pressure due to its lack of alpha activity.
- ACE inhibitor therapy for symptomatic as well as asymptomatic congestive cardiac failure is very beneficial, particularly in patients with an ejection fraction of less than 40%. All patients treated with ACE inhibitors should be monitored for hypotension, hyperkalaemia and progression of renal failure.
- Angiotensin-II receptor inhibitors can be used with equal efficacy for symptomatic cardiac failure where there is ACE inhibitor intolerance.

BOX 25.5 BNP levels in the management of heart failure

- Plasma BNP > 500 ng/L is diagnostic of severe heart failure.
- If plasma BNP < 100 ng/L, heart failure is unlikely.
- Moderately elevated BNP level (100–350 ng/L) in a dyspnoeic patient may also suggest right heart failure, pulmonary embolism or chronic renal failure.
- Elevated BNP level has a diagnostic as well as prognostic value.
- BNP levels help distinguish between cardiac failure and other causes of acute dyspnoea.

BNP: B-type natriuretic peptide.

- Hydralazine combined with isosorbide dinitrate is a proven alternative for the ACE inhibitor-intolerant, symptomatic patient.
- Amlodipine is a dihydropyridine calcium channel blocker that has been shown to be useful in patients who do not tolerate ACE inhibitor therapy. This agent has also shown proven survival benefits.
- Digoxin is useful in persistent congestive cardiac failure despite ACE inhibitor therapy. This is of benefit to patients in AF as well as to those in sinus rhythm.
- Oral anticoagulation is indicated for patients with a history of previous thromboembolism, chronic or paroxysmal AF or a left ventricular thrombus.
- Aldosterone receptor antagonists such as spironolactone (and eplerenone) administered long-term have been shown to minimise the aldosterone-mediated myocardial fibrosis in patients with chronic congestive cardiac failure; a cardiac failure patient has high levels of aldosterone in the circulation as a compensatory response.
- Intravenous loop diuretics infusion and intravenous inotropic (dobutamine) therapy may be useful in refractory fluid retention and refractory cardiac failure.
- Cardiac resynchronisation with biventricular pacing is beneficial to the patient in sinus rhythm, in particular those who have a prolonged QRS complex in the ECG (> 130 ms).
- An implanted cardiac defibrillator has been shown to be protective for patients who suffer from recurrent symptomatic sustained VT and episodes of ventricular fibrillation.
- Highly specialised centres offer left ventricular assist devices (LVADs) that can be implanted to assist the pump function of the left ventricle. These battery operated devices can be used as bridging therapy prior to cardiac transplantation and in selected groups of patients as destination (definitive) therapy. In very refractory cases, cardiac transplantation should be considered.
- All patients require ample education on this chronic disease and instructions on how to live with it. Self-monitoring of weight and fluid intake is very important. Most patients require fluid restriction to about 1.5 L a day and limits on salt ingestion. The patient should be advised on how to identify early signs of decompensation and an action plan should be given.
- Patients benefit from regular, gentle physical exercise, preferably with advice from an exercise physiologist.
- Patients should be referred to a community-based multidisciplinary heart failure management program.
- Most benefit from psychiatric and occupational counselling and help.
- In all cardiac failure patients, consider vaccination against *Pneumococcus* as well as seasonal influenza virus.
- Evidence suggests that CoQ10 and the herb hawthorn are of benefit for cardiac failure. These were discussed at length earlier in this chapter.

DIASTOLIC CARDIAC FAILURE / HEART FAILURE WITH NORMAL SYSTOLIC FUNCTION

Diastolic cardiac failure is the most common cause of heart failure in the elderly (> 75-year age group). The pathology is related to the build-up of fluid in the lungs due to impaired cardiac filling.

Common causes of diastolic failure are:

- chronic ischaemic heart disease
- left ventricular hypertrophy due to chronic hypertension
- restrictive cardiomyopathy, which could be due to amyloidosis, haemochromatosis or sarcoidosis
- hypertrophic obstructive cardiomyopathy
- constrictive pericarditis
- pericardial effusion
- persistent or recurrent tachyarrhythmias
- diabetes mellitus.

Examination should show evidence of pulmonary congestion, elevated JVP and an S4 gallop on auscultation.

Investigations that should be requested for patients with diastolic cardiac failure are:

- chest X-ray—there would be no evidence of cardiomegaly
- echocardiography—may show left ventricular hypertrophy and also quantify the ventricular chamber dimensions and wall thickness
- if the chest X-ray suggests calcific pericarditis, a CT scan or an MRI scan of the chest would be useful to confirm the diagnosis of constrictive pericarditis
- cardiac catheterisation—may further help, by chamber pressure assessment, in diagnosing as well as distinguishing between restrictive cardiac pathology and constrictive pericarditis
- stress electrocardiography, nuclear medicine stress perfusion scanning and stress echocardiography—can be done to exclude cardiac ischaemia
- right ventricular cardiac biopsy—if amyloidosis, haemochromatosis or sarcoidosis is suspected as the causative mechanism.

Management of diastolic heart failure

- Loop diuretic and topical or oral nitrate therapy.

- If in AF, the ventricular rate should be controlled to facilitate adequate diastolic filling of the ventricle, which already has a compromised filling capacity.
- Control hypertension to prevent further progression of the disease.
- Beta-blocker or verapamil therapy is useful in hypertrophic obstructive cardiomyopathy.
- Other non-pharmacological management is similar to that of systolic heart failure.

ACUTE DECOMPENSATED CARDIAC FAILURE (ACUTE PULMONARY OEDEMA)

Acute decompensated cardiac failure is a clinical emergency. Decompensation can be recognised by the presence of features of acute pulmonary oedema with severe dyspnoea, orthopnoea and desaturation. It may be triggered by an insult such as sepsis, myocardial infarction, arrhythmia (often it is AF with a rapid ventricular response) or excess fluid intake. Management requires first stabilising the patient. Then the underlying cause can be addressed.

- First ensure that the patient is haemodynamically stable and in a stable cardiac rhythm.
- Sit the patient upright and provide oxygen via the Hudson mask. Severe cases may require oxygen via the non-rebreather mask or non-invasive ventilation in the way of continuous positive airway pressure (CPAP) or bilevel positive airways pressure (BiPAP).
- Administer intravenous frusemide 80–120 mg, and observe the response by monitoring the urine output. Administer subcutaneous or intravenous morphine at an initial dose of 5 mg. Morphine therapy helps reduce load on the heart. In addition the anxiolytic effect of it helps in the stabilisation of the patient.
- Intravenous or topical nitrate therapy helps preload reduction as well as after-load reduction. Ensure that the blood pressure is satisfactory.
- Once the patient is stable, perform a 12-lead ECG, a chest X-ray and the standard battery of blood tests (full blood count, electrolyte profile, renal function indices and cardiac biomarkers).
- Echocardiogram is important to define the biventricular function and cardiac anatomy (including the valvular function).
- Those with severe hypotension (cardiogenic shock) may progress to rapid multi-organ failure due to hypoperfusion. Therefore these patients require therapy with intravenous inotropic agents (adrenaline, dopamine, dobutamine). These agents should be administered via a centrally placed venous catheter and the patient should be monitored closely in an intensive care ward or the coronary care ward.
- Some patients may need the placement of an intraaortic balloon pump to improve coronary perfusion.
- Levosimendan is a calcium sensitiser that has shown benefit in the treatment of acute decompensated heart failure. It improves cardiac output and decreases pulmonary capillary wedge pressure. This is an expensive drug that has proven survival benefits for the patient.

INTEGRATIVE MANAGEMENT OF HEART FAILURE

The first effective therapy to help patients with cardiac failure was digitalis leaf. This was in the eighteenth century, when William Withering noted that the local herbalist was having good results in patients with 'dropsy' using a combination of herbs. Using his knowledge of botany, he predicted that it was the digitalis leaf that was the most effective component of the herbal preparation. Using pure digitalis extract, he was able to get similar results.

The most recent effective therapy in patients with heart failure is another herbal preparation, hawthorn. Over the past few decades many small trials have shown improved symptoms and heart function with various hawthorn preparations.[37] More specifically, a highly purified extract, Crataegus (WS1442), at a dose of 450 mg b.i.d. in addition to standard drug therapy, reduced cardiac-related deaths by 20%. This was in the SPICE trial, which was inducted in 156 centres in Europe and involved 2681 patients with severe impairment of left ventricular function documented by echocardiography.[38] Background therapy included ACE inhibitor therapy in greater than 80%, beta-blocker in greater than 60%, α_2-antagonists in approximately 70% and spirinolactone in approximately 40%. The beneficial results in addition to standard therapy were on a background of a number of small randomised trials which showed improvements in patients with heart failure. Hawthorn extract has many potential compounds responsible for the beneficial outcome, including ACE inhibitor type activity and anti-inflammatory action.

Coenzyme Q10 has also been used for more than 20 years, and in a number of small randomised trials many patients showed subjective improvement in symptoms, and in earlier studies showed improvement in heart function, although its role in benefiting heart function is still being fully established.[39] However, the most rigorous newer trials have not shown benefit in heart function. In one trial that involved patients with significant heart failure, the addition of coenzyme Q10 led to a 38% reduction in the need for hospitalisation

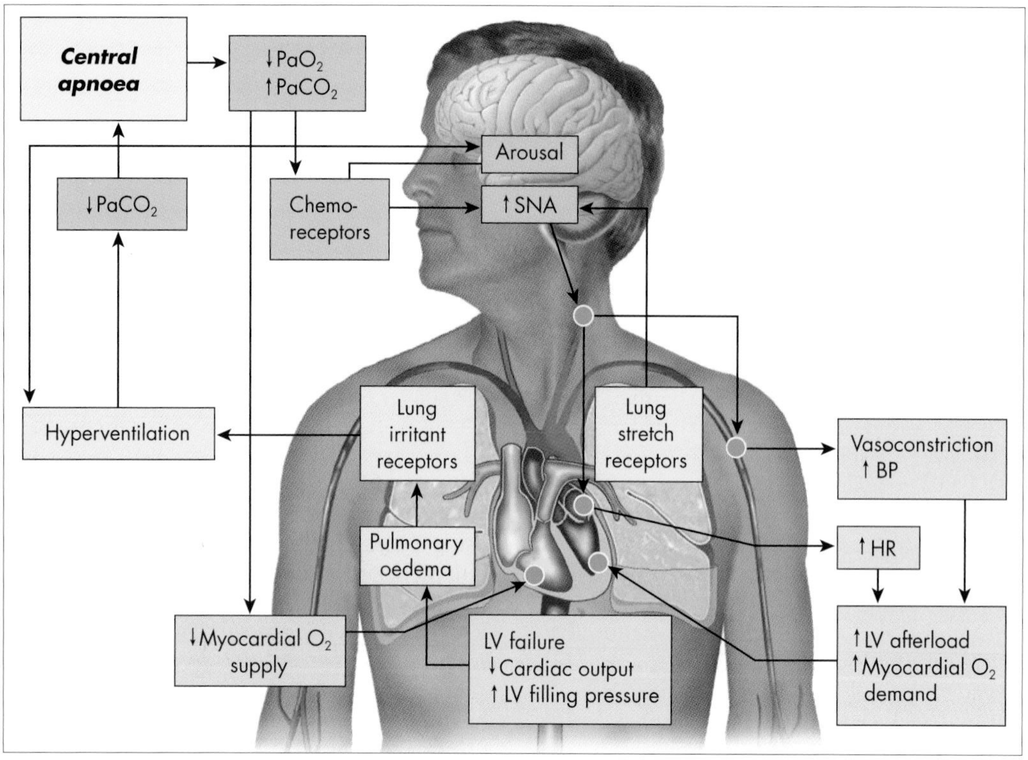

FIGURE 25.10 The clinical features of left heart failure

due to heart failure during the trial period. Coenzyme Q10 may also be useful as an antihypertensive agent.[40,41]

Until recently, there has been considerable controversy regarding the need for coenzyme Q10 supplementation in patients on statins. There is no doubt that statin therapy lowers serum coenzyme Q10, as the carrier molecule LDL cholesterol is lowered by statin therapy. Patients on statins, however, have a lower incidence of heart failure, and a recent randomised trial in patients with heart failure showed decrease in cardiovascular events, although no improvement in heart failure.[42] Occasionally in patients on statin therapy, coenzyme Q10 supplementation eases aches and pains. Interestingly, in the Australian Lipid Trial, serum coenzyme Q10 levels did not predict cardiovascular outcomes during the 6-year follow-up after the index coronary event.[40]

ANTIBIOTIC PROPHYLAXIS AGAINST ENDOCARDITIS

- Current recommendation is to give antibiotics cover to patients who are at high risk of infective endocarditis due to bacteraemia associated with contaminable invasive procedures. Maintaining optimal oral hygiene is more effective in preventing bacteraemia-associated complications than prophylactic antibiotics. Patients at the highest risk of infective endocarditis are those with a past history of endocarditis, prosthetic cardiac valves, cyanotic congenital heart disease (unrepaired) or some native valvular heart diseases. Most authorities do not recommend antibiotic prophylaxis for bicuspid aortic valve, mitral valve prolapsed with regurgitation, repaired mitral disease, hypertrophic obstructive cardiomyopathy, aortic stenosis and mitral regurgitation.
- For dental and other oral procedures, and procedures on the upper respiratory tract: a single dose of amoxicillin 2 g orally 60 minutes prior to the procedure. Patients allergic to penicillin can be treated with azithromycin or clarithromycin 500 mg or clindamycin 600 mg stat.
- For those maintained nil by mouth, parenteral ampicillin 2 g; or for those allergic to penicillin, 600 mg parenteral clindamycin.
- For genitourinary and lower gastrointestinal tract procedures: amoxicillin 2 g orally 60 minutes prior to the procedure (for low-risk patients with an active infection) or ampicillin 2 g parenterally together with gentamycin 1.5 mg/kg parenterally 30 minutes before the procedure. This should be

followed by 1 g of ampicillin parenterally 6 hours after the procedure.
- Penicillin-allergic patients can be given vancomycin 1–2 g parenterally.
- In pregnant women, normal vaginal delivery or caesarean section do not warrant routine antibiotic prophylaxis. However, if there are high-risk features, amoxycillin and vancomycin should be considered.
- A probiotic should be recommended for patients who take antibiotics.

CONGENITAL HEART DISEASE

Heart defects are among the most common congenital abnormalities of the newborn. The incidence of congenital heart disease is observed to be around 8% per 1000 births. The majority of the congenital heart defects are ventricular septal defect (VSD) (30%), atrial septal defect (ASD) (10%), patent ductus arteriosus (PDA) (10%), pulmonary stenosis (7%), coarctation of aorta (7%), aortic stenosis (6%), tetralogy of Fallot (6%) and transposition of great arteries (4%).

Predisposing genetic conditions include trisomy 21 (Down syndrome, associated with AV canal defect), trisomy 18 (Edwards' syndrome, associated with VSD, PDA) and trisomy 13 (Patau's syndrome, associated with VSD, PDA, dextrocardia), XO (Turner's syndrome, associated with coarctation of aorta, aortic stenosis) and familial ASD with heart block. Other causes include maternal infections such as rubella or mumps, maternal exposure to substances such as warfarin, alcohol, lithium, phenytoin or thalidomide, and maternal illnesses such as systemic lupus erythematosus (SLE).

There are two types of congenital heart defects: cyanotic and non-cyanotic. Some congenital heart defects demonstrate a familial clustering. With most children with congenital cardiac anomalies surviving to adulthood due to improved means of management, there is a growing population of patients with adult congenital heart disease.

Non-cyanotic congenital heart defects are VSD, ASD, PDA, aortic stenosis and pulmonary stenosis. Cyanotic congenital heart defects include tetralogy of Fallot and transposition of great arteries, persistent truncus arteriosus, total anomalous pulmonary venous connection and tricuspid atresia.

Investigations in the setting of congenital heart defects include chest X-ray, ECG, echocardiogram and cardiac catheterisation.

With ASD, small defects can close spontaneously. Larger defects can manifest in adulthood. The larger the defect, the worse the prognosis. Issues related to ASD include pulmonary hypertension, right ventricular failure and paradoxical embolism. Surgical closure or percutaneous device closure is superior to conservative management. Increased pulmonary vascular resistance (> 10 units/m^2) is a contraindication to closure in adulthood.

Small VSDs close spontaneously during childhood. Large VSDs are usually repaired during childhood. Unrepaired VSD can lead to left heart failure, right heart failure and Eisenmenger's syndrome (shunt reversal to right to left). Patients have a pansystolic murmur. Patients are at risk of infective endocarditis, and hence require prophylactic antibiotics when predisposed to bacteraemia. VSD closure is performed surgically; however, muscular VSD can be repaired with percutaneous device closure.

PERIPHERAL VASCULAR DISEASE

Two herbal preparations have been thoroughly investigated recently regarding management of claudication. These preparations are *Ginkgo biloba* and the Tibetan herbal preparation PADMA® 28.

Ginkgo has been used for the relief of intermittent claudication. In a meta-analysis of eight randomised trials, a dose ranging from 120 to 600 mg per day was used, and overall there are reports of a significant increase in pain-free walking distance.[43] The clinical relevance of this increase is unclear, but it is similar to drug therapy, which has not been very successful in this difficult group of patients. Some studies have shown improvement in lipid profile and, surprisingly, it may increase blood pressure in patients taking thiazide diuretics.

PADMA® 28 is a traditional Tibetan preparation. Seven randomised clinical trials have shown significant improvement in walking distance with this preparation. Many studies have shown improvement in lipid profile, and lowering of blood pressure may occur.[44] No significant drug interactions are known. There is also some evidence that it may reduce angina.

CARDIAC REHABILITATION

Cardiac rehabilitation involves graded physical activity and lifestyle modification after a cardiovascular event, for the purpose of secondary prevention. The fundamental elements of cardiac rehabilitation include patient education, counselling, physical therapy and physical exercise. The programs are run by a multidisciplinary team which may consist of nurse practitioner, physiotherapist, dietician, nurse educator, psychologist, pharmacist, occupational therapist and exercise physiologist.

In phase 1 of the program, which takes place immediately after the index event (often at the hospital), a nurse educator provides essential information and education to the patient on the disease condition, risk factor control and lifestyle modification. The patient may undergo an exercise stress test to ascertain the level of effort tolerance that helps develop individualised exercise prescription.

Phase 2 of the program is run at a designated centre, usually over a period of 6 weeks, where the patient is taken through a graded series of physical exercises while under close supervision. In addition, structured educational sessions and counselling on lifestyle modification and coping strategies are provided by the other members of the professional team. Often the patient's partner is also invited to participate in the education sessions.

Phase 3 of the program involves self-directed and unsupervised physical exercise upon discharge from the program. However, patients are provided with ongoing support and access to advice and services for healthy living in the community.

There is convincing evidence in the clinical literature of the enormous benefits of cardiac rehabilitation in the secondary prevention of cardiovascular disease. In some facilities rehabilitation is offered to individuals at very high risk of cardiovascular disease for the purpose of primary prevention ('prehabilitation').

THE ESSENCE MODEL IN MANAGING CARDIOVASCULAR DISEASE

Education

Patients obviously need to be educated about heart disease, its causation, lifestyle factors and medical management. Also important is to understand the major principles of behaviour change and stress management.

Stress management

Information on the effects of stress on the heart and cardiovascular system is given in preceding sections of this chapter. Sympathetic nervous system (SNS) over-activation, acutely and chronically, increases the risk of cardiac events and accelerates the progression of cardiovascular disease. Autonomic nervous system activation in negative emotional states is an unbalanced one, being nearly all SNS, whereas in positive emotional states it is a far more balanced one between SNS and parasympathetic nervous system (PNS), which is cardio-protective.[45] Anger, for example, was reported by over one in six heart attack patients in the 1–2 hours before a cardiac event. Acute anger more than doubled the risk of having a heart attack. It was also found that anger is more common in younger and socioeconomically disadvantaged patients who present with heart attacks.[46] Stroke is also closely related to levels of anger, especially for men who are not able to control their anger. Men who express more anger have double the chance of having a stroke, but the risk grows to seven-fold for men with a previous history of heart disease.[47] There is also an increased risk of stroke for those with chronic anxiety, panic disorder[48] and depression.[49]

The term 'vital exhaustion' is used to denote the long-term effects of over-activation of the SNS. Vital exhaustion among men was gauged by their response to the statement, 'At the end of the day I am completely exhausted mentally and physically.' This is an extremely useful question to add to the history-taking of a person at risk of CVD. If a man said that that statement accurately described his typical daily experience, then over the following 10 months he would be nearly nine times as likely to die from a cardiac event. Even three and a half years later the risk was still three times higher.[50] The figures for women may be similar, although they are unlikely to be as high. When followed for 18 months after coronary angioplasty, the risk for new cardiac events for those with vital exhaustion is tripled.[51]

Reviews of the medical literature find consistent data linking chronic depression, anxiety, work stress and social isolation to heart disease risk and progression.[52,53] Rosanski and colleagues relate CVD risk to five specific psychosocial domains: depression, anxiety, personality factors and character traits (principally anger and hostility), social isolation and chronic life stress.[47] The relationship is less strong for type A personality.[54]

More importantly, this increased risk is reversible. A review of 23 studies on including psychological and social support in the management of heart disease clearly showed major reductions in morbidity and mortality if people had psychological and emotional support as a part of their management.[55] Compared with those who were given psychosocial support, those with no such support were 70% more likely to die from their heart disease and 84% more likely to have a recurrence. The researcher's conclusion was unambiguous: 'The addition of psychosocial treatments to standard cardiac rehabilitation regimens reduces mortality and morbidity, psychological distress, and some biological risk factors. ... It is recommended to include routinely psychosocial treatment components in cardiac rehabilitation.'

Although being unemployed is associated with a higher incidence of heart disease, so too is having long working hours, especially under high pressure. The effects of over-employment can be as harmful as those of under-employment.[56] Low job control, often associated with low socioeconomic status, and ongoing work stress produce the biochemical and physiological changes which make heart attacks more likely to happen.[57–59]

Meditation, as a means of activating the relaxation response, is also being investigated as a treatment for CVD and risk-factor reduction. A series of studies on the effects of transcendental meditation (TM) over 7 months found not only a significant reduction in blood pressure[60,61] but also reversal of atherosclerosis over the following 9 months.[62] The improvements were not attributable to changes in other cardiovascular risk factors such as diet and exercise. The effects of just 9 months of practice translated into reductions in the risk of heart attack by 11% and of stroke by 15%. In another study on the 7-year effects of TM on the elderly[63] it was found that the TM group had a 23% reduction in the risk of death from any cause, a 30% decrease in risk of death specifically from CVD and a 49% decrease in risk of death from cancer.

Spirituality

Spirituality is an important part of many people's ability to deal with stress, depression and hostility. It has been found to be associated with a significant reduction in allostatic load, biological markers of stress and cardiovascular risk factors such as blood pressure, waist/hip ratio, blood fats, markers of diabetes, cortisol and adrenaline levels.[64] The effect was much more prominent among women. Among religious attenders there is also a lower level of inflammatory markers relevant for CVD such as C-reactive protein and fibrinogen.[65] Reviews of the research suggest that overall religious attendance promotes better health, including a reduced risk of heart disease,[66] although some studies have raised doubts about whether there is a cardiovascular protective effect for religious attendance that is independent of lifestyle and social factors.[67] If indeed there is an effect, it is probably a combination of lifestyle, social support, better emotional health in terms of coping with anger or depression and the protective effect of religious practices such as prayer or meditation.

Exercise

Cardiovascular disease is the number one cause of death in the industrialised/affluent world. Inactivity by itself results in a 1.5 to two-fold rise in the risk of CVD[68] and a three-fold increased risk of stroke.[69] Physical exercise protects the heart in a number of ways, apart from helping to facilitate other healthy lifestyle choices. In the long term it leads to:

- improvement in lipid profiles[70,71]
- better blood flow and reduced thrombogenesis[72]
- improved blood glucose and improved responsiveness to insulin[73]
- reduced blood pressure[74,75]
- improved endothelial function
- reductions in inflammatory markers.[76,77]

Being fit also helps in the case of having an acute cardiac event. The risk of death from that heart attack is halved if the person has recently been involved in regular, moderate physical activity. Although regular exercise in the long term clearly reduces the chances of having a heart attack, very vigorous physical exertion, particularly in those not used to it, increases the risk by three and a half times.[21,78,79] It is therefore important, especially if older, unfit or unaccustomed to regular exercise, to initially take things gently and build up slowly.

For each MET (metabolic equivalent: a measure of energy expenditure) increase there is an approximate 4% reduction in cardiac risk. Walking slowly consuming roughly 2 MET per hour, walking briskly 4 MET and jogging nearly 9 MET. Higher-intensity activities are associated with lower risk of heart disease.[80] The Women's Health Initiative Observational study looked at over 70,000 postmenopausal women and found that the number of MET-hours per week was inversely associated with heart disease risk.[81,82] Most of the emphasis has previously been on the importance of aerobic exercise but the risk of heart disease is reduced by nearly a quarter if weight or resistance training as well as aerobic exercise is included in one's exercise routine.[83] Resistance training is particularly helpful in metabolic syndrome because it helps to build muscle mass, which is like a 'metabolic sink' for blood fats and glucose. It may also be the preferred option to aerobic training for those who have a low threshold for inducing angina.

Heart failure is the most common reason for hospitalisation in people over 60 years of age. Traditionally, bed rest was advised for heart failure but we now know that a graded exercise program is associated with better vitality, reduced disability, fewer symptoms and better quality of life for heart failure patients.[84] In heart failure patients, exercise also results in improved blood flow, reduced enlargement of the heart, improved heart output, improved function of blood vessel lining and better autonomic function.[85,86] The recommended intensity for heart failure patients is 50–70% of VO_2 max—that is, 'walk & talk' level. If a patient cannot talk while they walk, they should slow down a little.

Although physical activity may not be as dramatic as many drugs in lowering blood pressure or lipids, it is because it acts via many complementary mechanisms that it has such a beneficial overall effect. Exercise can also help to facilitate other healthy lifestyle changes.

Nutrition

Examples of an overall approach to nutrition—such as the Ornish diet (described below), the Mediterranean diet, calorie restriction and the Polymeal diet—have been found to be clearly helpful, independent of their effects on weight loss. Individual dietary constituents such as omega-3 fatty acids are discussed extensively below.

Nutrition and supplements

Coronary heart disease is almost entirely due to atherosclerosis in the coronary arteries. Rupture of a plaque in the coronary arteries is a pathological event underlying key coronary syndromes, sudden death, acute myocardial infarction or unstable angina. Lifestyle factors, particularly diet, play a role in the pathogenesis of coronary atherosclerosis. Diet has a significant effect on serum lipids and can affect other risk factors such as blood pressure and haemostatic factors. In the 1950s it was clearly documented that saturated fat is the major dietary macronutrient that modifies serum cholesterol and particularly LDL cholesterol.

An elevated LDL cholesterol level is the sine qua non for the development of atherosclerosis. Approximately 30 trials have now demonstrated by repeat angiography with or without intravascular ultrasound that lowering LDL cholesterol stabilises plaques and can lead to regression of atherosclerosis.[87] When on treatment, LDL cholesterol is < 2 μmol/L. After 2 years, two-thirds of patients show regression of plaque volume of more than 10%. This translates into fewer coronary events and fewer strokes, and greater survival.

There are a number of healthy diets, with the best-researched being the Mediterranean diet. A Mediterranean diet low in saturated fat, rich in monounsaturated fat, fibre, vegetable proteins, regular nut consumption and with moderate intake of alcohol not only lowers LDL cholesterol but independently of this can decrease the risk of coronary events. The famous Lyon Diet Trial of the Mediterranean diet showed a decrease in mortality of 56% compared with the usual low-fat diet.[88] The benefit was independent of drug therapy and is in fact greater than seen with cholesterol reduction using statin therapy. However, more long-term follow-up data is required, to confirm these findings. In contrast, the larger Lipid Trial is a typical statin trial with follow-up to 6 years. A 20% cholesterol reduction was associated with a 24% reduction in mortality.[89]

When a total-diet approach is used, such as in Jenkins' Portfolio Diet, which used the Mediterranean diet plus use of plant sterol enriched food, a 20–25% reduction of LDL cholesterol is seen, which is similar to that for low dose of statins.

Nutraceuticals were first defined in 1979 by Steven DeFelice as:

> food, or part of food, that provides medical and health benefits to cumulative prevention and/or treatment of disease. Such products may range from isolated nutrients, diet supplements and foods that are genetically engineered, herbal products.[90]

Nutraceuticals have been endorsed by the American Heart Association (Adult Treatment Panel III) as lowering LDL cholesterol, plant sterols/stenols and soluble fibre.[91] Plant sterols and stenols are available in margarine, yoghurt and milk. The dose is 2–4 g per day, and on average the LDL decreases by 10%. Some patients may have zero response and others may have up to 30% lowering of LDL. Plant sterol enrichment also has an additive effect to statin therapy. Soluble fibre (most commonly *Psyllium* husk) at a dose of 2 tablespoons per day can lower LDL by about 5%. It can be combined with other nutraceuticals and/or statins.

Garlic potentially affects serum lipids, platelet aggregation, blood pressure and blood glucose. In recent reviews, moderate short-term effects of diet supplementation were noted, although findings in all trials have not always been consistent.[92,93] This may relate to the differences in concentration of active components between test substances. Soy-based foods have cholesterol-lowering effects and antioxidant properties. A meta-analysis of 38 trials of soy protein demonstrated a reduction of LDL cholesterol of 12% and lowering of triglycerides by 10%.[94] Extracts of soy, and in particular isoflavones, seem to have no effect on serum lipids.

In the literature there are many extravagant claims of the beneficial effects of various citrus flavonoids, mushroom extract, olive leaf extract, guggulipid, artichoke, spirulina and policosanol. Almost all the supporting data come from small studies using various animals; randomised clinical controlled trials have rarely been conducted in humans. Policosanol is a sugar cane extract and contains a mixture of aliphatic alcohols. A number of published trials initially showed significant benefit in lipid lowering with 15–20 mg per day.[95] LDL decreased by 20–30%, and HDL increased from 8% to 15%, although more recent trials have cast doubt on those initial findings.

Fish oil or, more specifically, eicosapentaenoic acid (EPA) and docosapentanoic acid (DPA) is effective in lowering triglycerides. Marine lipids have no benefit in lowering LDL. High doses of marine ω-3 lipids may increase LDL. The usual-strength fish oil capsules contain 300 mg of combined EPA and DPA. A more concentrated super-strength form, containing 600 mg or more of combined EPA and DPA, is now available. The starting dose for lowering triglycerides is four 1 g capsules, up to 12 capsules per day.[96] Fish oil used in this combination is as effective as fibrates in lowering triglycerides and has an additive effect.

Fish oil prevents sudden death in patients post infarction, and at a dose of two 1 g fish oil capsules per day there is significant decrease in sudden death within a few months post infarction. In the GISSI-P trial 11,324 patients within 3 months of a heart attack were randomised to fish oil (one superstrength capsule) per day or not, and followed for 3.5 years.[97] Independent of drug therapy, diet or any other risk factors, those randomised to fish oil had a 41% reduction of mortality in 3 months due to a large reduction of sudden death (53% reduction at 4 months).

These favourable results were confirmed by the Japanese JELIS trial.[98] In this trial, 18,645 patients, 2500 of whom had a history of heart disease, were commenced on statin therapy and randomised to high-dose EPA or not. At a 4.6 year follow-up there was a significant 20% reduction in the combined cardiovascular end point of sudden death, myocardial infarction, unstable angina or revascularisation, with fish oil supplementation. This was on the background of a group of patients with a high intake of fish. Fish oil has a number of potential mechanisms for cardiovascular prevention, including an antiarrhythmic effect, triglyceride-lowering effect, anti-inflammatory effects, and it improves mood, endothelial function, lowers blood pressure and slows heart rate.

The American Heart Association in 2002 recommended that all patients with coronary heart disease have at least 1 g of combined EPA and DPA per day, which in practice means supplementation.[99] The Australian National Heart Foundation's position, released in 2008, is consistent with that of the United States.[19]

Vitamins

The best-studied vitamins in relation to vascular disease are vitamins E and C, folic acid[100] and vitamin B_3. Vitamin B_3 (or nicotinic acid, or niacin) is a mainstream therapy for LDL reduction. Nicotinic acid was noted in the 1950s to be effective in lowering serum cholesterol, lowering triglycerides and increasing HDL. Unfortunately, the therapeutic dose is 3 g per day, and 75% or more of patients cannot tolerate this dose, due to severe flushing.[101] In addition, the tablet size is 250 mg and is not as widely available. It is still popular in the United States, particularly in slow-release preparations, because it is relatively cheaper to prescribe.

The most recent update on vitamin supplements in cardiovascular disease by the American Heart Association was in 2004. Epidemiological studies have suggested potential benefit with high natural vitamin E intake or supplements, although the overview by the American Heart Association was that the existing database did not justify routine use of antioxidant supplements for the prevention and treatment of cardiovascular disease.[102] However, specific trials that have used natural vitamin E at high dose (greater than 500 IU per day)—and composed of alpha-tocopherol and various levels of gamma-tocopherol and perhaps tocotrienols—have shown a decrease in cardiovascular events in patients on renal dialysis and regression of carotic and coronary heart disease. In contrast, when vitamin E is used in combination with beta carotene, other studies suggest there may even be an increase in mortality.

Elevated homocysteine is associated with increased risk of cardiovascular disease. However, more than five large randomised trials have not shown a benefit, despite significant lowering of homocysteine by 20% or more, with combination B vitamin therapy.[103] There is general consensus now that homocysteine is a marker of increased cardiovascular disease, but it is no longer a target for therapy.

A few years ago, a comparison was made of major mainstream drug therapy and complementary therapies in the prevention of recurrent coronary events in patients with cardiovascular disease. In fact, the most effective therapies were the Mediterranean diet and fish oil supplementation (see Table 25.1).

Connectedness

Cardiovascular risk reduction is taken up differently by different social groups, with the taking up of healthier behaviour conferring greater benefits on those in higher socioeconomic groups.[105] Those from lower socioeconomic groups are far less likely to make healthy lifestyle changes, perhaps because of lower autonomy, greater job stress, less education and greater exposure to negative influences such as the higher concentration

TABLE 25.1 Odds ratios comparing interventions aimed at lowering the risk of coronary heart disease

		Annual risk of CHD		
Therapy	**OR**	**0.5%**	**3%**	**6%**
Aspirin	0.82	222	37	18
Beta-blocker	0.78	181	30	15
Statins	0.74	154	26	13
Smoking advice	0.68	125	21	10
Fish (± fish oil)	0.65	114	19	9
Mediterranean diet	0.24	52	9	4

Low-fat diet odds ratio (OR) = 0.96:95% confidence interval 0.89–1.04.

NB: The lower the odds ratio, the more protective the intervention.

Source: Ebrahim et al 1998[104]

of fast-food outlets in lower socioeconomic areas.[106] A US taskforce looking into predictors for CVD found that job dissatisfaction and unhappiness are stronger predictors than the usually accepted risk factors.[107]

Some social factors have protective effects on the risk of CVD, including being married (provided it is at least moderately happy), having an extended network of friends and family, church membership and group affiliation.[108] Social disadvantage and social isolation are not only predictors of CVD but are also predictors of poor outcomes post-stroke.[109] The risk for CVD in later life may be significantly affected by our social and emotional circumstances early in life.[110] A study of childhood loss found that the effect of relationships early in life affects how we respond to stressors and the level of SNS activation later in life.

Furthermore, social circumstances have a profound effect upon other lifestyle factors, like whether we exercise or not, and our use of healthcare resources.

Environment

Environment can affect CVD in many ways. For example, living in a heavily air-polluted urban environment significantly increases the risk of CVD,[111] whereas regular moderate levels of sun exposure are associated with a reduced risk of CVD, probably because of increased levels of vitamin D.[112] The risk of heart disease can be increased by exposure to various chemicals at home, including arsenic,[113] endocrine disruptors and pesticides,[114] lead[115] and mercury.[116] If there are concerns in this area, it is useful to perform tests to measure the levels of such chemicals and heavy metals.

Environment can be conducive or not conducive to a healthy lifestyle. Having access to attractive and safe parks, for example, increases the likelihood of being physically active. Our social environment at work or home, and the advertising we are subject to, all have their effects. For example, employees who experience a 'just' work environment had a 35% lower risk of heart disease than employees with low or intermediate level of justice, independent of other lifestyle and risk factors.[117] Chronic noise exposure can also be a stressor, and living in a noisy environment increases the risk of heart disease, mostly among those who tend to be annoyed by the noise.[118]

THE ORNISH PROGRAM FOR HEART DISEASE

Dean Ornish is a US cardiologist who pioneered an integrated approach to cardiac rehabilitation, which serves as an excellent model for holistic care.[119] Although it is not based on the ESSENCE model discussed above (and in Ch 6), it includes all the elements in a systematic and cohesive way. The Ornish program was the first demonstration ever that, given the right conditions, cardiovascular disease is a reversible illness. Importantly, the program improved quality of life as well as producing better clinical outcomes.[120] In the first landmark study published in *The Lancet*, people with already well-established heart disease were divided into two groups. The control group had conventional medical management only and the intervention group had the usual medical management plus the Ornish lifestyle program. The program consisted of:

- group support
- stress management including meditation and yoga
- a low-fat vegetarian diet
- moderate exercise
- no smoking.

Patients were followed with regard to angina frequency, duration and severity. They also had angiograms before the program and 12 months later, to measure whether their coronary arteries were becoming more or less blocked. The findings are summarised in Table 25.2. Basically, the cardiovascular health of patients in the Ornish program improved significantly.

In both groups, improvement was directly related to lifestyle change in a so-called 'dose–response' manner, meaning that the more the person put lifestyle change into effect in their day-to-day life, the greater the improvement in their condition. Another important point is that the program saved a huge amount of money by reducing cardiac events, hospitalisations, medications and the need for invasive procedures.[121] The observation that enhancing mental health and coping with stress were great contributors to good

TABLE 25.2 Summary of the results of the Ornish program on progression of atherosclerosis, and symptom frequency, duration and severity

	Intervention group	Control group
Progression	82% regressed	53% progressed
Symptom:		
• frequency	91% ↓	165% ↑
• duration	42% ↓	95% ↑
• severity	28% ↓	39% ↑

outcomes and healthy lifestyle change is not surprising, as we know that poor mental health and high stress are significant predictors of relapse to unhealthy lifestyle.[122]

Five-year follow-up of Ornish program participants showed that the divergence between the two groups had widened even further.[123] The Ornish group continued to reverse their disease angiographically and symptomatically. Furthermore, the usual-care group had had nearly 2½ times as many major cardiac events over the follow-up period.

SUMMARY

Various complementary and alternative medicines are frequently used by patients with or without their physician's knowledge. Comprehensive treatment of patients to improve cardiovascular outcomes involves lifestyle measures and certain complementary and medical treatments. The American Heart Association has embraced high intake of omega-3 in all patients with coronary heart disease, and the ATP3 (Expert Panel on Detection, Evaluation, and Treatment of High Blood Cholesterol in Adults (Adult Treatment Panel III)) has embraced plant sterols and soluble fibre as treatments after nutrition to lower cholesterol. Fish oil supplementation can be considered standard alternative first-line therapy for managing triglycerides, mandatory in all patients with coronary disease and, interestingly, can also be useful for improving mood or depression. Other lipid-lowering complementary medicines are less well documented. A Mediterranean-type diet, regular exercise and cessation of smoking are all important components of improving cardiovascular outcome with a similar magnitude to standard drug therapy. There is emerging data that patients who are encouraged to follow lifestyle measures are also more adherent to drug therapy.

Hawthorn or, more specifically, the preparation Crataegus 1442 can be considered an important add-on to standard drug therapy to improve cardiovascular outcomes. There is conflicting evidence regarding the value of coenzyme Q10 and at present it cannot be recommended.

There is considerable heterogeneity regarding the results of vitamin therapy, but it is reasonable to recommend natural vitamin E in patients with coronary heart disease. There is consensus that beta-carotene as a supplement is contraindicated, and B vitamin therapy to lower homocysteine is ineffective.

RESOURCES

American Heart Association, http://www.americanheart.org

National Heart Foundation of Australia, http://www.heartfoundation.org.au

Preventive Medicine Research Institute, http://www.pmri.org

REFERENCES

1 National Heart Foundation of Australia. The shifting burden of cardiovascular disease. Access Economics; 2005.

2 Australian Institute of Health and Welfare (AIHW) 2004. Heart, stroke and vascular diseases—Australian facts 2004. AIHW Cat. No. CVD 27. Canberra: AIHW and National Heart Foundation of Australia (Cardiovascular Disease Series No. 22). Online. Available: http://www.heartfoundation.com.au

3 Vogel JHK, Bolling SF, Costello RB et al. Integrating complementary medicine into cardiovascular medicine. A report of the American College of Cardiology foundation. J Am Coll Cardiol 2005; 45:184–221; a p 187.

4 Rozanski A, Blumenthal JA, Kaplan J. Impact of psychological factors on the pathogenesis of cardiovascular disease and implications for therapy. Circulation 1999; 99:2192–2217.

5 Jackson R. Updated New Zealand cardiovascular disease risk–benefit prediction guide. Editorial. BMJ 2000; 320:709–710.

6 Wilson PWF, D'Agostino RB, Levy D et al. Prediction of coronary heart disease using risk factor categories. Circulation 1998; 97:1837–1847.

7 Wei ZH, Wang H, Chen XY et al. Time- and dose-dependent effect of psyllium on serum lipids in mild-to-moderate hypercholesterolemia: a meta-analysis of controlled clinical trials. Eur J Clin Nutr 2009; 63(70):821–827.

8 Vale MJ, Jelinek MV, Best JD. How many patients with coronary artery disease are not achieving their risk-factor targets? Experience in Victoria 1996–1998 versus 1999–2000. Med J Aust 2002; 176:211–215.

9 National Heart Foundation of Australia and Cardiac Society of Australia and New Zealand. Position Statement on Lipid Management; 2005.

10 National Prescribing Service Ltd. Clinical audit. Management of hypertension. New South Wales: NPS Ltd. Online. Available: http://www.nps.org.au/__data/assets/pdf_file/0004/22837/Hypertension2007ClinicalAuditPack.pdf

11 Rosenfeldt FL, Hilton D, Pepe S et al. Systematic review of effect of coenzyme Q10 in physical exercise, hypertension and heart failure. Biofactors 2003; 18:91–100.

12 Stevinson C, Pittler MH, Ernst E. Garlic for treating hypercholesterolemia. A meta-analysis of randomized clinical trials. Ann Intern Med 2000; 133(6):420–429.

13 Pittler MN, Ernst E. Clinical effectiveness of garlic (*Allium sativum*). Mol Nutr Food Res 2007; 51(11):1382–1385.

14 Reid K. Effect of garlic on blood pressure: a systematic review and meta-analysis. BMC Cardiovascular Disord 2008; 16(8):13.

15 Reinhart KM, Coleman CI, Teevan C et al. Effects of garlic on blood pressure in patiens with and without systolic hypertension: a meta-analysis. Ann Pharmacother 2008; 42(12):1766–1771.
16 Antonello M, Montemurro D, Bolognesi M et al. Prevention of hypertension, cardiovascular damage and endothelial dysfunction with green tea extracts. Am J Hypertens 2007; 20(12):1321–1328.
17 Nakachi K, Matsuyama S, Miyake S et al. Preventive effects of drinking green tea on cancer and cardiovascular disease: epidemiological evidence for multiple targeting prevention. Biofactors 2000; 13 (1–4):49–54.
18 Jee SH, Miller ER III, Guallar E et al. The effect of magnesium supplementation on blood pressure: a meta-analysis of randomised clinical trials. Am J Hypertens 2002; 15(8):691–696.
19 National Heart Foundation. Guidelines; 2008. Online. Available: http://www.heartfoundation.org.au/Search/Pages/Results.aspx?k=management%20guidelines%20for%20hypertension
20 Linden W, Stossel C, Maurice J. Psychosocial interventions for patients with coronary artery disease: a meta-analysis. Arch Int Med 1996; 156(7):745–752.
21 Cherchi A, Lai C, Angelino F et al. Effects of L-carnitine on exercise tolerance in chronic stable angina: a multi-center, double blind, randomized, placebo controlled crossover study. Int J Clin Pharmacol Ther Toxicol 1985; 23(10):569–572.
22 Overvad K, Diamant B, Holm L et al. Coenzyme Q10 in health and disease. Eur J Clin Nutr 1999; 53(10): 764–770.
23 Kamikawa T, Kobyashi A, Yamashita T et al. Effects of coenzyme Q10 on exercise tolerance in chronic stable angina pectoris. Am J Cardiol 1985; 56(4):247–251.
24 Rosenfeldt FL, Pepe S, Linnane A et al. Coenzyme Q10 protects the aging heart against stress: studies in rats, human tissues, and patients. Ann NY Acad Sci 2002; 959:355–359.
25 Rosenfeldt F, Marasco S, Lyon W et al. Coenzyme Q10 therapy before cardiac surgery improves mitochondrial function and in vitro contractility of myocardial tissue. J Thorac Cardiovasc Surg 2005; 129(1):25–32.
26 Rosenfeldt FL, Pepe S, Linnane A et al. The effects of ageing on the response to cardiac surgery: protective strategies for the ageing myocardium. Biogerontology 2002; 3(1/2):37–40.
27 Rosenfeldt FL, Korchazhkina OV, Richards SM et al. Aspartate improves recovery of the recently infarcted rat heart after cardioplegic arrest. Eur J Cardiothorac Surg 1998; 14(2):185–190.
28 Munsch CM, Rosenfeldt FL, O'Halloran K et al. The effect of orotic acid on the response of the recently infarcted rat heart to hypothermic cardioplegia. Eur J Cardiothorac Surg 1991; 5(2):82–92.
29 Munsch C, Williams JF, Rosenfeldt FL. The impaired tolerance of the recently infarcted rat heart to cardioplegic arrest: the protective effect of orotic acid. J Mol Cell Cardiol 1989; 21(8):751–754.
30 Hadj A, Esmore D, Rowland M et al. Pre-operative preparation for cardiac surgery utilising a combination of metabolic, physical and mental therapy. Heart Lung Circ 2006; 15(3):172–181.
31 Cutshall SM, Fenske LL, Kelly RF et al. Creation of a healing enhancement program at an academic medical center. Complement Ther Clin Pract 2007; 13(4): 217–223.
32 Anderson PG, Cutshall SM. Massage therapy: a comfort intervention for cardiac surgery patients. Clin Nurse Spec 2007; 21(3):161–165.
33 Pepe S, Marasco SF, Haas SJ et al. Coenzyme Q10 in cardiovascular disease. Mitochondrion 2007; 7(Suppl):S154–S167.
34 Rosenfeldt FL, Haas SJ, Krum H et al. Coenzyme Q10 in the treatment of hypertension: a meta-analysis of the clinical trials. J Hum Hypertens 2007; 21(4): 297–306.
35 Gage BF, Waterman AD, Shannon W et al. Validation of clinical classification schemes for predicting stroke: results from the National Registry of Atrial Fibrillation. JAMA 2001; 285(22):2864–2870.
36 Sali A. Integrative medicine and arrhythmias. Aust Fam Physician 2007; 36(7):527–528. Online. Available: http://www.racgp.org.au/afp/200707/200707sali.pdf
37 Holubarsch CJF, Colucci WS, Meinertz T et al. Survival and prognosis: investigation of Crataegus extract WS1442 in congestive heart failure (SPICE)—rationale, study design and study protocol. Eur J Heart Fail 2000; 2(4):431–437. (Results presented at American College of Cardiology meeting March 2007.)
38 Pittler MH, Guo R, Ernst E. Hawthorn extract for treating chronic heart failure (review). Cochrane Database Syst Rev 2008; 1:CD005312.
39 Singh U, Devaraj S, Jialal I. Coenzyme Q10 supplementation and heart failure. Nutr Rev 2007; 65(6/1):286–293.
40 Morisco C, Trimarco B, Condorelli M. Effect of coenzyme Q10 therapy in patients with congestive heart failure: a long-term multicentre randomised study. Clin Investig 1993; 71(8 Suppl):S134–S136.
41 Sinatra ST. Metabolic cardiology: the missing link in cardiovascular disease. Altern Ther Health Med 2009; 15(2):48–50.
42 Stocker R, Pollicino C, Gay P et al. Neither plasma coenzyme Q10 concentration, nor its decline during pravastatin therapy, is linked to recurrent cardiovascular disease events: a prospective case-control

study from the LIPID study. Atherosclerosis 2006; 187(1):198–204.
43 Pittler MH, Ernst E. *Ginkgo biloba* extract for the treatment of intermittent claudication: a meta-22 analysis of randomised trials. Am J Med 2000; 108: 276–281.
44 Blumenthal M, The American Botanical Council. The ABC clinical guide to herbs. New York: Thieme; 2003:383–385.
45 McCraty R, Atkinson M, Tiller W et al. The effects of emotions on short-term power spectrum analysis of heart-rate variability. Am J Cardiol 1995;76(14): 1089–1093.
46 Strike PC, Perkins-Porras L, Whitehead DL et al. Triggering of acute coronary syndromes by physical exertion and anger: clinical and sociodemographic characteristics. Heart 2006; 92:1035–1040.
47 Everson S, Kaplan G, Goldberg D et al. Anger expression and incident stroke: prospective evidence from the Kuipio ischaemic heart disease study. Stroke 1999; 30(3):523–528.
48 Weissman M, Markowitz J, Ouellette R et al. Panic disorder and cardiovascular/cerebrovascular problems: results from a community survey. Am J Psych 1990; 147(11):1504–1508.
49 Simonsick E, Wallace R, Blazer D et al. Depressive symptomatology and hypertension-associated morbidity and mortality in older adults. Psychosom Med 1995; 57(5):427–435.
50 Appels A, Otten F. Exhaustion as precursor of cardiac death. Br J Clin Psych 1992; 31(3):351–356.
51 Appels A, Kop W, Bar F. Vital exhaustion, extent of atherosclerosis, and the clinical course after successful percutaneous transluminal coronary angioplasty. Eur Heart J 1995; 16(12):1880–1885.
52 Hemingway H, Marmot M. Evidence-based cardiology: psychosocial factors in the aetiology and prognosis of coronary heart disease. BMJ 1999; 318(7196): 1460–1467.
53 Rozanski A, Blumenthal J, Kaplan J. Impact of psychosocial factors on the pathogenesis of cardiovascular disease and implications for therapy. Circulation 1999; 99(16):2192–2217.
54 Rugulies R. Depression as a predictor for coronary heart disease. a review and meta-analysis. Am J Prev Med 2002; 23(1):51–61.
55 Linden W, Stossel C, Maurice J. Psychosocial interventions for patients with coronary artery disease: a meta-analysis. Arch Intern Med 1996; 156(7):745–752.
56 Sokejiana S, Kagamimori S. Working hours as a risk factor for acute myocardial infarction in Japan: a case control study. BMJ 1998; 317(7161):775–780.
57 Steptoe A, Kunz-Ebrecht S, Owen N et al. Socioeconomic status and stress-related biological responses over the working day. Psychosom Med 2003; 65(3):461–470.
58 Steptoe A, Kunz-Ebrecht S, Owen N et al. Influence of socioeconomic status and job control on plasma fibrinogen responses to acute mental stress. Psychosom Med 2003; 65(1):137–144.
59 Ishizaki M, Martikainen P, Nakagawa H et al. The relationship between employment grade and plasma fibrinogen level among Japanese male employees. YKKJ Research Group. Atherosclerosis 2000; 151(2):415–421.
60 Wenneberg SR, Schneider RH, Walton KG et al. A controlled study of the effects of the Transcendental Meditation program on cardiovascular reactivity and ambulatory blood pressure. Int J Neurosci 1997; 89:15–28.
61 Alexander CN, Schneider R, Claybourne M et al. A trial of stress reduction for hypertension in older African Americans, II: sex and risk factor subgroup analysis. Hypertension 1996; 28:228–237.
62 Castillo-Richmond A, Schneider R, Alexander C et al. Effects of stress reduction on carotid atherosclerosis in hypertensive African Americans. Stroke 2000; 31:568–573.
63 Schneider RH, Alexander CN, Staggers F et al. Long-term effects of stress reduction on mortality in persons > or = 55 years of age with systemic hypertension. Am J Cardiol 2005; 95(9):1060–1064.
64 Maselko J, Kubzansky L, Kawachi I et al. Religious service attendance and allostatic load among high-functioning elderly. Psychosom Med 2007; 69(5):464–472.
65 King DE, Mainous AG III, Steyer TE et al. The relationship between attendance at religious services and cardiovascular inflammatory markers. Int J Psychiatry Med 2001; 31(4):415–425.
66 Powell LH, Shahabi L, Thoresen CE. Religion and spirituality. Linkages to physical health. Am Psychol 2003; 58(1):36–52.
67 Obisesan T, Livingston I, Trulear HD et al. Frequency of attendance at religious services, cardiovascular disease, metabolic risk factors and dietary intake in Americans: an age-stratified exploratory analysis. Int J Psychiatry Med 2006; 36(4):435–448.
68 Berlin J, Colditz G. A meta analysis of physical activity in the prevention of coronary heart disease. Am J Epidemiol 1990; 132:612–628.
69 Shinton R, Sagar G. Lifelong exercise and stroke. BMJ 1993; 307:231–234.
70 Moore S. Physical activity, fitness and atherosclerosis. In: Bouchard C, Shepherd R, Stephens J, eds. Physical activity, fitness and health. Illinois: Human Kinetics; 1994:570–577.
71 Sdringola S, Nakagawa K, Nakagawa Y et al. Combined intense lifestyle and pharmacologic lipid treatment

further reduce coronary events and myocardial perfusion abnormalities compared with usual-care cholesterol-lowering drugs in coronary artery disease. J Am Coll Cardiol 2003; 41:263–272.

72 Eliasson M, Asplund K, Evrin P. Regular leisure time physical activity predicts high levels of tissue plasminogen activator. Int J Epidemiol 1996; 25:1182–1188.

73 Tsatsoulis A, Fountoulakis S. The protective role of exercise on stress system dysregulation and comorbidities. Ann NY Acad Sci 2006; 1083:196–213.

74 Fagard R, Tipton C. Physical activity, fitness and hypertension. In: Bouchard C, Shepherd R, Stephens J, eds. Physical activity, fitness and health. Illinois: Human Kinetics; 1994:633–655.

75 Kelley G, McClellan P. Antihypertensive effects of aerobic exercise—a brief meta-analytic review. Am J Hypertens 1994; 7:115–119.

76 Hamer M. Exercise and psychobiological processes: implications for the primary prevention of coronary heart disease. Sports Medicine 2006; 36(10):829–838.

77 Edwards KM, Ziegler MG, Mills PJ. The potential anti-inflammatory benefits of improving physical fitness in hypertension. J Hypertens 2007; 25(8):1533–1542.

78 American College of Sports Medicine, American Heart Association. Exercise and acute cardiovascular events: placing the risks into perspective. Med Sci Sport Exerc 2007; 39(5):886–897.

79 Thompson PD, Franklin BA, Balady GJ et al. American Heart Association Council on Nutrition, Physical Activity, and Metabolism. American Heart Association Council on Clinical Cardiology. American College of Sports Medicine. Exercise and acute cardiovascular events placing the risks into perspective: a scientific statement from the American Heart Association Council on Nutrition, Physical Activity, and Metabolism and the Council on Clinical Cardiology. Circulation 2007; 115(17):2358–2368.

80 Tanasescu M, Leitzmann MF, Rimm EB et al. Exercise type and intensity in relation to coronary heart disease in men. JAMA 2002; 288:1994–2000.

81 Manson JE, Greenland P, LaCroix AZ et al. Walking compared with vigorous exercise for the prevention of cardiovascular events in women. N Engl J Med 2002; 347:716–725.

82 Owen N, Bauman A. The descriptive epidemiology of physical inactivity in adult Australians. Int J Epidemiol 1992; 21:305–310.

83 Braith RW, Stewart KJ. Resistance exercise training: its role in the prevention of cardiovascular disease. Circulation 2006; 113(22):2642–2650.

84 Fleg JL. Exercise therapy for elderly heart failure patients. Clin Geriatr Med 2007; 23(1):221–234.

85 Maiorana A, O'Driscoll G, Cheetham C et al. Combined aerobic and resistance exercise training improves functional capacity and strength in CHF. J Appl Physiol 2000; 88:1565–1570.

86 Maiorana A, O'Driscoll G, Dembo L et al. Effect of aerobic and resistance exercise training on vascular function in heart failure. Am J Physiol Heart Circ Physiol 2000; 279(4):1999–2005.

87 Chatriwalla AK, Nicholls SJ, Wang TH et al. Low levels of low-density lipoprotein cholesterol and blood pressure and progression of coronary atherosclerosis. J Am Coll Cardiol 2009; 53(13):1110–1115.

88 de Lorgeril M, Salen P, Martin J-L et al. Mediterranean diet, traditional risk factors and the rate of cardiovascular complications after myocardial infarction. Final report of the Lyon Diet Heart Study. Circulation 1999; 99:779–785.

89 Lipid Study Group. Prevention of cardiovascular events and death with prevention in patients with coronary heart disease and a broad range of initial cholesterol levels. N Engl J Med 1998; 339:1349–1357.

90 Biesaeski HK. Nutraceuticals, the link between nutrition and medicine. In: Kramer K, Hoppe PP, Packer L, eds. Nutraceuticals in health and disease prevention. New York: Marcel Dekker; 2001:1–26.

91 National Cholesterol Education Program Expert Panel on Detection, Evaluation and Treatment of High Blood Cholesterol in Adults (Adult Treatment Panel III). Third Report of the National Cholesterol Education Program (NCEP) Expert Panel on Detection, Evaluation and Treatment of High Blood Cholesterol in Adults (Adult Treatment Panel III) final report. Circulation 2002; 106:3143–3421.

92 Butt MS, Sultan MT, Iqbal J. Garlic: nature's protection against physiological threats. Crit Rev Food Sci Nutr 2009; 49(6):538–551.

93 Reinhart KM, Talati R, White CM et al. The impact of garlic on lipid parameters: a systematic review and meta-analysis. Nutr Res Rev 2009; 22(1):39–48.

94 van Ee JH. Soy constituents: modes of action in low-density lipoprotein management. Nutr Rev 2009; 67(4):222–234.

95 Chen JT, Wesley R, Shamburek RD et al. Meta-analysis of natural therapies for hyperlipidemia: plant sterols and stanols versus policosanol. Pharmacotherapy 2005; 25(2):171–183.

96 Harris WS. N-3 fatty acids and serum lipoproteins: human studies. AJM Clin Nutr 1197; 65:1645S–1654S.

97 Marchioli R, Schweiger C, Tavazzi L et al. Dietary supplementation with n-3 polyunsaturated fatty acids and vitamin E after myocardial infarction: results of the GISSI-Prevenzione Trial. Lancet 1999; 354(9177):447–455.

98 Yokoyama M, Origasa H, Matsuzaki M et al. Effects of eicosapentaenoic acid on major coronary events in hypercholesterolaemic patients (JELIS): a randomized

open-label, blinded endpoint analysis. Lancet 2007; 369(9567):1090–1098.

99 Kris-Etherton PM, Harris, WS, Appel LJ (American Heart Association Nutrition Committee). Fish consumption, fish oil, omega-3 fatty acids and cardiovascular disease. Circulation 2002; 106:2747–2757.

100 Wang X, Qin X, Demirtas H et al. Efficacy of folic acid supplementation in stroke population: a meta-analysis. Lancet 2007; 369:1876–1882.

101 Kamanna VS, Kashyap ML. Mechanism of action of niacin on lipoprotein metabolism. Curr Atheroscler Rep 2000; 2:36–46.

102 Kris-Etherton PM, Lichtenstein AH, Howard BV et al. American Heart Association Scientific Statement. Antioxidant vitamin supplements and cardiovascular disease. Circulation 2004; 110:637–641.

103 Sánchez-Moreno C, Jiménez-Escrig A, Martín A. Stroke: roles of B vitamins, homocysteine and antioxidants. Nutr Res Rev 2009; 22(1):49–67.

104 Ebrahim S, Smith GD, McCabe C et al. Cholesterol and coronary heart disease: screening and treatment. Quality in Health Care 1998; 7:232–239.

105 Bartley M, Fitzpatrick R, Firth D et al. Social distribution of cardiovascular disease risk factors: change among men in England 1984–1993. J Epidemiol Comm Health 2000; 54(11):806–814.

106 Bosma H, Marmot MG, Hemingway H et al. Low job control and risk of coronary heart disease in the Whitehall II (prospective cohort) study. BMJ 1997; 314:558–565.

107 Work in America: report of a Special Task Force to the Secretary of Health, Education and Welfare. Cambridge, MA:MIT Press; 1973.

108 Berkman L, Syme S. Social networks, host resistance and mortality: a nine-year follow-up study of Alameda County residents. Am J Epidemiol 1979; 109:186–204.

109 Boden-Albala B, Litwak E, Elkind MS et al. Social isolation and outcomes post stroke. Neurology 2005; 64(11):1888–1892.

110 LJ Luecken. Childhood attachment and loss experiences affect adult cardiovascular and cortisol function. Psychosom Med 1998; 60:765–772.

111 Cancado JE, Braga A, Pereira LA et al. Clinical repercussions of exposure to atmospheric pollution. Jornal Brasileiro De Pneumologia: Publicacao Oficial Da Sociedade Brasileira De Pneumologia E Tisilogia 2006; 32(Suppl 2):S5–S11.

112 Holick MF. Vitamin D: importance in the prevention of cancers, type 1 diabetes, heart disease, and osteoporosis. Am J Clin Nutr 2004; 79(3):362–371.

113 Wang CH, Hsiao CK, Chen CL et al. A review of the epidemiologic literature on the role of environmental arsenic exposure and cardiovascular diseases. Toxicol Appl Pharmacol 2007; 222(3):315–326.

114 Newbold RR, Padilla-Banks E, Snyder RJ et al. Developmental exposure to endocrine disruptors and the obesity epidemic. Reprod Toxicol 2007; 23(3):290–296.

115 Navas-Acien A, Guallar E, Silbergeld EK et al. Lead exposure and cardiovascular disease—a systematic review. Environ Health Perspect 2007; 115(3):472–482.

116 Virtanen JK, Rissanen TH, Voutilainen S et al. Mercury as a risk factor for cardiovascular diseases. J Nutr Biochem 2007; 18(2):75–85.

117 Kivimaki M, Ferrie JE, Brunner E et al. Justice at work and reduced risk of coronary heart disease among employees: the Whitehall II Study. Arch Intern Med 2005; 165(19):2245–2251.

118 Willich SN, Wegscheider K, Stallmann M et al. Noise burden and the risk of myocardial infarction. Eur Heart J 2006; 27:276–282.

119 Ornish D. Dr Dean Ornish's program for reversing heart disease: the only system scientifically proven to reverse heart disease without drugs or surgery. New York: Random House; 1990.

120 Ornish D, Brown SE, Scherwitz LW et al. Can lifestyle changes reverse coronary heart disease? The Lifestyle Heart Trial. Lancet 1990; 336:129–133.

121 News. US insurance company covers lifestyle therapy. BMJ 1993; 307:465.

122 Penninx BW, Beekman AT, Honig A et al. Depression and cardiac mortality: results from a community-based longitudinal study. Arch Gen Psych 2001; 58(3):221–227.

123 Ornish D, Scherwitz L, Billings J et al. Intensive lifestyle changes for reversal of coronary heart disease. JAMA 1998; 280:2001–2007.

chapter 26

Diabetes

INTRODUCTION AND OVERVIEW

Diabetes mellitus is classified into several types:

- *type 1 diabetes*—constitutes about 5–10% of cases of diabetes, with onset at any age, but predominantly under the age of 30 years
- LADA (latent autoimmune diabetes of adulthood) or 'type 1.5 diabetes'—a slowly progressive form of type 1 diabetes mellitus. Patients are often diagnosed as type 2 diabetes, but have positive pancreatic islet antibodies, especially to glutamic acid decarboxylase (GAD). They do not immediately require insulin for treatment, are often not overweight, and have little or no resistance to insulin
- *type 2 diabetes*—a growing global epidemic linked to overweight and obesity, calorie-dense foods, physical inactivity and increasing levels of stress. It is closely associated with an increased risk of cardiovascular disease. Although historically type 2 diabetes has been a condition of the elderly, because of changing lifestyle patterns we are now seeing type 2 diabetes in preteens. The long-term health and economic implications of the rising incidence and falling age of onset are enormous
- *gestational diabetes*—a transient but significant form of diabetes; 3–5% of pregnant women will develop gestational diabetes at week 24–28 of pregnancy. Blood glucose levels usually return to normal after the delivery, but women who have gestational diabetes have a 30–50% chance of developing type 2 diabetes within 20 years.[1]

The role of the general practitioner is in identifying those at risk of diabetes and advising on preventive and early intervention strategies when impaired glucose tolerance, prediabetes or diabetes is identified.

Once a diagnosis of diabetes is established, management of diabetes is aimed at secondary prevention strategies through control of blood sugar levels, correction of micronutrient deficiencies and active risk factor management. The long-term effects of diabetes are largely due to its effect on blood vessels leading to both micro and macro vascular disease.

RISK FACTORS AND PRIMARY PREVENTION

In order to establish advice for patients on how to prevent or delay the onset of diabetes, it is important to:

- understand the aetiology, and
- identify and assess any avoidable or modifiable risk factors.

AETIOLOGY

Type 1 diabetes

Type 1 diabetes constitutes around 5–10% of diabetes cases. Aetiological factors are the following:

- *autoimmune response*—thought to be triggered by exposure to environmental agents such as viruses and toxins in individuals with an inherited predisposition
- *genetic factors*—there is some association of type 1 diabetes with other autoimmune conditions within individuals and families, such as coeliac disease, autoimmune thyroiditis,[2] Addison's disease and pernicious anaemia. Human leucocyte antigen (HLA) class II association: HLA DR4-DQ8 and/or DR3-DQ2 are positively associated with diabetes type 1, while DR15-DQ6 (B*0602) is negatively associated.

Type 2 diabetes

Type 2 diabetes constitutes around 90–95% of cases of diabetes. Aetiological factors are the following:

- overweight

- physical inactivity
- inherited predisposition
- stress (allostatic load)
- inflammation
- environmental factors
- calorie-dense diet.

Type 2 diabetes, being strongly related to lifestyle, is most common in affluent countries, where there is abundant food along with sedentary occupations and a significant uptake of labour-saving devices. Within those affluent countries, however, type 2 diabetes is more common among lower socioeconomic groups, where poor-quality food, social disadvantage and poorer education have their impact. In either case, the cause of the condition being largely lifestyle related also means that it is preventable and can be managed with appropriate and sustained lifestyle change. To illustrate how important simple lifestyle factors are in diabetes prevention, never smoking, having a BMI < 30, exercising moderately for 3.5 hours per week and following a few healthy dietary principles (high intake of fruit, vegetables and wholegrain bread, and low meat consumption) compared with not having any of those four factors was associated with a 93% reduced risk of developing type 2 diabetes over 8 years of follow-up.[3]

The challenge in type 2 diabetes management, as with other chronic illnesses related to lifestyle, is to motivate the patient to make the necessary changes. From a sociological perspective, the solution also requires that we address the social, economic and educational conditions that make it easier for a condition like type 2 diabetes to flourish. This needs motivated healthcare practitioners as well as educators, health promoters, legislators and policy makers. No single solution will work in isolation from the others.

Gestational diabetes

The hormones responsible for promoting fetal growth and development increase markedly in the last 20 weeks of pregnancy. Human placental lactogen in particular has anti-insulin effects. Despite higher insulin levels in the last trimester, there is a reduction in peripheral insulin sensitivity and higher basal hepatic glucose output.

Prediabetes and metabolic syndrome

Prediabetes is a state in which the body does not respond properly to insulin, so blood glucose levels are higher than normal, but not in the range for a diagnosis of diabetes. It is generally asymptomatic. Progression to a diagnosis of diabetes is not inevitable.

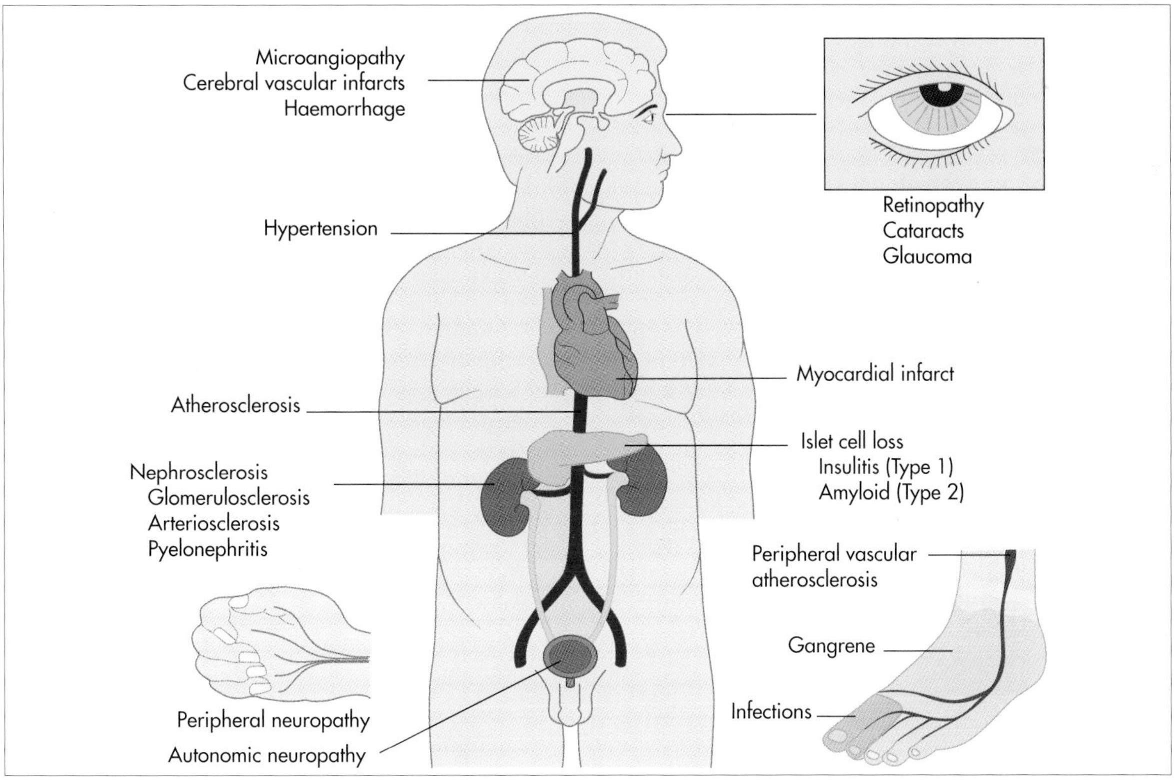

FIGURE 26.1 Long-term complications of diabetes

BOX 26.1 Definition of metabolic syndrome

- Abdominal obesity with waist circumference:
  - > 102 cm in men
  - > 88 cm in women
- Waist–hip ratio
  - > 1.0 for women
  - > 0.9 for men
- BMI > 30 kg/m^2
- TG > 1.69 mmol/L
- HDL:
  - < 1.03 mmol/L in men
  - < 1.29 mmol/L in women
- BP > 135 systolic and > 85 diastolic or treated hypertension
- Fasting glucose > 6.11 mmol/L

BMI: body mass index; BP: blood pressure; HDL: high-density lipoprotein; TG: triglycerides

Metabolic syndrome is a recognised precursor to the development of type 2 diabetes. A diagnosis of metabolic syndrome requires three of the risk factors listed in Box 26.1 to be present.[4]

Significance of metabolic syndrome

Metabolic syndrome is a cluster of risk factors that increase the risk of developing diabetes, heart disease and stroke. It is also known as syndrome X, dysmetabolic syndrome and insulin resistance syndrome. Incidence increases with age. It is thought to be the result of a combination of genetic predisposition and lifestyle factors, including dietary and exercise habits.

PRIMARY PREVENTION

Nutritional and environmental

Pre-conception counselling and pregnancy

Maternal malnutrition and overnutrition during pregnancy are associated with subsequent type 2 diabetes in the offspring.[5] Primary prevention needs to start with pre-conception counselling of women planning pregnancy, with advice on exercise and nutrition to maintain optimal weight and nutritional status during the pregnancy.

Infant supplements

A systematic review of observational studies found that giving infants vitamin D supplements could protect them from type 1 diabetes.[6] Infants given the supplement had an almost 30% reduced risk of diabetes compared with those who were not supplemented. This is particularly important in breastfed infants of vitamin-D-deficient mothers.

Weight management

Preventing or reversing metabolic syndrome involves weight loss and waist circumference reduction through diet and increased activity, and maintaining goal levels of blood pressure, lipids and lipoproteins and blood glucose. BMI per se is now seen as a less accurate marker of cardiovascular risk. It is not just the presence of excess weight but the pattern of weight distribution that is important. Abdominal or 'apple' obesity is the pattern associated with greater risk. The so-called 'pear' distribution of fat, mostly around the hips and legs, is less of a problem than the apple distribution. The measurement to determine which category a patient falls into is the waist–hip ratio. If this is above 1.0 for women or 0.9 for men, the person is said to have the apple distribution of fat; below these figures the person would be classified as having the pear distribution.

The mainstays of primary prevention of diabetes are:

- a healthy diet from conception onwards, including a wide range of regular physical activity
- avoidance of sedentary activities
- maintenance of a healthy weight
- moderate alcohol consumption
- avoidance of smoking
- avoidance of environmental toxins.

Case detection

Proactive screening of asymptomatic patients

There is an asymptomatic phase of undetected diabetes mellitus that provides an opportunity for early detection, reducing the incidence of long-term complications. Microvascular complications such as retinopathy, neuropathy and renal disease are commonly already present at the time of diagnosis of type 2 diabetes.

The following groups of asymptomatic patients should be tested:[7]

- individuals over 55 years of age
- people aged 45 or older who have one or both of the following risk factors:
  - obesity with BMI > 30
  - hypertension
- Aboriginals and Torres Strait Islanders aged 35 or older
- certain high-risk non-English-speaking background groups aged 35 or older (specifically Pacific Island people, people from the Indian subcontinent or of Chinese origin)
- all people with impaired glucose tolerance or impaired fasting glucose
- all people with clinical cardiovascular disease (myocardial infarction, stroke, angina)
- women with polycystic ovary syndrome who are obese
- patients taking antipsychotic drugs
- women with a past history of gestational diabetes.

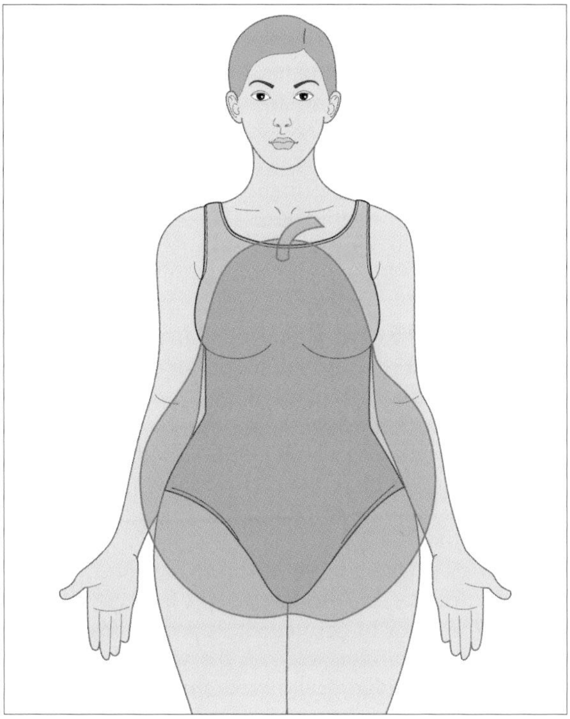

FIGURE 26.2 Pear body

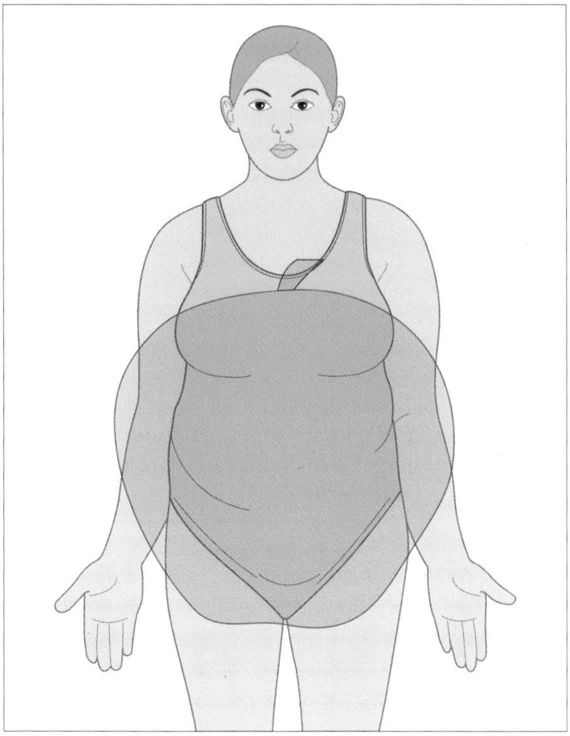

FIGURE 26.3 Apple body

Blood glucose level

The test of choice for diagnosis is fasting plasma glucose performed in an accredited laboratory. Random measures may be used.

Interpretation of blood glucose level (BGL) results:

- < 5.5 mmol/L—diabetes unlikely
- ≥ 7.0 mmol/L or more fasting or ≥ 11.1 mmol/L random—diabetes likely
- 5.5–6.9 mmol/L fasting, or 5.5–11.0 mmol/L random—perform a glucose tolerance test (GTT).

Re-testing should be performed under the following circumstances:

- on a different day, to confirm a BGL test suggesting a diagnosis of diabetes
- 1 year later for people who have an initial test suggesting diabetes that is not confirmed on the subsequent test
- each year for people with impaired GTT or impaired fasting glucose
- every 3 years for people in high-risk groups with negative screening tests.

People in high-risk groups with negative screening blood glucose tests are also at high risk for cardiovascular disease and should be encouraged to reduce their cardiovascular risk factors.

Glucose tolerance test

People found to have impaired glucose tolerance, where glucose levels are above normal but fall short of a diagnosis of diabetes, are at higher risk of later developing type 2 diabetes and also at higher risk of cardiovascular disease. Approximately one-third of people with impaired glucose tolerance will develop type 2 diabetes.

SYMPTOMS

Symptoms of diabetes mellitus include:

- polydipsia
- polyuria
- recurrent infections
- recurrent vaginal candidiasis
- tiredness, fatigue
- visual changes
- paraesthesia or numbness of feet
- neuropathic pain
- erectile dysfunction
- coronary artery disease
- peripheral vascular disease
- weight loss—may be evident in the presentation of type 1 diabetes
- overweight or obese—may be in type 2 diabetes.

MANAGEMENT

INITIAL ASSESSMENT

History

Initial assessment of the patient with diabetes involves a comprehensive medical, social and lifestyle history:

- food diary for 3–7 days to assess current eating patterns
- exercise diary—including current patterns of exercise frequency, duration and intensity
- psychosocial assessment (stress, anxiety, depression)
- current medication and supplements
- tobacco and alcohol consumption
- family history of diabetes, cardiovascular disease, osteoporosis, coeliac disease and hyperlipidaemia
- review results of recent investigations where available.

Examination

Comprehensive physical examination, including:

- blood pressure, cardiovascular assessment
- peripheral neurological assessment
- height, weight, BMI
- waist circumference
- feet—ulcers, neuropathy, peripheral vascular disease
- urinalysis (especially looking for asymptomatic urinary tract infection and microalbuminuria)
- visual acuity, retinal fundoscopy
- ECG.

Laboratory tests and further investigations:

- fasting BGL
- HbA_{1c} every 6 months
- urinary albumin/protein
- full blood examination including haemoglobin and white cell count
- C-reactive protein
- homocysteine (cardiovascular risk)
- thyroid function tests (TFT) (TSH and free T_4)
- fasting lipids (cholesterol and HDL)
- micronutrient assessment (especially iron, folate, vitamin B_{12}, B_6)
- coeliac serology (association between type 1 diabetes and coeliac disease—1 in 20 people with type 1 diabetes have coeliac disease and as many as 1 in 10 test positive for transglutaminase IgA autoantibodies)
- baseline retinal and visual assessment
- bone densitometry for patients aged over 40.

Type 1 or type 2?

Blood tests can help distinguish between type 1 and type 2 diabetes.

- Tests for islet cell and anti-GAD antibodies are positive in 90% of patients with type 1 diabetes.
- C-peptide levels would be abnomally low in type 1 and normal in type 2 diabetes.

INITIAL MANAGEMENT

The aim of initial management is to establish glycaemic control, normalise lipid and lipoprotein levels and motivate the patient to make significant and lasting changes to their lifestyle, including exercise and weight control.

A significant feature of the initial management phase includes patient education in self-monitoring, symptom awareness (including signs of hypoglycaemia), diet and exercise, and self-care.

A decision needs to be made about appropriate medication and supplements (see below).

Education

As is the case with the successful management of any chronic disease, the healthcare professional acts as informed advisor to the patient. It is the person living with diabetes who has to 'walk the walk', deciding on their level of compliance with recommended treatments. This involves 'big picture' decisions like starting oral hypoglycaemic agents or insulin treatment, or wholesale lifestyle adjustment, as much as the micromanagement of individual risk factors, such as choice of exercise program and the finer details of dietary components. For this reason, management plans must have mutually agreed, achievable goals.

The primary aim of treatment of diabetes is to optimise blood sugar control in order to increase longevity and quality of life, and to minimise complications of the disease. When devising a management plan, you will need to consider the patient's level of education, cultural beliefs, preferences and financial resources. For example, although a personal trainer might be a desirable way to motivate a person to exercise regularly, this would not be affordable for many. A walking group might be an option.

Education also needs to include significant others in the patient's life. Whoever has responsibility for food shopping and preparation in the household will need to be involved in education about dietary changes. Exercise programs will need to involve the encouragement of significant others, to aid compliance.

Home blood glucose monitoring is an essential part of the management of diabetes, initially under close supervision. In the early stages after diabetes is diagnosed, BGL readings three or four times a day are recommended. Once blood glucose levels stabilise, monitoring can be reduced to once or twice a day, one or two days a week.

Symptoms of hypoglycaemia

Patients diagnosed with diabetes will need to be aware of the early signs of hypoglycaemia so they can take steps to correct their BGL. Symptoms occur when the BGL falls too low (below about 4.0 mmol/L). They include:

- shaking
- hunger
- rapid heartbeat /palpitations
- tingling around the mouth and lips
- lethargy
- headache
- dizziness.

If not corrected, this can proceed to confusion, slurred speech, unsteady gait and drowsiness leading to unconsciousness.

If a patient is hypoglycaemic but conscious and able to drink, a sweet drink such as fruit juice is simplest and will help to correct the problem within minutes.

If the patient is unconscious, administration of glucagon 1 mg SC, IV or IM will be necessary. People with diabetes, and their families and associates, should be instructed in the use of a 'hypo kit'.

If this fails to restore consciousness, follow glucagon with IV 50% glucose 20–30 mL.

ONGOING MANAGEMENT

Successful long-term management of diabetes requires a commitment by the patient to lifelong healthy lifestyle measures. Management programs need to be negotiated with the patient so that realistic goals can be set which take into account the patient's current state of health and fitness, their individual food and activity preferences, their financial status and their access to healthcare professionals and facilities.

The general practitioner is most often where the initial diagnosis and investigation occurs and plays a central role in coordinating care involving other healthcare professionals. This coordinating role requires excellent communication between all professionals involved in care. It also depends upon a reliable and efficient recall and reminder system.

Once the initial diagnosis and management are in place, the patient needs to be linked up with other healthcare professionals, ideally including:

- endocrinologist
- diabetes education clinic
- dietician
- podiatrist
- optometrist/ophthalmologist
- community pharmacist
- fitness professional
- appropriate complementary practitioner(s).

Goals of management

People with diabetes and prediabetes should be encouraged to achieve and maintain the following targets:

- fasting BGL 4.0–6.0 mmol/L
- HbA_{1c} 7.0–7.9% (over-zealous management below these levels increases the risk of severe hypoglycaemia and may be associated with increased mortality)
- total cholesterol < 4.0 mmol/L
- HDL cholesterol > 1.0 mmol/L
- LDL cholesterol < 2.5 mmol/L
- triglycerides < 1.5 mmol/L
- blood pressure $\leq 130/80$ mmHg
- BMI ≤ 25 kg/m^2 where appropriate
- urinary albumin excretion < 20 mg/L (spot collection)
- cigarette consumption zero
- alcohol consumption 2 standard drinks/day or less
- exercise 30–45 minutes/day minimum, total > 150 minutes/week.

The ACCORD study reported by the NIH in 2008 suggests that aiming for stricter control for type 2 diabetics in the range of a HbA_{1c} of ≤ 6.5 was associated with higher mortality than those controlled in the range of 7.0–7.9.[8]

Secondary prevention

Secondary prevention in diabetes refers to the management of risk factors, and prevention or early intervention in the event of complications (see Box 26.2).

Immunisation

Consider influenza vaccination annually and pneumococcal vaccination every 5 years.

Diet

Careful and well-informed dietary management is central to the management of all types of diabetes mellitus and prediabetic states, with the aim of achieving targets for BGL, lipids, waist circumference and weight. Consultation with a qualified dietician is highly recommended.

Box 26.2 Complications of diabetes

- Myocardial infarction
- Stroke
- Retinopathy and visual impairment
- Renal disease
- Neuropathy
- Foot ulcers
- Limb amputation
- Erectile dysfunction
- Depression

Principles of dietary management in diabetes:

- patient is encouraged to keep a detailed food diary in the early stages of their management and if BGL or weight management is an issue
- low saturated fats
- low-glycaemic-index, high-soluble-fibre carbohydrates
- avoid sugary sweets and soft drinks
- emphasis on fresh whole foods, fruit and vegetables and whole grains
- quality protein sources such as soy foods, organic lean meat or chicken, including at least two meals of oily fish per week (salmon, herring, trout, mackerel, sardines); protein should contribute 10–20% of total energy
- portion control
- regular mealtimes during the day
- limit alcohol to one to two drinks per day maximum, with at least two alcohol-free days a week.

Glycaemic index

The glycaemic index (GI) is a ranking of carbohydrates from 0 to 100, based on the extent to which they raise blood glucose levels after ingestion. High-GI foods (white bread, white rice, potatoes) are rapidly digested and absorbed, and result in higher fluctuations of BGL. A predominantly high-GI diet is associated with a higher risk of obesity, type 2 diabetes and cardiovascular disease. Low-GI foods (most fruits and vegetables, whole grains) cause gradual increases in BGL and insulin levels. The presence of soluble fibre reduces the GI of foods by slowing the gastric emptying rate.

A low-GI diet is recommended for primary prevention of type 2 diabetes and cardiovascular disease, in the management of diabetes and prediabetes and for maintenance of general health. A low-GI diet is part of the story, but the glycaemic load is an important marker of how good or bad a food is for blood glucose control, insulin level and diabetic control. The high GI of foods such as parsnip and dates is offset by their high dietary

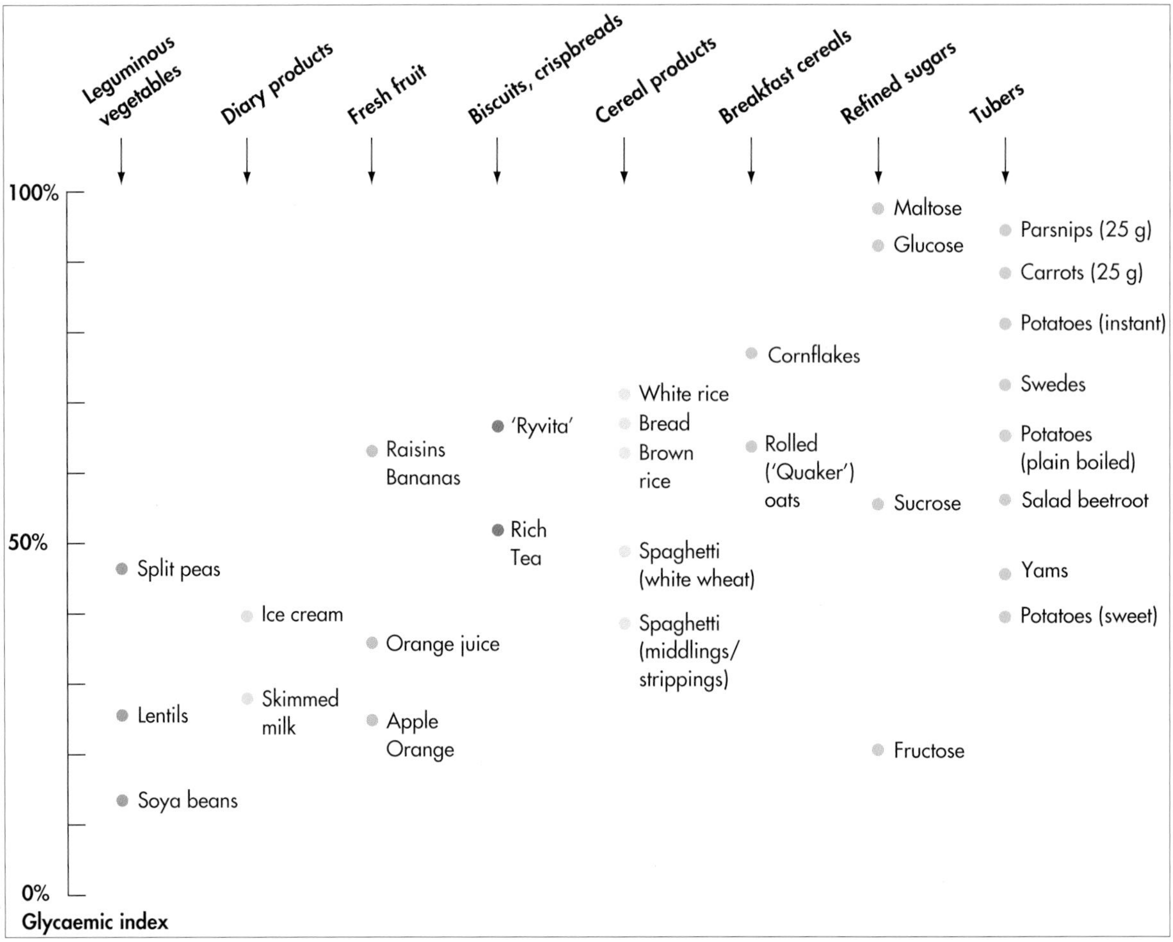

FIGURE 26.4 Glycaemic index chart for some common foods

fibre content, meaning that they have a relatively low total glycaemic load. Hence, although many fruits and vegetables have a relatively high sucrose content, they are nevertheless good for diabetics because of their high natural levels of fibre. Sucrose, a form of sugar made up of glucose and fructose, has a moderate GI. Many commercially produced foods contain high levels of refined sucrose (sugar) but very low fibre content and therefore have a high glycaemic load. Hence, it is not 'sugar' per se that is problematic for diabetics, but *refined* sugar. Many commercially produced fruit-juice drinks and foods are labelled as having 'no added sugar' but actually have high levels of sucrose through the addition of things such as fruit juice concentrate or corn syrup. Many 'low-fat' foods also masquerade as being healthy for diabetics but often have high levels of refined sucrose. It is therefore important for patients to cultivate their ability to read and understand the contents on food labels in order to understand what they are eating. A dietician can help with this.

Exercise

Regular exercise improves metabolism of glucose and lipids. If a patient is aged over 40 and leads a sedentary lifestyle, has a family history of heart disease and/or other risk factors for cardiovascular disease, a medical assessment including stress ECG is advisable before a specific exercise program is recommended.

For a walking program, a pair of correctly fitting shock-absorbing sports shoes and diabetic socks is an important prerequisite. Commence with brisk walking for 30–45 minutes every day, and build up intensity and time gradually as exercise tolerance improves.

Resistance (weight) training increases basal metabolic rate, maintains lean muscle mass, improves muscle glycogen uptake and reduces the risk of osteoporosis.

Avoidance of tobacco smoke

Apart from stating the obvious—that every patient needs to be encouraged to avoid tobacco smoke—the increased risk for people with diabetes makes it an imperative because of its strong association with cardiovascular disease and microvascular complications of diabetes. Patients should be offered counselling and advised, if necessary, on nicotine replacement, hypnotherapy and acupuncture to help reduce craving.

Supplements

There is no international consensus on a protocol of supplements for diabetes management, and decisions will need to be made on an individual basis. The following guide will assist decision-making and can form a part of initial integrative lifestyle and nutritional management.

Fish oil

Omega-3 polyunsaturated fatty acid (PUFA) supplementation in type 2 diabetes lowers triglycerides and VLDL cholesterol, but may raise LDL cholesterol (although results were non-significant in subgroups) and has no statistically significant effect on glycaemic control or fasting insulin. Trials with vascular events or mortality-defined endpoints are needed. No adverse effects of the intervention were reported.[9]

Recommendation: 2–3 g per day.

Multivitamins

A high-quality daily multivitamin and mineral may be the most convenient and cost-effective way to ensure compliance and adequate daily vitamin intake.

Antioxidants

Patients with type 1 diabetes have a higher level of free radicals than non-diabetics.

Vitamin C

People with diabetes, both type 1 and type 2, have lower levels of Vitamin C. Vitamin C can improve glucose tolerance in type 2 diabetes.

Recommendation: 1–2 g vitamin C per day.

B vitamins

Vitamin B_1—correction of thiamine deficiency in experimental diabetes by high-dose therapy with thiamine and the thiamine monophosphate prodrug, benfotiamine, was found to prevent multiple mechanisms of biochemical dysfunction: activation of protein kinase C, activation of the hexosamine pathway, increased glycation and oxidative stress. Consequently, the development of incipient diabetic nephropathy, neuropathy and retinopathy was prevented. Both thiamine and benfotiamine produced other remarkable effects in experimental diabetes: marked reversals of increased diuresis and glucosuria without change in glycaemic status. High-dose thiamine also corrected dyslipidaemia in experimental diabetes—normalising cholesterol and triglycerides. Dysfunction of beta-cells and impaired glucose tolerance in thiamine deficiency, and suggestion of a link of impaired glucose tolerance with dietary thiamine, indicates that thiamine therapy may have a future role in prevention of type 2 diabetes.[10]

Vitamin B_3 (nicotinamide)—500 mg daily for a month, followed by 250 mg daily helps reduce BGL in some diabetics. By the time insulin-dependent diabetes mellitus (IDDM) is diagnosed, 80–90% of pancreatic beta islet cells have already been destroyed. Nicotinamide has been shown to protect pancreatic beta cells from inflammation leading to their destruction and to improve remaining beta cell function after the onset of IDDM.[11,12] The extended release form has a lower incidence of flushing as a side effect. Higher doses may cause insulin resistance and increase fasting blood glucose in patients with non-insulin-dependent diabetes mellitus (NIDDM), so it should be used with caution in this group of patients.

Recommendation: recently diagnosed IDDM: 1500–2000 mg extended-release nocte. NIDDM: use only with caution, monitor requirement for hypoglycaemic agents and fasting BGL.

Vitamin B_6—low levels of vitamin B_6 are common in people with type 2 diabetes.

Recommendation: 50–100 mg daily.

Chromium

Chromium is an essential trace mineral, and a key component in glucose tolerance factor. It is essential for normal carbohydrate metabolism and insulin sensitivity, and reduces insulin resistance. Chromium also inhibits the pro-inflammatory cytokine tumour necrosis factor alpha, which reduces the activity of insulin. It seems to be more effective in non-insulin-dependent diabetes mellitus (NIDDM) than in IDDM.

Recommendation: There is strong evidence that 200–1000 μg of chromium picolinate daily in two divided doses improves glycaemic control. Biotin might enhance its effects, but this combination requires further s tudy.

Magnesium

Magnesium deficiency is common in people with diabetes and may be protective against the development of early-stage type 2 diabetes in individuals with normal renal function.[13]

Recommendation: Increase consumption of major food sources of magnesium, such as whole grains, nuts and green leafy vegetables. Supplement where renal function is normal and diet is deficient.

Zinc

Zinc deficiency is common in type 1 and type 2 diabetes. Diabetes decreases zinc absorption and increases urinary excretion, decreasing total body zinc. It is particularly common in vegetarians. Production, storage and secretion of insulin requires zinc. Zinc supplementation therefore is a reasonable strategy for prevention of zinc deficiency in diabetes.[14] Zinc used as therapy in obese women with normal glucose tolerance has been shown to decrease insulin resistance.

Recommendation: 30 mg elemental zinc daily (check renal function).

HERBAL

Gymnema sylvestre

Gymnema sylvestre suppresses perception of 'sweet' taste and reduces sweet craving.[15] It reduces intestinal absorption of glucose and inhibits active glucose transport in the small intestine, stimulates insulin secretion and increases the number of islets of Langerhans and pancreatic beta cells.[16] Doses of hypoglycaemic medication may need to be adjusted, as it can reduce BGL.

Dose: When used to regulate BGL, to be given in divided doses with meals. Extract standardised to contain 24% gymnemic acids: 400–600 mg/day. Liquid extract (1:1): 3.6–11.0 mL/day.

Fenugreek

Fenugreek has been used traditionally to regulate BGL levels by delaying glucose absorption and enhancing its utilisation.[17] It has mild hypoglycaemic, lipid-lowering and anti-inflammatory effect. Forms and treatment regimens vary. Doses of hypoglycaemic medication may need to be adjusted, as it can reduce BGL.

Dose: 50–100 g seed daily in divided doses with meals, or 1 g/day ethanolic seed extract.

Evening primrose oil

Evening primrose oil is useful in treating mild to moderate diabetic neuropathy.[18] It may be combined with fish oil.

Dose: 360–480 mg gamma linoleic acid (GLA) (equivalent to 4–6 × 1 g capsules per day).

Cinnamon[19]

Cinnamon has been used for thousands of years to treat diabetes and other conditions. The aqueous extract appears to activate the insulin receptor by multiple mechanisms, and also increases glycogen synthase activity. Overall, there is moderate evidence that cinnamon lowers blood glucose levels. Its effect on HbA_{1c} appears negligible, but long-term studies are required to properly evaluate this outcome.

ACUPUNCTURE

Acupuncture may help improve local microcirculation and delay progression of neurological or circulatory complications such as retinopathy, intermittent claudication and peripheral vascular disease.

MENTAL HEALTH, STRESS AND DIABETES

Diabetes can predispose a patient to poor mental health, and poor mental health can predispose patients to diabetes as well as increasing comorbidity, negatively affecting the person's lifestyle and also making it harder for patients with diabetes to cope with their condition.

People living with diabetes have at least double the risk of depression compared with individuals without diabetes.[20] Depressive symptoms in initially non-diabetic adults have also been shown to be predictive of later development of type 2 diabetes,[21] with a 63% increased risk of diabetes in subjects demonstrating depressive symptoms (including recent fatigue, sleep disturbance, feelings of hopelessness, loss of libido and increased irritability) at baseline.

Psychological stress can precipitate a range of autoimmune conditions including type 1 diabetes[22] through the process of dysregulation of the immune system. Stress increases blood sugar and fat levels and so can also destabilise type 2 diabetes and increase the chances of diabetic complications such as heart disease. It can also contribute to the destabilisation of diabetes via secondary effects such as:

- making it more likely that the person will not follow a healthy and disciplined lifestyle
- leading to poorer maintenance and monitoring
- increasing susceptibility to infections or other illnesses.

Research on diabetes shows that stress management leads to a significantly better level of diabetic control and lower rate of complications,[23] making for more stable control, healthier lifestyle and better compliance with treatment and monitoring. Stress management is therefore a core element in diabetes management.

Chronic or long-term activation of the stress response leads to high 'allostatic load',[24] a form of prolonged wear and tear on the body. High allostatic load is found in chronic stress and anxiety, and depression, and is associated with poor immunity, acceleration of atherosclerosis, 'metabolic syndrome' and chronically high cortisol levels. Stress in the workplace has been shown to be an important risk factor for metabolic syndrome.[25] This is thought to be associated with high basal secretion of cortisol.

YOGA

A systematic review of studies examining the effect of yoga on diabetes suggest beneficial changes in several risk indices, including glucose tolerance and insulin sensitivity, lipid profiles, anthropometric characteristics, blood pressure, oxidative stress, coagulation profiles, sympathetic activation and pulmonary function, as well as improvement in specific clinical outcomes.[26] Yoga may improve risk profiles in adults with type 2 diabetes, and may have promise for the prevention and management of cardiovascular complications in this population. However, the limitations characterising most studies preclude any firm conclusions being drawn.

MEDICATION

Trial of lifestyle measures first

If a 6-week trial of lifestyle and nutritional measures fails to control blood glucose levels in an asymptomatic person with type 2 diabetes, pharmaceutical oral hypoglycaemic agents may be indicated. Start with small doses and increase weekly, depending on response.

Oral hypoglycaemic agents

If symptomatic or if BGL at diagnosis is > 20 mmol/L, medication is indicated to reduce BGL and relieve symptoms at the time of diagnosis.

- *Metformin*—first-line for the overweight person with type 2 diabetes. Raised serum creatinine is an absolute contraindication. Caution in patients with heart or liver disease or heavy alcohol intake. Usual starting dose is 500 mg twice a day or 850 mg once daily. Gradually increase by 500 mg per day at weekly intervals or 850 mg per day at intervals of 2 weeks as tolerated and based on the blood glucose response.
- *Sulfonylureas* (tolbutamide, gliclazide)—stimulate the pancreas to produce insulin. Special care is needed in the elderly with regard to precipitating hypoglycaemia. May cause weight gain, nausea, diarrhoea.
- *Glitazones*—reduce insulin resistance. Pioglitazone and rosiglitazone can be used with insulin or other hypoglycaemic agents. However, there have been reports of rates of myocardial infarction increasing by 40% with rosiglitazone, and both rosiglitazone and pioglitazone have been reported to precipitate heart failure, cause peripheral fractures and possibly cause or worsen macular oedema.

INITIATION OF INSULIN

The decision to commence insulin, and the choice of insulin to prescribe, depends on the level of glycaemic control, and the patient's eating and exercise patterns.

The types of insulin include:

- *rapid-onset, fast-acting insulin* (Lispro and Aspart)—onset of action within 1–20 minutes. Peaks after 1 hour and lasts 3–5 hours. Patient must eat immediately after injecting
- *short-acting insulin* (neutral)—peak effect at 2–4 hours, and lasts for 6–8 hours
- *intermediate-acting insulin* (Isophane)—begins to work after about 90 minutes, peaks at 4–12 hours and lasts for 16–24 hours
- *mixed insulin*—pre-mixed combination of either a rapid-onset, fast-acting or a short-acting insulin, and intermediate-acting insulin. The numbers written after the brand name show the mix of the two types of insulin. For example, Humulin

30/70 contains 30% short-acting insulin and 70% intermediate-acting insulin. Mixtard 50/50 contains 50% short-acting insulin and 50% intermediate-acting insulin
- *long-acting insulin* (insulin glargine or insulin detemir)—releases insulin into the bloodstream at a fairly constant rate over 24 hours.

TYPE 1 DIABETES

Initial assessment by an endocrinologist is advisable, to establish a program of shared care and to arrange diabetes education.

- Insulin initiation is most commonly with Isophane insulin twice daily (or Isophane Insulatard for pens) subcutaneously at a dose of 5 units b.i.d. (or 6 units for a pen that delivers in multiples of 2 units) if random blood glucose level is below 15 mmol/L.
- Starting dose is 10 units b.i.d. if blood glucose is 15 mmol/L or above.
- Insulin to increase by 2 units b.i.d until blood glucose readings are under 10 mmol/L.
- Insulin can be increased by 4 units b.i.d. if blood glucose level remains above 17 mmol after 48 hours of insulin therapy.
- If daily insulin requirements increase to 20 units in a single dose of intermediate-acting insulin, mixed insulin may be introduced.
- A combination of pre-prandial soluble (Actrapid) insulin, given with a background of medium-/long-acting insulin taken at bedtime may give greater flexibility of mealtimes and food types.

TYPE 2 DIABETES

Establish that lifestyle measures have been adequate, and exclude intercurrent infection or other complicating medical conditions.

While intensive lifestyle management and/or oral hypoglycaemic agents are first-line treatments for type 2 diabetes, many patients with type 2 diabetes will eventually fail to respond adequately to oral hypoglycaemic drugs and will require insulin therapy.

The United Kingdom Prospective Diabetes Study (UKPDS)[27] showed that most people with type 2 diabetes will experience progressive pancreatic beta-cell dysfunction despite excellent control, and become refractory to oral hypoglycaemic agents.

Some patients will require insulin early in the course of the disease if they fail to respond to lifestyle management and oral hypoglycaemic agents. This may indicate that they in fact had type 1 diabetes.

People with type 2 diabetes requiring insulin can often be managed with a single daily dose of intermediate- or long-acting insulin added to their oral hypoglycaemic schedule. Quick-acting insulin is not necessarily needed.

A regimen of intermediate-acting insulin (10 units) at bedtime in combination with daytime oral drugs is usually acceptable to patients, simple to start and results in rapid improvement in glycaemic control.[28]

The aim is to 'start low and go slow'. Doses can be increased in increments of 10–20% at intervals of 2–4 days.

The basal insulin can be isophane or glargine. Glargine may cause less hydroglycaemia than isophane. In the long term, metformin can be continued or added, to reduce insulin resistance (and dose) and to help reduce weight gain.

Insulin can be delivered in syringes, pens or insulin pumps.

Sites for insulin injections:

- abdominal wall—generally fastest and the most uniform rate of absorption
- legs—slowest absorption (unless exercising); acceptable site
- arms—not recommended; injections should be subcutaneous.

REGULAR DIABETES REVIEW

Checklist of regular monitoring:

- HbA_{1c}: every 6 months
- blood pressure: every 6 months or opportunistically
- lipids: annually
- microalbuminuria: annually
- BMI (height, weight, BMI): every 6 months or opportunistically
- waist circumference: every 6 months
- examine feet: every 6 months
- eye referral: annually
- check smoking status: every opportunity
- review medication: annually once stable, or as required.

MANAGEMENT OF A HYPERGLYCAEMIC EMERGENCY

Absolute insulin deficiency results in diabetic ketoacidosis. This is a life-threatening emergency that requires acute stabilisation and transfer to a specialist endocrine unit. There may be a precipitating cause, such as urinary tract infection, gastroenteritis, chest infection or myocardial infarction.

Symptoms and signs may develop over hours or days:

- polyuria, polydipsia resulting in dehydration
- hyperventilation
- ketotic breath odour
- ketonuria
- drowsiness, progressing to lowered state of consciousness

- potassium and phosphate depletion
- shock.

Acute management:

- Arrange emergency hospital admission.
- Give 10 units rapid-acting insulin intramuscularly.
- Establish IV access and start infusion of IV normal saline.

RESOURCE

Diabetes Australia. Diabetes management in general practice. Guidelines for type 2 diabetes, 2009/10, http://www.diabetesaustralia.com.au/PageFiles/763/Diabetes%20Management%20in%20GP%2009.pdf

REFERENCES

1 Hoffman L, Nolan C, Wilson JD et al. Gestational diabetes mellitus—management guidelines. Med J Aust 1998; 169:93–97.

2 Humber A, Menconi F, Coathers S et al. Joint genetic susceptibility to type 1 diabetes and autoimmune thyroiditis: from epidemiology to mechanism. Endocr Rev 2008; 29(6):697–725.

3 Ford ES, Bergmann MM, Kröger J et al. Healthy living is the best revenge: findings from the European Prospective Investigation Into Cancer and Nutrition—Potsdam Study. Arch Intern Med 2009; 169(15): 1355–1362.

4 Expert Panel on Detection. Executive summary of the Third Report of the National Cholesterol Education Program (NCEP) Expert Panel on Detection, Evaluation, and Treatment of High Blood Cholesterol in Adults (Adult Treatment Panel III). JAMA 2001; 285:2186–2197.

5 Juvanovic L. Nutrition and pregnancy: the link between dietary intake and diabetes. Curr Diab Rep 2004; 4(4):266–272.

6 Zipitis C, Akobeng A. Vitamin D supplementation in early childhood and risk of type 1 diabetes: a systematic review and meta-analysis. Arch Dis Child 2008; 93:512–517. Online. Available: http://adc.bmj.com/cgi/content/abstract/adc.2007.128579v1

7 Evidence-based guideline for case detection and diagnosis of type 2 diabetes. Online. Available: http://www.diabetesaustralia.com.au/_lib/doc_pdf/NEBG/CD/Part3-CaseDetection-311201.pdf

8 National Heart, Lung and Blood Institute, National Institutes of Health. Action to Control Cardiovascular Risk in Diabetes (ACCORD) Trial. Questions and answers. Online. Available: http://www.nhlbi.nih.gov/health/prof/heart/other/accord/q_a.htm

9 Hartweg J, Perera R, Montori V et al. Omega-3 polyunsaturated fatty acids (PUFA) for type 2 diabetes mellitus. Cochrane Database Syst Rev 2008; 1:CD003205 .

10 Thornalley PJ. The potential role of thiamine (vitamin B_1) in diabetic complications. Curr Diabetes Rev 2005; 1(3):287–298.

11 Lampeter EF, Klinghammer A, Scherbaum WA et al. The Deutche Nicotinamide Intervention Study. DENIS group. Diabetes 1998; 126(4):435–438.

12 Gale EA. Theory and practice of nicotinamide trials in pre-type 1 diabetes. J Pediatr Endocrinol Metab 1996; 9(3):375–379.

13 Ruy LR, Willett W, Rimm E et al. Magnesium intake and risk of type 2 diabetes in men and women. Diabetes Care 2004; 27(1):134–140.

14 Cunningham JJ, Fu A, Mearkle PL et al. Hyperzincuria in individuals with insulin-dependent diabetes mellitus: concurrent zinc status and the effect of high-dose zinc supplementation. Metabolism 1994; 43:1558–1562.

15 Frank RA, Mize SJS, Kennedy LM et al. The effect of *Gymnema sylvestre* extracts on the sweetness of eight sweeteners. Chem Senses 1992; 17(5):461–479.

16 Prakash AO, Mathur S, Mathur R et al. Effect of feeding *Gymnema sylvestre* leaves on blood glucose in beryllium nitrate treated rats. Ethnopharmacol 1986; 18(2): 143–146.

17 Al Habori M, Raman A, Lawrence MJ et al. In vitro effect of fenugreek extracts on intestinal sodium-dependent glucose uptake and hepatic glycogen phosphorylase A. Int J Exp Diabetes Res 2001; 2(2):91–99.

18 Jamal GA, Carmichael H. The effect of gamma linoleic acid on human diabetic peripheral neuropathy: a double blind placebo-controlled trial. Diabet Med 1990; 7(4):319–323.

19 Nahas R. Complementary and alternative medicine for the treatment of type 2 diabetes. Can Fam Physician 2009; 55(6):591–596.

20 Anderson RJ, Freedland K, Clouse RE et al. The prevalence of comorbid depression in adults with diabetes: a meta-analysis. Diabetes Care 2001; 24:1069–1078.

21 Golden S, Williams JE, Ford DE et al. Depressive symptoms and the risk of type 2 diabetes. Diabetes Care 2004; 27:429–435.

22 Sepa A, Ludvigsson J. Psychological stress and the risk of diabetes-related autoimmunity: a review article. Neuroimmunomodulation 2006; 13(5/6):301–308.

23 Surwit RS, van Tilburg MA, Zucker N et al. Stress management improves long-term glycemic control in type 2 diabetes. Diabetes Care 2002; 25(1):30–34.

24 McEwen BS. Protection and damage from acute and chronic stress: allostasis and allostatic overload and relevance to the pathophysiology of psychiatric disorders. Ann NY Acad Sci 2004; 1032:1–7.

25 Chandola, T, Brunner E, Marmot M. Chronic stress at work and the metabolic syndrome: prospective study. BMJ 2006; 332:521–525.

26 Innes KE, Vincent HK. The influence of yoga-based programs on risk profiles in adults with type 2 diabetes mellitus: a systematic review. Evid Based Complement Alternat Med 2007; 4(4):469–486.

27 UK Prospective Diabetes Study (UKPDS) Group. Intensive blood-glucose control with sulphonylureas or insulin compared with conventional treatment and risk of complications in patients with type 2 diabetes (UKPDS 33). Lancet 1998; 352:837–853.

28 Wong J, Yue D. Starting insulin treatment in type 2 diabetes. Australian Prescriber 2004; 27:93–96.

chapter 27

Ear, nose and throat

INTRODUCTION AND OVERVIEW

This chapter is a brief summation of commonly encountered otolaryngology, head and neck issues in general practice. It is not exhaustive but, rather, aims to give the reader an understanding of common problems and assist in management.

THE EAR

The ear is the organ of hearing. In medicine it is divided for descriptive and functional purposes into an outer, middle and inner ear (Fig 27.1). The ear amplifies sound, converting it from mechanical energy into an electrical impulse, which the individual translates. It is unusual for any disease process to affect more than one component at any one time.

OUTER EAR

The outer ear acts as a funnel, collecting sound waves and concentrating them onto the tympanic membrane (eardrum). It includes the pinna (auricle) and external

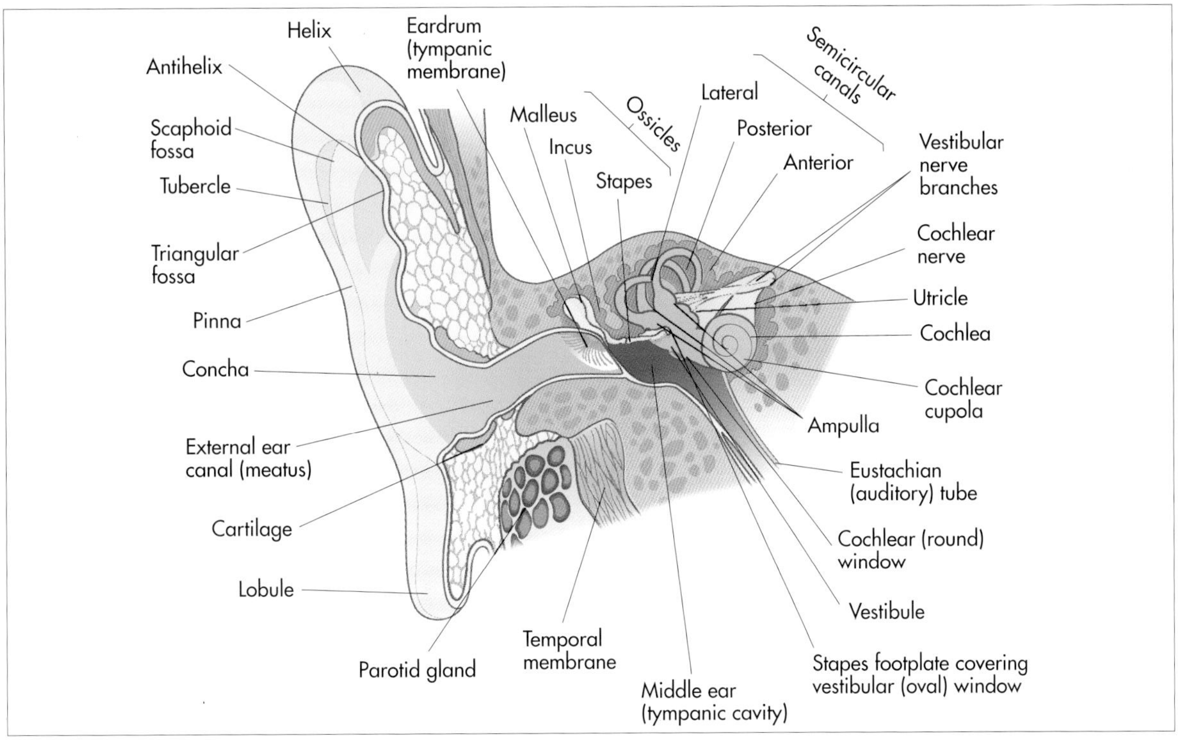

FIGURE 27.1 Anatomy of the ear

auditory canal (EAC), and it represents the part accessible to examination, and is not uncommonly an area of decoration by piercing. The EAC is cylindrical in shape, and approximately 2.5 cm long. The lateral EAC is composed of cartilage, and the medial part is bony. The cartilaginous aspect contains hair, and cerumen (earwax) is produced here. The canal is lined with very specialised squamous epithelium, which self-cleans in a migratory pattern from inside to out. It is important at this stage to understand the harm caused by cotton buds in inhibiting this process. Cotton buds tend to compress wax and can cause occlusion, deafness and infection.

Ear wax

Excess ear wax may present as loss of hearing acuity, tinnitus, a sense of fullness in the ear or dizziness.

The chemical basis of cerumen, or ear wax, is a fat. Like all body fats, the fluidity is affected by the ratio of omega-3 to omega-6 fatty acids and saturated fats.

Although genetic factors are thought to be involved, hard wax (inviting medical removal) may simply reflect a lack of omega-3s in the person's diet. Hence, increasing omega-3 intake may help to prevent the problem. In the acute situation, treatment is with drops to soften the ear wax. This may need to be followed by syringing or suction aural toilet.

Trauma

'Cauliflower ear'

'Cauliflower ear' is a commonly seen injury endured by rugby players caused by blunt trauma to the ear. The shearing forces cause a sub-perichondrial haematoma, (Fig 27.2) which compromises the diffusion nutrient supply to the cartilage. The haematoma is susceptible to infection, which can further deplete nutrient supply to the cartilage. The cartilage is replaced with fibrous scar tissue and deformity results. Therefore immediate haematoma evacuation is required in cases of acute trauma.

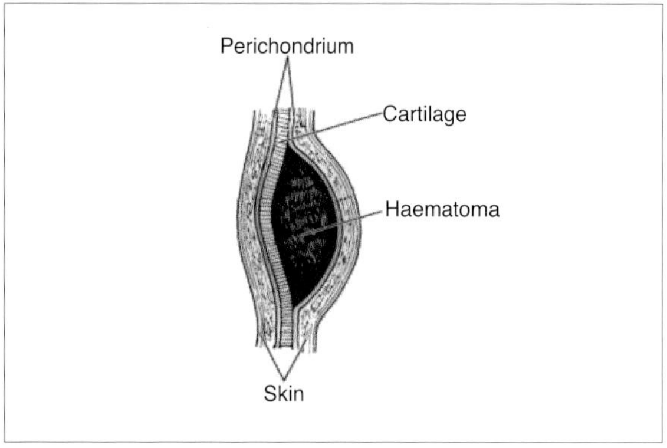

FIGURE 27.2 Haematoma in cauliflower ear

Foreign body

Festive seasons and birthdays often herald the season of foreign bodies in the ears of children (Fig 27.3). Anything small enough, from beads to batteries, has been found there. The deeper the foreign body, the more difficult and painful it is to remove. In children a general anaesthetic may be required. In general, appropriate equipment allows easy removal with a compliant child. The hardest to remove is often the foreign body that others have attempted to remove. It may be associated with tympanic membrane perforation, although this is unlikely and depends largely on the mechanism of trauma. If associated with a perforated eardrum, it is reassuring to know that most heal spontaneously. Water precautions should be adhered to until the eardrum heals, and an audiogram is recommended (in a perforated tympanic membrane).

One unpleasant type of foreign body is an insect near or attached to the tympanic membrane. As first aid, instant pain relief and destruction of the creature, olive oil poured straight into the ear is safe and effective.

Otitis externa

Ear infections are particularly common in cultures where swimming is popular. Otitis externa (OE) refers to infection of the EAC (Fig 27.4). It is commonly caused by *Pseudomonas*, *Staphylococcus aureus* or fungal species. However, because the EAC is just like skin, other causes of OE include viral infection and allergy (seborrhoeic).

Otitis externa is often preceded by a combination of maceration (cotton buds) and water trapping. Dermatological conditions of the ear canal also predispose to OE. It is not uncommon to have exostoses, which can predispose to OE by water trapping. In OE the canal is typically oedematous and reddened. The diagnosis is made clinically with discharge, deafness and severe otalgia. In fungal infections, spores may be encountered. Compared with otitis media, otitis externa is exquisitely tender, esapecially with traction of the pinna, or there is pain with movement of the jaw, and the patient can therefore be difficult to examine.

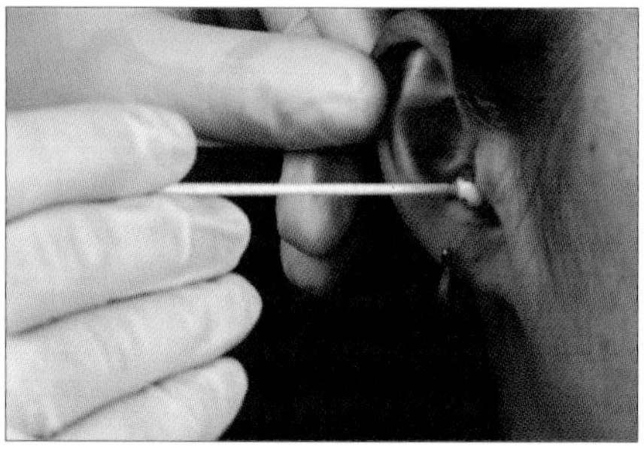

FIGURE 27.3 Removal of foreign body from the ear

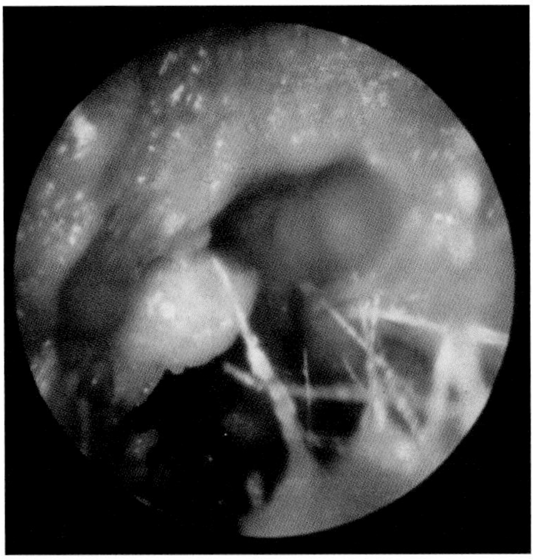

FIGURE 27.4 Otitis extema

A swab for culture and sensitivity of causative organisms can guide therapy decisions. The recalcitrant nature of OE is often due to inadequate use of ototopical medication. Oral antibiotics are rarely warranted for OE and reserved for systemic illness, severe surrounding cellulitis and recalcitrant infections. Topical preparations are far more effective in attaining higher antibiotic concentration at the infected site, and minimise the risk of antimicrobial resistance. It is important to perform a micro-ear toilet to clear the EAC of debris, to allow greater penetration of the antibiotics/antifungals. This is also possible with 'tissue spears'—the corners of a tissue may be rolled and gently inserted into the ear in a twisting motion, to absorb moisture. This also allows better penetration of antibiotics and antifungals. A cotton bud has rigidity and therefore causes more trauma, whereas the tissue spear acts purely as absorbent. In severe cases of occlusion, an otowick is used. This is a cottonoid pledget that expands with ototopical antibiotic/antifungal preparations to allow delivery of the ototopical preparation to the area of inflammation/infection.

Ototopical medication has recently come under close scrutiny because of the potential toxic effect of the aminoglycosides in some ototopical medications. The Australasian Society of Otolaryngology, Head and Neck Surgeons recently published guidelines on their use.[1]

- When possible, topical antibiotic preparations that are free of potential ototoxicity are preferable to those that do have the potential for otologic injury in patients with an open middle ear or mastoid.
- When a potentially ototoxic antibiotic is chosen, it should be used only in infected ears and it should be discontinued shortly after the infection has resolved.
- When a potentially ototoxic antibiotic drop is prescribed for a patient with an open middle ear or mastoid, the patient or parent should be warned of the risk of ototoxicity.
- The patient or parent should be specifically instructed to call the physician or return to the office if the patient develops dizziness or vertigo, hearing loss or a worsening of hearing if such an impairment was already present, or tinnitus.
- If the tympanic membrane is known to be intact and the middle ear and mastoid are closed, then the use of potentially ototoxic preparations presents no risk of ototoxic injury.

Prevention: Keep the ear dry, especially with swimming and water sports. This can be achieved with fitted earplugs and a bathing cap. If the canal becomes wet, apply spirit drops to help dry the canal. Dry canal with a hair dryer held about 30 cm from the ear.

Malignant otitis externa

What may seem a simple ear infection in an immunocompromised patient (commonly the diabetic or elderly patient) can rapidly deteriorate into a life-threatening condition. A *Pseudomonas* infection can colonise and spread into the temporal bone and become very difficult to eradicate. The patient presents with severe otalgia, aural discharge and progressive cranial nerve neuropathies. These patients warrant urgent referral to otolaryngology services.

Tumours

Basal cell carcinoma and squamous cell carcinoma (melanoma is less likely) must not be forgotten in consideration of ongoing discharge and eczema of the pinna in elderly patients, especially as the area is prone to UV sun exposure. Initially superficial, these lesions tend to ulcerate and weep. They require definitive surgical management.

Prevention: Everyday sun protection with sunscreen, including the ears, and a hat with a broad brim.

Exostoses

Exostoses are a benign condition of the EAC seen frequently in avid swimmers, culminating over many years. They are more commonly associated with cold water exposure and are well represented in surfing communities. An *osteoma* is a single, solitary lump, whereas *exostoses* are multiple. They are smooth bony protuberances of the ear canal. Although benign in nature, they become problematic when they are large enough to inhibit the ear's natural self-cleaning. Water trapping occurs on repeated swimming, and the ear canal becomes irritated, and macerated with attempted cleaning, and it is then only a matter of time before repeated infections occur. It is more a problem in this population as it limits the joy of the aetiology: swimming and water sports. Most are observed until they become problematic and then are surgically reduced.

Prevention: Fitted earplugs can be worn for swimming, and the ear canal should be dried with a hairdryer after swimming and hair washing.

TYMPANIC MEMBRANE

The tympanic membrane (eardrum) is the Rolf Harris of the ear. It is a thin membrane separating the external auditory canal from the middle ear, approximately 10 mm in diameter (Fig 27.5). It vibrates (wobbles) in response to mechanical energy from sound waves. It is attached to the ossicles (ear bones), which together amplify sound energy to the inner ear. The tympanic membrane is important not only in sound transmission but also in preventing water entering the middle ear cleft. The respiratory epithelium of the middle ear cleft differs from the squamous epithelium of the external auditory canal. Impaired function consequently has profound effects on the hearing ability of the affected ear. Various conditions can affect the tympanic membrane, and include:

- *myringitis*—infection of the tympanic membrane; may be viral or bacterial; treated with ototopical antibiotics
- *bulla myringitis*—an acutely painful condition characterised by bulla formation on the tympanic membrane; often caused by a virus and as such supportive therapy is required, although superimposed bacterial infection is not uncommon
- *myringosclerosis*—scarring of the tympanic membrane in the form of collagen deposits; appears as 'clouds' or 'chalk marks' on otoscopy and is often a result of trauma from infection or previous grommet insertion; intervention is rarely necessary unless the condition is causing conductive hearing loss.

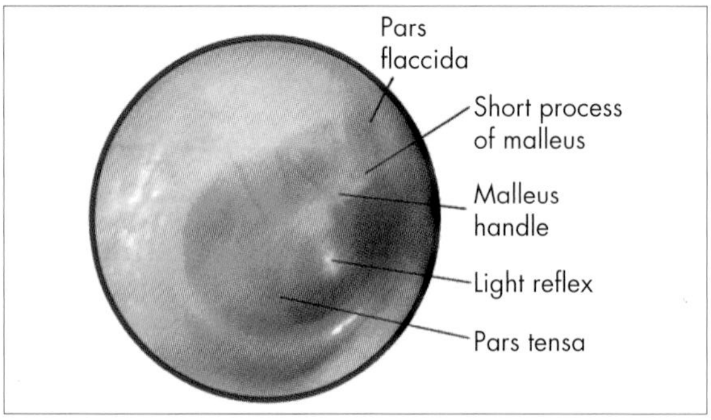

FIGURE 27.5 The tympanic membrane

Tympanic membrane perforation

Tympanic membrane perforation (Fig 27.6) may result from trauma (personal or surgical), infection or pressure changes. It may be *marginal*, involving part of the tympanic membrane annulus, or *central*, involving any other part. It needs to be distinguished from a retraction.

Examine by removing the blood clot by suction or by gentle mopping. Exclude any foreign body and check the hearing, as perforation can cause hearing loss.

The mainstay of treatment is supportive, maintaining water precautions (to prevent infection) and obtaining an audiogram. Prescribe a broad-spectrum antibiotic and adequate analgesia. Review in two days, then weekly until healed. Perforations tend to heal spontaneously over days to months in a non-infected ear with good eustachian tube function. Hearing should be rechecked two months after the injury.

Non-healing perforations may require surgical repair with a myringoplasty. Referral is warranted earlier if suspicious of complications such as inner ear involvement expressed as tinnitus, vertigo, sensorineural hearing loss, bleeding, otalgia or facial nerve paralysis.

Prevention: Discourage any objects being inserted into the ear canal except by trained professionals.

MIDDLE EAR

The middle ear is a collective term describing the space bounded by the tympanic membrane laterally and the inner ear medially. It houses the ossicles, the bones of sound conduction. It is lined by respiratory mucosa and has a connection to the posteriorly based mastoid air cells, and is drained by the eustachian tube antero-inferiorly. The external ear collects the sound waves, while the middle ear amplifies the sound transmission

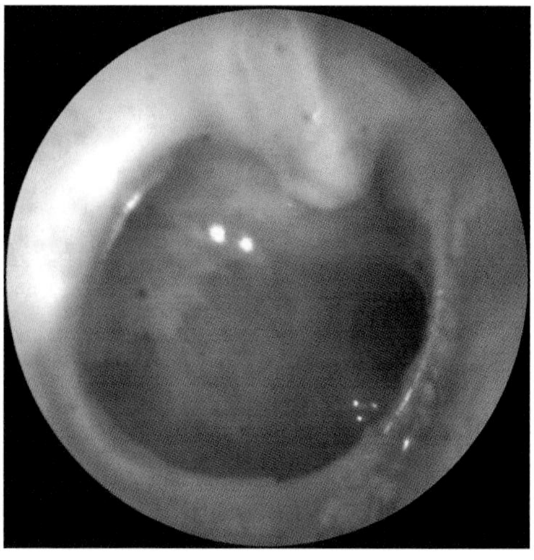

FIGURE 27.6 Tympanic membrane perforation

to the inner ear. The eustachian tube's primary function is to allow equalisation of pressure, to maximise sound transmission.

Middle ear effusion

Failure of adequate drainage is not uncommon in children, as the eustachian tube is shorter, the diameter is thinner and it lies in a more horizontal plane than the adult eustachian tube (Table 27.1). The narrow lumen is easily obstructed in upper respiratory tract infections, there is less capacity for natural drainage, and its length is thought to allow more exposure to reflux and, hence, inflammation. Adenoidal hypertrophy may predispose to lower eustachian tube obstruction. (In the adult population, one must be wary of neoplastic postnasal obstruction.)

Failure of drainage leads to accumulation of fluid, as water is absorbed through the middle ear mucosa, the tympanic membrane is retracted or the fluid thickens. Consequently, the ossicles fail to vibrate, and lack of aeration of the middle ear cleft leads to dampening of the sound waves and conductive hearing loss.

Surgical treatment (grommets ± adenoidectomy) is usually reserved for non-resolving effusions causing developmental delay such as speech and learning. Most will, spontaneously, resorb or drain within 4–6 weeks. Referral is indicated if there is persistent middle ear effusion three months after an attack of acute otitis media, or if there are signs of hearing loss, frequent recurrences or severe complications (e.g. mastoiditis).

Acute otitis media

Accumulation and contamination of middle ear fluid, which is normally sterile, leads to infection, otitis media. It is a common disease of the paediatric population. The patient typically presents as a febrile, runny-nose mouth breather. Again, this is because of the special relationship of the eustachian tube with the post-nasal space. Because of this relationship it may also be associated with rhinitis, sinusitis, snoring, obstructive

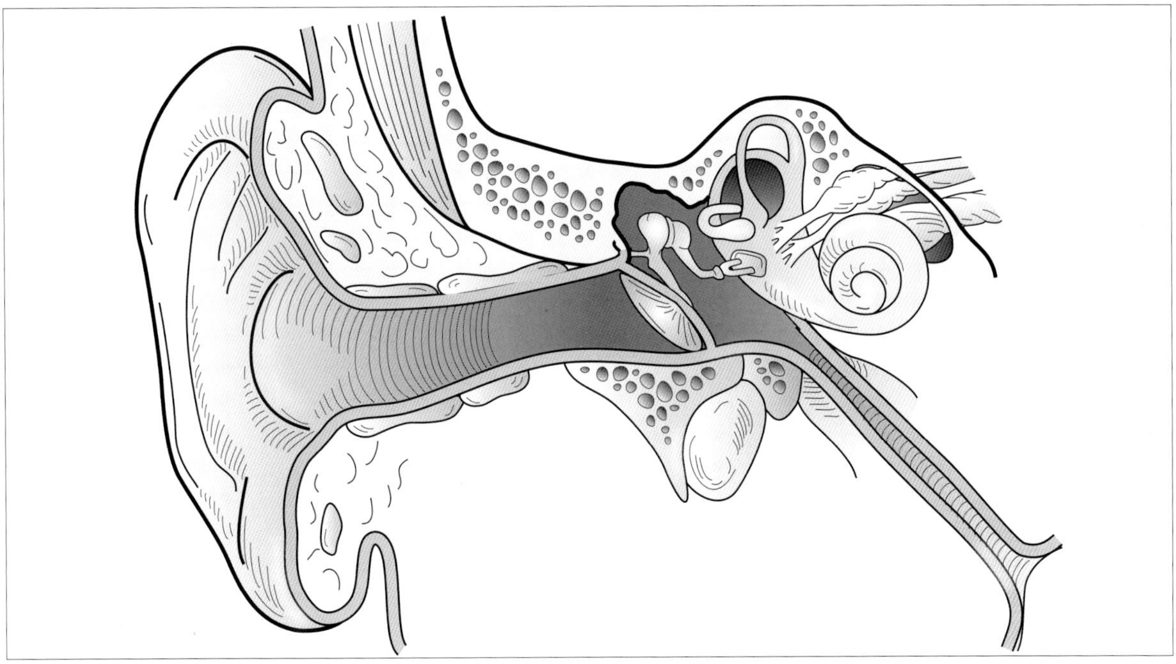

FIGURE 27.7 Middle ear with Eustachian tube

TABLE 27.1 Issue in a child's eustachian tube, compared with an adult

Anatomy	Consequence
More horizontal lie	Less capacity to drain
Smaller diameter	More easily occluded
Shorter	Easier to reflux More prone to inflammation

sleep apnoea and asthma-like associations. It has an increased incidence in lower socioeconomic groups, and an alarmingly high prevalence in the Australian Indigenous population.

The common organisms found in infection of the middle ear include *Streptococcus pneumoniae*, *Haemophilus influenzae* and *Moraxella catarrhalis*. A less likely cause of infection is gram-negative bacteria or a viral aetiology.

The controversy surrounding the use of oral antibiotics in acute otitis media has been noted. In a meta-analysis it was found that the NNT (number needed to treat to benefit one patient) was 17. The benefit was small—a reduction in pain by 12 hours. In this study, the likelihood of complications was not increased in the non-treated group.[2,3] Against this, the cost of increasing antibiotic resistance, and the disruption to the ecosystem of the gut flora, have to be counted.

Pain relief in otitis media can be as simple as showing the parent how to use a 2 mL syringe to put olive oil into the child's ear.

Complicated otitis media (see below) requires full medical treatment.

Recurrent otitis media has been considered a response to food allergy. The theory is that cytokines released when problem foods are eaten results in oedema of membranes in the respiratory tract. Easy blockage of small passages, such as the eustachian tube, ensues.

It can be a useful trial of therapy to put all children on a strict one-month dairy-free diet before sending them for tonsillectomy, grommets or other surgical interventions. Many respond to this diet, and a few respond once gluten/wheat, citrus and other food allergens are also withdrawn. It should be noted that such 'allergic' responses are not usually mediated through the immunoglobin E (IgE) arm of the immune system and as such should not, strictly speaking, be called allergies.

The immune mechanisms involved may be IgG or IgA mediated, or a direct cytokine response not involving any immune globulin. Inhalant allergens must also be considered; and, of course, a marked and statistically significant association has been found between the incidence of otitis media and tonsillectomy in children and parental smoking in the home environment.

Otitis media, along with chronic sinusitis, recurrent tonsillitis and migraine, all tend to cluster within individuals and families. Understanding the biochemistry helps us see them as systemic problems, and rationalises the approach.

In babies and children, a red tympanic membrane does not necessarily mean otitis media. The tympanic membrane can appear red if the child is crying.

Complications of otitis media

Acute otitis media generally responds well to adequate analgesia with or without oral antibiotics. Most effusions will resolve within 3–6 months with active non-intervention. Surgical intervention is reserved for chronicity, recurrence or impending complication of otitis media. There is much debate surrounding absolute indications for intervening.

Under pressure, several sequelae may occur in otitis media. By far the most important implications of prolonged or recurrent infections are the serious consequences for the growth and learning of a child. Complications of otitis media are associated with direct spreading of infection, and include:

- mastoiditis
- meningitis
- Bezold's abscess (neck abscess)
- sigmoid sinus thrombosis
- apicitis
- tympanic membrane perforation.

All these are, hopefully, prevented with early intervention. Prompt otolaryngological referral is advised.

Chronic otitis media with effusions (OME)

Most effusions will resolve within 3–6 months with active non-intervention. Surgical intervention is reserved for chronicity, recurrence or impending complication of otitis media. There is much debate surrounding absolute indications for intervening.

TABLE 27.2 Complications of cholesteatoma

Pathology	Symptom/sign
Erosion of ossicles	Deafness
Erosion of facial nerve	Facial palsy
Sigmoid sinus thrombosis/hydrocephalus	Meningism
Erosion of labyrinth	Balance difficulties
Infection petrous apex	Gardener's sign
Tegmen bone erosion	Brain abscess/meningitis

Cholesteatoma

A cholesteatoma is a benign skin growth in an abnormal location within the ear. The skin-lined sac increases in size, leading to infection and bony destruction. It is dangerous because of its location near the tympanic membrane and its tendency to expand and cause destruction of neighbouring structures. Its clinical significance is in recalcitrant discharging ears and its destructive process.

Complications of untreated cholesteatoma include those listed in Table 27.2. Complete surgical removal is urgent, essential and unavoidable.

Bell's palsy

Bell's palsy is the most common palsy. Full recovery is the normal outcome with active non-intervention. It is important to note that it is a diagnosis of exclusion, and therefore a careful history and examination is paramount. The aetiology is thought to be viral (herpes virus) in nature; however, steroids and anti-viral medication are still controversial in the literature.

Therapeutic approaches include:[4]

- acyclovir plus prednisolone
- vitamin therapy (including vitamin B_{12}, B_6 and zinc), which may help nerve growth
- relaxation techniques
- electrical stimulation acupuncture (more trials needed).

Otosclerosis

Otosclerosis is a bone disease of the otic capsule resulting in abnormal deposition of bone around the otic capsule. The presenting symptom is deafness, more commonly from stapes fixation (preventing ossicular mobility). More rare is ossification of the cochlea, which renders the hair cells inactive. There is a slight female preponderance and it is therefore thought to be associated with hormonal fluctuation. When suspected, audiogram and referral are warranted.

RHINOLOGY

The nose is the organ of olfaction (smell), and has several important functions besides olfaction, including cleansing inspired air, humidification and warming. Functionally it has an external and an internal part (Fig 27.8). The external part contains bone and cartilage and acts to prop open the portal for air movement. The internal nose is highly vascular, particularly over the turbinates, to allow warming of air, and plays a role in nasal defence. Unfortunately, engorgement may also cause obstruction. Problems of the nose surround difficulties in the normal physiology of the nose. The two most commonly dealt with by doctors include epistaxis and sinusitis.

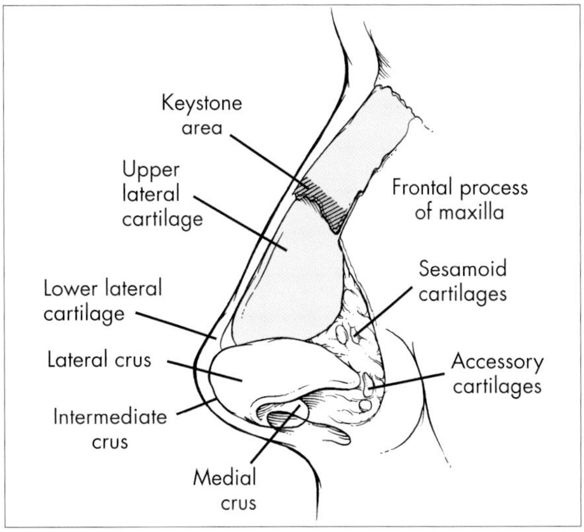

FIGURE 27.8 Anatomy of the nose

EPISTAXIS

Otherwise known as nose bleeding, epistaxis is a common problem. It is most commonly idiopathic in origin. In very basic terms, it may be divided into anterior and posterior bleeding. Anterior bleeding is by far the most common presentation and can be precipitated in children by nose picking, repeated blowing or other trauma. Most anterior bleeding will stop spontaneously with pressure alone (with or without cotton wool pledget). A confluence of small vessels on the anterior septum, known as Little's area, is the most common site of bleeding, and is very amenable to cauterisation in the absence of any bleeding diathesis.

Posterior bleeding is more common in older hypertensive patients and is more difficult to manage, not uncommonly requiring hospital admission and review. Neoplastic cause or coagulation defect should be considered.

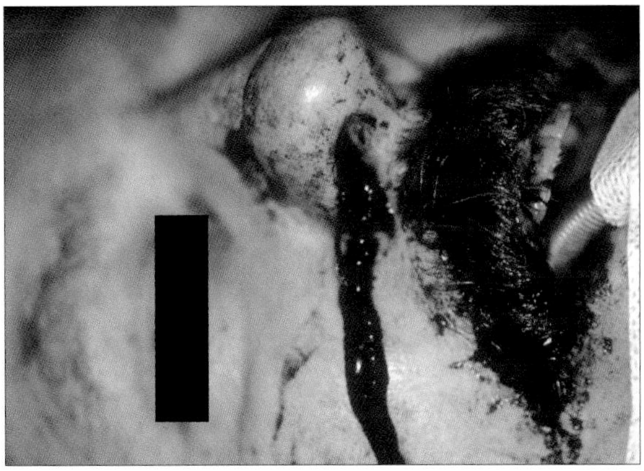

FIGURE 27.9 Severe postoperative epistaxis

SINUSITIS

The sinuses are located in the bony make-up of the face, and include the paired maxillary, ethmoid, frontal and sphenoid sinuses. Their role continues to be debated in the literature and includes resonance of sound, facial strength without mass, humidification and warming of inspired air, and other functions. The clinical significance is vastly different and focuses on pain and discharge. Sinusitis may be acute or chronic and in simple terms occurs after mucus accumulation in the sinuses, which often becomes infected, leading to pain, discharge and nasal obstruction. Odontogenic origin must also be a consideration. The mechanism of blockage may be due to obstruction of the natural sinus drainage pathway, failure of muco-ciliary clearance or thickened inspissated mucus. The most common infection is bacterial, with *Streptococcus pneumoniae* and *Haemophilus influenzae* the most common. Viral infection can implicate narrow drainage pathways in sinusitis. Fungal infection warrants urgent referral.

Acute treatment centres on supportive therapy with fluid, antibiotics and nasal irrigation. Severe cases and any complications may require surgical intervention. Complications involve surrounding structures such as the orbit (periorbital cellulitis) and brain (meningitis, abscess). The timing and type of surgery depends on the individual case presented. The aim is to relieve pain, prevent complications and restore the sinus to its natural function. Functional endoscopic sinus surgery (FESS) has revolutionised surgical access, minimising external scarring and allowing greater access to all the sinuses.

Food and inhalant sensitivity can present as chronic sinusitis, with comparable culprit lists. Once again, dairy is a common food culprit, along with oranges, nuts and seeds. Only a small proportion of cases will be identified on IgE testing.

It should be noted that IgA-deficient patients have more allergies/sensitivities, and IgA deficiency should be excluded in all patients with chronic sinusitis.

Herbal treatments

Herbal medicines have a role to play in reducing symptoms from both acute and chronic respiratory conditions. Gathering evidence suggests that herbs have antiviral and antimicrobial activity to assist in the management of infection, antipyretic and diaphoretic activity to manage fevers, and anti-inflammatory activity. Mucillaginous herbs soothe and repair mucous membranes. Immunomodulatory activity is a common feature.

Common herbs used are:[5,6]

- licorice root (*Glycyrrhiza glabra*)—antiviral, anti-inflammatory
- *Echinacea* spp whole plant (*Echinacea* spp)—immunomodulating
- thyme leaf (*Thymus vulgaris*)—antimicrobial, antiviral
- sage leaf (*Salvia officinalis*)—antiseptic
- olive leaf (*Oleo europa*)—antimicrobial, antiviral
- yarrow (*Achillea millefolium*)—diaphoretic.

VESTIBULAR DISORDERS

HISTORY

Vestibular disorders are difficult to pinpoint, and history remains the best tool for diagnosis. It includes conditions such as benign paroxysmal positional vertigo (BPPV), vestibular neuronitis, migrainous vertigo and Ménière's disease. The history should consider periodicity, duration and associated and possible precipitating factors. It is important to distinguish true vertigo from lightheadedness, generalised malaise and blackouts.

True vertigo is *always*:

- due to asymmetry in vestibular apparatus
- transient
- worse with head movement.

Periodicity of attacks:

- Single episode versus recurrent attacks.

Duration of attacks:

- True vertigo lasting seconds to a minute is virtually pathognomonic of BPPV.
- First ever episode of true vertigo with nausea/vomiting lasting 24–72 hours is likely to be vestibular neuronitis.
- Recurrent episodes of vertigo lasting hours to days is likely to be endolymphatic hydrops (e.g. Ménière's disease) or migraine, depending on associated symptoms and past history.

Associated symptoms:

- Endolymphatic hydrops includes episodes of vertigo with low-frequency hearing loss, tinnitus and aural fullness.
- Past history of migraine may be associated with vestibular migraine.
- Cerebellar infarction may not have associated neurological signs, and if presenting as isolated vertigo needs to be distinguished from vestibular neuronitis.

Precipitating factors:

- BPPV is always induced by head movement (vertigo induced by rolling over in bed is the most classic).

EXAMINATION

Eye movements should be followed closely. Check visual smooth pursuits and saccades (rapid eye movements). An abnormality suggests central cause of vertigo.

Other tests:

- *high-frequency head impulse test*—abnormality is pathognomonic of peripheral vestibular disorder (vestibular neuronitis in the acute setting)

- *head shake test*—enhances ability to detect unidirectional nystagmus
- *cerebellar testing*—standard assessment (e.g. past-pointing, heel–shin, dysdiadochokinesis)
- *hyperventilation test*—excludes anxiety disorder or may be concomitant
- *Unterberger (Fukuda stepping) test*—diagnostic of peripheral vestibulopathy
- *ability to stand*:
  - with eyes open, in acute setting, usually excludes cerebellar disorder
  - when absent with eye closure but present with eyes open, suggests vestibular disorder
- *Dix-Hallpike manoeuvre*—pathognomonic of BPPV when positive with classical torsional nystagmus and vertigo following a brief latency period (Fig 27.10).

Organise formal audiology in all cases.

BENIGN PAROXYSMAL POSITIONAL VERTIGO

Benign paroxysmal positional vertigo (BPPV) is the most common cause of recurrent vertigo. It is seen more often in females than in males, and occurs in all ages. In the elderly population it commonly occurs spontaneously; in younger patients it is more common after traumatic injury. The feeling commonly occurs after rapid head movement leading to movement of loose otoconia in the posterior semicircular canal, resulting in a brief transient episode of vertigo lasting only seconds. Episodes recur with any movement that causes fluid shift in the affected canal—rolling in bed, hanging out the washing on the line, opening a high cupboard, and so on.

Generally there are no examination findings apart from positive Dix-Hallpike manoeuvre.

The treatment uses the Epley manoeuvre, with a good cure rate (80%+). This often expedites recovery rather than waiting for spontaneous remission (up to 18 months).

It may recur months to decades later and is treated in the same manner.

Rarely, surgical intervention is required, to occlude the posterior semicircular canal.

VESTIBULAR NEURONITIS AND LABYRINTHITIS

Vestibular neuronitis is a relatively sudden onset of unilateral vestibulopathy presenting with vertigo and nausea/vomiting. It is the most common cause of first ever acute fulminant episode of vertigo with nausea and vomiting.

Vertigo with nausea and vomiting with the additional symptoms of hearing loss with or without tinnitus indicates acute labyrinthitis.

There is no gender predilection, and the average age of presentation is approximately 40 years.

The aetiology is likely to be viral or ischaemic, but is largely uncertain. It disrupts the superior and/or inferior vestibular nerve input to one vestibule, resulting in sudden severe vertigo with nausea.

There are no cochlear symptoms or signs, no neurological symptoms or signs, and a positive high-frequency head impulse test (diagnostic). The patient usually recovers completely within weeks. Recovery requires good compensation (by normal proprioception, vision and other inputs).

Treatment is to encourage compensation with early mobilisation once the vertigo and nausea settle.

Symptomatic relief with medications such as PR stemetil, p.o. or sublingual benzodiazepine or prochloroperazine should be limited, to avoid lack of compensation, toxicity and suppression of contralateral vestibular apparatus.

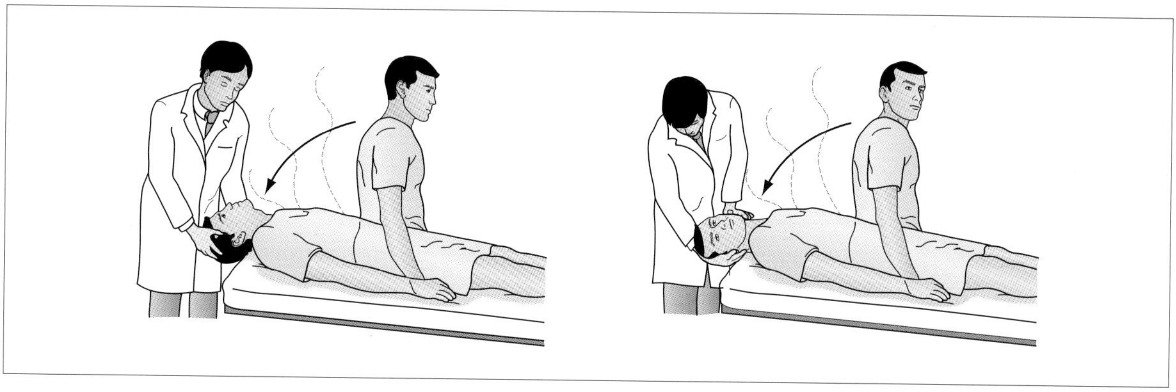

FIGURE 27.10 Dix-Hallpike manoeuvre. The patient's head is turned 45° to the right. The patient is then brought into the supine position with the neck extended below the level of the examination table and observed for nystagmus and symptoms of vertigo.

The patient is often referred for vestibular physiotherapy if not compensated within 4–6 weeks or if the patient has poor compensatory mechanisms (e.g. patient with walking stick, poor eyesight).

MIGRAINOUS VERTIGO

Migrainous vertigo is more difficult to manage, with a recurrent type of vertigo with or without headache. It is often associated with a family history of migraines, and is a common cause of recurrent vertigo (variably described as second or third behind BPPV). It occurs in all ages, with a predilection for migraine sufferers.

Comments about food-related reactions and cytokines also apply in migrainous vertigo. Inhalants such as cigarette smoke and petrochemicals in the form of cosmetics and perfume should also be considered. Fumes travel up the nose and through the cribriform plate directly to the brain. For the chemically sensitive, and/or those with migraine genes, migrainous vertigo is a common and distinctly unpleasant experience.

Like migraines, migrainous vertigo is thought to be a vascular phenomenon, with the vertigo lasting minutes to days with or without headache. The patient shows only transient neurological signs, with possible central signs on visual assessment. There are often very different serial electronystagmography (ENG) and caloric testing.

A trial of classic migraine management is best for prevention, including trigger identification and lifestyle modification.

One retrospective review found that migraine treatments were effective in about 90% of patients with migraine-associated vertigo.[7] Treatments included:

- dietary changes—reduction or elimination of aspartame, chocolate, caffeine or alcohol
- lifestyle changes—exercise, stress reduction and relaxation techniques, improvements in sleep patterns
- vestibular rehabilitation exercises.

Migraine medications including pizotifen or propranolol can help in repeat events. Other medications that may be useful include benzodiazepines, tricyclic antidepressants, selective serotonin reuptake inhibitors (SSRIs), calcium channel blockers and antiemetics.

MÉNIÈRE'S DISEASE

Ménière's disease is a disorder of the inner ear caused by endolymphatic hydrops (increased volume and pressure of the endolymphatic sac). Its incidence is approximately 100/100,000, with a usual onset in early to mid-adulthood, with no male/female preponderance. There are multiple postulated theories (e.g. viral infection causing release of saccin, leading to fluid retention and endolymphatic hydrops, expressing as clinical episodes), but the common feature is an enlarged endolymphatic sac.

During an episode, the patient classically has:

- low-frequency hearing loss
- tinnitus
- aural fullness
- vertigo (often of hours' duration).

The prognosis is variable, with contralateral involvement in 20% of patients by 20 years of age. The condition rarely reaches the stage of Tumarkin crises or Lermoyez syndrome.

Confirming the diagnosis includes obtaining an audiogram, caloric testing, MRI (to exclude other inner ear pathology) and ENT referral. Treatment centres on reducing the absorption of fluid into the endolymphatic sac.

For an acute attack:

- diazepam 5 mg IV with or without prochlorperazine 25 mg suppository, or IM
- betahistine 8 mg p.o. t.d.s. if persistent.

Example of a stepwise approach:

- low-sodium diet (< 1500–2000 mmol/day)—Ménière's disease has many features in common with migrainous vertigo. It is a hybrid allergic disorder, but is also subject to many of the problems afflicting the modern Western diet. The role of sodium is significant; however, the dietary balance of sodium and potassium is a consideration. In a primitive diet, the ratio of potassium to sodium was 10:1 *or more*. The modern diet has reversed this and it is now 1:2 at the very best. For those with salt-retaining genes and an allergic diathesis, Ménière's is a logical consequence
- magnesium supplementation—magnesium deficiency is made all the worse by the consumption of calcium tablets without magnesium balance. Magnesium depletion is a common agricultural problem in the developed world. The ideal dietary ratio of calcium to magnesium is 3:2. In dairy products, the balance is closer to 8:1 or even 16:1. This adds a relative magnesium deficiency to an already absolute deficiency. Magnesium supplements have a distinct role to play in Ménière's disease
- avoidance/treatment of precipitants in some cases (e.g. food additives, antihistamines)
- avoidance of tobacco and coffee
- diuretics—hydrochlorothiazide/amiloride
- vestibular suppressants
- ventilation tube ± Meniett® device
- intratympanic gentamicin
- anxiety management
- surgical options for intractable cases.

TONSILLAR AND PERITONSILLAR DISORDERS

The tonsils and adenoids are congregations of lymphoid tissue in the oropharynx. They play an important role in immunology and memory for infection and, consequently, are implicated in mucosal defence. They are most active in childhood and therefore are often considered an entity of childhood illness.

Most commonly, tonsillar and peritonsillar disorders are part of a child's development, and surgical intervention is not often required. Infection or tonsillitis is the most common complaint of the tonsils. Symptoms and their frequency and severity often dictate treatment. It is important to assess for obstructive symptoms and, in children, for poor behaviour with morning 'hang-over', and in adults, for daytime somnolence, poor sleep hygiene, cardiovascular comorbidity and Epworth Sleepiness Scale (Fig 27.11). Formal sleep studies may be required before making a decision on surgery.

In patients who 'rebound' or re-present with tonsillitis, it is important to consider the likelihood of being 'under-antibioticised', or the likelihood of being 'under-analgesed'. A duration of more than 3–4 days, trismus, referred unilateral otalgia and/or previous peritonsillar abscess may suggest peritonsillar abscess (quinsy).

For patients with these conditions presenting less acutely, consider sleep-disordered breathing, recurrent tonsillitis affecting school/university or work, recurrent peritonsillar abscess or suspicion of malignancy, as key reasons for referral to ENT.

THE EPWORTH SLEEPINESS SCALE

Name: ______

Today's date: ______ Your age (years): ______

Your sex (male–M; female–F): ______

How likely are you to doze off or fall asleep in the following situations in contrast to feeling just tired? This refers to your usual way of life in recent times. Even if you have not done some of these things recently, try to work out how they would have affected you. Use the following scale to choose the *most appropriate number* for each situation:

0 = would *never* doze
1 = *slight* chance of dozing
2 = *moderate* chance of dozing
3 = *high* chance of dozing

Situation	Chance of dozing
Sitting and reading	______
Watching TV	______
Sitting inactive in a public place (e.g., a theater or a meeting)	______
As a passenger in a car for an hour without a break	______
Lying down to rest in the afternoon when circumstances permit	______
Sitting and talking to someone	______
Sitting quietly after a lunch without alcohol	______
In a car, while stopped for a few minutes in traffic	______

FIGURE 27.11 Epworth Sleepiness Scale

On examination, general signs of infection or inflammation are evident, with fever and tachycardia the most common. The patient may have cervical lymphadenopathy, trismus (moderate to severe increases suggestive of quinsy in acute setting), erythema of tonsils, crypt debris in tonsils or purulence of tonsils. Confluent slough over the tonsils increases the suggestion of Epstein-Barr virus (EBV; mononucleosis).

Abdominal (spleen/liver) examination and generalised lymphadenopathy is palpated for when suspicious of EBV mononucleosis.

Severe infections should be referred, and flexible nasopharyngolaryngoscopy by an ENT surgeon is possible if there is concern regarding obstructed breathing, deep neck space infection, supraglottitis, epiglottitis or lingual tonsillitis.

PERITONSILAR ABSCESS (QUINSY)

Quinsy is inflammation of the peritonsillar space with suppuration. Classically it occurs between the ages of 15 and 40 years, but it is possible at any age. Inflammation of the tonsils can lead to peritonsillar space infection adjacent to acute tonsillitis. This may lead to abscess formation, with resultant swelling of the unilateral peritonsillar space, oedema, fluctuance, deviation of uvula and trismus.

If untreated, extension of infection into any of the other deep neck spaces is possible. Prompt treatment is therefore recommended. After the first quinsy, there is a 25% risk of subsequent quinsy; a second quinsy increases that risk to 50% risk of subsequent quinsy. A third quinsy almost always (90% risk) gives a subsequent quinsy.

Treatment is by acute drainage (incisional drainage or repeated aspiration under local anaesthetic).

'Hot' tonsillectomy (removal of the tonsils while they are acutely infected) is controversial and rarely seen these days. Supportive therapy must include antibiotics (with a probiotic), fluids and analgesia. More recently, the use of steroids has helped settle severe infections more rapidly.

LARYNGITIS

Laryngitis is an acute inflammation of the larynx due to overuse, inflammation or infection. It may be acute or chronic, and presents with hoarseness. The patient may also complain of sore throat, fever, dry cough, trouble swallowing and trouble breathing.

Acute laryngitis

Causes of acute laryngitis incude viral URTI, vocal abuse and irritants such as cigarette smoke. Treatment includes the following:

- resting the voice
- hot lemon and honey drinks
- avoidance of tobacco and alcohol
- steam inhalation
- simple analgesia for pain.

Referral is required if symptoms persist for longer than four weeks.

Chronic laryngitis

Risks for chronic laryngitis include smoking, excessive alcohol consumption and overuse of the voice. Chronic hoarseness requires examination of the vocal cords to exclude benign nodules or carcinoma.

Benign nodules may respond to conservative measures such as ceasing smoking, voice rest and speech therapy. They may require surgical removal.

Exclude gastro-oesophageal reflux disease, a common hidden cause of hoarseness. Refer for specialist assessment.

Herbal treatments

Common herbs used are similar to those for sinusitis.[8]

Traditional Chinese medicine

Laryngitis refers to inflammation of the larynx, which can be acute or chronic. For both conditions, in TCM they fall into the category of 'Hou Yin', which means 'loss of voice due to throat problem'. For acute conditions, the invasion of pathogenic wind-cold or wind-heat is the major cause of blockage at the throat area. In chronic conditions, it is due to a yin deficiency failing to nourish the throat area. The primary treatment for acute laryngitis is to expel wind-cold or wind-heat; for chronic laryngitis the treatment is nourishing yin.

TCM herbs:[9,10]

- platycodon root (*Platycodon grandiflorum*)
- figwort root (*Scrophularia ningpoensis*)
- dwarf lilyturf tuber (*Ophiopogon japonicus*)
- Vietnamese sophora root (*Sophora tonkinensis*)
- isatis root (*Isatis indigotica*).

INFECTIOUS MONONUCLEOSIS

An acute inflammation of the tonsils often caused by Epstein-Barr virus (classical) is called infectious mononucleosis. There are two peaks of primary infection: at age 1–5 years and in adolescence. Most children seroconvert by 5 years of age, so clinical disease usually manifests in adolescents or young adults who failed to seroconvert in childhood.

As with tonsillitis, a prodromal fever or malaise accompanied by odonyphagia is common. Confluent exudative and sloughy tonsillitis is classic. Cervical and generalised lymphadenopathy is noted, along with the possibility of a rash, jaundice and/or hepatosplenomegaly. Usually it is self-limiting and very rarely causes significant airway, neurological, cardiovascular or haematological sequelae.

The diagnosis should be confirmed with blood tests for:

- Epstein-Barr virus (EBV) titre IgM and IgG
- full blood examination—lymphocytosis and atypical lymphocytes
- C-reactive protein (CRP)
- liver function tests.

The virus is generally spread among children, adolescents and young adults through salivary contact, and only causes clinical illness when primary infection is delayed until adolescence or beyond. Symptomatic infectious mononucleosis occurs in approximately 50% of young adult cases of EBV infection.

While most people with EBV infection recover fully within a few weeks, Epstein-Barr virus may cause long-term fatigue and is known to be able to induce tumours such as B-lymphoproliferative disease and Hodgkin's disease.

Prevention

There is no droplet transmission, so isolation is not necessary. Transmission is through saliva, and the virus may be present for months or years after clinical infection.

Advise household contacts to avoid kissing the infected person or sharing cups, eating utensils or toothbrushes with them. Learning stress management techniques helps improve the immune system and may help reduce the risk of viral infection such as EBV.

Acute stage

Rest is essential in the early stages. Graduated increase in activity is to be encouraged after two weeks as tolerated. Splenomegaly occurs in about 50% of cases, so contact sports and heavy lifting should be avoided for two months because of the risk of splenic rupture.

Medication

- Paracetamol or aspirin (not in children).
- Corticosteroids may be needed to relieve obstructive symptoms from tonsillar hypertrophy or neurological complications.
- Prescription of amoxicillin or ampicillin should be avoided if EBV is suspected, as it can cause a pink maculopapular rash if given to a patient with EBV.
- Steroids and antibiotics are reserved for severe cases with superimposed bacterial infection.

Nutrition

- Sore throat and tonsillar hypertrophy can make adequate nutrition difficult to achieve. Soups, soft foods and purees may be needed in the acute phase.
- Avoid fatty foods.

- Avoid coffee and other stimulants, alcohol and tobacco. Alcohol should be avoided completely, particularly if transaminases are elevated.
- Drink 6–8 glasses of fluids, including herbal teas, broths and filtered water daily.
- Eat a predominance of antioxidant-rich fruits and vegetables.
- Eat tofu, fish or legumes for protein.

Supplements

Supplements help to ensure nutritional adequacy and immune support, and may include:

- a multivitamin daily, containing the antioxidant vitamins A, C, E, the B-vitamins, and trace minerals, such as magnesium, calcium, zinc and selenium
- intravenous vitamin C administered by a doctor experienced in the procedure—can be very effective in the acute phase, and will reduce the risk of chronic fatigue syndrome when recovery is prolonged
- omega-3 fatty acids, such as fish oil and flaxseed oil, to help decrease inflammation and improve immunity
- coenzyme Q10, 100–200 mg at night, for antioxidant effect and to counter fatigue and myalgia
- probiotic (containing *Lactobacillus acidophilus*) for maintenance of gastrointestinal and immune health.

Herbs

A variety of herbs can be useful support for management of infectious mononucleosis. These include:

- *Glycyrrhiza glabra* (licorice root) 5–15 g daily. In vitro studies suggest that glycyrrhizin may interfere with an early step of the EBV replication cycle.[11] It must be used with caution and under professional supervision. If used in high doses for more than two weeks it can cause hypertension, fluid retention and hypokalaemia.
- green tea (*Camellia sinensis*) (caffeine free)[12]
- rhodiola (*Rhodiola rosea*) standardised extract, 100–600 mg daily, for antioxidant, anti-stress and immune activity[13]
- milk thistle (*Silybum marianum*) seed standardised extract, 80–160 mg two to three times daily, for liver support, especially if transaminases are elevated[14]
- elderberry (*Sambucus nigra*) extract, 1 tablespoonful twice daily, for antiviral and immune activity[15]
- reishi mushroom (*Ganoderma lucidum*), 150–300 mg two to three times daily, or tincture of this mushroom extract, 30–60 drops two to three times daily[16]
- cat's claw (*Uncaria tomentosa*) standardised extract, 20 mg three times daily, for inflammation and antiviral activity.[17]

RESOURCES

Information and patient education

Information and images of ear, nose and throat, http://www.google.com.au/images?client=safari&rls=en&q=ear+nose+and+throat&oe=UTF-8&redir_esc=&um=1&ie=UTF-8&source=univ&ei=M8fcS5T5FNCgkQX1kOjBBw&sa=X&oi=image_result_group&ct=title&resnum=11&ved=0CDUQsAQwCg

Medline Plus, Ear, nose and throat, http://www.nlm.nih.gov/medlineplus/earnoseandthroat.html

Queensland Government, Ear, nose and throat health, http://access.health.qld.gov.au/hid/EarNoseandThroatHealth/index.asp

ENT colleges

American Academy of Otolaryngology—Head and Neck Surgery, http://www.entnet.org/

Australian Society of Otolaryngology, Head and Neck Surgery, http://www.asohns.org.au/

American Academy of Otolaryngology—Head and Neck Surgery, http://www.entnet.org/

Royal College of Surgeons of Edinburgh, http://www.rcsed.ac.uk/site/630/default.aspx

ENT UK, http://www.entuk.org/patient_info/

REFERENCES

1 Black RJ, Cousins V, Chapman P et al. Ototoxic ear drops with grommet and tympanic membrane perforations: a position statement. Med J Aust 2007; 187(1):62.

2 Taylor PS, Faeth I, Marks MK et al. Cost of treating otitis media in Australia. Expert Rev Pharmacoecon Outcomes Res 2009; 9(2):133–141.

3 Glasziou PP, Del Mar CB, Sanders SL et al. Antibiotics for acute otitis media in children. Cochrane Database Syst Rev 2004; 1:CD000219.

4 National Institute of Neurological Disorders and Stroke. Bell's palsy fact sheet. Last updated 2009. National Institutes of Health. Online. Available: http://www.ninds.nih.gov/disorders/bells/detail_bells.htm#109663050

5 Mills S, Bone K. Principles and practice of phytotherapy: modern herbal medicine. London: Churchill Livingstone; 2000.

6 Weiss RF, Fintelmann V. Herbal medicine. 2nd edn. Stuttgart: Thieme; 2000.

7 Johnson GD. Medical management of migraine-related dizziness and vertigo. Laryngoscope 1998; 108(1 pt 2):1–28.

8 Blumenthal M, Goldberg A, Brinckmann J, eds. Herbal medicine. Expanded Commission E Monographs. Austin, Texas: American Botanic Council; 2000.

9 Kim H-Y, Shin H-S, Kim Y-C et al. In vitro inhibition of coronavirus replications by the traditionally used

medicinal herbal extracts, *Cimicifuga rhizoma*, *Meliae cortex*, *Coptidis rhizoma*, and *Phellodendron cortex*. J Clin Virol 2008; 41(2):122–128.
10 Maclean W, Taylor K. The clinical manual of Chinese herbal patent medicines. Sydney: Pangolin Press; 2000.
11 Lin JC. Mechanism of action of glycyrrhizic acid in inhibition of Epstein-Barr virus replication in vitro. Antiviral Res 2003; 59(1):41–47.
12 Chang L-K, Wei T-T, Chiu Y-F et al. Inhibition of Epstein-Barr virus lytic cycle by (–)-epigallocatechin gallate. Biochem Biophys Res Commun 2003; 301(4):1062–1068.
13 Kelly G. *Rhodiola rosea*: a possible plant adaptogen. Altern Med Rev 2001; 6(3):293–302.
14 Pradhan S, Girish C. Hepatoprotective herbal drug, silymarin from experimental pharmacology to clinical medicine. Indian J Med Res 2006; 124(5):491–504.
15 Barak V, Halperin I, Kalickman I. The effect of Sambucol, a black elderberry-based, natural product, on the production of human cytokines: I. Inflammatory cytokines. Eur Cytokine Netw 2001; 12(2):290–296.
16 Sanodiya BS, Thakur GS, Baghel RK et al. *Ganoderma lucidum*: a potent pharmacological macrofungus. Curr Pharm Biotechnol 2009; 10(8):717–742.
17 Williams J. Review of antiviral and immunomodulating properties of the plants of the Peruvian rain forest with a particular emphasis on Una de Gato and Sangre de Grado. Altern Med Rev 2001; 6(6):567–579.

chapter 28

Eyes

INTRODUCTION

Essential ocular conditions likely to present to a general practitioner also overlap to some extent with those seen in the emergency department. We start with important definitions, a list of basic equipment, tips on a focused ocular history and a concise and appropriate examination of the eye, and then discuss conditions that are common and/or serious (sight- or even life-threatening). It is important to have confidence with diagnosis and management, including prompt referral when required. This is by no means an all-inclusive list. Syndromes and ocular complications of systemic diseases are not covered.

The aim is to provide a practical and accessible guide for the general practitioner. Ocular conditions are divided into four main overlapping sections according to patient presentation to a general practitioner: red eye, loss of vision in the white eye, painful eye, and double vision. For example, a red eye is commonly painful as well, but by following the main symptom it is possible to exclude several diagnoses. Diagnostic summary flow charts can be used for quick reference.

HISTORY

The history involves both a specific ocular history and a comprehensive general history. Often the patient is distressed: they greatly fear losing their sight, and having the eyes touched is often psychologically threatening and physically uncomfortable.

HISTORY OF PRESENTING ILLNESS

What is the main or most serious complaint?

- Is the eye painful—duration, severity, associated and relieving features.
- Is the vision abnormal—missing letters or field, misty, coloured rings around lights, distance or near.
- Is the vision double—vertical, horizontal or torsional.
- Is the eye red—discharge, pain, location of redness: conjunctiva, limbus, sclera, sectoral or diffuse.
- Is there discharge—white versus yellow, sticky versus pus.

If there are multiple complaints, prioritise and address each one separately. Try to determine the order of events. Note symptom duration and any associated features such as ocular discharge, headache or cranial nerve palsy.

How did the patient attempt to treat the problem? A popular home remedy is to wash the open eye with tap water or weak tea. This can introduce bacteria and complicate the findings.

Over-the-counter (OTC) preparations often contain an antihistamine and/or a vasoconstrictor, which may mask conjunctival injection without treating the underlying condition.

PAST OCULAR HISTORY

Determine the pre-morbid level of vision, past acute and chronic conditions, which may recur. Note previous ocular:

- hospitalisations—corneal abscess, trauma, endophthalmitis
- surgery—cataract, glaucoma, strabismus, retinal detachment
- diseases—cataract, glaucoma, age-related macular degeneration
- need for glasses and/or contact lenses
- childhood strabismus ('squint' or 'turn')/amblyopia ('lazy eye')
- use of drops—OTC and prescription.

FAMILY OCULAR HISTORY

Familial diseases include:

- glaucoma
- age-related macular degeneration
- cataract (especially juvenile)
- ocular dystrophies and syndromes.

MEDICAL HISTORY

Systemic diseases with possible ocular manifestations include: diabetes, thyroid disease, autoimmune disease, coronary and/or carotid artery disease, infections.

Systemic diseases that affect adherence to topical treatment: arthritis, dementia, tremor, stroke.

Systemic diseases that may be exacerbated by topical beta blockers: congestive heart failure, asthma, heart block.

A systemic disease whose management may be affected by topical beta blockers is insulin-dependent diabetes (may mask incipient hypoglycaemia).

MEDICATIONS

Medications with ocular side effects include: steroids, amiodarone, chlorpromazine, anti-TB and anti-HIV medications, beta-blockers, anticholinergics, tricyclic antidepressants, anticonvulsants and selective serotonin reuptake inhibitors.

Systemic medications that may be potentiated by topical beta-blockers are: beta-blockers, calcium channel blockers.

Potential systemic side effects from eye drops include: reactive airways disease, cardiac block, congestive cardiac failure (beta-blockers), allergic reactions (any drop), dry mouth, drowsiness, hypotension (alpha-2 agonists).

Ask specifically about eye drops—patients often forget to mention them. Look for overlap between topical and systemic drug classes and concurrent inappropriate use of both new and old drops (e.g. simultaneous use of two preparations, each containing beta-blockers).

Ask about allergy and/or adverse reactions to drops, sulfonamides, antibiotics and anaesthetic agents.

FAMILY HISTORY

Ask about diabetes, heart disease and problems with anaesthetics.

SOCIAL HISTORY

The social history will affect all aspects of patient care, from the ability to seek medical care, through follow-up, to adherence to a management program. Identifying and modifying risk factors is vital, to prevent or to minimise morbidity.

Ask whether the patient is:

- living alone
- able to access transport
- able to afford treatment
- able, from a visual perspective, to shop, cook, clean, work, read, drive, play sport
- a recent traveller (think unusual infections)
- a smoker and/or illicit drug user
- using complementary medicines.

OCULAR EXAMINATION FOR GENERAL PRACTITIONERS

Equipment required:

- visual acuity chart—distance and near
- plastic occluder (large)
- red-topped bottle or hatpin
- torch with bright light (ensure ongoing fresh/rechargeable batteries!)
- ophthalmoscope / cobalt blue light
- cotton buds to evert eyelids, remove subtarsal foreign body
- drops: fluorescein, short-acting anaesthetic (benoxinate, tetracaine, proxymetacaine).

STRUCTURED EXAMINATION

Visual acuity

Distance visual acuity (Snellen VA)—expressed as a fraction, x/y where x is fixed as the distance the patient sits from chart and y is the line read. For example, if a patient sits at 6 metres and can read the '18' line, VA is 6/18.

Occlude one eye at a time carefully and completely, and measure each eye separately. The vision should be measured with and without distance glasses (best corrected visual acuity: BCVA). A pinhole can be used if glasses have been forgotten or are not current. By eliminating non-paraxial rays, pinholes act as a 'universal' lens, indicating potential BCVA.

Visual acuity near (NA)—ask the patient to read letters at 30 cm, with reading glasses if required.

Note: glasses or the pinhole will correct refractive errors. Glasses won't improve vision decreased by ocular conditions requiring treatment, so have the patient wear glasses for testing.

Pupil examination

Direct reflex to light—constricts the illuminated pupil. This measures ipsilateral optic nerve function (light going in) and oculomotor nerve function (pupil constriction) in that eye.

Consensual reflex to light—constricts the contralateral pupil, testing ipsilateral optic nerve function and contralateral oculomotor nerve function.

Relative afferent defect (RAPD)—there is paradoxical *initial* pupil dilatation in the illuminated eye when the torch is swung across from the other eye. With the patient fixating steadily at an object across the room, shine the light steadily for a few seconds into one eye, then swing it across to the second eye, watching the movement of that (second) pupil. If the first movement

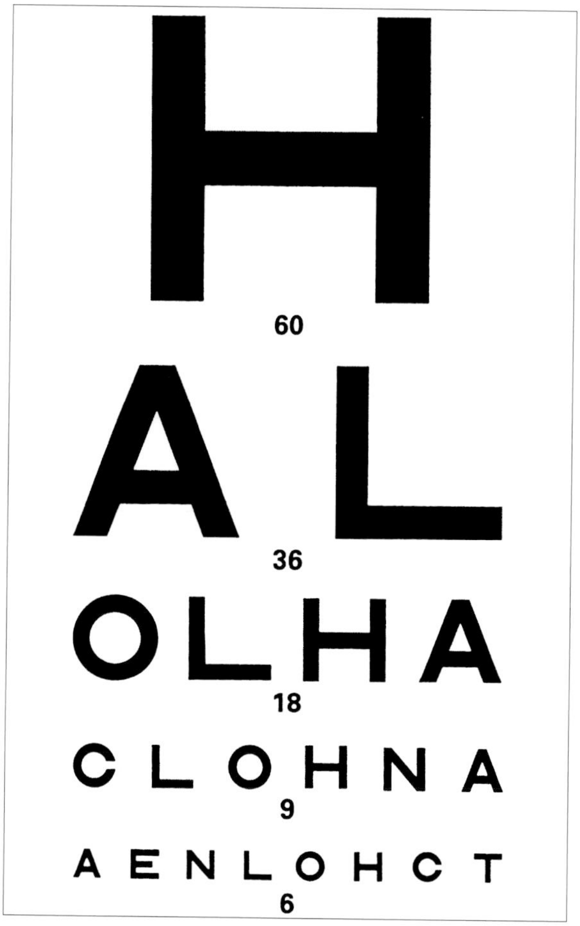

FIGURE 28.1 Snellen Visual Acuity Chart

is constriction, the pupil response is normal; if the first movement is dilatation (and then constriction), that demonstrates a defect. Such a defect means that there is a relative abnormality in that optic nerve (compared with its fellow). It suggests optic neuropathy, such as optic neuritis or glaucoma (early to moderate loss is usually asymmetric).

Horner's pupil—on the affected side there is miosis, dilatation lag in dark, and mild upper eyelid ptosis.

The *red reflex* is the reflection of light off the retina through the pupil. It can be seen as 'red eye' on photographs and is diminished or abnormal with media opacities, such as cataract or vitreous haemorrhage.

Extraocular movements

With the patient's head steady, ask them to watch the red bottle top or hatpin carefully while you draw a large, wide 'H' in the air. Corneal light reflexes indicate symmetrical movement.

Confrontation visual fields

Face the patient at a distance of about two arms' length. Using a red top or hatpin, bring the object into view from four oblique directions. Initially test with both eyes open for a gross defect (such as hemianopia), then each eye individually.

Ocular examination

Always compare one side with the other, and use adequate illumination and magnification.

- Face—rash, asymmetry, trauma.
- Eyelids—rash, position, trauma, evert if foreign body is suspected.

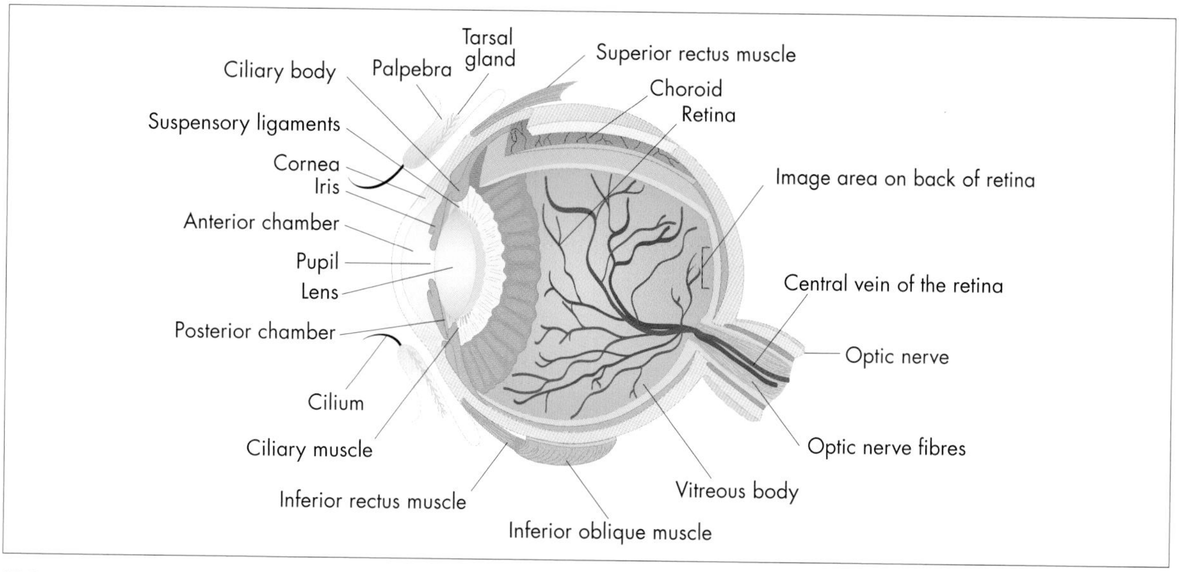

FIGURE 28.2 Anatomy of the globe

- Test cranial nerves.
- Look at globe systematically—position, presence/location of any injection.
- Look at all layers of globe individually.
- Conjunctiva—pull down lower eyelids, evert upper eyelids.
- Cornea—with magnification, white light, fluorescein and cobalt blue light for abrasions.
- Episclera/sclera—redness, haemorrhage, ulceration, pallor (presence, extent, location).
- Iris and pupil—irregularity, asymmetry, reflexes.
- Lens—look at red reflex through ophthalmoscope to evaluate media opacities.
- Fundus—ask patient to look straight ahead to examine optic nerve head, at the light to see macula, up/down/side to side for mid-peripheral retina.
- Gently ballotte both eyeballs through relaxed upper eyelids (with patient looking down) and compare intraocular pressures between the eyes.
- Do not compare digital eye pressures with your own if you suspect infection!

OCULAR CONDITIONS

PREVENTION

As with other aspects of health, preventing eye disease is preferable to treating it. Simple preventive measures include:

- measures to prevent the spread of infection
- avoid eye trauma e.g. wear appropriate eye protection
- maintain a healthy lifestyle and avoid smoking, to reduce the risk of conditions such as diabetic retinopathy, retinal vein occlusions and macular degeneration
- adequately manage systemic conditions associated with eye complications
- secondary preventive measures with regular eye checks, especially in the presence of a family history for conditions such as glaucoma or diabetes
- adequate sun protection with protective eyewear, especially for those who are regularly outdoors in sunny environments
- low-fat diet (elevated cholesterol is a risk factor for macular degeneration[1] and diabetic complications)
- high dietary intake of lutein/zeaxanthin[3]—carotenoids in plants with orange, red or yellow colour, fish and green leafy vegetables. Also high intakes of omega-3 polyunsaturated fatty acids may decrease the incidence of nuclear cataract and higher intake of protein may decrease the risk of posterior subcapsular cataract.[2]

RED EYE

Red eye is very common and covers a broad spectrum of anterior segment diagnoses.

Conjunctivitis

Conjunctival inflammation is the predominant feature. Patients present with a red eye and mucopurulent discharge. The eyelids commonly become 'stuck together' overnight and difficult to open on waking. Ocular discomfort varies from surface irritation (e.g. sandiness/grittiness) to pain.

Signs include generalised conjunctival erythema, swelling and discharge. The conjunctiva develops distinct papillae (lymphoid tissue with a central vascular core) or follicles (collection of chronic inflammatory cells), depending on the aetiology. Vision is usually unaffected.

The multiple aetiologies, often separable by history, symptoms and discharge, include those described below.

Common

Bacterial conjunctivitis

(*Staphylococcus epidermidis/aureus, Streptococcus pneumoniae, Haemophilus influenzae*)

The conjunctiva appears 'beefy red' with yellow/green and mucopurulent discharge.

Treatment—antibiotic drops (e.g. chloramphenicol) initially every 2 hours during waking hours if severe, then q.i.d. for 1 week. Heat and lubricants can relieve symptoms. Antibiotic ointment can be used at bedtime.

The second eye usually becomes involved within a few days. Complete resolution is common within 1–2 weeks.

Viral conjunctivitis (predominantly adenovirus)

Follows contact with an affected person in epidemics, less commonly after a viral illness. Patients present with very red eye(s), lid swelling, watering and photophobia, and discomfort may be severe.

On examination there is marked conjunctival erythema and a clear watery discharge, pseudomembranes and subconjunctival haemorrhages if severe, and tender pre-auricular and cervical lymphadenopathy.

Treatment is symptomatic—cold or warm compresses and lubricant tear drops. For most patients this is adequate.

The condition is typically unresponsive to antibiotics and often worse in the first 3–7 days before slow resolution, which takes 2–3 weeks. It is rarely complicated by corneal inflammation (keratitis), which may lead to a longer duration and visual compromise through corneal scarring. These patients need to be referred to an ophthalmologist, who may prescribe weak steroid drops.

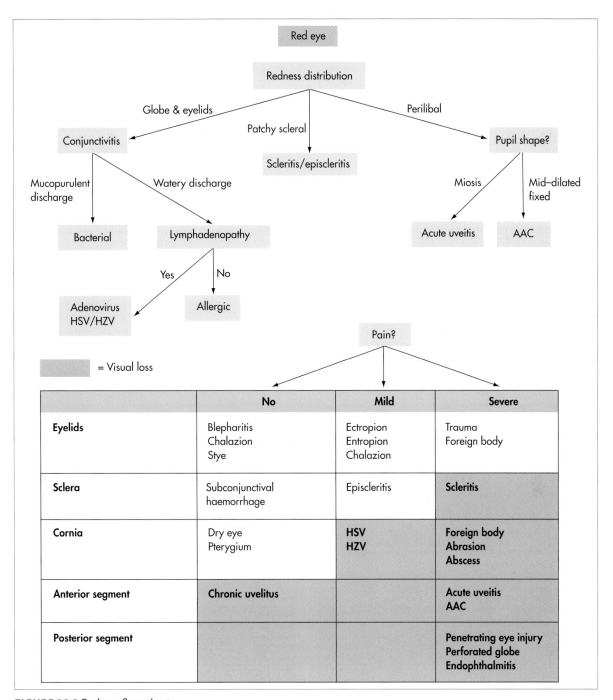

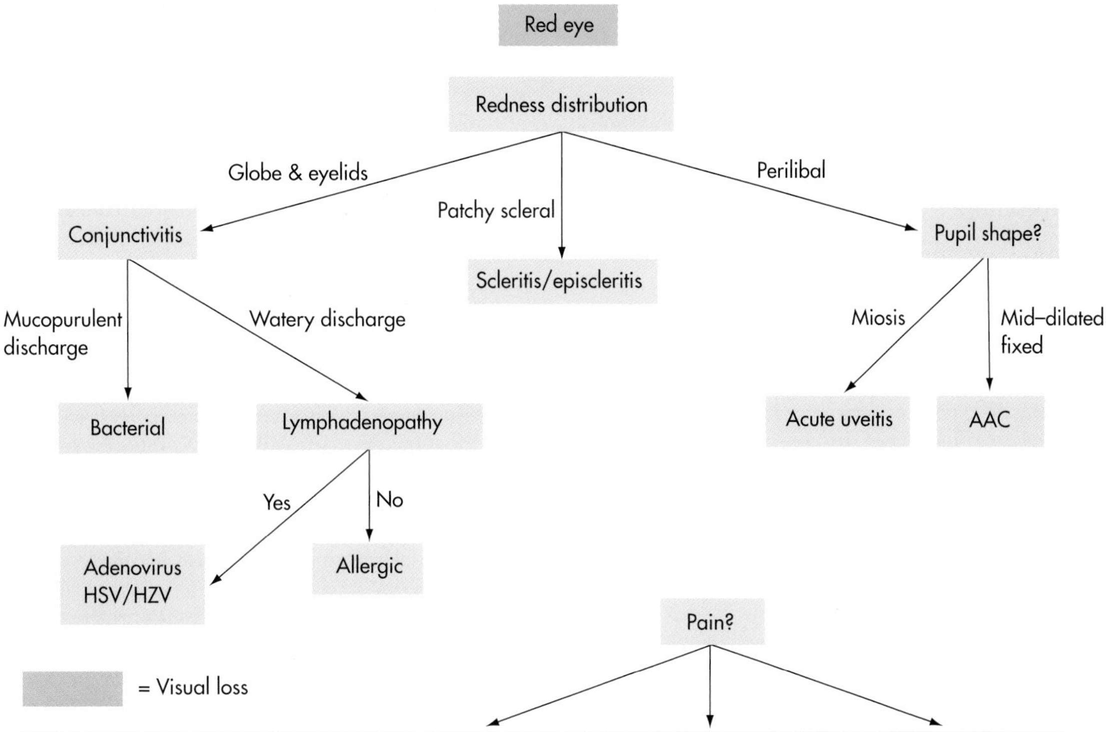

	No	Mild	Severe
Eyelids	Blepharitis Chalazion Stye	Ectropion Entropion Chalazion	Trauma Foreign body
Sclera	Subconjunctival haemorrhage	Episcleritis	**Scleritis**
Cornia	Dry eye Pterygium	**HSV** **HZV**	**Foreign body** **Abrasion** **Abscess**
Anterior segment	**Chronic uvelitus**		**Acute uveitis** **AAC**
Posterior segment			**Penetrating eye injury** **Perforated globe** **Endophthalmitis**

FIGURE 28.3 Red eye flow chart

Allergic conjunctivitis

This is usually seasonal (often with hay fever) or there is a known history of allergy. Patients present with red eyes, swollen eyelids, itching and watering. Conjunctival erythema is mild and pink, rather than red. The discharge may be whitish mucus, or clear and watery.

Treatment—involves flushing out the allergen with frequent use of unpreserved lubricant drops.

If severe, the patient should be referred to an ophthalmologist for anti-inflammatory and mast cell stabiliser drops such as fluorometholone and olopatadine or ketotifen.

The prognosis is usually good: most patients do not require long-term medication.

Uncommon

Patients with the conditions described below should be referred to an ophthalmologist for diagnosis, swabs and treatment co-managed with a sexually transmitted disease specialist.

Chlamydia

(*Chlamydia trachomatis*)

Patients complain of longstanding ocular symptoms, unresponsive to different treatments. A history of sexually transmitted disease is not always apparent, and the patient may be asymptomatic.

On examination there is conjunctival erythema, eyelid swelling, mucopurulent discharge and pre-auricular lymphadenopathy.

Treatment—includes systemic antibiotics (e.g. doxycycline for 3–6 weeks).

Gonorrhoea

(*Neisseria gonorrhoeae*)

While men may have urethral discharge, it is often asymptomatic in women.

The ocular symptoms and signs are florid. Patients present with red eye and creamy discharge. On examination there is profuse, thick, white purulent discharge and pre-auricular lymphadenopathy.

Keratitis occurs in severe infection and is vision threatening. It requires urgent referral to an ophthalmologist and hospital admission for intravenous antibiotic (e.g. ceftriaxone).

Prevention

This must be reinforced by the general practitioner. Infective conjunctivitis is highly contagious: make patients aware of this!

Patients should avoid touching their eyes and avoid sharing towels and pillow cases. They should wash their hands frequently, and every time after touching their face or eyes.

Patients should be given a medical certificate for a week, or while the eyes are red and discharging, occasionally longer in the case of viral conjunctivitis.

Sexually transmitted infection requires co-management and education with a specialist in this field.

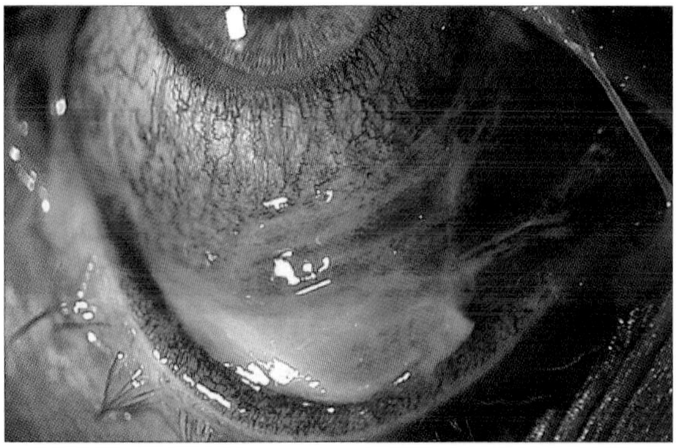

FIGURE 28.4 Infective conjunctivitis

Blepharitis

Blepharitis is a very common condition, with flaky deposits and crusting on the eyelashes. Patients complain of gritty, sandy and irritated eyes. Deposits and oil droplets can be seen with magnification or, if severe, with the naked eye, over the meibomian gland orifices.

An ophthalmologist usually diagnoses these patients and the treatment needs to be reinforced by the general practitioner.

Lid and lash hygiene techniques involve washing the eyelashes with baby shampoo, with eyes closed, and topical lubricants. As this is often ongoing, the frequency of washing is tailored to control the symptoms.

If severe or associated with acne rosacea, the ophthalmologist may prescribe doxycycline 50 mg daily for at least 6 weeks. Tetracycline antibiotics alter the lipid chemistry of the eyelid glands and the protective effect may last for up to a year.

Chalazion

A chalazion is an eyelid inflammatory mass caused by blockage of meibomian glands.

Treatment—massage with a hot wash cloth, and lid and lash hygiene as above. Surgical incision and curettage under local anaesthetic if conservative treatment fails.

Episcleritis and scleritis

Episcleritis and scleritis are inflammatory conditions affecting the episclera and the sclera.

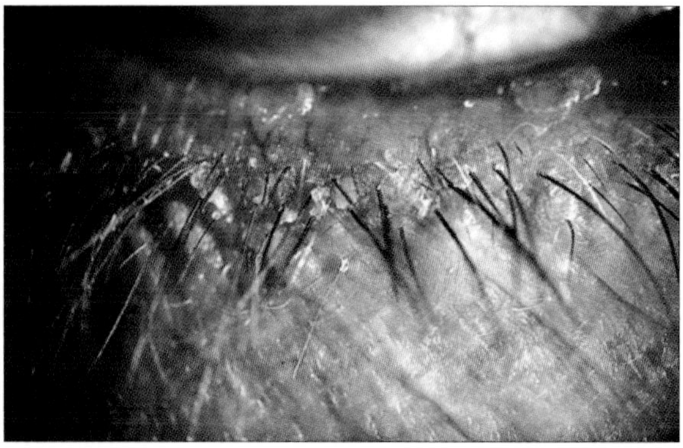

FIGURE 28.5 Blepharitis

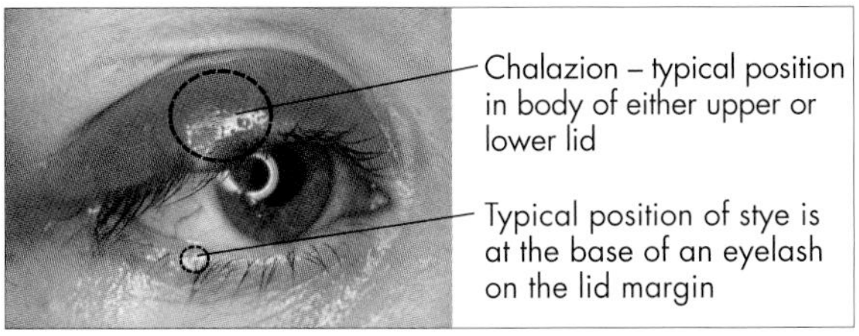
Chalazion – typical position in body of either upper or lower lid
Typical position of stye is at the base of an eyelash on the lid margin

FIGURE 28.6 Eyelid chalazion and lid margin stye

Episcleritis causes a tender red eye. The redness is over the bulbar sclera and maybe localised, sectoral or diffuse. There are no other ocular signs. It is rarely associated with an underlying systemic condition. Symptomatic treatment with lubricants and/or non-steroidal anti-inflammatory drops leads to complete resolution.

Scleritis is uncommon and characterised by a deep, severe ocular pain. This needs to be referred to an ophthalmologist for management, as it may be vision threatening. Scleritis may be associated with autoimmune disease (rheumatoid arthritis, Wegener's granulomatosis, systemic lupus erythematosus, scleroderma) and treatment may involve systemic immunosuppression.

Pterygium and pinguecula

A pathologically identical, fleshy conjunctival overgrowth changes from *pinguecula* to *pterygium* when it extends onto the cornea.

Damage occurs to the conjunctival basal cells as a result of sun exposure.

Patients present with ocular irritation, redness and, rarely, altered vision from corneal indentation, impingement on the visual axis or dry eye.

Treatment—ocular lubricants and protection from sun exposure. Patients should be encouraged to wear a hat and wraparound sunglasses. Patients predisposed to pterygium (blue eyes, fair complexion) are also at increased risk of skin cancers and should be warned about this.

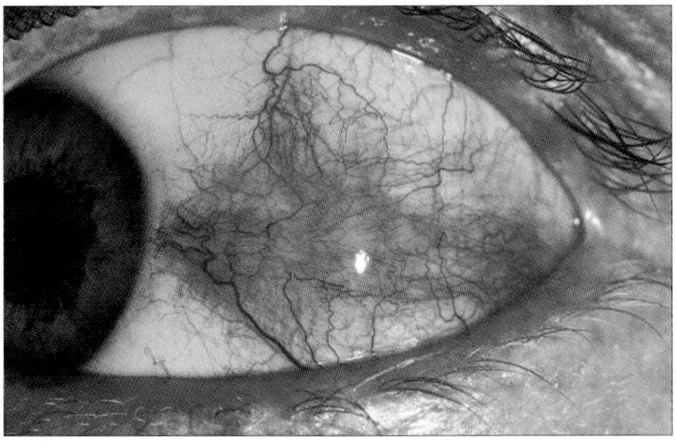

FIGURE 28.7 Episcleritis

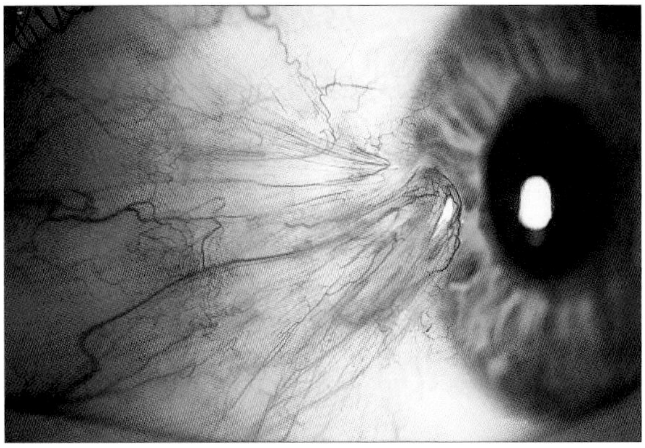

FIGURE 28.8 Pterygium

If symptoms are severe and unresponsive to lubricants, the ophthalmologist may prescribe a weak steroid for a short time to control inflammation, or recommend surgical excision. The pterygium is excised and a conjunctival graft is sutured onto the defect to decrease the chance of recurrence. Surgery has a high success rate.

Occasionally, precancerous dysplasia and frank squamous cell carcinoma may mimic a pterygium.

Corneal disease

Abrasion, foreign body

A corneal abrasion, usually from trauma, is an epithelial defect that stains with fluorescein.

Check the cornea for a foreign body. A metallic foreign body rapidly forms a rust ring and requires prompt removal with adequate anaesthesia, movement control, magnification and illumination.

Patients present with a history of trauma and a painful, watery and red eye. Depending on the location of the defect (central or peripheral) and the size, vision might be affected.

Treatment—prevention and detection of infection while healing occurs, usually within several days. A topical antibiotic (e.g. gtt chloramphenicol q.i.d.) is used until healing is complete. Daily follow-up may be necessary until resolution. Lubricant drops should be used for at least a month to minimise risk of recurrent corneal erosion.

Keratitis (bacterial, viral)

A corneal abscess usually follows corneal trauma, except in contact lens wearers, where microtrauma routinely occurs during insertion and removal; this favours bacterial infection.

A corneal abscess is seen as an area of white cell infiltrate, with an overlying epithelial defect and an inflammatory reaction in the anterior chamber (even to the extent of hypopyon). It is usually extremely painful and if not treated promptly may result in permanent visual loss, secondary to scarring, especially if central.

All contact lens wearers with an acute red eye should be referred to an ophthalmologist that day.

Depending on the size and location of the abscess, an ophthalmologist will perform corneal scrapings to send for urgent microscopy, culture and sensitivity testing. After this, antibiotic treatment with fortified and broad-spectrum antibiotics is commenced. As drops are administered every 15 minutes including overnight, these patients usually require hospital admission.

Prognosis is variable, depending on the organism isolated and abscess location. *Pseudomonas*, common in contact lens wearers, is extremely aggressive.

Prevention of corneal infection is achieved through patient education, nightly contact lens removal and cleaning with an approved sterilising agent. Contact lenses should be checked regularly for deposits and tears prior to insertion and should be removed from the eyes immediately when ocular pain, redness or decreased vision occurs.

Viral keratitis, usually due to herpes simplex virus (HSV) or herpes zoster virus (HZV), forms a dendrite (branching structure) on the cornea that stains with fluorescein. Corneal sensation is absent when tested with a wisp of cotton, and vision is reduced.

These viruses have a number of ocular (e.g. conjunctivitis, keratitis, uveitis, scleritis, glaucoma, retinitis) and systemic (e.g. cranial nerve palsy, meningitis, stroke) complications.

Avoid and remove all steroid drops if you suspect viral keratitis.

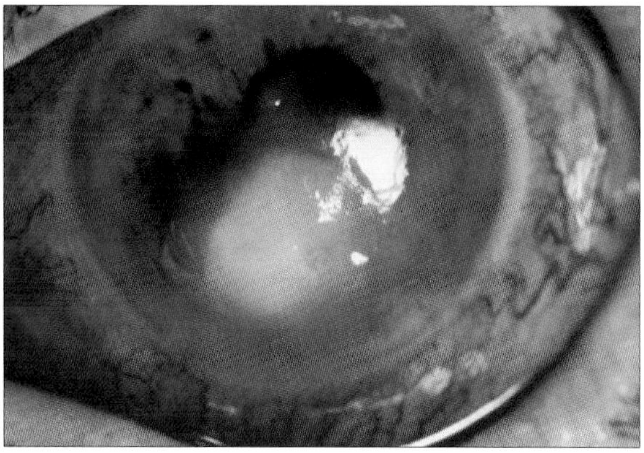

FIGURE 28.9 Bacterial keratitis with abscess

Patients should be referred to an ophthalmologist for assessment and treatment with topical aciclovir 5 times a day. Steroid drops may be added by an ophthalmologist, once the infection is controlled, to minimise scarring.

If the condition is systemic or the patient is immunosuppressed, oral aciclovir/famciclovir/valaciclovir is indicated.

Trauma

Chemical injury

The eyelids, conjunctiva and cornea are commonly affected. Alkali injuries may continue to penetrate deeper tissues even after removal of the toxin.

Treatment should be initiated immediately—lavage with normal saline until pH is neutral. Local anaesthetic may be required. Transfer to hospital with continued irrigation if necessary en route.

Carefully remove particulate matter with a moist cotton bud, check conjunctival fornices to their depths. Assess the depth and extent of injury. Patients with severe injuries are hospitalised and treated with intensive drops to prevent infection and scarring while promoting healing.

Blunt trauma

Blunt trauma sends a shock wave though the globe, which may affect all ocular structures. A systematic examination, from anterior (corneal abrasion, hyphaema, traumatic mydriasis, uveitis) to more posterior (cataract, vitreous haemorrhage, commotio retinae, choroidal rupture, retinal detachment, optic nerve avulsion, ruptured globe) will reveal the damage sustained. Any patient with a history of significant trauma or any signs should be referred to an ophthalmologist. Place a protective shield over the eye without pressure, once the eyelids have been closed gently. Complications (e.g. glaucoma) may occur decades later.

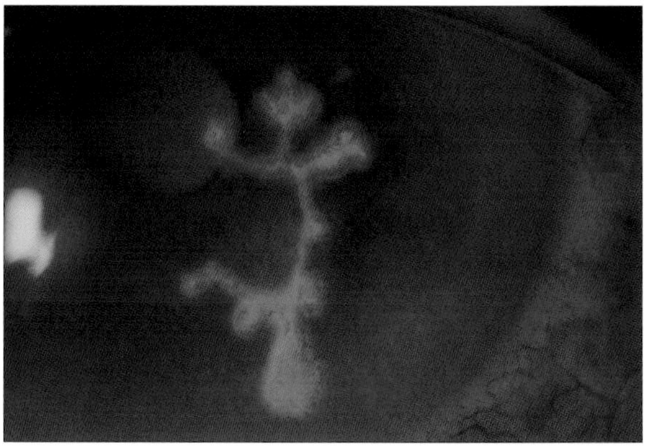

FIGURE 28.10 Corneal dendrite stained with fluorescein

Penetrating eye injury

Patients present with a history of trauma with a sharp object or a small high-speed projectile (e.g. hammering metal on metal). Suspect a penetrating injury or intraocular foreign body from grinding or hammering metal. The signs maybe subtle, but vision is reduced and the iris appears abnormal.

If a ruptured globe, penetrating eye injury or intraocular foreign body is suspected:

- Do not press on the globe.
- Protect the eye with a plastic shield.
- Give analgesia, antiemetic, antibiotic and tetanus booster as appropriate.
- Keep patient fasted.
- Refer to an ophthalmologist as soon as possible for examination, imaging and surgical repair.

Uveitis

Uveitis is inflammation of the uveal tract of the eye, affecting the iris (anterior uveitis), ciliary body (intermediate uveitis) or choroid (posterior uveitis).

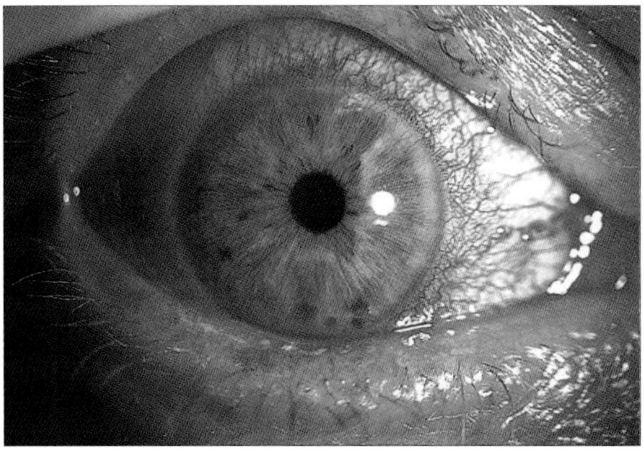

FIGURE 28.11 Anterior uveitis with red eye and miosis

Anterior uveitis or iritis is the most common. The patient presents with red eye, photophobia, ocular pain and decreased vision.

On examination there is decreased visual acuity, ciliary injection (perilimbal redness) and pupillary

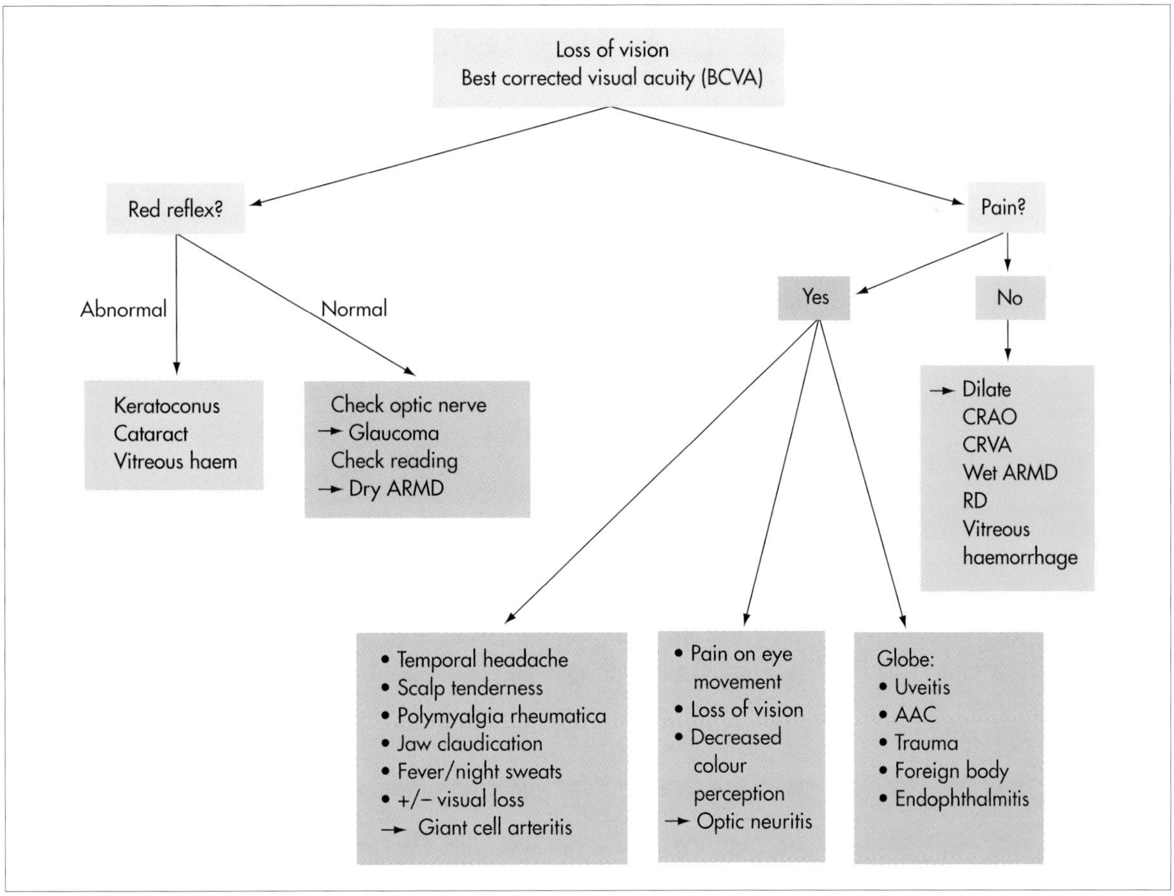

FIGURE 28.12 Loss of vision flow chart

constriction (miosis). Slit lamp examination reveals anterior chamber cells and flare (white blood cells and protein).

Half of anterior uveitis cases are idiopathic.

Associations include:

- systemic diseases
  - ankylosing spondylitis (most common) and other HLA B27 positive disease
  - sarcoidosis
  - juvenile rheumatoid arthritis
- infectious diseases
  - toxoplasmosis
  - tuberculosis
  - syphilis
  - HIV
- drugs
  - HIV medications (rifabutin, cidofovir)
- ocular syndromes
- trauma.

The general practitioner should be involved in the systemic work-up of a uveitis patient. Investigations include blood tests (antinuclear antibody (ANA), antineutrophil cytoplasmic antibody (ANCA), ESR, C-reactive protein, syphilis test, rheumatoid factor, HLA B27, HIV) and a chest X-ray (tuberculosis and sarcoidosis).

Ocular treatment, initiated by an ophthalmologist, involves steroids and mydriatics. The iris is dilated to prevent central posterior internal adhesions.

In the absence of systemic disease, most patients achieve complete resolution following an episode of acute anterior uveitis. An appropriate referral should be made to a physician if an underlying cause is found or if anterior uveitis becomes recurrent or chronic.

Acute angle closure

Acute angle closure occurs in the presence of an anatomically narrow anterior chamber angle. It is more common in older individuals (larger crystalline lens), females (smaller eyes) and especially people of Chinese descent. It is often precipitated in semi-dark conditions, when the pupil is mid-dilated.

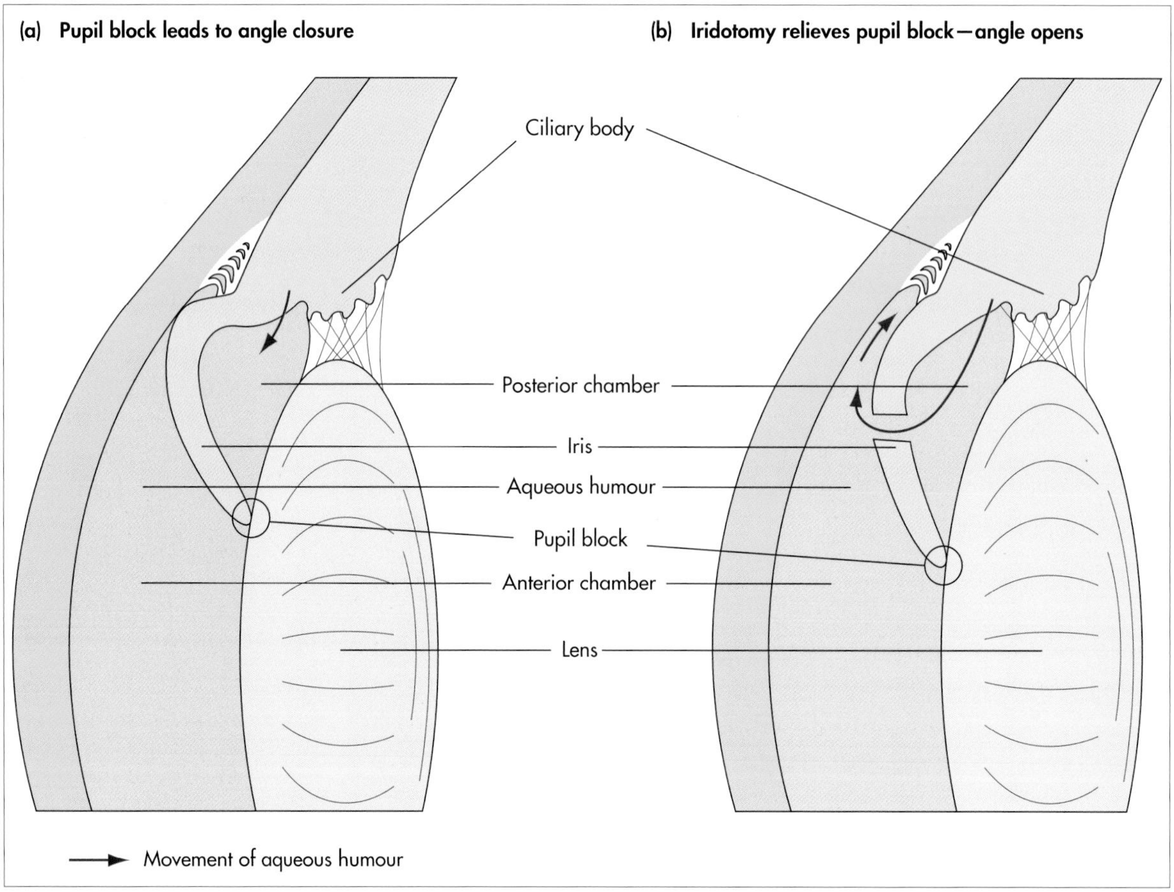

FIGURE 28.13 Acute angle closure

Warning signs may precede full closure: intermittent episodes of ocular pain and redness, with blurred vision and coloured rings around lights. In an acute angle closure crisis, pain is often severe and there may be nausea and even vomiting. Vision blurs as the cornea becomes cloudy, there is perilimbal injection, the pupil is mid-dilated and non-reactive to light, and digital eye pressure is extremely high.

Refer the patient urgently for treatment, to minimise irreversible damage to the anterior and posterior segments of the eye.

Definitive treatment eliminates pupil block and re-establishes aqueous outflow through the trabecular meshwork. A hole is made in the peripheral iris with a laser (laser iridotomy). After the attack has been broken, the patient is assessed and treated if needed, as per primary open-angle glaucoma (see below).

LOSS OF VISION IN THE WHITE EYE

Loss of vision is a common presentation to the general practitioner. On examination the external eye appears normal. Speed of referral to an ophthalmologist depends on the duration and onset of symptoms. Sudden visual loss should be referred promptly and is usually due to a vascular or retinal cause.

Gradual vision loss (BCVA) can be due to cataract and, more rarely, glaucoma. A slow onset of loss may be discovered suddenly by a patient (usually by covering the other eye for the first time).

Cataract

Cataract is opacification of the crystalline lens. It is most commonly related to age ('senile' cataract). Other types are congenital, drug-related (steroids, amiodarone, chlorpromazine, anti-glaucoma drops), traumatic, and related to ocular (e.g. uveitis, retinitis pigmentosa) and systemic diseases (e.g. diabetes, atopy, neurofibromatosis, myotonic dystrophy).

Many causes for senile cataract have been investigated, without a single cause found. Sunlight exposure may contribute. Wearing sunglasses and a hat is a relatively simple protective measure. Diet has also been extensively studied, with varied results. In a recent paper, high dietary intake of lutein/zeaxanthin and vitamin E seem to be partly protective.[3] Smoking is an independent risk factor.

Visual complaints from cataracts depend on morphology, location and type of lens opacities present. There is commonly a decrease in visual clarity (distance and near, and not correctable with glasses), foggy or misty vision, glare especially associated with driving at night (from oncoming car headlights) and a paradoxical improvement in near vision (nuclear sclerosis increases lens dioptric power, thus possibly facilitating close work focus).

On examination there is decreased BCVA and opacity on red reflex in the visual axis.

A dilated slit lamp examination determines the type, severity and associated ocular conditions requiring management. An assessment is made of the need for and risks of surgery for that individual eye and patient.

Cataracts do not 'damage' the eye unless they precipitate angle closure or are allowed to become hypermature. A decision to extract a cataract depends on the patient's symptoms, visual needs and lifestyle. Poor vision in the elderly is related to depression and an increased risk of falls.

Any surgical procedure should be conducted only when the possible benefits outweigh the risks to an individual patient. In cataract surgery, the cataractous lens is removed and replaced by an artificial one. This is usually conducted under assisted local or topical anaesthesia and most patients are awake but comfortable.

Cataract surgery is generally safe and successful. Complications occur rarely; the most serious include infection (endophthalmitis), intraocular haemorrhage, retinal detachment and decreased vision in the fellow eye from a very rare autoimmune condition (sympathetic ophthalmia). Other complications (raised intraocular pressure, macular oedema, a second-stage operation if zonules or posterior capsule have torn) may lead to a prolonged and difficult postoperative course but often do not prevent good long-term results.

Most patients will need to use antibiotic and steroid drops for around 1 month postoperatively, and attend follow-up with their ophthalmologist during this time. Even years later, opacification of the 'bag' (posterior

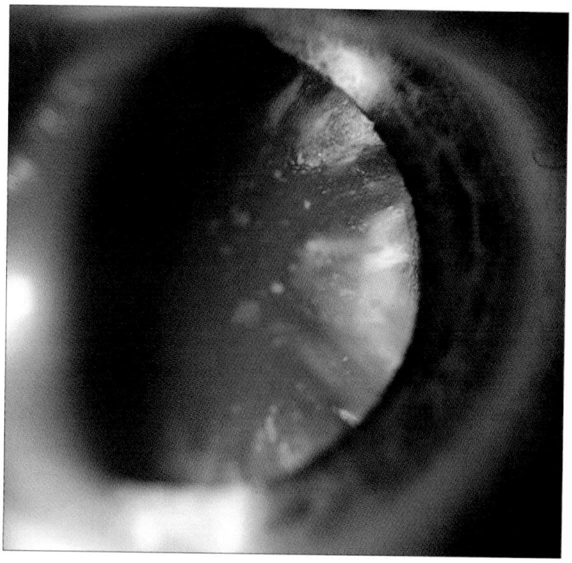

FIGURE 28.14 Cataract

capsule) in which the artificial lens sits may diminish vision. This is treated with a laser posterior capsulotomy.

The general practitioner and the ophthalmologist together facilitate the patient's readiness for and recovery from surgery.

Glaucoma

Glaucoma is a group of diseases which cause progressive optic neuropathy. They are classified into primary (absence of other conditions) and secondary (known cause). Open versus angle closure describes aqueous dynamics and depends on the gonioscopic appearance of the anterior chamber drainage angle. The most common type of glaucoma in our community is primary open-angle glaucoma.

Primary open-angle glaucoma

The main risk factors for primary open-angle glaucoma (POAG) are advancing age, family history and an elevated intraocular pressure.

The condition is usually asymptomatic in the early stages. As the glaucoma advances, the patient increasingly loses visual field and may complain of bumping into things or falling. Glaucoma causes irreversible visual loss, and is the leading cause of preventable blindness globally.

The key to management is early diagnosis by opportunistic screening, followed by regular monitoring and appropriate treatment.

Diagnosis is made by optic nerve examination and visual field assessment. In a general practice office, a decrease in visual acuity can be measured (not usually from the glaucoma itself), and a visual field defect elicited if sufficiently extensive. A relative afferent pupillary defect (see pupil examination, earlier) detects optic nerve function asymmetry between the two eyes.

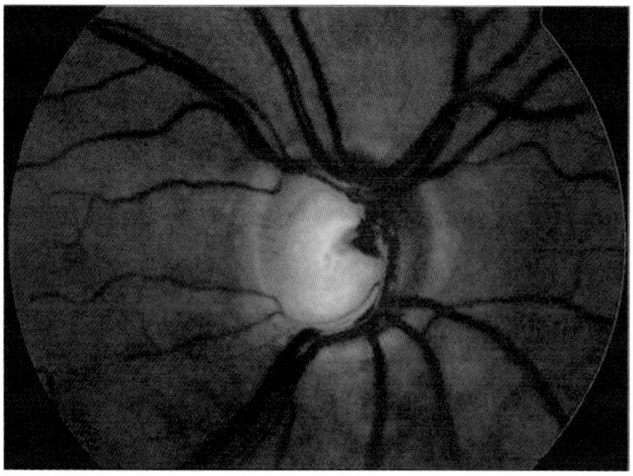

FIGURE 28.15 Glautomatous optic disc with inferior and superior rim thinning

This is usually the case in early to moderate glaucoma, and is a very useful way for general practitioners to detect this progressive disease simply and quickly while it is asymptomatic.

An ophthalmologist will measure intraocular pressure, and evaluate and record the appearance of the optic nerve head. Diagnostic tests (perimetry) are performed to determine optic nerve function.

Treatment, initiated by an ophthalmologist, involves intraocular pressure reduction, usually at first with drops, but sometimes with laser trabeculoplasty. There are five classes of ocular hypotensive medications: alpha-adrenergic agonists (brimonidine, apraclonidine), beta-blockers (timolol, betaxolol), carbonic anhydrase inhibitors (topical dorzolamide and brinzolamide, systemic acetazolamide), cholinergics (pilocarpine) and lipid receptor agonists (latanoprost, bimatoprost, travoprost). There are also fixed combinations of timolol with some of these, such as with latanoprost (Xalacom™), with travoprost (DuoTrav™), with bimatoprost (Ganfort™), with dorzolamide (Cosopt™) and with brimonidine (Combigan™).

Medications are tailored to the individual patient. All may have local side effects and many have the potential for systemic side effects, as drops can enter the systemic circulation directly through the nasopharyngeal mucosa. In this way, topical medications can mimic intravenous medications.

To widen the systemic safety of topically applied agents, patients should be guided to adopt the 'double DOT' instillation technique (Digital Occlusion of the Tear Duct, and Don't Open Technique). After instilling drops, the lacrimal sac should be occluded steadily with index finger digital compression and the eye closed for 3 minutes. This reduces systemic absorption by two-thirds. If more than one drug is used, wait at least 5 minutes between drops to obtain maximal advantage from each.

Eye pressure can also be reduced by laser and surgical treatments.

Retinal and vitreous detachment

Posterior vitreous detachment (PVD) is part of normal ageing. As the vitreous liquefies and separates from the retina, a peripheral retinal tear can form. If fluid enters through the tear, a retinal detachment follows.

Vitreous detachment causes floaters, seen as black spots that move with the eye in the vision. Symptoms of *retinal detachment* include new floaters, flashes of light, decreased vision or a new scotoma (area of missing vision). All patients with these symptoms should be referred that day.

Symptoms associated with PVD usually settle spontaneously within months. However, the retina needs to

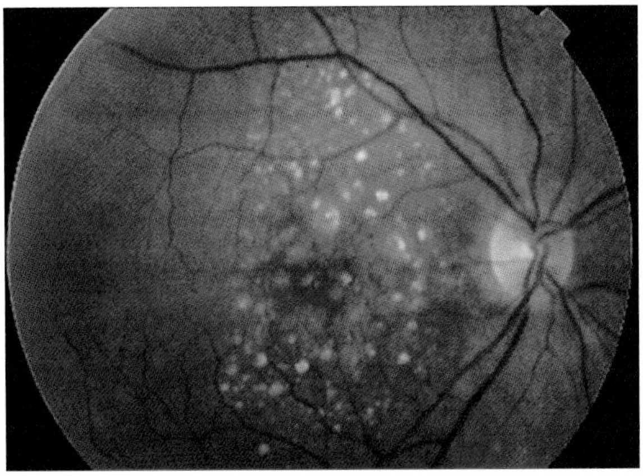

FIGURE 28.16 Dry macular degeneration with drusen and atrophy

be checked for tears and holes—these can be treated with laser. Retinal detachment often requires surgery.

Age-related macular degeneration

Age-related macular degeneration (ARMD) is a condition affecting the macula (the area for central vision) of patients aged over 50, with characteristic slit lamp features. This leads to a decrease in central vision (reading, writing, recognising faces, watching television).

There are two types, based on morphology. *Dry or atrophic* type comprises 80–90% of cases, and is characterised by retinal drusen (deposits of lipid waste products) and areas of atrophy. This leads to a gradual decline in central vision.

Wet or neovascular type occurs in only 10–20% of cases, but is responsible for most severe and sudden visual loss. Retinal features include choroidal neovascular membrane formation, areas of haemorrhage and scarring.

Patients present with a decrease in reading vision, not correctable with reading glasses, distortion of straight lines (metamorphopsia) or missing letters (scotoma) and difficulty recognising faces. These symptoms can occur gradually over years as in the dry form, or suddenly over days in the wet variety.

There is no specific treatment for dry macular degeneration but much research is being conducted in this area. Treatment targets other reversible ocular conditions contributing to visual loss, such as cataract, and monitoring for neovascular changes. Education is provided regarding risk factors, provision of visual aids, support groups and information (see below).

Wet ARMD needs early referral, diagnosis and intervention. Retinal bleeding commonly obscures the neovascular membrane. Ocular coherence tomography (OCT) and fluorescein angiography permit diagnosis and guide management. Neovascular membranes are classified according to proximity to the fovea (subfoveal, juxtafoveal and extrafoveal), type of vascular pattern (e.g. classic or occult) and size.

Juxtafoveal or extrafoveal membranes may be treated with thermal argon laser, as the resulting scotoma is not at the centre of vision.

Subfoveal and some juxtafoveal lesions can be treated with intravitreal injections of an antivascular endothelial growth factor (anti-VEGf). These agents may maintain or even improve vision, and have revolutionised management over the past few years. Injections may be needed every 4–6 weeks while the vascularisation process is active; monitoring is lifelong. The most serious risk of intravitreal injections is intraocular infection (endophthalmitis), with a reported prevalence of less than 1%.

Early diagnosis and treatment in wet ARMD is essential to improve prognosis. Patients are asked to monitor their central vision daily, using an Amsler grid: they look steadily at the central dot, one eye at a time, with reading glasses on, noting any new or changed patches of metamorphopsia. In this way, even mild retinal oedema can be recognised early by the apparent distortion of lines and areas of absent lines. If this occurs, treatment should be initiated within a few days.

The important risk factors for ARMD are increasing age, smoking and family history. Cardiovascular risk factors such as hypertension also contribute.

There are no definitive dietary guidelines. A healthy diet low in animal fat and high in fish is recommended.

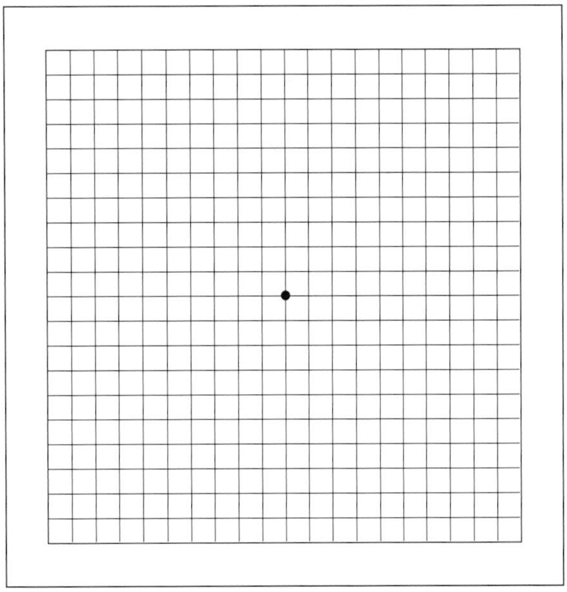

FIGURE 28.17 Amsler grid

A variety of vegetables of different colours, especially green leafy ones, may be beneficial.

Specific ARMD vitamin formulations are available over the counter, and these may help to slow the progression of already established ARMD; however, they have not been shown to affect early disease or prevent disease occurring.

The Age-Related Eye Disease Study (AREDS)[4] found that a combination of antioxidant vitamins plus zinc helped slow the progression of intermediate macular degeneration to an advanced stage, which is when most vision loss occurs. The US National Eye Institute recommends that people with intermediate ARMD in one or both eyes or with advanced ARMD (wet or dry) in one eye but not the other take this formulation each day.[5] However, this combination of nutrients did not help prevent ARMD, nor did it slow progression of the disease in those with early ARMD. The doses of nutrients are:

- vitamin C (500 mg per day)
- vitamin E (400 IU per day)
- beta-carotene (15 mg per day, or 25 000 IU of vitamin A)
- zinc (80 mg per day)
- copper (2 mg per day, to prevent copper deficiency that can occur when taking extra zinc).

Any patient already taking other supplements needs to consider correct total doses of nutrients. Beta-carotene increased the rate of lung cancer in smokers and for this reason has been omitted in commonly available commercial preparations.

A patient qualifies for a blind pension if 'legally blind'—this means BCVA of 6/60 in the better eye and/or less than 10 degrees of visual field around fixation in both eyes. All medical practitioners caring for a patient should be aware of community support available from government departments and non-government organisations, and should ensure that the patient is receiving appropriate assistance, not only financially, but also to maintain their safety and maximise their visual performance and, thus, their independence and dignity.

Retinal vascular disease

Diabetic retinopathy

Diabetes affects the microcirculation of the eyes, just as it does elsewhere in the body. Diabetic retinopathy is classified as non-proliferative/background (NPDR) or proliferative (PDR), which can be mild, moderate or severe. *Maculopathy* refers to disease affecting the macula (area for central vision) and can occur in both NPDR and PDR.

As retinopathy is commonly asymptomatic, patients need to be referred for regular screening. At a minimum this should occur annually. Severe retinopathy can lead to blindness through vitreous and retinal haemorrhage(s), retinal scarring and detachment.

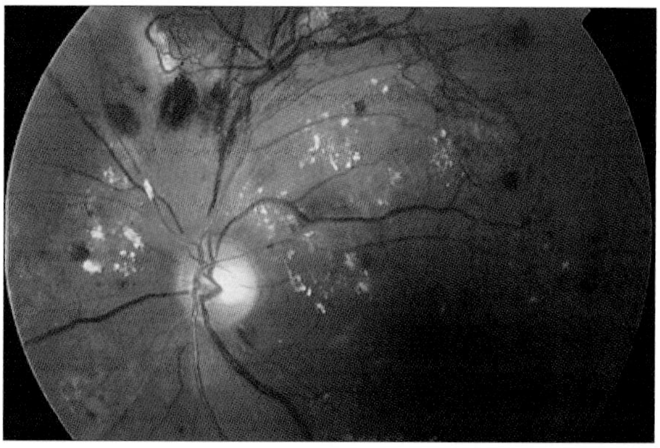

FIGURE 28.18 Proliferative diabetic retinopathy—superior neovascularisation, cotton wool spots, dot and blot haemorrhages

Patients with diabetes may have decreased visual acuity for a number of reasons, the most common being cataract and maculopathy.

A dilated fundus examination needs to be performed by an ophthalmologist.

Retinal fluorescein angiography determines the presence and location of abnormal vessels, areas of ischaemia and macular swelling. Increasingly, macular images with ocular coherence tomography are facilitating management.

The ischaemic retina releases angiogenic factors that promote inappropriate neovascularisation. These new vessels are leaky and prone to haemorrhage; this in turn causes scarring, retinal contraction and detachment.

PDR is treated with thermal laser to destroy ischaemic retina and stop the release of angiogenic factors. The new vessels regress, but laser treatment reduces the visual field, which can be significant when driving. In advanced cases, vitreoretinal surgery may remove vitreous scaffolding, clear haemorrhage and repair detachment. Gentle laser over the macular area decreases macular swelling. There is ongoing research into intravitreal agents also.

The key to successful management is prevention. The patient's general practitioner is paramount in educating, treating and coordinating management. Patients need help to accept responsibility for and control of their blood sugar levels, to stop smoking, to exercise, to adhere to a diabetic diet and to reduce cardiovascular risk factors. The general practitioner coordinates appropriate referral to subspecialists.

Vein occlusion

Vein occlusion occurs in patients with cardiovascular risk factors, and coagulative and autoimmune disorders.

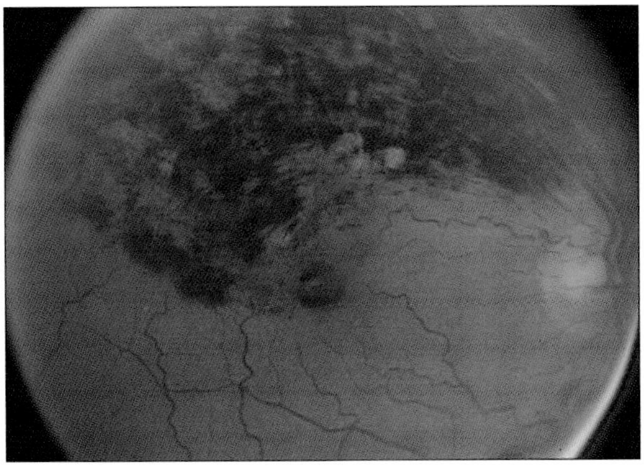

FIGURE 28.19 Branch retinal vein occlusion

Central vein occlusion results in significant visual loss; branch occlusions may be asymptomatic.

Treatment, initiated by the ophthalmologist, is guided by the type and severity of occlusion, with laser to areas of ischaemia and macular swelling.

The prognosis is best for small branch occlusions with good vision and no ischaemia.

Treatment of underlying systemic risk factors is coordinated with the general practitioner and subspecialists. Control of the risk factors minimises the risk of retinal venous disease, and control after a vein occlusion minimises the risk of recurrence.

Arterial occlusion

Arterial occlusion is commonly due to emboli and is associated with other cardiovascular risk factors. It may be central retinal or branch retinal, with visual sequelae dependent on the location and extent.

These patients require a comprehensive cardiovascular work-up, in particular echocardiography and carotid duplex Doppler.

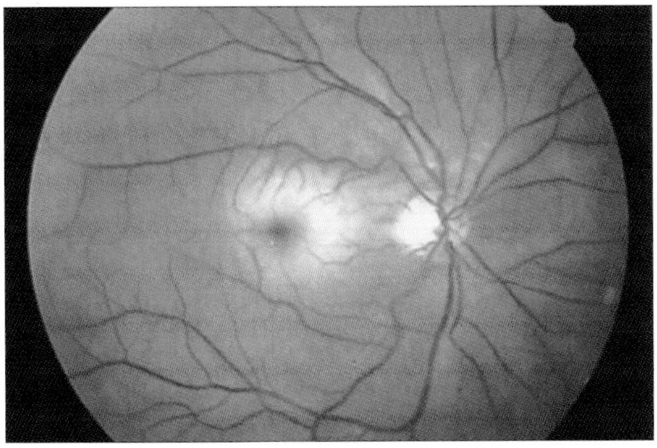

FIGURE 28.20 Central retinal artery occlusion with cherry red spot

Patients present with sudden severe visual loss or 'a curtain coming down' over the vision (amaurosis fugax). The fundus appears pale and infarcted, with a 'cherry red spot' at the macula.

Treat cardiovascular risk factors. The ocular prognosis is poor. If referred and treated early, a few cases have benefited from ocular massage, paracentesis and/or hyperbaric oxygen.

Temporal or giant cell arteritis

Temporal or giant cell arteritis (GCA) can progress very rapidly. It is a systemic vasculitis that can be life threatening as well as blinding. A key feature is pain.

Important associated features of GCA are:

- scalp tenderness
- temporal headache
- jaw claudication—difficulty and pain when chewing
- polymyalgia rheumatica—proximal muscle pain and stiffness
- fevers, night sweats, weight loss, depression.

GCA can affect vision by causing anterior ischaemic optic neuropathy, central retinal artery occlusion, ocular ischaemia, cranial nerve palsy and stroke. Patients with suspected GCA should be referred urgently to an ophthalmologist. Once a clinical diagnosis of GCA is made, patients are commenced on high-dose steroids. Urgent blood tests for ESR and CRP are taken to confirm the diagnosis. Later a temporal artery biopsy is performed for histological confirmation.

PAINFUL EYE

There is much overlap between red and painful eyes. Take a thorough pain history to elicit the differential diagnoses. The diagnoses may not be ocular (Fig 28.21).

DOUBLE VISION

Is the diplopia (double vision) monocular (still seen with one eye closed) or binocular (only present with both eyes open)? (See Fig 28.22.) Monocular diplopia is usually caused by an anatomical change such as refractive error, cataract or retinal pathology in that eye. Binocular diplopia is discussed below.

Neuro-ophthalmology and squint

A true squint is an ocular misalignment where the corneal light reflexes are asymmetrical (Fig 28.23).

Squint in children is asymptomatic. Screening is necessary to avoid permanent visual loss from amblyopia (reduced BCVA despite normal visual pathways). In children, a white pupil reflex (leucocoria) is a very significant sign (Fig 28.24) and must be referred.

Important causes of leucocoria include retinoblastoma, cataract and high refractive error.

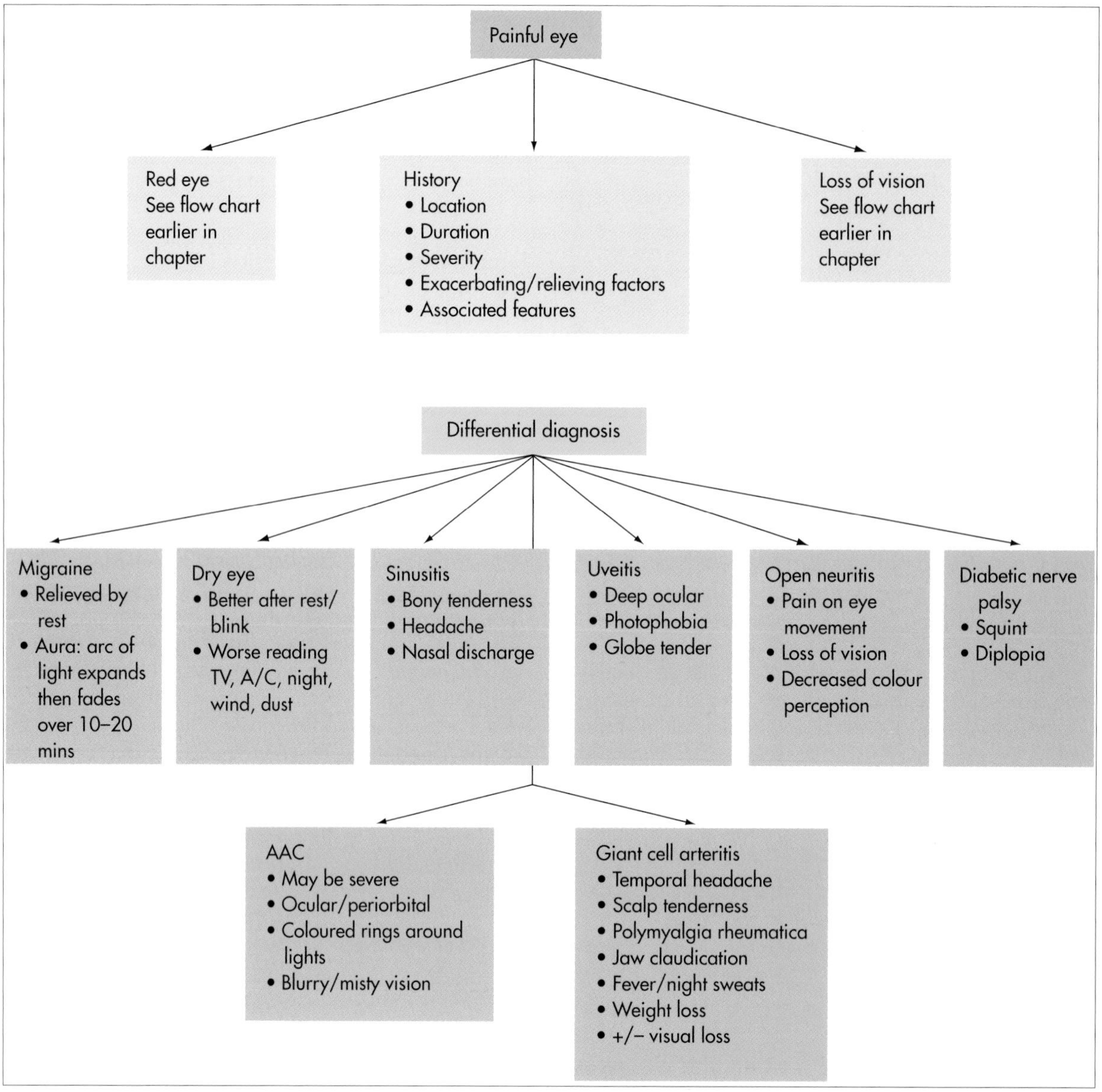

FIGURE 28.21 Painful eye flow chart

New-onset adult squint causes diplopia. Important causes include:

- *cranial nerve (CN) palsies*
  - should be referred to a neurologist or an ophthalmologist
  - *oculomotor CN III*—the eye looks 'down and out' (unopposed lateral rectus and superior oblique muscle action), pupillary dilation and ptosis. Palsy may be complete, partial, involve the pupil or not. If the pupil is involved, a cerebral aneurysm must be excluded. Patient requires an urgent neurosurgical referral. A complete palsy is usually due to a microvascular cause (e.g. hypertension, diabetes).
  - *trochlear CN IV*—the eye is elevated and the patient tilts the head to the affected side to try to compensate for torsion
  - *abducens CN VI*—the eye is unable to turn out (abduction). Look for evidence of raised intracranial pressure, papilloedema and cerebral lesion (see Fig 28.25).
- *thyroid eye disease*
  - causes a vertical squint. Vision is affected from corneal exposure and/or optic neuropathy.

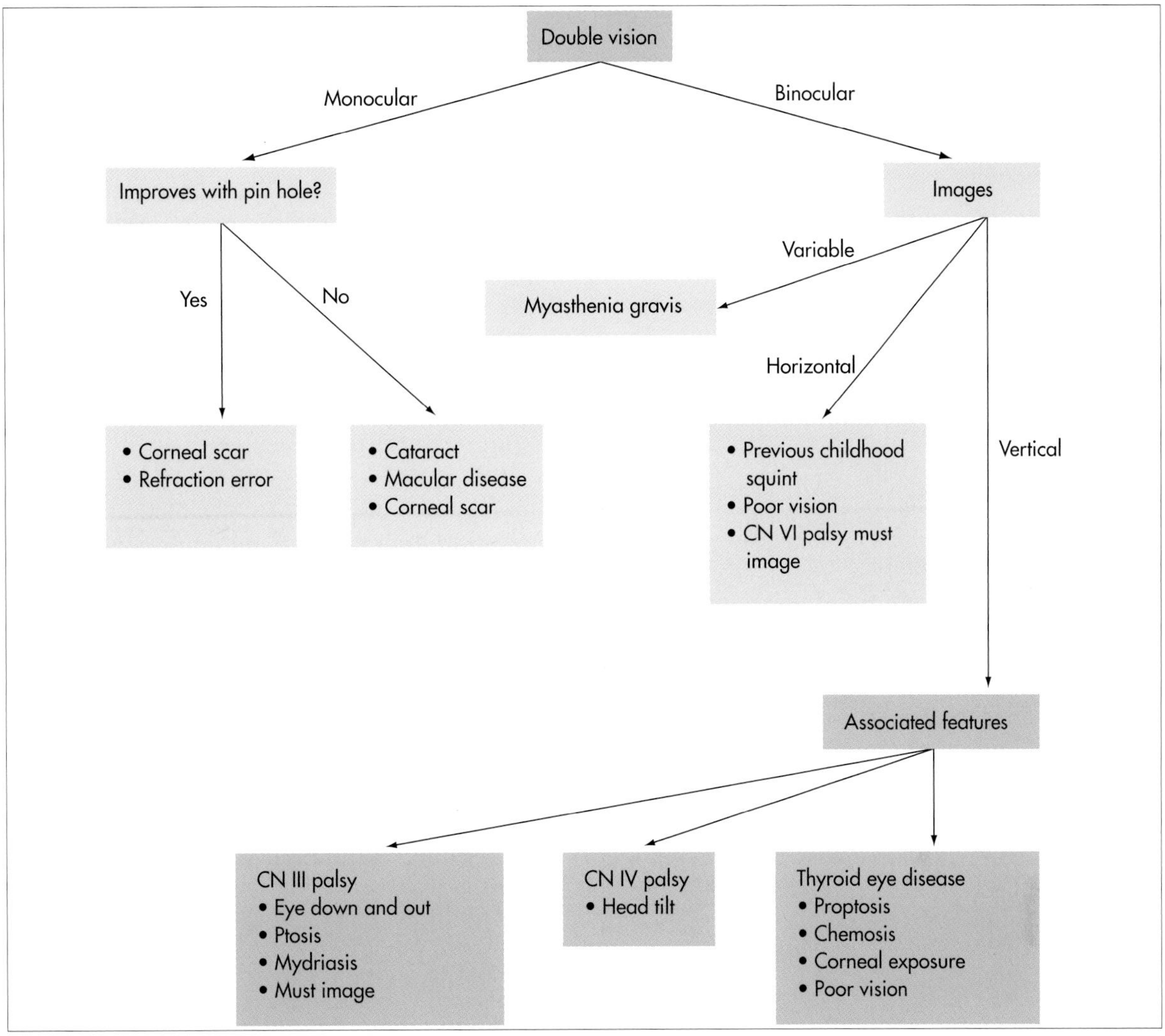

FIGURE 28.22 Double vision flow chart

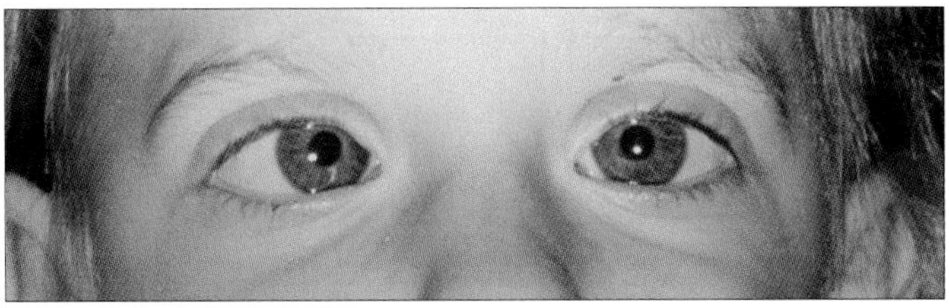

FIGURE 28.23 Strabismus—note asymmetric corneal reflexes

Intraocular pressure may become raised, especially on upgaze (from tight extraocular muscles).

- *myasthenia gravis*
  - causes a squint that varies in type and 'fatigues' throughout the day. Can be life threatening if it affects breathing, talking and swallowing. Requires urgent referral to a neurologist for a Tensilon test and treatment with pyridostigmine bromide (Mestinon®).

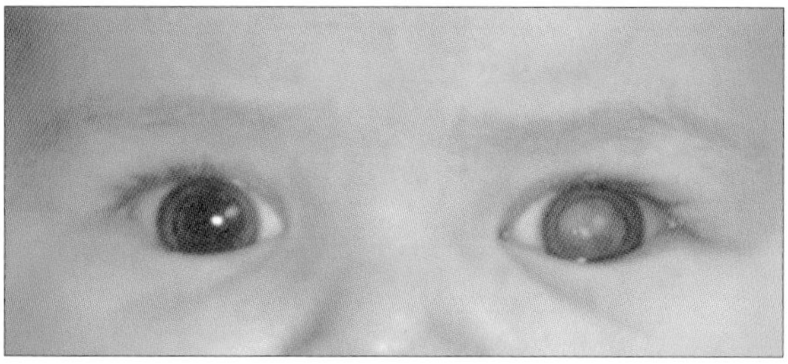

FIGURE 28.24 Leucocoria

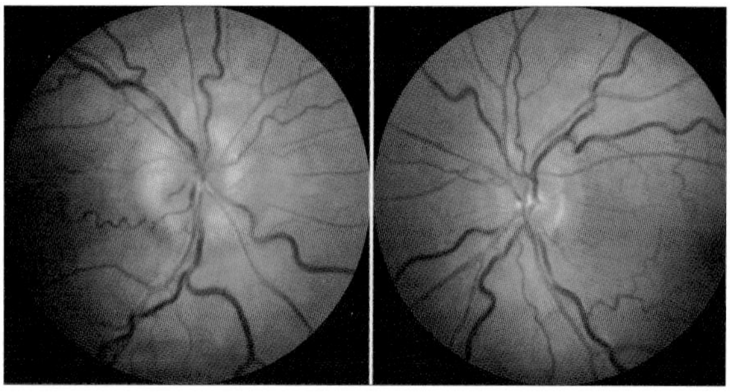

FIGURE 28.25 Papilloedema with disc elevation and indistinct margins

RESOURCES

Glaucoma Australia, www.glaucoma.org.au

Macular Degeneration Foundation www.mdfoundation.com.au

South East Asia Glaucoma Interest Group (SEAGIG), www.seagig.org

Vision Australia, www.visionaustralia.org.au

FURTHER READING

American Academy of Ophthalmology Focal Points. San Francisco: American Academy of Ophthalmology; 2000–2007.

Batterbury M, Bowling B. Ophthalmology: an illustrated colour text. 2nd edn. Edinburgh: Elsevier; 2005.

Kanski J. Clinical ophthalmology, 5th edn. Edinburgh: Butterworth–Heinemann; 2003.

Kanski J. Clinical diagnosis in ophthalmology. Philadelphia: Elsevier; 2006.

Rhee M, Pyfer M. The Wills eye manual. 3rd edn. Philadelphia: Lippincott Williams & Wilkins; 1999.

South East Asia Glaucoma Interest Group (SEAGIG). Asia Pacific Glaucoma Guidelines. Singapore: SEAGIG; 2004.

Webb LA. Manual of eye emergencies diagnosis and management. 2nd edn. Oxford: Butterworth–Heinemann; 2004.

REFERENCES

1 Cho E, Hung S, Willet WC et al. Prospective study of dietary fat and the risk of age-related macular degeneration. Am J Clin Nutr 2001; 73(2):209–218.

2 Townend BS, Townend ME, Flood V et al. Dietary macronutrient intake and five-year incident cataract: the blue mountains eye study. Am J Ophthalmol 2007; 143(6):932–939.

3 Moeller SM, Voland R, Tinker L et al. Associations between age-related nuclear cataract and lutein and zeaxanthin in the diet and serum in the Carotenoids in the Age-Related Eye Disease Study, an Ancillary Study of the Women's Health Initiative. Arch Ophthalmol 2008; 126(3):354–64.

4 Age-Related Eye Disease Study Research Group. A randomized, placebo-controlled, clinical trial of high-dose supplementation with vitamins C and E, beta carotene, and zinc for age-related macular degeneration and vision loss: AREDS Report No. 8. Arch Ophthalmol 2001; 119(10):1417–1436.

5 National Eye Institute, National Institutes of Health. Age-related macular degeneration. Online. Available: http://www.nei.nih.gov/health/maculardegen/armd_facts.asp

chapter 29

Endocrinology

INTRODUCTION AND OVERVIEW

Endocrine problems are important in the general practice setting, for a range of reasons. First, they are common enough to occur regularly, either as new cases or in patients managing a chronic illness. Secondly, they can cause serious and life-threatening complications if not diagnosed and treated. Thirdly, they often present a challenging diagnostic problem because of their often slow onset and their capacity to produce non-specific symptoms such as weakness, tiredness or weight change, particularly in the early stages.

This chapter explores the endocrinological disorders that are important for a GP to know about and to manage. The common model of managing endocrine problems is as a shared-care model with an endocrinologist.

PITUITARY DISORDERS

The pituitary is the 'master controller' of hormone function in the body, converting signals from the brain and hypothalamus to actions via hormones.

The pituitary normally sits in the sella turcica at the base of the middle cranial fossa (Fig 29.1). It is covered by a dural layer known as the diaphragma sella. The pituitary is joined to the hypothalamus by the infundibulum or pituitary stalk, in front of which sits the optic chiasm. The sella turcica is bounded laterally by the cavernous sinuses and their contents, and the sphenoid sinus antero-inferiorly. The anterior pituitary is embryologically derived from the posterior pharynx and secretes prolactin follicle-stimulating hormone (FSH), luteinising hormone (LH), growth hormone (GH), thyrotropin-stimulating hormone (TSH) and adrenocorticotrophic hormone (ACTH) in response to trophic-releasing hormones from the hypothalamus via a portal blood flow system. The posterior pituitary secretes oxytocin and vasopressin under neural control from the hypothalamus.

PITUITARY TUMOUR

Tumours in the pituitary are common and have been found to occur in around 10% of people in autopsy studies.[1] Various series have reported rates of up to 24%. With the high background rate of pituitary masses seen on MRI, clinical questions about how to proceed are likely to occur. Unless the brain is imaged for another reason, it is more prudent to have a clinical diagnosis and confirmatory tests of a pituitary disorder before requesting a CT or MRI of the pituitary.

Tumours of the pituitary may be developmental cysts, blood or infarcted tissue, physiological hyperplasia or adenomas.

Adenomas may be functioning or non-functioning. Physiological effects may be excess autonomous secretion of hormones or trophic hormones, loss of normal pituitary function or mass effects that include compression of nearby structures such as the optic chiasm.

Tumours smaller than 10 mm in size are called *microadenomas*, and those bigger than 10 mm, *macroadenomas*. Compressive effects of a pituitary tumour normally occur when the adenoma grows to > 10 mm and enlarges beyond the pituitary fossa. Common symptoms of a mass effect are headaches and loss of peripheral vision that correlates with a bitemporal hemianopia as the optic chiasm is compressed.

As an adenoma grows, there may be loss of function of the normal anterior pituitary in a typical order. The mnemonic: 'Go Looking For That Adenoma' is a good aide memoire for the order of loss of pituitary function:

- **g**rowth hormone
- **l**uteinising hormone
- **f**ollicle-stimulating hormone
- **t**hyroid-stimulating hormone
- **a**drenocorticotrophic hormone.

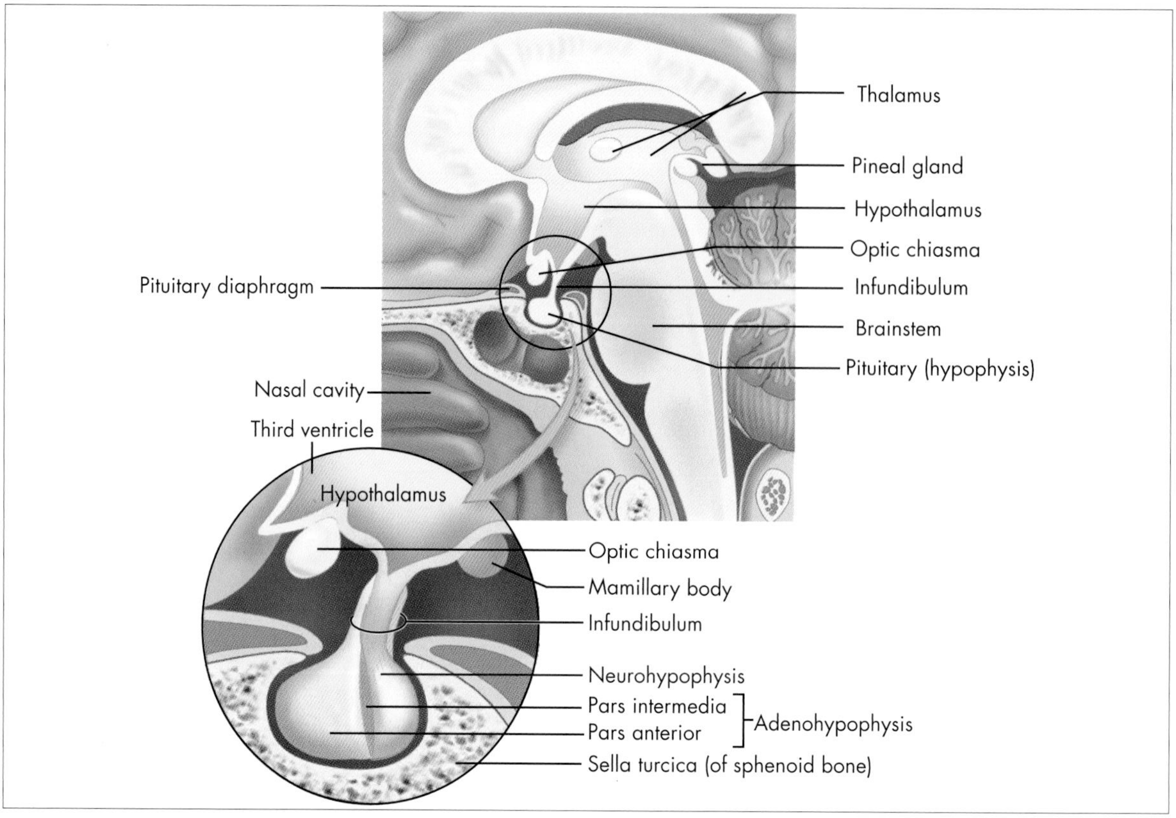

FIGURE 29.1 Anatomy of the pituitary gland and surrounding structures

Aetiology

Pituitary tumours can be:

- primary, as are the majority
- secondary, such as in the case of severe long-standing hypothyroidism where there is growth of the thyrotroph cells in response to a lack of negative feedback from T_3
- very rarely due to metastatic deposits or manifestations of diseases such as Wegener's granulomatosis or histiocytosis X.

Simple developmental cysts account for around 40% of pituitary tumours. Around 20% are adenomas, of which the majority are prolactin-secreting tumours known as prolactinomas. The ACTH-secreting tumours of Cushing's disease or the GH-secreting tumours of acromegaly and gigantism are much rarer. Non-functioning adenomas are also quite common, and may still impair normal anterior pituitary function.

Pathology

It is thought that somatic mutations in cell signal pathways are the cause of primary pituitary tumours, with growth of monoclonal cells. The minority of tumours have a germline mutation aetiology, such as in the case of multiple endocrine neoplasia (MEN-1) and Carney complex.

Diagnostic approach

The most important thing is that the diagnosis of a pituitary hormone-stimulated excess or deficiency is made, or at least suspected, and then the pituitary may be imaged. Tumours are sometimes found when a CT head or MRI brain is performed for another reason. In this case, careful history and examination needs to be done, and then testing for any anterior pituitary hormone deficiencies or excesses may be done.

Tumours are defined by their size and secretion of hormones. Tumours do not tend to invoke a mass-related loss of function of other anterior pituitary hormones until they tend toward macroadenomas. The exception to this is a prolactinoma, which will suppress the gonadotrophs in a normal physiological way even when it is a microprolactinoma.

Prolactinomas tend to produce prolactin in a linear relation to their size. Macroadenomas therefore tend to produce levels of prolactin greater than 10 times the upper limit of the reference range. Microadenomas tend to produce levels of prolactin from 1–10 times the upper limit of normal. Other causes of prolactin in this range include medications with a dopamine antagonistic effect, such as antipsychotics and antiemetics. Stress may cause a transient increase in prolactin, as will physical causes such as nipple stimulation and lesions that affect the T_4 dermatome, including *Varicella zoster*. Masses that result in compression or loss of function of the pituitary stalk also limit the inhibitory signals from the hypothalamus and result in microadenoma-level hyperprolactinaemia.

History

Cushing's disease and TSH-omas tend to present with microadenomas, while acromegaly tumours are more often macroadenomas than they are microadenomas. Prolactinomas can be either, and tend to present as microadenomas in women, due to the objective problems of loss of regular periods.

Apart from pressing on the optic chiasm, prolactinomas may invade laterally into the bones and cavernous sinuses, as they may produce enzymes that erode the bones of the sella. These large tumours therefore may produce mass effects of headaches and visual field losses as well as the symptoms of hormone excesses and losses as noted above.

A family history can be helpful, especially in younger patients, due to the fact that pituitary tumours run together with the almost ubiquitous primary hyperparathyroidism, and also pancreatic endocrine tumours such as insulinomas. This is an autosomal-dominant condition.

TABLE 29.1 Signs, symptoms and tests for pituitary tumours

Condition	Symptoms	Signs	Tests
Acromegaly (gigantism if occurring before closure of epiphyses)	• Hyperhidrosis • Arrhythmias • Ring, glove and shoe size increases • Symptoms of hyperglycaemia • Bone and joint pains • Obstructive sleep apnoea symptoms • Carpal tunnel syndrome	• Macroglossia • Underbite with mandibular prominence • Frontal bone bossing • Left ventricular hypertrophy • Skin tags • Acanthosis nigricans	GH, IGF-1 and OGTT with lack of suppression to < 1 ng/mL
Prolactinoma	• Amenorrhoea • Galactorrhoea • Infertility • Sexual dysfunction (men) • Headache • Visual disturbance	• Few specific • Visual field defect	Serum prolactin
Cushing's disease	• Bruising • Weight gain • Proximal myopathy symptoms • Infections • Symptoms of hyperglycaemia • Fragility fractures	• Violaceous striae • Central obesity • Buffalo hump • Moon facies • Proximal myopathy • Purpura and bruising • Thin skin	• 24 hr urinary free cortisol and creatinine • 1 mg dexamethasone suppression test with ACTH
TSH-oma (very rare)	Hyperthyroid symptoms	Hyperthyroidism	• High TSH • High T_4 • Blunted response to TRH • High alpha-1 glycoprotein subunit
Gonadotroph-oma (rare)	Very few	Very few	

Examination

Target the examination to the symptoms and manifestations of hormone excesses or deficiencies as outlined in Table 29.1. Check for galactorrhoea as well as back and skin lesions in patients suspected with hyperprolactinaemia. Galactorrhoea from one breast in the absence of hyperprolactinaemia requires careful examination to ensure that there is no local breast pathology. Always check visual fields to confrontation.

Investigations

Pathology

In a pituitary mass, checking paired trophic hormones and their target hormones is essential for proper interpretation. Check ACTH and cortisol at around 8–9 am, together with FSH, LH and testosterone (oestrogen in females), which also has a diurnal variation, with higher levels in the morning, TSH and thyroxine (T_4), prolactin (with dilution in macroadenomas), GH and insulin-like growth factor 1 (IGF-1). Non-functioning adenomas tend to produce higher levels of alpha-1 glycoprotein subunit, which may be requested on a sample of serum. Be aware that ACTH in particular degrades quickly, and so informing the laboratory beforehand of an impending test can help ensure it is put on ice and sent to the central laboratory quickly.

The above are static tests. If both results are normal, beware of the inappropriate levels such as a T_4 at the lower limit of normal, with a lower limit of normal TSH (inappropriately normal).

If there are any concerns, dynamic tests may be ordered, although these are often ordered by a specialist and/or in a hospital environment. Of the dynamic test, the oral glucose tolerance test (OGTT) to suppress GH to < 1.0 ng/mL is the only one that is reliable and may safely be done as an outpatient. Twenty-four hour urinary free cortisol and 1 mg overnight dexamethasone suppression tests may also be performed as an outpatient, to help with the investigation of cortisol excess. If an excess is confirmed, then a high-dose dexamethasone suppression test will help delineate whether the problem is Cushing's disease or ectopic ACTH production.

Special tests

Insulin tolerance tests to look for adequate ACTH and GH release can be done, but should be done by an experienced endocrine unit as an inpatient.

Rarely, pituitary adenomas produce central diabetes insipidus, and a water deprivation test needs to be done as an inpatient, to ensure a safe and reliable answer to the test.

Perimetry testing or neuro-ophthalmology should be organised for all patients, especially those with a macroadenoma.

Integrated management

Active surveillance

In microadenomas that have been confirmed to be both non-functioning and not affecting normal pituitary function, it may be appropriate to watch at intervals, monitoring for signs of growth or endocrine disturbances.

Pharmacological and surgical

Prolactinomas are usually medically treated, even if they exhibit mass effects. Dopamine agonists such as cabergoline and bromocriptine can be used to suppress the production of prolactin and to shrink the tumour.

Acromegaly, Cushing's disease and the rare TSH-omas should be considered for surgical treatment in the first instance by an experienced neurosurgeon, although there have been some advances in medical technology with new drugs such as pasireotide, which have a better blockade of the somatostatin 5 and 3 receptors. These receptors are more commonly expressed in acromegaly, and Cushing's/non-functioning adenomas respectively.

There may be some benefit in blocking both D2 and somatostatin receptors together in acromegaly, even though only 20–25% of tumours tend to co-secrete both growth hormone and prolactin.

Other medical

In surgically and medically refractory conditions, radiotherapy may be used to try to control mass and growth, and function of pituitary tumours. The effect is more gradual and also tends to result in panhypopituitarism at a rate of around 5–8% per year. Often, maximal medical therapy needs to be continued while awaiting the radiotherapy effects.

If control cannot be achieved, blocking the production of the target hormone, or blocking its effects, may be an option. Ketaconazole and metyrapone have been used to block the production of cortisol in surgical and medically refractive Cushing's disease. This may also be done in acromegaly with pegvisomant, although with the loss of feedback of IGF-1 on the pituitary, there is the potential for growth of the pituitary tumour.

Ongoing review and/or monitoring

Any patient with a pituitary adenoma should be co-managed by a GP and an endocrinologist. Interval hormone anterior pituitary hormone testing and MRI scans should be organised at intervals that are patient specific.

Important pitfalls

Be wary of the 'normals' in paired pituitary and target hormone testing. Pituitary drive of a particular hormone may be normal but inappropriately low for the level of the target hormone.

Testosterone and gonadotrophs, and the hypothalamic-pituitary-thyroid axis, are the two axes that may be affected most by patient conditions and stressors. If the tests don't make sense, seek endocrinological clarification.

Consider also that sometimes testosterone and growth hormones have been used by athletes to enhance sports performance.

ACROMEGALY

Acromegaly is a condition of monoclonal growth of pituitary somatotrophs that produces excess growth hormone in a non-regulated way. It has a prevalence of around three per million.[2]

GH is normally secreted in a diurnal and metabolic fashion, with pulsatile release that is highest during sleep. Amino acids and ghrelin from the gut are also stimuli to its release via the hypothalamus.

GH stimulates the production of IGF-1 and IGFBP-3 (insulin-like growth factor binding protein-3) on binding to the receptors in the liver. There are some direct effects on the cartilage but, other than that, the majority of the physiological effects of GH are mediated via IGF-1. The liver's ability to produce IGF-1 in response to GH is blunted in liver disease, hypothyroidism and poorly controlled diabetes mellitus. Interestingly, malnutrition reduces IGF-1 production, and obesity inhibits GH pulses from the pituitary.

Aetiology and pathology

There are several somatic mutations that confer autonomous monoclonal cell signal proliferation, or loss of apoptosis that may result in somatotroph growth in the person with other genetic predispositions. The growth is a benign monoclonal expansion that results in the excess secretion of GH, in a non-physiological, non-pulsatile fashion.

The excess IGF-1 and IGFBP-3 that result stimulate the growth of tissues through stimulation of cell proliferation and inhibition of apoptosis. The clinical features are listed below.

If excess GH is produced before the closing of the epiphyses, gigantism occurs and the diagnosis is made relatively quickly with overt clinical signs. In adults the diagnosis may be delayed, due to slow insidious changes in appearance and the overlap with the common primary conditions of diabetes, weight gain, obstructive sleep apnoea and osteoarthritis.

Diagnostic approach

If the clinical diagnosis is suspected on clinical grounds, then testing the visual fields to confrontation and measurement of a static GH and IGF-1 should be done. If the levels are normal but the clinical suspicion is high, then an OGTT suppression test should be performed, to confirm that the GH can suppress to < 1 ng/mL. This is a very sensitive test, with about 85% specificity if > 2 ng/mL after 2 hours.

History

The onset of the separate symptoms may be insidious. Symptoms include:

- symptoms of diabetes mellitus
- arthralgias
- hyperhidrosis
- palpitations and arrhythmias
- reduced exercise tolerance
- increase in shoe, ring, hat or glove size
- symptoms of nerve entrapment such as carpal tunnel syndrome
- symptoms of obstructive sleep apnoea
- weight gain.

Examination

- Visual fields
- Arrhythmias
- Shoe size and weight, head circumference
- Tinels and Phalen's sign of carpal tunnel syndrome
- Greasy skin
- Skin tags in the axillae and acanthosis nigricans
- Signs of pulmonary hypertension, diastolic heart failure or valvular heart disease
- Macroglossia
- Prognathism (prominent mandible with underbite malocclusion)
- Acral bone growth of frontal bone bossing
- Blood pressure
- Goitre.

Investigations

Consulting room:

- An ECG should be performed and a spot capillary glucose with a glucometer may be performed.

Pathology:

- GH, IGF-1
- Remaining anterior pituitary tests with target hormones including prolactin, given acromegaly commonly is a macroadenoma and may therefore exhibit mass effects on the remainder of the anterior pituitary cells.
- Corrected calcium, which may be increased.

Special tests:

- Once the diagnosis has been made, an MRI of the pituitary, a colonoscopy, echocardiogram and staging of the diabetes mellitus should be done.

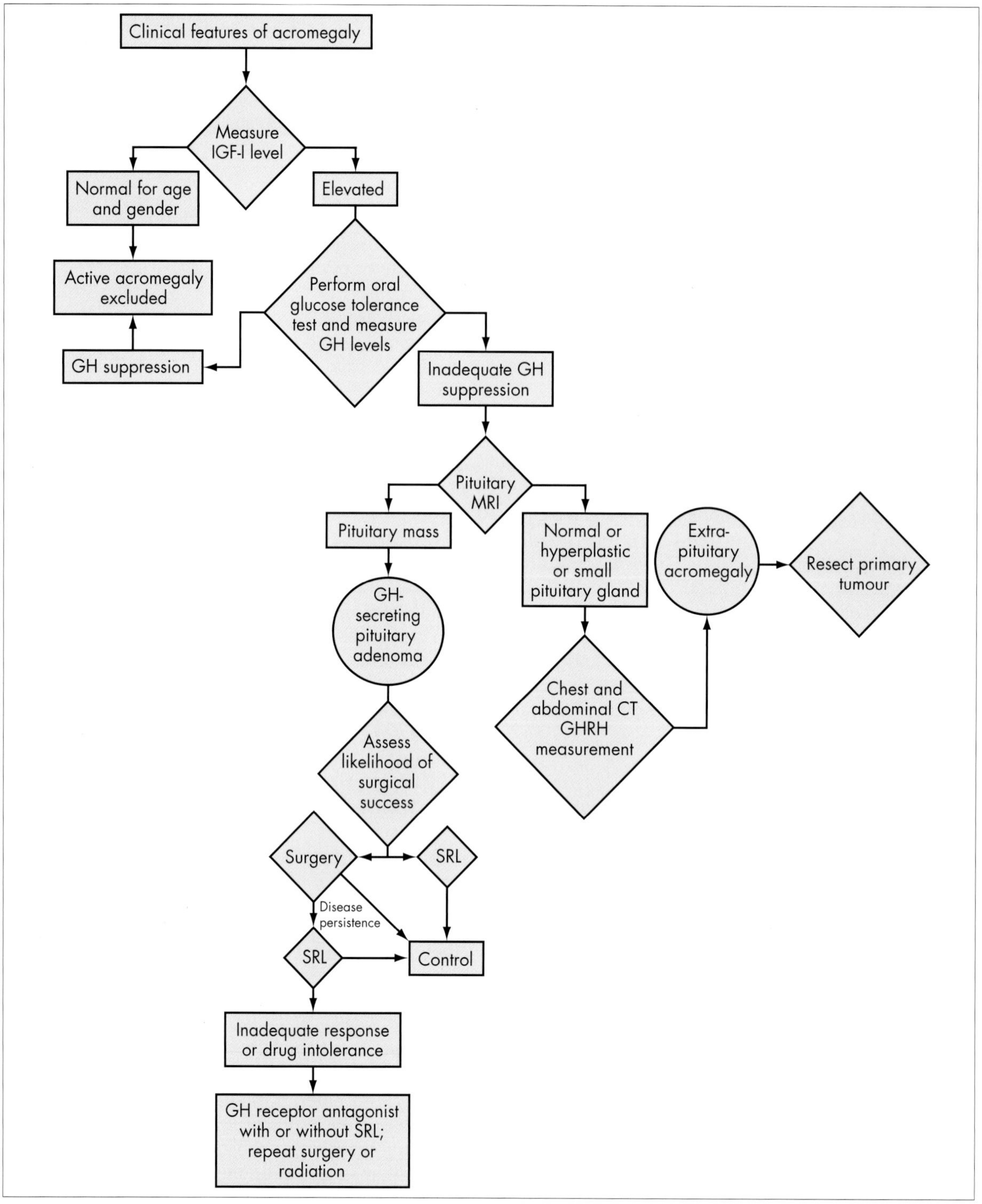

FIGURE 29.2 Integrated management of acromegaly

Integrated management

See Fig 29.2 for an overview of management.

Active surveillance

The patient's preference may be to not have surgery at the time. Acromegaly has been shown to confer an increased mortality, which may limit lifespan by approximately 10 years. This is mainly due to increased cardiovascular morbidity and mortality, and cancer-related mortality.

With either surgical or medical treatment, there is a reduction in mortality back to the baseline with cure.

The metabolic manifestations such as diabetes, hypertension, diastolic heart failure, arrhythmias and hyperhidrosis are all improved with treatment, but patients should be warned that much of the soft tissue growth will not regress, but neither will it progress further. Obstructive sleep apnoea may improve but is often not cured. The longer the patient waits, the more soft tissue will grow.

Surgical

Surgical management is the currently accepted primary treatment for the majority of acromegalic adenomas. Macroadenomas have a lower cure rate and higher complication rate than microadenomas, on the whole. Complications include diabetes insipidus or syndrome of inappropriate antidiuretic hormone hypersecretion (SIADH), and hypopituitarism, including panhypopituitarism. Immediate surgical risks include bleeding and CSF leaks.

Pharmacological

While surgical management is still thought to be the primary option for acromegaly, there are some data indicating that long-acting octreotide, in the form of octreotide LAR, shrinks acromegalic adenomas without complete regression. This takes several months of treatment and the effects are modest. At this stage there are no outcome data indicating that this improves surgical outcomes when used in this neo-adjuvant way. Microadenomas do have a higher surgical cure rate and lower complication rate than do macroadenomas.

Somatostatin analogues or SRIFs (somatomedin-releasing inhibitory factors) currently on the market are octreotide, octreotide LAR and lanreotide. These three tend to be more active against the SST-2 receptors expressed in lower levels on acromegalic tumours, and less active at blocking the SST-5 receptors, which are more prevalent. Pasireotide has a stronger effect at blocking SST-5 receptors and less effect at SST-2, so as it becomes available, medical therapy may become more successful at controlling acromegaly. Octreotide or lanreotide ± D2 agonist is the current medical treatment. The somatostatin analogues may be given as injections once a month and should be started at the lowest dose, warning the patient of diarrhoea, nausea and cholecystitis as possible complications of therapy. Dopamine agonists (DA) may produce nausea and peripheral vasodilatation, resulting in postural hypotension on the days it is given.

Ongoing review and/or monitoring

Given that the majority of acromegalic tumours are macroadenomas at the time of diagnosis, complete surgical cure is not a certainty. Confirmation of cure should be carried out with a measurement of GH in the perioperative period together with confirmation of pituitary reserve.

Cure and return to background-for-age mortality risk occurs when an OGTT is able to suppress GH to a level of < 1 ng/mL. Yearly MRI is prudent for a few years, to ensure no recurrence of the tumour, together with biochemical testing as required.

For those with improved but not cured acromegaly, medical management should be aimed at the same GH target. The interval for re-imaging the pituitary with contrast will be patient specific, depending on the size and location of residual tumour and symptomatology, but should be at least yearly as a default. The neurosurgeons or endocrinologists will provide guidance if different from this.

Important pitfalls

Acromegaly may be missed by even the most astute clinicians, and unless the diagnosis is entertained, a history checked and the tests done, it will not be discovered.

Prognosis

The prognosis depends on whether the GH levels return to normal. If so, the mortality, which is mainly due to cardiovascular disease, returns to the background for non-acromegalic patients. There may be some residual medical morbidity associated with the irreversible issues of joint pains and osteoarthritis, OSA and cosmetic changes.

HYPOPITUITARISM

Hypopituitarism may be complete (pan-) or partial. It may be congenital, acquired or iatrogenic.

Congenital problems are many and rare, and such things as PIT-1 gene mutations cause a loss of lactotrophs (prolactin), thyrotrophs (TSH) and somatotrophs (GH). Others, such as Kallmann's syndrome, result in loss of the gonadotrophs and a normal male phenotype but hypogonadotrophic hypogonadism and a degree of olfactory deficit.

Acquired hypopituitarism may occur due to problems such as trauma affecting the pituitary stalk (infundibulum), apoplexy or infarction in Sheehan's syndrome. Other issues such as lymphocytic hypophysitis are being increasingly recognised with higher-teslar MRI machines. Infections and inflammatory lesions such as sarcoid and histiocytosis may affect the pituitary, as well as intra- and extrasellar masses.

Iatrogenic causes include radiation-associated pituitary damage or surgical complication after attempted removal of a macroadenoma.

Lastly, hypopituitarism can be secondary to hypothalamic disease.

Diagnostic approach

Screening for hypopituitarism should be thought of in those with developmental problems such as:

- failure to start puberty
- lack of linear growth

or those with:

- significant head trauma
- postpartum haemorrhage or sudden drop in blood pressure post-partum
- brain tumours that proximate the hypothalamus or pituitary

or those who have had pituitary surgery or cranial radiation.

Once suspected, paired trophic hormones and their target hormones should be checked, being careful not to miss the inappropriately normal trophic hormone level, but with low normal target hormone.

History

Depending on the suspected aetiology, a developmental, pubertal and menstrual history should be taken. Some of the symptoms of each of the trophic deficiencies are listed in Table 29.2.

Special tests

- Imaging of the brain and pituitary with MRI may be indicated, depending on the suspected cause.
- Measurement of testes size and checking of genitalia is important in children thought to be hypopituitary.
- Plotting growth, weight and developmental milestones should be done in children.

Integrated management

Pharmacological

Many of the deficiencies of the hypothalamic-pituitary axis are life threatening. Replacement of glucocorticoids, if these are thought to be deficient, should be done prior to thyroxine replacement and would generally be instigated by an endocrinologist and in hospital. If

TABLE 29.2 Symptoms of trophic deficiencies

Trophic hormone	History/symptoms	Tests
LH/FSH	• Pubertal and developmental history • Inability to adequately lactate post partum • Erections/shaving • Menstrual history • Height	• FSH, LH and oestradiol or testosterone • Bone age
GH	• Failure of linear growth • Neonatal hypoglycaemia (with ACTH and TSH deficiency)	• GH, IGF-1 IGFBP-3 • Provocative test (insulin tolerance test) not used in children • Bone age
ACTH	• Hypotension • Lethargy ± hyponatraemia • Hypoglycaemia • Abdominal pains, nausea and diarrhoea • Weight loss	• 0800 ACTH/cortisol • Insulin tolerance test (often manifestations of complete loss are clear and life threatening, but insufficiency may require an ITT • Treat with steroids after blood has been taken, if clinical concern is high
TSH	• Lethargy • Weight gain • Heart failure • Dry hair and skin • Hypotension and coma	
ADH/vasopressin	• Polyuria and polydipsia • Lethargy • Coma	• Water-deprivation test

a patient is in a critical condition, then 200 mg of IV hydrocortisone should be given. Otherwise 100 mg of IV hydrocortisone with 50 mg q6h can be started and blood tests awaited. Maintenance doses of glucocorticoids are not fully elucidated but hydrocortisone equivalent 20–30 mg given in 2–3 divided doses, or cortisone acetate at 25–37.5 mg per day in two divided doses for adults, is a good place to start. The goal is to very slowly and carefully titrate down to the lowest dose that keeps the patient well. Thyroxine may then be replaced if necessary at a dose of 1.6 μg/kg.

Taking a child through puberty requires slow introduction of oestrogen and progesterone in girls and testosterone in boys. This should be done by a paediatrician.

Central diabetes insipidus may be treated by dDAVP® (desmopressin) administration via oral tablet or nasal spray. Starting dose should be 50 μg per day for the tablet and 10 μg a day for the nasal spray.

Surgical

If a mass is blocking normal pituitary function, neurosurgical opinion may be sought as to whether pituitary surgery may help. Normally, 90% of the pituitary mass has to be lost, to render the patient panhyopituitary.

Ongoing review and/or monitoring

Hypogonadotrophic hypogonadal patients may be able to successfully become parents with assisted reproductive technologies.

Discussion about a Medicalert bracelet, and teaching the patient and carer how to administer intramuscular glucocorticoids, are critical. Teaching the patient about sick-day management is also very important. A minor illness such as a respiratory virus would require a doubling of the dose for at least 3 days and then decreasing to normal dose. In an illness significant enough to make the patient bed-bound, a tripling of the dose for at least 3 days, or for as long as the condition remains, is advisable. A vomiting illness preventing the patient from taking their glucocorticoids requires administration of IM glucocorticoids and attendance at a hospital.

Long-term slow-down titration of the glucocorticoids to the lowest dose that keeps the patient well is the goal. Seek expert endocrine advice if necessary.

Important pitfalls

Measurement of trophic hormones without their paired target hormones makes the interpretation very difficult and will miss many cases of relative deficiency.

Prognosis

While the reason is not known, there is an increase in the mortality in panhypopituitary patients after pituitary surgery of about double that of the normal population. This is even after replacement therapy was instituted. Further information and evidence is still being gathered on adult replacement of growth hormone, and the physiological replacement doses of glucocorticoids.

PARATHYROID DISORDERS

Located generally behind the thyroid gland are the four parathyroid glands, which have the role of producing parathyroid hormone (PTH). PTH is the main controller of calcium levels within the blood and bones, and this of course has important implications for neuromuscular function.

HYPERCALCAEMIA

Extracellular calcium is a tightly controlled electrolyte. Significant symptoms, including life-threatening conditions, occur when control is lost and the levels of calcium in the body go outside the tightly controlled range. The largest store of calcium within the body is in the bones, but calcium is stored within skeletal and cardiac muscle, and within the neuronal signalling and neuromuscular junctions.

The most common symptoms of hypercalcaemia are the classic 'stones, bones, moans and groans' of kidney stones, bone pains, mood changes including depressive symptoms and abdominal pains including constipation. Polyuria and dehydration can occur secondary to high serum calcium. The most common cause for congenital hypercalcaemia is familial hypocalciuric hypercalcaemia. The most common acquired causes of hypercalcaemia are hyperparathyroidism and malignancy. A useful thought map to think about acquired hypercalcaemia is to think about PTH-dependent and PTH-independent causes of hypercalcaemia (see Fig 29.3).

Aetiology

Extracellular calcium is normally controlled very tightly by two interrelated hormones, namely parathyroid hormone (PTH) and vitamin D. There is a sigmoidal inverse relationship between serum calcium levels and PTH levels, such that a decrease in serum calcium results in increased PTH and vice versa.

Familial hypocalciuric hypercalcaemia is a congenital variation in the sensitivity of the calcium-sensing receptor, with a reduced sensitivity to serum calcium and so a higher set point of serum calcium at which the PTH is turned down. Serum calcium is high, as is PTH, but urine 24-hour calcium excretion is low.

Milk–alkali syndrome is less common now that histamine receptor antagonists and proton pump inhibitors are the mainstay treatment of hyperacidity syndromes of the stomach. The use of antacids together with the ingestion of milk products results in increased

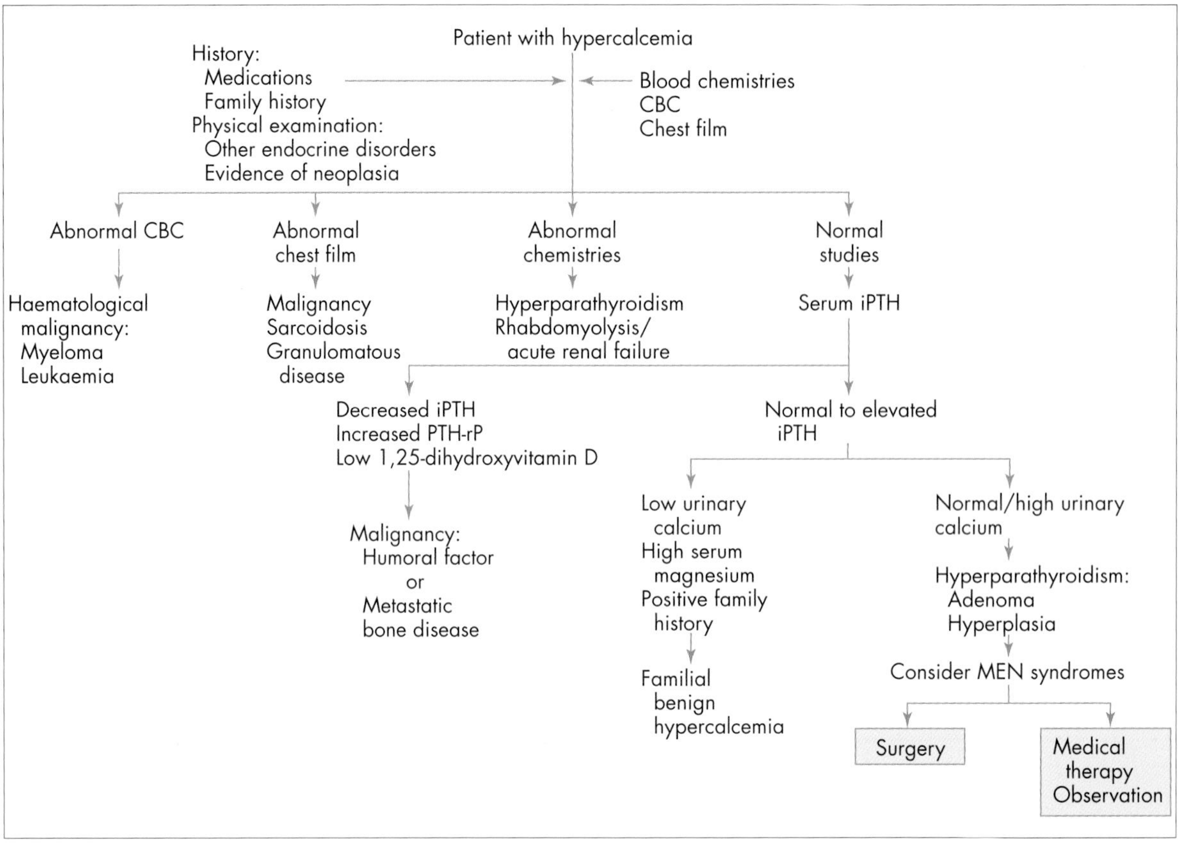

FIGURE 29.3 Integrative management of hypercalcaemia

absorption and mild hypercalcaemia. While there has been a reduction in the presentation of milk–alkali syndrome from these less-used drugs, there have been a number of case reports of similar presentations in those using large doses of calcium carbonate, which provides both calcium and alkali. High calcium level together with high bicarbonate and perhaps some renal impairment should prompt the GP to ask about calcium carbonate intake.

PTH-dependent hypercalcaemia can be due to primary hyperparathyroidism, less commonly secondary hyperparathyroidism, or tertiary hyperparathyroidism. Secondary hyperparathyroidism often does not result in hypercalcaemia alone, as it is an appropriate response to maintain calcium levels. This occurs in the situation of vitamin D deficiency, where high parathyroid levels maintain serum calcium when vitamin D levels are insufficient to provide enough gut and renal absorption to do so. Primary hyperparathyroidism may be due to a parathyroid adenoma, or adenomas on their own or in the setting of MEN1 syndrome of pituitary tumours, hyperparathyroidism and pancreatic tumours, or MEN2 with medullary thyroid cancer and phaeochromocytoma. Parathyroid adenomas are most commonly sporadic and not part of another syndrome, and are mostly single-gland adenomas. Less commonly, PTH-secreting thymus tumours can produce the parathyroid hormone excess. Tertiary hyperparathyroidism is thought to occur through long-standing secondary hyperparathyroidism, which then causes irreversible parathyroid gland hyperplasia and autonomous function.

PTH-independent causes of hypercalcaemia are usually due to excesses in active vitamin D, or lytic lesions of the bone. The far less common production of PTHrp (PTH-related protein) is usually associated with squamous cell carcinomas, or renal, bladder, breast or ovarian cancers. The conditions that result in excess active vitamin D (1,25-dihydroxy vitamin D) are excess intake of calcitriol, or granulomatous diseases such as sarcoid, tuberculosis and lymphoma, both non-Hodgkins and Hodgkins. In these conditions the macrophages in the granulomata convert the inactive vitamin D to active vitamin D without the need for PTH, which normally carries this out by stimulating the 1-alpha-hydroxylase enzyme in the kidneys.

Other causes such as multiple myeloma and breast cancer are the two more common malignancies that can lead to lytic bone lesions and uncontrolled release of calcium into the extracellular fluid, independently of a suppressed PTH level.

Diagnostic approach

The first thing to do is to try to ameliorate the symptoms and effects of the hypercalcaemia. In many cases there is a degree of dehydration from polyuria. Correction of the volume status will often correct some of the hypercalcaemia.

Thinking of the causes, checking the PTH together with 25 OH vitamin D, calcium and phosphate, electrolytes and liver function tests, and a full blood count, is a good place to start. If the PTH is normal or high with a high calcium, think of familial hypocalciuric hypercalcaemia (FHH) or hyperparathyroidism, whether it be primary or tertiary. Hyperparathyroidism will have a high 24-hour urinary calcium, whereas FHH will not, and so this is the next test.

If PTH is low, the cause is high calcium with an appropriately suppressed PTH. Check active vitamin D (1,25 dihydroxycholecalciferol), PTHrp, selenoprotein P (sEPP), ask for a chest X-ray and, if the sEPP shows a monoclonal protein band, a skeletal survey for lytic lesions. These tests are best done stepwise, to avoid unnecessary tests and costs, although the patient's condition and preference may dictate otherwise.

History

- First ask about symptoms and history suggestive of hypercalcaemia and duration of these. Ask about symptoms of nocturia or polyuria and dehydration.
- Ask about any specific areas of bone pains, with nocturnal inflammatory rest bone pains being the most discriminatory.
- Ask about risk factors for breast, ovarian, head and neck or lung cancer.
- Check for other medical conditions, notably renal failure or osteoporosis.
- Check medications, most notably calcitriol, caltrate and antacids.
- Ask about a family history of hypercalcaemia and its manifestations, and MEN1 or MEN2 conditions.

Examination

- Examine the patient's volume status and fluid balance.
- Examine the abdomen for signs of constipation or faecal loading.
- Examine any bones described as painful by the patient.
- Examine for peripheral lymphadenopathy.
- Examine the neck for any masses, particularly anterior neck masses. With hypercalcaemia, a palpable neck mass may be lymphadenopathy of lymphoma, granulomatous disease or a parathyroid carcinoma. Parathyroid adenomas are not often palpable.
- Examine the patient for a peripheral mononeuropathy of sarcoid, or a painful peripheral neuropathy of a hypergammaglobulinaemia of multiple myeloma.
- Breast exam if appropriate for a breast cause of PTHrp.

Investigations

Pathology:

- PTH with Ca, PO_4 (phosphate) and vitamin D (25-OH Vit D)
- Chest X-ray, ECG
- TFT, FBC electrolytes and LFTs
- sEPP and urine EPP with Bence Jones protein detection
- ACE only if lymphadenopathy detected
- Whole LN excisional biopsy if palpable lymph node and concern about lymphoma or PTH-independent hypercalcaemia.
- Skeletal survey if there is evidence on sEPP of multiple myeloma.

Special tests:

- Bone mineral density (BMD) in a postmenopausal woman to help guide treatment of any primary hyperparathyroidism.
- 24-hour urine calcium and creatinine if there is PTH-dependent disease.
- Nuclear medicine parathyroid scan to localise the adenoma if it is found to be primary hyperparathyroidism and surgery is an option for the patient.

Integrative management

Surgery is indicated for primary hyperparathyroidism in symptomatic disease. In the case of asymptomatic primary hyperparathyroidism, surgery can be considered if:

- serum calcium is >0.25 mmol/L higher than the upper limit of normal of your assay
- age < 50 years
- osteoporosis established by minimal trauma fracture or BMD
- renal failure with eGFR < 60 mL/min.

If the patient is not a surgical candidate, due to frailty, then Cinacalcet, a calcium sensing receptor agonist, may be an option, but at the time of publication is only indicated for secondary hyperparathyroidism in renal failure and parathyroid cancer.

Pharmacological

While determining the cause of hypercalcaemia, it is important to treat the symptoms. Ensure good hydration, which will help with kaliuresis. IV fluids can be given in hospital and, if need be, the addition of a loop diuretic can help lower serum calcium and make the patient feel much better. In the case of severe hypercalcaemia not adequately treated with IV fluids and frusemide, bisphosphonates can be used, particularly in hypercalcaemia of malignancy, with the normal precautions in their use. There have been concerns over osteonecrosis of the jaw with bisphosphonate treatment in those who then undergo dental treatment, mostly teeth extractions. This is estimated to be 1:250 to 1:1000 with IV bisphosphonates treatment and much lower with oral treatment, in the order of 1:100,000 to 1:250,000. It is wise to ensure, where possible, that the patient has had a dental review prior to starting IV bisphosphonates treatment particularly. Sometimes this is not practicable. Treating the root cause of the hypercalcaemia is the basis for definitive treatment.

Self-help

If no treatment for the primary hyperparathyroidism is given, make sure the person stays well hydrated, to prevent renal stones and help with natural diuresis, which will minimise excess serum calcium.

Ongoing review and/or monitoring

By far the most common problem associated with hyperparathyroidism is vitamin D deficiency. Checking for vitamin D deficiency particularly in those at high risk is important to prevent secondary hyperparathyroidism. Elderly people in nursing homes, and those whose cultural dress requires total cover, are worth assessing for vitamin D deficiency. With the high use of sunscreens and avoidance of direct exposure to sunlight in countries such as Australia and New Zealand, it can occur even in children.

Pitfalls

Don't forget that mild hypercalcaemia may occur in cases of prolonged bed rest or immobility, and marked hypercalcaemia may occur in Graves' disease, due to increased turnover of bone, and in Addison's disease.

HYPERPARATHYROIDISM

Most of the investigation and treatment of hyperparathyroidism is covered above, in the hypercalcaemia section. Brief further information is given below.

Hyperparathyroidism can be primary, secondary or tertiary.

Primary hyperparathyroidism (PHPTH) is due to between one and four functioning adenomas of the parathyroid glands. In 85% of cases there is a single parathyroid gland adenoma, which secretes PTH independent of the serum calcium. It is most common in women over the age of 55 years. The remainder of PHPTH is due to multiple adenomas, hyperplasia and, very rarely, parathyroid carcinoma. The incidence of PHPTH is around 4 per 100,000.

Secondary hyperparathyroidism is usually found in the setting of vitamin D deficiency. With the strength of the sun and concerns about skin cancer, in some countries such as Australia and New Zealand, and the increasingly indoor lifestyle of the population in developed countries, vitamin D deficiency can be very common. Those at highest risk are the elderly, such as those in institutional care, dark-skinned races and societies where it is culturally appropriate to wear head-to-toe clothing.

In vitamin D deficiency, the control of serum calcium falls back onto PTH, which stimulates renal absorption of calcium, liberation of calcium from the mineralised bone at the expense of bone mineral density, and increased hydroxylation of the low levels of 25-OH Vit D to 1,25-OH Vit D. These patients are normally eucalcaemic. Secondary hyperparathyroidism can also occur in the setting of renal failure, with loss of kidney parenchyma to convert 25-OH Vit D to 1,25-OH Vit D under the control of PTH. As such, the patient has reduced active vitamin D, and PTH predominates. 1,25-OH Vit D actively inhibits the growth of the PTH glands. The renal physician may elect to give the patient active vitamin D in the form of calcitriol, but it depends on the levels of calcium and phosphate. Elective parathyroidectomy may be indicated at very high levels of secondary hyperparathyroidism, depending on the stage of their chronic kidney disease.

Tertiary hyperparathyroidism usually occurs in renal patients who have had long-standing secondary hyperparathyroidism. With low levels of active vitamin D, there is loss of inhibition of parathyroid gland hyperplasia, and autonomous PH secretion results from the hyperplastic glands, even when the cause of the secondary hyperparathyroidism is corrected.

Diagnostic approach

Endocrinologists are friendly people who like to do things in pairs, including measuring hormone-releasing hormones, hormones and their targets. In the setting of calcium, and parathyroid hormone, corrected calcium, phosphate, 25-OH Vit D and PTH should be measured together. The results may then be interpreted properly.

History

Tertiary hyperparathyroidism should be evident with a patient who has chronic kidney disease being managed by a renal physician. Treatment and management of this condition should be discussed with that specialist physician.

Secondary hyperparathyroidism may be a surprising finding in a patient for whom the only real risk factors are avoidance of sunlight, increasing age, and culture in which patients tend to cover up. Asking about fragility fractures is wise, as these patients may have a low BMD from long-standing high levels of PTH.

Primary hyperparathyroidism can occur as part of a genetic syndrome, the most common of which is MEN1, where it clusters with pituitary tumours, and pancreatic/neuroendocrine tumours. PHPTH is the predominant finding in this condition, being present in 90% of cases of MEN1. It can also occur in MEN2A, with medullary thyroid cancer and phaeochromocytoma being the other components. Medullary thyroid cancer occurs in > 90% of MEN2A, and PHPTH occurs only in 10–20%. Asking about a family history of PHPTH and these associated endocrine problems is appropriate in the family history.

Asking about urolithiasis and fragility fractures is important in the diagnosis of PHPTH and in consideration of surgical treatment.

Examination

One finding not to miss is a noticeable or palpable tumour in the anterior triangle of the neck, as a palpable tumour and primary hyperparathyroidism should raise concern about a parathyroid carcinoma, and a biopsy should be obtained. Other examination should be targeted based on the history obtained.

Investigations

The triad of PTH, 25-OH Vit D and corrected calcium are the three investigations that should be ordered together, to interpret the result properly. Although not as common as it used to be, osteitis fibrosis cystica is the classic manifestation of hyperparathyroidism of the bones. While the radiological findings of subperiosteal erosions on the radial side of the middle phalanges, erosion of the tips of the distal phalanges and lateral clavicles, brown tumours of the long bones and 'salt and pepper skull' are not used in diagnosis, their appearance on imaging of the bones should prompt a check of the intact PTH, corrected calcium and vitamin D.

In order to differentiate between familial hypocalciuric hypercalcaemia and primary hyperparathyroidism, 24-hour urinary calcium and creatinine should be collected.

Checking the renal function and phosphorus, as well as magnesium, can be done but is not necessary for diagnosis. It is useful for screening for complications.

Special tests

With hyperparathyroidism, either primary or secondary, a bone mineral densitometry should be estimated with a DEXA scan. If primary hyperparathyroidism is confirmed, an ultrasound and sestamibi technetium scan to localise the parathyroid adenoma can be requested, if the patient would be considered for surgical removal of the adenoma.

Pitfalls

A normal level of PTH with a high corrected serum calcium is in fact hyperparathyroidism, as it is inappropriately normal.

PTH is very unstable, and when blood is taken it must be processed and frozen immediately, otherwise it breaks down and gives a low level. It is not uncommon for a result to come back with normal calcium and phosphate with a very low or un-recordable level of PTH. Before being alarmed, request the vitamin D, corrected calcium and PTH again.

Integrative management

Active surveillance

There is a case for conservative management of primary hyperparathyroidism if there are no symptoms of hypercalcaemia, the hypercalcaemia is mild, there is no loss of BMD, the renal function is normal or the patient is older. They should be advised to keep well hydrated, to minimise the extent of hypercalcaemia, and to avoid thiazide diuretics. This decision can be made in conjunction with a specialist, in order to ensure ongoing follow-up.

Lifestyle

Lifestyle factors are as listed above, in the section on 'history'.

To prevent the complications of secondary hyperparathyroidism and the resulting loss of bone density to maintain serum calcium, a check and replacement of low 25-OH Vit D is suggested. This is normally achieved with 5–7 minutes in the sun each day, with increasing requirements in older and darker-pigmented patients. If regular moderate sun exposure is not desired, a loading dose then 1000 IU of cholecalciferol is appropriate treatment for lower serum levels.

Surgical

In primary hyperparathyroidism, the newer imaging techniques and newer surgical approaches have meant that, for experienced surgeons, the parathyroid adenoma that has been identified pre-surgery may be excised through a limited neck dissection. If surgery is not indicated or not chosen, then good hydration and maintaining 25-OH Vit D > 50 nmol/L should be pursued. Cinacalcet is currently indicated for parathyroid carcinoma, and secondary hyperparathyroidism of renal disease with hypercalcaemia. It may be possible to consider the use of Cinacalcet in non-surgical PHPTH patients.

Other medical

Frusemide may be added to a forced increased water intake to minimise the degree of hypercalcaemia. Care must be taken to ensure that pre-renal renal failure does not ensue.

Ongoing review and/or monitoring

Serum calcium and renal function should be checked each year, with a 2-yearly BMD, and surgery considered each time.

There have been some benefits in reduction of serum calcium with drugs used to treat osteoporosis with primary hyperparathyroidism. These include oestrogen/medroxyprogesterone therapies, bisphosphonates and the selective oestrogen receptor modulator, raloxifene.

HYPOPARATHYROIDISM

Hypoparathyroidism is most commonly acquired, with transient or permanent hypoparathyroidism post surgery for thyroid disorders. Aside from surgery, there are several causes of hypoparathyroidism that arise due to aplasia of the glands, autoimmune destruction or inhibition of the release of PTH by activating antibodies to the calcium-sensing receptor. Many of the causes of hypoparathyroidism that appear in childhood are parts of rare but important syndromes, which should be managed by a paediatric endocrinologist. The more common cause for childhood hypoparathyroidism, as part of the autoimmune polyglandular syndrome type 1, is discussed in this section.

Aetiology

Normally, as extracellular calcium drops, there is less activation of the calcium-sensing receptor on the surface of the parathyroid cells, and thus less inhibition of PTH synthesis and release. PTH action requires adequate magnesium, and results in the stimulation of the 1-alpha hydroxylase of the kidney to activate 25-OH Vit D to its active form, 1,25-OH Vit D. The active vitamin D then stimulates renal resorption of calcium cations, and gut absorption of calcium, to raise serum calcium. The PTH directly stimulates the kidney to resorb calcium ions, secrete phosphate ions and stimulate osteoclasts to resorb calcium from mineralised bone. PTH secretion is thus stimulated by low extracellular levels of calcium and high levels of phosphate. Hypoparathyroidism therefore results in hypocalcaemia, due to lack of direct effects of PTH and the effects on activating vitamin D.

Pathology

Congenital and genetic:

- X-linked and autosomal-recessive conditions occur where there is aplasia of the parathyroid glands.
- Aplasia of the parathyroid glands occurs in rare syndromes such as DiGeorge's syndrome, where there is failure of development of the third and fourth pharyngeal pouches.
- Congenital and genetic problems with the parathyroid gland are detected early in life, and are so rare and complex that they will be managed by specialist paediatricians.

PTH release problems:

- There have been point mutations of the PTH gene that result in aberrant production of PTH and therefore hypoparathyroidism.
- Severe hypermagnesaemia and hypomagnesaemia are associated with reduced release of PTH and also end-organ resistance to PTH, in the case of hypomagnesaemia.

Surgery:

- Surgical manipulation of the thyroid gland, especially in total or subtotal thyroidectomy, can result in transient hypoparathyroidism in around 20% of cases, and permanent hypoparathyroidism in less than 1% of cases.

Autoimmune:

- Autoimmune hypoparathyroidism is mostly associated with activating antibody production to the calcium sensing receptor, mimicking calcium and providing a signal to suppress PTH release. This is most commonly found as part of polyglandular autoimmune syndrome type 1, which consists classically of the triad of hypoparathyroidism, mucocutaneous candidiasis and autoimmune hypoadrenalism. Other immune endocrinopathies and autoimmune conditions have also been associated with APS-1 (autoimmune polyglandular syndrome type 1).
- It is much rarer for destructive antibodies to the parathyroid gland to be the cause of autoimmune hypoparathyroidism.

Pseudohypoparathyroidism:

- American endocrinologist Fuller Albright described a condition of short-statured patients with distinctive morphological features such as shortened third metacarpals and hypocalcaemia together with hyperphosphataemia, which was then found to be due to parathyroid hormone resistance. These will usually come to attention of specialist paediatricians.

History

Asking about symptoms of hypocalcaemia such as paraesthesias, inability to open the mouth normally (trismus), breathing problems and twitching is an important first step. Some patients will have no symptoms with hypocalcaemia. The duration is important, to try to establish whether it may be a long-standing congenital condition, or acquired. Given that the most common cause is surgical, the onset should be clear with the surgery.

Ask about any candidiasis or symptoms of adrenal insufficiency, such as syncope, prolonged recovery from illnesses, or postural hypotension particularly, thinking of autoimmune polyglandular syndrome type 1 (APS1). A family history of the same is important. APS1 usually presents in the first years of life and, if it has not occurred by the age of 20 years, is not likely to be a possibility.

Examination

Chvostek's sign is elicited by tapping the facial nerve just in front of the tragus of the ear—if positive, this results in a twitch of the corner of the mouth on the same side.

Trousseau's sign occurs when a blood pressure cuff is inflated above the systolic blood pressure for 3 minutes, and is positive when there is carpal spasm shown in 'Le Main d'Accoucheur' or the hands of the obstetrician. There is forced adduction of the thumb, flexion of the metacarpophalangeal (MCP) joints and extension of the proximal interphalangeal (PIP)/distal interphalangeal (DIP) joints.

Look for involuntary muscle twitches and listen for stridor.

Investigations

Consulting room:

- ECG—looking for prolonged QTc interval
- Flow-volume loop—looking for extrathoracic obstruction.

Pathology:

- PTH, vitamin D, corrected calcium and phosphate. If the symptoms are transient, an arterial blood gas can be useful to look for respiratory alkalosis, which can lead to a lower ionised calcium level and symptoms that are the same as those of prolonged hypocalcaemia.

Integrative management

Active surveillance

Active surveillance alone is not a valid option. Hypoparathyroidism and the resulting hypocalcaemia may result in coma and death if not treated, so once identified, it should be treated promptly.

Pharmacological

In hospital, IV calcium gluconate should be given by a central line, to minimise the chance of tissue necrosis, which can occur if there is extravasation. If given quickly it may result in nausea and flushing, and risk cardiac arrest.

- Symptomatic patients with tetany, laryngeal spasm, prolonged QTc or reduced level of consciousness with a low corrected calcium should be given calcium gluconate as an infusion. Use 10 mL of 10% calcium gluconate in 100 mL of 5% dextrose running over an hour, or 100 mL of 10% calcium gluconate in 1000 mL running over 24 hours.
- Patients with surgically induced hypoparathyroidism will need calcitriol and calcium carbonate. Typical doses are 0.5 μg calcitriol b.i.d and 1200 mg b.i.d. of calcium carbonate. These may be started 1–2 days before high-risk thyroid surgery, as the half-life of calcitriol is about 1 day and it will therefore take around 5 days to reach a steady level. If there is sufficient PTH demonstrated by blood test on day 1 post surgery, the calcitriol and calcium carbonate may be stopped.
- Teriparatide, a recombinant portion of human PTH, is not yet indicated for treatment of transient or permanent hypoparathyroidism (only for osteoporosis).
- Cholecalciferol or 25-OH Vit D_3 is of no benefit to correct hypocalcaemia secondary to hypoparathyroidism, as the enzyme required to activate vitamin D is PTH dependent.

Important pitfalls

Transient low ionised calcium may occur with symptoms of hypocalcaemia in respiratory alkalosis of hyperventilation.

Always measure PTH, vitamin D, corrected calcium and phosphate together for correct interpretation. PTH is very unstable and may degrade before being assayed, leading to a falsely low PTH. If the patient has a normal calcium level, consider repeating the test before investigating further.

Prognosis

If the patient has hypoparathyroid hypocalcaemia, they will need ongoing calcitriol treatment to maintain corrected calcium levels in the lower normal range, to prevent nephrolithiasis.

PARATHYROID TUMOUR

Parathyroid adenoma and carcinoma are difficult to differentiate clinically. Parathyroid carcinoma is an uncommon but important condition occurring in around 2% of investigated hyperparathyroidism. With a different prognosis and natural history, it is important to identify. Typically, parathyroid carcinomas tend to cause higher levels of hyperparathyroidism and hypercalcaemia than primary hyperparathyroidism.

Aetiology

Parathyroid carcinomas are often associated with a germline mutation of a gene on chromosome 1, known as HRPT2, which is a tumour suppressor gene. The gene encodes a protein called parafibromin, which is expressed in parathyroid carcinomas but not in adenomas, and this makes it a useful diagnostic tool in histopathological analysis of a parathyroid tumour.

Diagnostic approach

Patients who present with a neck mass and primary hyperparathyroidism should be suspected for parathyroid carcinoma, especially if they have PTH levels greater than five times the upper limit of normal, or a corrected calcium greater than 3.5 mmol/L. Referral to a surgeon and endocrinologist with concerns about parathyroid carcinoma should prompt appropriate surgical therapy and pathological testing.

Patients will often be symptomatic of severe hypercalcaemia, including the bone complications of hyperparathyroidism, and will often need hospitalisation for treatment of the hypercalcaemia. The parathyroid carcinomas are rarely non-functioning with normal levels of parathyroid hormone and calcium.

History

Assessing for symptoms of hypercalcaemia is important, as correction of this will improve the patient's wellbeing.

Anyone who presents with a neck mass and hyperparathyroidism should be considered to possibly have a parathyroid carcinoma. Parathyroid carcinoma is more common in patients aged 45–55 years, in equal male:female ratio. Parathyroid carcinoma is more likely to have a PTH level greater than five times the upper limit of normal, with a corrected calcium level > 3.5 mmol/L.

A patient with a neck mass, hyperparathyroidism and symptoms of local invasion such as a change in voice and signs of a laryngeal nerve palsy should be suspected of a parathyroid carcinoma.

Examination

Hypercalcaemia and a neck mass may represent a lymphoma or a chronic granulomatous disease such as sarcoid or tuberculosis. Examination for other signs of these conditions, such as generalised lymphadenopathy, hepatosplenomegaly, nerve palsies and CNS findings and rashes may be helpful. Biochemical testing will help differentiate between PTH-dependent hyperparathyroidism that occurs in parathyroid carcinoma and the PTH-independent hypercalcaemia that occurs in the granulomatous diseases, lymphomas and other cancers.

Examine the jaw for bone tumour, which may occur with parathyroid carcinoma in the parathyroid carcinoma–jaw tumour syndrome.

Investigations

Pathology

The first step is to confirm the extent of the hypercalcaemia and establish that it is PTH-dependent hypercalcaemia. Use the flow diagram and work-up algorithm in Fig 29.3 (in the section on hypercalcaemia).

Special tests

One of the very useful tests to differentiate parathyroid adenoma from parathyroid carcinoma is parafibromin on immunohistochemical staining.

An ultrasound of the neck or CT scan may be helpful to confirm the location and extent of the mass, and any involved structures.

Once a parathyroid carcinoma has been histologically diagnosed, genetic testing for HRPT gene mutation is useful for monitoring the patient and for investigation and surveying the patient's family members.

Integrative management

Pharmacological

The patient's first concern will be that of the symptoms of their hypercalcaemia. Rehydration, forced diuresis and loop diuretics are necessary, and hospitalisation may be required. Bisphosphonates may be useful, such as pamidronate given as an IV infusion.

Cinacalcet, a calcimimetic, has been approved for use in parathyroid carcinoma for symptomatic control of hypercalcaemia.

There is little data on adjuvant chemotherapy or radiotherapy for parathyroid carcinoma.

Surgical

Surgical management is the mainstay of a parathyroid adenoma with symptomatic hypercalcaemia or parathyroid carcinoma. Once the diagnosis of parathyroid carcinoma is confirmed, a significant proportion of patients will need further neck surgery.

Ongoing review and/or monitoring

About one-third of patients will be cured with surgical treatment, one-third will have recurrence requiring further surgery and one-third will have a poor prognosis.

Patients should have their calcium, PTH and vitamin D levels checked every 6 months, unless earlier is clinically indicated. With a high rate of recurrence, and increased possibility of transformation of normal parathyroid tissue to parathyroid carcinoma in those who carry the HRPT gene mutation, recurrence may be detected early.

Family members of those with HRPT mutations should be screened for the mutation. If negative, screening for hyperparathyroidism may not be necessary. Referral to a clinical geneticist may be helpful to guide screening and follow-up.

THYROID DISORDERS

The thyroid gland is a butterfly-shaped gland that sits in the neck around the thyroid and cricoid cartilages of the larynx and trachea. It is primarily responsible for producing the hormone thyroxine, which accelerates or brakes the body's metabolic processes. The symptoms of an over- or underactive thyroid vary, and can be quite different between patients.

HYPERTHYROID DISORDERS

Symptoms of hyperthyroidism are those of a metabolism that is sped up, and include symptoms resembling anxiety and agitation, tremors, weight loss despite an increased appetite, palpitations, a syncopated heartbeat, spread out or absent periods, frequent opening of bowels, heat intolerance and lethargy. There is often a family history of thyroid problems, either hyperthyroidism or hypothyroidism. There are a few common causes for an overactive thyroid, described below.

Diagnosis

The first challenge in diagnosing a thyroid disorder is to consider it. It may not always be obvious, as the symptoms can creep up over a prolonged period, or they may imitate other health problems such as anxiety or stress, or they may aggravate other health problems such as ischaemic heart disease. It should also be mentioned that significant and prolonged emotional stress can produce a mildly elevated level of thyroid hormones. When suspected, or when needing to exclude it as a possible diagnosis, the following tests are recommended:

- T_4 (thyroxine) and T_3 (triiodothyronine)—raised
- TSH—low due to suppression in the presence of raised T_4 and T_3
- radioisotope scan—evidence of diffuse and uniform overactivity in Graves' disease, and irregularly increased uptake seen in multinodular goitre.

Graves' disease

Normally the thyroid gland's production is controlled by the pituitary gland. The control is finely tuned. Graves' disease is an autoimmune condition and is the most common cause of hyperthyroidism, affecting up to 2% of women—it is approximately four times more common in women than in men. In Graves' disease, the immune response, rather than destroying the thyroid gland, stimulates it, making it grow in both size and production of thyroxine. This creates a goitre, which is typically painless, and the symptoms of thyrotoxicosis mentioned above.

The antibodies or proteins that stimulate the thyroid gland may also stimulate the tissues behind the eyes, and the anterior tibial region. If these antibodies stimulate the tissues behind the eyes it leads to exophthalmos, creating an impression of staring, and may affect vision if extreme. Referral to an ophthalmologist is appropriate. Eye problems in Graves' disease seem to be more common in smokers.

Treatment

Carbimazole (Neomercazole®) 10–45 mg orally daily blocks the thyroid's ability to make thyroxine. Surgery to remove the thyroid, or radioactive iodine, which selectively destroys the thyroid gland, may also be used, more commonly if carbimazole is contraindicated or ineffective. An endocrinologist's guidance will be helpful in determining which management approach will suit the patient, and to monitor the effectiveness of treatment.

Medication may need to be continued for at least 12–18 months. There is some chance that, with a 12–18 month treatment with tablets, the thyroid will settle down and not need further treatment.

Toxic multinodular goitre

Toxic multinodular goitre is a condition in which overactive nodules in the thyroid overproduce thyroxine, producing the symptoms of hyperthyroidism.

The nodules are common, and tend to grow slowly over time and become a little more active. As they get bigger they may produce a noticeable goitre. Carbimazole can be effective in treating these nodules, but sometimes surgery or radioactive iodine may be needed if the goitre grows large enough to cause dyspnoea, dysphagia or breathing problems. Surgery can be used if the goitre is cosmetically disfiguring to the patient, or if there are concerns about whether the nodule is neoplastic. Fine-needle biopsy is indicated if a nodule grows or has atypical features on ultrasound.

Subacute (de Quervain's) thyroiditis

In subacute thyroiditis there is inflammation of the thyroid, often post viral infection, which typically results in symptoms of hyperthyroidism and a painful neck. The thyroid will be tender to palpation. This condition may be transient and follow a viral illness such as a common cold, and tends to settle down over several weeks. Analgesia is commonly required. Steroids may be used if aspirin or anti-inflammatory medications are not effective. Beta-blockers may be used to treat the symptoms of hyperthyroidism if they are significant. The condition tends to resolve spontaneously over a few weeks to months, and may be followed by a short period of hypothyroidism, as it recovers and reverts to normal.

Commonly used medications for thyrotoxicosis

Carbimazole or methimazole, and propylthiouracil, block the production of thyroid hormone by the thyroid gland, and are typically used in Graves' disease or toxic multinodular goitre. They can take a few weeks to get the thyroxine levels under control. Thyroid function tests will need to be checked every few weeks to make sure the doses are correct.

Precautions:

- If a rash develops, medication will need to be ceased.
- Immune function may be affected.
- Liver function should be monitored.
- Women of childbearing age should be advised not to become pregnant during treatment.

Symptoms associated with anxiety and stress can mimic symptoms associated with hyperthyroid disorders, and vice versa. Furthermore, significant and chronic stress can lead to an elevation in thyroid activity and even trigger the activation of autoimmune thyroiditis. Therefore it is advisable to always consider the potential diagnosis of thyroid problems in patients who present complaining of stress-related symptoms, and to consider the role of psychological factors in the management of hyperthyroid disorders.

HYPOTHYROID DISORDERS

The symptoms associated with an underactive thyroid gland and low levels of thyroxine include tiredness, weight gain and reduced appetite, dyspnoea on exertion, peripheral oedema, dry skin and hair, cold intolerance, menorrhagia and easy bruising. The most common cause is autoimmune destruction of the thyroid gland, Hashimoto's thyroiditis.

Hashimoto's thyroiditis

This is an autoimmune condition resulting in destruction of the thyroid gland and consequently a low level of thyroid hormone. It is not uncommon, tending to be more prevalent in women, and tending to run in families. There may or may not be a noticeable goitre.

The rate of loss of function of the thyroid may be rapid, but function can also decline slowly over months. The treatment is to replace the missing hormone with thyroxine, starting at 50–100 μg and increasing to 100–150 μg once daily. For the elderly and those with a history of arrhythmias or ischaemic heart disease, it would be useful to commence with a lower dose of 25–50 μg, to avoid the precipitation of palpitations. TSH levels and resolution of symptoms are monitored, to ensure the right maintenance dose of thyroxine. Any symptoms from the low levels of thyroid hormone will respond very effectively to replacement with normal levels of thyroxine. The dose may need some adjustment as the function of the thyroid gland declines, but once the correct dose is found, the dose generally does not need to be altered through life, except in the case of pregnancy.

Thyroid nodules

Thyroid nodules are common and it is estimated that they occur in around two-thirds of people normally. Most nodules are benign and do not produce excess thyroid hormone, and need no active management. In fact, 95–99% of found nodules in the thyroid are benign nodules, cysts or adenomas. The most appropriate test for thyroid nodules is fine-needle biopsy. If a nodule is found to contain thyroid cancer cells on biopsy (papillary carcinoma is the most common thyroid malignancy), the management generally includes total thyroidectomy and radioactive iodine, and replacement of thyroxine. The prognosis is very good. Post-surgical follow-up and monitoring, including nuclear scans, is recommended.

Thyroid nodules may be detected in several ways: the patient may present with a lump or pain in the neck; it may be noticed on an ultrasound or CT scan that includes the thyroid; or it may be felt by palpation of a patient's neck.

A thyroid nodule may be investigated in several ways:

- blood tests
- thyroid function tests (TSH, free T_3, free T_4)
- ultrasound—can be very sensitive; can find nodules 2 mm in size
- fine needle aspiration and biopsy—usually done when ultrasound suggests atypical features
- nuclear scan—to assess whether the nodule in question is functioning normally.

THYROID DISEASE: SUMMARY OF THERAPEUTICS

Hypothyroidism:

- Medication—thyroxine, commence on 100 μg, lower dose in the elderly.
- Test urinary iodine levels—if deficient, correct iodine deficiency. Food sources include seaweed, crustaceans, sardines and other saltwater fish and

iodised salt. Iodine supplements are available in tablets and drops.
- Screen for coeliac disease.
- Ensure sufficient dietary zinc, vitamins E, C, A and B, to metabolically support the thyroid gland. Supplement if necessary.
- Fresh wholefoods.
- Strict low-cholesterol diet is important, because of the association between hypothyroidism and hypercholesterolaemia.
- Foods that depress thyroid activity by blocking iodine utilisation include turnips, soybeans, peanuts, pine nuts, mustard, broccoli, cabbage, brussel sprouts, cauliflower, kale and spinach. These foods should be avoided in a hypothyroid condition.
- Supplements:
  - *Vitamins* C (1 g per day), A (10,000–25,000 IU per day), B complex (50–100 mg per day), augmented with B_2 (riboflavin, 10–15 mg), B_3 (niacin, 10–25 mg), and B_6 (pyridoxine, 25–50 mg), selenium (200 µg per day), vitamin E (400 IU per day) and zinc (30 mg per day) are necessary for normal thyroid hormone production.
  - *Calcium* (1000 mg per day) and *magnesium* (200–600 mg per day) may help metabolic processes function correctly.
  - *Selenium* status influences thyroid hormone production, particularly in the elderly. Recommended dose is 200–300 µg daily. Selenium and iodine also have an antagonistic relationship. It is theoretically dangerous to give selenium supplements by themselves in iodine-deficient areas. Correct iodine levels first.
  - *Essential fatty acids* (1000–1500 mg three times per day), found in flaxseed oil and fish oil, in the management of hypercholesterolaemia.
  - *Iron* may interfere with absorption of thyroid hormone medication, so if supplementation is needed, take at different times of the day.
  - *Zinc* and *copper*—either copper deficiency or copper excess can affect thyroid chemistry. As a broad generalisation: in hypothyroidism, zinc deficiency is a common problem; in hyperthyroidism, it is often copper deficiency. Copper and zinc have an antagonistic effect on each other. At the very least, it is easy to check serum copper levels, but for accuracy you should also do ceruloplasmin levels. Red cell zinc levels can also be tested.
- Exercise—stimulates thyroid hormone secretion and raises metabolic rate. *Recommendation*: 30–60 minutes per day of aerobic exercise and resistance (weight) training.
- Herbs:
  - *Coleus forskohlii* (50–100 mg 2–3 times per day) may stimulate thyroid function, to increase thyroid hormone.
  - Guggul (*Commiphora mikul*) and hawthorn (*Crataegus monogyna*) (500 mg twice a day) help to lower high cholesterol.

Thyroiditis:
- Avoid refined foods, sugar, dairy products, wheat, caffeine, alcohol.
- Essential fatty acids (1000–1500 mg three times per day), found in flaxseed oil and fish oil, are anti-inflammatory and necessary for hormone production.
- Bromelain (250–500 mg three times per day between meals) may reduce inflammation in thyroiditis.
- Turmeric (*Curcuma longa*) enhances the effect of bromelain and should be taken between meals, 500 mg t.d.s.
- Carefully monitor any intervention, because thyroiditis may convert from hyperthyroidism to hypothyroidism very quickly.

Hyperthyroidism:
- Foods that depress thyroid activity by preventing iodine utilisation include turnips, soybeans, peanuts, pine nuts, mustard, broccoli, cabbage, brussel sprouts, cauliflower, kale and spinach. These foods should be included in the diet of patients with overactive thyroid.
- Check whether the patient is taking any herbs or supplements that may affect thyroid function. For example, ashwagandha (*Withania somnifera*) and bladderwrack (*Fucus vesiculosus*) should be avoided in thyroid disease, as they can stimulate hyperthyroidism.

ADRENAL GLAND DISORDERS

The adrenal glands sit atop the kidneys and are primarily responsible for releasing a range of chemical mediators of the stress response, such as glucocorticoids (e.g. cortisol) from the outer cortex. The cortex is also responsible for releasing mineralocorticoids such as aldosterone, which has an important role in regulating blood pressure, and androgens such as dehydroepiandrosterone (DHEA). Catecholamines such as adrenaline and noradrenaline are released from the central area of the gland, called the medulla.

ADDISON'S SYNDROME

Adrenal insufficiency is an important treatable condition, and can be life-threatening if not identified and treated properly. The incidence varies between developed and developing countries, due to the higher incidence of infective diseases affecting the adrenal gland, in the latter—it is estimated at 1 in 100,000 in developed countries and up to 11 per 100,000 in developing countries, and is likely to increase in the latter in line with the incidence of *Mycobacterium tuberculosis* disease and HIV/AIDS.

Aetiology

Adrenal insufficiency may be secondary, due to pituitary disease. It usually occurs in panhypopituitary patients after surgery, trauma affecting the stalk, hypothalamic disease or radiotherapy. ACTH chromophobe cells of the pituitary are usually the last cells to lose their function in the setting of a compressing macroadenoma. ACTH may be selectively lost in isolation, as in lymphocytic hypophysitis. These patients differ clinically in that they do not have typical hyperkalaemia, due to the fact that they have an intact renin-angiotensin-aldosterone system.

More commonly, adrenal insufficiency is primary, due to diseases that directly affect the adrenal gland itself. These patients are more likely to be hyperkalaemic, with loss of the mineralocorticoid as well as the glucocorticoid production. Primary adrenal diseases may be congenital anatomical problems such as adrenal hypoplasia, or congenital enzyme problems, as in congenital adrenal hyperplasia where the genes encoding enzymes involved in the production of cortisol are defective.

Infections such as *Mycobacterium tuberculosis* may produce a granulomatous destruction of the adrenal cortex and medulla, usually in the setting of disseminated tuberculosis. Syphilis and HIV have been documented to result in adrenal insufficiency. *Neisseria meningitidis* septicaemia may result in adrenal infarction and the Waterhouse-Friderichsen syndrome of associated adrenal insufficiency. Infarction may occur in any form of septicaemia, as can haemorrhage due to disseminated intravascular coagulation (DIC) and coagulopathy. Supratherapeutic anticoagulation may also result in adrenal haemorrhage and insufficiency.

Fungal infections with *Histoplasmosis* and *Cryptococcus* may result in adrenal insufficiency, which may or may not recover with appropriate treatment.

Ketaconazole, which may be used for its antifungal effects or for metastatic prostate cancer, may also block enzymes in the steroidogenesis pathway of cortisol and result in reversible loss of adrenal cortisol production. It and other drugs such as metyrapone etomidate and mitotane may be used with the indication of medically and surgically resistant Cushing's syndrome, due to their effects on decreasing cortisol production from the adrenal cortex.

The very common but often forgotten cause of adrenal insufficiency is withdrawal of corticosteroids too quickly after a course long enough and at high enough dose to suppress ACTH stimulation of the adrenal cortices, and thus atrophy, and poor ACTH response when exogenous steroids are withdrawn. The static laboratory test of adrenal function with an early-morning cortisol and ACTH or the dynamic short synacthen test are identical, and history should point to the cause. Steroids must then be reintroduced and tapered at a slower rate. It is variable but a prednisone equivalent dose to around 10 mg per day for approximately 3 weeks should be assumed to suppress the adrenal cortex, and will require a slower taper. Adrenocortical suppression is more likely in elderly patients and those with dexamethasone or nocturnal doses of steroids. The nocturnal doses more effectively suppress the early morning peak of ACTH and thus lead more quickly to adrenal cortex atrophy and blunted ACTH response.

Adrenal cortical dysfunction is most commonly autoimmune in the developed world. It may occur in isolation or in the setting of APS types 1 and 2. Type 1 APS is characterised by mucocutaneous candidiasis, hypoparathyroidism and autoimmune adrenalitis that usually occurs in the first years of life and almost invariably occurs before the age of 20 years. APS Type 2 is more common than type 1 and occurs later in life than type 1, with autoimmune adrenalitis, autoimmune thyroid disease (hypo- more than hyperthyroidism) and type 1 diabetes mellitus. Adrenalitis usually occurs first but may follow the other manifestation in a good proportion of patients.

Other congenital causes of adrenal insufficiency such as adrenoleukodystrophy are more rare.

Infiltration from amyloid or metastatic breast or lung cancer is also rare.

Diagnostic approach

History and examination will often lead to a feeling for whether there is a problem with adrenocortical function, and may point to a possible cause. (See the section on history, below, for common symptoms and signs.)

Hyponatraemia is common in adrenal insufficiency, but hyperkalaemia is less common and does not occur in secondary adrenal insufficiency due to intact aldosterone production. An early-morning paired cortisol and ACTH will indicate whether there is a problem with primary or secondary hypoadrenalism. A cortisol peak of 400 nmol/L has a high specificity for adequate adrenal function. Regardless of ACTH levels, there is no need to further investigate adrenocortical insufficiency.

ACTH is released in a peak and is relatively unstable if not collected properly, but, those issues aside, a low cortisol with a low or inappropriately normal ACTH would tend to point to secondary adrenal insufficiency. A high ACTH at any time of the day with a less than adequate cortisol is very indicative of primary adrenal problems. In the indeterminate range, a short synacthen test of 250 μg of synacthen given as an intramuscular injection with cortisol measured at 0, 30 and 60 minutes can be performed. If done at 0800 with a morning ACTH and cortisol, a basal result of > 400 nmol/L or a stimulated rise of about 550 nmol/L indicates adequate adrenal function. Check with your local laboratory as to the normal cut-offs for its particular assay. The short synacthen test does not differentiate between primary and secondary adrenal insufficiency in the chronic setting, where there is inadequate ACTH drive with resulting adrenal atrophy and blunting of adrenal response, as one would see in primary disease.

Some have argued that this is a supraphysiological test, which may not properly assess for partial adrenal insufficiency. It has been suggested that a 1 μg synacthen test may be more of a physiological test dose.

History

The diagnosis of adrenal insufficiency may become apparent during an adrenal crisis with an intercurrent illness. As well as looking for the aetiological factors listed above, symptoms of weight loss, anorexia, fatigue, vomiting, abdominal pains, fevers, joint pains, recurrent illnesses that have a prolonged recovery phase, and postural symptoms, should be asked about. If the history points to a secondary cause, ask about menstrual history, hypothyroid symptoms and galactorrhoea.

Examination

Check the patient for signs of shock. Check for signs of hyperpigmentation, which should only occur in chronic primary adrenal insufficiency. Check the palms, new scars and wounds, pressure areas such as the elbows and knees, and the mucosal surfaces of the lips, buccal surfaces, anus and labia for signs of hyperpigmentation. Check postural blood pressure, including the pulse rate in each position. Examination of the abdomen may reveal what appears to be a surgical abdomen. It is important to investigate this, but also consider adrenal problems if any of the other features on history or exam point to adrenal insufficiency. In secondary adrenal insufficiency, visual fields should be checked with confrontation testing using a red hatpin.

Investigations

Consulting room:

- postural hypotension
- capillary glucose for hypoglycaemia.

Pathology:

- FBC for lymphocytosis and eosinophilia
- eLFTs for hyponatraemia, hyperkalaemia and hypercalcaemia
- random ACTH or 0800 ACTH and cortisol
- coagulation profile.

Special tests:

- These depend on the suspected cause. Anti-adrenal antibodies are not particularly sensitive but may be done if the cause clinically is thought to be autoimmune.

Integrative management

Prevention

Treat any secondary causes such as tuberculosis or HIV before adrenal involvement.

Active surveillance

Active surveillance alone is not a valid option. Adrenal insufficiency is a life-threatening condition and should be treated promptly, including admission to hospital and specialist assessment.

Lifestyle

The replacement with glucocorticoids is an estimation and therefore may be initially a higher dose than physiologically required. Maintaining a healthy diet and exercise, and being aware that excess steroids will stimulate appetite, will help the patient maintain a healthy weight.

Pharmacological

If the patient has presented unwell, hypotensive and shocked, and you suspect adrenal insufficiency, establish large-bore IV access and take blood for FBC, eLFT, ACTH and cortisol, and then commence treatment for shock, as well as giving 100 mg of IV hydrocortisone. The patient should be transferred to care in hospital. If the cortisol result returns as adequate in 1–2 days, then the steroids treatment may be stopped.

All steroids except dexamethasone have mineralocorticoid effects. Patients with secondary adrenal insufficiency will have an intact mineralocorticoid output, so addition of any extra mineralocorticoid in the form of fludrocortisone is not necessary.

In chronic adrenal insufficiency, replacement regimens are many but the aim is to try to provide enough glucocorticoid replacement in a normal physiological pattern that follows a diurnal variation, with a peak early in the morning that then tapers through the day. This may be achieved with hydrocortisone 20–30 mg per day in 2–3 divided doses in a regimen such as 12 mg on waking, 8 mg at lunch and 4 mg at afternoon tea. A simpler strategy is hydrocortisone 20 mg mane and 10 mg in the early afternoon, or cortisone acetate

25 mg mane and 12.5 mg in the early afternoon. The afternoon dose may be brought closer to midday if the patient reports difficulty sleeping. If the patient reports feeling unwell and quite fatigued in the early evening, then using a three-times-a-day split dose with a smaller proportion in the late afternoon can be trialled.

Be aware that fatigue as a symptom of inadequate replacement may lead to excessive replacement. There are many causes of fatigue. If hydrocortisone is used, checking a 24-hour urine collection for free cortisol may be used to assess whether the replacement is excessive.

In the setting of adrenal suppression from long-term steroids, treatment for other conditions in someone who should otherwise have an intact hypothalamic–pituitary–adrenal (HPA) axis, then a slow taper of the steroids, should allow for recovery of their normal axis function. The longer the patient has been on steroids, and the older the patient, the slower the taper. This may require a taper over several months to a year. Adequacy of their axis may be checked with a morning ACTH and cortisol prior to their normal dose, noting that the dexamethasone with its longer duration of action is likely to interfere with this technique.

If patients with primary adrenal insufficiency have documented postural hypotension or symptoms, and are on adequate glucocorticoid replacement, fludrocortisones 0.05–0.1 mg/day may be added.

Other medical and complementary therapies

There are some data indicating that in secondary hypoadrenalism in panhypopituitary women, replacement of adrenal androgens with DHEA 25–50 mg per day has some beneficial effects on quality of life and libido. This has only been shown in women so far. Men have their own stronger androgens in the form of testosterone, either from their own testes or from replacement in hypopituitary patients.

Some advocate the benefits of DHEA in patients with otherwise normal steroid production. At this stage there is no evidence that there is objective benefit with treatment. Be aware also that many of the forms of DHEA that are available have a very variable content. DHEA can be obtained by prescription from compounding pharmacies. The forms available may vary in the quantities of active substance. Further studies are ongoing to assess any benefits of adrenal androgen replacement.

Paramedical

- Patients should be advised about sick-day management. For a minor illness the replacement dose should be doubled for 3 days.
- For illnesses that require the patient to be bed-bound, a tripling of the dose for 3 days can be advised.
- If the patient has a vomiting or diarrhoeal illness, an IM dose of 100 mg hydrocortisone should be given and the patient should then go to the nearest hospital immediately. The injection is available as Solu-Cortef® as a powder for reconstitution, in many but not all countries.
- The patient should be educated about self-injection techniques, to ensure they can manage in a crisis. The partner or significant other should also be involved in the education.
- A MedicAlert bracelet is recommended, in case the patient is hospitalised or is found unwell or unconscious.

Ongoing review and/or monitoring

Titration of maintenance dose based on symptoms with the use of signs and objective biochemical tests can be done over time, with the goal being to work out the lowest effective dose for the patient to try to prevent iatrogenic Cushing's syndrome.

Important pitfalls

Glucocorticoids given at night for inflammatory conditions in a patient with normal HPA axis are more likely to suppress the axis in long term, due to suppression of the 0500 ACTH surge.

Dexamethasone will not be picked up on an assay of cortisol at all and prednisone only around 25%. Hydrocortisone has a 100% cross-reactivity with the cortisol assay.

Prognosis

Recovery of adrenal function is possible in cases of treated infectious adrenalitis, but does not usually happen.

CUSHING'S SYNDROME

Cushing's disease is the disorder described by Harvey Cushing, with pituitary disease with ACTH-dependent hypercortisolism. *Cushing's syndrome* describes the other forms of cortisol excess. (See Table 28.3 for a list of other causes of hypercortisolaemia.) The incidence of Cushing's disease or syndrome is difficult to quantify. There is significant overlap between the manifestation of Cushing's disease, and that of obesity and its complications. European series have estimated the incidence at 1–3 per million patients.

Establishing the diagnosis of hypercortisolaemia involves establishing a clinical likelihood or pre-test probability, establishing the biochemical excess of glucocorticoids, and then establishing the cause, in order to plan effective treatment.

The diagnosis may be perplexing, given that there is much overlap between normal levels in biochemical

TABLE 28.3 Causes of hypercortisolaemia

Name	Cause
Cushing's disease	ACTH-dependent pituitary disease
Pseudocushing's disease	• Obesity • Alcohol use (rarely causes) • Cushing's syndrome depression—rare cause of Cushing's syndrome but common elevator of UFC or 1 mg DST
Factitious Cushing's	Iatrogenic or surreptitious glucocorticoid excess
Ectopic ACTH	Bronchogenic tumours producing ACTH
Primary hypercortisolism	Cortisol-secreting adrenal tumour

testing and levels in those with true glucocorticoid excess.

Aside from iatrogenic Cushing's syndrome, Cushing's disease accounts for the majority of cases of Cushing's syndrome, at 60–70%. Adrenal disease is also not uncommon, accounting for approximately 20% of cases. Ectopic ACTH secretion and resultant Cushing's syndrome accounts for approximately 10–15% of cases, with the other causes responsible for the few remaining per cent.

Aetiology

Excessive glucocorticoids may be due to excessive ACTH drive, excessive adrenal glucocorticoid or iatrogenic administration of glucocorticoids.

With ACTH-driven disease, there is bilateral adrenal hypertrophy as well as excessive glucocorticoids. In Cushing's disease there is also excessive stimulation of the melanocytes via melanocyte-stimulating hormone. Pro-opiomelanocortin (POMC) is secreted form the pituitary under stimulation by CRH (corticotropin-releasing hormone). POMC is then cleaved into ACTH, with ACTH stimulating the cells of the zona fasciculata of the adrenal cortex, and melanocyte-stimulating hormone (MSH). Thus, ACTH-independent hypercortisolism of a cortisol-secreting tumour of the adrenal gland does not result in hyperpigmentation.

Pathology

Excessive cortisol has many effects:

- hyperglycaemia—increased gluconeogenesis and insulin resistance
- hypertension—excessive stimulation of the mineralocorticoid receptor in the kidney, with high levels of glucocorticoids
- osteoporosis—inhibition of proliferation of osteoblasts, apoptosis of osteoblasts, antagonisation of PTH effects on bone, and hypogonadism
- proximal myopathy
- central obesity with overall weight gain and moon facies
- thin skin and fragile microvasculature—loss of subcutaneous fat and thinning of subcutaneous tissues
- mood changes
- increased appetite
- hypogonadotrophic hypogonadism, with menstrual irregularities in women.

Diagnostic approach

Question 1: Do the history and examination point to glucocorticoid excess?

Most of the features of Cushing's syndrome are very similar to those of obesity and its complications. Of the clinical features, the most discriminatory for Cushing's syndrome over simple obesity are:

- in children:
  - slow growth with weight gain
  - osteoporosis
  - hypertension
  - thin skin
- in adults:
  - easy bruising
  - facial plethora
  - proximal myopathy
  - striae—violaceous > 1 cm wide.

Think about how high your pre-test probability/clinical suspicion is, based on these discriminatory features and other non-discriminatory symptoms.

Question 2: Is there glucocorticoid excess?

The Endocrine Society has released guidelines for investigation of Cushing's Syndrome and Cushing's disease.[3]

- For initial investigation:
  - 2 × 24-hour urinary free cortisol (UFC)
  - 1 mg overnight dexamethasone suppression test (DST)
  - DST
    - longer low-dose 0.5 mg q6h 48-hour DST
    - midnight salivary cortisol—the results of the 1 mg DST will give varying sensitivities and

specificities, depending on the cut-offs used for a normal suppression
 - < 50 mmol/L (2 μg/dL) at 8 am has a sensitivity of 92% and is the recommended cut-off.
- Midnight serum cortisol should be low in those without Cushing's syndrome, including obese or depressed patients. Midnight salivary cortisol, if available, may be used, and the normal levels are assay-dependent.
- If there are two normal tests and the pre-test probability is low, then testing need only be done in the future if the signs and symptoms that initially caused clinical suspicion progress, and it has been more than 6 months since the normal test results.
- If the pre-test probability is high, repeating the tests to gather more evidence for or against the diagnosis is warranted. Consider referral to an endocrinologist at this point. If the repeated tests are abnormal, Cushing's syndrome is likely.

See Figure 29.4 for an overview.

Note: Conditions that may lead to abnormal results with few features of Cushing's syndrome clinically include:

- pregnancy
- depression and significant mental illness, including eating disorders
- alcohol excess
- glucocorticoid resistance
- morbid obesity
- poorly controlled diabetes
- physical stress, including illness
- malnutrition
- high-intensity consistent exercise
- hypothalamic amenorrhoea
- capillary blood glucose (CBG) excess in hyperoestrogenic states (urine results not affected).

Question 3: Is the cortisol excess ACTH dependent?

Two measurements randomly of the ACTH and cortisol in a patient with established Cushing's syndrome should be taken:

- ACTH:
  - < 5 pg/mL (1.1 pmol/L) represents ACTH-independent hypercortisolism, and a CT scan with thin slices of the adrenal glands should be performed
  - 5–20 pg/mL (1.1–4.4 pmol/L) is less reliable but probably indicates ACTH dependence, as it is inappropriately normal level, and not suppressed
  - > 20 pg/mL (4.4 pmol/L) indicates clear ACTH-dependent hypercortisolism.
- Most cases of ACTH-dependent Cushing's syndrome are pituitary in aetiology:
  - To establish this, an 8 mg overnight DST can be performed, on the basis that nearly all pituitary ACTH-secreting tumours may be suppressed by high-dose glucocorticoids, but most ectopic sources of ACTH will not.
  - Inferior petrosal sinus sampling with CRH stimulation may be done after an MRI of the pituitary, if it is thought to be Cushing's disease.

History

Clinical suspicion may be increased and testing performed in those with:

- hypertension or osteoporosis at an early age
- multiple and progressive signs and symptoms, particularly thin skin and bruising that are otherwise unexplained, facial plethora, proximal myopathy, or fresh violaceous striae
- an adrenal mass—for investigation as part of the work-up, to assess whether it is hormonally functional
- (in children) increasing weight but decreasing height
- a smoking history
- use of inhaled or other exogenous steroids
- menstrual irregularities ± hirsutism.

Examination

- Typical body habitus:
  - centripetal obesity with relatively thin limbs
  - easy bruising and thin skin
  - facial plethora
  - buffalo hump, supraclavicular fat pad
  - moon facies
- Proximal myopathy
- Blood pressure
- Visual fields
- Mucosal pigmentation including the buccal surfaces and lips
- Striae—abdomen, buttocks and legs > 1 cm and violaceous
- Peripheral stigmata of lung cancer (if appropriate):
  - supraclavicular lymph nodes
  - Horner's sign
  - Pancoast tumour
  - clubbing
  - hypertrophic pulmonary osteoarthropathy.

Investigations

- Consulting room—capillary glucose
- Pathology—see Fig 29.4.

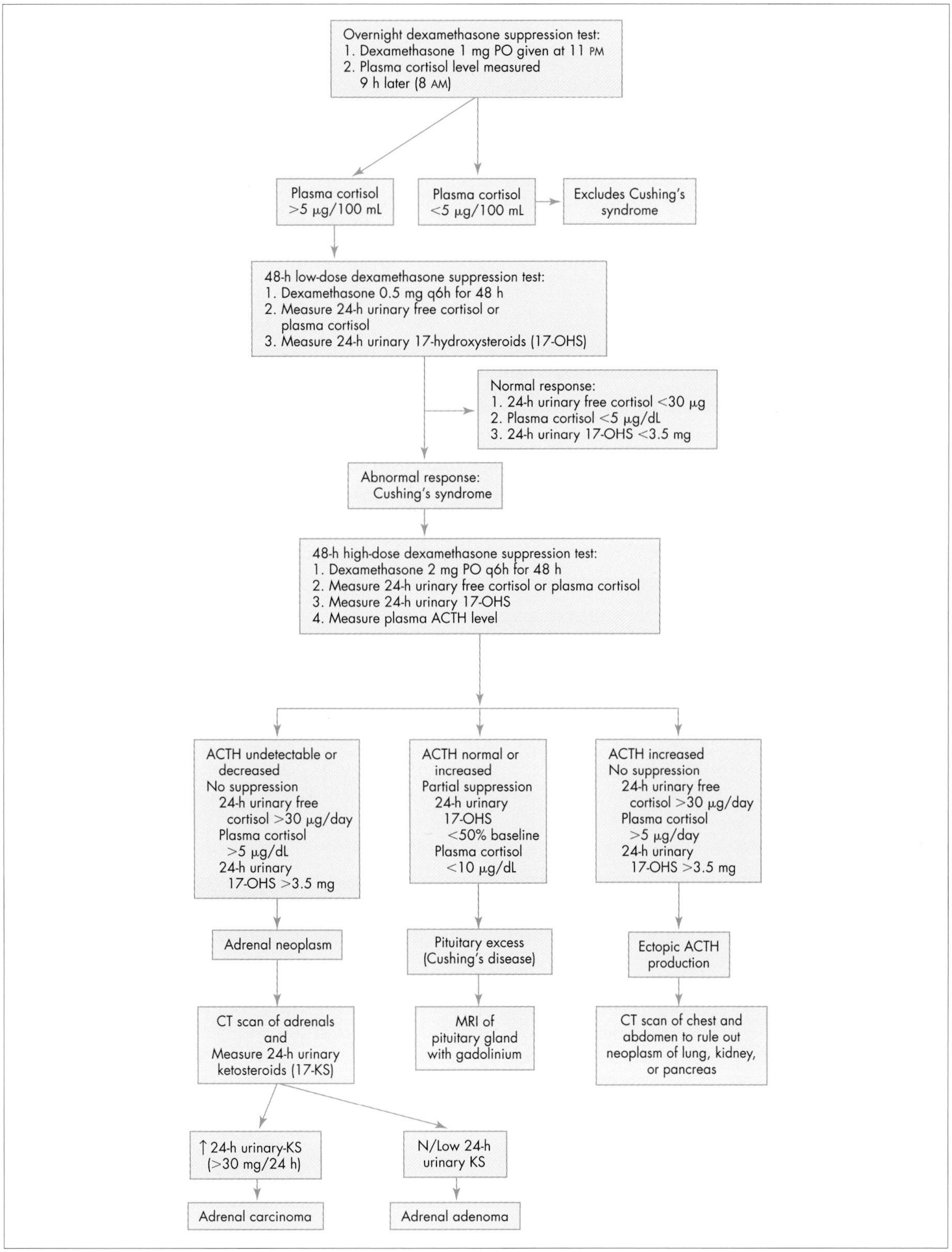

FIGURE 29.4 Diagnosing Cushing's syndrome

Integrative management

Active surveillance

- While the diagnosis is being investigated, treatment of the metabolic complications should be initiated as with non-Cushingoid patients.
- The prognosis used to be poor, prior to good therapies for the metabolic complications, with survival usually limited to around 5 years. Modern diabetes, hypercholesterolaemia and hypertension therapies have made little improvement.
- The diagnosis must be made biochemically and clinically before organising imaging and localising studies.

Lifestyle

Maintaining good physical activity can help limit insulin resistance, hypertension, dyslipidaemia and proximal myopathy.

Pharmacological

Medical therapies are aimed at the two different parts of the problem.

- Metabolic complications:
  - antidiabetic drugs
  - antihypertensives
  - anti peptic ulcer drugs
  - dyslipidaemia drugs
  - osteoporosis treatments if indicated.
- Aetiology:
  - cortisol may be blocked in production by ketaconazole, which blocks some of the stages of steroidogenesis
  - metyrapone may be used to block adrenal production of steroids. Effective medical therapy may result in enlargement of the tumour in Cushing's syndrome, a problem known as Nelson's syndrome. This is more common when bilateral adrenalectomy is performed to control Cushing's disease
  - etomidate
  - mitotane
  - somatostatin agonists:
    - octreotide and lanreotide have little effect in Cushing's disease but pasireotide with greater binding to sst-3 receptors may be more useful
    - octreotide has shown some biochemical benefit in ectopic ACTH-secreting tumours.

Surgical

- Trans-sphenoidal surgery of an established Cushing's disease—tumours tend to be more commonly microadenomas at diagnosis. Microadenomas are more successfully cured and with fewer complications of pituitary insufficiencies than macroadenomas.
- Adrenalectomy for a cortisol-secreting tumour established by adrenal vein sampling.
- Bilateral adrenalectomy for non-operatively curable ACTH-dependent Cushing's syndrome. In the case of an inoperable Cushing's disease, there is a risk of Nelson's syndrome, with lack of negative feedback on the tumour leading to increasing tumour growth and mass effects.

Paramedical

- Physiotherapy to maintain muscle strength and function.
- Dietician to help with healthy weight range.

Complementary therapies

There is little data on therapies that may be of use in humans.

Ongoing review and/or monitoring

Surgically 'cured' Cushing's disease patients should be monitored periodically on an ongoing basis for clinical and biochemical recurrence of their disease.

Prognosis

- Effective treatment of hypercortisolaemia results in the correction of many of the complications within 6–12 months.
- BMD may improve but osteoporotic crush fractures cannot be reversed.
- The metabolic consequences will be improved but may not be 'cured', although they may return to background levels for the patient if they had normal levels of cortisol.

RESOURCES

Endocrine Society, http://www.endo-society.org
Endocrineweb, http://www.endocrineweb.com/

REFERENCES

1 Molitch ME, Russell EJ. The pituitary 'Incidentaloma'. Ann Intern Med 1990; 112(12):925–931.

2 Holdaway IM, Rajasoorya C. Epidemiology of acromegaly. Pituitary 1999; 2:29–41.

3 Endocrine Society. The diagnosis of Cushing's syndrome: an Endocrine Society practice guideline. J Clin Endocrin Metab 2008; 93(5):1526–1540.

chapter 30

Gastroenterology

INTRODUCTION AND OVERVIEW

The adage 'you are what you eat' is only partly true. In fact, you are what you eat, manage to digest and absorb across the gastrointestinal tract into the bloodstream, and which you are not intolerant of or allergic to. The gastrointestinal tract is the interface with the ingested environment, and dysfunction in the gut may affect any or every vital function.

In the process of diagnosing and formulating a management plan for patients with gastrointestinal problems, it is essential to keep in mind not just the gut symptoms, but the lifestyle factors affecting gut function, and the systemic and nutritional consequences of gut dysfunction.

COMMON PRESENTATIONS

ACUTE ABDOMINAL PAIN[1,2]

Acute abdominal pain is pain of recent onset, which can vary in severity from mild and self-limiting to severe and life-threatening. Episodes may resolve spontaneously or require medical assessment and intervention. It is important to assess the site, chronicity, severity and nature of the pain and any associated signs and symptoms.

The patient's general condition and the urgency of intervention will need to be assessed before investigations are arranged. If the patient is haemodynamically stable and there are no signs of sepsis, judiciously selected investigations may be arranged in the community setting. In an emergency or potential emergency situation, it may well be prudent to transfer the patient to hospital and have investigations carried out there.

Nature of pain

- *Visceral pain*—abdominal organs are not sensitive to touch. However, stretching or distending the bowel does cause pain that is poorly localised, usually to the midline. Distension of the capsule of the liver also causes pain.
- *Peritoneal pain*—the parietal peritoneum has pain fibres, but the visceral peritoneum does not. Pain from inflammation of the parietal peritoneum is well-localised to the area of inflammation. It is exacerbated by movement such as coughing or respiration.
- *Referred pain*—referred pain is pain felt distant from the site of the problem that is causing the pain. For example, right shoulder tip pain is referred from the parietal peritoneum under the diaphragm, with these areas both innervated by somatic C4 nerves. Cardiac pain may be felt in the epigastrium, and pelvic pain in the umbilical area.

Abdominal guarding is a significant sign, due to reflex contraction of muscles in the abdominal wall in response to stimulation of pain fibres of the same dermatome.

Mechanisms of abdominal pain

Acute inflammation produces pain whose features depend on whether the organ affected is intraperitoneal or extraperitoneal. Intraperitoneal inflammation causes peritonitis that is well-localised, aggravated by sudden movement and relieved by being still. Inflammation restricted to bowel mucosa does not cause peritonism.

- *Obstruction*—pain tends to be colicky unless there is a complication such as secondary infection or perforation, when it becomes continuous.
- *Ischaemia* (including torsion)—arterial ischaemia is sudden in onset, severe and continuous. Venous ischaemia is slower in onset.
- *Increased pressure in a solid organ*—pain tends to be dull and constant (e.g. haemorrhage into an ovarian cyst).

Site of pain

(See Fig 30.1)

- Generalised
- Localised to:
  - epigastrium
  - right upper quadrant (RUQ)
  - left upper quadrant (LUQ)
  - central (periumbilical)
  - right iliac fossa (RIF)
  - left iliac fossa (LIF)
  - hypogastrium

Type and chronicity of pain

- Constant
- Peritoneal
- Colicky—felt in the midline, associated with forceful smooth muscle contraction related to stomach (epigastric), intestine (small bowel and right hemicolon colic felt periumbilically; left hemicolon colic felt suprapubically) or uterus (suprapubic). Repetitive cyclic pattern of intense pain, then relief.

Biliary 'colic' is continuous rather than intermittent, in the epigastrium or RUQ.

Associated features

- Fever, nausea, vomiting, micturition difficulty, bowel habit, menstruation and gynaecological history, obstetric history, medication and supplements
- Mass, rebound tenderness, guarding, signs of dehydration or blood loss (tachycardia, hypotension, pallor, reduced level of consciousness)

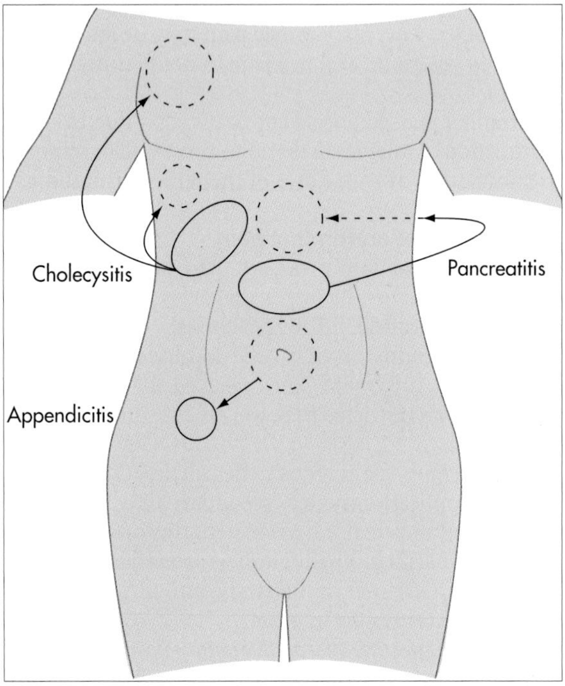

FIGURE 30.1 Sites of abdominal pain

GENERALISED ABDOMINAL PAIN

Severe generalised abdominal pain requires rapid and accurate assessment, resuscitation and transfer to hospital.

Signs of serious abdominal pathology include generalised peritonitis with rebound, guarding and absence of bowel sounds. Signs of shock (tachycardia, hypotension, oliguria, peripheral vasoconstriction) may be evident if there has been dehydration, haemorrhage or severe allergic reaction.

Consider:

- *Perforated appendix*—history suggestive of appendicitis: initially central colicky abdominal pain later localising to the RIF, fever, tachycardia. Tenderness and rebound in RIF. Tenderness on the right on digital rectal examination. Neutrophilia and raised C-reactive protein. Requires immediate surgical referral.
- *Perforated peptic ulcer*—sudden prostration with severe generalised peritoneal-type abdominal pain. Symptoms may improve after 2–6 hours. Peritonitis develops after 6–12 hours with generalised tenderness and guarding, maximal in the epigastrium, board-like rigidity, loss of bowel sounds and loss of liver dullness to percussion. Gas under diaphragm may be seen on erect abdominal X-ray. Limited gastrograffin meal may help diagnosis. Initial treatment: resuscitation, nasogastric suction, antibiotics. Urgent surgical referral.
- *Perforated diverticulum*—history of diverticular disease or preceding undiagnosed pain in LIF. Tenderness and rebound in LIF, gas under diaphragm in erect abdominal X-ray.
- *Ruptured ectopic pregnancy*—suspect in a woman of childbearing age with a late period and sudden onset of pelvic or lower abdominal pain. Symptoms and signs are maximal in the pelvis; sometimes pain is felt in region of rectum. This is sometimes reported as increase in pain when woman tries to sit down. Tender mass may be evident on vaginal examination. Shock is common. Usually elevated β-hCG levels are found and ectopic implantation seen on ultrasound at 5–6 weeks of amenorrhoea. Urgent gynaecological surgery referral.
- *Ruptured solid organ*—a history of trauma is usually present. Symptoms and signs will include significant blood loss and also be organ-specific.

- *Ruptured aortic aneurysm*—patient usually elderly with risk factors for cardiovascular disease. Pain is central, constant and radiates through to the back. Not usually signs of peritonism, as bleeding is retroperitoneal. Pulsatile mass in central abdomen. May sometimes present with sudden pain followed by shock and loss of consciousness. Surgical emergency.
- *Strangulated bowel*—site of pain depends on area of strangulation. Is there a history or signs of a hernia or previous abdominal surgery? May be associated signs and symptoms of small bowel obstruction. Urgent surgical referral required.
- *Superior mesenteric artery thrombosis or embolism*—causes massive small bowel ischaemia. Often preceded by a history of atrial fibrillation or myocardial infarction. CT scan will define the problem but should not delay urgent surgical referral.
- *Ischaemic colitis*—associated bloody diarrhoea, signs maximal in LIF. Colonoscopy may assist diagnosis. Urgent hospital referral, although surgery usually not required.
- *Pancreatitis*—check for history of alcoholic binges, gallstones, trauma or medication known to cause pancreatitis.

LOCALISED ACUTE ABDOMINAL PAIN

Epigastrium

Causes

- Cardiac referred pain
- Oesophagus (GORD)
- Stomach—peptic ulcer
- Pancreatitis (pain may radiate to the back)
- Biliary pain
- Abdominal aortic aneurysm.

Investigation

- Plain X-ray of chest and abdomen (erect and supine)
- Full blood count
- Liver function tests
- Serum amylase/lipase
- If indicated: upper abdominal ultrasound; endoscopy of upper gastrointestinal tract (GIT), electrocardiogram (ECG) and cardiac work-up.

Right upper quadrant

Causes

- Gallstones (biliary colic)
- Cholecystitis
- Cholangitis
- Hepatitis or other liver pathology
- Renal colic
- Pyelonephritis
- Right lung/pleural pathology (basal pulmonary consolidation).

Investigation

- Plain X-ray of chest and abdomen
- Full blood count
- Liver function tests
- Amylase/lipase
- Blood culture if features of sepsis
- If indicated: upper abdominal ultrasound.

Left upper quadrant

Causes

- Renal colic
- Pyelonephritis
- Splenic infarct
- Left lung/pleural pathology.

Investigation

- Plain X-ray of chest and abdomen
- Full blood count
- Amylase/lipase
- Blood culture if features of sepsis
- If indicated: upper abdominal ultrasound.

Central (periumbilical)

Causes

- Appendicitis (early)
- Mesenteric artery embolism
- Ruptured aortic aneurysm
- Large bowel obstruction (bowel cancer, volvulus)
- Irritable bowel syndrome
- Gastroenteritis
- Constipation.

Investigation

- Plain X-ray of abdomen
- Full blood count
- Blood culture if features of sepsis
- Stool cultures
- If indicated: abdominal ultrasound
- Angiography if indicated.

Right iliac fossa

… think gut and gynaecology.

Causes

- Appendicitis (late presentation)
- Crohn's disease
- Mesenteric adenitis (common in children and adolescents, presumed viral cause, self-limiting)
- Ureteric colic

- Terminal ileitis (associated diarrhoea, culture for *Yersinia enterocolitica*)
- Caecal carcinoma
- Acute Meckel's diverticulum inflammation
- Ovarian pathology (ruptured/haemorrhage into ovarian cyst)
- Mittelschmerz (ovulation)
- Acute salpingitis
- Endometriosis
- Ectopic pregnancy
- Urinary tract infection.

Investigation

- Plain X-ray of abdomen
- Full blood count
- Blood culture if features of sepsis
- Stool cultures
- Pregnancy test
- Midstream urine (MC&S)
- Colonoscopy ± bowel biopsy
- Intravenous pyelogram (IVP)
- If indicated: pelvic ultrasound
- Angiography if indicated.

Left iliac fossa

… think gut and gynaecology.

Causes

- Ureteric colic
- Diverticulitis
- Colitis
- Bowel cancer
- Constipation
- Ovarian pathology (ruptured/haemorrhage into ovarian cyst)
- Mittelschmerz (ovulation)
- Acute salpingitis
- Endometriosis
- Ectopic pregnancy
- Urinary tract infection.

Investigation of left and right iliac fossa pain

- CT scan if appendicitis suspected (periumbilical pain initially, later localising to RIF, point tenderness over McBurney's point, mild fever)
- Urinalysis/urine microscopy and culture
- Women:
  - pregnancy test (women of childbearing age)
  - pelvic ultrasound
- Laparoscopy may be necessary.

Hypogastrium

Causes

- Urinary tract infection
- Ruptured ectopic pregnancy
- Ovarian pathology
- Mittelschmerz
- Acute pelvic infection
- Period pain
- Labour pains
- Acute urinary retention—severe lower abdominal pain, usually from prostatomegaly, bladder neck obstruction, pelvic mass or anticholinergic drugs.

Investigation

- Plain X-ray of abdomen
- Full blood count
- Blood culture if features of sepsis
- Pregnancy test
- Midstream urine (MC&S)
- If indicated: pelvic ultrasound.

CHRONIC ABDOMINAL PAIN

Consider:

- Subacute appendicitis
- Adhesions
- Irritable bowel syndrome
- Chronic pancreatitis
- Peptic ulcer
- Gallstones
- Malignancy
- Mesenteric vascular insufficiency
- Gastroparesis
- Abdominal wall pain (e.g. Spigelian or umbilical hernia)
- Crohn's disease
- Food intolerance
- Medication side effect.

Investigation

Investigations will be determined by the site of pain and the most likely diagnoses, and may include:

- stool microscopy and culture
- abdominal and pelvic ultrasound
- endoscopy (endoscopy or colonoscopy or both)
- CT scan
- laparoscopy.

CONSTIPATION

Constipation refers to difficulty in passing small, hard stools. If a patient presents with 'constipation', it is important to find out exactly what they mean. Question the patient about their bowel motions' frequency, volume, colour and consistency, and the presence or absence of blood. Lifestyle factors are also an important contributor to or exacerbating factor for constipation.

While the cause of constipation may be a simple matter of diet, drug side effect or behavioural bowel habit, constipation may be an indication of a serious underlying disorder.

Aetiology

Miscellaneous:

- Lifestyle
  - dietary inadequacy (fibre and fluids)
  - physical inactivity
- Irritable bowel syndrome
- Slow transit (may run in families)
- Pelvic floor dysfunction (woman may manually disimpact with digital pressure in vagina)
- Painful bowel motions, e.g.
  - anal fissure
  - strangulated haemorrhoid.

Structural:

- Colon cancer
- Colonic stricture
- Megacolon
- Abnormal myenteric plexus (Hirschsprung's disease, Chagas' disease)
- Perianal infection
- Anal stenosis
- Dystrophia myotonica
- Systemic sclerosis
- Crohn's disease.

Neurological:

- Diabetic autonomic neuropathy
- Sacral parasympathetic damage
- Spinal cord damage
- Spinal cord disease (e.g. multiple sclerosis)
- Parkinson's disease
- Psychosis.

Metabolic:

- Hypothyroidism
- Hypercalcaemia
- Porphyria
- Pregnancy.

Psychological:

- Depression
- Anorexia nervosa
- Dementia.

Drug side effects:

- Narcotics
- Antihypertensives
- Antidepressants
- Iron supplements.

Diagnosis

Ascertain frequency, volume, colour and consistency of bowel motions and whether there has been any bleeding or mucus per rectum. Enquire about the duration of the problem and previous attempts to relieve it, such as use of laxatives, herbal therapies or dietary adjustment. Sometimes severe and chronic constipation can present with loose bowel motions and faecal leakage. Ask about associated bloating, pain or weight loss.

A full dietary history is necessary, preferably with a food diary recorded over a week.

Complete physical examination including abdominal examination and digital rectal examination is necessary, including examining for fissures, fistulae, abscesses or signs of neoplasm in the anal area. Sigmoidoscopy may be helpful. In women examine for rectocele.

Investigation

- History, diet assessment and physical examination may be all that is required to elucidate the cause of constipation.
- Further investigation will be guided by likely aetiology based on history and examination.
- Blood tests—check for anaemia (FBC), iron studies, CRP, thyroid function, serum calcium.
- Plain abdominal X-ray
- Colonoscopy—to identify or exclude cancer, Crohn's disease or stricture
- Anorectal manometry

Therapeutics

- Treat any underlying medical cause if present, such as hypothyroidism or hypercalcaemia.
- Dietary fibre 20–30 g per day, especially fresh fruit and vegetables and whole cereals (especially oatmeal).
- Prunes may help.
- Supplement with psyllium husks or Metamucil.
- Increase water intake.
- Drink warm lemon water before meals.
- Take time to eat slowly.
- Replace or remove medications that have constipation as a side effect.
- Avoid stimulant laxatives.
- Use stool softener, such as Coloxyl.
- In high doses, magnesium exerts a laxative effect (Epsom salts or milk of magnesia) for short-term relief.
- Lactulose (osmotic laxative) is useful for chronic constipation.
- Glycerin suppositories before bowel motion may assist passage of stool.
- Enemas may be required as an occasional emergency measure.
- Establish a regular toilet routine. Hypnotherapy or behavioural therapy may assist with relaxation.
- Regular physical exercise.
- Probiotic supplement.

DIARRHOEA

Diarrhoea refers to frequent loose or watery stools. History taking should include duration and severity of symptoms and systemic features (fever, myalgia, malaise, arthralgia), and presence of blood or mucus in the stool.

Acute diarrhoea

Patient should be questioned about pain, stool frequency, colour and consistency, presence of blood, and incidence of vomiting.

- Acute watery diarrhoea is most often due to viral or bacterial gastroenteritis/enteritis or protozoal infection.
- Frothy, windy, smelly stools may indicate malabsorption of fats and/or giardiasis.
- Bloody diarrhoea may be a result of infectious colitis, drug-induced colitis, inflammatory bowel disease, ischaemic colitis or antibiotic-associated diarrhoea.
- Acute diarrhoea may be a first presentation of coeliac disease, Crohn's disease or inflammatory bowel disease.
- History should elicit symptoms of volume depletion such as dry mouth, orthostatic hypotension, tachycardia, especially when vomiting is associated.
- Questions about systemic symptoms will include fever, malaise, myalgia and arthralgia.
- History should include recent travel, medications (especially antibiotics and vitamin supplements), dietary history, consumption of fast food or leftovers and whether other members of family or a dining group developed diarrhoea, and any history of immune deficiency.

Investigation

- General physical examination will include cardiovascular assessment, signs of toxicity (fever, tachycardia, shock), abdominal palpation for mass or tenderness, and digital rectal examination for tenderness, mass or faecal impaction.
- Patients presenting with diarrhoea will need to be assessed for volume depletion, and this is particularly important in children and the elderly.
- For minor resolving episodes of diarrhoea without systemic features, no investigations will be necessary.
- Stool examination for blood, and stool culture looking for ova, cysts and parasites, may help to target therapy in cases of severe or prolonged acute diarrhoea. However, standard stool examination can be unreliable. Special requests for identification of pathogens may need to be made for suspected *Campylobacter*, *Clostridium difficile* and toxin, *Yersinia*, and *Cryptosporidium* or amoebic dysentery.
- Blood tests can give valuable information about the cause and/or the effects of the diarrhoea. These might include full blood count, ESR, iron studies, folate, vitamin B_{12}, calcium, electrolytes and thyroid function.
- Sigmoidoscopy or colonoscopy may be indicated where colitis or inflammatory bowel disease is suspected.
- Initial treatment for most cases is to support hydration and relieve symptoms (see below). Where a treatable cause of diarrhoea can be established or a presumptive diagnosis made, treatment should be targeted at the cause.
- Hospitalisation is indicated for patients with sepsis or severe dehydration.

Viral gastroenteritis/enteritis

The usual cause is infection with rotavirus or noravirus. Viral gastroenteritis/enteritis generally presents with acute onset of watery diarrhoea with or without vomiting.

Treatment

- Rehydrate with fluid and electrolyte solution, and monitor fluid balance. Use the simplest route where possible (oral) but sometimes the nasogastric or IV route may be required in emergency situations (e.g. infants) or where oral rehydration is not possible. Avoid rehydration with sweet drinks such as lemonade unless diluted to one-third to one-quarter normal strength.
- Low-fibre diet (soups, diluted fruit juice, white rice)
- Exclude lactose until diarrhoea settles.
- Exclude drinks containing sorbitol.
- Antiemetic injection if required for severe vomiting (metoclopramide or prochlorperazine), or ondansetron waters.
- Probiotic (*Lactobacillus* spp) particularly for prolonged and antibiotic-induced diarrhoea[3].

Prevention

- Immunisation of babies against rotavirus (responsible for 50% of children's hospital admissions).
- Maintain strict hand washing after nappy changing and toileting. Infected individuals should avoid handling food.

Bacterial gastroenteritis

Nausea, vomiting, diarrhoea and abdominal pain are common to most. Neurological, hepatic and renal complications can also occur. Rapid onset (hours) after ingestion of contaminated food suggests a pre-formed toxin, while a longer incubation period (1–3 days) suggests a bacterial or viral cause.

Pathogens include: enterotoxigenic *Escherichia coli*, *Campylobacter*, *Salmonella*, *Shigella*, *Entamoeba histolytica*, *Clostridium perfringens*, *Bacillus cereus*, *Vibrio parahaemolyticus*.

Enterotoxigenic *E. coli*

A leading cause of traveller's diarrhoea. Adheres to the gut wall and produces enterotoxins.

Symptoms

- Watery diarrhoea, cramping abdominal pain, nausea.

Treatment

- Maintain hydration; general supportive advice.
- Norfloxacin 400 mg b.i.d. p.o. or ciprofloxacin may be used for moderate to severe symptoms. Cotrimoxazole can be used for children.

Campylobacter jejuni

A common cause of food-borne illness from contaminated milk, sick pets, poorly stored food and contaminated water.

After an incubation period of 2–6 days, symptoms include: malaise, fever, myalgia, headaches and acute diarrhoea. Stools are initially watery and progress to blood and mucus. Severe cramping abdominal pain is common.

Diagnosis

- Stool culture with special request.

Treatment

- Maintain hydration; general supportive advice.
- If symptoms fail to settle: erythromycin 500 mg q.i.d. for 7 days or norfloxacin 400 mg b.i.d for 7 days.

Salmonella

Salmonella are gram-negative bacilli that can cause a range of clinical pictures including gastroenteritis, typhoid fever, bacteraemia and localised infection.

Complications include osteomyelitis, bacteraemia, abscesses, meningitis and pneumonia.

Antibiotics are generally not advised.

Treatment

If required, when disease is severe or patient is at risk of complications:

- Ciprofloxacin 500 mg p.o. b.i.d. for 2 weeks
- Probiotics.

Shigella

Highly contagious; transmission is by the faecal–oral route. Symptoms include diarrhoea with blood and pus, cramping abdominal pain, frequently with tenesmus. Invasion of colonic epithelium and production of an enterotoxin causes intestinal damage resulting in oedema, crypt abscesses and mucosal ulceration.

Complications

- Rectal prolapse, toxic megacolon, colonic perforation, haemolytic uraemic syndrome, reactive arthritis, pneumonia.

Diagnosis

- Stool culture and antibiotic sensitivity
- Sigmoidoscopy and biopsy to exclude inflammatory bowel disease and ameobic colitis.

Therapeutics

- Maintain hydration.
- Antibiotic treatment may be necessary: co-trimoxazole b.i.d. for 7–10 days or ciprofloxacin 500 mg b.i.d. for 2 weeks.
- Probiotic with bovine colostrum.

Entamoeba histolytica

Entamoeba histolytica is a protozoan parasite that exists as an invasive trophozoite and as an infective cyst. Spread by the faecal–oral route, it can reside in asymptomatic form in the large intestine, but can become invasive, resulting in colitis, or spread to involve the liver and other organs. Transmission is person-to-person, or by contaminated food and water.

Symptoms range from mild diarrhoea to fulminating amoebic dysentery with fever, profuse bloody diarrhoea and abdominal pain and tenderness.

Complications include perforation, strictures, amoeboma and involvement of other organs, such as liver abscess.

Diagnosis

- Stool culture
- Indirect haemagglutination assay
- Liver ultrasound.

Treatment

- Metronidazole 600–800 mg t.d.s. for 6–10 days plus diloxanide furoate 500 mg t.d.s. for 10 days.

Clostridium perfringens

A common food-borne pathogen with an incubation period of 8–24 hours. Usually the result of eating contaminated meat or poultry.

Symptoms

- Watery diarrhoea, cramping abdominal pain
- Usually resolves after 24 hours.

Treatment

Hydration and supportive treatment.

Bacillus cereus

A form of food poisoning, usually related to ingestion of contaminated fried rice or rice that is cooked then improperly refrigerated, although a wide variety of foods have been implicated. Infection is associated with two distinct syndromes: a vomiting syndrome (ingestion of a pre-formed toxin) and a diarrhoeal syndrome resulting from the production of an enterotoxin.

Usually self-limiting over 20–36 hours, but will respond to quinolones if necessary.

Yersinia enterocolitica

Transmission is via the faecal–oral route through contaminated food and water and by person-to-person transmission. Symptoms include diarrhoea and vomiting. Bloody diarrhoea is more common in children than adults, and infection usually resolves after 2 weeks.

Diagnosis

- Stool culture or serology.

Treatment

- Antibiotic treatment is usually not required.
- If required, cotrimoxazole or one of the quinolones is usually effective.

Cryptosporidium parvum

This is a protozoan parasite causing diarrhoea in normal and immunocompromised people. Transmission is via the faecal–oral route through contaminated food and water and by person-to-person transmission. Outbreaks of cryptosporidiosis have been associated with childcare centres, public swimming pools and contaminated water.

Symptoms

- Profuse watery diarrhoea, abdominal pain, nausea
- May have vomiting and low-grade fever
- Usually abates after 1–2 weeks, but diarrhoea and weight loss may persist in some people.

Diagnosis

- Stool culture
- Colonic biopsy
- Enzyme immunoassay.

No specific treatment is available.

Giardiasis

Giardia lamblia is a flagellated protozoon. The cystic form is shed in the stool and can survive in the environment. Transmission is through contaminated food or water, or person-to-person contact.

Infection is characterised by colicky abdominal pain, pasty or frothy foul-smelling stools that may be paler than usual, anorexia, malaise and excess flatus. May present as an acute diarrhoeal illness or chronic diarrhoea. Blood in the stool and fever are not features of giardiasis. Symptoms may resolve after 1–3 weeks but can persist for many months.

Diagnosis

Usually made clinically, as stool examination is not very sensitive.

Treatment

- Therapeutic trial of tinidazole 500 mg × 4 stat or metronidazole 400 mg p.o. t.d.s. for 7 days
- Probiotic (*Lactobacillus* spp).

Pseudomembranous colitis

Pseudomembranous colitis is usually due to overgrowth of *Clostridium difficile*. This may be a result of antibiotics when a probiotic is not co-prescribed. Features include profuse watery diarrhoea, cramping abdominal pain and tenesmus ± fever within days or weeks of taking an antibiotic.

Treatment

- Cease the offending antibiotic
- Metronidazole 400 mg p.o. t.d.s. for 7–10 days plus a probiotic; *OR*
- Vancomycin 125 mg p.o. q.d. for 10 days plus a probiotic.

A probiotic supplement (*Lactobacillus* spp and *Saccharomyces boulardii*) has been shown to prevent antibiotic-associated diarrhoea.[4] The *S. boulardii* strain is used to restore microbial balance and inhibit *C. difficile* proliferation.[5]

Traveller's diarrhoea

Common in visitors to developing countries. The most common pathogen is enterotoxigenic *E. coli*, although other pathogens can be responsible, including *Shigella* (10%), *Salmonella* (5%), *Campylobacter* (3%), *Yersinia* (2%), *G. lamblia* (4%), *E. histolytica* (1%), *Cryptosporidium* (3%) and viruses (3%).[1]

Onset is abrupt, with up to six bowel movements a day, lasting for 3–4 days in most cases. Symptoms may be more severe, with profuse watery diarrhoea. Blood in the stool suggests invasive disease.

Treatment

- Maintain fluid and electrolyte intake. If rehydration sachets are not available, add one teaspoon of sugar and a pinch of salt to a 250 mL glass of filtered, boiled or bottled water. Soups with added salt and diluted fruit juices and low-fibre bland foods until diarrhoea settles.
- Norfloxacin 400 mg p.o. b.i.d. for 3 days for suspected bacterial gastroenteritis.
- Tinidazole or metronidazole for suspected giardiasis.
- Antiemetic for severe vomiting (metoclopramide).

- Loperamide (Imodium®) can be used two caps stat then one after each unformed stool to a maximum of eight per day.
- Probiotic.
- Small amounts of low-fibre food until diarrhoea settles.
- Avoid alcohol, coffee, raw fruit and vegetables and wholegrain cereals until diarrhoea settles.
- Medical assistance should be sought in the event of bloody diarrhoea, persisting severe symptoms, abdominal pain or high fever, and special caution should be exercised with children, the frail elderly and immunocompromised individuals.

Prevention

- Drink filtered or bottled water only.
- When travelling, avoid tap water, ice in drinks, dairy products, peeled fruit, uncooked vegetables and salads, and raw seafood.
- Safe food storage and preparation
- Antibiotic prophylaxis is not routinely recommended.

Herbs and supplements for diarrhoea[6]

- *Bilberry*—astringent activity, traditional use in acute non-specific diarrhoea. Approved by Commission E for this indication.[7]
- *Chamomile*—used to relieve stomach cramps, dyspepsia and flatulence. A study of chamomile and pectin in children aged between 6 months and 5.5 years with diarrhoea showed reduced duration and severity of diarrhoea.[8] Approved by Commission E for gastrointestinal spasms and inflammatory diseases of the gastrointestinal tract.[7]
- *Colostrum*—bovine colostrum is derived from cow's milk. Hyperimmune bovine colostrum is produced by immunising cows with either specific pathogens or their antigens. It has been shown to be highly effective in prophylaxis and treatment of infectious diarrhoea caused by rotavirus.[9]

  Dose: 100 mL t.d.s. for 3 days with bovine colostrum from cows immunised with the four serotypes of human rotavirus.
- *Goldenseal*—used traditionally as an antidiarrhoeal agent. Much of the research has been done on the chief constituent, berberine. Supplements should be standardised to contain at least 8 mg/mL of berberine and 8 mg/mL of hydrastine. It acts by decreasing intestinal activity and inhibiting toxin formation from microbes.

Ciguatera fish poisoning

Results from ingestion of a fish containing a neurotoxin (ciguatoxin) that originates in algae living in tropical waters, particularly the Pacific and Caribbean. Ciguatoxin is very heat resistant, so ciguatoxin-laden fish cannot be detoxified by conventional cooking. Symptoms start within 5 minutes to 30 hours of ingestion: nausea, vomiting, diarrhoea, photophobia, blurred vision, ataxia and paraesthesiae. Bradycardia, hypotension and heart block may occur. There is no proven effective treatment or antidote for ciguatera poisoning. The symptoms can last from weeks to years, and in extreme cases as long as 20 years, often leading to long-term disability.[10] Most people do recover slowly over time. Often patients recover but redevelop symptoms in the future. Relapses can be triggered by consumption of nuts, alcohol, fish or fish-containing products, chicken or eggs, or by exposure to fumes such as those of bleach and other chemicals. Exercise is also a possible trigger.[11]

Chronic diarrhoea

Frequent or urgent passing of unformed stools for more than a month can be referred to as chronic diarrhoea. It should be distinguished from faecal incontinence or tenesmus.

Diagnosis

History and investigations are directed at finding a treatable cause of chronic diarrhoea.

- Patient should be questioned about pain, stool frequency and timing, colour and consistency, and presence of blood, flatus or mucus.
- A history of travel to developing countries, even several months or years before, may assist diagnosis.
- A comprehensive dietary history should be ascertained, including all foods, alcohol, soft drinks, fruit juices and milk.
- Medication history, including antibiotics and antacids, herbs and supplements.
- Inquire specifically about weight loss, mouth ulceration, joint pain, visual problems and emotional health.
- Family history may suggest suspicion of coeliac disease, inflammatory bowel disease or bowel cancer.

Physical examination should be comprehensive, bearing in mind the possibility that diarrhoea could be a result of local gastrointestinal inflammation or infection, gastrointestinal manifestation of systemic disease such as thyrotoxicosis or an adverse drug effect, or that the diarrhoea will have systemic and nutritional consequences such as malabsorption, anaemia, dehydration or nutritional deficiencies.

Abdominal palpation, rectal examination and examination of stool are essential.

Diagnostic clues:

- Tenesmus suggests rectal involvement.
- Small-volume frequent stools suggest large bowel disease.
- Steatorrhoea (pale, bulky, greasy, floating stools) suggests small bowel or pancreatic disease.
- Large-volume watery stools suggest small bowel disease or laxative overuse.
- Bright red blood suggests local anal bleeding, or rectal or low colonic disease.
- Altered blood, or blood mixed with stool, suggests problems higher in the colon.
- Weight loss suggests an underlying organic disease, malabsorption, colon cancer or thyrotoxicosis.
- Arthritis or sacroiliitis suggests inflammatory bowel disease or hypogammaglobulinaemia.
- Central abdominal pain suggests small bowel origin.
- Iliac fossa pain suggests large bowel origin.
- Diarrhoea waking the patient from sleep at night, or blood in stools, excludes functional bowel disease.
- Skin rash may suggest coeliac disease (dermatitis herpetiformis) or inflammatory bowel disease (erythema nodosum or erythema multiforme).
- Abdominal bloating is non-specific.
- Diarrhoea in association with certain food types suggests food intolerance or reaction (e.g. milk and lactose intolerance, gluten and coeliac disease, sorbitol in chewing gum or drinks).
- Sexual history may lead to HIV testing, with diarrhoea a common symptom.

Diagnostic possibilities:

- Coeliac disease (see p. 392)
- Giardiasis (see p. 372)
- Irritable bowel syndrome (see p. 389)
- Inflammatory bowel disease (see p. 390)
- Crohn's disease (see p. 390)
- Dietary intolerance
- Malabsorption
- Overuse of laxatives.

Investigations

Investigations for chronic diarrhoea need to be carefully selected to target the most probable diagnosis and to assess any consequences.

- Stool examination and culture
- Full blood count and ESR to assess for possibility of anaemia
- Iron studies, folate, vitamin B_{12}
- Albumin
- Calcium, electrolytes
- Thyroid function and hormone-secreting tumours (gastrin, vasoactive intestinal polypeptide)
- HIV antibody
- Malabsorption studies
- Coeliac serology, IgA and tissue typing
- Endoscopy (proctosigmoidoscopy, small bowel biopsy and disaccharidase assay, colonoscopy).

If small bowel pathology is suspected, a Pillcam® (endoscopic capsule) may identify the cause.

A supervised exclusion diet may be helpful in cases of suspected food intolerance.

Therapeutics

Identify and treat any underlying cause.

- Probiotic—*Lactobacillus acidophilus* and/or bifidobacteria taken as powder or in capsules helps normalise bowel flora.
- Bovine colostrum is a component in some probiotic supplements and helps treat some kinds of infectious diarrhoea.
- Maintain hydration.
- Maintain nutrition. Rice or barley water, fresh vegetable juices, miso broth, or other clear broths with added Celtic sea salt help restore fluid and electrolyte balance.
- Avoid coffee, chocolate, dairy products and strong spices.
- Multivitamin supplement.
- Protein supplement may be necessary for malabsorption.

Herbs

- Blackberry leaf (*Rubus fruticosus*) or raspberry leaf (*Rubus idaeus*) teas.
- Bilberry (*Vaccinum myrtillus*) also has astringent properties (4 g per day in divided doses).
- Agrimony (*Agrimonia eupatorium*) is a traditional remedy for diarrhoea. Usual dosage is about ½ teaspoon per day.

For relieving gut inflammation:

- Quercetin (250–500 mg 2–4 times per day) to be taken with bromelain as this improves its digestion. They commonly come together in formulas and bromelain is also an anti-inflammatory. (*Caution*: Commission E states that hypersensitivity to bromelain can cause diarrhoea.)
- Chamomile (*Matricaria recutita*) tea.
- Marshmallow root (*Althea officinalis*) as cold-water tea.
- Slippery elm powder (*Ulmus fulva*) or marshmallow root powder (*A. officinalis*). Plants containing berberine can be used for infectious diarrhoea. These include barberry (*Berberis vulgaris*) 250–500 mg three times per day, goldenseal (*Hydrastis canadensis*) 250–500 mg three times per day and Oregon grape (*Berberis aquifolium*) 250–500 mg three times per day.

ALTERNATING DIARRHOEA AND CONSTIPATION

Consider irritable bowel syndrome, carcinoma of colon, diverticular disease, giardiasis, food intolerance.

FAECAL INCONTINENCE

Faecal incontinence, or involuntary leakage of faecal material, is thought to occur in about 10% of adults but is reported in only one in eight cases.[12] It can cause severe restriction of social interaction and lifestyle, and is a common precipitant for admission to residential aged care.

Clinical features

Risk factors include advancing age, debility with faecal impaction with spurious diarrhoea, perianal or rectal injury from childbirth or radiotherapy, anal surgery, irritable bowel syndrome, chronic constipation (and laxative abuse), neurological disorders and psychiatric disorders.

History will often lead you to the underlying cause. A rectal examination is necessary to assess sphincter tone, and proctoscopy to examine rectal mucosa.

Investigations

- Sigmoidoscopy.
- Patients with advanced incontinence or those resistant to initial treatment should be evaluated by anorectal physiology testing to establish the severity and type of incontinence (e.g. anorectal manometry, nerve conduction studies for suspected neurogenic incontinence).
- Endoanal ultrasound to identify defect in the internal or external sphincter.
- CT scan of pelvic or lumbosacral spine in suspected cases of spinal cord lesion.
- Stool examination for chronic diarrhoea.

Therapeutics

Treatment will be determined by the cause. Try dietary modification and treatment of diarrhoea or constipation.

Proper clinical assessment followed by conservative medical therapy leads to improvement in more than 50% of cases,[13] including patients with severe symptoms.

Patients with gross sphincter defects should undergo surgical repair. Those who fail to respond to sphincteroplasty and those with no anatomical defects have the option of sacral nerve stimulation or other advanced procedures.

GLOSSODYNIA (PAINFUL TONGUE)

'Glossodynia' refers to persistent burning or pain in the mouth, which may be accompanied by dryness, paraesthesia and altered taste or smell. It may be a result of altered oral sensory function but the mechanism is unknown. It is two to three times more common in women and mostly occurs in middle age.

Aetiology

- Poor-fitting dentures
- Dental plaque
- Candidiasis
- Lichen planus
- Nutritional deficiency: iron, vitamin B_{12}, folate, riboflavin (B_2), pyridoxine (B_6), zinc
- Endocrine—diabetes (oral sensory neuropathy or candidiasis), hypothyroidism, menopause
- Neurological—referred from pharynx, referred from teeth, lingual nerve neuropathy, glossopharyngeal neuralgia (paroxysmal pain in the nerve distribution), oesophageal reflux
- Crohn's disease, coeliac disease
- Reaction to mouthwash or medication
- Xerostomia
- Trauma (bitten tongue)
- Herpes simplex (acute primary herpetic gingivostomatitis in children)
- Psychogenic—depression
- Idiopathic
- Consider neoplasia, immunosuppression or HIV
- Erythema migrans (geographical tongue).

Diagnosis

History and full physical examination should aim to elicit symptoms and signs of any systemic disease. Mouth, pharynx, tongue and teeth should be examined under good light.

Ask about lifestyle and mind–body factors such as stress, depression, tobacco or cannabis use, spicy foods, oral hygiene.

Investigations may include:

- full blood count and ESR
- serum iron, B_{12} and folate, riboflavin, B_6
- blood glucose
- thyroid function tests
- zinc taste test
- swabs for microbiology
- antinuclear antibodies (ANA)
- coeliac serology, total IgA and coeliac tissue typing may be indicated
- dental opinion
- nutritional assessment.

Therapeutics

- Exclude or assess and treat any underlying causes.

- Correct nutritional deficiencies with diet and supplementation.
- Assess and advise on stress management. Psychological assessment and counselling may benefit.

HICCUPS

Hiccups are a reflex muscular contraction causing sudden inspiration against a closed glottis. It usually responds to simple measures. Persistent or intractable hiccups (present for over 24 hours) may come to the attention of a healthcare professional and can be a sign of serious underlying disease.

Persistent hiccup can result from direct stimulation or irritation of the afferent or efferent vagal or phrenic nerve pathways, from lesions in the medulla or be secondary to metabolic disturbances.

Aetiology

Self-limited episodes:

- Gastro-oesophageal reflux disease (GORD) (may be cause or effect)
- Gastric distension
- Alcohol
- Sudden temperature change.

Persistent or intractable hiccups:

- Medullary lesion—infarction, tumour, abscess, aneurysm, haematoma, syrinx, demyelination etc
- CNS infection—viral encephalitis, syphilis, HIV encephalopathy, meningitis
- Irritation of neuronal pathway—oesophageal or small bowel obstruction, achalasia, pancreatic or biliary disease, foreign body in external auditory meatus (auricular branch of vagus nerve)
- Mediastinal disease—tumour, thoracic aortic aneurysm, diaphragmatic irritation from subphrenic or hepatic disease, pleural or pericardial effusion, myocardial infarction
- Metabolic/endocrine—diabetes, uraemia, hypocalcaemia, hyponatraemia, Addison's disease
- Medication side effect—alcohol, general anaesthetic, corticosteroids, benzodiazepines, barbiturates, etoposide
- Idiopathic.

Diagnosis

Investigation of persistent hiccups is directed at identifying an underlying cause.

History should include close questioning about neurological, gastrointestinal, cardiac and respiratory symptoms and drug and alcohol use.

Physical examination should include full neurological assessment, cognitive assessment, cardiopulmonary examination, examination of auditory canals, and abdominal examination.

Investigations will be guided by symptoms and physical findings. Initial investigations will include:

- metabolic screen (serum electrolytes, serum calcium, blood glucose, liver function tests)
- full blood count
- chest X-ray and ECG if a cardiopulmonary cause is suspected
- thoracic CT scan if mediastinal disease is suspected
- upper abdominal ultrasound or CT scan if hepatic or subdiaphragmatic pathology suspected
- endoscopy if oesophageal or gastric cause is suspected
- oesophageal motility studies.

Therapeutics

Brief episodes:

- Try: holding the breath, Valsalva manoeuvre, rebreathing in a paper bag, drink ice water, eat coarse grained sugar, pressure on eyeballs, pass nasogastric tube quickly in and out.

Persistent episodes:

- Identify and treat underlying cause
- Acupuncture
- Hypnotherapy.

Drug therapy:

- Baclofen 5–15 mg t.d.s. orally. If unsuccessful add nifedipine 5–10 mg t.d.s.; *OR*
- Chlorpromazine 20–50 mg intravenous infusion (IVI). If unsuccessful, add metoclopramide 10 mg IVI
- Sodium valproate
- Phrenic nerve block.

MOUTH ULCERS

Oral ulcers are extremely common and usually limited to 5–10 days duration. Serious or recurrent painful ulceration can be an indicator of underlying systemic or gastrointestinal disease requiring further investigation.

Differential diagnosis

- Idiopathic aphthous ulcers
- Trauma (toothbrush, hard foods, biting buccal mucosa, sharp or malaligned dentition or poorly fitting denture)
- Reaction to chemical in mouthwash
- Poor oral hygiene
- Excessive stress
- Crohn's disease, ulcerative colitis
- Coeliac disease
- Pernicious anaemia
- Iron deficiency

- Herpes simplex (begins as clusters of vesicles and transforms into small punctuate ulcers mainly on the hard palate, gingival and alveolar ridges)
- Oral candidiasis
- Blood dyscrasia
- Autoimmune disease (e.g. lichen planus)
- Erythema multiforme (preceded by vesicles)
- Pemphigus and pemphigoid (preceded by bullae)
- Behçet's syndrome (oral ulceration occurs in conjunction with ocular and genital ulceration; can also affect skin, joints and gut)
- Xerostomia
- Neoplasm—biopsy if solitary ulcer not healed in 3 weeks.

Treatment of aphthous ulceration

- First-line—cooled, wet, squeezed-out, black teabag applied directly to the ulcer. Tannic acid in the tea promotes healing.
- Avoid acidic foods until the ulcers heal.
- Drink plenty of fluids and prefer soft foods.
- Maintain oral hygiene.
- Pain relief—topical lignocaine jelly or SM-33 gel as required.

Healing:

- Triamcinolone acetonide 0.1% paste or hydrocortisone hemisuccinate lozenges applied to the ulcers q.d.
- 1 g sucralfate dissolved in 30 mL water as a mouth wash.
- Honey-based preparations topically.

Prevention

- Establish or exclude underlying disease
- Regular dental checks
- Maintain oral hygiene
- Stress management.

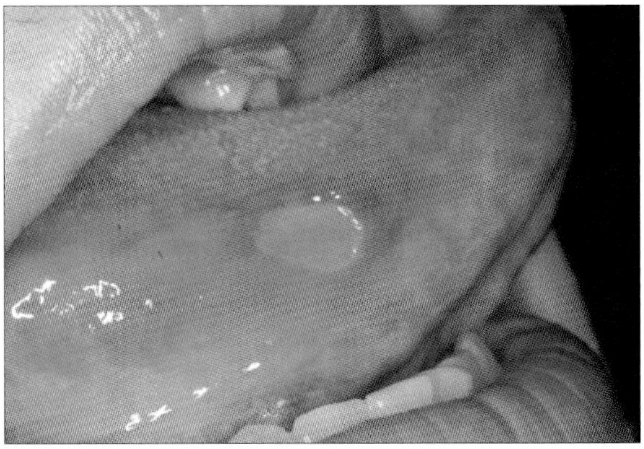

FIGURE 30.2 Aphthous ulcer

DYSPHAGIA

Dysphagia refers to difficulty swallowing, frequently associated with pain. It can be caused by structural or neuromuscular oesophageal problems in the oropharynx or oesophagus.

Aetiology

Structural:

- Foreign body
- Neoplasia in pharynx, oesophagus or stomach
- Extrinsic compression—left atrial enlargement, tumour, goitre
- Benign peptic stricture
- Head/neck surgery or radiotherapy
- Pharyngeal pouch
- Oesophageal web
- Eosinophilic oesophagitis.

Functional:

- Xerostomia
- Eating too fast
- Oesophageal spasm
- Reflux oesophagitis
- Achalasia
- Scleroderma
- Neurological—stroke, head injury, Parkinson's disease, motor neurone disease, multiple sclerosis, myasthenia gravis, cerebral tumour
- Drug side effect, e.g. phenothiazines
- Muscular—autoimmune myopathy, thyrotoxic myopathy, Guillain-Barré syndrome, muscular dystrophy.

Diagnosis

Comprehensive questioning and physical examination are required to identify the nature of any underlying cause.

- Exclude globus sensation, which is usually a painless sensation of a lump in the throat, felt between meals and often relieved by food.
- Progressive dysphagia predominantly for solids indicates a structural disorder. Malignant dysphagia is usually a short history of progressive difficulty with swallowing over weeks or months, and may be associated with weight loss.
- Sudden onset in association with other neurological symptoms may indicate a cerebrovascular cause.
- Intermittent dysphagia for liquids and solids, look for a motility disorder such as oesophageal spasm or pharyngeal cause.
- The patient's perception of the site of the hold-up of the bolus is notoriously unreliable.
- Associated symptoms such as dry mouth, heartburn, cough, nausea, weight loss or skin changes may provide clues to any underlying cause.

Investigation

- Barium swallow to assess motility and identify structural lesion. Should precede endoscopy.
- Endoscopy required in most cases to detect mucosal disease and obtain biopsies. Enables dilatation where indicated. Cannot diagnose motility disorders or external structural problems.
- Oesophageal manometry—for cases where endoscopy and barium swallow have failed to confirm a diagnosis. Required for definitive diagnosis of achalasia.
- ENT assessment may be necessary to exclude pharyngeo-laryngeal malignancy.
- Nutritional assessment, particularly where diet has become limited by inability to swallow solids.
- Blood tests may be helpful where indicated: CPK, FBC, ESR, ANA, thyroid function tests (TFT).

Therapeutics

- Identify and treat any underlying cause.
- Establish a safe means of nutrition.

INDIGESTION, DYSPEPSIA AND HEARTBURN

A detailed history is needed to find out exactly what a patient means when they complain of 'indigestion'. Find out if they are referring to regurgitation, epigastric burning or pain, eructation (burping), bloating or something else.

Dyspepsia generally refers to persistent or recurrent pain or discomfort in the upper abdomen, and may include heartburn or acid regurgitation. 'Discomfort' may also embrace sensations such as postprandial fullness, early satiety, nausea and upper abdominal bloating.

Heartburn and regurgitation imply oesophageal disease and often occur together.

Heartburn is described as a burning lower retrosternal pain that radiates upwards as far as the neck. It occurs intermittently, often 5 to 30 minutes postprandially or when the patient bends forward or lies flat in bed.

Larger meals can be an exacerbating factor, and certain foods can precipitate an attack. It is usually relieved by antacid medication within several minutes.

'Waterbrash' is a symptom describing the appearance of a volume of salty-tasting or tasteless fluid in the mouth. It is the result of salivary gland stimulation in response to gastro-oesophageal reflux or peptic ulcer disease.

Regurgitation of acid or stomach contents can be associated with dry cough, vocal hoarseness (chemical laryngitis), asthma, halitosis, choking attacks, glossodynia, dental caries and nasal aspiration. Patients may wake in the night with a choking sensation.

Symptoms of dyspepsia and GORD often overlap.

Causes of dyspepsia/indigestion

The causes of dyspepsia are many and varied, so precise elicitation of symptoms is important. Differential diagnosis includes:

- chronic peptic ulcer—duodenal ulcer pain is localised, worst at night and relieved by food; gastric ulcer pain is aggravated by food
- non-ulcer dyspepsia
- GORD
- oesophagitis (pain on swallowing hot or cold liquids)
- *H. pylori* gastritis
- hepatobiliary—hepatitis, biliary dyskinesia, cholelithiasis
- chronic pancreatitis
- giardiasis
- Crohn's disease
- upper GI malignancy
- mesenteric vascular insufficiency—diarrhoea 30 minutes after a meal
- metabolic—renal failure, hypercalcaemia, gastroparesis or gastric hypomotility
- irritable bowel sndrome
- psychosocial factors (stress, anxiety, depression)
- myocardial ischaemia
- referred back pain
- drug side effect (especially non-steroidal anti-inflammatory drugs (NSAIDs), antibiotics, antidepressants, digoxin, potassium, iron, zinc)
- alcohol-related.

Red flag features

Red flag features indicate organic disease warranting further investigation:

- Unexplained weight loss
- Dysphagia
- Vomiting
- Bleeding
- Family history of oesophageal or gastric cancer
- Pain waking patient at night
- Pain radiating to back
- Anaemia
- Lymphadenopathy
- Abdominal mass
- Retrosternal pain exacerbated by exercise.

Investigation

The aim of investigation is to identify any underlying treatable cause for the heartburn, indigestion or dyspepsia. Detailed history and physical examination will direct the choice of investigations.

- Test for *H. pylori* with serology (blood test) and C14 breath test.

- In the absence of associated 'red flag' symptoms, a trial of treatment such as lifestyle modification and antacid therapy may provide relief (see GORD).
- Upper gastrointestinal endoscopy is indicated if symptoms do not resolve after 8 weeks. The aim is to exclude peptic ulcer, significant reflux oesophagitis and malignancy.
- Epigastric or retrosternal pain, especially if precipitated by exercise, needs to be investigated for coronary ischaemia.

GASTRO-OESOPHAGEAL REFLUX DISEASE

A typical history of heartburn or acid regurgitation is usually sufficient to satisfy a diagnosis of gastro-oesophageal reflux disease (GORD). There are no specific signs on physical examination to support the clinical diagnosis.

Aetiology

Conditions that increase intraabdominal pressure and reduce the pressure of the lower oesophageal sphincter can cause reflux of stomach contents into the oesophagus. These factors include:

- overweight and obesity
- pregnancy
- hiatus hernia
- recurrent or persistent vomiting
- tobacco smoking
- alcohol
- caffeine
- some medicines, including calcium channel blockers, NSAIDs, potassium, dopamine, sedatives, bisphosphonates and beta-blockers
- psychological stress.

Barrett's oesophagus

A complication of gastro-oesophageal reflux, Barrett's oesophagus is a metaplastic transformation (intestinal metaplasia) of the stratified squamous epithelium in the lower oesophagus. It is a precursor to malignant adenocarcinoma of the distal oesophagus. Patients with high-risk dysplasia need to be monitored with surveillance endoscopy and biopsy every 2 years.

Guidelines

- No dysplasia: 3-yearly
- Low-grade dysplasia: yearly
- High-grade dyaplasia: repeat ~ 1 month (definitive treatment).

Investigation of symptoms suggesting GORD

- Trial of therapeutics.
- Upper gastrointestinal endoscopy if symptoms do not resolve after 8 weeks. The aim is to exclude peptic ulcer, significant reflux oesophagitis and malignancy.

Therapeutics

First-line

Aims of treatment are to reduce regurgitation, reduce stomach acid content, improve stomach emptying, and protect the lining of the oesophagus.

- Weight loss, if overweight
- Small light meals, avoiding eating close to bedtime
- Elevate the head of the bed with a house brick
- Avoid cigarettes, caffeine, alcohol and carbonated drinks
- Avoid foods that trigger symptoms
- Avoid carbonated drinks
- Reduce or exclude coffee, tea and chocolate
- Remove or replace medications or supplements possibly responsible for symptoms
- Relaxation and stress management including exercise, yoga, t'ai chi and meditation
- Deglycyrrhizinated licorice (DGL) (*Glycyrrhiza glabra*) has anti-inflammatory, mucoprotective and anti-ulcer effects. Approved by Commission E for treatment of gastric and duodenal ulcers.

  Dose: standardised extract, 250–500 mg three times daily, chewed either 1 hour before or 2 hours after meals
- Ginger—approved by Commission E for treatment of dyspepsia
- Slippery elm bark powder—half teaspoon in one cup of hot water three times a day
- Chamomile—widely used as a tea for treatment of dyspepsia
- Lemon balm—has antispasmodic activity and is approved by Commission E for functional gastrointestinal conditions
- Globe artichoke leaf extract—reduces symptoms of non-ulcer dyspepsia.[14]

Second-line

- Antacids as required for symptomatic relief, e.g. liquid alginate/antacid mixture
- Prokinetic agents such as metoclopramide
- Regular proton pump inhibitors if symptoms are persistent or frequent.

Prevention

- Maintain healthy body weight and waist circumference
- Do not smoke or drink alcohol excessively
- Small, regular meals
- Manage stress.

NAUSEA AND VOMITING

Precise definition of terms is important in establishing the nature and cause of symptoms, as patients will often adopt a common-language term to describe a symptom, rather than the correct descriptor.

- *Nausea* is a sensation of wanting to vomit and is painless but unpleasant.
- *Vomiting* is the forceful expulsion of stomach or intestinal contents through the mouth. It may be preceded by autonomic symptoms of various intensity, including salivation, bradycardia, sweating, pallor and hypotension.
- *Retching* is the repetitive contraction of stomach muscles associated with vomiting, but without the expulsion of stomach contents.
- *Regurgitation* is the effortless appearance of stomach contents in the mouth without nausea or diaphragmatic contractions.
- *Haematemesis* is vomiting of blood.

The history should include questions about duration, frequency and intensity of nausea and vomiting and any relationship to eating, and the nature of the vomitus. A comprehensive medical history including any medications or supplements is essential.

Causes

Intestinal obstruction:

- Small bowel obstruction—vomitus is usually bile-stained if the obstruction is below the level of the duodenal ampulla. Faecal vomiting would indicate distal small bowel obstruction. Malignant obstruction is usually associated with anorexia and weight loss.
- Gastric outlet obstruction—vomiting of partially digested gastric contents without the presence of bile.
- Pyloric stenosis—neonate, sudden onset of projectile vomiting week 3–6, failure to thrive, metabolic alkalosis sodium usually under 130 mol/L, more often male (5:1). Clinically may feel a pyloric tumour, or require ultrasound to confirm.
- Gastroparesis—may be associated with long-standing diabetes, often intense nausea, anorexia, postprandial fullness and early satiety. May be associated with peripheral or autonomic neuropathy.
- Chronic intestinal pseudo-obstruction.

Infection:

- Food poisoning
- Viral or bacterial gastroenteritis—acute onset, usually associated with headache, fever, myalgia and diarrhoea, and tends to settle within 5 days
- Acute viral hepatitis
- Urinary tract infection in children.

Central nervous system disorders:

- Migraine
- Meningitis
- Raised intracranial pressure—vomiting, sometimes projectile, on waking in the morning. Likely other neurological signs present. Space-occupying lesions may cause vomiting without nausea.
- Ménière's disease—associated tinnitus and vertigo
- Motion sickness.

Metabolic and endocrine disorders:

- Renal failure
- Diabetic ketoacidosis
- Hypercalcaemia
- Addison's disease—characteristic pigmentation
- Hyperthyroidism.

Drugs:

- Alcohol
- Digitalis
- Theophylline
- Morphine and opiate derivatives
- Chemotherapy
- NSAIDs
- Oral contraceptive pill
- Other.

Visceral pain:

- Peritonitis
- Cholecystitis
- Pancreatitis.

Emotional disorders:

- Anorexia or bulimia nervosa—repeated bouts of vomiting (self-induced) soon after meals with associated features which may include impaired body image, vigorous exercise, and laxative and diuretic abuse, amenorrhoea, binge eating.
- Panic attacks.

Pregnancy:

- Common in the first trimester of pregnancy but can persist throughout the gestation period. Pregnancy should be excluded in every female patient of childbearing age presenting with nausea and/or vomiting.

Cyclical vomiting syndrome:

- Asymptomatic periods between bouts of nausea and vomiting; often associated history of migraine. Can be associated with significant cannabis use (cannabinoid hyperemesis).

Functional vomiting:

- Conditioned reflexes to offensive sights or smells
- GORD
- Acute myocardial infarction.

Examination

Thorough physical examination is necessary to identify underlying causes for nausea and vomiting and to assess clinical consequences of vomiting, such as dehydration and malnutrition.

- Examine for dental caries.
- Careful neurological examination is required, including examination of the fundi for signs of raised intracranial pressure.
- If fever is present, examine for focus of infection, including urinalysis and middle ear.
- Note any scars from previous surgery.

Investigation

Investigations are directed at diagnosing the cause of the nausea and vomiting and assessing the health consequences, and may include:

- pregnancy test if appropriate
- stool microscopy and culture
- serum electrolytes
- serum albumin
- haemoglobin and white cell count
- liver function tests
- *H. pylori* serology
- pancreatic enzymes (if upper abdominal pain)
- supine and upright abdominal X-ray if small bowel obstruction is suspected
- upper endoscopy—especially if other GIT symptoms or gastric outlet obstruction suspected
- if endocrine cause is suspected—thyroid function tests, blood glucose test and serum cortisol
- CT or MRI of brain if a CNS cause is suspected.

Therapeutics

- Identify and treat any underlying cause.
- Identify and correct dehydration and electrolyte disturbances.
- Nutritional support.
- IV fluids or nasogastric tube if indicated.
- Acupuncture and acupressure.
- Psychotherapy—hypnotherapy, relaxation exercises and other psychotherapies can be useful adjuncts, particularly where psychological or emotional factors are contributing to the presentation or when a patient is having to cope with an unpleasant symptom like chronic nausea and vomiting.
- Antiemetic medication for symptomatic relief:
  - pregnancy-associated nausea—ginger and vitamin B_6/pyridoxine (10–25 mg t.d.s.)
  - ginger used preoperatively can reduce post-operative and chemotherapy-induced nausea[15,16]
  - ginger is approved by Commission E for prevention of motion sickness (see below)
  - baiacal skullcap—pretreatment may reduce nausea and vomiting of chemotherapy
  - prochlorperazine (oral, IV or PR) 5–10 mg t.d.s. p.r.n.
  - chlorpromazine
  - metoclopramide p.o. or IM
  - promethazine 25 mg q.i.d. p.r.n.
  - ondansetron 8 mg p.o., wafers or IV (for severe postoperative and chemotherapy-induced nausea).

Motion sickness:

- Ginger; or scopolamine transdermal patch; or promethazine 25 mg p.o. 1 hour before travel and repeated 4–6 hourly during trip
- Prokinetic agents (where delayed gastric emptying is a feature):
  - metoclopramide (5–20 mg q.i.d.) may cause tardive dyskinesia
  - erythromycin (accelerates gastric emptying)—high doses induce nausea. Will need to include a probiotic.
  - domperidone (Motilium®) 10 mg t.d.s.

HALITOSIS

Halitosis is an unpleasant odour on the breath that may be physiological or pathological (Box 30.1). Physiological causes may include ingestion of particular foods or medications. It is most commonly caused by action of microflora on oral debris around the teeth and gums. Gram-negative organisms cause putrefaction and release of chemicals, particularly sulfide compounds, in the alkaline oral environment.

The odour can vary depending on diet, time of day, time of menstrual cycle and state of hunger.

BOX 30.1 Differential diagnosis of halitosis

- Foods—garlic, onion, peppers, broccoli, radish, leek, salami, strong cheeses
- Drugs—isosorbide dinitrate, disulfiram, dimethyl sulfoxide, alcohol, tobacco
- Poor oral hygiene
- Dental decay
- Oral inflammation—gingivitis, periodontal disease, ulceration, candidiasis, dehydration
- Tumour or infection in the nasopharynx, tonsils, sinuses or respiratory tract
- Nasal foreign body
- Inhaled steroids for asthma causing candidiasis
- Lower respiratory tract—bronchitis, bronchiectasis, lung abscess, pneumonia, lung cancer, tuberculosis
- Xerostomia
- Pharyngeal pouch (stagnation and regurgitation of food)
- Oesophageal or gastric neoplasm
- Systemic—diabetic ketoacidosis, uraemia, hepatic failure, starvation, inborn errors of metabolism (aminoacidurias)
- Giardiasis
- Idiopathic

Treatment

- Identify and treat underlying cause, if identified.
- Dental referral for treatment of gingival or periodontal disease. Severe cases may require metronidazole for 5–10 days.
- Treat oral candidiasis with topical antifungal (nystatin) or oral fluconazole 150 mg stat.
- Improve dental hygiene, reduce tongue biofilm by brushing off tongue coating.
- Eliminate offending foods from diet.

Prevention

- Eat regularly, low-fat diet high in fruit and vegetables
- Increase fluid intake
- Reduce alcohol and eliminate smoking
- Brush after every meal, and floss between teeth daily
- Mouthwash containing chlorhexidine
- Regular dental checks
- Eliminate or substitute drugs likely to cause xerostomia, e.g. antihistamines, antidepressants, anticholinergics, anorexiants, antihypertensives, antipsychotics, antiparkinsonian agents, diuretics and sedatives. Other drug classes that commonly cause xerostomia include antiemetics, antianxiety agents, decongestants, analgesics, antidiarrhoeals, bronchodilators and skeletal muscle relaxants.

PERIANAL PAIN

Consider severity, duration, timing, relationship to defecation, rectal bleeding or prolapse. Examination needs to be focused on the perianal region but include abdominal and general examination.

Causes to consider are described below.

Anal fissure

Pain with defecation and bright red bleeding are common. Usually associated with intense spasm of internal anal sphincter muscle and initially produced by splitting from passage of a hard stool. Internal sphincter spasm results in ischaemia in anal mucosa. Avoid digital rectal examination because of pain.

Secondary fissures may be due to Crohn's disease, ulcerative colitis or immunosuppression. Assess for HIV or syphilis testing if indicated.

Treatment

- Topical 0.2% glyceryl trinitrate ointment.
- Treat constipation with a bulking agent and adequate fluid intake.
- Surgery if fissure fails to heal and remains painful.

Haemorrhoids

The main symptom is rectal bleeding. Uncomplicated haemorrhoids may be painless, cause itch or cause discomfort with defecation. Thrombosed or prolapsed haemorrhoids cause acute severe pain. With internal haemorrhoids, bleeding may be a more prominent symptom than pain. Bleeding is bright red and may be seen on toilet paper or in the bowl.

Treatment

- Initial treatment: topical.
- Acute thrombosis can be relieved by surgical incision.
- May require injection, rubber band ligation or surgical excision.
- Treatment includes dietary modification to ensure adequate fibre and fluid intake. Prolonged sitting on toilet or straining should be discouraged.

Anal abscess

An extremely tender perianal lump will be evident. There may be fever if the abscess is large. In most cases an anal abscess develops from a primary infection in an anal gland and may progress to perianal abscess, ischiorectal abscess or supralevator abscess.

May be secondary to Crohn's disease or ulcerative colitis. Patients should be checked for immune deficiency, immunosuppression and diabetes. Look for evidence of a fistula. Rectal carcinoma should be excluded.

Treatment

Anal abscess requires surgical referral for exploration and drainage. Underlying pathology needs to be identified and treated.

Anal fistula

Mild, dull, localised pain. Look for a sinus opening.

Pruritis ani

Anal itch, usually worse at night, in hot weather and after exercise. Causes include dermatitis, psoriasis, fungal infection (tinea or *Candida albicans*), haemorrhoids, anal fissure, anal warts, skin tags, anal carcinoma.

In children, threadworm infestation is a possible cause. Consider sensitivity to washing powders, soaps or bubble bath.

Treatment

- Identify and treat any underlying cause such as diabetes or fungal infection. Simple initial management might include a cream containing hydrocortisone 1% with clotrimazole 1%.
- Wash anal area three or four times daily with a mild soap substitute, dab dry.
- Avoid scratching.
- Apply a zinc oxide powder or cream.

- Eliminate possible chemicals that may cause sensitivity.
- Wear cotton underwear.
- Use soft, uncoloured toilet tissue.
- Keep bowel habit regular, with adequate fibre and fluids in the diet.
- Reduce weight if overweight.
- Manage stress and anxiety.
- Idiopathic cases not responding to simple measures may respond to acupuncture.

Proctalgia fugax

Presents as a history of severe pain in anal canal lasting 5–30 minutes. May wake patient from sleep. Can occur day or night. Affects adults, males more often than females. Thought to be due to spasm of levator ani muscles.

Treatment

- May respond to inhaled salbutamol (2 puffs stat).
- Difficult cases may respond to excision of prolapsing rectal mucosa.

RECTAL BLEEDING

Severity of bleeding varies from a small amount of blood on the toilet paper to heavy bleeding. History should include amount and colour of blood, whether it is on toilet paper only (suggesting local anal pathology) or mixed with stool, associated perianal pain, pattern of bowel habit, diet and family history of colorectal cancer.

Gastrointestinal bleeding should be considered in any patient aged over 40 years with iron deficiency anaemia. Menstrual bleeding and dietary deficiency in young women are common causes of iron deficiency.

Melaena

The passage of dark altered blood is a sign of bleeding in the upper gastrointestinal tract (usually peptic ulceration but may be a result of portal hypertension or portal enteropathy). It has a strong odour. It is an indication for urgent referral for hospital admission.

Black motions can also be the result of ingestion of liquorice or oral iron supplementation.

Bright bleeding

Causes include haemorrhoids, anal fissure, inflammatory bowel disease (proctitis), rectal polyps, infective colitis, Meckel's diverticulum, intussusception, colorectal cancer, diverticular disease, ischaemic colitis.

Investigation

Examination should include anal, rectal and abdominal examination as well as proctoscopy or sigmoidoscopy.

A bleeding source may be clearly identified (e.g. bleeding haemorrhoids or fissure).

Do not assume that haemorrhoids are the cause of bleeding, especially in an elderly patient. Persistent or recurrent bleeding or any uncertainty regarding the cause warrants a colonoscopy.

Positive faecal occult blood test (FOBT)—population testing for faecal occult blood yields some positive results. The test will detect 40–80% of asymptomatic colorectal cancers and 30–40% of large colorectal adenomas. A positive FOBT is a trigger for colonoscopy.

ESTABLISHED DIAGNOSIS

GASTRITIS

Gastritis can be acute, chronic or asymptomatic, an incidental finding on endoscopy. Patients may present with:

- loss of appetite
- epigastric pain
- nausea or dyspepsia
- hiccups
- vomiting, possibly haematemesis
- melaena
- weight loss.

Aetiology

- Infection with *H. pylori*
- Alcohol excess
- Tobacco smoking
- Medications, particularly aspirin and NSAIDs
- Emotional stress
- Backflow of bile
- Allergy
- Autoimmune conditions such as pernicious anaemia.

Investigations

- *H. pylori* serology or C14 urea breath test
- Endoscopy.

Prevention

- Avoidance of gastric irritants
- Stress management.

Therapeutics

- Remove or treat any identified cause.
- Find alternative treatments for conditions requiring aspirin or NSAIDs.
- *Helicobacter* eradication (antibiotics and proton pump inhibitor), probiotic therapy with *Lactobacillus acidophilus*.

Diet

- Dietary modification—exclude alcohol and caffeine.
- Fibre-rich diet (especially as fruits and vegetables).

- Avoid high-fat foods (from animal studies, high-fat foods increase inflammation in the stomach lining).
- Patients with pernicious anaemia and *H. pylori* infection are deficient in vitamin B_{12}.[17] Supplementation may be used to treat both.[18] Good dietary sources of vitamin B_{12} include fish, dairy products, organ meats (particularly liver and kidney), eggs, beef, and pork. Vitamin B_{12} supplementation can be administered sublingually or injected intramuscularly.
- *H. pylori* appears to impair absorption of vitamin C, so vitamin C supplementation may be necessary in the presence of *H. pylori*.[19]

Herbal

- Slippery elm bark powder (*Ulmus fulva*)—has a long history of use based on clinical experience. Gastritis and peptic ulcer are among the conditions that respond to slippery elm.
- *Astragalus*—used traditionally to treat stomach ulcers. May also prevent chemotherapy- or radiotherapy-induced gastritis.
- Chamomile (*Chamaemelum nobile*)—traditionally used to treat nausea, vomiting, heartburn and excess intestinal gas.
- Ginger—used in Chinese medicine to aid digestion and treat stomach upset.
- Green tea (*Camellia sinensis*)—population studies in Japan suggest that regular green tea drinkers have lower rates of chronic atrophic gastritis.[20]
- Licorice (*Glycyrrhiza glabra*)—this herb is a demulcent (soothing, coating agent). Licorice root extracts, known as deglycyrrhizinated licorice (DGL), may be as effective as some prescription drugs for stomach ulcers.

Medication

- Antacids—liquid alginate/antacid mixture
- Proton pump inhibitors—esomeprazole, lansoprazole, omeprazole, pantoprazole, rabeprazole.

PEPTIC ULCER

- Peptic ulceration is characterised by dyspepsia with intermittent bouts of more severe, burning epigastric pain within hours of a meal.
- Ulcers can be located in the lower oesophagus, stomach and duodenum.
- Duodenal ulcers are four times more common than gastric ulcers.

Investigations

- *H. pylori* serology or C14 urea breath test.
- Endoscopy will confirm presence and nature of ulceration, including neoplastic ulceration.
- Urease testing for *H. pylori* is done at the time of an endoscopy.

Aetiology

Peptic ulcers are more common in males than females. Risk factors include presence of *H. pylori* infection, smoking, family history of ulcer disease, stress, blood type O, and use of NSAIDs.

Prevention

Avoid or eliminate NSAIDs, smoking, alcohol abuse and excessive stress.

Therapeutics

First-line

The first aim of treatment is to eliminate causative or exacerbating agents such as NSAIDs, smoking, alcohol abuse and stress. Factors which cause recurrent inflammation and/or impair the body's healing capacity need to be eliminated if an optimal outcome is to be achieved. Then treatment is aimed at relieving symptoms and preventing recurrence.

NSAID-related ulcers with no presence of *H. pylori* can be treated with acid suppression to accelerate healing.

Provide alternative treatments for conditions requiring NSAIDs.

H. pylori is responsible for 90% of duodenal ulcers and 70% of gastric ulcers, so if *H. pylori* is present, eradication is necessary with triple therapy (two antibiotics and a proton pump inhibitor), which has a 75% success rate. Proton pump inhibitors: esomeprazole, lansoprazole, omeprazole, pantoprazole, rabeprazole.

Treatment failure may be due to poor compliance with the full treatment regimen or antibiotic resistance.

Second-line

Second-line treatment is with alternative antibiotics to eradicate *H. pylori*, and proton pump inhibitor.

Adjunctive

Adjunctive treatment is aimed at reducing gut inflammation, accelerating healing and relieving symptoms. These should be discussed with the patient regardless of which other medical therapies are being employed.

Diet

- Prevention—reduced risk of duodenal ulcers in individuals with high intake of fruit and vegetables, total fibre and soluble fibre[21]
- Adequate dietary vitamin A
- Reduce refined sugars
- Avoid tobacco smoke
- Reduce coffee and carbonated drinks
- Reduce excessive alcohol consumption

- There is little evidence indicating that fat, type of fat, protein intake or consumption of alcohol or caffeine affect the aetiology of duodenal ulcer
- Foods containing flavonoids, like apples, celery, cranberries (including cranberry juice), onions and tea may inhibit the growth of *H. pylori*.

Probiotics

- Assist with *H. pylori* eradication through inhibitory action, reducing gastric inflammation and preventing adhesion of *H. pylori* to stomach and gut lining.
- Addition of probiotics to standard antibiotic treatment improved *H. pylori* eradication rates (81% *vs* 71%, for combination treatment *vs* *H. pylori*-eradication treatment alone).[22]
- Counter side effects of antibiotics.
- Dose—according to manufacturer's instructions; the most effective strains are *Lactobacillus caseii* and *L. johnsonii* La1.

Vitamin C

- Assists with prevention of *H. pylori* infection.
- Assists with eradication of *H. pylori* by inhibiting bacterial growth.
- Dose: 1 g t.d.s.

Cranberry

- Prevents *H. pylori* bacteria adhering to gut-lining mucosa.
- Dose: 250 mL b.i.d.

Lactoferrin (bovine)

- Antimicrobial activity assists with *H. pylori* eradication.
- Dose: 200 mg b.i.d.

Slippery elm bark powder (*Ulmus fulva*)

- There is traditional evidence of symptomatic relief by coating the stomach.
- Dose: 1 tspn (5 g) q.d. before meals and at bedtime.

Licorice (*Glycyrrhiza glabra*)

- Traditional use as a soothing, coating agent in the treatment of ulcers. Assists *H. pylori* eradication through bacterial inhibition. Some licorice root extracts (DGL) have the healing properties of licorice without the harmful effects (such as hypertension).
- Dose: 1–3 mL t.d.s. or 2–4.5 g/day of DGL.

Sucralfate

- Sucralfate can coat the ulcer, protecting the mucosa during healing.

Stress management

Yoga, biofeedback and stress management programs can not only improve coping but also enhance immunity and healing rates, as well as reduce inflammation. They can also assist in facilitating healthy lifestyle change.

Risks

- People with peptic ulcers should not take the herbs devil's claw (*Harpagophytum procumbens*) or green tea (*Camellia sinensis*).
- High-dose licorice can cause hypertension.
- High-dose vitamin A supplementation can cause toxicity. Avoid in pregnant women.

STOMACH CANCER

Clinical features

Early stages of stomach cancer are generally asymptomatic and diagnosed incidentally at gastroscopy.

Symptoms often indicate the presence of more advanced disease and include upper abdominal pain, weight loss, anorexia and nausea (± early satiety). Dysphagia may be a feature if the cancer is located around the cardia.

Typically, spread is to local lymph nodes and/or liver.

Investigations

Stomach cancer is diagnosed by gastroscopy with biopsy. Stage of disease is the most important determinant of prognosis. Staging is done with CT scanning, looking for lymph node metastases, liver metastases and ascites. Laparoscopy can identify smaller liver and peritoneal metastases. PET scanning may be used.

Aetiology

Chronic atrophic gastritis begins as a multifocal process. In patients predisposed to intestinal metaplasia and dysplasia it can progress to cancer.

H. pylori is a carcinogen associated with gastric adenocarcinoma and lymphoma, increasing cancer incidence three to six times.

Note: Despite the epidemiological association between *H. pylori* and gastric cancer, only a minority of infected individuals will actually develop cancer—population screening for *H. pylori* has therefore not been recommended.

Risk factors for gastric adenocarcinoma[1] include:

- genetic—blood group A, family history, hereditary non-polyposis colon cancer syndrome
- environmental—low consumption of fruit, vegetables and vitamin C, high consumption of smoked or salted foods
- precursor conditions—untreated *H. pylori* infection, pernicious anaemia, gastric polyps, previous partial gastrectomy.

Prevention

- Healthy diet with diverse types of fruit and vegetables
- Eradication of *H. pylori*
- Gastroscopy for persistent symptoms suggesting gastric cancer.

Therapeutics

Treatment is determined by stage of cancer at the time of diagnosis.

Complete surgical resection of the tumour and adjacent lymph nodes may cure early-stage disease. Adjuvant chemotherapy and radiotherapy may improve survival.

More advanced cancer is usually treated with palliative surgery to relieve gastric outlet obstruction or control significant bleeding. Combination chemotherapy may be used where surgery is contraindicated.

Following gastrectomy, patients will require:

- vitamin B_{12} injections
- management of bile reflux—options include slippery elm bark powder, *Aloe vera* juice, ursodeoxycholic acid, proton pump inhibitors, low-fat diet, avoid alcohol and smoking, raise the head of the bed, relaxation techniques
- management of 'dumping syndrome'—postprandial nausea, dizziness and abdominal pain; patients are advised to eat smaller, more frequent meals with a diet low in sugar and high in fats and protein; may be transient or permanent
- referral to a dietician for nutritional support.

OESOPHAGEAL CANCER

Clinical features

Oesophageal cancer may be squamous cell carcinoma or adenocarcinoma. Suspicion should be raised in patients with dysphagia of recent onset, or weight loss with progressive dysphagia.

Investigations

- Symptoms should be investigated with gastroscopy.
- CT chest and upper abdomen and PET scanning to assess tumour extent.

Aetiology

- Barrett's oesophagus is a premalignant condition caused by chronic long-term acid reflux in the lower oesophagus, which is lined with gastric mucosa.
- Based on fair evidence, serum CagA antibodies and gastric atrophy are associated with an increased risk of oesophageal squamous cell carcinoma.[23]
- Smoking, excess alcohol, ingestion of nitrites and fungal toxins are risk factors for squamous cell cancers.
- Gastro-oesophageal reflux and obesity are risk factors for adenocarcinoma.

Prevention

- Avoiding tobacco and alcohol reduces the risk of squamous cell carcinoma.
- Diets high in cruciferous (cabbage, broccoli, cauliflower) and green and yellow vegetables and fruits are associated with a decreased risk of oesophageal cancer.[24,25]
- Investigation of dyspepsia[26]
- It is not known whether elimination of gastro-oesophageal reflux by surgical or medical means reduces the risk of oesophageal adenocarcinoma.
- Two-yearly surveillance endoscopies in patients with previously noted Barrett's oesophagus allows early detection of adenocarcinoma. Early treatment of high-grade dysplasia in Barrett's oesophagus should be considered because of the poor survival rate of patients with oesophageal cancer.

Therapeutics

Surgery

Surgery is the treatment of choice for small localised cancers or to bypass the lower oesophagus to relieve dysphagia. Once dysphagia is present, there is a high likelihood that the cancer has already metastasised.

Chemotherapy and radiotherapy may improve survival.

Photodynamic therapy

Photodynamic therapy (PDT) can be performed as an outpatient procedure to treat or relieve the symptoms of oesophageal cancer. An intravenous photosensitising agent (porfimer sodium) is injected, and 24–72 hours later the cancer is exposed to light from a laser source. The photosensitiser in the tumour absorbs the light and produces an active form of oxygen that destroys nearby cancer cells. It can be used repeatedly and in combination with surgery, radiotherapy and chemotherapy.

Patients treated with porfimer sodium should avoid direct sunlight and bright indoor light for at least 6 weeks after treatment.

Adjunctive therapies

- Nutritional support is essential for patients with dysphagia and undergoing treatment for cancer.
- Referral to a dietician is advisable.
- Mind–body treatments.

COLORECTAL CANCER

Colorectal cancer is the most common internal cancer, and the second most common cause of cancer death in Western countries. Most are adenocarcinomas.

Aetiology

Inherited or acquired mutations in genes coding for proteins that regulate cell growth and behaviour cause dysplastic proliferation leading to polyp formation. Most colon cancers arise from pre-existing adenomatous polyps.

Gut health is directly affected by food, and colorectal cancer is more commonly associated with Western diets high in fat and low in protein and fibre.

Other predisposing factors include:

- sporadic colon cancer in a first-degree relative above age 55 years—doubles population risk; first-degree relative under 55 years or two first/second-degree relatives on the same side of the family at any age increases risk six-fold
- inflammatory bowel disease, particularly long-standing ulcerative colitis over 8 years, increases risk
- untreated coeliac disease increases risk
- familial adenomatous polyposis (FAP)
- hereditary non-polyposis colorectal cancer (autosomal dominant disease characterised by multiple cancers and early age of onset).

The last two conditions in the list above are specific but uncommon genetic syndromes that are not applicable to the general population. They require different surveillance and treatment approaches (e.g. prophylactic colectomy in FAP, as cancer risk = 100%).

Clinical features

Clinical presentation of a colorectal cancer can be varied and a high risk of suspicion is warranted.

- Recent change in bowel habit (constipation or diarrhoea)
- Abdominal pain or rectal discomfort, including a sensation of incomplete rectal emptying
- Occult or frank bleeding and/or mucus in stools
- Faecal incontinence

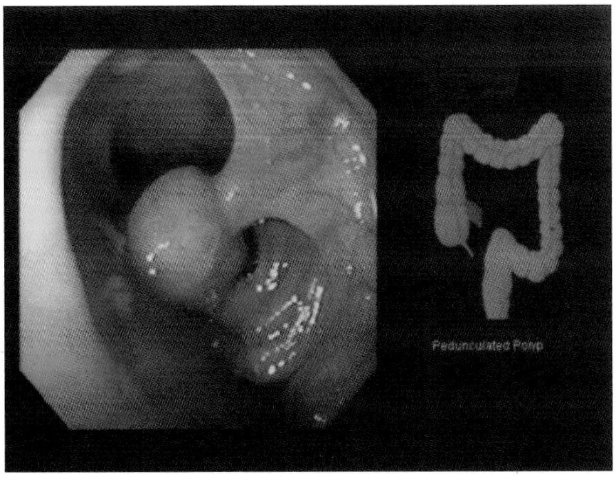

FIGURE 30.3 Bowel polyp

- Weight loss
- Lethargy
- Perforation or obstruction of bowel
- Symptoms of anaemia
- Signs of metastatic disease (jaundice, bone pain, pathological fracture, paraneoplastic syndromes).

Investigations

- FOBT is of little value in the presence of symptoms (although it has been evaluated as screening tool in normal populations).
- Sigmoidoscopy will identify colorectal cancers in the sigmoid colon and rectum.
- Colonoscopy is essential if there is suspicion of colorectal cancer.
- Preoperative assessment may include:
  - full blood examination
  - electrolytes
  - liver function tests
  - baseline chorioembroyonic antigen (CEA) (but is of no use and often misleading as a cancer screening test)
  - chest X-ray
  - CT scanning or PET scanning to assess metastases.

Staging

Staging is a guide to prognosis.

- *Duke's classification*:
  - Stage A: cancer limited to mucosa or submucosa (5-year survival > 90%)
  - Stage B: cancer extends into muscularis or serosa (5-year survival 70–80%)
  - Stage C: cancer involves regional lymph nodes (5-year survival 30–60%)
  - Stage D: distant metastases (5-year survival 5%).
- The *TNM staging system* is another approach that assesses stage by histology of the primary tumour, degree of involvement of regional lymph nodes and presence of metastases.

Prevention

- FOBT screening (reduces population incidence of colorectal cancer through earlier detection of GI bleeding) followed up with colonoscopy for any positive results
- Surveillance colonoscopy with removal of polyps is the gold standard
- High-fibre, low-fat diet
- Regular exercise
- Maintain healthy weight and waist circumference
- Avoid smoking
- Avoid excess alcohol
- Limit fatty foods, fried foods and red meats

- Ensure adequate vitamin D levels—patients with higher vitamin D levels have been found to have 50% reduced risk of developing colorectal cancer, and patients with higher vitamin D levels before a diagnosis of colorectal cancer have significantly higher survival rates.[27]

Therapeutics

- Cancer can be prevented by removal of polyps found at colonoscopy.
- Colorectal cancer has a good prognosis if detected and treated at an early stage with surgical resection of any cancer found, preferably by laparoscopically assisted hemicolectomy.
- Chemotherapy and radiotherapy may be indicated as adjunctive therapies in advanced disease. Hepatic metastases may be resectable.
- Regular follow-up colonoscopy
- Probiotic supplement with lactobacillus acidophilus may help reduce recurrence of tumours.
- Vitamin D supplement if levels inadequate
- Antioxidant and selenium supplementation
- Green tea (*Camellia sinensis*) standardised extract, 250–500 mg daily (caffeine free).[28]
- Reishi mushroom (*Ganoderma lucidum*) standardised extract, 150–300 mg two to three times daily, or tincture of reishi mushroom extract, 30–60 drops two to three times daily.
- Maitake mushroom (*Grifola frondosa*)[29] standardised extract (D-fraction), 600 mg twice daily or tincture of maitake mushroom extract, 30–60 drops two to three times a day.
- Turmeric (*Curcuma longa*)[30] standardised extract, 300 mg three times a day.

Diet suggestions to assist postoperative rehabilitation

- Organic foods where possible (especially meat, vegetables and fruit).

If nausea is present or digestion impaired:

- keep food simple and bland—nutritionally as well as being easy to prepare
- vegetable juices (mild)—carrot, celery, apple (beetroot if tolerated), small quantity of ginger (cinnamon, coriander, mint)
- fruit such as watermelon, grapes, pears, paw paw (not if taste is too strong)
- stewed fruit
- vegetable soups—more broths than thick soups, with legumes such as barley and a mix of vegetables; miso soup may also be a good option
- plain yoghurt or sheep's yoghurt (use organic if not intolerant)
- plain toast or biscuits
- smoothies—whey protein, rice milk or coconut milk, fruit, honey or maple syrup, or apple juice concentrate
- vegetables—sweet potatoes, pumpkin, zucchini, squash, greens (if desired), peas, and so on
- meat—white fish, lamb (particularly stewed or shanks), veal, osso bucco, chicken (organic where possible).

Following postoperative recovery:[31]

- Specific foods to include are:
  - *cruciferous vegetables*—broccoli, cabbage, cauliflower, brussel sprouts, radish
  - *high-fibre foods*—legumes, vegetables, whole grains such as oats, quinoa, buckwheat, barley, rye, spelt; be careful with quantity, to maintain good consistency to stool
  - continue with *vegetable juice*
  - continue with *fruit* but increase the range of berries, cherries, ripe bananas, paw paw, rockmelon, figs, persimmon, goji and blueberries
  - *whole grains*—sourdough, wholemeal bread (rye, wheat or spelt), porridge, oats soaked overnight, quinoa, buckwheat, millet, cous cous, brown rice, black rice and so on
  - *vegetables*—emphasis on high-coloured vegetables; lots of greens, broccoli, cauliflower, cabbage, sweet potato, pumpkin, carrot, turnips; eating beetroot improves liver function
  - *seafood*—oysters, mussels; also salmon, sardines, herrings, cod and other white fish (no flake, mackerel, swordfish or bluefin tuna); eat fish three times a week (cod, tuna, salmon, sardines)
  - *meat*—any good-quality organic, but keep red meat to once or twice per week; veal, lamb, chicken, pork, turkey, duck; not beef
  - *vegetarian protein*—legumes, beans, nuts, seeds are important in a vegetarian diet; if taking protein powder use once or twice per day for maximum absorption and utilisation of amino acids (i.e. half dose at morning and afternoon teas)
  - *water*—2 to 3 litres of filtered water plus herbal teas such as green tea (*Sencha*); filter water where possible with a high-grade carbon filter
  - *fats*—cold-pressed extra virgin olive oil (normal, not 'lite'), flaxseed oil, coconut oil, butter, small amount of sesame oil, etc.
  - *spices*—garlic, onions, turmeric, rosemary, parsley and ginger in cooking
  - *dairy*—if eating dairy, have organic milk, yoghurt, matured cheese, feta, etc

  - *nuts and seeds*—use tahini or nut butters; chew nuts well; also have flaxseed
  - *legumes*—soaked; such as chickpeas, adzuki beans, lentils, lima beans, broad beans, etc; watch portion size and chew well
- Vitamin D foods:
  - fish such as cod, halibut, herring, tuna, salmon
  - eggs, dairy, sprouted seeds
- Selenium foods:
  - whole wheat, garlic, brazil nuts, organ meats
  - very small amounts in fish, seafood, some cereals, broccoli, onions, alfalfa etc
- Mushrooms:
  - shiitake, reishi, maitake
- Foods to avoid:
  - all simple carbohydrates (cakes, biscuits, etc)
  - potato and corn
  - no deli meats and preferably not bacon (organic and preservative-free if possible, if going to have any, or just as a treat).

Tips:
- Reduce refined and processed carbohydrate—no cakes, sweets, soft drinks, lollies, sugar, coffee.
- Eat 5–6 small meals per day.
- Use butter and virgin olive oil in cooking.
- Reduce consumption of cured meats such as ham, bacon, sausage (high nitrates).
- Avoid any food sensitivities, in particular wheat, gluten (oats, rye, barley) and dairy foods.
- Avoid chemical exposure to tobacco, paint fumes, car fumes etc.
- Wash all fruit and vegetables to remove pesticide residue.

IRRITABLE BOWEL SYNDROME

Clinical features

Symptoms include abdominal pain and bloating, often provoked by eating; diarrhoea, or alternating diarrhoea and constipation. There may be nausea and anorexia, bloating and abdominal distension.

Symptoms can be exacerbated premenstrually and at times of stress.

Irritable bowel syndrome (IBS) is a diagnosis of exclusion. This is not to say there is an absence of organic pathology. It means that diseases such as colon cancer, pancreatic cancer, ovarian cancer, Crohn's disease, diverticular disease, active infection, abdominal aortic aneurysm, adhesions, food intolerance and coeliac disease need to be excluded and treated.

Red flag symptoms warranting investigation include: unexplained weight loss, fever, rectal bleeding or steatorrhoea, new symptoms in an older patient, exacerbation of existing symptoms, elevated CRP, dysphagia.

Investigations

Investigations will be guided by history of symptoms and findings on clinical examination to confirm or exclude alternative diagnosis. Patients who have been diagnosed with irritable bowel syndrome in the past need to be reassessed if their pattern of symptoms changes.

- Stool examination and culture
- Coeliac serology, particularly tissue transglutaminase (strongly recommended)
- Lactose tolerance test
- Full blood count
- CRP
- Iron, folate and vitamin B_{12} levels
- Liver function, serum albumin, electrolytes and urea (usually unhelpful)
- Sigmoidoscopy/colonoscopy if colonic disease suspected
- Abdominal and/or pelvic ultrasound
- Laparoscopy if a gynaecological cause for symptoms is suspected.

Aetiology

The exact aetiology is unknown. Dysmotility and hypersensitivity of the gut is thought to be a mechanism.

Visceral hypersensitivity results in heightened perception of gut sensations arising from intestinal distension and contractions. This may also trigger disordered gut motility and/or altered gut secretion and absorption, resulting in the erratic bowel habit seen in IBS.

In up to 25% of patients, IBS is preceded by an attack of gastroenteritis or infective diarrhoea, possibly as a result of damage to the enteric nervous system.

There is a common association with stress, anxiety and depression. There is no predisposing personality type.

Therapeutics

First-line

- Avoid known food allergens or irritants. High-fat foods move slowly through the gut and may exacerbate bloating and constipation. Excessive bloating and flatus can be exacerbated by cabbage, brussel sprouts, baked beans, fructose and sorbitol. Dairy products, caffeine, onion, tomato and citrus fruits may trigger symptoms.
- Trial gluten and dairy-free, low-fat diet for one month.
- Ensure adequate soluble fibre in the diet, and slowly add a stool-bulking fibre supplement (*Psyllium*, slippery elm, marshmallow root).
- Probiotic supplement with *Lactobacillus plantarum* twice daily to rebalance normal bowel flora.
- A single dose of tinidazole 500 mg × 4 stat p.o. may help correct intestinal dysbiosis or undetected chronic giardiasis.

- Eliminate/avoid laxatives and codeine-containing preparations.

Second-line

- A formal supervised elimination/challenge diet may be necessary to identify foods which exacerbate symptoms.
- Enteric-coated peppermint oil capsules or tablets; dose 0.2–0.4 mL t.d.s. after meals.
- Drink a tea of peppermint leaf, fennel seed or ginger root after meals.
- Artichoke leaf extract, dose 640 mg/day.
- Drug therapies are of limited usefulness in IBS but might include: anticholinergic agents (e.g. Colofac®), antiflatulents, antidiarrhoeal medication (e.g. loperamide) or laxative/stool-softening agents.

Adjunctive

- Stress reduction techniques (biofeedback, meditation, counselling).
- Acupuncture to relieve pain and reduce bloating.
- Herbal—tincture of equal parts of: *Valeriana officinalis*, passionflower (*Passiflora incarnata*), anise seed (*Pimpinella anisum*) extract, meadowsweet (*Filipendula ulmaria*), wild yam (*Dioscorea villosa*), and milk thistle (*Silybum marianum*).

  Dose: 30 drops three times per day before meals.
- *Aloe vera*—may be effective for patients with diarrhoea-predominant IBS (43% responders *vs* 22% for placebo).[32]

Risks

Since IBS is a diagnosis of exclusion, other conditions such as coeliac disease, Crohn's disease, endometriosis or bowel cancer need to be excluded by comprehensive investigation.

It is important to keep the diagnostic radar on in patients with long-standing presumed IBS and re-investigate if their symptoms change or substantially worsen.

Interactions

Concentrated peppermint oil may increase bioavailability of felodipine, simvastatin and cyclosporin. It is contra-indicated in biliary duct occlusion, gallbladder inflammation and severe liver disease.

Artichoke should not be used by people with known allergy to globe artichoke or members of the Asteraceae/Compositeae family of plants. It should be used with caution by people with disease of the liver or gallbladder. Its safety in pregnancy is not established.

INFLAMMATORY BOWEL DISEASE

Ulcerative colitis and Crohn's disease are collectively known as *inflammatory bowel disease*.

Crohn's disease

Crohn's disease causes inflammation of the full thickness of the bowel wall and can affect any part of the gastrointestinal tract. Inflammation affects the absorption of nutrients. It is also a systemic disease with prominent gastrointestinal features and extra-intestinal manifestations.

Clinical features

Features vary according to the part of the gastrointestinal tract affected and the degree of activity of the disease.

- Small bowel disease—postprandial abdominal pain, diarrhoea and weight loss, vomiting ± features of small bowel obstruction
- Terminal ileal disease—fever, right iliac fossa pain
- Large bowel disease—diarrhoea and rectal bleeding
- Systemic features—fever, malaise, weight loss
- Perianal disease—fissure, fistulae, abscess.

GIT complications:

- Toxic megacolon
- Perforation
- Haemorrhage
- Colorectal cancer
- Stricture
- Abscess
- Fistula (Crohn's disease).

Extra-intestinal manifestations of inflammatory bowel disease:

- Systemic—fever, malaise and weight loss
- Arthritis—reactive arthritis, ankylosing spondylitis
- Mouth—aphthous ulcers
- Skin—erythema nodosum, pyoderma gangrenosum
- Eyes—conjunctivitis, episcleritis, uveitis, iritis
- Liver—fatty infiltration, sclerosing cholangitis, chronic hepatitis, cholangiocarcinoma, gallstones, granulomatous hepatitis, amyloidosis
- Blood—iron deficiency, folate deficiency, B_{12} deficiency, haemolytic anaemia, thrombosis
- Renal—oxalate renal stones, renal amyloidosis.

Aetiology

The cause is not known but current knowledge suggests that Crohn's disease is due to an abnormal immune response to an environmental antigen or to abnormal exposure of the immune system to that antigen due to an excessively permeable mucosal barrier.

Gene mutations have been identified which result in an increased susceptibility to Crohn's disease in some populations (such as Ashkenazi Jews and people of Scandinavian heritage).

Smoking doubles the risk.

Emotions have a powerful impact upon immunity. Psychological stress, anxiety and depression, for example, are all associated with immune dysregulation. In practical terms this means a greater tendency to inflammation and exacerbation of autoimmune conditions, including inflammatory bowel diseases, as well as poorer immune defences against infections and cancer.

Investigations

- Stool culture and examination (including *Clostridium difficile* assay if there is a recent history of antibiotic use) to exclude infective causes of diarrhoea and bleeding on the initial presentation. Even after diagnosis, you will need to be aware that during relapses, diarrhoea or bleeding could be related to infection, especially if diarrhoea is watery or there has been a recent overseas trip.
- Full blood examination, C-reactive protein—may show evidence of iron, folate or vitamin B_{12} deficiency, neutrophilia. thrombocytopenia, high ESR or C-reactive protein.
- Serum albumin levels may be low if there is associated nutritional deficiency.
- Antibody testing—anti-*Saccharomyces cerevisiae* antibody (ASCA) positive and antineutrophil cytoplasmic antibody (p-ANCA) negative suggest Crohn's disease but are not diagnostic.
- Screen for coeliac disease with coeliac serology (antigliadin, antiendomysium and antitransglutaminase antibody tests) and serum IgA, as there is a significant degree of comorbidity.[33]
- Colonoscopy—investigation of choice for diagnosis of Crohn's disease.
- Small bowel radiology or wireless capsule study may be required, to document Crohn's disease in the small intestine.

Therapeutics for inflammatory bowel disease (Crohn's disease and ulcerative colitis)

- Correct anaemia, malnutrition and fluid balance
- Cease smoking if patient is a smoker
- Nutritional advice with diet and supplementation (especially iron, folate, vitamin B_{12}, zinc, calcium and protein)
- Selenium 200 mcg daily
- Magnesium
- Omega-3 supplementation (3 g/day)
- Commence low-fibre, gluten-free diet
- A low-amine diet may help a significant number of people with Crohn's disease to relieve symptoms and maintain remission
- Avoid caffeine and alcohol
- Eliminate all sulfur preservatives (E220–227)[34]
- Psychological support, particularly at the time of diagnosis
- Relaxation techniques and mind–body exercises such as yoga, t'ai chi, meditation and hypnotherapy may improve immune function and ease anxiety.

Medication

- 5-amino salicylates: sulfasalazine (more effective in active colonic disease); mesalazine (more effective for active terminal ileal disease)
- Corticosteroids—start at high dose (40–60 mg/day and taper down) to induce remission. Not useful for preventing relapse.
- Budesonide (for treatment of active terminal ileal disease)
- Oral metronidazole may be useful in treating complicated perianal disease.
- Azathioprine, 6-mercaptopurine, methotrexate—monitoring with monthly blood count is essential.
- Infliximab infusions or Humira® (adalimumab) injections
- Probiotics—*Saccharomyces boulardii*
- Monoclonal antibodies—under evaluation
- Surgery—may be required for abscesses, fistulae, stricture or resection of severe disease.

Herbal

- Slippery elm (*Ulmus fulva*)—1 teaspoon of powder mixed with water three to four times a day
- Marshmallow (*Althacea officinalis*) soothes mucous membranes. One cup of tea three times per day. Avoid marshmallow if diabetic.
- Curcumin or turmeric (*Curcuma longa*, 1–2 g per day)
- Cat's claw (*Uncaria tomentosa*, 250 mg per day).
- Boswellia (*Boswellia serrata*, 1200 mg three times per day for up to 8 weeks) has anti-inflammatory properties, and a few small studies have suggested that it may help in treating Crohn's disease.
- *Aloe vera* gel has been shown in a small trial to induce clinical remission in 30% of subjects with mild to moderate ulcerative colitis compared with 7% for placebo, and symptom improvement in 37% versus 7% for placebo. Histological disease activity was reduced.[35]

  Dose: fresh from living plant or as stabilised juice 25 mL, 4.5:1 up to q.d.

  Extracts standardised to acemannan: preparation containing up to 800 mg/day.

Acupuncture

Acupuncture has been used traditionally to treat inflammatory bowel conditions and has been shown to be a helpful adjunctive treatment in active Crohn's disease.[36]

Prevention
- Avoid smoking.
- Eat a diet low in sugar and saturated fat and high in fruit and vegetables.
- Options for prevention of relapse include immunomodulating drugs such as 6-mercaptopurine and infliximab.
- Steroids and 5-ASA drugs are not helpful for preventing relapse.

Ulcerative colitis
A form of inflammatory bowel disease, ulcerative colitis is mainly a disease of Western societies and is most commonly seen in young adults.

Clinical features
Ulcerative colitis affects only the colon and rectum, and inflammation is usually limited to the mucosa and crypts. Inflammation is continuous rather than patchy.

Symptoms depend on the degree of inflammatory change and include:
- diarrhoea
- per rectum bleeding and mucus in stools
- abdominal pain, which may be eased by defecation
- tenesmus if there is rectal involvement
- systemic symptoms—fever, weight loss, anorexia, tachycardia, anaemia
- severe attacks—toxic megacolon. Extensive mucosal ulceration exposes the muscle layer, causes colonic atony and dilatation, which can lead to perforation.
- extra-intestinal manifestations—as for Crohn's disease. May precede the colonic manifestations or occur even after total colectomy.

Investigations
- Stool microscopy and culture—to exclude active infection as a diagnosis or as a cause of exacerbation of symptoms in a confirmed case. *Clostridium difficile* culture and toxin specifically requested in appropriate cases where there has been a recent history of hospitalisation or antibiotic use.
- Full blood count—may be elevated white cell count, ESR or CRP
- Haemoglobin and serum albumin—may be reduced in more severe cases
- Liver function tests
- Sigmoidoscopy and biopsy—will demonstrate the changes of ulcerative colitis
- Colonoscopy—to determine the extent of the disease and for surveillance for colorectal cancer. Often delayed in cases of severe active colitis because of increased risk of perforation.

Aetiology
The cause of ulcerative colitis remains unknown. It is thought to be an inflammatory immune response to infection. There is a family history in up to 20% of cases. Cigarette smoking lowers the risk but is not advised as a preventive measure.

Prevention
- High-fibre diet
- Stress management.

Therapeutics
As for Crohn's disease. *Note*: General principles are much the same, although specific approaches may differ.
- Treatment of flare:
  - ASA (mild to moderate)
  - steroids (moderate to severe)
  - infliximab or cyclosporin (very severe)
- Maintenance:
  - ASA (more established and useful than in Crohn's)
  - azathioprine if ASA unsuccessful.

Patients with ulcerative colitis are less likely to require surgery than patients with Crohn's disease but it may be necessary where medical measures fail. Surgery ± pouch may be curative.

COELIAC DISEASE AND GLUTEN SENSITIVITY
Coeliac disease (CD) is a systemic immune response to the presence of ingested gluten. Gluten is a protein found in many grains, including wheat, oats, rye and barley. Susceptibility is inherited. Virtually all affected individuals are HLA-DQL or DQ8 tissue type. Until recent years the most often-quoted incidence of CD was around one in 1000; now it appears that the incidence is closer to 1 in 100 to 150.

In addition to the well-described gut symptoms of CD, gluten intolerance and gluten allergy, there are many other ways that gluten sensitivity or intolerance can present. Coeliac disease can affect all organs, and can have an effect on moods and personality as well as work, friendships and family relationships.

There was a time when gluten sensitivity was not taken as seriously as it should be, by the medical profession, the food industry and the general public, who were all largely unaware of the potential dangers of gluten exposure for some people.

A high index of suspicion will lead to a diagnosis of a disease which can be managed to eliminate symptoms and consequences in most people.

Investigation and diagnosis

Features that should raise suspicion of CD:

- Infancy and childhood:
  - previously thriving infant who becomes unwell after introduction of solids
  - diarrhoea or constipation
  - abdominal distension (enlarged abdomen, malabsorption)
  - failure to thrive (pallor, low weight, lack of fat, hair thinning)
  - anorexia, vomiting
  - irritability
  - rashes
  - mouth ulcers
  - psychomotor developmental impairment (muscle wasting)
  - anaemia (especially iron deficiency, vitamin B_{12} deficiency)
  - short stature
  - delayed puberty.
- Adulthood:
  - diarrhoea or constipation (may not be present)
  - anaemia
  - iron, B_{12}, folate deficiencies
  - aphthous ulcers, sore tongue and mouth (mouth ulcers, glossitis, stomatitis)
  - dyspepsia, abdominal pain, bloating
  - weight loss
  - infertility
  - unexplained fatigue, anxiety, depression
  - bone pain (osteoporosis)
  - rash (dermatitis herpetiformis)
  - weakness (myopathy, neuropathy)
  - family history of gut or unexplained health problems
  - family history of autoimmune cluster conditions (type 1 diabetes, Addison's disease, thyroid disease).

Investigation

If you suspect CD as a differential diagnosis, arrange blood tests for:

- anti-tissue transglutaminase antibodies (tTGA)
- endomysial antibody (Ab) (EMA)
- antigliadin Ab
- total IgA—up to 5% of individuals have IgA deficiency and will have false negative screening tests to IgA antigliadin antibody, EMA and tTGA
- coeliac tissue typing.

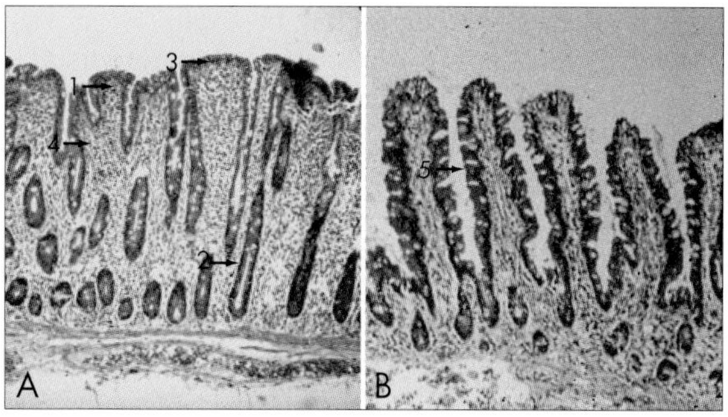

FIGURE 30.4 Coeliac disease—flattened villi

The 'gold standard' for diagnosis is an endoscopic biopsy of the small intestine to identify the characteristic flattened villi.

Once the diagnosis of CD is confirmed, patients need to develop an instant zero tolerance response to gluten in the diet. Even minute exposure to gluten can cause symptoms or gut damage.

There is an additional group of patients who cannot be diagnosed with coeliac disease as they are sero-negative and/or biopsy-negative, but whose symptoms suggest gluten intolerance and resolve with a gluten-free diet.

Emotional reactions to a diagnosis of food intolerance

Emotional reactions are to be expected:

- grief, particularly if favourite foods are to be excluded from the diet for life
- frustration at being 'different', having to make special arrangements and needing to be constantly vigilant
- sense of isolation
- anxiety and depression—may be a feature of the gluten exposure or a reaction to the diagnosis and its implications
- fear of accidental exposure
- mistrust of food safety and people preparing food
- disruption of family activities.

Reduced health-related quality of life in coeliac disease is associated with:

- other physical and emotional comorbidities
- non-compliance with gluten-free diet
- dissatisfaction with doctor–patient communication.[37]

Clinical features

Coeliac disease can present with the classic gut symptoms of abdominal bloating, abdominal pain, occasional diarrhoea, indigestion and consequences of malabsorption of nutrients such as iron, vitamin B_{12} and folate.

However, gut symptoms may be absent or accompanied by a variety of other systemic symptoms and signs.

Neurological

- Gluten ataxia—cells in the cerebellum can be susceptible to damage from gluten. It is a serious, progressive and permanent impairment of neurological function. A strict gluten-free diet can prevent further deterioration, so early diagnosis is extremely important.
- Gluten headaches—worth considering in patients with unexplained headaches. May also be associated with gluten ataxia (causing unsteadiness and clumsiness).
- 'Brain fog'—many patients describe a 'brain fog', a blunting of their ability to think and concentrate if they are exposed to gluten. It can take several days to clear completely. This can be misunderstood as depression or cognitive impairment.

'Behavioural problems' in children

- Refusing to eat
- Lethargy
- Crankiness and irritability
- Poor attention span and learning difficulties
- 'Hyperactivity'—the data indicate that ADHD-like symptomatology is markedly overrepresented among untreated CD patients and that a gluten-free diet may improve symptoms significantly within a short period of time.

ADHD-like symptoms

ADHD-like symptomatology is markedly overrepresented among untreated CD patients and a gluten-free diet may improve symptoms significantly within a short period of time.[38] Coeliac disease should be included in the list of differential diagnoses in presentations of ADHD-like symptomatology.

An Israeli study found that the variability of neurological disorders that occur in children with CD is broader than previously reported and includes 'softer' and more common neurological disorders, such as chronic headache, developmental delay, hypotonia and learning disorders or ADHD.[39]

Psychiatric symptoms

Several neurological, psychiatric (including schizophrenia) and mood disorders have been reported in coeliac patients; these complications occur in approximately 8–10% of subjects affected by CD, although the cause is not yet known.

In patients with both CD and schizophrenia, the CD-associated schizophrenia may respond dramatically to a gluten-free diet.

In a 2004 study, regional cerebral perfusion was assessed by single-photon emission computed tomography (SPECT) in untreated CD patients, comparing them with CD patients on a gluten-free diet (GFD) and with healthy controls. The study showed the presence of regional cerebral hypoperfusion in 73% of the untreated CD patients, compared with only 7% of CD patients on a GFD and none of the controls.[40]

Considering each single region, a significantly lower cerebral perfusion was found in untreated coeliac patients compared to controls in seven of the 26 cerebral regions evaluated. There were no significant differences in cerebral perfusion between untreated patients and those on a GFD, or between patients on a GFD and healthy controls, reflecting a beneficial effect of a GFD on these alterations. Perfusion defects were predominant in the superior and anterior areas of the frontal cortex with the involvement of the adjacent anterior cingulated cortex. Similar cerebral blood flow changes have been reported in patients suffering from different psychiatric disorders.

Psychiatric and/or neurological disorders in CD patients could be related, in part, to brain perfusion alterations. These haemodynamic changes seem to be linked to disease activity, and resolve some months after commencement of a strict gluten-free diet.

Fatigue

Tiredness/fatigue/irritability can be related to the multiple nutritional (iron, vitamin B_{12}, folate) deficiencies, muscle weakness or neurological complications of gluten sensitivity.

Skin

Dermatitis herpetiformis—look for gluten antibodies. Appears as a skin rash on the elbow, knees and buttocks that is associated with CD which can appear with gluten exposure and disappears once a GFD has been in place for some time. It occurs in 15–25% of people with coeliac disease.

If the antibody tests are positive and the skin biopsy has the typical findings of dermatitis herpetiformis, the patient does not need to have an intestinal biopsy.

Bones

Fracture from minimal trauma or an incidental finding of osteoporosis should trigger testing for CD.

Gut malignancy

The malignancy associated with untreated CD is a lymphoma of the small intestine, 'enteropathy-associated T-cell lymphoma'.

Cancers of the small intestine, mouth, oesophagus or pharynx are also recognised malignancies associated with untreated CD.

A strict gluten-free diet can protect against these malignancies. Long-term follow-up indicates that for coeliac patients who have maintained a GFD for 5 years or more, the risk of developing cancer over all sites is not increased compared with the general population.[41]

Autoimmune cluster

Coeliac disease is associated with a cluster of other hereditary autoimmune diseases and patients will need to be monitored for these:

- type 1 diabetes
- autoimmune chronic active hepatitis
- Addison's disease
- Hashimoto's thyroid disease
- pernicious anaemia / vitamin B_{12} deficiency
- systemic lupus erythematosus
- Raynaud's syndrome
- Sjögren's syndrome
- myasthenia gravis.

Therapeutics

Diet

Referral to a dietician with special skill in managing CD is recommended.

Patients should be encouraged to join their local coeliac society or support group for information and advice.

Education

Patients and their families will need detailed advice on gluten-free alternatives (buckwheat, corn, rice, quinoa) and hidden sources of gluten such as stock cubes, soups, gravy mixes, sauces, soy sauce, malt on cornflakes, additives to some medications, some teabags, communion wafers.

Where a child has been diagnosed with CD, it may be advisable for the household to go gluten free.

Gluten-free diet

Regardless of the presence of gut symptoms, gluten can still cause damage to villi and affect nutrient absorption, and cause neurological consequences. Gluten exposure also increases the risk of cancer (intestinal T-cell lymphoma) unless the person sticks to their GFD.

The average gluten-containing diet includes roughly 10–40 g of gluten per day. The smallest amount of gluten that has been shown by biopsy to cause damage to a coeliac is 0.1 g per day.[42]

Lactose-free diet

Lactose intolerance is frequently a side effect of CD. Coeliacs who eat gluten become lactose intolerant, after the villi and microvilli in their small intestine become damaged and are no longer capable of catching and breaking down the lactose molecule. The problem usually disappears when the coeliac removes gluten from their diet, which allows the damaged villi and microvilli to eventually grow back. Lactose intolerance symptoms can continue for a significant period after the introduction of a 100% GFD. In some cases the damaged villi and microvilli can take up to 2 years to heal completely after a person with CD has started a GFD, but in most cases it takes between 6 months and a year.

Nutritional supplementation

The patient will need to be assessed for nutritional deficiencies and supplemented accordingly, particularly in the months following diagnosis when the gluten-free, lactose-free diet is initiated.

A quality multivitamin is appropriate, with iron, vitamin B_{12}, iron, folate and zinc. Protein supplementation may be indicated.

Exercise

Exercise including weight training is essential to assist rehabilitation for muscle wasting.

DIVERTICULAR DISEASE

Diverticular disease (*diverticulosis*) occurs when mucosal pouches form in the large intestine. It becomes more common with increasing age and is associated with a low-fibre diet, obesity and a sedentary lifestyle. *Diverticulitis* is infection or inflammation of those pouches.

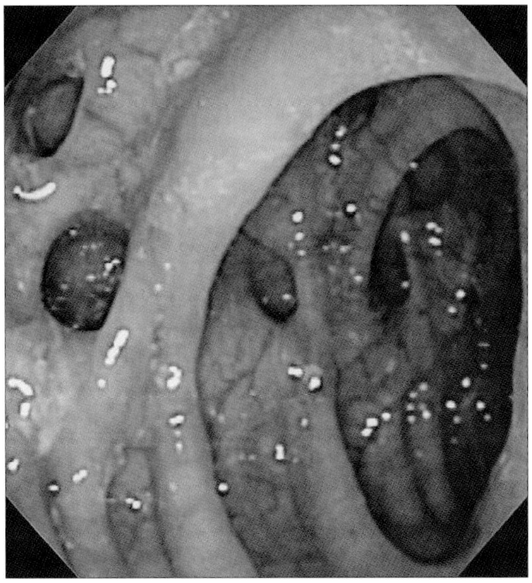

FIGURE 30.5 Diverticular disease

Clinical features

Diverticular disease occurs most commonly in the sigmoid colon. There may be associated muscular hypertrophy of the muscularis propria of the sigmoid colon. Uncomplicated diverticular disease is usually asymptomatic. If diverticulosis is extensive it can affect bowel function.

Diverticulitis

- Peritoneal-type pain in the LIF and fever
- May be a tender mass in the LIF
- May include pain, bloating, fever, nausea, altered bowel habit, blood in stool, flatulence.

Complications occur when the neck of a diverticulum becomes obstructed and contents of the sac become infected: include acute diverticulitis, abscess, perforation, obstruction, fistula formation (bladder, vagina, small bowel).

Investigations

- Abdominal ultrasound / CT scan
- Full blood count for anaemia or leucocytosis, ESR
- Colonoscopy to confirm diagnosis and exclude sigmoid bowel cancer
- CT scan may be indicated if unresolving abscess is suspected
- Stool culture to exclude bowel infection.

Prevention

- High-fibre diet
- Regular bowel habit.

Therapeutics

Uncomplicated diverticular disease:

- Increase dietary soluble fibre (fresh vegetables) and psyllium husks
- Avoid nuts and seeds
- Regular exercise.

Acute diverticulitis:

- Bowel rest with oral fluids
- Broad-spectrum antibiotics (cephalexin 500 mg and metronidazole 400 mg t.d.s. for 5–7 days)
- Severe cases—intravenous ceftriaxone and metronidazole
- Analgesia
- Probiotics such as *Lactobacillus acidophilus*, *L. plantarum*, *Saccharomyces boulardii* and bifidobacteria
- Multivitamin supplement while diet is restricted
- Hemicolectomy—may be required in extensive symptomatic disease.

Herbal

- Flaxseed (*Linum usitatissimum*) contains fibre and works as a bulk-forming laxative and stool softener.
  Dose: use ground flaxseed, 15 g per day.
- Slippery elm (*Ulmus fulva*) as a demulcent.
- Marshmallow (*Althacea officinalis*) is a demulcent and emollient. Drink one cup of tea. Steep 2–5 g of dried leaf or 5 g dried root in one cup boiling water, strain and cool.
- Chamomile (*Matricaria recutita*), 1–3 cups of tea per day. To make tea, steep 3 g flower heads in one cup boiling water, strain and cool.
- Licorice (*Glycyrrhiza glabra*) can reduce spasms and inflammation in the gastrointestinal tract. Look for products that contain mostly DGL, which is less likely to raise blood pressure. *Dose*: 380–1140 g per day.
- Diverticular abscess—surgical drainage.

ISCHAEMIC COLITIS

Main features are sharp lower abdominal pain with bloody diarrhoea (may also be painless), usually in an elderly patient, or periumbilical pain and diarrhoea 15–30 minutes postprandially.

Enquire about a history of cardiovascular disease or arrhythmia, as it usually occurs on a background of significant existing cardiovascular disease.

There may be a loud bruit in the central abdomen.

Investigations

- Plain abdominal X-ray shows gross oedema in the left colon.
- The definitive test is selective angiography of the mesenteric vessels.
- Colonoscopy may help, as there are characteristic changes at the splenic flexure and descending colon.

Therapeutics

Managed conservatively and medically as an inpatient under specialist care, unless signs of sepsis develop or perforation or stricture is suspected.

LIVER DISEASES

The liver is responsible for:

- synthesis and metabolism of essential proteins
- synthesis of blood coagulation factors
- synthesis of cholesterol and triglycerides
- storage of vitamins, minerals and iron
- glucose metabolism
- metabolism of food
- detoxification of blood
- production of substances responsible for immune function
- production of bile for fat digestion.

The assessment and management of a patient with liver disease will need to take into account abnormalities relating to these important functions.

Symptoms and signs of liver disease

Attention may be directed to investigation for liver disease in an asymptomatic patient by the finding of abnormal results of routine liver function tests.

Symptoms and signs of liver disease may be the presenting features. These include:

- symptoms:[1]
  - fatigue
  - pruritis
  - bleeding
  - RUQ pain
  - nausea
  - anorexia
  - myalgia
  - jaundice
  - dark urine
  - pale stools
  - fever
  - weight loss
- peripheral signs of chronic liver disease:
  - spider naevi
  - palmar erythema
  - white nails
  - gynaecomastia
  - loss of body hair
  - testicular atrophy
  - hepatomegaly (see 'Hepatomegaly' below)
- signs of portal hypertension:
  - splenomegaly
  - ascites
  - peripheral oedema
- end-stage liver failure:
  - wasting
  - severe fatigue
  - encephalopathy—asterixis, fetor, coma
- other signs:
  - hepatic rub—peritoneal inflammation from underlying infarction or malignancy
  - RUQ bruit—alcoholic hepatitis, malignancy, intrahepatic shunting, large haemangioma.

Hepatomegaly

Enlargement of the liver may be uniform or irregular. Differential diagnosis of diffuse uniform enlargement:

- metastatic disease
- alcoholic liver disease with fatty infiltration
- myeloproliferative or haematological diseases (leukaemia, lymphoma)
- haemochromatosis
- fatty liver from diabetes mellitus or obesity (classic associations but not exclusive—most common cause of hepatomegaly)
- amyloidosis
- hepatitis
- cirrhosis (strictly speaking, the liver shrinks, but cirrhosis can be associated with fatty liver and/or inflammation, leading to increased size)
- biliary obstruction
- sarcoidosis
- HIV infection.

Differential diagnosis of irregular or patchy enlargement:

- metastatic disease
- cirrhosis
- hydatid disease
- polycystic liver disease.

Localised swellings:

- cystic—likely to be a simple cyst or hydatid cyst
- solitary solid lesion—likely to be a hepatoma or solitary metastasis
- multiple solid lesions—metastatic liver disease is the most likely cause, with primary in the colon, pancreas, stomach, breast or lung
- liver abscess.

Interpreting liver function test abnormalities[1]

Abnormal liver function profiles may not be clinically apparent and may appear in routine biochemical testing. The significance or otherwise of abnormal liver function tests (LFTs) needs to be assessed in the clinical context.

Abnormalities fall into two groups: hepatocellular and cholestatic.

Abnormal LFTs generally indicate some hepatic pathology, although some hepatic diseases such as chronic hepatitis C, well-compensated cirrhosis and some space-occupying lesions of the liver may have normal-range LFTs despite the presence of significant pathology.

Liver imaging is an important tool in the assessment of abnormal LFTs. Ultrasound can ascertain liver and spleen size and presence of mass lesions. Abdominal CT scans may help diagnose the neoplasm.

MRI/MRCP

All patients with abnormal LFTs need to be regarded as having significant liver disease, and causes sought. The assessment and therapeutic management of liver disease and abnormal LFTs needs to address the implications of disruption of normal liver function.

Tests reflecting hepatic function

Bilirubin

Elevated serum bilirubin levels can occur in all forms of liver disease. Jaundiced patients (bilirubin > 19 μmol/L) do not necessarily have significant hepatic disease. Serum bilirubin reflects production, hepatic uptake, processing and secretion.

- Conjugated bilirubin levels are highest in cholestatic disease and fulminant hepatic failure.
- Unconjugated hyperbilirubinaemia may reflect haemolysis, neonatal physiological jaundice or genetic defects in bilirubin transport and conjugation (Gilbert's syndrome and Crigler-Najjar Syndrome). Haemolysis rarely produces a bilirubin level over 50–90 μmol/L.
- In acute liver disease, bilirubin level is of little prognostic significance. However, in chronic liver disease, rising bilirubin indicates the approach of end-stage disease.
- In the presence of cholestasis, renal failure will reduce the clearance of conjugated bilirubin sufficiently to increase serum levels.

Serum albumin

Serum concentration of this protein depends on nutritional state, hepatic synthesis and losses—e.g. renal (nephritic syndrome) or gut (e.g. protein-losing enteropathy).

In chronic liver disease, low serum albumin is an important prognostic indicator. It can reflect paucity of functioning hepatocytes to maintain albumin production. Malnutrition can be a major contributor to low albumin in chronic liver disease.

Alcohol excess can reduce albumin synthesis. Albumin concentration can be reduced by the diluting effect of ascites and oedema.

Albumin has a half-life of 17–26 days, so low levels reflect chronic rather than acute hepatic dysfunction.

Prothrombin time

As with albumin, the vitamin-K-dependent clotting factors are synthesised by the liver and may fall in the presence of significant liver disease. Prothrombin time assesses the activity of these coagulation factors. It is a useful test of function and prognostic in both acute and chronic liver disease (once vitamin K deficiency is excluded—that is, prothrombin does not correct after 10 mg IV vitamin K).

Transaminases

Serum transaminases are a measure of hepatocellular damage or injury rather than functional capacity of the liver. Transaminases enter the circulation as a result of hepatocellular lysis or damage. Marked elevation of transaminases (> 1000 U/L) occurs in acute viral hepatitis, drug reactions and acute exacerbation of chronic autoimmune hepatitis.

- Non-hepatic causes of raised transaminases—acute cholestasis, shock, cardiac failure.
- Persistent elevation—chronic viral or autoimmune hepatitis, hepatic metastases.
- *Alanine aminotransferase (ALT)*—liver-specific. Isolated ALT elevation is highly suggestive of liver disease. Usually higher than AST levels in viral liver injury.
- *Aspartate aminotransferase (AST)*—found in liver, skeletal muscle, myocardium, kidney, pancreas and red blood cells. Damage to any of these cell types can cause elevation of serum AST.
- Consider alcoholic liver disease if AST is more than twice the level of ALT.
- Mitochondrial isoenzyme of AST is especially elevated in alcoholic liver injury.
- *Alkaline phosphatase (ALP)*—in the liver, ALP is localised to the biliary membrane of hepatocytes. Raised ALP is a marker of biliary disease or a hepatic infiltrative disorder.
- Mild elevation of ALP is often seen in hepatocellular injury.
- ALP is also found in bone, intestine, kidney and placenta. Damage to any of these organs will elevate ALP. Pregnancy and rapid growth in adolescence may increase ALP.
- If other liver function tests are normal, consider a non-hepatic cause such as Paget's disease of bone, bone tumour, acromegaly or fracture. Milder ALP rises are seen in myocardial infarct.
- Gamma-glutamyl transpeptidase (GGT)—this membrane-bound enzyme is present in liver, pancreas, kidney, intestine and prostate. Raised GGT is seen in biliary disorders, obesity, hyperlipidaemia, anorexia nervosa, diabetes mellitus, hyperthyroidism, porphyria, myocardial infarction, enzyme-inducing drugs and liver disease. It is particularly useful in association with ALP in cholestatic disorders. Serum GGT is not raised in pregnancy or bone disorders, so raised GGT supports a hepatic cause of raised ALP.
- Not all heavy alcohol drinkers will have a raised GGT, although it is a prognostic marker.
- Lactate dehydrogenase (LDH)—present in all cells. When LDH level is elevated out of proportion to transaminases, consider ischaemic liver injury or secondary neoplasia.

Cirrhosis

Clinical features

- Anorexia, nausea, vomiting
- Peripheral oedema
- Spider naevi
- Palmar erythema

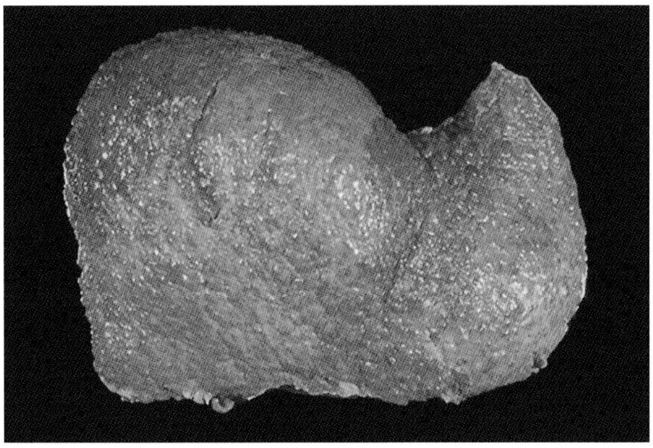

FIGURE 30.6 Cirrhosis

- Jaundice
- Tender hepatomegaly
- Gynaecomastia
- Ascites
- Bleeding
- May be splenomegaly
- Drowsiness, confusion, coma.

Causes of hepatic cirrhosis

- Excess alcohol
- Chronic viral hepatitis
- Autoimmune chronic active hepatitis
- Primary biliary cirrhosis
- Haemochromatosis
- Wilson's disease
- Drugs
- Idiopathic.

Non-alcoholic fatty liver disease

Non-alcoholic fatty liver disease (NAFLD) is the most common cause of abnormal liver function tests in Australia, the United States and the United Kingdom. Increasing prevalence has been associated with increased incidence of overweight and obesity and there is an association with type 2 diabetes, dyslipidaemia and hypertension (metabolic syndrome). NAFLD is actually associated with increased cardiovascular risk. There may be a family history of type 2 diabetes and evidence of insulin resistance. A percentage of individuals develop non-alcoholic steatohepatitis (NASH), which can progress to cirrhosis, liver failure and liver cancer (HCC).

Clinical features

Usually asymptomatic, but patients may complain of fatigue, malaise and dull right upper quadrant abdominal discomfort. Patients are usually overweight. It can (unusually does) progress to hepatic fibrosis and cirrhosis (NASH).

Investigations

- Liver function tests—usually mild increases in transaminases, often with elevated GGT.
- Careful history to clarify alcohol intake and medications.
- Viral serology (hepatitis A, B, C, EBV, CMV and herpes viruses, rubella) to exclude viral cause of abnormal liver function tests.
- Fatty infiltration of the liver may be seen on ultrasound. Strictly speaking, increased echogenicity is seen on ultrasound; this is consistent with or suggestive of fatty infiltration.
- Blood glucose, HbA_{1c} or glucose tolerance test to identify coexisting diabetes.
- Thyroid function tests—NASH is significantly higher in patients with hypothyroidism than the general population.[43]
- NASH resembles alcoholic liver disease histologically, but liver biopsy is usually not necessary.

Therapeutics

- Low-fat diet, kilojoule-restricted diet to reduce body weight by 0.5 to 1.0 kg per week
- Regular exercise
- Optimal diabetes control
- Management of hyperlipidaemia
- Limit alcohol consumption to 10 g or less per day
- Vitamin C (1000 mg daily) and vitamin E (1000 IU daily) for 6 months has been shown to be effective in improving fibrosis scores in NASH patients.[44] (However, the evidence presented in that study is not overwhelming—small *n*; lack of improvement in LFTs and steatosis; fibrosis changes post treatment were not statistically different between vitamin and placebo groups.)

Herbal

- *Silybum marianum* (St Mary's thistle) has a hepatoprotective effect.[45] *Dose*: 600–1800 mg daily.
- Omega-3 essential fatty acids.

Alcoholic liver disease

The most recognised forms of alcoholic liver disease are fatty liver, alcoholic hepatitis and alcoholic cirrhosis.

Aetiology

Alcoholic liver disease is the result of hepatocellular injury caused by excessive consumption of alcohol (acetaldehyde toxicity). Genetic factors and nutritional status will determine the degree of liver damage.

Poor nutrition results in reduction of antioxidant defence mechanisms.

Hepatitis C is more prevalent in alcoholics than the general population. Alcohol consumption accelerates hepatitis-C-associated liver disease.

Fatty liver

Fatty liver is reversible if abstinence from alcohol can be maintained. If drinking continues, fatty liver is a prognostic indicator for the development of long-term liver damage.

Clinical features

- Hepatomegaly
- Elevated transaminases (especially GGT) common but not inevitable. When serum AST levels are at least double the ALT level, alcoholic liver disease is likely.
- GGT levels can be used to monitor abstinence.
- Ultrasound may show fatty infiltration.

Therapeutics

- Reversible with abstinence from alcohol
- Counselling to achieve and maintain alcohol abstinence
- Healthy diet
- Thiamine, multivitamins
- *Silybum marianum* (St Mary's Thistle)[45] has hepatoprotective and hepatic repair effect. *Dose*: 600–1800 mg daily.

Alcoholic hepatitis

Alcoholic hepatitis involves active inflammatory injury to the liver. When severe, features may include weakness, anorexia, weight loss, nausea and diarrhoea. Fever, jaundice (cholestasis is common), neutrophilia, elevated transaminases and tender hepatomegaly may also be present.

Other liver stigmata: spider telangiectasia, parotid enlargement, gynaecomastia.

Signs of hepatic failure: encephalopathy, ascites, gastrointestinal bleeding.

It is a precursor to alcoholic cirrhosis or can occur in the presence of underlying cirrhosis. Severe alcoholic hepatitis has a high mortality rate (≥40%).

Investigations

Common laboratory findings include:

- LFTs—AST 2–3 times higher than ALT (both usually < 500 IU/L), raised serum bilirubin
- prolonged prothrombin time, especially if severe or underlying cirrhosis
- decreased serum albumin
- decreased IgA and IgG but may have polyclonal gammopathy
- decreased cholesterol
- decreased T_3 (triiodothyronine)
- leucocytosis with left shift
- liver ultrasound
- liver biopsy—may be necessary to assess severity of hepatic injury and determine prognosis.

Therapeutics

- Abstinence from alcohol
- Counselling to achieve and maintain alcohol abstinence
- High-kilojoule, high-protein diet
- Nutritional supplementation
- Corticosteroids may improve short- (to medium-) term survival (up to 1 year) in severe disease
- Pentoxifylline 400 mg t.d.s. may reduce development of hepatorenal syndrome (not overwhelming evidence).

Cirrhosis

This condition has a high mortality rate, usually over years.

Prevention

Lifelong safe alcohol consumption. Liver transplantation is a possibility if there is no other end-organ damage (brain and heart) and the patient remains abstinent from alcohol.

Alpha$_1$-antitrypsin deficiency

Alpha$_1$-antitrypsin deficiency is an uncommon cause of cirrhosis as a single pathology in adults. An autosomal-recessive disorder, it may be present in childhood or adult life, with features of chronic hepatitis or cirrhosis. The person may have emphysema (especially adults).

Investigations

- Abnormal LFTs
- Serum alpha$_1$-antitrypsin level
- Liver biopsy to assess extent of hepatic damage and presence of cirrhosis.

Therapeutics

Liver transplant (unless precluded by emphysema in adults).

Viral hepatitis

Hepatitis A

Hepatitis A is a viral infection with hepatitis A virus. Transmission is via the faecal–oral route from the ingestion of contaminated food or water. Liver injury occurs as a result of T-lymphocyte activity rather than a direct hepatocyte injury.

Clinical features

- Incubation period is 15–45 days.

- Prodromal illness involves anorexia and nausea (with or without vomiting), malaise, headache, right upper quadrant discomfort, mild fever.
- Once jaundice develops, patients develop pale stools, dark urine, hepatomegaly. Some will have splenomegaly.
- Viral shedding occurs late in the incubation period and persists for about 2 weeks. It tends to be a self-limiting acute illness and does not cause chronic liver disease. However, about 10–20% of cases will follow a relapsing course over several months.
- The severity of symptoms tends to increase with age. Fulminant hepatic failure is possible but rare.

Investigations

- Liver function tests—serum transaminases in the 1000s
- IgM antibodies to hepatitis A—elevated in acute infection
- IgG antibodies to hepatitis A—indicate past infection or immunity
- Ultrasound—to exclude biliary obstruction as a cause of jaundice (especially in the elderly).

Therapeutics

- Abstinence from alcohol
- Withdraw medications known to cause hepatic damage
- Rest as required
- Low-fat diet
- Avoid tobacco
- Advice on hygiene to prevent spread to others
- Do not allow patient to handle food for others
- Do not share crockery or cutlery.

Nutritional supplements

- Multivitamin daily
- Omega-3 EFA, 1000–2000 mg t.d.s.
- Vitamin C, 500–3000 mg daily
- Vitamin E
- Coenzyme Q10, 100–200 mg daily
- Zinc
- Magnesium
- S-adenosylmethionine, 400–1600 mg daily in divided doses (evidence weak).

Herbal

Caution needs to be exercised as some herbal preparations may affect liver function adversely. Herbal treatments are aimed at reducing oxidative stress, reducing inflammation and supporting the immune system.

- St Mary's thistle—milk thistle (*Silybum marianum*) seed standardised extract, 80–160 mg 2–3 times daily. Commission E approves the use of standardised St Mary's thistle (70–80% silymarin content) as supportive treatment in chronic inflammatory liver disease and hepatic cirrhosis.[7]
- Green tea (*Camellia sinensis*) standardised extract, 250–500 mg daily or as a tea
- Cat's claw (*Uncaria tomentosa*) standardised extract, 20 mg three times daily
- Garlic (*Allium sativum*), standardised extract, 400 mg 2–3 times daily
- Glycyrrhizin
- Reishi mushroom (*Ganoderma lucidum*), 150–300 mg 2–3 times daily
- Maitake mushroom (*Grifola frondosa*) standardised extract (D-fraction), 600 mg twice daily.

Prevention

- Immunisation against hepatitis A, especially in travellers to endemic regions, plumbers, child-care and healthcare workers
- Effective public health measures (sewer and garbage disposal)
- Regular hand washing
- Immune serum globulin for passive immunity for close contacts of infected individuals.

Hepatitis B

Hepatitis B is a highly infectious viral infection with hepatitis B virus. Transmission is parenteral, mostly intravenous drug use with shared or re-used needles and equipment or sexual transmission, and also unsterile tattooing, body piercing or blood transfusion prior to routine testing of donated blood.

Clinical features

- Incubation period is 30–180 days. Most cases are asymptomatic and recover completely.
- It is possible for most adults to spontaneously clear the virus.
- Acute hepatitis develops in 25% of cases, and 1% develop fulminant hepatic failure. Liver injury is mediated by T-lymphocytes.
- Less than 10% of adults progress to chronic infection (70–90% develop a carrier state) and develop varying amounts of liver damage over time.
- In neonates, 95% progress to chronic infection; in infants/children, 50% progress to chronic infection.
- Vitamin and mineral deficiencies are common in patients with chronic liver disease.
- Worldwide, chronic hepatitis B infection is the major cause of hepatocellular carcinoma.

Investigation

- Liver function tests—raised transaminases
- HBV antigens:

- HBsAg = surface (coat) protein. Its presence in serum indicates that virus replication is occurring in the liver. Put simply, it is consistent with infection (does not indicate degree of activity).
- HBcAg = inner core protein
- HBeAg = presence in serum indicates a high level of viral replication in the liver
- Surface antibody (anti-HBs) becomes detectable late in convalescence, and indicates immunity following infection. It remains detectable for life and is not found in chronic carriers.
- e antibody (anti-HBe) becomes detectable as viral replication falls. It may indicates low infectivity in a carrier (see below).
- HBV DNA (viral load) is especially useful in chronic infection and correlates with activity, risk of liver damage and eventual complications. It also differentiates between low-activity eAg-negative disease (+anti-HBe pos) and high-activity eAg-negative disease (previously known as pre-cor mutants).

Therapeutics

Chronic hepatitis B:

- lamivudine, adefovir, entecavir, tenofovir and/or interferon alpha.

Nutritional supplements:

- vitamin E
- vitamin C
- grapeseed extract, 300–400 mg daily
- CoQ10, 300–400 mg daily
- zinc
- magnesium
- S-adenosylmethionine
- whey protein, as a meal supplement
- alpha lipoic acid, 250–500 mg daily.

Herbal

Commission E approves the use of standardised St Mary's thistle (70–80% silymarin content) as supportive treatment in chronic inflammatory liver disease and hepatic cirrhosis.[7] See Hepatitis A, 'Herbal' (above).

Prevention

- Immunisation of uninfected individuals, particularly household contacts and sexual partners, healthcare workers.
- Passive immunity with hyperimmune immunoglobulin within 72 hours of exposure.
- Safe sexual practices.
- Avoid high risk-practices such as sharing intravenous needles, unsterile tattooing and body piercing.
- Safe disposal of needles, syringes, blood products and medical equipment and dressings.

Hepatitis C

Hepatitis C is a viral infection caused by the hepatitis C virus. The virus is directly cytopathic to the hepatocyte. There are (at least) six main genotypes, named genotypes 1 to 6, and the clinical course and therapeutic decisions are influenced by the genotype identified. Particular genotypes are prevalent in different parts of the world.

Clinical features

Incubation period is 15–160 days. Of people exposed to the virus, 25–30% can clear it from their blood within 6 months of infection, without treatment. The remainder proceed to chronic hepatitis C infection.

Symptoms include fatigue, malaise, sleep disturbance, dry mouth, dry eyes, poor concentration, forgetfulness, nausea, anorexia, right upper quadrant discomfort, intolerance to fatty foods and alcohol.

Hepatic failure and hepatocellular carcinoma can be long-term complications of chronic hepatitis C infection.

Transmission

Hepatitis C is spread by blood-to-blood contact but the source may never be known.

- High risk:
  - sharing or re-using equipment used for injecting drugs
  - unsterile tattooing practices
  - unsterile body piercing practices

Moderate/low risk:

  - mother to baby during pregnancy or childbirth (6%)
  - needlestick injury
  - shared personal hygiene items (razors, toothbrushes, nail clippers, nail files)
  - blood transfusion or infected blood products prior to February 1990 (moderate to high risk).
- Very low risk.
  - sexual contact
  - blood products since 1990.

Investigations

A number of investigations are used to diagnose and monitor hepatitis C.

- Liver function tests—especially ALT.
- Hepatitis C antibody—initial test to identify hepatitis C antibodies. Indicates past exposure or current infection. Can take 6 months after infection to become positive.
- PCR test—detects presence of viral RNA. Qualitative PCR detects presence of virus.

Quantitative PCR used to assess viral load and monitor treatment response.
- Genotype—used to determine duration of treatment and assess prognosis.
- Liver biopsy—assesses degree of hepatic damage.
- Hepatitis B antigen and HIV antibody—to identify cases of co-infection because of similar routes of transmission.

Therapeutics

- Complete abstinence from alcohol (ideal, otherwise limit to 3–4 standard drinks per week)
- Low-fat diet
- Stress management and lifestyle modification
- Cease and avoid any medications that may affect the liver.

Pegylated interferon and ribavirin

Pegylated interferon is given subcutaneously once a week for 24–48 weeks, determined by genotype and degree of liver damage. It stops the hepatitis C virus from replicating, boosts the body's immune system and slows or stops progression of hepatocellular damage.

Currently, genotypes 1, 4, 5 and 6 are treated for 48 weeks provided there is a treatment response after 12 weeks (i.e. PCR undetectable or 2 log drop; if still positive at 12 weeks, treatment is continued and PCR tested again at 24 weeks to assess response). If still positive at 24 weeks, treatment is ceased. If negative at 24 weeks, treatment continues to 48 weeks. Genotypes 2 and 3 require 24 weeks of treatment unless there is evidence of cirrhosis or bridging fibrosis.

Ribavirin is given daily orally throughout the course of treatment. An antiviral drug, it boosts the effectiveness of pegylated interferon. PCR is tested at 72 weeks as follow-up. Strictly speaking, 24 weeks after completion of the antiviral course.

Viral eradication is successful in 50–80% of cases. Treatment with pegylated interferon and ribavrin is effective against both hepatitis B and C in cases of co-infection.

Pregnancy should be avoided during treatment with pegylated interferon and ribavirin and for 6 months after treatment has concluded.

Consider immunisation against hepatitis A and B (recommended).

Nutritional supplements

- Multivitamin daily
- Vitamin E, 1000 IU daily
- Vitamin C, 500–3000 mg daily
- Grapeseed extract, 300–400 mg daily
- CoQ10, 300–400 mg daily
- Zinc
- Magnesium
- S-adenosylmethionine
- Whey protein, as a meal supplement
- Alpha lipoic acid, 250–500 mg daily.

Herbal

Commission E approves the use of standardised St Mary's thistle (70–80% silymarin content) as supportive treatment in chronic inflammatory liver disease and hepatic cirrhosis.[7] See 'Herbal', under 'Hepatitis A' (above).

Prevention

- Avoid risk factors.
- Carefully dispose of needles, syringes, dressings and blood spills.
- Even if patients have hepatitis C or have had it in the past, they can become reinfected with another genotype.

Other causes of viral hepatitis

Hepatitis D and E

Hepatitis D virus can only occur in the presence of hepatitis B. The virus uses the hepatitis B surface antigen as part of its own structure, making it totally dependent on hepatitis B. It occurs as a concomitant infection or as a super-infection with modes of transmission similar to hepatitis B. Combined infection causes more severe liver injury and worse prognosis.

Hepatitis E virus is transmitted by the faecal–oral route. It is endemic in India, South-East Asia and Africa, and the Northern Territory in Australia. Illness is self-limiting and no chronic carrier form exists. There is a risk of fulminant hepatic failure, particularly in pregnancy.

Investigation

- Liver function tests
- IgM antibodies to hepatitis E in a patient with hepatitis who has been in an area where the disease is known to occur.

Other viral causes of hepatitis

Acute hepatitis may also occur as part of the clinical course of a number of viral infections, including human cytomegalovirus, Epstein-Barr virus, herpes simplex virus, yellow fever virus and rubella.

Wilson's disease

Wilson's disease is a genetic defect causing defective copper metabolism, resulting in the progressive accumulation of copper, with ongoing liver injury. There are 60 polymorphisms, so genetic testing is not practical in general practice.

Clinical features

- Presentation may be acute hepatic illness complicated by neurological abnormalities (psychiatric symptoms, dysarthria, ataxia, tremor).
- Kaiser-Fleischer rings (brown deposits around the periphery of the iris)
- There is an elevated risk of intraabdominal malignancy.

Investigations

- Low serum caeruloplasmin levels
- Urinary copper excretion
- Liver biopsy may show excessive copper staining.

Therapeutics

- D-penicillamine chelates copper and allows its removal from the body.
- Alternatively, triethylenetetramine dihydrochloride as a chelating agent.
- Zinc supplementation orally inhibits intestinal copper absorption.
- In early presymptomatic Wilson's disease, zinc (50 mg b.i.d.) can prevent progression to clinical disease.

Haemochromatosis

Haemochromatosis is a common autosomal-recessive condition resulting in deregulation of metabolism and/or intestinal absorption of iron, resulting in iron overload.

People who are homozygous for the C282Y mutation and compound heterozygotes with C282Y and H63D mutations are at highest risk of iron overload. Individuals who are heterozygous for C282Y can also develop iron overload.

Clinical features

Unexplained fatigue is one of the most common presenting symptoms. Patients often present because of an incidental finding of iron overload or abnormal liver function tests or request testing because a relative has been diagnosed with the condition.

Undiagnosed and untreated, haemochromatosis may lead to chronic iron overload resulting in hepatomegaly, cirrhosis or hepatocellular carcinoma, diabetes, bronze skin pigmentation, arthropathy (hands, knees, wrists and hips), cardiac failure and hypogonadism.

Investigations

- Iron studies—serum iron, transferrin and ferritin. Normal transferrin saturation makes haemochromatosis unlikely.
- Haemochromatosis gene test (C282Y and C282Y H63D, S63D).
- Liver function tests (diagnosis not excluded by normal LFTs).
- Diagnosis is confirmed on liver biopsy.

Therapeutics

The aim is to identify individuals by screening of first- and second-degree relatives of patients with haemochromatosis and following up patients found to have abnormal iron studies.

Treatment is phlebotomy. Frequency is determined by response, monitored by serial haemoglobin levels and iron studies with the aim of achieving and maintaining normal range iron studies.

If iron levels are reduced to normal and maintained before there is any end-organ damage, life expectancy is normal.

Haemochromatosis may be complicated by a 20-fold increased risk of hepatocellular carcinoma. This is more likely to occur in males aged over 50 years with a history of cirrhosis, chronic alcoholism and smoking.

Autoimmune liver diseases

Autoimmune liver diseases are not common but they are not rare (autoimmune hepatitis, primary biliary cirrhosis ± primary sclerosing cholangitis).

Hepatocellular carcinoma

Hepatocellular carcinoma is the most common primary malignancy of the liver.

Clinical features

- Hepatocellular carcinoma usually arises in a cirrhotic liver, so signs of chronic liver disease (see p. 396), ascites or portal hypertension may be present.
- There may be a history of chronic active hepatitis B or C infection, alcohol abuse, autoimmune liver disease or haemochromatosis.
- Right upper quadrant pain (as a result of tissue expansion, rupture or haemorrhage).
- Bruising or bleeding.
- Onset of abdominal pain, weight loss, early satiety, jaundice and a palpable mass in the upper abdomen usually indicate an advanced cancer or any worsening of hepatic function in a known cirrhotic.

Median survival following diagnosis is 6–20 months.

Investigations

- Liver function tests
- Abdominal ultrasound
- If a mass is detected, abdominal CT scan (triple phase) or MRI
- Liver biopsy (usually not required or indicated—potential for HCC rupture, seeding of biopsy tract)

- Tumour marker—serum alpha-fetoprotein (AFP). Note, however, that mild increases are often seen in hepatic inflammation (AFP marker of regeneration) and are non-diagnostic; conversely, small hepatomas may have normal AFP.

Therapeutics
- Treatment may involve surgical excision of resectable tumours, or liver transplantation, which may be curative if the diagnosis is early and the tumour small.
- Radiofrequency ablation (palliation) or may be useful prior to transplantation.
- Percutaneous ethanol injection.
- Transarterial embolisation.
- Chemotherapy—sorafenib, a multikinase inhibitor recently approved by the TGA for treatment of advanced HCC in compensated liver disease. Survival increased from 7.9 to 10.7 months (median).
- Nutritional support.
- Mind–body.

Prevention
- Childhood immunisation against hepatitis B
- Public health education to reduce transmission of hepatitis B and C
- Avoid excessive alcohol consumption
- Identify and treat cases of haemochromatosis
- Regular ultrasound monitoring and alpha-fetoprotein screening of at-risk patients.

> **Medications and the liver**
> Any assessment of abnormal liver function tests must include a careful assessment of consumption of medication, supplements, herbs, illicit drugs and alcohol. Reactions affecting the liver can be toxic and dose-dependent or idiosyncratic. Mechanisms vary and are complex.

GALLBLADDER
Cholelithiasis
Gallstones may be an asymptomatic incidental finding on abdominal ultrasound. Only 10% of gallstones are detectable on X-ray.

Clinical features
Biliary colic is severe pain of gradual onset in the right upper quadrant or epigastrium. It may peak for minutes to hours, then slowly resolve. It characteristically radiates around the right side to the scapular area. There may be associated nausea and vomiting.

Gallstone complications
- Acute cholecystitis
- Empyema of gallbladder (abscess of gallbladder)
- Mucocoele of gallbladder
- Acute cholangitis
- Obstructive jaundice
- Acute pancreatitis
- Gallstone ileus.

Investigations
- Upper abdominal ultrasound
- White cell count (leucocytosis indicating cholecystitis)
- Serum amylase and lipase to exclude pancreatitis
- Liver function tests.[46]

Therapeutics
- Asymptomatic gallstones are usually managed by observation
- Low-fat diet
- Magnesium supplementation, 400–600 mg daily
- Avoid tobacco and alcohol
- Nutritional support:
  - a multivitamin daily, containing the antioxidant vitamins A, C, E, the B-complex vitamins and trace minerals such as calcium, zinc and selenium
  - vitamin C, 500–1000 mg daily
  - alpha-lipoic acid, 25–50 mg twice daily
- Prophylactic cholecystectomy may be offered to patients with diabetes or where the stone size is > 2.5 cm
- Laparoscopic cholecystectomy is indicated if gallstones become symptomatic. Operative cholangiogram is performed at the time of surgery to ensure that no stones are retained in the common bile duct, and that the duct has not been damaged.

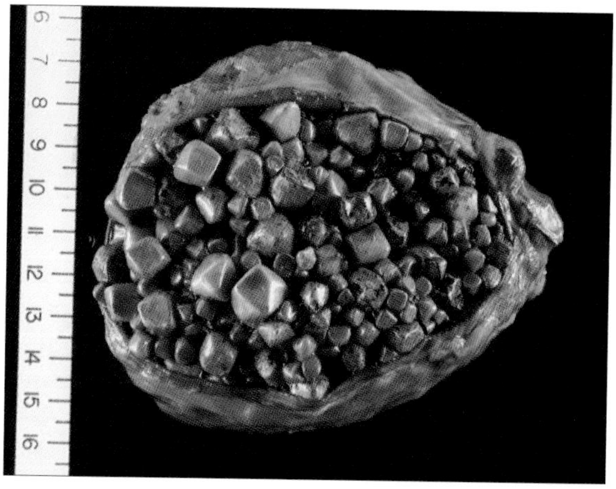

FIGURE 30.7 Gallstones

Acute cholecystitis

Obstruction of the outlet of the gallbladder causes biliary colic. Obstruction causes inflammation of the gallbladder, which may be complicated by secondary bacterial infection.

Clinical features

- Constant severe right upper quadrant/epigastric pain
- Nausea and vomiting bile
- Tenderness over gallbladder and guarding
- Gallbladder may be palpable
- ± Fever.

Investigations

- Upper abdominal ultrasound
- HIDA scan (demonstrates obstructed cystic duct)
- White cell count and C-reactive protein.

Therapeutics

- Bed rest
- IV fluids
- Analgesia
- Antibiotics
- Probiotic
- Cholecystectomy once acute inflammation has settled.

Nutritional support

- Low-fat diet
- A multivitamin daily, containing the antioxidant vitamins A, C, E, the B-complex vitamins, and trace minerals such as calcium, zinc and selenium
- Vitamin C, 500–1000 mg daily
- Alpha-lipoic acid, 25–50 mg twice daily.

Herbal

- Green tea (*Camellia sinensis*) standardised extract, 250–500 mg daily or as a tea
- Milk thistle (*Silybum marianum*) seed standardised extract, 80–160 mg two to three times daily
- Globe artichoke (*Cynara scolymus*) standardised extract, 250–500 mg two to three times daily
- Turmeric (*Curcuma longa*) standardised extract, 300 mg three times daily.

Gallbladder polyps

Gallbladder polyps are usually asymptomatic and detected during upper abdominal ultrasound. Polyps should be monitored for increase in size after 3–6 months. Polyps will not increase significantly in size. A malignancy will.

Cholecystectomy is considered for polyps over 1 cm because of the possibility of gallbladder malignancy.

PANCREAS

Acute pancreatitis

Clinical features

Acute pancreatitis is characterised by sudden onset of severe central epigastric pain, with nausea and vomiting. Pain may radiate to the back. Sweating and weakness are common.

Signs include sweating and pallor, and epigastric tenderness without guarding or rebound. Fever and tachycardia may be noted and abdominal distension may be a feature.

Aetiology

- Gallstones causing pancreatic duct obstruction
- Infection with mumps, hepatitis virus, rubella, Epstein-Barr virus (the cause of mononucleosis) and cytomegalovirus
- Acute abdominal trauma
- Excessive alcohol
- Drug reaction—steroids, sulfonamides, azathioprine, NSAIDs, diuretics such as furosemide and thiazides, and didanosine.

Investigation

- Full blood examination—leucocytosis
- Serum amylase and serum lipase elevated; if the lipase level is about 2.5–3 times that of amylase, it is an indication of pancreatitis due to alcohol
- CRP elevated
- Blood glucose level elevated
- Serum calcium reduced
- Liver function tests may show an obstructive pattern (especially if gallstone-induced)
- Plain X-ray may display a sentinel loop
- CT scan
- Ultrasound to exclude pancreatic cyst or gallstone.

Therapeutics

- Urgent hospital admission
- Nil by mouth
- Parenteral or post-pyloric enteral feeding
- IV fluids and analgesia
- Avoid coffee, stimulants, alcohol and tobacco
- Cease drugs that may cause pancreatitis
- Consider IV vitamin C.

Chronic pancreatitis

Clinical features

- Upper abdominal pain is deep and boring, and intermittent or more persistent. It is usually post-prandial and often radiates to the back.
- Pain may be relieved by sitting up and leaning forward. May be exacerbated by fatty meals or alcohol ingestion.

- Malabsorption and secondary diabetes may develop.
- Weight loss, muscle wasting and steatorrhoea can be features.
- If the common bile duct is obstructed the patient may be jaundiced.
- Necrotising pancreatitis can lead to development of pseudocysts and abscesses.

Aetiology

Excessive alcohol consumption is by far the most common cause of chronic pancreatitis. Smoking also increases the risk. Other causes include:

- hypertriglyceridaemia
- hypercalcaemia
- trauma
- autosomal-dominant inherited
- cystic fibrosis
- nutritional
- haemochromatosis
- prolonged parenteral nutrition
- obstruction (benign or malignant)
- autoimmune
- medication adverse effect (e.g. steroids)
- sphincter of Oddi dysfunction.

Investigation

- Amylase and lipase levels are unhelpful in chronic pancreatitis.
- Secretin stimulation test.
- Plain abdominal X-ray or abdominal CT scan may show pancreatic calcification and exclude pancreatic cancer.
- Consider cystic fibrosis (sweat electrolytes) if the patient is a child or young adult.
- Check serum calcium and triglycerides.

Therapeutics

- Analgesia for pain management.
- Oral pancreatic enzymes with meals (relieve pain because they reduce cholecystokinin secretion and relieve steatorrhoea). *Dose*: Viokase® or Cotazyme® or enteric-coated pancreases.
- Patients with refractory steatorrhoea may benefit from the addition of an H_2 antagonist or proton-pump inhibitor with pancreatic enzyme replacement.
- Micronutrients, including antioxidants, should be replaced if serum levels suggest a deficiency.
- Complete alcohol abstinence.
- Small, low-fat meals.
- Stenting or surgical relief of obstruction if present
- If high triglyceride levels: lose weight, exercise and avoid medications such as thiazide diuretics and beta-blockers that increase triglyceride levels.
- Blood glucose control (may need insulin).
- Consider IV vitamin C.

Adjunctive therapies for acute and chronic pancreatitis

- Intravenous vitamin C, 15 g starting dose
- Selenium.

After the nil by mouth phase in acute pancreatitis has passed and in the management of chronic inflammation, some herbs may be helpful along with conventional medical treatment:

- Green tea (*Camellia sinensis*) standardised extract, 250–500 mg daily, or as a tea
- Holy basil (*Ocimum sanctum*) standardised extract, 400 mg daily
- Rhodiola (*Rhodiola rosea*) standardised extract, 150–300 mg one to three times daily, for immune support. Rhodiola is an 'adaptogen' and helps the body adapt to various stresses.
- Cat's claw (*Uncaria tomentosa*) standardised extract, 20 mg three times a day
- Reishi mushroom (*Ganoderma lucidum*), 150–300 mg two to three times daily, for inflammation and for immunity
- Indian gooseberry (*Emblica officinalis*) powder, 3–6 g daily; a traditional ayurvedic medicinal plant used to treat pancreatic disorders
- Grape seed extract (*Vinis vinifera*) standardised extract, 100–300 mg daily

Prevention

- Alcohol moderation or abstinence
- Not smoking
- Healthy general nutrition

Pancreatic cancer

Pancreatic cancer is the second most common gastrointestinal malignancy after colorectal cancer. It is more common in males than females. Prognosis is poor.

Aetiology is unknown but risk factors include increasing age, smoking, diabetes mellitus, chronic pancreatitis, some familial cancer syndromes, *Helicobacter pylori*, obesity and high-fat diet.

Clinical features

Pancreatic cancer often presents at a late stage with features such as upper abdominal pain, malaise, weight loss and anorexia. Gastric outlet obstruction with vomiting may occur. Jaundice occurs where there is biliary obstruction, and generalised pruritis without a rash is common.

Gallbladder is usually enlarged and may be palpable (if biliary obstruction).

Uncommon presentations may include migratory thrombophlebitis, venous thrombosis, acute pancreatitis, and recent onset of diabetes mellitus.

Metastasis may be evident in supraclavicular gland of Virchow.

Investigation

- Upper abdominal ultrasound
- Abdominal CT scan
- Endoscopic retrograde cholangiopancreatography (ERCP) / magnetic resonance cholangiopancreatography (MRCP).

PREBIOTICS AND PROBIOTICS

Prebiotics are defined as non-digestible food ingredients that selectively stimulate the growth or activity of one or a limited number of probiotic bacterial species in the colon. Most are soluble carbohydrate fibres and oligosaccharides. Sources of oligosaccharides include fruits, legumes and whole grains.

Probiotics are live microorganisms that, when taken in adequate doses, confer a health benefit on the human host.[47] Furthermore, probiotics can lessen the severity of several conditions and may also enhance immunity and the general health of people requiring gastrointestinal and immune support.[48] A recent extensive review has suggested that combining probiotics and prebiotics into *synbiotics* may enhance the immunosupportive effects.[48]

For a strain to be considered 'therapeutic' it must be:

- stomach acid resistant
- bile resistant
- pepsin and pancreatin resistant
- able to adhere to human intestinal cells
- able to inhibit the growth of pathogenic organisms
- of human origin.

Over the past 10 years there has been considerable research into probiotics and their effects on the human body, particularly the function and integrity of the gut and associated immune function,[49] and clinical applications are increasingly being clarified.

It is estimated that the human gastrointestinal tract is composed of approximately 100 trillion microbial symbiont cells, and that the human cells are outnumbered by gut flora by at least 10 to 1. Recent studies have indicated that the human gut may contain at least 500 different phylotypes (species of microorganisms). This extensive microbiome is dominated by two main phyla, namely Firmicutes (with members such as Lactobacillales and Clostridia) and Bacteriodetes (with members such as Bacteriodes), which contribute to maintaining an ecological balance in the gastrointestinal tract. Beneficial bacterial species, such as lactobacilli and bifidobacteria, colonise different regions of the gastrointestinal tract. Lactobacilli primarily colonise the distal part of the small intestine, while bifidobacteria are found predominately in the large intestine. These probiotic bacteria adhere to the intestinal wall, competitively inhibiting adhesion of pathogens, including *Candida* species, and inhibiting their growth. Low levels of these beneficial bacteria can lead to a dysbiotic gut, which can favour an overgrowth of pathogens, which may result in sustained gut dysfunction.

Intestinal microflora are able to influence immune function[50] through a number of actions:

- preventing pathogen-induced membrane damage—by inhibiting pathogen adhesion and maintaining the correct organisation of the tight junction and cytoskeleton proteins
- preventing or reducing allergic disease—maintenance of oral tolerance has been postulated to be a cause of food allergy; feeding probiotic bacteria may prevent or ameliorate the onset of allergic disease and the associated inflammatory reactions, through mechanisms involving modulation of T regulatory cells
- repairing intestinal barrier function
- normalising gut flora through competitive colonisation and pathogen eradication
- enhancing IgA immune response
- stimulating T-cell populations by antigen presenting cells
- competitively excluding pathogens.

Regardless of its genus and species, each probiotic strain is unique, and therefore the properties and the human health effects of each strain must be assessed in a case-by-case manner.[51]

Different probiotics have different functions and activity, and so the selection of the type of probiotic will influence the immuno-regulatory outcome. Some examples are discussed below.

LACTOBACILLUS ACIDOPHILUS

The *Lactobacillus* species are a group of Gram-positive rods that are indigenous inhabitants of the human intestine and vagina. The primary benefit of *L. acidophilus* and other indigenous microflora is that they reinforce the protective barrier of the mucosal surfaces and prevent the attachment of pathogenic microorganisms. They accomplish this through several mechanisms, including competing with pathogens for epithelial space and nutrients, and maintaining the epithelial surface at a slightly acidic pH, which is inhibitory to pathogenic bacteria.

Lactic acid bacteria, including *L. acidophilus*, metabolise carbohydrates and produce lactic acid, acetic acid, hydrogen peroxide and short-chain fatty acids such as propionate and acetate. Lactic acid and the short-chain fatty acids help reduce the pH of the mucosal surface, while hydrogen peroxide inhibits growth of pathogenic bacteria and yeasts. *L. acidophilus* also produces natural antimicrobial substances called *bacteriocins*. Together these chemicals produce an environment that inhibits the growth of potentially pathogenic microorganisms, such as staphylococci, *Pseudomonas* and *Salmonella*.[52]

BIFIDOBACTERIUM LACTIS

The predominant probiotic bacteria in the large intestine are *Bifidobacterium lactis. B. lactis* is able to survive gut transit to ensure delivery to and colonisation of the large intestine.[53] *B. lactis* inhibits growth of pathogenic organisms, such as *Salmonella* spp, *Bacillus cereus, Staphylococcus aureus, Campylobacter* spp, *E. coli, Shigella dysenteria, Listeria* spp and *Vibrio cholerae*.[54,55]

Antibiotic treatment may destroy beneficial bacteria in the colonic and vaginal epithelium, creating an environment in which pathogenic organisms can flourish.[56,57] If patients have been prescribed antibiotics, it is recommended that bacteria-derived probiotics be taken twice a day, at least 2 hours away from the antibiotic dose, so as to minimise the amount of probiotics that are killed by the antibiotics.[58]

Research supports the need for a minimum daily oral dose of over 10 billion live organisms, to effectively recolonise the intestines and vagina. It is generally recommended that the probiotics be taken for at least 4 weeks, to ensure adequate colonisation.

LACTOBACILLUS PLANTARUM

Lactobacillus plantarum 299v improves the gut's defensive barrier, reduces bloating in patients with symptoms of irritable bowel syndrome,[59] and reduces mucosal inflammation. It increases the production of anti-inflammatory cytokines produced by regulatory T-cells (Th3) in the mucosal immune system. These cytokines maintain the Th1/Th2 balance and, it is thought, restore oral tolerance to microbial and environmental antigens. This results in an overall reduction in the production of excessive innate inflammatory cytokines, including IL-1, IL-6 and tumour necrosis factor. These cytokines are responsible for initiating the vascular changes associated with the development of cardiovascular disease, diabetes and cancer.

L. plantarum 299v is the most studied strain. It has been shown to reduce inflammation with experimentally induced enterocolitis[60] and minimise inflammation in the intestinal mucosa of rats after radiation.[61]

L. plantarum 299v has application in the treatment of low-grade inflammatory diseases (irritable bowel syndrome, cardiovascular disease, osteoarthritis) and autoimmune conditions.

LACTOBACILLUS RHAMNOSUS GG

When administered orally, *Lactobacillus rhamnosus* GG adheres to the mucous membrane of the intestine and may help to restore the balance of the gastrointestinal microflora, promote gut-barrier functions, diminish the production of carcinogenic compounds by other intestinal bacteria and activate the innate immune response and enhance adaptive immunity, especially during infections.[62]

SACCHAROMYCES BOULARDII

Saccharomyces boulardii is a strain of yeast that has been studied extensively for its probiotic effects. The clinical activity of *S. boulardii* is especially relevant to antibiotic-associated diarrhoea,[63] and recurrent *Clostridium difficile* intestinal infections.[64] Although generally safe and well tolerated, *S. boulardii* should be used cautiously in severely immunocompromised patients.

RESOURCES

Coeliac Society of Australia, http://www.coeliacsociety.com.au/
Hepatitis Australia, http://www.hepatitisaustralia.com/
Talley N, Martin C. Clinical gastroenterology. A practical problem-based approach. 2nd edn. Sydney: Elsevier; 2006.

REFERENCES

1 Talley N, Martin C. Clinical gastroenterology. A practical problem-based approach. 2nd edn. Sydney: Elsevier; 2006.
2 Murtagh J. General practice. 3rd edn. Sydney: McGraw Hill; 2007.
3 Allen SJ, Okoko B, Martinez E et al. Probiotics for treating infectious diarrhoea. Cochrane Database Syst Rev 2 2004:CD003048.
4 D'Souza AL, Rajkumar C, Cooke J et al. Probiotics in prevention of antibiotic-associated diarrhoea: meta-analysis. BMJ 2002; 324:1361.
5 Elmer GW. Probiotics: living drugs. Am J Health Syst Pharm 2001; 58(12):1101–1109.
6 Braun L, Cohen M. Herbs and natural supplements. An evidence-based guide. Sydney: Elsevier; 2007.
7 Blumenthal M, Goldberg A, Brinckmann J eds. Herbal medicine: expanded commission E monographs. Austin, TX: Integrative Medicine Communications; 2000.
8 De la Motte, Bose-O'Reilly S, Heinisch M et al. Double blind comparison of an apple pectin–chamomile extract preparation with placebo in children with diarrhoea. Arzneimittelforschung 1997; 47(11): 1247–1249.
9 Davidson GP, Whyte PB, Daniels E et al. Passive immunization of children with bovine colostrums containing antibodies to human rotavirus. Lancet 1989; 2:709–712.

10 Gillespie N, Lewis R, Pearn J et al. Ciguatera in Australia. Occurrence, clinical features, pathophysiology and management. Med J Aust 1986; 145(11/12):584–590.

11 Swift A, Swift T. Ciguatera. J Toxicol Clin Toxicol 1993; 31(1):1–29.

12 Kalantar JS, Howell S, Talley NJ et al. Prevalence of faecal incontinence and associated risk factors. An underdiagnosed problem in the Australian community? Med J Aust 2002; 176(2):54–57.

13 Maslekar S, Gardiner A, Maklin C et al. Investigation and treatment of faecal incontinence. Postgrad Med J 2006; 82:363–371.

14 Holtmann G, Adam B, Haag S et al. Efficacy of artichoke leaf extract in the treatment of patients with functional dyspepsia: a six week placebo controlled, double-blind, multicentre trial. Aliment Pharmacol Ther 2003; 18:1099–1105.

15 Sontakke S, Thawani V, Naik MS et al. Ginger as an antiemetic in nausea and vomiting induced by chemotherapy: a randomized crossover double blind study. Indian J Pharmacol 2003; 35(1):32–36.

16 Mausirivithaya S, Sripamote M, Tangitgamol S et al. Antiemetic effect of ginger in gynecologic oncology patients receiving cisplatin. Int J Gynecol Cancer 2004; 14(6):1063–1069.

17 Kaptan K, Beyan C, Ural AU et al. *Helicobacter pylori*—is it a novel causative agent in vitamin B_{12} deficiency? Arch Intern Med 2000; 160(9):1349–1353.

18 Lederle FA. Oral cobalamin for pernicious anemia. Medicine's best kept secret? JAMA 1991; 265:94–95.

19 Woodward M, Tunstall-Pedo H, McColl K. *Helicobacter pylori* infection reduces systemic availability of dietary vitamin C. Eur J Gastro Hepatol 2001; 13(3):233–237.

20 Shibata K, Mariyama M, Fukushima T et al. Green tea consumption and chronic atrophic gastritis: a cross-sectional study in a green tea production village. J Epidemiol 2000; 10(5):310–316.

21 Aldoori WH, Giovannucci EL, Stampfer MJ et al. Prospective study of diet and the risk of duodenal ulcer in men. Am J Epidemiol 1997; 145:42–50.

22 Lesbros-Pantoflickova D, Corthésy-Theulaz I, Blum AL. *Helicobacter pylori* and probiotics. J Nutr 2007; 137(3 Suppl 2):812S–818S.

23 Ye W, Held M, Lagergren J et al. *Helicobacter pylori* infection and gastric atrophy: risk of adenocarcinoma and squamous-cell carcinoma of the esophagus and adenocarcinoma of the gastric cardia. J Natl Cancer Inst 2004; 96(5):388–396.

24 Chainani-Wu N. Diet and oral, pharyngeal, and esophageal cancer. Nutr Cancer 2002; 44(2):104–126.

25 Boeing H, Dietrich T, Hoffmann K et al. Intake of fruits and vegetables and risk of cancer of the upper aero-digestive tract: the prospective EPIC-study. Cancer Causes Cont 2006; 17(7):957–969.

26 Lagergren J, Bergström R, Lindgren A et al. Symptomatic gastroesophageal reflux as a risk factor for esophageal adenocarcinoma. N Engl J Med 1999; 340(11):825–831.

27 Ng K, Meyerhardt J, Wu K et al. Circulating 25-hydroxyvitamin D levels and survival in patients with colorectal cancer. J Clin Oncol 2008; 26:2984–2991.

28 Shimizu M, Fukutomi Y, Ninomiya M et al. Green tea extracts for the prevention of metachronous colorectal adenomas: a pilot study. Cancer Epidemiol Biomarkers Prev 2008; 17(11):3020–3025.

29 Kodama N, Komuta K, Nanba H. Effect of maitake (*Grifola frondosa*) D-fraction on the activation of NK cells in cancer patients. J Med Food 2003; 6(4): 371–377.

30 Kawamori T, Lubet R, Steele VE et al. Chemopreventive effect of curcumin, a naturally occurring anti-inflammatory agent, during the promotion/progression stages of colon cancer. Cancer Res 1999; 59:597–601.

31 Flood A, Schatzkin A. Colorectal cancer: does it matter if you eat your fruits and vegetables? J Natl Cancer Inst 2000; 92(21):1706–1707.

32 Davis K, Philpott S, Kumar D et al. Randomised, double-blind placebo-controlled trial of aloe vera for irritable bowel syndrome. Int J Clin Pract 2006; 60:1080–1086.

33 Tursi A, Giorgetti GM, Branimarte G et al. High prevalence of celiac disease among patients affected by Crohn's disease. Inflamm Bowel Dis 2005; 11(7): 662–666.

34 Vines G. A gut feeling. New Scientist 1998; 159(2146):26–30.

35 Langmead L, Feakins RM, Goldthorpe S et al. Randomized, double-blind, placebo-controlled trial of oral aloe vera gel for active ulcerative colitis. Aliment Pharmacol Ther 2004; 19(7):739–747.

36 Joos S, Brinkhaus C, Maluche N et al. Acupuncture and moxibustion in the treatment of active Crohn's disease: a randomized controlled study. Digestion 2004; 69(3):131–139.

37 Häuser W, Stallmach A, Caspary WF. Predictors of reduced health-related quality of life in adults with coeliac disease. Alim Pharmacol Ther 2007; 25(5): 569–578.

38 Niederhofer H, Pittschieler K. A preliminary investigation of ADHD symptoms in persons with celiac disease. J Atten Disord 2006; 10(2):200–204.

39 Zelnik N, Pacht A, Obeid R et al. Range of neurologic disorders in patients with celiac disease. Pediatrics 2004; 113(6):1672–1676.

40 Addolorato G, DiGiuda D, DeRossi G et al. Regional cerebral hypoperfusion in patients with celiac disease. Am J Med 2004; 116:312–317.

41 Holmes GK, Prior P, Lane MR et al. Malignancy in coeliac disease—effect of a gluten-free diet. Gut 1989; 30(3):333–338.

42 Catassi C, Fabiani E, Iacono G et al. A prospective, double-blind, placebo-controlled trial to establish a safe gluten threshold for patients with celiac disease. Am J Clin Nutr 2007; 85:160–166.

43 Liangpunsakul S, Chalasani N. Is hypothyroidism a risk factor for non-alcoholic steatohepatitis? J Clinical Gastroenterol 2003; 37(4):340–343.

44 Harrison S, Torgerson S, Hayashi P et al. Vitamin E and vitamin C treatment improves fibrosis in patients with nonalcoholic steatohepatitis. Am J Gastroenterol 2003; 98(11):2485–2490.

45 Hajaghamohammadi AA, Ziaee A, Rafiei R et al. The efficacy of silymarin in decreasing transaminase activities in non-alcoholic fatty liver disease: a randomized controlled clinical trial. Hepatitis Monthly 2008; 8(3):191–195. Online. Available: http://hepmon.com/view/?id=343

46 Tsai CJ, Leitzmann MF, Willett WC et al. Long-term effect of magnesium consumption on the risk of symptomatic gallstone disease among men. Am J Gastroenterol 2008; 103(2):375–382.

47 Bruce AW, Reid G. Probiotics and the urologist. Can J Urol 2003; 10(2):1785–1789.

48 Vitetta L, Sali A. Probiotics and prebiotics and gastro-intestinal health. Medicine Today 2008; 9(6):65–70.

49 Isolauri E, Sütas Y, Kankaanpää P. Probiotics: effects on immunity. Am J Clin Nutr 2001; 73(2):S444–S450.

50 Mengheri E. Health, probiotics, and inflammation. J Clin Gastroenterol 2008; 42:S177–S178.

51 Salminen SJ, Gueimonde M, Isolauri E. Probiotics that modify disease risk. J Nutr 2005; 135(5): 1294–1298.

52 Tlaskalova-Hogenova H, Stepankova R, Hudcovic T et al. Commensal bacteria (normal microflora), mucosal immunity and chronic inflammatory and autoimmune diseases. Immunol Letters 2004; 93(2004):97–108.

53 Probiotic Identity Card: Bifidobacterium lactis BI-07. Flora Fit. Rhodia Probiotics. Version 6-D-04.

54 Shu Q, Qu F, Gill HS. Probiotic treatment using Bifidobacterium lactis HNO19 reduces weanling diarrhea associated with rotavirus and *Escherichia coli* infection in a piglet model. J Ped Gastroenterol Nutr 2001; 33:171–177.

55 Gill HS, Rutherfurd KJ, Cross ML et al. Enhancement of immunity in the elderly by dietary supplementation with the probiotic *Bifidobacterium lactis* HN019. Am J Clin Nutr 74(6):833–839.

56 Wren SM, Ahmed N, Jamal A et al. Preoperative oral antibiotics in colorectal surgery increase the rate of *Clostridium difficile* colitis. Arch Surg 2005; 140(8): 752–756.

57 Schumann A, Nutten S, Donnicola D et al. Neonatal antibiotic treatment alters gastrointestinal tract developmental gene expression and intestinal barrier transcriptome. Physiol Genomics 2005; 23(2): 235–245.

58 Reid G, Beuerman D, Heinemann C et al. Probiotic *Lactobacillus* dose required to restore and maintain a normal vaginal flora. FEMS Immunol Med Microbiol 2001; 32(1):37–41.

59 Nobaek S, Johansson ML, Molin G et al. Alteration of intestinal microflora is associated with reduction in abdominal bloating and pain in patients with irritable bowel syndrome. Am J Gastroenterol 2000; 95:1231–1238.

60 Mao Y, Yu J-L, Ljungh A et al. Intestinal immune response to oral administration of *Lactobacillus reuteri* R2LC, *Lactobacillus plantarum* DSM 9843, pectin and oatbase on methotrexate-induced enterocolitis in rats. Microb Ecol Health Dis 1996; 9:261–270.

61 Liu Q, Nobaek S, Adawi D et al. Administration of *Lactobacillus plantarum* 299v reduces side effects of external radiation on colonic anastomatic healing in an experimental model. Colorectal Dis 2001; 3: 245–252.

62 National Cancer Institute. Online. Available: http://www.cancer.gov/drugdictionary/?CdrID=468840

63 Katz JA. Probiotics for the prevention of antibiotic-associated diarrhea and *Clostridium difficile* diarrhea. J Clin Gastroenterol 2006; 40(3):249–255.

64 Czerucka D, Piche T, Rampal P. Review article: yeast as probiotics—*Saccharomyces boulardii*. Aliment Pharmacol Ther 2007; 26(6):767–778.

chapter 31

Genetic conditions

INTRODUCTION AND OVERVIEW

Genetic conditions are those that are directly or indirectly due to a pathogenic variation in a person's genome that is present at birth. The variant may be inherited from a parent, or occur for the first time in the family in that person in the production of the egg or sperm or at conception (spontaneous mutation or chromosomal change).

Until recently, the focus has been on genetic conditions, usually rare, that are directly due to a genetic variation. There are many thousands of these conditions, and they include changes to chromosome number and structure, pathogenic variants in single genes. For example, around 2300 comparatively rare conditions are now known to be primarily due to an inherited mutation in a single gene.[1] As they follow a pattern of inheritance in families first defined by Mendel over 100 years ago, these conditions are often referred to as Mendelian. Still, the genes and mutations causing around 1600 or so Mendelian conditions remain to be identified.[1] Also, more than one gene can be involved in the causation of some Mendelian conditions.

For all these genetic conditions, treatment is limited and symptomatic. Gene therapy—treatment to correct the underlying genetic change—is still in its infancy and research is continuing, to ensure its safety and efficacy.[2] Currently the only preventive strategy is detection through genetic testing prenatally and termination of an affected pregnancy or pre-implantation. These strategies can only be used where pregnancies are identified as at-risk. This determination results from genetic counselling and genetic testing where appropriate, and may be available based on a positive family history or ethnicity.

An emerging area is the use of DNA genetic testing to guide prescribing and drug response (pharmacogenomics).[3] This field epitomises the move to tailored medicine.

EPIGENETICS

For decades, our view of heredity has been rather fixed and one-dimensional. It was written in the language of DNA—and genetic mutations and recombinations have driven most descriptions of how phenotypic traits are handed down from one generation to another. However, recent discoveries in the field of *epigenetics*—the study of heritable changes in gene function that occur without a change in the DNA sequence—have blurred this picture, and are changing the way we think about heredity.

Increasingly there is recognition of the significant contribution to many common conditions of the interaction between the person's inherited genome and factors in their fetal, childhood and/or adult environment. Despite the presence of the predisposing mutation since birth, a person will remain asymptomatic unless further acquired genetic variations or other interactions occur during the person's lifetime that lead to disease onset. Identification of the factors that lead to the variants or interactions is crucial for prevention.

In practical terms it means that non-genetic factors such as drugs, diet, exercise, stress responses and environmental factors can cause an organism's genes to behave (or 'express themselves') differently and even pass that expression on to the next generation. In other words, Nurture can alter Nature.

Epigenetic mechanisms, and their effects in gene activation and inactivation, are increasingly being found to play a critical role in phenotype transmission and development. The study of epigenetics is therefore telling us much about the mechanisms whereby lifestyle, environmental and psychosocial factors can influence the activation and progression of chronic illnesses, including cancer,[4] dementia[5] and ageing.[6] But, more optimistically, it also tells us much about the potential for lifestyle and environmental modification to alter disease progression.

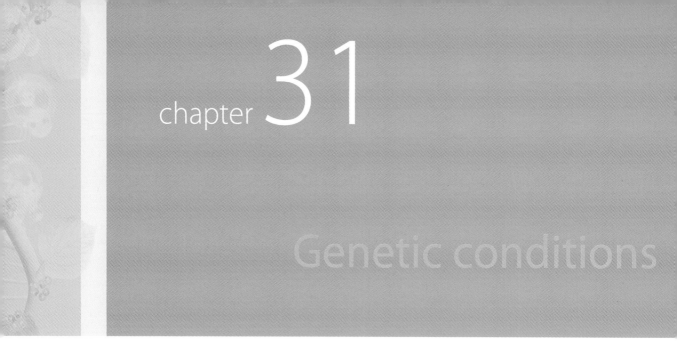

LIFESTYLE FACTORS AND GENETICS

Our genes are programmed not just by the DNA but also by the 'epigenome', which is the chemicals and proteins laid down over the genes and which alter their expression. Epigenetic patterns are sculpted during fetal development, and are affected by maternal nutrition and exposure to environmental toxins as well as psychological stress.[7] It is now also known that extensive lifestyle changes, such as those undertaken in the Ornish program, are associated with alterations of cancer gene expression[8] and improved telomerase-based genetic repair.[9] Thus, alterations in genetic function and repair probably explain a significant amount of the benefit of lifestyle-based interventions.

Some further examples and implications are explored below.

Mind–body and DNA modulation

An important but possibly under-recognised factor in determining the development, expression and repair of genes is our mental and emotional state.

Psychological stress increases DNA damage[10] in animal studies[11,12] and studies on humans. There is an increase in DNA damage in humans under stress—in students taking examinations, for example—and stress increases the number of genetic mutations and probably impairs the body's ability to repair them[13] (due to the effect of the mediators of the stress response[14]), increases oxidation and affects DNA repair enzymes.

DNA damage stimulates the body's DNA repair mechanisms in order to compensate for the damage.[15] A study of healthy medical students showed that during the exam period, compared with low-stress periods after vacations, there was an increase in DNA repair capacity (DRC) in nearly all the study participants.[16] Students who had higher and more consistent levels of stress and mood disturbance during exam periods had a reduction in DRC, or no change when they needed it most, suggesting that the response had been impaired in some way due to emotional stress. The implications of DRC are important. A study comparing DRC in women with breast cancer and in cancer-free women found significant differences.[17] Women with breast cancer have a lower DRC (5.6% DRC) than women without breast cancer (8.7% DRC). Younger breast cancer patients had a more significant reduction in DRC. A low DRC increased susceptibility to breast cancer, with a 1% decrease in DRC corresponding to a 22% increase in breast cancer risk.

Not only is DNA function, damage and repair affected by psychological states, but the mind also affects genetic ageing. Telomeres are segments of DNA at the ends of the DNA strands that help the DNA to not 'unravel', which would cause the cell to die. A study of healthy premenopausal women who were carers for someone with a major disability found that psychological stress, in terms of both perception and duration, was significantly associated with markers of cell death and longevity. The women who were coping least well with the demands showed higher oxidative stress, lower telomerase activity (the enzyme that repairs telomeres) and shorter telomere length. Women with the highest levels of perceived stress, compared with those with the lowest, had telomeres shorter on average by the equivalent of 9–17 years of additional ageing.[18] A similar finding has been demonstrated for people with depression.[19] Low telomerase activity is associated with high allostatic load and also with other risk factors for cardiovascular disease, such as smoking, lipids, high blood pressure, high fasting glucose, and metabolic syndrome.[20]

Much work is now going into investigating whether practices such as mindfulness training, which have been found to reduce stress and improve mental health, can also slow the ageing process, measured by markers such as telomere length and telomerase activity. Interestingly, the research is suggesting that ageing may be able to be slowed, or even reversed to an extent, through the use of these practices. 'We review data linking telomere length to cognitive stress and stress arousal and present new data linking cognitive appraisal to telomere length. Given the pattern of associations revealed so far, we propose that some forms of meditation may have salutary effects on telomere length by reducing cognitive stress and stress arousal and increasing positive states of mind and hormonal factors that may promote telomere maintenance. Aspects of this model are currently being tested in ongoing trials of mindfulness meditation.'[21]

Psychological states also affect genetic expression in conditions as varied as addictive behaviours,[22] cardiovascular disease,[23] mental health problems such as depression[24] and schizophrenia,[25,26] and asthma,[27] which goes some way to explaining why stress is such a common trigger for many diseases. For example, chronic pain is associated with depression, but it is the emotional reactivity to chronic pain that can sensitise the brain to pain messages, increase the likelihood of a genetic disposition to depression activating itself, and impair the ability of the brain to make new neurons (neurogenesis).[28]

Spirituality and religion may have important effects on lifestyle, including assisting in lowering rates of substance abuse in those genetically at risk.[29] For example, this may be mediated by the reduced risk of expressing a genetic disposition to smoking and other addictive behaviours in those with a high level of self-rated religiosity.[30]

Exercise

Physical activity levels have been linked with genetic function, expression and repair.[31] How exercise does this is coming to be understood, but it is not necessary to understand how it works in order to enjoy the benefits. Regular moderate exercise helps to reduce oxidative damage and is associated with improved DNA repair, which may be one of the reasons that exercise is associated with slower ageing and cell death.[32] Extreme training, on the other hand, is associated with more oxidative damage,[33] although it does stimulate DNA repair.[34] These effects can be seen for a week after extreme exertion, such as after a marathon.[35] Part of the protective effect of exercise may relate to it producing a similar effect to calorie restriction—that is, it helps to change the balance of calories and exceeding calories out.[36] The anti-inflammatory effect of exercise may also be a factor. Exercise also has beneficial effects on mental health which, bearing in mind the preceding section on stress management and genetics, may be an important factor in protecting our genes. All in all, healthy genes are just another reason to exercise regularly.

Nutrition

Nutrition has an important role in the function, repair, expression and ageing of DNA.[37–39] Various micronutrients, vitamins and minerals are required for DNA synthesis, prevention of oxidative damage and DNA maintenance. For example, low levels of folate are associated with increased risk for a baby with a neural tube defect, whereas increasing folate is associated with better DNA repair.[40] Also, the minerals selenium, manganese and zinc minerals are cofactors for DNA repair enzymes.[41] The Mediterranean diet, rich in olive oil and vegetables, is associated with a reduced incidence of cancer, which is postulated to be partly because of effects on DNA damage and repair.[42]

GENETIC COUNSELLING AND GENETICS SERVICES

Genetic counselling is provided as part of a comprehensive genetics service[43,44] whose elements include clinical, laboratory and education. Genetic counselling provides information, supportive counselling regarding the diagnosis and risk for a genetic condition in the family, genetic testing where appropriate and management of rare conditions in some cases. The healthcare professional team providing genetic counselling may consist of clinical geneticists or other medical specialists, genetic counsellors and social workers. Internationally, genetic counselling is increasingly provided by genetic counsellors working as part of mainstream medicine.

Taking and verifying the family history is at the core of genetic counselling and the provision of appropriate genetic testing. The history is, optimally, collected by the general practitioner at the first visit and updated regularly as it can provide information for preventive strategies. The family history changes with time, and ideally the patient should maintain their own copy of their family health history, update it opportunistically and be able to answer the question: 'Do you have a family history of XX condition?'. For example, the family health record can be downloaded from the NSW Health (New South Wales government) Centre for Genetics Education website.[45]

While it may not always be possible, the record of the family history will optimally be three-generational, including primary relatives (children, siblings, parents) and secondary relatives (aunts, uncles and grandparents) on both sides of the family, and noting in particular: ethnic background (ancestry and culture); adoption; age at diagnosis; age and cause of death; birth defects, stillbirths and miscarriages. It is not always possible to assume ethnicity from country of birth or surname. More information can be obtained by asking patients where their parents, grandparents or great-grandparents were born.[46] There are no privacy implications in taking a family history.

GENETIC TESTING

Genetic testing for changes in chromosome number and structure traditionally used cytogenetic karyotyping, but increasingly will rely on molecular cytogenetic testing, which can reveal very small changes not identifiable under the light microscope.[47] DNA genetic testing also is changing rapidly, with increased use of sequencing of parts, or the whole, of a patient's genome.

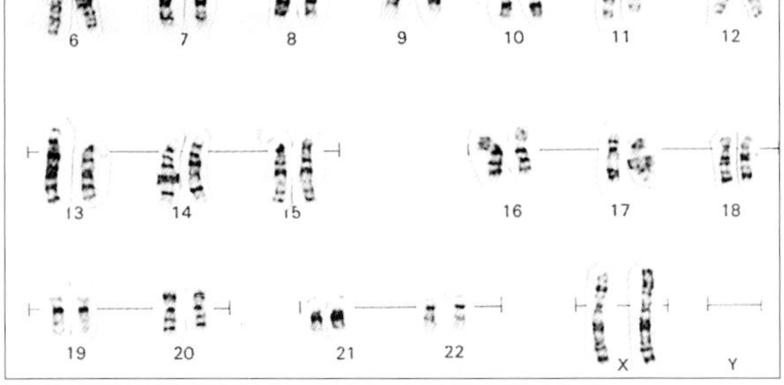

FIGURE 31.1 Karyotype of a normal individual

Genetic screening is done for a particular condition in individuals, groups or populations without family history of the condition (e.g. genetic carrier screening for genetic conditions common in the Ashkenazi Jewish population[48]). Usually, a panel of mutations that are common to the population group will be tested for, so rarer mutations will not be detected.

Genetic testing is done for a particular condition where an individual is suspected of being at increased risk due to their family history or as the result of a genetic screening test. *Direct DNA gene testing* looks at the presence or absence of a known mutation in the gene. The mutation may be family-specific. The test is very accurate and is used for diagnosis and screening, including prenatal, genetic carrier testing, cascade testing, and presymptomatic and predictive testing (Table 31.1). Limitations of direct DNA genetic testing include the following:

- Interpretation of the test result—for example, finding that a person has a mutated gene does not always relate to how a person is, or will be, affected by that condition.
- The testing may be time-consuming and expensive—for the health service, if not for the patient.
- For some complex conditions (e.g. cancer), the testing may have to be done on a family member with the condition, to identify a family-specific mutation in the gene (mutation searching) before unaffected family members can be offered predictive testing.

ORDERING GENETIC TESTS

Costs to the patient of genetic testing vary according to how pathology testing is funded in each country—that is, whether there is a national health system or private health insurance. With developments in technology, such as sequencing the patient's whole DNA, rather than just looking at specific genes using direct gene testing, costs are expected to decrease in the next few years.[49]

Before obtaining consent, the patient should be informed about the purpose and personal/family implications of a genetic test. Patients who have had a predictive or presymptomatic genetic test have a duty to inform life insurers of the test result when applying for a new, or altering an existing, policy.[50]

The patient should be encouraged to share the information with their relatives, and supported in doing so.[46] Changes to the Australian National Privacy Act in 2006 allow, in appropriate exceptional circumstances, for a healthcare professional working in the private sector to release information to genetic relatives without the consent of the person being tested.[51] However, this should only be seen as the last resort after counselling patients to inform their relatives where there is a serious risk to their life, health or safety. When such action is considered, guidelines are available.[52] A general practitioner has no duty to inform a patient's relatives about a positive genetic test result.[53]

A number of ethical issues arise from genetic testing that are relevant not only for individuals and families but for society in general as well.[54] These issues have been addressed internationally[55–57] and include:

- predictive and presymptomatic genetic testing for disorders for which there are currently no treatments, especially in children and adolescents
- privacy and confidentiality, especially when the privacy of the individual is to be balanced against the needs of other family members
- the necessity to ensure that all decision-making regarding genetic testing is made, as far as possible, on an informed basis
- the implications of genetic testing for those wishing to take out superannuation, or life or disability insurance
- the effect that genetic information will have on the concept of 'disability'.

TABLE 31.1 Uses of genetic testing

Type of test	Use
Genetic carrier testing	Testing an individual to determine whether they are a carrier of a faulty, or mutated, gene for a particular condition
Cascade testing	Testing of blood relatives when a mutation has been identified in a family member
Pre-implantation testing	Testing an at-risk embryo for a genetic condition, prior to implantation, thereby obviating the need to terminate an affected pregnancy
Prenatal testing	Testing to detect fetal abnormalities
Diagnostic testing	Specific testing in an individual who has symptoms suggestive of a genetic condition
Presymptomatic testing	Testing to determine, prior to any sign of the condition, whether an individual will, without appropriate intervention, develop the condition in the future
Predictive testing	Testing prior to any sign of the presence of the condition, to determine whether an individual is at risk for developing the condition in the future

Increasingly, genetic tests are being marketed directly to consumers through the internet (direct to consumer (DTC) genetic testing). Laboratories conducting DTC genetic testing are largely based in the United States[58,59] as regulation in countries such as Australia allows laboratories to conduct tests for health conditions only when referred from a medical practitioner.[60] DNA samples are collected at home using kits provided (a cheek swab or saliva sample) and sent to the laboratory through the mail. Payment is made via the internet. Support may or may not be available for explanation of the results, again via the internet. Concern has been raised about the marketing and scientific credibility of these DTC genetic tests internationally.[61,62] Further, for genetic tests that purport to provide evidence for lifestyle and dietary modification, caution should be exercised in interpreting the results and recommendations provided, on the basis that analysis of the person's DNA is in a non-holistic context.[63]

CHROMOSOMAL CONDITIONS

While chromosomal conditions due to a change in the number of chromosomes in the cells are rare overall, some are encountered more commonly. These include trisomy 21 (Down syndrome), XXY syndrome (Klinefelter syndrome) and 45,X syndrome (Turner syndrome.

TRISOMY 21, DOWN SYNDROME[64–66]

Incidence: 1 in 660 births.

Aetiology

- Extra copy of chromosome 21 (trisomy 21) in all cells of the body (about 95% of cases)
- Extra copy of chromosome 21 in some cells of the body (mosaic trisomy 21; about 1%) and clinical features may be less severe
- Or chromosomal translocation involving chromosome 21 (about 4%).

History

Associated with increased maternal age (Fig 31.2). A family history may indicate the translocation type of trisomy 21.

Examination

Features may include:

- hypotonia
- facial characteristics such as short, sometimes webbed neck, low nasal bridge, epicanthal folds, upward-slanting eyes
- cardiac and/or gastrointestinal manifestations and brachycephaly
- intellectual disability
- cardiac and gastrointestinal malformations
- auditory and/or visual deficits
- hypothyroidism
- epilepsy
- respiratory problems
- immunodeficiency
- leukaemia.

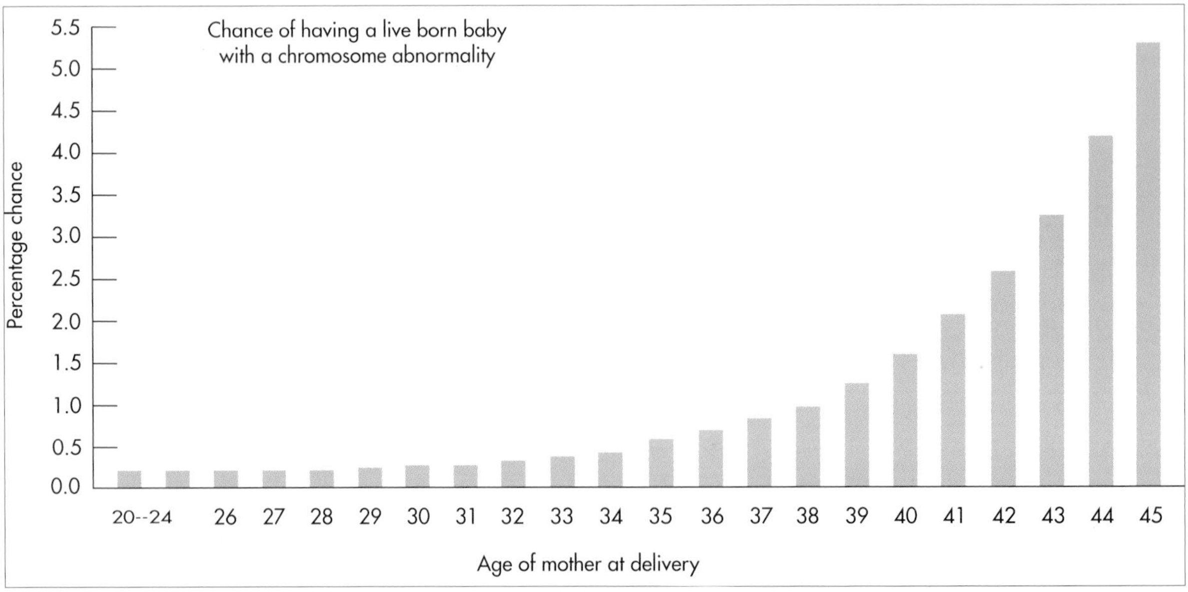

FIGURE 31.2 Chance of having a live-born baby with Down syndrome (trisomy 21) according to the mother's age at the time of delivery of the baby (source: Morris et al,[67] adapted from Barlow-Stewart 2007[68])

Investigations
For the neonate/infant: cytogenetics.
For the parents:
- personal/family history of recurrent miscarriage, infertility or developmental delay
- consider cytogenetics pre-conception or in the prenatal period as appropriate.

Management
Prevention
The recurrence risk in a family with a child with standard non-translocation trisomy 21 is about 1% in addition to the age-related risk. There is no detectable increase in risk for second-degree relatives. Where a parental karyotype shows a translocation, refer to a genetics service for genetic counselling and risk assessment. If detected prenatally, genetic counselling is important, to discuss the condition and options. Pre-implantation genetic diagnosis can prevent implantation of an affected embryo.

Self-help
Referral to Down syndrome support group (see Resources list).

Medical referral
Referral to medical specialists for interventions related to syndrome-associated medical issues.

Complementary therapies
Early intervention services including physiotherapy, occupational and speech therapies can optimise potential. Most people with Down syndrome can learn to read, write, handle money, do simple maths, use a calculator and become competent and independent.

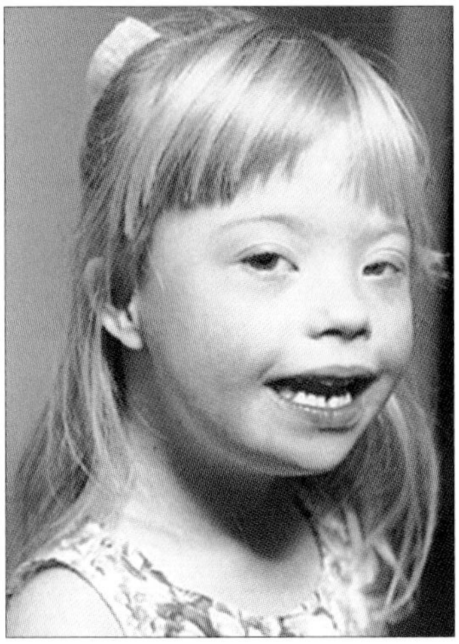

FIGURE 31.3 Down syndrome

Important pitfalls
Not all individuals will have all the clinical features. The number of physical characteristics present does not have any relationship to intellectual ability or vice versa.

Prognosis
Average life expectancy is 55+ years. Dementia of the Alzheimer type is a common feature with increasing age.

47,XXY KLINEFELTER SYNDROME[69]
Incidence: 1 in 500 total births (1 in 1000 male births).

Aetiology
Boys who have:
- two copies of the X chromosome instead of the usual one copy (47,XXY) in all cells of their body—about 80% of cases
- three or four extra X chromosome copies in all cells (48,XXXY or 49,XXXXY)—very rare, but the clinical features may be more exaggerated
- two or more copies of the X chromosome in some of the cells of the body (mosaic XXY syndrome)—about 6% of cases, and the clinical features may be less severe.

History
Does not appear to be related to maternal or paternal age.

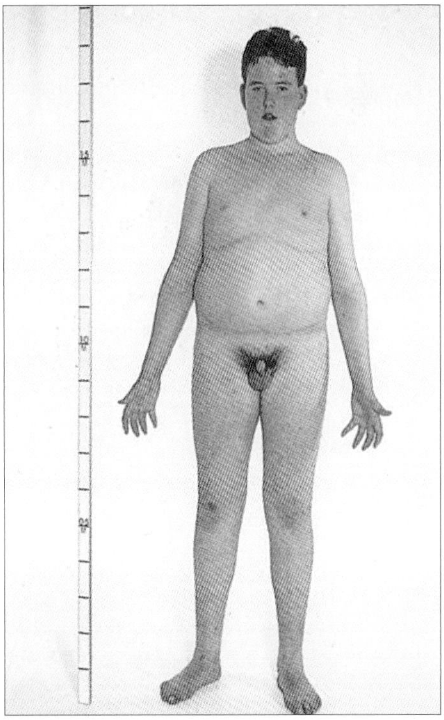

FIGURE 31.4 Klinefelter syndrome

Examination

Features likely to be present include:

- primary hypogonadism
- pubertal gynaecomastia
- small testes (generally < 6 mL)
- relatively tall stature
- infertility
- often shy, apprehensive and passive personality with delayed language development.

Investigations

Diagnosis by cytogenetics may first be made when the development of secondary sexual characteristics is delayed and incomplete.

Management

Prevention

Recurrence risk is low. If detected prenatally, genetic counselling is important, to discuss options and the condition.

Self-help

Refer to Klinefelter syndrome support group.

Medical referral

Refer to paediatric endocrinologist for treatment with testosterone to promote virilisation, including growth of the testes. Hormone therapy usually starts at around 11 or 12 years of age. Gynaecomastia may require surgery.

Complementary therapies

The use of testosterone therapy has secondary benefits in helping to improve self-image and self-esteem. This in turn will affect a boy's performance at school and his ability to form friendships. Learning problems and language deficits can be helped with expert intervention following a thorough assessment. The personality and language delay may lead to the learning difficulties experienced at school. Intervention services (including physiotherapy, occupational and speech and reading therapies) can be helpful.

Important pitfalls

Sexuality is normal, although men with the syndrome may be infertile. Not all features may be present.

Prognosis

Testosterone treatment (available using patches) does not restore the function of the testes, and infertility will persist. Testicular sperm aspiration and intracytoplasmic sperm injection of the egg at IVF have resulted in some pregnancies.

45,X TURNER SYNDROME[70]

Incidence: 1 in 2000 total births.

Aetiology

Girls are missing:

- one (or part of one) of their two X chromosome copies (45,X) in all cells of their body—about 50% of cases
- the X chromosome in some cells of the body (mosaic Turner syndrome)—about 20% of cases.

Or: two copies of the X chromosome are present but with a number of possible rearrangements of the second X chromosome—about 30% of cases.

History

Does not appear to be related to maternal or paternal age.

Examination

Poor growth or pubertal delay is highly characteristic. Other features include:

- short stature (average adult height is 143 cm)
- otitis media
- lack of sexual development at puberty and streak ovaries
- primary amenorrhoea

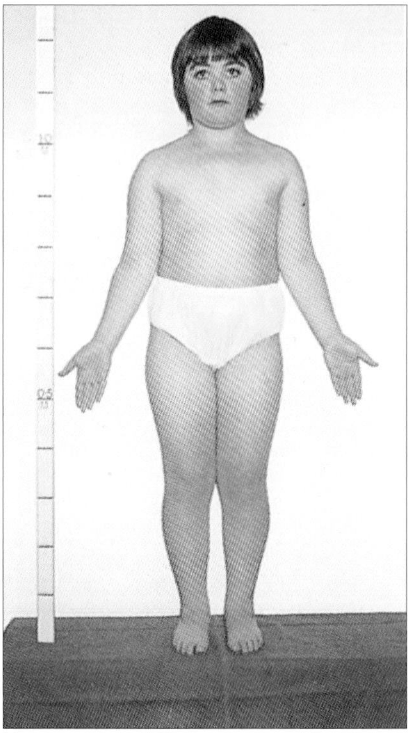

FIGURE 31.5 Turner syndrome

- infertility
- webbed neck
- various malformations including cardiac and renal
- high-arched palate, which may lead to sucking and feeding problems in infancy
- sleeping problems related to high activity levels as well as emotional immaturity and learning problems in the area of non-verbal or spatial learning, such as mathematics.

Adults have an increased risk of chronic inflammatory bowel disease, hypothyroidism, diabetes mellitus.

Investigations

Diagnosis by cytogenetics may be made in the neonatal or infancy period, or when the development of secondary sexual characteristics is delayed and incomplete. Elevated circulating follicle-stimulating hormone (FSH) levels in girls in infancy or adolescence indicates gonadal failure.

Management

Prevention

Recurrence risk is low. If detected prenatally, genetic counselling is important, to discuss options and the condition.

Self-help

Referral to Turner syndrome support group.

Medical referral

Refer to paediatric endocrinologist for oestrogen and growth hormone treatments. Frequent otitis media can cause deafness and predispose to cholesteatoma. Close monitoring and treatment are required. Hypertension requires treatment.

Complementary therapies

Feeding difficulties sometimes require specific intervention due to physical problems such as the high-arched palate, requiring special teats, or Rosti (cleft palate) feeding bottles, and advice from an infant feeding consultant or speech therapist. Assistance in addressing the associated sleeping problems and specific learning difficulties is warranted.

Important pitfalls

Most girls with Turner syndrome do not have all the features. Most will be mosaic for 45,X. Intellectual disability is not part of the syndrome.

Prognosis

About 5% of girls of will menstruate but the period of fertility will be short and pregnancy is very rare. Women with other arrangements of the X chromosome can occasionally be fertile. However, the rate of miscarriage and birth abnormalities in the children of women with Turner syndrome is likely to be higher than average. Referral for IVF (GIFT) may be considered.

SINGLE GENE CONDITIONS

Of the 20,000 or so human genes identified, pathogenic variants in about 12,000 of these result in a genetic condition that follows a clear pattern of inheritance in families.[1] Again, each one is individually rare but several are more commonly found in particular population groups—these include cystic fibrosis and haemoglobinopathies such as alpha and beta forms of thalassaemia and sickle cell anaemia.

CYSTIC FIBROSIS[71–74]

Incidence: 1 in 2500 births. Of the population with Northern European ancestry, 1 in 25 carry a cystic fibrosis mutation. It is less frequent in southern European and Middle-Eastern populations, and is rare or absent in Asians.

Aetiology

Cystic fibrosis (CF) is caused by mutations in the CFTR (cystic fibrosis transmembrane regulator) gene. It follows an autosomal recessive pattern of inheritance (Fig 31.6), so both parents must carry the mutated gene. There is often no family history of the condition, because the mutation has previously only been present in healthy carriers on each side of the family. CFTR regulates the transport of chloride and sodium ions in the epithelial surfaces of the airway, pancreatic and biliary ducts, gastrointestinal tract, sweat ducts and vas deferens. Pathogenic mutations either remove or reduce the function of the CFTR gene. There are more than 1500 known CFTR mutations, but not all are associated with classic CF (see below).[75] A genetic carrier for CF—that is, a person carrying only one mutated copy of the CFTR gene—will still produce sufficient amounts of the salt-transport protein for normal body function.

History

Ninety-five per cent of new cases will be detected by newborn screening.

Examination

Features of classic CF include:

- sweat gland salt loss (100% of cases)
- chronic suppurative lung disease (95%)
- pancreatic exocrine insufficiency, leading to malabsorption (85%)
- male infertility due to congenital absence or altered bilateral vas deferens (CABVD) (99%)
- meconium ileus (20%)

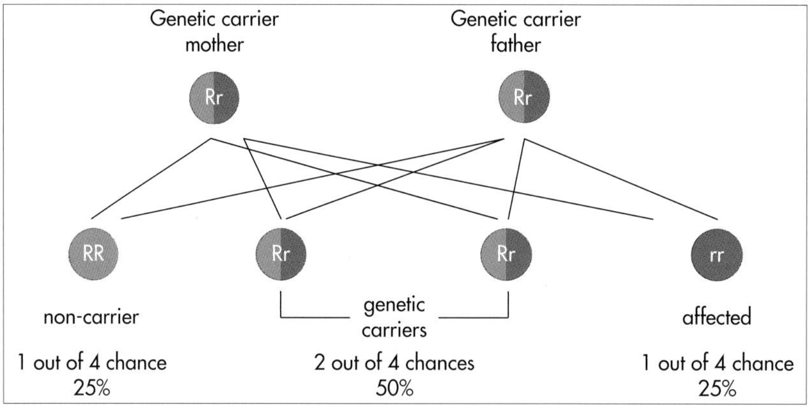

FIGURE 31.6 Autosomal-recessive inheritance when both parents are unaffected genetic carriers for the condition. The mutated copy of the gene containing a recessive mutation is represented by 'r', the working copy of the gene by 'R' (adapted from Barlow-Stewart 2007[76])

- distal intestinal obstruction syndrome (20%)
- CF-related diabetes (20%)
- CF liver disease (20%)
- nasal polyps (10%).

Some clinical features of CF seem to be mediated by the specific mutations in the CFTR gene that an individual inherits.

Investigations

Refer to a paediatrician/respiratory physician for a sweat test where there is clinical suspicion of CF, regardless of the newborn screening result. Diagnosis may be made on the presentation of male infertility due to CABVD. All primary relatives of an affected family member should be referred to genetics services for cascade testing. Carrier testing is accurate if the CFTR gene mutation in the family is known.

Management

Prevention

Pre-conceptional cascade genetic carrier testing and screening in appropriate population groups to identify mutation carriers enables prenatal testing and reproductive choice. The most common mutation in the CFTR gene is known as p.Phe508del (traditionally known as ΔF508 or dF508), which accounts for approximately 70% of all CF gene mutations in those of northern European ancestry. Laboratories test for varying numbers of the common mutations. Testing for 12 or more mutations covers at least 80% of possible mutations in Australians of northern European ancestry.[77] The rest of the mutations are extremely rare. Mutations that are common in populations other than those whose ancestry is northern European may not be included in the panel of mutations that are routinely tested for by laboratories.

Self-help

Referral to cystic fibrosis association.

Medical

Under-treated bacterial infection is responsible for destruction of the airways in CF patients. Antibiotics are usually started early and continued until symptoms improve. Prolonged therapy might be required in some patients. Sputum culture is important in guiding antibiotic therapy. Pancreatic enzyme replacement is necessary in most people with CF prior to all meals and snacks. A DEXA scan should be performed during puberty, to determine bone mineral density.

Lifestyle

Daily chest physiotherapy is usually performed. Salt replacement is necessary during periods when there is a risk of salt depletion. Patients with CF have an increased basal metabolic rate requiring 120–150% of the recommended daily calorie intake. This requirement increases if there are additional persistent lung infections. A diet high in fat and protein is required.

Complementary therapies

Most patients require fat-soluble vitamin supplements (principally vitamins A and E, and some will require vitamin D). Serum levels should be measured annually.

Important pitfalls

In the absence of a family history of CF, a negative screen for CFTR gene mutations is reassuring, but cannot absolutely rule out the possibility of being a carrier, as not all mutations can be tested. Therefore if a couple choose screening for CF there is still a small risk of having a baby with CF if their carrier test is negative. The major selection criterion for lung transplantation is a life expectancy predicted to be 50% or less at 2 years. This can be indicated by increasing decline in respiratory function, quality of life and weight, and more frequent need for IV therapy.

Prognosis

Life expectancy is improving and is now up to the third or fourth decade. Lung transplantation is currently the only available efficient treatment of life-threatening CF, and it can improve quality of life and long-term survival. Regardless of the form of transplant (single lung, double lung, or heart and double lung), the majority of patients (approximately 90%) will live for at least a year or more following their transplant, and 80% will live for four or more years. Quality of life, measured by ability to exercise and attend educational courses, is significantly improved.

HAEMOGLOBINOPATHIES

(including alpha- and beta-thalassaemia and sickle cell disease)[78–80]

Incidence

Incidence varies depending on ancestry. Globally, at least 5% of adults are carriers for a haemoglobin condition: approximately 2.9% for thalassaemia and 2.3% for sickle cell disease. Carriers of a haemoglobinopathy mutation are most common in those with any of the following ethnic backgrounds: southern European, Middle Eastern, African, Chinese, South-East Asian, Indian sub-continent, Pacific Islander, New Zealand Māori, South American and some northern Australian Indigenous communities.

Aetiology

Haemoglobinopathies are caused by mutations in the genes of the 'alpha-globin chain' and/or the 'beta-globin chain' of haemoglobin. They follow an autosomal-recessive pattern of inheritance (Fig 31.6), so both parents must carry the mutated gene.

- *Alpha-thalassaemia major* (also known as Hb Barts hydrops fetalis) is caused by absence of production of the alpha-globin chains in the haemoglobin protein, due to deletion of or a change in the alpha-globin chain genes. This condition is fatal at or around the time of birth.
- *Beta-thalassaemia major* is caused by reduced or absent production of the beta-globin chain of the haemoglobin, due to deletion or change in both copies of the beta-globin chain gene. The main symptom is severe anaemia requiring lifelong blood transfusions.
- *Sickle cell disease* is caused by changes in the structure of the beta-globin chains of haemoglobin, resulting in red blood cells that form an irreversible sickle shape and leading to severe anaemia and other problems.

History

Carriers are often detected following routine blood screening. Carriers for a thalassaemia have the minor form of the disease and can have mild anaemia. Carriers for sickle cell disease are healthy and are not affected by anaemia; rarely (e.g. under anaesthesia), the red blood cells of a carrier can undergo sickling. Anaesthetists should be informed when a patient is a carrier for sickle cell disease.

Examination

- Alpha-thalassaemia major—fatal at or around the time of birth.
- Beta-thalassaemia major—severe anaemia, pallor, lethargy, poor appetite, developmental delay, failure to thrive, irritability, splenomegaly, growth failure with bone changes and fractures.
- Sickle cell disease—anaemia, failure to thrive, repeated infections, painful swelling of the hands or feet, infarction, asplenia, abdominal and chest pain.

Investigations

- Undertake full blood evaluation (FBE), iron studies (ferritin) and haemoglobin electrophoresis, especially in women of reproductive age.
- Indications for DNA testing:
  - possible carrier for alpha-thalassaemia (low-borderline MCV or MCH, normal ferritin and normal haemoglobin electrophoresis)
  - proven carrier for beta-thalassaemia and partner is also a carrier for thalassaemia or other haemoglobinopathy
  - confirmation of carrier status for a haemoglobin variant.

Management

Prevention

Screening pre-conception to identify mutation carriers enables prenatal testing and reproductive choice. Those most likely to be carriers are those:

- with a family history of anaemia/thalassaemia/abnormal haemoglobin variant
- from the ethnic groups listed above
- whose partners are known or identified haemoglobinopathy carriers, and when their mean corpuscular volume (MCV) < 80 fL or mean cell haemoglobin (MCH) < 27 pg. If both partners of a couple are carriers, refer to a genetics service and/or haematology clinic for genetic counselling and testing. *This is particularly urgent for pregnant couples.*

Self-help

Refer to a thalassaemia association (see Resources list).

Medical

- Beta-thalassaemia major—require lifelong blood transfusions every 3–4 weeks with iron chelation.
- Sickle cell disease—usually have chronic anaemia due to increased destruction of red blood cells and may also experience sickle cell crises due to blockage of blood vessels by these cells, causing bone and chest pain and damage to other organs. These crises require immediate treatment in the emergency department of a hospital for administration of IV fluids, pain relief and other treatment if indicated, which may include regular blood transfusions. Usually autosplenectomise within the first 10 years of life.

Lifestyle

Carriers for beta-thalassaemia and alpha-thalassaemia should avoid high altitudes.

Complementary therapies

Carriers for beta-thalassaemia should have folic acid (5 mg) daily throughout all pregnancies, and must not have long-term iron treatment to attempt to cure microcytosis, unless they are also iron deficient.

Important pitfalls

A haematologist or thalassaemia service should be consulted for assistance in interpreting haemoglobinopathy testing results, as interpretation is influenced by the clinical picture (Table 31.2). Prenatal diagnosis is available to couples where there is a risk of having a child affected by a haemoglobinopathy and the causative globin mutations carried by the parents are known. Because of the time-consuming nature of DNA testing to identify causative gene mutations, it is important that, wherever possible, DNA studies are carried out pre-pregnancy.

Prognosis

The life expectancy of well-treated, compliant patients for both Beta-thalassaemia major and sickle cell disease is likely to be normal or near normal. Bone marrow transplantation may cure Beta-thalassaemia major but has a significant risk of complications and mortality.

INHERITED GENETIC SUSCEPTIBILITY

Many of the more common adult-onset conditions seen in general practice may be indirectly due to an inherited mutation. These conditions, such as some forms of cancer, cardiac and haematological conditions, involve inherited predisposition and are usually associated with a positive family history. Where the family history is suggestive of an inherited predisposition, genetic counselling and, where appropriate and available, genetic testing may identify the causative predisposing inherited

TABLE 31.2 Interpretation of haemoglobinopathy carrier testing results[77]

MCH (pg)	Ferritin	Haemoglobin electrophoresis	Interpretation
≥ 27	Normal	Normal	Thalassaemia unlikely but single gene deletion alpha-thalassaemia not excluded
	Normal	HbS present	Carrier for sickle cell disease
	Low	Normal	Reduced iron stores or iron deficiency, thalassaemia unlikely but single gene deletion alpha-thalassaemia not excluded
< 27	Normal	HbA2 increased HbF increased	Carrier for beta-thalassaemia
		HbA2 normal HbH present	Carrier for alpha-thalassaemia
		HbS present	Carrier for sickle cell disease Possible coexistent thalassaemia carrier state
		Normal	Possible carrier for alpha-thalassaemia DNA testing indicated
	Low	Normal	Iron deficiency Thalassaemia may coexist If woman is pregnant, seek advice about DNA testing; test partner for full haemoglobinopathy screen

MCH: mean cell haemoglobin

mutation. National guidelines have been produced for healthcare professionals to triage on the basis of the family history into those who are at potentially high risk for the condition running in the family due to an inherited predisposition. For example, those whose family history suggests they are at potentially high risk for breast, ovarian or colorectal cancer could be referred to a family cancer service.[43] If appropriate, genetic testing may then be used to identify the family-specific mutation and enable predictive genetic testing for other blood relatives.

BREAST AND OVARIAN CANCER INHERITED SUSCEPTIBILITY[81]

Incidence: About 5% of all breast and ovarian cancers.

Aetiology

A mutation in either the BRCA1 or the BRCA2 gene is identified in a blood relative who has or had breast and/or ovarian cancer and who was identified at potentially high risk on the basis of her family history. Inheritance of the mutated gene follows a pattern of autosomal-dominant inheritance (Fig 31.7). The BRCA1 or BRCA2 genes are tumour suppressor genes that normally function in both breast and ovarian tissues as 'cancer protection' genes in the cell, contributing to the maintenance of controlled cell growth. The woman's breast and/or ovarian cancer is due to her having inherited a mutation in one copy of her BRCA1 or BRCA2 gene in her cells. For breast and/or ovarian cancer to develop, other mutations must build up over time in other 'cancer protection' genes in the cells of the breast and/or ovary. The mutation is family-specific, and now predictive genetic testing for the mutation can be offered to unaffected blood relatives.

History

The BRCA1 or BRCA2 mutations can be inherited from either the mother or the father. The inheritance pattern is described as autosomal-dominant (Fig 31.7). A child of a parent who carries the mutated gene has a 1 in 2, or 50%, chance of inheriting the mutation and being predisposed to develop breast and/or ovarian cancer.

Examination

These are unaffected patients with an identified inherited predisposing mutation.

Investigations

It is recommended that an individual surveillance program be developed in consultation with a cancer genetics specialist. Although this should be determined on an individual basis, it is generally accepted practice to begin screening at least 5 years prior to the age of diagnosis of the closest relative.

Management

Prevention

Early detection using screening strategies. For breast cancer, regular breast examinations, mammography (with or without breast ultrasound) and breast magnetic resonance imaging (MRI) may be beneficial for women at high risk of breast cancer, as they can help to detect breast cancer at an early stage. Prophylactic mastectomy is an option for some women.[82] Ovarian cancer surveillance is not recommended for women at high or potentially high risk. Evidence shows that ultrasound or CA125, singly or in combination, is not effective at detecting early ovarian cancer. The most effective risk-reducing strategy for ovarian cancer is bilateral salpingo-oophorectomy.[83,84]

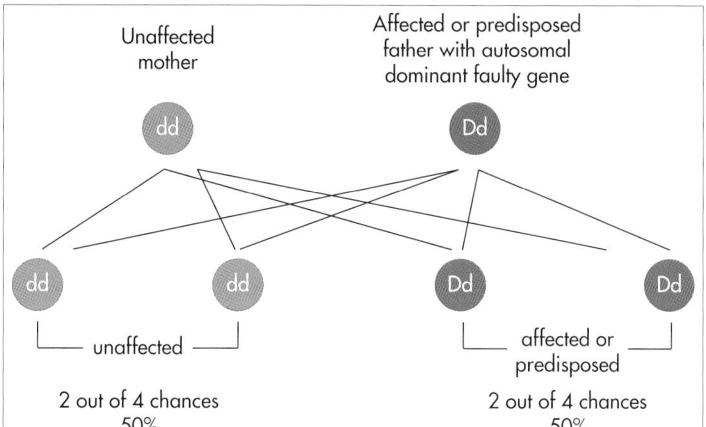

FIGURE 31.7 Autosomal-dominant inheritance when one parent carries the autosomal-dominant faulty gene copy. The autosomal-dominant mutated gene copy is represented by 'D', and the working copy of the gene by 'd' (adapted from Barlow-Stewart 2007[76]).

Self-help
Refer to relevant cancer services. Psychosocial support through contact with others at identified genetic high risk may be available.

Complementary therapies
There are currently no recommendations for the prevention of breast or ovarian cancer.

Lifestyle
Moderate to vigorous physical activity for 30–60 minutes per day, maintain a healthy body weight, avoid or limit alcohol consumption (no more than two standard drinks per day for men and no more than one standard drink per day for women) and do not smoke. Current smokers should quit smoking.

Important pitfalls
Cancer will not develop in a woman who is a carrier of a mutated BRCA1 or BRCA2 gene unless further mutations occur in additional other 'cancer protection' genes in the cells during her life. Women who have not inherited a mutated BRCA1 or BRCA2 gene are not at increased risk of developing breast and/or ovarian cancer in their lifetime and cannot pass the faulty gene on to their own children. However, they still have the same risk for developing breast and/or ovarian cancer as the average woman in the Australian population. Recommendations for early detection and prevention for the general population should be followed.

Prognosis
Inheriting a mutated BRCA1 gene means women have a 40–80% risk to age 75 years of breast cancer and 10–60% for ovarian cancer; for men there is a small lifetime increased risk of prostate cancer. Inheriting a mutated BRCA2 gene means women have a 40–80% risk to age 75 years of breast cancer and 10–40% for ovarian cancer; for men there is a small lifetime increased risk of male breast, prostate and pancreatic cancers.

LYNCH SYNDROME INHERITED SUSCEPTIBILITY[85,86] (formerly hereditary non-polyposis colorectal cancer, HNPCC)
Incidence: Between 1% and 4% of all colorectal cancers.

Aetiology
In Lynch syndrome, a small number of polyps develop in the bowel and can develop into bowel cancer. Cancers in both men and women can also occur in the kidney, ureter and parts of the gut such as the small bowel, stomach or pancreas. Women also have an increased risk of cancer of the inner lining of the uterus and the ovaries, although the risk of bowel cancer is higher. Age of onset is very variable (from 20s to 80s). The condition is due to an inherited mutation in one of the copies of one of their mismatch repair (MMR) genes. Inheritance of the mutated gene follows a pattern of autosomal-dominant inheritance (Fig 31.3). The MMR genes normally function as 'cancer protection' genes in the cell, contributing to the maintenance of controlled cell growth by repairing any changes in the DNA that occur as the cells are copied. Genetic testing to identify the mutated MMR gene involved is undertaken in a family member who has or had colorectal cancer and who is identified as potentially high risk on the basis of their family history. For the colorectal cancer to have developed, other mutations must build up over time in other 'cancer protection' genes in the cells of the colon. The mutation is family-specific, and now predictive genetic testing for the mutation can be offered to unaffected blood relatives.

History
The MMR mutation can be inherited from either the mother or the father. The inheritance pattern is described as autosomal dominant. A child of a parent who carries the mutated gene has a 1 in 2, or 50%, chance of inheriting the mutation and being predisposed to develop Lynch syndrome.

Examination
These are unaffected patients with an identified inherited predisposing mutation.

Investigations
Colonoscopy every 1–2 years from age 25, or 5 years earlier than the youngest diagnosis in the family (whichever comes first). Faecal occult blood testing may be offered in alternate years or to subjects unwilling to accept colonoscopy. There are options for surveillance at other sites, usually starting from age 25–35 years.

Management
Prevention
- Early detection using screening strategies as above.
- Prophylactic surgery may be appropriate for some.
- Although HRT may reduce the risk for colorectal cancer in women, its use for that purpose is not recommended, because of possible increased risk for breast cancer, stroke and pulmonary embolism.
- Because of uncertainty about dose and side effects, aspirin and non-steroidal anti-inflammatory drugs are also not recommended for prevention of colorectal cancer. However, in people who have had an adenoma removed, aspirin should be considered as prophylaxis against further adenoma development.

Self-help
Refer to the relevant cancer services. Psychosocial support through contact with others at identified genetic high risk may be available.

Complementary therapies
Folate, phytonutrients, antioxidant vitamins and selenium supplements are not currently recommended for the prevention of colorectal cancer.

Lifestyle
- Moderate to vigorous physical activity for 30–60 minutes per day.
- Maintain a healthy body weight.
- Avoid or limit alcohol consumption (no more than two standard drinks per day for men and no more than one standard drink per day for women)
- Do not smoke. Current smokers should quit smoking.
- It is recommended that daily energy intake be restricted (< 2500 calories for men and < 2000 calories for women) and intake of dietary fat be reduced (< 25% of total energy).
- It is also advised that vegetables (five or more serves), fruit (two serves) and dietary calcium (1000–1200 mg) be consumed each day.
- Consumption of poorly soluble cereal fibres (e.g. wheat bran) is encouraged.
- A moderate intake of lean red meat can be eaten as part of a mixed diet. Charring of red meat is best avoided, and consumption of processed meats should be limited.

Important pitfalls
Cancer will not develop in a person who has inherited a mutated MMR gene unless further mutations occur in additional other 'cancer protection' genes in the cells during their life. People who have not inherited the mutated MMR gene copy will not develop Lynch syndrome, but they still have the same chance of developing cancer as others in the general population and should follow the recommendations for early detection and prevention for the general population.

Prognosis
Inheriting a mutated MMR gene confers a risk for colorectal cancer to age 75 years of 70–90%, and a lifetime increased risk for cancer of the endometrium (40%), ovary and stomach (10%), urinary tract, small intestine, pancreas, biliary tree and brain.

RESOURCES
Association of Genetic Support of Australasia Inc, http://www.agsa-geneticsupport.org.au

Australasian Genetic Alliance, http://www.australasiangeneticalliance.org.au

Cancer Council Australia, http://www.cancer.org.au

Centre for Genetics Education, NSW Health (Australia), http://www.genetics.edu.au

Cystic Fibrosis Australia Inc, http://www.cysticfibrosisaustralia.org.au

Down Syndrome NSW, Australia, http://www.dsansw.org.au

House of Lords Science and Technology Committee, Subcommittee Report, Genomic Medicine (2009), http://www.publications.parliament.uk/pa/ld200809/ldselect/ldsctech/107/10702.htm.

March of Dimes, Genetics and your practice, http://www.marchofdimes.com/gyponline/index.bm2

National Human Genome Research Institute, Frequently asked questions about genetic testing, http://www.genome.gov/19516567.

NHMRC, eGenetics, http://www.nhmrc.gov.au/your_health/egenetics/

Thalassaemia Society of New South Wales, http://www.thalnsw.org.au

Turner Syndrome Association of Australia Ltd, http://www.turnersyndrome.org.au

REFERENCES

1 John Hopkins University. Online Mendelian inheritance in man. Online. Available: http://www.ncbi.nlm.nih.gov/sites/entrez?db=OMIM&itool=toolbar

2 Barlow-Stewart K. Gene therapy. In: Barlow-Stewart K, ed. The Australasian genetics resource book. Royal North Shore Hospital, Sydney: Centre for Genetics Education; 2007. Online. Available: http://www.genetics.edu.au/factsheet/fs27.html Feb 2008.

3 Stanford University, Pharmacogenomics knowledge base. Online. Available: http://www.pharmgkb.org/index.jsp

4 Nise MS, Falaturi P, Erren TC. Epigenetics: origins and implications for cancer epidemiology. Med Hypotheses 2010; 74(2):377–382.

5 Johnson W, Deary IJ, McGue M et al. Genetic and environmental transactions linking cognitive ability, physical fitness, and education in late life. Psychol Aging 2009; 24(1):48–62.

6 Ostojić S, Pereza N, Kapović M.A current genetic and epigenetic view on human aging mechanisms. Coll Anthropol 2009; 33(2):687–699.

7 Szyf M, Weaver I, Meaney M. Maternal care, the epigenome and phenotypic differences in behavior. Reprod Toxicol 2007; 24(1):9–19.

8 Ornish D, Magbanua MJ, Weidner G et al. Changes in prostate gene expression in men undergoing an intensive nutrition and lifestyle intervention. Proc Natl Acad Sci USA 2008; 105(24):8369–8374.

9 Ornish D, Lin J, Daubenmier J et al. Increased telomerase activity and comprehensive lifestyle changes: a pilot study. Lancet Oncol 2008; 9(11):1048–1057. Erratum in: Lancet Oncol 2008; 9(12):1124.
10 Gidron Y, Russ K, Tissarchondou H et al. The relation between psychological factors and DNA damage: a critical review. Biol Psychol 2006; 72(3):291–304.
11 Adachi S, Kawamura K, Takemoto K. Oxidative damage of nuclear DNA in liver of rats exposed to psychological stress. Cancer Research 1993; 53(18):4153–4155.
12 Fischman H, Pero R, Kelly D. Psychogenic stress induces chromosomal and DNA damage. Int J Neurosci 1996; 84(1–4):219–227.
13 Kiecolt-Glaser J, Glaser R. Psychoneuroimmunology and immunotoxicology: implications for carcinogenesis. Psychosom Med 1999; 61(3): 271–272.
14 Flint MS, Baum A, Chambers WH et al. Induction of DNA damage, alteration of DNA repair and transcriptional activation by stress hormones. Psychoneuroendocrinology 2007; 32(5):470–479.
15 Oldham KM, Wise SR, Chen L et al. A longitudinal evaluation of oxidative stress in trauma patients. J Parenteral Nutr 2002; 26(3):189–197.
16 Cohen L, Marshall G, Cheng L et al. DNA repair capacity in healthy medical students during and after exam stress. J Behav Med 2000; 23(6):531–545.
17 Ramos JM, Ruiz A, Colen R et al. DNA repair and breast carcinoma susceptibility in women. Cancer 2004; 100(7):1352–1357.
18 Epel ES, Blackburn EH, Lin J et al. Proc Natl Acad Sci USA 2004; 101(49):17312–17315.
19 Simon NM, Smoller JW, McNamara KL et al. Telomere shortening and mood disorders: preliminary support for a chronic stress model of accelerated aging. Biol Psychiatry 2006; 60(5):432–435.
20 Epel ES, Lin J, Wilhelm FH et al. Cell aging in relation to stress arousal and cardiovascular disease risk factors. Psychoneuroendocrinology 2006; 31(3):277–287.
21 Epel E, Daubenmier J, Moskowitz JT et al. Can meditation slow rate of cellular aging? Cognitive stress, mindfulness, and telomeres. Ann NY Acad Sci 2009; 1172:34–53.
22 Self D, Nestler E. Relapse to drug seeking: neural and molecular mechanisms. Drug Alcohol Depend 1998; 51(1–2):49–60.
23 Cui Y, Gutstein W, Jabr S et al. Control of human vascular smooth muscle cell proliferation by sera derived from 'experimentally stressed' individuals. Oncol Rep 1998; 5(6):1471–1474.
24 Lopez J, Chalmers D, Little K et al. Regulation of serotonin 1A, glucocorticoid, and mineralocorticoid receptor in rat and human hippocampus: implications for the neurobiology of depression. Biol Psychiatry 1998; 43(8):547–573.
25 Benes F. The role of stress and dopamine-GABA interactions in the vulnerability for schizophrenia. J Psychiatr Res 1997; 31(2):257–275.
26 Kato T. Epigenomics in psychiatry. Neuropsychobiology 2009; 60(1):2–4.
27 Mrazek DA, Klinnert M, Mrazek PJ et al. Prediction of early-onset asthma in genetically at-risk children. Pediatr Pulmonol 1999; 27(2):85–94.
28 Duric V, McCarson KE. Persistent pain produces stress-like alterations in hippocampal neurogenesis and gene expression. J Pain 2006; 7(8):544–555.
29 Kendler KS, Liu XQ, Gardner CO et al. Dimensions of religiosity and their relationship to lifetime psychiatric and substance use disorders. Am J Psychiatry 2003; 160(3):496–503.
30 Timberlake DS, Rhee SH, Haberstick BC et al. The moderating effects of religiosity on the genetic and environmental determinants of smoking initiation. Nicotine Tob Res 2006; 8(1):123–133.
31 Teran-Garcia M, Rankinen T, Bouchard C. Genes, exercise, growth, and the sedentary, obese child. J Appl Physiol 2008; 105(3):988–1001.
32 Radak Z, Chung HY, Goto S. Exercise and hormesis: oxidative stress-related adaptation for successful aging. Biogerontology 2005; 6(1):71–75.
33 Pittaluga M, Parisi P, Sabatini S et al. Cellular and biochemical parameters of exercise-induced oxidative stress: relationship with training levels. Free Radic Res 2006; 40(6):607–614.
34 Radák Z, Apor P, Pucsok J et al. Marathon running alters the DNA base excision repair in human skeletal muscle. Life Sci 2003; 72(14):1627–1633.
35 Tsai K, Hsu TG, Hsu KM et al. Oxidative DNA damage in human peripheral leukocytes induced by massive aerobic exercise. Free Radic Biol Med 2001; 31(11):1465–1472.
36 Kritchevsky D. Caloric restriction and experimental carcinogenesis. Hybrid Hybridomics 2002; 21(2): 147–151.
37 Tyson J, Mathers JC. Dietary and genetic modulation of DNA repair in healthy human adults. Proc Nutr Soc 2007; 66(1):42–51.
38 Mathers JC, Coxhead JM, Tyson J. Nutrition and DNA repair—potential molecular mechanisms of action. Curr Cancer Drug Targets 2007; 7(5):425–431.
39 Mathers JC. Nutritional modulation of ageing: genomic and epigenetic approaches. Mech Ageing Dev 2006; 127(6):584–589.
40 Wei Q, Shen H, Wang LE et al. Association between low dietary folate intake and suboptimal cellular DNA repair capacity. Cancer Epidemiol Biomarkers Prev 2003; 12(10):963–969.

41 Sheng Y, Pero RW, Olsson AR et al. DNA repair enhancement by a combined supplement of carotenoids, nicotinamide, and zinc. Cancer Detect Prev 1998; 22:284–292.
42 Machowetz A, Poulsen HE, Gruendel S et al. Effect of olive oils on biomarkers of oxidative DNA stress in Northern and Southern Europeans. FASEB J 2007; 21(1):45–52.
43 Centre for Genetics Education. Find a genetics service; 2008. Online. Available: http://www.genetics.edu.au/services/index.html Feb 2008.
44 Human Genetics Society of Australasia. Certification in genetic counselling. Online. Available: http://www.hgsa.com.au/index.cfm?pid=111440 May 2010.
45 Centre for Genetics Education, NSW Health. Family history; 2007. Online. Available: www.genetics.com.au/publications/family_history.asp May 2010.
46 Barlow-Stewart K, Emery J, Metcalfe S. Genetics in practice (Ch 17). In: Genetics in family medicine: the Australian handbook for general practitioners. Biotechnology Australia, Commonwealth Department of Industry, Tourism and Resources; 2007. Online. Available: http://www.nhmrc.gov.au/your_health/egenetics/practitioners/gems.htm May 2010.
47 Saam J, Gudgeon J, Aston E et al. How physicians use array comparative genomic hybridisation results to guide patient management in children with developmental delay. Genet Med 2008; 10(3):181–186.
48 Pacific Laboratory Medicine Services. Fact sheets on genetic conditions in the Ashkenazi Jewish community; 2007. Online. Available: http://www.palms.com.au/Education/Genetics/genlist.shtml May 2010.
49 Tucker T, Marra M, Friedman JM. Massively parallel sequencing: the next big thing in genetic medicine. Am J Hum Gen 2009; 85(2):142–154.
50 Centre for Genetics Education, NSW Health. Life insurance products and genetic testing in Australia; 2007. Online. Available: http://www.genetics.com.au/factsheet/fs23a.asp May 2010.
51 Privacy Legislation Amendment Act 2006. Online. Available: http://www.comlaw.gov.au/ComLaw/Legislation/Act1.nsf/all/search/592A1E3B62096FD6CA2571ED0012E038 May 2010.
52 National Health & Medical Research Council. Guidelines approved under Section 95AA of the Privacy Act 1988 (Cth); 2009. Online. Available: http://www.nhmrc.gov.au/publications/synopses/e96syn.htm May 2010.
53 Otlowski MFA. Disclosure of genetic information to at-risk relatives: recent amendments to the Privacy Act 1988 (Cth). Med J Aust 2007; 187(7):398–399.
54 Barlow-Stewart K, Christadoulou J. It's all in our genes. In: Oates K, Currow K, Hu W et al, eds. Child health: a manual for general practice. Sydney: MacLennan & Petty; 2001.
55 Australian Law Reform Commission. Essentially yours: the protection of human genetic information in Australia; 2003. Online. Available: http://www.austlii.edu.au/au/other/alrc/publications/reports/96/index.htm May 2010.
56 National Institute for Health and Clinical Excellence. NHS evidence: genetic conditions. Ethical, legal and social implications (ELSI) of genetic information. Online. Available: http://www.library.nhs.uk/GENETICCONDITIONS/ViewResource.aspx?resID=59911 May 2010.
57 US Department of Energy Office of Science, Office of Biological and Environmental Research, Human Genome Program. Online. Available: www.ornl.gov/sci/techresources/Human_Genome/elsi/elsi.shtml May 2010.
58 23andMe. Choose the DNA test that's right for you. Online. Available: http://www.23andme.com/ May 2010.
59 Genetics and Public Policy Center, Washington DC, USA. Direct-to-consumer genetic testing companies. Online. Available: http://www.dnapolicy.org/resources/DTCcompanieslist.pdf May 2010.
60 National Pathology Accreditation Advisory Council (NPAAC). Laboratory accreditation standards and guidelines for nucleic acid detection and analysis; 2006. Online. Available: http://www.health.gov.au/internet/main/publishing.nsf/Content/npaac-nucleic-acid-toc~npaac-nucleic-acid-diag~npaac-nucleic-acid-gen
61 National Health & Medical Research Council. Direct to consumer (DTC) DNA tests. Online. Available: http://www.nhmrc.gov.au/your_health/issues/genetics/testing/dtc.htm May 2010.
62 Hunter D, Khoury M, Drazen J. Letting the genome out of the bottle—will we get our wish? N Engl J Med 2008; 358(2):105–107.
63 Saukko P. Pitching products, pitching ethics: selling nutrigenetic tests as lifestyle or medicine. In: Castle D, Ries N, eds. Nutrition and genomics: issues of ethics, law, regulation and communication. Sydney: Elsevier; 2009.
64 Gardner RJM, Sutherland G. Chromosome abnormalities and genetic counselling. 3rd edn. New York: Oxford University Press; 2004.
65 Morris JK, Mutton DE, Alberman E. Recurrences of free trisomy 21: analysis of data from the national Down syndrome cytogenetic register. Prenat Diagn 2005; 25:1120–1128.
66 Australian Institute of Health and Welfare. Australia's babies, their health and wellbeing. Bulletin Issue 21; 2004. Online. Available: http://www.aihw.gov.au/publications/aus/bulletin21 Jan 2008.
67 Morris JK, Mutton DE, Alberman E. Revised estimates of maternal age specific live birth prevalence of Down syndrome. J Med Screen 2002; 9:2–6.

68 Barlow-Stewart K. Trisomy 21—Down syndrome. In: Barlow-Stewart K, ed. The Australasian genetics resource book. Sydney: Centre for Genetics Education, Royal North Shore Hospital; 2007. Online. Available: http://www.genetics.edu.au/factsheet/fs28.html Feb 2008.

69 Barlow-Stewart K, Emery J, Metcalfe S. Chromosomal conditions (Ch 7). In: Genetics in family medicine: the Australian handbook for general practitioners. Biotechnology Australia, Commonwealth Department of Industry, Tourism and Resources; 2007. Online. Available: http://www.nhmrc.gov.au/your_health/egenetics/practitioners/gems.htm May 2010.

70 Neilsen J, Naeraa R. Turner's syndrome and Turner contact groups: an orientation. 3rd edn, rev. Denmark; 1991. Online. Available: http//www.aaa.dk/TURNER/ENGELSK/TURN_ORI.HTM May 2010.

71 Barlow-Stewart K, Emery J, Metcalfe S. Cystic fibrosis (Ch 9). In: Genetics in family medicine: the Australian handbook for general practitioners. Biotechnology Australia, Commonwealth Department of Industry, Tourism and Resources; 2007. Online. Available: http://www.nhmrc.gov.au/your_health/egenetics/practitioners/gems.htm May 2010.

72 Cystic Fibrosis Mutation Database. Online. Available: http://www.genet.sickkids.on.ca/cftr/ May 2010.

73 Massie J, Clements B. Diagnosis of cystic fibrosis after newborn screening: the Australasian experience—twenty years and five million babies later: a consensus statement from the Australasian Pediatric Respiratory Group. Pediatr Pulmonol 2005; 39:440–446.

74 Wilcken B, Wiley V. Newborn screening. Pathology 2008; 40:104–115.

75 Human Genetics Society of Australasia. Cystic fibrosis population screening position paper; 2009. Online. Available: http://www.hgsa.com.au/index.cfm?pid=111468. May 2010.

76 Barlow-Stewart K. Autosomal recessive inheritance—traditional patterns of inheritance (Ch 1). In: Barlow-Stewart K, ed. The Australasian genetics resource book. Sydney: Centre for Genetics Education, Royal North Shore Hospital; 2007. Online. Available: http://www.genetics.edu.au/factsheet/fs8.html Feb 2008.

77 Massie Rj, Delayticki MB, Bankier A. Screening couples for cystic fibrosis status: why are we waiting? Med J Aust 2005; 183:501–502.

78 Barlow-Stewart K, Emery J, Metcalfe S. Haemoglobinopathies (Ch 12). In: Genetics in family medicine: the Australian handbook for general practitioners. Biotechnology Australia, Commonwealth Department of Industry, Tourism and Resources; 2007. Online. Available: http://www.nhmrc.gov.au/your_health/egenetics/practitioners/gems.htm May 2010.

79 Bowden DK. Screening for thalassaemia. Australian Prescriber 2001; 24:120–123.

80 Trent R, Webster B, Bowden D et al. Complex phenotypes in the haemoglobinopathies: recommendations on screening and DNA testing. Pathology 2006; 38:507–519.

81 National Breast and Ovarian Cancer Centre. Advice about familial aspects of breast cancer and epithelial ovarian cancer; 2006. Online. Available: http://www.nbocc.org.au/view-document-details/bog-advice-about-familial-aspects-of-breast-cancer-and-ovarian-cancer May 2010.

82 Centre for Genetics Education, NSW Health. Information for women considering preventive mastectomy because of a strong family history of breast cancer. Online. Available: http://www.genetics.com.au/publications/cancer.asp

83 National Breast and Ovarian Cancer Centre Position Statement. Surveillance of women at high or potentially high risk of ovarian cancer; 2009. Online. Available: http://www.nbocc.org.au/our-organisation/position-statements/surveillance-of-women-at-high-or-potentially-high-risk-of-ovarian-cancer May 2010.

84 Centre for Genetics Education, NSW Health. Risk management options for women at increased risk of developing ovarian cancer. Online. Available: http://www.genetics.com.au/publications/cancer.asp May 2010.

85 Cancer Institute NSW. Hereditary non-polyposis colon cancer (HNPCC). Online. Available: http://www.cancerinstitute.org.au/cancer_inst/programs/hnpcc.html May 2010.

86 Australian Cancer Network and NHMRC. Clinical practice guidelines for the prevention, early detection and management of colorectal cancer; 2006. Online. Available: http://www.cancer.org.au/Healthprofessionals/clinicalguidelines/cancergenetics.htm May 2010.

Acknowledgment

The content of this chapter has drawn heavily upon *Genetics in family medicine: the Australian handbook for general practitioners* (2007), produced with Kristine Barlow-Stewart's colleagues A/Professor Sylvia Metcalfe, University of Melbourne, and Professor Jon Emery, University of Western Australia, following a national needs assessment conducted with general practitioners.

chapter 32

Principles of the immune system

INTRODUCTION AND OVERVIEW

The human immune system is extremely complex, with intricate multidirectional connections between our gastrointestinal, psychological, endocrinological and other systems, and communication via various neurotransmitters, cytokines and other immune system messengers. This chapter presents a simplified view of the principles of immunology, with specific focus on some of the most recently researched complementary therapies known to improve immune system health. For more comprehensive information, please refer to the resources and references listed at the end of this chapter.

Our immune system consists of two basic types of immunity: innate (or natural) immunity and adaptive (or acquired) immunity.

TYPES OF IMMUNITY

INNATE IMMUNITY

Innate immunity primarily refers to our body's first line of defence and includes physical barriers, such as the skin and cilia, and the corresponding inflammatory markers that are produced in response to tissue injury. These may involve both cellular and humoral mediators.

The main leucocyte cells in this system are phagocytes, which include the polymorphonucleoleucocytes and macrophages.[1]

ADAPTIVE IMMUNITY

Adaptive immunity is antigen-specific and may take days or weeks to develop. Depending on the antigen and the route of presentation, the response can be either cellular (e.g. cytotoxic T-cells), humoral (e.g. antibodies) or both (as may be induced by viral antigens). Different protein antigens can produce different classes of specific antibodies or immunoglobulins, such as IgA, IgG and IgM.[2]

There are two types of lymphocytes (B-cells and T-cells) that can be activated by these antigens, with both being produced in the bone marrow. B-lymphocytes (plasma cells) mature here, whereas T-cells mature within the thymus. After initial antigen exposure, immune memory develops and can subsequently result in early recognition and stronger reactions to repeat exposures.[1,2]

GASTROINTESTINAL-ASSOCIATED LYMPHOID TISSUE

The state of our digestion is extremely important to the health of our immune system, as the gastrointestinal mucosa is the major contact area between the human body and the external world of microflora. Over 400 square metres in size, it is colonised by an immense number of bacteria that are in constant communication with our immune cells.[3,4]

Within the gastrointestinal-associated lymphoid tissue (GALT) is the largest number of immune cells (70–80%) in the entire body. It consists of discrete sites, known as inductive and effector sites, which can discriminate between harmful and harmless antigens while maintaining homeostasis. Inductive sites are organised into specialised aggregations of lymphoid follicles, called Peyer's patches; effector sites are more diffusely dispersed throughout the gut tissue.[5]

In addition to this distinct architecture, the gastrointestinal tract has specialised immune cells that aid in promoting a tolerogenic response to orally induced antigens.[5] Cytotoxic $CD4^+$ T-cells are subdivided into Th1 and Th2 cells, and their relative presence or activation is thought to have a regulatory effect on immune behaviour.[4]

Th1 cells produce cytokines with pro-inflammatory activities that stimulate the proliferation of cytotoxic

T-cells, with the role of providing host defence against viral, bacterial and fungal infections. They are also thought to be critically involved in some hyperinflammatory conditions, such as autoimmune (rheumatoid) arthritis, where over-activity is detrimental.

Th2 cells produce cytokines that are responsible for the activation of the humoral immune response in healthy people, primarily in response to allergens, chemicals and parasites.[6] Some of the cytokines produced by Th2 cells (IL-4, IL-5, IL-10, IL-13) also have immune regulatory qualities, and hence excess Th2 activity can cause an imbalance and may lead to particular clinical conditions.

This has led to the perception that the balance between Th1 and Th2 cells is the prime denominator of tolerance, with the breakdown of this tolerance leading to disease.[4] As this is a developing area of immune system science, it is possible that, in the future, the immune system may be manipulated by balancing the Th1/Th2 cell ratio—further work is required, however, to verify the specific Th1/Th2 relationships in particular medical conditions and, additionally, which therapeutic agents (pharmacological and nutriceutical/herbal) may be most effective in re-establishing normal balance in the individual patient.

IMMUNE DEFICIENCY VERSUS IMMUNE HYPER-REACTIVITY (AUTOIMMUNE DISEASE)

Both immune deficiency and autoimmune disease—two sequelae of immune dysregulation—are primarily due to an imbalance in the function of our immune system, which may occur through a variety of mechanisms. Immune deficiency can ultimately result in illnesses such as infections and cancer. In the case of autoimmunity, the body produces substances that attack our own body cells, resulting in disease. Box 32.1 provides some examples of the consequences of immune dysregulation.

BOX 32.1 The sequelae of immune dysregulation

- Immune deficiency:
  - recurrent acute infections—respiratory tract infections, urinary tract infections, thrush,
  - chronic infections—e.g. HIV/AIDS, sinusitis
  - cancer
- Immune hyper-reactivity/autoimmune:
  - asthma
  - Hashimoto's disease, Graves' disease
  - rheumatoid arthritis
  - type 1 diabetes
  - psoriasis
  - ankylosing spondylitis
  - Crohn's disease

IMMUNE DISEASES

BACKGROUND AND PREVALENCE

Unfortunately, the incidence of many atopic diseases (asthma, allergies, eczema, food intolerances) and autoimmune diseases is continuing to increase. Likewise, despite advances in medical technology and treatments, many chronic diseases (such as diabetes, metabolic syndrome, cardiovascular diseases, attention deficit disorder (ADD), attention deficit hyperactivity disorder (ADHD) and cancer) are also on the rise. We are also now faced with a plethora of other syndromes with likely immune system links, such as autistic spectrum disorder, chronic fatigue and multiple chemical sensitivity syndromes, all of which as yet have no specific diagnostic tests or pharmaceutical treatments. It is therefore our duty to investigate the multifactorial origins of such diseases and to aim to treat in the least harmful ways possible. Complementary therapies have a particular role in the management of these debilitating conditions.

Defined disorders of the immune system are usually genetic, such as severe combined immunodeficiency or selective IgA deficiency. The International Union of Immunological Societies recognises eight classes of primary immunodeficiencies, with a total of over 120 conditions.[7]

The suspicion of a primary immune deficiency disease should be raised in the event of infections that are unusually persistent, recurrent or resistant to treatment, or when infections involve unexpected spread or severity, or unusual organisms.

The treatment of primary immunodeficiencies is the domain of the immunologist and is specific to the nature and severity of the deficiency. Treatment options include immunoglobulin replacement therapy, immunomodulation (e.g. interferon gamma) or stem cell transplant, reducing exposure to potential pathogens and early intervention in infections.

Immunodeficiency may be secondary to infection (HIV/AIDS), ageing, malnutrition or reaction to pharmaceuticals (disease-modifying antirheumatic drugs (DMARDs), immunosuppressive drugs or chemotherapy).

Common autoimmune diseases include Hashimoto's thyroiditis, rheumatoid arthritis, diabetes mellitus type 1 and systemic lupus erythematosus (SLE).

AETIOLOGY

The importance of breastfeeding

Although the intestinal immune system is fully developed after birth, the actual protective function of the gut requires the microbial stimulation of bacterial colonisation. Breast milk contains prebiotic oligosaccharides, designed to feed and proliferate specific resident bacteria with important protective functions (probiotics), primarily *Lactobacillus* and *Bifidobacterium*, in the infant's gut.[8] However, the nature and species of microflora are also determined by many other factors, including external environment microflora, use of antibiotics and immunomodulatory agents, and early introduction of cow's milk.[9]

Developmental immunotoxicology and early-life immune insult

Many chronic diseases of increasing incidence are now recognised as having immune dysregulation as an important underlying component.[10] These include many childhood illnesses such as asthma, allergic disease, leukaemia, autoimmunity and certain infections.[11]

The developing immune system is extremely sensitive to environmental toxins, such as infectious agents, allergens, maternal smoking, maternally administered drugs, exposure to xenobiotics, diesel exhaust and traffic-related particles, antibiotics, environmental oestrogens, heavy metals and other prenatal/neonatal stressors.[10–16] It has been postulated that dysfunctional immune responses to infections in childhood play a role in childhood leukaemia.[11,15] Evidence for an association between environmentally associated childhood immune dysfunction and autistic spectrum disorders also suggests that early-life immune insult (ELII) and developmental immunotoxicology (DIT) may contribute to these conditions.[13,16]

Indeed, it has been proposed that ELIIs are pivotal in producing chronic symptoms in later life. In particular, the period from mid-gestation until 2 years of age seems to be of particular concern, with this critical maturational window displaying a heightened sensitivity to chemical disruption, with the outcome of persistent immune dysfunction and/or misregulation.[10] The same toxin may result in different immune maturational processes, depending on the dose and timing of the insult.[10,14]

Available data indicate that ELIIs result in a shift from Th1 towards Th2 predominance, alterations in regulatory T-cell function and problematic regulation of inflammatory cell function, leading to hyperinflammatory responses and perturbation of cytokine networks. The resulting health risks may extend far beyond infectious diseases, cancer, allergy and autoimmunity to pathologies in the neurological, cardiovascular, endocrinological, respiratory and reproductive systems.[12–16]

Epigenetics, nutrigenomics, psychoneuroimmunology and psychoneuroendocrinology

The important emerging fields of *epigenetics* (combined environmental and genetic history) and *nutrigenomics* (combined nutritional status and genetic history) are also extremely relevant with regard to how our nutritional status and environmental influences may alter how particular genes associated with disease may be expressed in an individual. We now know that not everyone with a genetic make-up predisposing them to a particular disease will develop that disease. Lifestyle and psychological factors can explain much of this difference in terms of phenotypic expression. Therefore, avoiding potentially negative psychological, environmental and nutritional triggers of disease through optimal preventative medicine is an extremely significant factor in immune system health. Conversely, we have come to understand in more detail how unhealthy lifestyle and environment, and poor mental health, can predispose a person to a range of immunologically based illnesses. There is a wealth of evidence regarding the profound impact that psychological stress can have, not only upon our immune system but upon every system of the body. As such, the specialty fields of *psychneuroimmunology* (PNI) and *psychoneuroendocrinology* have now been created to further elucidate the significant connections that exist between mind, body and spirit.[17–19] Further discussion of PNI can be found in the chapter on mind–body medicine (Ch 8).

PATHOLOGY

The diagnosis of immune deficiency is primarily determined by comprehensive history taking and examination. Pathological investigations are more pertinent to the investigation of specific immune system disorders. In order to save critical consultation time, detailed questionnaires may be provided to the patient before the initial consultation.

DIAGNOSTIC APPROACH

History

- Birth history:
  - normal vaginal delivery versus caesarean section
  - prematurity
  - time in neonatal intensive care unit
  - early use of antibiotics
  - breastfeeding versus formula feeding
  - presence of colic, reflux, irritability, difficulty sleeping—exclude lack of probiotics and/or food intolerances
- Maternal history—concurrent illnesses, pre-eclampsia, gestational diabetes, vegetarian diet, specific food allergies, intolerances, nutritional imbalances (deficiencies or excesses), heavy metals etc
- Family history—coeliac, pernicious anaemia, autoimmune disease etc
- Early childhood illness/insult:
  - location of childhood—farms etc

  - parental occupation/hobbies involving chemicals, heavy metals etc
  - reactions to vaccinations in susceptible individuals (Th 1 switch to Th2)
  - recurrent illnesses—ears, tonsils, asthma, eczema; exclude food intolerance, particularly dairy
- Other stressors:
  - bullying
  - emotional, physical, sexual assault
  - prolonged recovery time from viruses such as glandular fever
  - development of syndromes such as chronic fatigue
- Concomitant illnesses/diseases that may also compromise the immune system
- Past and current illnesses/symptoms:
  - digestive symptoms—abdominal bloating, discomfort, pain, diarrhoea, constipation, excessive burping and/or flatulence, reflux; exclude lack of probiotics and/or food intolerances
  - hormonal imbalances—amenorrhoea/dysmenorrhoea, irregular periods, mood changes, headaches, breast tenderness, acne, sinusitis, chocolate cravings, particularly before periods
  - nutritional deficiencies, for example:
    - iron, vitamin B_{12}—fatigue, lack of clarity of thought
    - magnesium—eyelid twitches, palpitations in the absence of cardiac disease, growing pains (child), tightness and/or cramps in calves/feet, restlessness and/or restless legs, anxiety, insomnia
  - infertility—exclude chronic infection with *Chlamydia* (PCR) or *Mycoplasma/Ureaplasma* by cervical swab

Other symptoms that need to be explored:

- Frequency of illnesses:
  - *Candida* infection—thrush, skin rashes, systemic
  - upper respiratory tract infections
  - urinary tract infections etc
- Toxin exposure:
  - work/home—chemicals, electromagnetic frequencies, moulds etc
  - alcohol, smoking, drugs (recreational and pharmaceutical)
  - food allergies/intolerances
    - pro-inflammatory environment
- Lifestyle factors (current and history):
  - sleep
  - exercise
  - weight
  - diet (vegetarian, food intolerances etc)
  - stress.

Examination

- Nails:
  - white marks—consider zinc deficiency
  - brittle, splitting—consider essential fatty acid deficiency
  - peeling skin (hands/feet)—consider yeast infection
  - nail ridges—consider mineral deficiency
  - pitting—consider autoimmune disease (e.g. psoriasis, ankylosing spondylitis)
  - biting—likely anxiety
  - fungal infections
  - paronychia
- Eyes:
  - pale conjunctiva—consider iron deficiency
  - injected sclera—consider vitamin C/bioflavonoid deficiency
  - yellow sclera—likely liver disease
  - dark circles under eyes—consider iron deficiency and/or food intolerances
  - dry eyes—exclude autoimmune disease
- Skin:
  - butterfly rash—exclude autoimmune disease
  - easy bruising—exclude haematological disease
  - acne—consider hormonal imbalances, food intolerances
  - rosacea—exclude chronic *Helicobacter pylori* infection
  - skin cancers
  - psoriasis
  - eczema—exclude lack of probiotics and/or food intolerances, particularly dairy
  - tinea versicolor—fungal infection
  - dry skin—likely essential fatty acid deficiency
  - goose flesh—likely essential fatty acid deficiency
  - facial hair—likely hormonal imbalance in women
- Mouth and tongue
  - lips (cheilosis, stomatitis)—consider B vitamin deficiency
  - mouth ulcers—consider autoimmune disease, B vitamin deficiency
  - purple, flattened tongue—consider vitamin B_{12} deficiency
  - dry tongue—exclude dehydration, diabetes, autoimmune disease
  - twitchy tongue—consider magnesium deficiency
  - midline fissure—consider B vitamin deficiency
  - geographical tongue—vitamin/mineral deficiency

- coated tongue/halitosis—digestive problems, poor dental health
- Neck:
  - cervical lymph nodes (acute)—consider infection
  - cervical lymph nodes (chronic)—exclude haematological disease or neoplasm, consider food intolerances
  - thyroid (nodules, goitre)—investigations required
- Cardiovascular/respiratory—exclude conventional illnesses
- Gastrointestinal:
  - abdominal bloating—consider dysbiosis, lack of probiotics and/or food intolerances; exclude gastrointestinal disease
  - right upper quadrant tenderness—likely liver inflammation
  - faecal impaction—constipation
  - generalised abdominal tenderness with/without guarding/rebound—consider lack of probiotics and/or food intolerances, exclude gastrointestinal disease.

INVESTIGATIONS

Consulting room

There are no specific investigations in the consulting room other than investigations that arise from and are related to specific history taking and examination findings.

Pathology

As always, pathological investigations are ordered with respect to particular findings at the initial consultation.

Unless the individual is suffering from a readily diagnosable clinical condition, such as hyperthyroidism, diabetes, UTI or URTIs, for example, many states of immune deficiency are not recognisable by conventional pathology testing.

Usual medical testing with respect to immunology includes a full blood count (including accurate lymphocyte and granulocyte counts) and immunoglobulin levels (the three major antibodies: IgG, IgA and IgM), CRP, ESR and fasting BSL, with more-specific tests such as serum protein EPG/IEPG (electrophoretogram and immunoelectrophoretogram), ANA (anti-nuclear antibody), ENA (extractable nuclear antigen), double-stranded DNA, rheumatoid factor, thyroid function tests (TFTs) ordered if indicated.

A sensitive way to diagnose a possibly underactive thyroid, which may be significant in immune system dysfunction, is to have the patient take three morning temperatures. If the patient is a woman who is pre/perimenopausal, this should be done during the follicular phase of her menstrual cycle (before ovulation). The patient sleeps with the thermometer next to their bed and takes their temperature before rising. Temperatures below 36 degrees may indicate an underactive thyroid, despite TFTs apparently being normal. Recently, the maximum reference range for TSH has been reduced to closer to the upper value of 2.0, which most nutritionally oriented doctors traditionally aim for. It is also important to attain a free T_3 level when possible, as this is the active form of thyroid hormone.

Other tests that may be ordered include levels of specific vitamins and minerals, such as iron studies, vitamin B_{12} and red cell folate. The normal ranges for such nutrients are quite wide (e.g. ferritin 30–300, vitamin B_{12} 140–1500) and it is important to note that individuals are often symptomatic when below mid-range. This is similar for other nutrients, including fasting 25-hydroxy vitamin D, urinary iodine, plasma zinc and plasma copper.

Special tests

There is a wide range of more comprehensive investigations that may assist in the diagnosis of suboptimal immune system health. Such tests are often performed by private laboratories and come with some cost to the patient. Depending upon the patient's history and current symptoms, these may include stool tests such as a comprehensive digestive stool analysis or bioscreen, anaerobic/aerobic microbial testing, heavy metal testing through the use of hair tissue, mineral analyses or urinary porphyrins, urinary kryptopyrroles to exclude zinc and/or vitamin B_6 deficiency.

INTEGRATED MANAGEMENT

Prevention and lifestyle management

Obesity

The prevalence of obesity has now reached epidemic levels in many parts of the world, and is a major public health problem.[20] The accumulation of visceral fat has well-established links with chronic low-grade systemic inflammation, oxidative stress and subsequent impaired immunity, which has been associated with the development and progression of many chronic diseases.[21–23] Such illnesses include metabolic syndrome, inflammatory diseases, bronchial asthma, type 2 diabetes and insulin resistance, depression, cardiovascular disease, osteoarthritis, fatty liver disease and cancer.[20,22,24–26]

Major endogenous endocrine and steroid hormones can combine with lifestyle factors (low exercise, excess weight, poor diet, etc) to heighten the risk of many diseases, including cancer.[27]

There are also complex links between the metabolic and immune systems, with multiple neuroendocrine peptides, cytokines and chemokines interacting to integrate energy balance with immune function.[28] Ghrelin and leptin are two important hormones and cytokines that regulate energy balance and influence immune function.[26] Obesity reduces ghrelin, contributing to inflammation by subsequently increasing proinflammatory cytokines. In contrast, caloric restriction, which increases ghrelin and reduces leptin, can reduce oxidative stress and is a potentially immune-enhancing state that has prolonged a healthy lifespan in all species studied to date.[23,28–30]

Sleep

Good sleep is essential for physical and mental health.[31] There is strong evidence that inadequate sleep is associated with a multitude of health problems, including cognitive impairment, mood disorders, parasitical infections, cardiovascular disease and compromised immunity.[32–35] Unfortunately, frequently disrupted and restricted sleep is a common problem in today's society, with more than 50% of adults aged over 65 years reporting at least one chronic complaint.[32,34] Both animal and human studies have revealed that sleep restriction/deprivation can result in mild temporary increases in the activity of the major neuroendocrine stress systems—the autonomic sympatho-adrenal system and the hypothalamic-pituitary-adrenal (HPA) axis. Chronic sleep deprivation may also affect the reactivity of these systems to future stresses and challenges, such as physical and mental illness.[33,36]

Sleep restriction alters the neurotransmission of serotonin, resulting in reduced production of melatonin, our natural sleep hormone.[37] Recent studies have shown that melatonin has an immune-modulating effect, stimulating the production of natural killer cells and $CD4^+$ cells and inhibiting $CD8^+$ cells. It also stimulates the production of granulocytes and macrophages, as well as the release of various cytokines from natural killer cells and T-helper lymphocytes.

Poor sleep quality has recently been confirmed to increase susceptibility to the common cold, and atypical time schedules such as shift work have also been associated with breast cancer, due to a circadian disruption and nocturnal suppression of melatonin production.[38,39] Thus, enhancement of the production of melatonin, or melatonin itself, has potential therapeutic value in enhancing immune function.[40]

The recognition and treatment of sleep dysfunction can therefore be an important part of management of many immune-related conditions.[38]

Stress management

There is a wealth of evidence that psychological stress can adversely affect the development and progression of almost every known disease. Both acute and chronic stressful states produce documentable changes in both our innate and our adaptive immune responses.[41–48]

In an elaborate multidirectional communication system, neurotransmitters, hormones and neuropeptides all regulate our immune system cells and subsequently communicate with all other systems through the secretion of a wide variety of cytokines.[49]

Acute stress has been shown to have a stimulating effect on the immune system, whereas chronic stress down-regulates the immune system.[47,50] Chronic stress has been associated with increased susceptibility to infectious diseases and cancer.[42,43,45] It is also linked with worse outcomes in many immune-related disorders, including cancer, and inflammatory and infectious diseases, indicating that the effects of our mental state on our immune system are directly and clinically relevant to disease expression.[46,50,51]

There is considerable variability in each individual's immune response to stress. Encouraging particular activities that increase that person's ability to cope with stress may therefore have a significantly beneficial effect on their immune system, with subsequent modification in the development and progression of many different diseases.[47,49,52,53]

It is also important to note that stress during fetal and neonatal development can alter the programming of the neuro-endocrine-immune axis, influencing stress, immune responsiveness and even disease resistance in later life.[54] Identification and treatment of suboptimal moods in pregnant women is therefore imperative.

Various behavioural strategies have demonstrated improved immune parameters, with reduced affective distress in many different diseases.[43,55] These include a systematic review of the beneficial effects of mindfulness-based stress reduction in the management of cancer, particularly breast and prostate, and HIV.[53–64]

Hypnosis, relaxation and guided imagery have been shown to be effective in cases of breast cancer, viral illnesses, including chronic herpes simplex, and the common cold.[65,66] Several studies have demonstrated the effectiveness of cognitive behaviour therapy with regards to immune parameters in HIV-positive men,[67–69] while autogenic training and group psychotherapy were effective for women with breast cancer.[70,71]

Exercise

There is a wealth of evidence supporting the beneficial effects of exercise upon the immune system. In particular, exercise has beneficial effects on many chronic diseases. It is known to have an anti-inflammatory effect, reducing body fat percentage and macrophage accumulation in adipose tissue.[72–74]

Natural killer cells have been found to be the most responsive immune cell to acute exercise. Their sensitivity to physiological stress and their important role in innate immune defences indicate that these cells are one link between regular physical activity and general health status.[75]

In animal studies, anaerobic exercise has been shown to increase both innate and adaptive immune function.[76] Secretory IgA, which is the predominant immunoglobulin in mucosal secretions providing first-line defence against pathogens and antigens presented at the mucosa, has also been shown to be increased after exercise in people aged over 75 years.[77,78]

Exercise needs to be performed in moderation, however. Multiple effects of over-training resulting in impaired immune responses have been documented.[78–83] In the short term, this can result in increased susceptibility to respiratory infections; in the longer term, more chronic conditions such as chronic fatigue syndrome may develop.[78,83]

Self-help

Yoga

There have been limited studies on the efficacy of yoga practice for the immune system. Most have focused on the breathing disciplines within yoga, namely Pranayama and Sudarshan Kriya, which are both rhythmic breathing processes traditionally used to reduce stress and improve the immune system.[84] Studies on both healthy individuals and those with cancer have shown increased antioxidant status and improved immune status in those practising these techniques, compared with controls.[85–88]

Qi gong

Qi gong is an ancient Chinese psychosomatic exercise that integrates movement, meditation and breathing into a single exercise. All studies have been on healthy people and most demonstrate that, after 1 month, there are significant changes in immune parameters.[89–92]

Although qi gong may regulate immunity, metabolic rate and apoptosis, further studies are required to validate these findings.[90]

Massage

There are mixed results as to the benefits of massage for immune enhancement. Two earlier studies noted increases in dopamine, serotonin, natural killer cells and lymphocytes in women with breast cancer after thrice weekly massage for 5 weeks.[93,94] However, a more recent RCT showed that effleurage massage had no significant effect on immune and neuroendocrine parameters.[95]

Nutrition/dietary modulation

Many natural foods are thought to balance the immune system and prevent excessive immune activity. These foods include fish, fruit and vegetables, and culinary herbs such as ginger, garlic and turmeric. In contrast, there is strong evidence regarding the pro-inflammatory effects of 'fast foods' that contain large amounts of saturated fatty and trans-fatty acids, refined carbohydrates with a high glycaemic index, and artificial colours, flavours and preservatives.

Box 32.2 lists the main foods thought to have an immune-modulating effect by altering the inflammatory reactivity of the human environment.

However, any food may be pro-inflammatory for an individual who is intolerant to that food. Adverse reactions to foods can have a significant impact on the immune system and general wellbeing of an individual. Immune-mediated adverse reactions may be roughly divided into IgE-mediated and non-IgE-mediated. Non-IgE-mediated food reactions are not well understood and their negative effects on wellbeing and immune efficiency may be greatly underestimated. In the first few years of life, humans gradually develop an intricate balance between tolerance and immune reactivity in the gut mucosa, along with a tremendous expansion of the GALT, which is profoundly affected by changes in commensal flora.[96]

The simplest test to determine which foods contribute to gastrointestinal or other symptoms is to perform a

BOX 32.2 Foods with an immune-modulating effect

Anti-inflammatory
- restricted energy intake
- low-GI foods
- antioxidant-rich foods
- omega-3-rich foods, e.g. fish
- monounsaturated fat
- lean game meats
- fruit and vegetables
- high-fibre foods
- herbs, e.g. garlic, ginger, curcumin
- nuts
- green tea
- moderate alcohol

Pro-inflammatory
- excess energy
- high-GI foods
- high trans fats foods
- saturated fats
- salt
- excessive alcohol
- refined carbohydrates
- dairy
- artificial colours/flavours/preservatives

food elimination diet (FED), with initial avoidance, then separate reintroduction of individual foods. Some of the most common dietary intolerances are to wheat, dairy and soy. However, seemingly innocuous foods such as apples and tomatoes may be associated with immune reactivity.[97]

Alcohol in light–moderate amounts (10 g for women, 20 g for men) has been shown to be particularly beneficial for the immune system when compared with both non-drinkers and heavy drinkers.[98] Resveratrol, a polyphenol from red wine, is able to stimulate both innate and adaptive immune responses such it that may be important for host protection in different immune-related disorders.[99–101]

Epigallocatechin-3-gallate (EPG), present in green tea, is well known for its ability to reduce the risk of a variety of immunodeficiency disorders.[102] Green tea possesses antioxidant, anti-inflammatory, anti-carcinogenic and immune-enhancing properties.[103]

Environment

As stated previously, many chronic diseases of increasing incidence, such as atopic illnesses, autoimmune diseases, certain infections and cancers are now recognised to have immune dysregulation as an important underlying component.[10,11]

The developing immune system is extremely sensitive to a wide range of environmental toxins, such that DIT and ELII are now important recognised aetiologies for many illnesses.[10–16]

There is also strong evidence that complex syndromes, such as multiple chemical sensitivity, Gulf War syndrome, sick building syndrome and chronic fatigue syndrome, which often have no clear underlying medical explanation, may have an environmental component to their aetiology.[104]

Such syndromes may be associated with exposure to electromagnetic radiation,[105–109] novel environmental chemicals,[110–112] moulds and other bio-aerosols[113–117] and/or heavy metals.[118–120]

Paramedical

Acupuncture

Acupuncture has been used for centuries to prevent and treat various conditions, and simply to maintain good health.[121] In addition to its known effects on the nervous system, emerging evidence suggests that it may also effectively modulate the innate immune system, which plays important roles in inflammation, pain, metabolism, cell proliferation and apoptosis.[122,123]

There is now experimental evidence that the electrical stimulation of the vagus nerve inhibits macrophage activation and the production of pro-inflammatory cytokines, including TNF, IL-1 beta, IL-6 and IL-18, indicating a possible underlying neuro-immune basis to acupuncture.[124] Such observations suggest that acupuncture may regulate the immune system by promoting both humoral and cellular immunity as well as natural killer cell activity.[125,126]

Acupuncture may therefore be used as an adjunct to conventional medical treatment for a number of chronic inflammatory and autoimmune diseases. More studies, however, are required.[124]

Pharmacological/surgical

There are no pharmaceutical medications that have been designed to generally enhance or balance the immune system, other than for conditions associated with specific immune deficiency (e.g. IgG deficiency). In a similar manner, certain surgical procedures such as thyroidectomy, tonsillectomy and tooth extractions may be necessary when indicated. In such cases, specialist referral is strongly recommended.

Complementary therapies

In light of the above, the use of an integrative approach that can specifically enhance our immune health is therefore of even greater relevance and importance. Indeed, to ignore the wealth of evidence regarding the efficacy of complementary therapies is to remove a vital tool from the doctor's armament and may prematurely lead to the use of pharmaceutical medications and the risk of unnecessary side effects.

Nutritional supplementation

Nutrition is a critical determinant of immunity, with malnutrition being the most common cause of immunodeficiency worldwide.[127] Nutrients either enhance or depress immune function, depending on the nutrient and level of its intake.[128] Indeed, both insufficient and excess nutrient intakes can have negative consequences for immune status and susceptibility to a variety of pathogens.[129] Deficiency of nutrients may suppress immunity by affecting innate, T-cell mediated and adaptive antibody responses, leading to dysregulation of the host response. This can lead to increased susceptibility to infections, which can then lead to further nutrient deficiency, and so on.[130]

Available data indicate that vitamins A, B_6, B_{12}, C, D, E, folic acid and the trace elements iron (Fe), zinc (Zn), copper (Cu) and selenium (Se) all work synergistically to support the protective activities of the immune cells. With the exception of iron and vitamin C, they are all also intricately involved in antibody production.[127,130] Antioxidant vitamins and trace elements (vitamins C, E, Se, Cu, Zn) counteract damage to tissues secondary to reactive oxygen species, while simultaneously modulating immune cell function by affecting the production of cytokines and prostaglandins.

Adequate intake of vitamins B_6, B_{12}, C, E, folic acid and trace elements Se, Zn, Cu and Fe all support a Th1 cytokine-mediated immune response with sufficient production of pro-inflammatory cytokines. This maintains an effective immune response, avoiding a shift to an anti-inflammatory Th2 immune state and an increased risk of extracellular infections. Supplementation with these nutrients can reverse the Th2-cell-mediated immune response to Th1, thereby enhancing innate immunity.[131]

Presented below is a summary of evidence for the most recently studied nutrients and herbs with regards to immune system enhancement.

Probiotics

Probiotics are recognised for their role in nutrient absorption, mucosal barrier function, angiogenesis, morphogenesis and postnatal maturation of intestinal cell lineages, intestinal motility and, most importantly, maturation of the GALT, which contains 70–80% of immune cells in the body.[132]

An important adjustment of the immune system to bacterial colonisation of the gut is the production of secretory IgA by B-cells in the GALT.[133–135] Probiotics stimulate both production and secretion of polymeric IgA, the antibody that coats and protects mucosal surfaces against harmful bacterial invasion.[8] Secretory IgA also promotes an anti-inflammatory environment by neutralising immune stimulatory antigens.[136] Thus, sIgA plays a significant role in the regulation of bacterial communities and maintenance of immune homeostasis.[134]

In addition, appropriate colonisation with probiotics helps to produce a balanced T-helper cell response and prevent an imbalance, which can contribute in part to clinical disease.

Thus, pre- and probiotics are attractive options for maintaining the steady nutritional state of the host with defective gut barrier functions. Prebiotics (inulin from chicory root, fructooligosaccharides, arabinogalactans) resist enzymatic digestion in the upper gastrointestinal tract and therefore reach the colon virtually intact, where they undergo bacterial fermentation. The consumption of prebiotics favours the growth of probiotics and impedes growth of pathogenic organisms, thereby modulating immune parameters in the GALT, secondary lymphoid tissues and peripheral circulation.[137] The change in gut microflora may reduce intestinal permeability, consequently influencing both intestinal and systemic body functions.[138] Further, gut microflora are able to modify the structure of potentially harmful food antigens and thereby alter their immunogenicity.[139]

Both inulin and oligofructose stimulate the colonic production of short-chain fatty acids and favour the growth of lactobacilli and/or bifidobacteria, which have all been associated with reduced mucosal inflammation.[140]

Zinc

Zinc is an essential trace element that is critical for cellular function and structural integrity.[141] Normal zinc homeostasis is required for a functional immune system (both innate and adaptive), metabolic homeostasis (energy utilisation and hormone turnover), antioxidant activity, glucose homeostasis and wound healing.[142,143] Zinc is known to regulate the immune system systemically as well as having direct T-cellular effects, resulting in the regulation of gene expression, bioenergetics, metabolic pathways, signal transduction and cell invasion, proliferation and apoptosis.[144,145]

Zinc is also an essential cofactor for the structure and function of a wide range of cellular proteins including enzymes, structural proteins, transcription and replication factors. It is now known that nearly 2000 of these transcription factors require zinc for their structural integrity.[144,146,147] Zinc also affects entire functional networks of genes that are related to pro-inflammatory cytokines and cellular survival.[141] An individual's zinc status therefore has a significant impact on their immune system, with zinc deficiency having the potential to profoundly modulate immune function, and zinc supplementation the potential to prevent and treat many acute and chronic diseases.[148–152]

Even a mild zinc deficiency in humans can result in immune dysfunction by shifting from a Th1 to a Th2 cell response.[146,153] This in turn can enhance susceptibility to malignancies and infections with viruses and bacteria.[146] Ageing is associated with the same Th1/Th2 imbalance, and moderate zinc supplementation has been shown to alter these proportions.[154–156]

Zinc also directly influences GALT, contributing to host defence by maintaining the integrity of the gut mucosal barrier and thereby controlling inflammatory cell infiltration.[157] Oxidative stress is known to be an important contributing factor in many chronic diseases, and zinc deficiency is constantly observed in states of chronic inflammation.[158] Zinc supplementation has been shown to decrease the gene expression and production of both pro-inflammatory cytokines and oxidative stress markers.[143,146,153] As such, zinc may be a useful chemopreventative agent for a range of chronic diseases, including neurodegenerative disorders such as Parkinson's disease and multiple sclerosis, autoimmune diseases such as rheumatoid arthritis and inflammatory bowel disease, as well as macular degeneration, and cancer.[146]

Many studies have also demonstrated the beneficial effects of zinc supplementation in the management of the common cold, cold sores, influenza, acute and chronic diarrhoea and acute respiratory infections.[146,159–163] Current evidence also shows that zinc (and selenium) improves humoral immunity in elderly subjects after an influenza vaccination.[143]

Several recent animal studies have also demonstrated a link between zinc deficiency and several autoimmune diseases, including systemic lupus erythematosus and type 1 diabetes.[164,165]

Vitamin A

Vitamin A has received particular attention in recent years. It is now known to modulate a wide range of immune functions, such as lymphocyte activation and proliferation, T-helper cell differentiation, tissue-specific lymphocyte homing, the production of specific antibody isotypes and regulation of the immune response.[166,167]

Retinoic acid is produced naturally from intestinal dendritic cells.[168] The presence of high levels of retinoic acid in the intestine and GALT can boost the production of IgA in the intestinal mucosa.[135] When B- and T-cells are activated in the GALT, gut-homing receptors are induced on these cells via the actions of retinoic acid. These gut-homing B- and T-cells play essential roles in protecting the digestive tract from pathogens—that is, in the development of 'oral tolerance'.[169] Vitamin A deficiency is also a risk factor for low antibody production. In countries where vitamin A deficiency is endemic, many children are receiving retinol as an adjunct in their vaccinations, especially polio, diphtheria/pertussis/tetanus (DPT) and measles. This is because vitamin A appears to promote the vaccine antibody response.[170]

Current recommendations for vitamin A intake are based simply on the maintenance of normal vision. However, it has been realised that higher levels may be necessary in order to optimise innate immune function.[171] Vitamin A supplementation above dietary requirements has been shown to enhance inflammatory responses, with decreased Th1 and increased mucosal responses in animals.[172]

Selenium

Selenium is a potent nutritional antioxidant that significantly influences both inflammatory and immune responses.[173,174] Selenium is known to be essential for the proper functioning of neutrophils, macrophages, natural killer cells and T-lymphocytes. However, there are many other proposed mechanisms for its protective effects.[174–178]

Evidence is accumulating that selenium levels lower than previously thought can cause adverse health effects, such that the recommended daily allowance (RDA) levels have recently been increased to 150 μg/day. It has also been demonstrated that higher levels of selenium may give additional protection from many diseases by significantly enhancing immune responses.[179]

Selenium is a key nutrient in protection from certain viral infections, including Coxsackie virus, influenza virus and HIV progression to AIDS.[175,179–183]

Just as an inadequate status of selenium is linked to an increased risk of cancer, there is also growing evidence that elevated selenium intake may be associated with a reduced risk of cancer.[175,179–181,184] Interventions with selenium (at least 200 μg/day) have shown benefit in reducing both the incidence of cancer and the mortality in all cancers combined. This has been shown to be particularly relevant in liver, prostate, colorectal, lung, oesophageal and stomach cancers, the effect of which is most pronounced in those who are most deficient in selenium. There is also some new evidence that selenium may also affect the risk of cancer progression and metastasis.[185,186]

Vitamin C

The human body is unable to synthesise vitamin C, and hence we are entirely dependent upon dietary sources and/or nutritional supplementation to maintain adequate levels of this important water-soluble antioxidant.[187,188] It has long been known that vitamin C concentrations in the plasma and leucocytes decline rapidly during infections and stress, resulting in reduced resistance to pathogens.[160,189] For this reason, vitamin C has traditionally been used as a 'cure for the common cold'.

Supplementation of vitamin C has, indeed, been found to improve components of the immune system, such as antimicrobial and natural killer cell activities, lymphocyte proliferation, chemotaxis and delayed-type hypersensitivity. It also contributes to the maintenance of the redox activity of cells, thereby protecting them from reactive oxygen species generated during the inflammatory response.[160]

A large number of RCTs have indicated that vitamin C supplementation (up to 1 g/day) with zinc (up to 30 mg/day) can ameliorate the symptoms and shorten the duration of respiratory infections when used prophylactically. A recent Cochrane review has concluded that supplementation of vitamin C is only effective in preventing the common cold in cases of excessive physical activity or in cold environments.[189,190]

While the efficacy of vitamin C supplementation is still controversial, it is argued by some authors that to achieve an optimal daily allowance of vitamin C, we require 1 g daily supplementation accompanied by a diet high in fruits and vegetables.[187]

Vitamin D

Vitamin D has been rediscovered in recent years and there have now been many studies of the serious health consequences of vitamin D deficiency. Very few foods naturally contain vitamin D, so sun exposure is the primary source.[191]

Indeed, vitamin D deficiency is a recognised global pandemic, in both developing and developed countries, including Australia.[191–193] As such, a growing number of diseases are now known to be associated with vitamin D deficiency.[194] Originally, vitamin D deficiency was only considered important for bone health; it is now understood that this 'vitamin' is actually a complex hormone that is intricately involved in the integrity of the innate immune system.[195]

The immune-regulatory role of vitamin D affects both the innate and the adaptive immune systems.[196] The discoveries that activated macrophages produce active vitamin D, and that immune system cells express the vitamin D receptor, first suggested how the vitamin D endocrine system influenced immune system function.[197] Autoimmune diseases occur because of an inappropriate immune-mediated attack against self-tissue. Without vitamin D, auto-reactive T-cells develop; whereas in the presence of vitamin D, the enhanced activity of immune cells is suppressed, balance in the T-cell response is restored and the process of autoimmunity is avoided.[198,199]

Vitamin D deficiency is strongly associated with an increased risk of 17 common cancers, autoimmune diseases (such as multiple sclerosis, type 1 diabetes, irritable bowel disease (IBD), rheumatoid arthritis), infectious diseases (tuberculosis), mental health disorders, cardiovascular disease (hypertension), skin disorders (psoriasis) and bone disorders (osteoporosis, osteomalacia and rickets).[193–195,192, 200–203]

It has recently been estimated that there is a 30–50% reduction in the risk of developing breast, colorectal and prostate cancer by increasing one's vitamin D intake to at least 1000 IU/day. Women who are vitamin D deficient are estimated to have a 253% increased risk for developing colorectal cancer. Women who consume 1500 mg/day of calcium and 1100 IU/day of vitamin D_3 for 4 years reduce their risk of developing cancer by more than 60%.[204]

There are a multitude of studies associating vitamin D deficiency with the development and progression of autoimmune diseases such as multiple sclerosis, rheumatoid arthritis, insulin-dependent diabetes mellitus and IBD. Recent evidence also strongly suggests that supplementation with vitamin D may be beneficial, especially for Th1-mediated autoimmune disorders. By decreasing the Th1-immune driven response, the severity of symptoms is decreased. Some reports indicate that vitamin D may even be preventative in such disorders as multiple sclerosis and type 1 diabetes mellitus.[196,205–209]

Maternal vitamin D supplementation is also extremely important, as low prenatal vitamin D levels may also increase susceptibility to the same diseases later in life.[210]

Iodine

There is emerging evidence regarding iodine deficiency and the state of our immune health, in particular with regards to thyroid and breast health. Iodine deficiency is very common in Australia, such that it has been determined that salt iodisation is now not considered an effective strategy to correct iodine deficiencies in this country.[211]

It has been specifically proposed that the reduction in risk of breast disease associated with increased levels of thyroid hormones, or iodine, may derive from the pro-oxidant properties of its compounds. Conversely, the increased risk from hypothyroidism may derive from its ability to inhibit this stress-mediated apoptotic process.[212]

The protective effects of iodine against breast cancer have been increasingly demonstrated through epidemiological evidence and animal models.[213] Iodine-deficient breast tissues are more susceptible to carcinogen action, and promote lesions earlier and in greater profusion.[214] Treatment with iodine can reverse this dysplasia.[215,216] Furthermore, molecular iodine has clear antiproliferative and apoptotic effects in the human breast cancer cell line, MCF-7.[217]

Reports have documented the antiproliferative properties of molecular iodine and the arachidonic acid derivative, 6-iodolactone (6-IL) in both thyroid and mammary glands. Recent data has shown that both molecular iodine and 6-IL trigger the same intracellular pathways and suggest that the antineoplastic effect of iodine in breast cancer involves the intracellular formation of 6-IL. Mammary cancer cells are known to contain high concentrations of arachidonic acid, which may explain why iodine exerts apoptotic effects at lower concentrations only in tumour cells.[218] Iodine may therefore be useful as an adjuvant therapy in the pharmacological manipulation of the oestrogen pathway in women with breast cancer.[213]

Herbal medicine

Astragalus

Astragalus membranaceus is a common traditional Chinese medicinal plant that has for centuries been widely used to enhance the body's natural defence mechanisms.[219]

There have been numerous studies demonstrating the immunomodulating and immunorestorative effects, both in vitro and in vivo, of the roots of *A. membranaceus*.[219–221] It appears that the immunopotentiating effect of *Astragalus* is primarily due to the polysaccharide fraction (APS), as it increases both cellular and humoral immune responses.[221]

Astragalus has been shown to be efficacious in infective, atopic and autoimmune health conditions by its ability to reverse the Th2-dominant status of many common illnesses.[222,223] Many studies have shown that *Astragalus* has the potential to reverse the Th2-predominant status in patients with asthma.[224–226]

Th2 cytokines are also predominant in cancer patients and have been found to be associated with tumour progression.[222] *Astragalus* has been shown to be capable of restoring the impaired T-cell functions in cancer patients. It exhibits anti-tumour effects, both in vitro and in vivo, which appear to be achieved through activating the host's anti-tumour immune mechanisms.[227] Therefore patients may use *Astragalus* to help inhibit tumour growth or to boost resistance to infections.[228,229]

A 2005 Cochrane review concluded that *Astragalus* can stimulate immunocompetent T-cells and significantly reduce side effects such as nausea and vomiting in patients treated with chemotherapy. There was no evidence of harm arising from the use of *Astragalus*.[230]

Other herbs

Many other herbs, European, Chinese and Ayurvedic, have a long history of traditional use for immune system enhancement. Recently, there have been more randomised, placebo-controlled quality studies regarding the immune-boosting effects of many of these herbs. Of particular note are studies involving echinacea, cranberry, manuka honey, garlic and ginger.

Many studies have demonstrated the protective effects of proanthocyanidins in cranberry (*Vaccinium macrocarpon*) in reducing susceptibility to urinary tract infections by preventing bacteria from attaching to uroepithelial cells.[231,232] This decrease in bacterial adherence has been noted to occur in a dose-dependent relationship in which *Escherichia coli* loses its adherence the higher the dosage of cranberry given to a subject (36 mg vs 108 mg of cranberry capsule).[233] A 2008 Cochrane review of the clinical efficacy of the use of cranberry juice for urinary tract infections concluded that use of cranberry over a 12-month period may reduce the incidence of recurrent infections among women.[234] It should be noted that many commercial cranberry juices contain high levels of sugar, a concern that can be avoided by using cranberry extract capsules.

Clinical evaluation of echinacea and its influence on the immune system are, unfortunately, problematic due to the disparate use of different preparations across studies. A 2006 Cochrane review suggested that use of the aerial component of *Echinacea purpurea* may be beneficial in the early treatment of the common cold in adults.[235]

Manuka honey has been found to have therapeutic effects on wound and ulcer healing when applied with dressings.[236,237] Due to its antibacterial quality, clinical evidence as reported by a 2008 Cochrane review indicates that honey may reduce wound healing times compared with conventional dressings in partial thickness burns[238]; however, it does not appear to provide additional benefit to compression bandages for leg ulcers when measured over a 12-week period.[239] Manuka honey also appears to have benefit in reducing MRSA infections in patients with sloughy venous leg ulcers, although the results of this RCT were derived from a small population. It must be noted that honey used in medical practice should be of 'medical grade'—that is, sterilised by gamma irradiation and having standardised antibacterial activity.[240]

ONGOING REVIEW AND MONITORING

As with any other illness, it is imperative to review the patient as often as is necessary. In general, nutritional/herbal therapies may take up to 3 months to reach maximum effect. Unless the condition requires urgent follow-up, it is advisable to review the patient at 1 month to discuss any investigation results and review any change in their symptoms. Usually, the patient will notice some improvement in their symptoms at 4 weeks, more at 8 weeks and the greatest difference at 12 weeks. If there are no obvious improvements at 8 weeks, the nutritional/herbal regimen is generally changed.

Just as nutritional/herbal supplementation is a valuable initial tool in the healthcare provider's armament, most supplements may be weaned or discontinued, generally after 3–6 months, without the patient's health suffering. It is at this time that the patient now has enough knowledge and wisdom to recognise whether their own body's specific signs of deficiency return. In this case, the patient will notice a return of their symptoms and can take more active control of the management of their condition.

It is also significant to note that, as the integrity of the gut strengthens, reactions to specific foods may change. It is therefore advisable to repeat a food elimination regimen at an appropriate time (at least 6 months) to be certain that the patient is not avoiding foods that they were originally intolerant of, thereby unnecessarily reducing their nutritional status and quality of life.

IMPORTANT PITFALLS

It is most important to remember to always treat the patient, and not the number on the investigation report before you. Unless there is an obvious abnormality that requires treatment, if the patient is feeling well, it does not necessarily always matter that all their levels are not within the ideal reference range.

It is also extremely important to know and accept your own limitations. This is relevant with respect to both complex medical history/investigations, where referral to specialists may be required, and to appropriately qualified complementary therapists who may be more experienced and qualified than yourself in determining specific complementary medicine regimens.

PATIENT EDUCATION: CLINICAL TIPS

Physical activity

- Both aerobic and anaerobic exercise (preferably outside) are important for the immune system. Aim for 30–60 minutes, 5–7 days per week. Yoga, t'ai chi and qi gong may also be beneficial.
- Excessive exercise can be detrimental for your immunity, increasing the risk of colds and other infective processes.

Diet

- Obesity lowers immunity. Consider checking thyroid function, oestrogen levels and fasting insulin if not losing weight despite a healthy diet and exercise regimen.
- Consider performing a food elimination regimen to kick-start weight loss and determine individual food intolerances.
- Consider cow's milk intolerance for presentations (particularly children) with recurrent tonsillitis, otitis media, asthma, eczema or adults with chronic sinusitis. Trial totally dairy-free for 1 month.
- Eat regular balanced, healthy meals; ideally three main meals and two snacks per day, each containing protein.
- Increase fish (sardines, tuna, salmon, cod, mackerel) intake, especially deep sea fish > three meals per week.
- Two small serves of lean red meat per week should be consumed, to ensure adequate iron levels, unless intolerant.
- Consume large quantities of coloured fruit and vegetables.
- Use extra virgin cold-pressed olive oil and avocado in dressings.
- Eat nuts (especially brazil nuts), seeds, bean sprouts (e.g. alfalfa, mung, bean, lentil), shiitaki and oyster mushrooms.
- Enjoy dark chocolate.
- Consume 1–2 glasses of red wine every other day.
- Drink green tea and 1–2 litres of water per day.
- Avoid hydrogenated fats, salt, fast foods, sugar (e.g. soft drinks, lollies/confectionery, biscuits and cakes) and other processed foods (e.g. white bread, white pasta, pastries).
- Avoid chemical additives—preservatives, colourings, flavours, artificial sweeteners.
- Moderate intake of caffeinated drinks and alcohol.

Smoking

- Quit smoking through whatever means are available. Support is often essential, as achieving long-term smoking cessation is a challenge.

Sunshine

- Aim for at least 15–30 minutes of sunshine daily for vitamin D and melatonin production—especially before 10 am and after 3 pm, when sun exposure is safest.
- Ensure adequate skin exposure (back of hands or face) during this period. Apply sun protection after this period is achieved.
- More time in the sun is required for dark-skinned people.

Sleep

- Healthy sleep patterns are essential for improving the immune system. Wake with the sun and go to sleep between 9 and 10 pm (see Ch 43, Sleep disorders).

Stress reduction

- Reduce stress in any way you can. Seek help from a psychologist or other professional if needed.
- Mindfulness-based stress reduction programs, meditation, prayer, hypnosis, relaxation, guided imagery and massage can all help.
- Have fun and enjoy all that life has to offer! Seek joy in the simple aspects of life.

Environment

- Reduce exposure to chemicals wherever possible, including household cleaning agents, paints and solvents, petrochemical fumes, passive smoking, over-medication with pharmaceutical drugs (review with your doctor), drinking water bottles exposed to the sun, and so on.
- Reduce your exposure to electromagnetic radiation wherever possible. Carry your mobile phone away from the body rather than in your pocket. Turn off home appliances at the power point when not in use.
- Investigate whether there are any sources of mould in your environment and remove wherever possible.

Acupuncture

- Acupuncture may be used as an additional therapy in instances of inflammatory or immune system disease.

Supplementation

Broad-based multivitamin with high antioxidant value

Because of the synergistic manner in which vitamins and minerals support the immune system, it is recommended that a broad-based high-strength multivitamin be used.

Vitamin A

Indications

Reducing infection severity (measles and infectious diarrhoea), very low birth weight infants, chemoprevention, night blindness, retinitis pigmentosa, xerophthalmia, glaucoma and cataract prevention, acne, psoriasis, ichthyoses, skin cancers, improving dental health, Crohn's disease, asthma, sinusitis, rhinitis.

Dosage

See Table 32.1 for recommended daily intakes.

Treatment doses

- 10,000–50,000 IU/day in short term
- 200,000 IU on two consecutive days can reduce secondary infection in children with measles who are vitamin A deficient
- 15,000 IU/day for retinitis pigmentosa

Results

Depend on form of vitamin A and condition being treated.

Contraindications

Caution with concurrent use of isotretinoin, minocycline, oral contraceptive pills, or with liver or renal disease. Toxicity may occur at doses > 10,000 IU vitamin A/day or > 2000 IU/day when pregnant. Early signs: dry rough skin, cracked lips, coarse or sparse hair, alopecia of eyebrows, diplopia, dryness of mucous membranes, peeling of skin, bone and joint pain, fatigue, nausea and vomiting.

TABLE 32.1 Recommended daily intake of vitamin A*

Age (years)	RDI (μg/day)**
1–3	300
4–8	400
9–13	600
14+ (females)	700
14+ (males)	900
Pregnancy < 18	700
Pregnancy > 18	800
Lactation	1100

*Australian RDI. **Upper level of intake 3000 μg/day.

Side effects

None at appropriate doses.

Vitamin C

Indications

Upper respiratory tract infections, sinusitis, atopy, asthma (exercise-induced), to enhance the efficacy of some medications (cisplatin, cyclophosphamide, doxorubicin, etoposide, fluorouracil, L-dopa, tamoxifen, vincristine), to improve connective tissue integrity, wound healing, sunburn prevention, antihistamine, cancer prevention and treatment, prevention of cardiovascular disease, diabetes complications.

Dosage

For acute infections, short-term use (3–6 g) or until bowel tolerance, then reduce dose. For cancer, 10–30 g vitamin C IV 2–3 times weekly.

Contraindications

Use with caution in haemachromatosis, thalassaemia major, sideroblastic anaemia, erythrocyte glucose-6 phosphate dehydrogenase (G6PD) deficiency.

Side effects

Reversible diarrhoea at high doses when given orally.

Vitamin D

Indications

Autoimmune diseases, inflammatory bowel disease, cancer, infectious diseases.

Dosage

In the absence of adequate sun exposure, at least 800–1000 IU vitamin D_3 per day may be needed for adequate vitamin D levels in children and adults. Treatment doses vary considerably depending on condition: generally, 2000–6000 IU per day vitamin D_3. Up to 50,000 IU vitamin D_2 twice weekly for 5 weeks has been shown to be safe. Loading doses of 600,000 IU IM can be used for deficiency states.

Contraindications

Hypersensitivity to vitamin D, SLE, hypercalcaemia. Caution in sarcoidosis and hyperparathyroidism. Possible interaction with calcium channel blockers and digitalis.

Results
Three-month trial.

Side effects
Mild and rare when used appropriately.

Zinc
Indications
To improve immunity, reduce severity and frequency of infections and reduce oxidative stress.

Dosage
Elemental zinc 35–45 mg nocte.

Results
Three-month trial—cease earlier if nausea occurs.

Side effects
Nausea, vomiting, reduced copper after long-term use.

Contraindications
High zinc levels, sideroblastic anaemia, severe kidney disease. Caution with amiloride.

Selenium
Indication
To improve immunity, chemoprevention.

Dosage
Up to 150 μg/day.

Results
Three-month trial.

Side effects
Nausea, vomiting, irritability, fatigue, nail changes at doses > 1 mg.

Contraindications
Sensitivity to selenium.

Astragalus
Dosage
Dried root 2–30 g/day.
Liquid extract or solid dose equivalent (1:2) 4.5–8.5 mL/day.
Decoction: 8–12 g divided into two doses daily on empty stomach.

Results
May notice effects within 2 weeks.

Contraindications
Caution with immunosuppressive agents. May have additive effects with inotropic drugs.

Side effects
Nil known.

Echinacea
Dosage
E. angustifolia or *E. purpurea*, 1–3 g/day.
E. purpurea dried aerial part, 2.5–6 g/day.
E. purpurea expressed juice of fresh plant, 6–9 mL/day.
E. pallida ethanolic extract of root, 2–4 mL/day.

Results
Early results for acute infections.

Contraindications
If allergic to Compositae family of plants (chamomile, ragweed). Caution with immunosuppressive medications and long-term use (> 8 weeks).

Side effects
Rash can occur if allergic.

Probiotics
Indications
To enhance GALT, thereby providing balance between Th1 and Th2 cytokines in order to prevent and treat autoimmune and infectious diseases.

Dosage
Depending on condition, different probiotics may be required. Generalised treatment dose before breakfast:
- *Lactobacillus rhamnosus*, 12 billion CFU
- *L. acidophilus*, 4 billion CFU
- *L. casei*, 2 billion CFU
- *Bifidobacterium bifidum*, 1 billion CFU
- *B. longum*, 1 billion CFU.

Contraindications
- True cow's milk allergy if contained in product.

Results
- Few days to few weeks, depending on condition.

Side effects
- Gastrointestinal disturbance if wrong probiotic.

RESOURCES
DrWeil.com, http://www.drweil.com
Integrative Medicine, http://www.integrative-medicine.com.au
Mercola.com, http://www.mercola.com

REFERENCES

1 Stambach M. The truth about your immune system: what you need to know. Stamford: Harvard Medical School; 2004.

2 Wahlquist ML, Kouris-Blazos A. Immune function, infection and diseases of affluence. Food and Nutrition. 2nd edn. Sydney: Allen & Unwin; 2002.

3 Tsuji M, Suzuki K, Kinoshita K et al. Dynamic interactions between bacteria and immune cells leading to IgA synthesis. Semin Immunol 2008; 20(1):59–66.

4 van Eden W, van der Zee R, van Kooten P et al. Balancing the immune system: Th1 and Th2. Ann Rheum Dis 2002; 61(Suppl 2):S25–S28.

5 Mason KL, Huffnagle GB, Noverr MC et al. Overview of gut immunology. Adv Exp Med Biol 2008; 635:1–14.

6 Becker Y. The changes in Th1 and Th2 cytokine balance during HIV-1 infection are indicative of an allergic response to viral proteins that may be reversed by Th2 cytokine inhibitors and immune response modifiers—a review and hypothesis. Virus Genes 2004; 28(1):5–18.

7 Notarangelo L, Casanova JL, Conley ME et al. Primary immunodeficiency diseases: an update from the International Union of Immunological Societies Primary Immunodeficiency Diseases Classification Committee Meeting in Budapest, 2005. J Allergy Clin Immunol 2006; 117(4):883–896.

8 Forschielli ML, Walker WA. The role of gut-associated lymphoid tissues and mucosal defence. Br J Nutr 2005; 93(Suppl 1):S41–S48.

9 Ogra PL, Welliver RC Sr. Effects of early environment on mucosal immunologic homeostasis, subsequent immune responses and disease outcome. Nestle Nutr Workshop Ser Pediatr Program 2008; 61:145–81.

10 Dietert RR. Developmental immunotoxicity: focus on health risks. Chem Res Toxicol 2009; 22(1):17–23.

11 Dietert RR. Developmental immunotoxicology (DIT) in drug safety testing: matching DIT testing to adverse outcomes and childhood disease risk. Curr Drug Saf 2008; 3(3):216–226.

12 Dietert RR, Zelikoff JT. Early-life environment, developmental toxicology and the risk of paediatric allergic disease including asthma. Birth Defects Res B Dev Reprod Toxicol 2008; 83(6):547–560.

13 Dietert RR, Dietert JM. Possible role for early life immune insult including developmental immunotoxicology in chronic fatigue syndrome (CFS) or myalgic encephalomyelitis (ME). Toxicology 2008; 247(1):61–72.

14 Dietert RR, Diertert JM. Early life immune insult and developmental immunotoxicity (DIT)-associated diseases: potential of herbal and fungal-derived medicinals. Curr Med Chem 2007; 14(10): 1075–1085.

15 Dietert RR. Developmental toxicology postnatal immune dysfunction and childhood leukaemia. Blood Cells Mol Dis 2009; 42(2):108–112.

16 Dietert RR, Dietert JM. Potential for early life immune insult including developmental immunotoxicity in autism and autism spectrum disorders: focus on critical windows of immune vulnerability. J Toxicol Environ Health B Crit Rev 2008; 11(8):660–680.

17 Irwen MR. Human psychoneuroimmunology: 20 years of discovery. Brain Behav Immun 2008; 22(2):129–139.

18 Ziemssen T, Kern S. Psychoneuroimmunology—cross-talk between the immune and nervous systems. J Neurol 2007; 254(Suppl 2):II/8–II/11.

19 Tausk F, Elenkov I, Moynihan J. Psychoneuro-immunology. Dermatol Ther 2008; 21(1):22–31.

20 Okamatsu Y, Matsuda K, Hiramoto I et al. Ghrelin and leptin modulate immunity and liver function in overweight children. Pediatr 2009; 51(1):9–13.

21 Epel ES. Psychological and metabolic stress: a recipe for accelerated cellular aging? Hormones (Athens) 2009; 8(1):7–22.

22 Miranda-Garduno LM, Reza-Albarran A. Obesity, inflammation and diabetes. Gac Med Mex 2008; 144(1):39–46.

23 Hofer T, Fontana L, Anton SD et al. Long-term effects of caloric restriction or exercise on DNA and RNA oxidation levels in white blood cells and urine in humans. Rejuvenation Res 2008; 11(4):793–799.

24 Benson S, Arck PC, Tan S et al. Effects of obesity on neuroendocrine, cardiovascular and immune cell responses to acute psychological stress in premenopausal women. Psychoneuroendocrinology 2009; 34(2):181–189.

25 Holvoet P. Relations between metabolic syndrome, on stress and inflammation and cardiovascular disease. Verh K Acad Geneeskd Belg 2008; 70(3): 193–219.

26 Martin SS, Qasim A, Reilly MP. Leptin resistance: a possible interface of inflammation and metabolism in obesity-related cardiovascular disease. J Am Coll Cardiology 2008; 52(15):1201–1210.

27 Fair AM, Montgomery K. Energy balance, physical activity and cancer risk. Methods Mol Biol 2009; 472:57–88.

28 Dixit VD. Adipose-immune interactions during obesity and caloric restriction: reciprocal mechanisms regulating immunity and health span. J Leukoc Biol 2008; 84(4):882–892.

29 Fontana L, Villareal DT, Weiss EP et al. Caloric restriction or exercise: effects on coronary heart disease risk factors. A randomized controlled trial. Am J Physiol Endocrinol Metab 2007; 293(1):E197–E202.

30 Crujeiras AB, Parra D, Milagro FI et al. Differential expression of oxidative stress and inflammation related

genes in peripheral mononuclear cells in response to a low-calorie diet: a nutrigenomics study. OMICS 2008; 12(4):251–261.
31 Imeri L, Opp MR. How (and why) the immune system makes us sleep. Nat Rev Neurosci 2009; 10(3):199–210.
32 Smyth CA. Evaluating sleep quality in older adults: the Pittsburgh Sleep Quality Index can be used to detect sleep disturbances or deficits. Am J Nurs 2008; 108(5):42–50.
33 Meerlo P, Sgoifo A, Suchecki D. Restricted and disrupted sleep: effects on autonomic function, neuroendocrine stress systems and stress responsivity. Sleep Med Rev 2008; 12(3):197–210.
34 Novati A, Roman V, Cetin T et al. Chronically restricted sleep leads to depression-like changes in neurotransmitter receptor sensitivity and neuroendocrine stress reactivity in rats. Sleep 2008; 31(11):1579–1585.
35 Preston BT, Capellini I, McNamara P et al. Parasite resistance and the adaptive significance of sleep. BMC Evol Biol 2009; 9:7.
36 Bentivoglio M, Kristensson K. Neural–immune interactions in disorders of sleep–wakefulness organisation. Trends Neurosci 2007; 30(12):645–652.
37 Roman V, Walstra I, Luiten PG et al. Too little sleep gradually desensitizes the serotonin 1A receptor system. Sleep 2005; 28(12):1505–1510.
38 Cohen S, Doyle WJ, Alper CM et al. Sleep habits and susceptibility to the common cold. Arch Intern Med 2009; 169(1):62–67.
39 Spaggiari MC. Sleep medicine in occupational health. G Ital Med Lav Ergon 2008; 30(3):276–279.
40 Cardinali DP, Esquifino AI, Srinivasan V et al. Melatonin and the immune system in aging. Neuroimmunomodulation 2008; 15(4–6): 272–278.
41 Kemeny ME, Schedlowski M. Understanding the interaction between psychological stress and immune-related diseases: a stepwise progression. Brain Behav Immun 2007; 21(8):1009–1018.
42 Reiche EM, Nunes SO, Morimoto HK. Stress, depression, the immune system and cancer. Lancet Oncol 2004; 5(10):617–625.
43 Reiche EM, Morimoto HK, Nunes SM. Stress and depression-induced immune dysfunction: implications for the development and progression of cancer. Int Rev Psychiatry 2005; 17(6):515–527.
44 Alves GJ, Palermo-Neto J. Neuroimmunomodulation: the cross-talk between nervous and immune systems. Rev Bras Psiquiatr 2007; 29(4):363–369.
45 Leonard B. Stress, depression and the activation of the immune system. World J Biol Psychiatry 2000; 1(1):17–25.
46 Mawdsley JE, Rampton DS. Psychological stress in IBD: new insights into pathogenic and therapeutic implications. Gut 2005; 54(10):1481–1491.
47 Olff M. Stress, depression and immunity: the role of defence and coping styles. Psychiatry Res 1999; 85(1):7–15.
48 Miller AH. Neuroendocrine and immune system interactions in stress and depression. Psychiatr Clin North Am 1998; 21(2):443–463.
49 Tausk F, Elenkov I, Moynihan J. Psychoneuro-immunology. Dermatol Ther 2008; 21(1):22–31.
50 Raison CL, Miller AH. The neuroimmunology of stress and depression. Semin Clin Neuropsychiatry 2001; 6(4):277–294.
51 Maunder RG, Levelstein S. The role of stress in the development and clinical course of irritable bowel disease: epidemiological evidence. Curr Mol Med 2008; 8(4):247–252.
52 Grippo AJ, Johnson AK. Stress, depression and cardiovascular dysregulation: a review of neurobiological mechanisms and the integration of research from preclinical disease models. Stress 2009; 12(1):1–21.
53 Gold SM, Irwin MR. Depression and immunity: inflammation and depressive symptoms in multiple sclerosis. Neurol Clin 2006; 24(3):507–519.
54 Karrow NA. Activation of the hypothalamic–pituitary–adrenal axis and autonomic nervous system during inflammation and altered programming of the neuroendocrine–immune axis during fetal and neonatal development: lessons learned from the model inflammagen, lipopolysaccharide. Brain Behav Immun 2006; 20(2):144–158.
55 McGregor BA, Antoni MH. Psychological intervention and health outcomes among women treated for breast cancer: a review of stress pathways and biological mediators. Brain Behav Immun 2009; 23(2):159–166.
56 Smith JE, Richardson J, Hoffman C et al. Mindfulness-based stress reduction as supportive therapy in cancer care: systematic review. J Adv Nurs 2005; 52(3): 315–327.
57 Witek-Janusek L, Albuquerque K, Chroniak KR et al. Effect of Mindfulness-based stress reduction on immune function, quality of life and coping in women newly-diagnosed with early stage breast cancer. Brain Behav Immun 2008; 22(6):969–981.
58 Carlson LE, Speca M, Faris P et al. One-year pre-post intervention follow-up of psychological, immune, endocrine and blood pressure outcomes of mindfulness-based stress reduction (MBSR) in breast and prostate cancer outpatients. Brain Behav Immun 2007; 21(8):1038–1049.
59 Carlson LE, Speca M, Patel KD et al. Mindfulness-based stress reduction in relation to quality of life, mood,

symptoms of stress and levels of cortisol, DHEA and melatonin in breast and prostate cancer outpatients. Psychoneuroendocrinology 2004; 29(4):448–474.
60 Carlson LE, Speca M, Patel KD et al. Mindfulness-based stress reduction in relation to quality of life, mood, symptoms of stress and immune parameters in breast and prostate cancer outpatients. Psychosom Med 2003; 65(4):571–581.
61 Ott MJ, Norris RL, Bauer-Wu SM. Mindfulness meditation for oncology patients: a discussion and critical review. Integr Cancer Ther 2006; 5(2):98–108.
62 Creswell JD, Myers HF, Cole SW et al. Mindfulness meditation training effects on CD4+ T lymphocytes in HIV-1 affected adults: a small randomized controlled trial. Brain Behav Immun 2009; 23(2):184–188.
63 Robinson FP, Mathews HL, Witek-Janusek L. Psycho-endocrine-immune response to mindfulness-based stress reduction in individuals infected with the human immunodeficiency virus: a quasiexperimental study. J Altern Comp Med 2003; 9(5):683–694.
64 Taylor DN. Effects of a behavioural stress management program on anxiety, mood, self-esteem and T-cell count in HIV-positive men. Psychol Rep 1995; 76(2):451–457.
65 Collins MP, Dunn LF. The effects of meditation and visual imagery on an immune system disorder: dermatomyositis. J Alt Comp Med 2005; 11(2):275–284.
66 Gruzelier J, Smith F, Nagy A. Cellular and humoral immunity, mood and exam stress: the influences of self-hypnosis and personality predictors. Int J Psychophysiol 2001; 42(1):55–71.
67 Cruess S, Antoni M, Cruess D et al. Reductions in HSV-2 Ab titres after CBT and relationships with neuroendocrine function, relaxation skills and social support in HIV-positive men. Psychosom Med 2000; 62(6):828–837.
68 Antoni MH, Cruess S, Cruess DG et al. Cognitive behaviour therapy reduces distress and 24-hour urinary cortisol output among symptomatic HIV-positive gay men. Ann Behav Med 2000; 22(1):29–37.
69 Antoni MH, Cruess DG, Cruess S et al. CBT effects on anxiety, 24-hour urinary norepinephrine output and T-cytotoxic/suppressor cells over time among symptomatic HIV-positive gay men. J Consult Clin Psychol 2000; 68(1):35–45.
70 Hidderley M, Holt M. A pilot RCT assessing the effects of autogenic training in early stage cancer patients in relation to psychological status and immune system responses. Eur J Oncol Nurs 2004; 8(1):61–65.
71 van der Pompe G, Antoni MH, Duivenvoorden HJ et al. An exploratory study into the effects of group psychotherapy on CV and immunoreactivity to acute stress in breast cancer patients. Psychother Psychosom 2001; 70(6):307–318.
72 Woods JA, Vieira VJ, Keylock KT. Exercise, inflammation and innate immunity. Immunol Allergy Clin North Am 2009; 29(2):381–393.
73 Schedlowski M, Schmidt RE. Stress and the immune system. Naturwissenschaften 1996; 83(5):214–220.
74 Kizaki T, Takemasa T, Sakurai T et al. Adaptation of macrophages to exercise training improves innate immunity. Biochem Biophys Res Commun 2008; 372(1):152–156.
75 Timmons BW, Cieslak T. Human NK cell subsets and acute exercise: a brief review. Exerc Immunol Rev 2008; 14:8–23.
76 de Lima C, Alves LE, Iagher F et al. Anaerobic exercise reduces tumour growth, cancer cachexia and increases macrophage and lymphocyte response in Walker 256 tumour-bearing rats. Eur J Appl Physiol 2008; 104(6):957–964.
77 Sakamoto Y, Ueki S, Kasai T et al. Effect of exercise, aging and functional capacity on acute sIgA response in elderly people over 75 years of age. Geriatr Gerontol Int 2009; 9(1):81–88.
78 Bishop NC, Gleeson M. Acute and chronic effects of exercise on markers of mucosal immunity. Front Biosci 2009;14:4444–4456.
79 Gleeson M, Pyne DB. Special feature for the Olympics: effects of exercise on the immune system: exercise effects on mucosal immunity. Immunol Cell Biol 2000; 78(5):536–544.
80 Moreira A, Arsati F, Cury PR et al. The impact of a 17-day training period for an international championship on mucosal immune parameters in top-level basketball players and staff members. Eur J Oral Sci 2008; 116(5):431–437.
81 West NP, Pyne DB, Kyd JM et al. The effect of exercise on innate mucosal immunity. Br J Sports Med 2010; 44:227–231.
82 Nieman DC, Henson DA, McMahon M et al. Beta-glucan, immune function and URTI in athletes. Med Sci Sports Exerc 2008; 40(8):1463–1471.
83 Close P, Thielen V, Bury T. Mucosal immunity in elite athletes. Rev Med Liege 2003; 58(9):548–553.
84 Kjellgren A, Bood SA, Axelsson K et al. Wellness through a comprehensive yogic breathing program: a controlled pilot trial. BMC Comp Altern Med 2007; 7:43.
85 Sharma H, Datta P, Singh A et al. Gene expression profiling in practitioners of Sudarshan Kriya (rhythmic breathing practice). J Psychosom Res 2008; 64(2):213–218.
86 Sharma H, Sen S, Singh A. Sudarshan Kriya practitioners exhibit better antioxidant status and lower blood lactate levels. Biol Psychol 2003; 63(3):281–291.
87 Kochupillai V, Kumar P, Singh D et al. Effect of rhythmic breathing (Sudarshan Kriya and Pranayam) on immune function and tobacco addiction. Ann NY Acad Sci 2005; 1056:242–252.

88 Rao RM, Telles S, Nagendra HR et al. Effects of yoga on natural killer cell counts in early breast cancer patients undergoing conventional treatment. Med Sci Monit 2008; 14(2):LE3–4.
89 Manzaneque JM, Vera FM, Maldonado EF et al. Assessment of immunological parameters following a qigong training program. Med Sci Monit 2004; 10(6):CR264–CR270.
90 Li QZ, Li P, Garcia GE et al. Genomic profiling of neutrophil transcripts in Asian qigong practitioners: a pilot study in gene regulation by MB interaction. J Altern Complement Med 2005; 11(1):29–39.
91 Jones BM. Changes in cytokine production in healthy subjects practicing Guolin qigong: a pilot study. BMC Comp Altern Med 2001; 1:8.
92 Manzanaque JM, Vera FM, Rodriguez FM et al. Serum cytokines, mood and sleep after a qigong program: is qigong an effective psychobiological tool? J Health Psychol 2009; 14(1):60–67.
93 Hernandez-Reif M, Field T, Ironson G et al. Natural killer cells and lymphocytes increase in women with breast cancer following massage therapy. Int J Neurosci 2005; 115(4):495–510.
94 Hernandez-Reif M, Ironson G, Field T et al. Breast cancer patients have improved immune and neuroendocrine functions following massage therapy. J Psychosom Res 2004; 57(1):45–52.
95 Billhult A, Lindholm C, Gunnarsson R et al. The effect of massage on cellular immunity, endocrine and psychological factors in women with breast cancer: a randomized controlled trial. Auton Neurosci 2008; 140(1/2):88–95.
96 Jyonouchi H. Non-IgE mediated food allergy. Inflamm Allergy Drug Targets 2008; 7(3):173–180.
97 Jyonouchi H, Sun S et al. Innate immunity associated with inflammatory responses with cytokine production against common dietary proteins in patients with autism spectrum disorder. Neuropsychobiology 2002; 46(2):76–84.
98 Diaz LE, Montero A, Gonzalez-Gross M et al. Influence of alcohol consumption on immunological status: a review. Eur J Clin Nutr 2002; 56(Suppl 3): S50–S53.
99 Magrone T, Candore G, Caruso C et al. Polyphenols from red wine modulate immune responsiveness: biological and clinical significance. Curr Pharm Des 2008; 14(26):2733–2748.
100 Putics A, Vegh EM, Csermely P et al. Resveratrol induces the heat-shock response and protects human cells from severe heat stress. Antiox Redox Signal 2008; 10(1):65–75.
101 Falchetti R, Fuggetta MP, Lanzilli G et al. Effects of resveratrol on human immune cell function. Life Sci 2001; 70(1):81–96.
102 Monobe M, Ema K, Kato F et al. Immunostimulating activity of a crude polysaccharide derived from green tea extract. J Agric Food Chem 2008; 56(4):1423–1427.
103 Katiyer SK. Skin photoprotection by green tea: antioxidant and immunomodulatory effects. Curr Drug Targets Immune Endocr Metabol Disord 2003; 3(3):234–242.
104 Kipen HM, Fiedler N. Environmental factors in medically unexplained symptoms and related syndromes: the evidence and the challenge. Environ Health Perspect 2002; 110(Suppl 4):597–599.
105 Krewski D, Glickman BW, Habash RW et al. Recent advances in research on radio frequency fields and health: 2001–2003. J Toxicol Environ Health B Crit Rev 2007; 10(4):287–318.
106 Valberg PA, van Deventer TE, Repacholi MH. Workgroup report: base stations and wireless networks RF exposures and health consequences. Environ Health Perspect 2007; 115(3):416–424.
107 Knave B. Electromagnetic fields and health outcomes. Ann Acad Med Singapore 2001; 30(5):489–493.
108 Bonhomme-Fivre L, Marion S, Bezie Y et al. Study of human neurovegetative and haematological effects of environmental low-frequency (50 Hz) electromagnetic fields produced by transformers. Arch Environ Health 1998; 53(2):87–92.
109 Hardell L, Sage C. Biological effects from electromagnetic field exposure and public exposure standards. Biomed Pharmacother 2008; 62(2):104–109.
110 Fukuyama T, Ueda H, Hayashi K et al. Detection of low-level environmental chemical allergy by a long-term sensitization method. Toxicol Lett 2008; 180(1):1–8.
111 Dietert RR, Hedge A. Chemical sensitivity and the immune system: a paradigm to approach potential immune involvement. Neurotoxicology 1998; 19(2):253–257.
112 Bernstein DI. MCS: state of the art symposium. the role of chemical allergens. Regul Toxicol Pharmacol 1996; 24(1 Pt 2):S28–S31.
113 Laumbach RJ, Kipen HM. Bioaerosols and SBS: particles, inflammation and allergy. Curr Opin Allergy Clin Immunol 2005; 5(2):135–139.
114 Gray MR, Thrasher JD, Crago R et al. Mixed mould mycotoxicosis: immunological changes in humans following exposure in water-damaged buildings. Arch Environ Health 2003; 58(7):410–420.
115 Lander F, Meyer HW, Norn S. Serum IgE specific to indoor moulds, measured by basophil histamine release, is associated with building-related symptoms in damp buildings. Inflamm Res 2001; 50(4):227–231.
116 Kilburn KH. Summary of the 5th International Conference on Bioaerosols, Fungi, Bacteria, Mycotoxins and Human Health. Arch Environ Health 2003; 58(8):538–542.

117 Edmondson DA, Nordness ME, Zacharisen MC et al. Allergy and toxic mould syndrome. Ann Allergy Asthma Immunol 2005; 94(2):234–239.
118 Miller R. Thimerosal, micromercurialism and chronic fatigue syndrome. Med Hypotheses 2005; 64(5): 1063–1064.
119 Uter W. Chronic fatigue syndrome and nickel allergy. Contact Dermatitis 2000; 42(1):56–57.
120 Hon KL, Wang SS, Hung EC et al. Serum levels of heavy metals in childhood eczema and skin diseases: Friends or foes. Pediatr Allergy Immunol 2010; 19 Mar. [Epub ahead of print]
121 Cabioglu MT, Cetin BE. Acupuncture and immune modulation. Am J Chin Med 2008; 36(1):25–36.
122 Peng G, Zhen Ci, Yan J. Acupuncture and innate immunity. 2008; 33(1):49–52.
123 Du J, Zhen Ci, Yan J. The messengers from PNS to CNS: involvement of neurotrophins and cytokines in the mechanisms of acupuncture. 2008; 33(1):37–40.
124 Kavoussi B, Ross BE. The neuroimmune basis of anti-inflammatory acupuncture. Integr Cancer Ther 2007; 6(3):251–257.
125 Yamaguchi N, Takahashi T, Sakuma M et al. A regulates leukocyte subpopulations in human peripheral blood. Evid Based Comp Altern Med 2007; 4(4):447–453.
126 Wang JR, Chen XR, Zhang Q et al. Effect of moxibustion on immunological function in the patient of AIDS in spleen-kidney yang deficiency. Zhongguo Zhen Jiu 2007; 27(12):892–894.
127 Chandra RK. Nutrition and the immune system: an introduction. Am J Clin Nutr 1997; 66(2):S260–S263.
128 Harbige LS. Nutrition and immunity with emphasis on infection and autoimmune disease. Nutr Health 1996; 10(4):285–312.
129 Ferencik M, Ebringer L. Modulatory effects of Selenium and Zinc on the immune system. Folia Microbiol (Praha) 2003; 48(3):417–426.
130 Maggini S, Wintergerst ES, Beveridge S et al. Selected vitamins and trace elements support immune function by strengthening epithelial barriers and cellular and humoral immune responses. Br J Nutr 2007; 98 (Suppl 1):S28–S35.
131 Wintergerst ES, Maggini S, Hornig DH. Contribution of selected vitamins and trace elements to immune function. Ann Nutr Metab 2007; 51(4):301–323.
132 Pai R, Kang G. Microbes in the gut: a digestable account of host–symbiont interactions. Indian J Med Res 2008; 128(5):587–594.
133 Tsuji M, Suzuki K, Kinoshita K et al. Dynamic interactions between bacteria and immune cells leading to IgA synthesis. Semin Immunol 2008; 20(1):59–66.
134 Suzuli K, Fagarasan S. How host–bacterial interactions lead to IgA synthesis in the gut. Trends Immunol 2008; 29(11):523–531.
135 Mora JR, von Andrian UH. Role of retinoic acid in the imprinting of gut-homing IgA-secreting cells. Semin Immunol 2009; 21(1):28–35.
136 Mason KL, Huffnagle GB, Noverr MC et al. Overview of gut immunology. Adv Exp Med Biol 2008; 635:1–14.
137 Bodera P. Influence of probiotics on the human immune system (GALT). Recent Pat Inflamm Allergy Drug Discov 2008; 2(2):149–153.
138 Bodera P, Chcialowski A. Immunomodulatory effect of probiotic bacteria. Recent Pat Inflamm Allergy Drug Discov 2009; 3(1):58–64.
139 Singh V, Singh K, Amdekar S et al. Innate and specific gut-associated immunity and microbial interference. FEMS Immunol Med Microbiol 2009; 55(1):6–12.
140 Guarner F. Inulin and oligofructose: impact on intestinal diseases and disorders. Br J Nutr 2005; 93(Suppl 1):S61–S65.
141 Mazzatti DJ, Uciechowski P, Hebel S et al. Effects of long-term zinc supplementation and deprivation on gene expression in human THP-1 mononuclear cells. J Trace Elem Med Biol 2008; 22(4):325–336.
142 Heyland DK, Jones N, Cvijanovich NZ et al. Zinc supplementation in critically ill patients: a key pharmaconutrient? J Parenter Enteral Nutr 2008; 32(5):509–519.
143 Mocchegiani E, Malavolta M, Muti E et al. Zinc, metallothioneins and longevity: inter-relationships with niacin and selenium. Curr Pharm Des 2008; 14(26):2719–2732.
144 Franklin RB, Costello LC. The important role of the apoptotic effects of zinc in the development of cancers. J Cell Biochem 2009; 106(5):750–757.
145 Prasad AS. Zinc in human health: effect of zinc on immune cells. Mol Med 2008; 14(5/6):353–357.
146 Prasad AS. Zinc: mechanisms of host defence. Am J Nutr 2007; 137:1345–1349.
147 Overbeck S, Uciechowski P, Ackland ML et al. Intracellular zinc homeostasis in leukocyte subsets is regulated by different expression of zinc exporters ZnT-1 to ZnT-9. J Leukoc Biol 2008; 83(2):368–380.
148 Haase H, Mazzatti DJ, White A et al. Differential gene expression after zinc supplementation and deprivation in human leukocyte subsets. Mol Med 2007; 13(7/8):362–370.
149 Haase H, Overbeck S, Rink L. Zinc supplementation for the treatment or prevention of disease: current status and future perspectives. Exp Gerontol 2008; 43(5):394–408.
150 Wang L, Wildt KF, Castro E et al. The zinc-finger transcription factor Zbtb7b represses CD8-lineage gene expression in peripheral CD4+ T-cells. Immunity 2008; 29(6):876–887.
151 Hermann-Kleiter N, Gruber T, Lutz-Nicoladoni C et al. The nuclear orphan receptor NR2F6 suppresses

lymphocyte activation and T-helper 17-dependent autoimmunity. Immunity 2008; 29(2):205–216.
152 Haase H, Ober-Blobaum JL, Engelhardt G et al. Zinc signals are essential for lipopolysaccharide-induced signal transduction in monocytes. J Immunol 2008; 181(9):6491–6502.
153 Prasad AS. Clinical, immunological, anti-inflammatory and anti-oxidant roles of zinc. Exp Gerontol 2008; 43(5):370–377.
154 Uciechowski P, Kahmann L, Plumakers B et al. Th1 and Th2 cell polarization increases with aging and is modulated by zinc supplementation. Exp Gerontol 2008; 43(5):493–498.
155 Varin A, Larbi A, Dedoussis GV et al. In vitro and in vivo effects of zinc on cytokine signalling in human T-cells. Exp Gerontol 2008; 43(5):472–482.
156 Mariani E, Neri S, Cattini L et al. Effect of zinc supplementation on plasma IL-6 and MCP-1 production and NK cell function in healthy elderly: interactive influence of +647 MT1a and −174 IL-6 polymorphic alleles. Exp Gerontol 2008; 43(5):462–471.
157 Finamore A, Massimi M, Conti Devirgillis L et al. Zinc deficiency induces membrane barrier damage and increases neutrophil transmigration in Caco-2 cells. J Nutr 2008; 138(9):1664–1670.
158 Vasto S, Mocchegiani E, Malavolta M et al. Zinc and the inflammatory/immune response in aging. Ann NY Acad Sci 2007; 1100:111–122.
159 Caruso TJ, Prober CG, Gwaltney JM Jr. Treatment of naturally acquired common colds with zinc: a structured review. Clin Infact Dis 2007; 45(5): 569–574.
160 Wintergerst ES, Maggini S, Hornig DH. Immune-enhancing role of vitamin C and zinc and effect on clinical conditions. Ann Nutr Metab 2006; 50(2):85–94.
161 Lukacik M, Thomas RL, Aranda JV. A meta-analysis of the effects of oral zinc in the treatment of acute and persistent diarrhoea. Pediatrics 2008; 121(2):326–336.
162 Scrimgeour AG, Lukaski HC. Zinc and diarrhoeal disease: current status and future perspectives. Curr Opin Clin Nutr Metab Care 2008; 11(6):711–717.
163 Cuevas LE, Koyanagi A. Zinc and infection: a review. Ann Trop Paediatr 2005; 25(3):149–160.
164 Zhu B, Symonds AL, Martin JE et al. Early growth response gene (Egr-2) controls the self-tolerance of T-cells and prevents the development of lupus-like autoimmune disease. J Exp Med 2008; 205(10): 2295–2307.
165 Rathinam C, Lassmann H, Mengel M et al. Transcription factor Gfi1 restricts B-cell mediated autoimmunity. J Immunol 2008; 181(9):6222–6229.
166 Moro JR, Iwata M, von Andriano UH. Vitamin effects on the immune system: vitamin A and D take centre stage. Nat Rev Immunol 2008; 8(9):685–698.
167 Pino-lagos K, Benson MJ, Noelle RJ. Retinoic acid in the immune system. Ann NY Acad Sci 2008; 1143:170–187.
168 Kim CH. Roles of retinoic acid in induction of immunity and immune tolerance. Endocr Metab Immune Disord Drug Targets 2008; 8(4):289–294.
169 Bos JD, Spuls PI. Topical treatments in psoriasis: today and tomorrow. Clin Dermatol 2008; 26(5):432–437.
170 Ross AC. Vitamin A supplementation and retinoic acid treatment in the regulation of antibody responses in vivo. Vitamin Horm 2007; 75:197–222.
171 Ahmad SM, Haskell MJ, Raqib R et al. Markers of innate immune function are associated with vitamin A stores in men. J Nutr 2009; 139(2):377–385.
172 Albers R, Bol M, Bleumink R et al. Effects of supplementation with vitamins A, C, E, selenium and zinc on immune function in a murine sterilised model. Nutrition 2003; 19(11/12):940–946.
173 Hoffman PR, Berry MJ. The influence of selenium on immune responses. Mol Nutr Food Res 2008; 52(11):1273–1280.
174 Hoffman PR. Mechanisms by which selenium influences immune responses. Arch Immunol Ther Exp 2007; 55(5):289–297.
175 Ferencik M, Ebringer L. Modulatory effects of selenium and zinc on the immune system. Folia Microbiol (Praha) 2003; 48(3):417–426.
176 Sinha R, El-Bayoumy K. Apoptosis is a critical cellular event in cancer chemoprevention by selenium compounds. Curr Cancer Drug Targets 2004; 4(1):13–28.
177 Naithani R. Organoselenium compounds in cancer chemoprevention. Mini Rev Med Chem 2008; 8(7): 657–668.
178 Rikiishi H. Apoptotic cellular events for selenium compounds involved in cancer prevention. J Bioenerg Biomembr 2007; 39(1):91–98.
179 Rayman MP. The argument for increasing selenium intake. Proc Nutr Soc 2002; 61(2):203–215.
180 Rayman MP. The importance of selenium to human health. Lancet 2000; 356(9225):233–241.
181 Luty-Frackiewicz A. The role of selenium in cancer and viral infection prevention. Int J Occup Med Environ Health 2005; 18(4):305–311.
182 Khalili H, Soudbakhsh A, Hajiabdolbaghi M et al. Nutritional status and serum zinc and selenium levels in Iranian HIV-infected individuals. BMC Infect Dis 2008; 8:165.
183 Mocchegiani E, Malavolta M, Muti E et al. Zinc, metallothioneines and longevity: interrelationships with niacin and selenium. Curr Pharm Des 2008; 14(26):2719–2732.
184 Naithani R. Organoselenium compounds in cancer chemoprevention. Mini Rev Med Chem 2008; 8(7): 657–668.

185 Rayman MP. Selenium in cancer prevention: a review of the evidence and mechanism of action. Proc Nutr Soc 2005; 64(4):527–542.
186 Combs GF Jr, Clark LC, Turnball BW. An analysis of cancer prevention by selenium. Biofactors 2001; 14 (1–4):153–159.
187 Deruelle F, Baron B. Vitamin C: is supplementation necessary for optimal health? J Altern Comp Med 2008; 14(10):1291–1298.
188 Padayatty SJ, Katz A, Wang Y et al. Vitamin C as an antioxidant: evaluation of its role in disease prevention. J Am Coll Nutr 2003; 22(1):18–35.
189 Strohle A, Hahn A. Vitamin C and immune function. Med Monatsschr Pharm 2009; 32(2):49–54.
190 Douglas RM, Hemilia H, Chalker E et al. Vitamin C for preventing and treating the common cold. Cochrane Database Syst Rev 2007; 3:CD000980.
191 Holick MF, Chen TC. Vitamin D deficiency: a worldwide problem with health consequences. Am J Clin Nutr 2008; 87(4):S1080–S1086.
192 Holick MF. Sunlight and vitamin D for bone health and prevention of autoimmune diseases, cancers and cardiovascular disease. Am J Clin Nutr 2004; 80(6 Suppl):S1678–S1688.
193 Holick MF. Vitamin D: importance in the prevention of cancers, type 1 diabetes mellitus, heart disease and osteoporosis. Am J Clin Nutr 2004; 79(3):362–371.
194 Kurylowicz A, Bednarczuk T, Nauman J. The influence of vitamin D deficiency on cancers and autoimmune disease development. Endokrynol Pol 2007; 58(2): 140–152.
195 Wagner CL, Taylor SN, Hollis BW. Does vitamin D make the world go round? Breastfeed Med 2008; 3(4):239–250.
196 Szodoray P, Nakken B, Gaal J et al. The complex role of vitamin D in autoimmune disease. Scand J Immunol 2008; 68(3):261–269.
197 Hayes CE, Nashold FE, Spach KM et al. The immunological functions of the vitamin D endocrine system. Cell Mol Biol 2003; 29(2):277–300.
198 Cantorna MT. Vitamin D and its role in immunology: multiple sclerosis and irritable bowel disease. Prog Biophys Mol Biol 2006; 92(1):60–64.
199 Lips P. Vitamin D physiology. Prog Biophys Mol Biol 2006; 92(1):4–8.
200 Holick MF. Vitamin D: important for prevention of osteoporosis, cardiovascular disease, insulin dependent diabetes mellitus, autoimmune diseases and some cancers. South Med J 2005; 98(10):1024–1027.
201 de Luca HF. Evolution of our understanding of vitamin D. Nutr Rev 2008; 66(10 Suppl 2):S73–S87.
202 Reichrath J. The challenge resulting from positive and negative effects of sunlight: how much solar ultraviolet exposure is appropriate to balance between risks of vitamin D deficiency and skin cancer? Prog Biophys Mol Biol 2006; 92(1):9–16.
203 Peyrin-Biroulet L, Oussalah A, Bigard MA. Crohn's disease: the hot hypothesis. Med Hypotheses 2009; 73(1):94–96.
204 Holick MF. Vitamin D and sunlight: strategies for cancer prevention and other health benefits. Clin J Am Soc Nephrol 2008; 3(5):1548–1554.
205 Arnson Y, Amital H, Shoenfeld Y. Vitamin D and autoimmunity: new aetiological and therapeutic considerations. Ann Rheum Dis 2007; 66(9):1137–1142.
206 Cantorna MT, Mahon BD. Mounting evidence for vitamin D as an environmental factor affecting autoimmune disease prevalence. Exp Biol Med 2004; 229(11):1136–1142.
207 Du T, Zhou ZG, You S et al. Regulation by vitamin D_3 on altered toll-like receptor expression and response to ligands of monocyte from autoimmune diabetes. Clin Chim Acta 2009; 402(1/2):133–138.
208 Smolders J, Damoiseaux J, Menheere P et al. Fok-1 Vitamin D receptor gene polymorphism and vitamin D metabolism in multiple sclerosis. J Neuroimmunol 2009; 207(1/2):117–121.
209 Cantorna MT: Vitamin D and autoimmunity: is Vitamin D status an environmental factor affecting autoimmune disease prevalence? Proc Soc Exp Biol Med 2000; 223(3):230–233.
210 Lucas RM, Ponsonby AL, Pasco JA et al. Future health implications of prenatal and early-life vitamin D status. Nutr Rev 2008; 66(12):710–720.
211 Uren LJ, McKenzie G, Moriarty H. Evaluation of iodine levels in the Riverina poulation. Aust J Rural Health 2008; 16(2):109–114.
212 Gago-Dominguez M, Castelao JE. Role of lipid peroxidation and oxidative stress in the association between thyroid diseases and breast cancer. Crit Rev Oncol Hematol 2008; 68(2):107–114.
213 Stoddard FR II, Brooks AD, Eskin BA et al. Iodine alters gene expression in the MCF-7 breast cancer cell line: evidence for an anti-oestrogenic effect of iodine. Int J Med Sci 2008; 5(4):189–196.
214 Eskin BA. Iodine and mammary dysplasia. Adv Exp Med Biol 1977; 91:293–304.
215 Eskin BA, Grotkowski CE, Connoly CP et al. Different tissue responses for iodine and iodide in rat thyroid and mammary glands. Biol Trace Elem Res 1995; 49:9–19.
216 Strum JM. Effect of iodide-deficiency on rat mammary gland. Virchows Arch B Cell Pathol Inc Mol Pathol 1979; 30:209–220.
217 Anguiano B, Garcia-Solis P, Delgado G et al. Uptake and gene expression with antitumoural doses of iodine in thyroid and mammary gland: evidence that chronic administration has no harmful effects. Thyroid 2007; 17(9):851–859.

218 Arroya-Helguera O, Rojas E, Delgado G et al. Signalling pathways involved in the antiproliferative effect of molecular iodine in normal and tumoural breast-cells: evidence that 6 IL mediates apoptotic effects. Endocr Relat Cancer 2008; 15(4):1003–1011.
219 Cho WC, Leung KN. In vitro and in vivo immunomodulating and imunorestorative effects of *A. membranaceus*. J Ethnopharmacol 2007; 113(1):132–141.
220 Tan BK. Immunomodulatory and antimicrobial effects of some traditional Chinese medicine herbs: a review. Curr Med Chem 2004; 11(11):1423–1430.
221 Shao BM, Xu W, Dai H et al. A study on the immune receptors for polysaccharides from the roots of *A. membranaceus*, a Chinese medicinal herb. Biochem Biophys Res Commun 2004; 320(4):1103–1111.
222 Wei H, Sun R, Xiao W et al. Traditional Chinese medicine *Astragalus* reverses predominance of Th2 cytokines and their up-stream transcript factors in lung cancer patients. Oncol Rep 2003; 10(5):1507–1512.
223 Mao SP, Cheng KL, Zhou YF. Modulatory effects of *Astragalus membranaceus* on Th1/Th2 cytokine in patients with herpes simplex keratitis. Zhongguo Zhong Xi Yi Jie He Za Zhi 2004; 24(2):121–123.
224 Wang G, Liu CT, Wang ZL et al. Effects of *Astragalus membranaceus* in producing T-helper cell type 1 polarization and IFN gamma production by upregulating T-bet expression in patients with asthma. Chin J Integr Med 2006; 12(4):262–267.
225 Shan HH, Wang K, Li W et al. *Astragalus membranaceus* prevents airway hyperreactivity in mice related to Th2 inhibition. J Ethnopharmacol 2008; 116(2):363–369.
226 Du Q, Chen Z, Zhou LF et al. Inhibitory effects of astragaloside IV on ovalbumin-induced chronic experimental asthma. Can J Physiol Pharmacol 2008; 86(7):449–457.
227 Cho WC, Leung KN. In vitro and in vivo anti-tumour effects of *Astragalus membranaceus*. Cancer Lett 2007; 252(1):43–54.
228 Block KI, Mead MN. Immune system effects of echinacea, ginseng and astragalus: a review. Integr Cancer Ther 2003; 2(3):247–267.
229 Dong J, Gu HL, Ma CT et al. Effects of large dose of AM on the dendritic cell induction of peripheral mononuclear cell and antigen-presenting ability of dendritic cells in children with acute leukaemia. Zhongguo Zhong Xi Yi Jie He Za Zhi 2005; 25(10): 872–875.
230 Taixang W, Munro AJ, Guanjian L. Chinese medical herbs for chemotherapy side-effects in colorectal cancer patients. Cochrane Database Syst Rev 2005; 1:CD004540.
231 Nergard CS, Solhaug V. Cranberries for prevention of recurrent urinary tract infections. Tidsskr Nor Laegoforen 2009; 129(4):303–304.
232 Feldman M, Weiss E, Shemesh M et al. Cranberry constituents affect fructosyltransferase expression in *Streptococcus mutans*. Altern Ther Health Med 2009; 15(2):32–38.
233 Lavigne JP, Bourg G, Combescure C et al. In-vitro and in-vivo evidence of dose-dependent decrease of uropathogenic *Escherichia coli* virulence after consumption of commercial *Vaccinium macrocarpon* (cranberry) capsules. Clin Microbiol Infect 2008; 14(4):350–355.
234 Jepson RG, Craig JC. Cranberries for preventing urinary tract infections. Cochrane Database Syst Rev 2008; 1:CD001321.
235 Linde K, Barrett B, Wolkart K. Echinacea for preventing and treating the common cold. Cochrane Database Syst Rev 2006; 1:CD000530.
236 Braun L. Honey: a sweet skin healer. J Complement Med 2003; 2(1):54–56.
237 Lusby PE, Coombes A, Wilkinson JM. Honey: a potent agent for wound healing? J Wound Ostomy Continence Nurse 2002; 29(6):296–300.
238 Jull, AB, Rodgers A, Walker N. Honey as a topical treatment for wounds. Cochrane Database Syst Rev 2008; 4:CD005083.
239 Jull AB, Rodgers A, Paraq V et al. Randomized trial of honey-impregnated dressing for venous ulcers. Br J Surg 2008; 95(2):175–182.
240 Evans J, Flavin S. Honey: a guide for healthcare professionals. Br J Nurs 2008; 17(15):S24, S26, S28–S30.

chapter 33

Joints and connective tissues

INTRODUCTION

In order to diagnose and manage the patient presenting with musculoskeletal symptoms, it is important to distinguish whether the pathology is arising primarily in the so-called hard tissues (such as bone) or the soft tissues (such as cartilage, disc, synovium, capsule, muscle, tendon, tendon sheath). It is also important to distinguish between the two most common causes of musculoskeletal symptoms, namely inflammatory and degenerative.

HISTORY AND EXAMINATION

The history and physical examination are the two most important components of the diagnostic process for identifying the cause of musculoskeletal symptoms, and pattern recognition is the key to diagnosis.

- *Do the symptoms arise in the musculoskeletal system, or from a disease in another system (e.g. neurological, vascular, endocrine)?* In some musculoskeletal conditions, the disease may be multi-system in origin—for example, carpal tunnel syndrome may be due to entrapment of the median nerve by tenosynovitis, or associated with hypothyroidism, diabetes, obesity or pregnancy.
- *Is it an articular or non-articular process?* Once the doctor has established that the disorder originates in the joints, the history and examination will help to identify a diagnostic pattern (see Box 33.1).

Some arthropathies present with an acute onset of pain, with peak intensity reached within hours or days; in others it occurs gradually over weeks to months. The clinical pattern may be monarticular, oligoarticular or polyarticular. Variations of these patterns may occur within the same disorder. For example, rheumatoid arthritis may present as an acute monarthritis of the knee before spreading to other joints, or as an acute polyarthritis. Although almost any arthropathy may begin as a monarthritis, the initial pattern of certain disorders is characteristically monarticular, with pain, redness and swelling. Certain diagnoses, such as infection or crystal arthritis, should be suspected in this situation (see Box 33.2). Infectious monarthritis is an important diagnosis to make early, as joint damage can occur if untreated.

Chronic monarthritis is the presenting manifestation of a variety of joint disorders, some of which are listed in Box 33.3. Involvement of two to four joints is usually

BOX 33.1 Major features for diagnosis of joint disease

Mode of onset
- acute

Duration of symptoms
- chronic

Number of affected joints
- monarthritis
- oligoarthritis (2–4 joints)
- polyarthritis

Distribution of joint involvement
- symmetric
- asymmetric

Localisation of affected joints
- axial
- peripheral
- both

BOX 33. 2 The acute hot joint

Infectious
- bacterial
- mycobacterial

Crystal-induced
- gout
- CPPD (pseudogout)

Traumatic

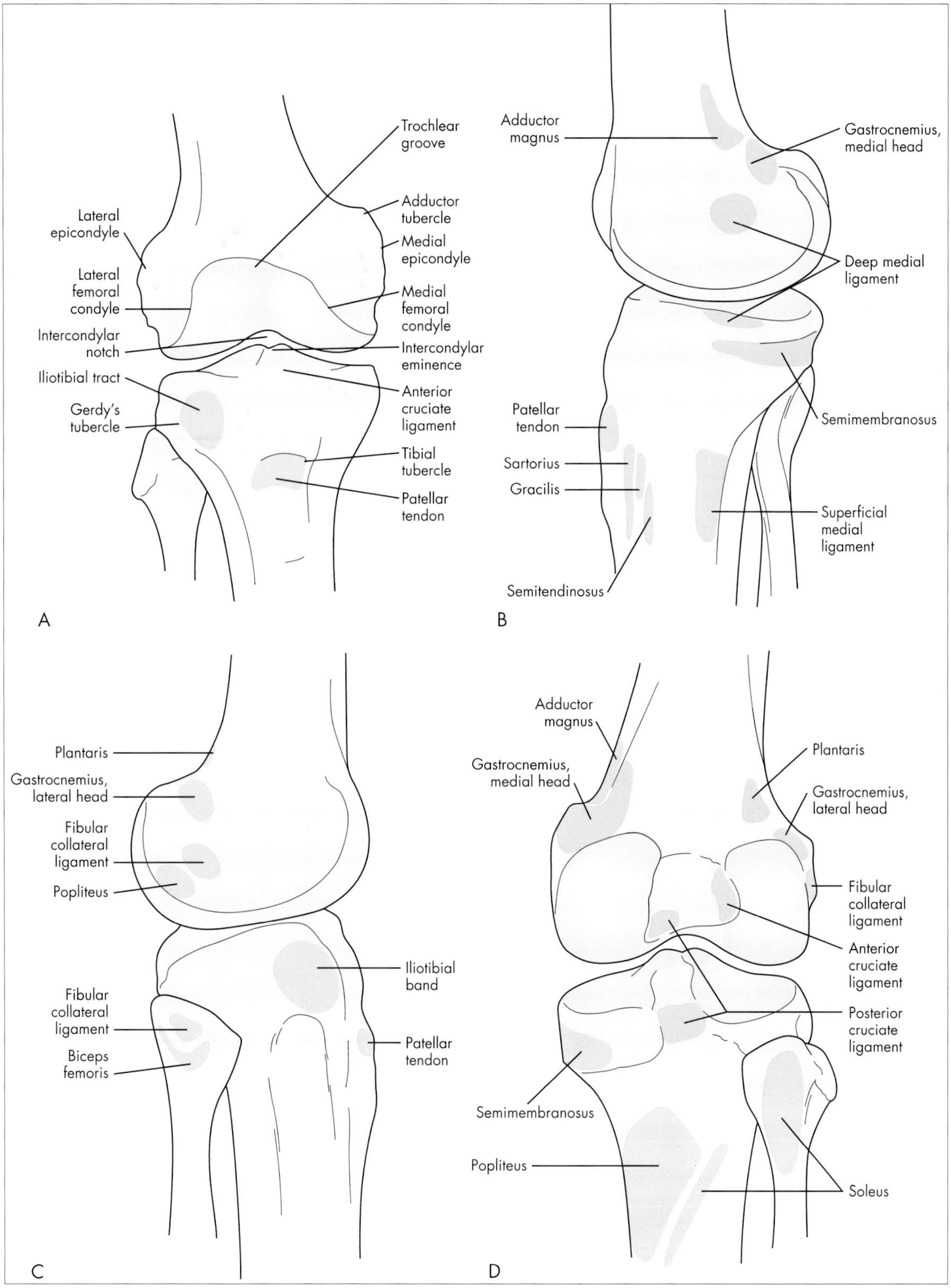

FIGURE 33.1 Anatomy of knee: **A** anterior, **B** medial, **C** lateral and **D** posterior views

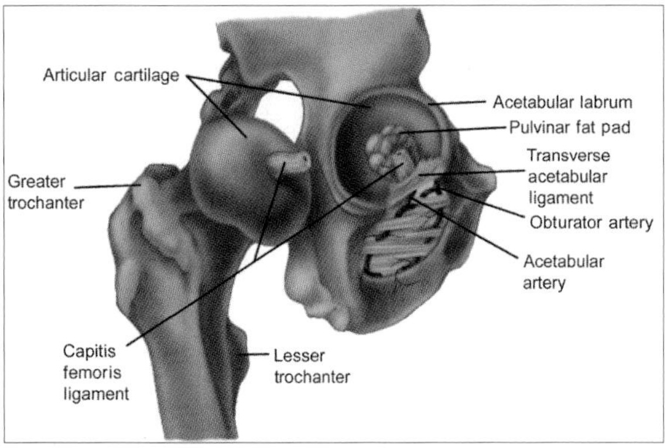

FIGURE 33.2 Anatomy of hip

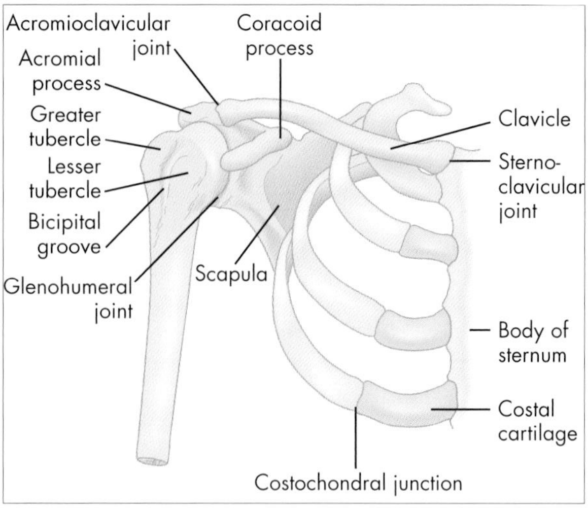

FIGURE 33.4 Anatomy of shoulder

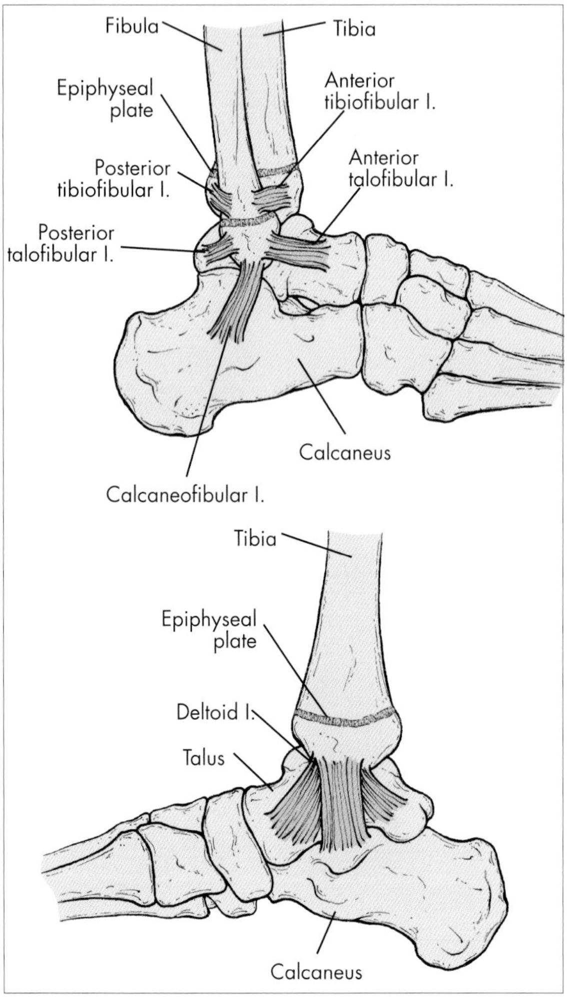

FIGURE 33.3 Anatomy of ankle

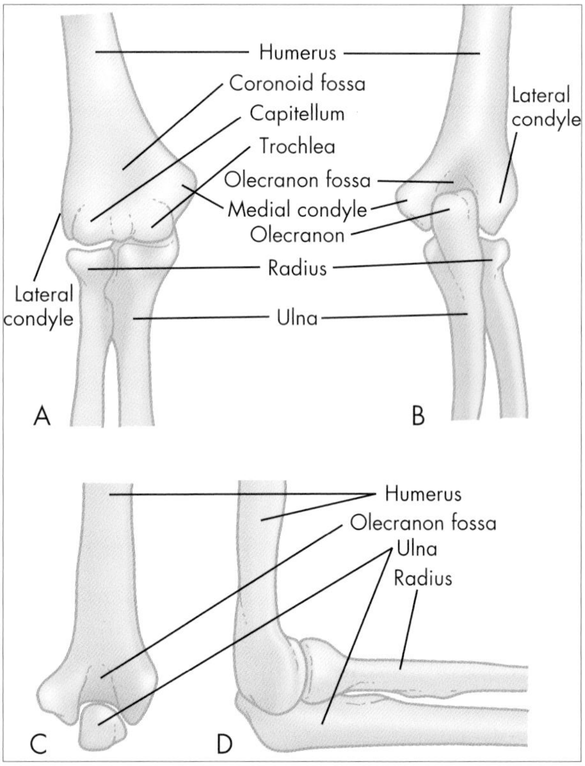

FIGURE 33.5 Anatomy of right elbow: **A, B** anterior and posterior views; **C** posterior view with 90° flexion; **D** lateral view

referred to as *oligoarthritis*. There are a number of conditions in which involvement of two or three joints rather than one may significantly narrow the differential diagnosis, including pseudogout and psoriatic arthritis.

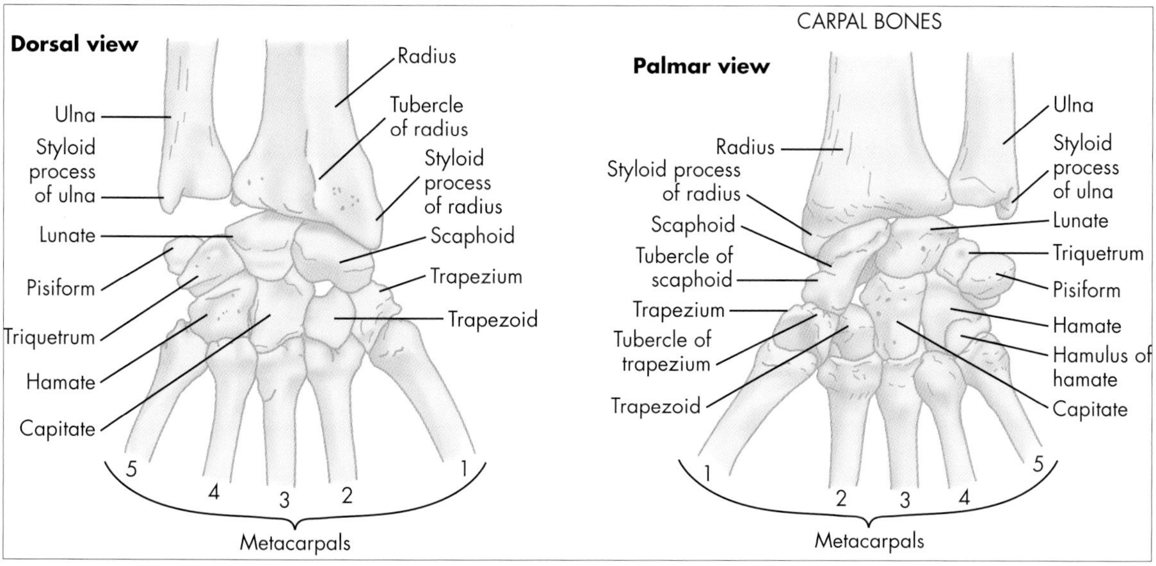

FIGURE 33.6 Anatomy of wrist

BOX 33.3 Common causes of chronic monarthritis

Inflammatory arthritis
- mycobacterial, bacterial
- crystal-induced
- monarticular rheumatoid arthritis (RA)
- seronegative spondyloarthropathies (ankylosing spondylitis, reactive arthritis, colitic arthritis)
- psoriatic arthritis
- foreign body synovitis (e.g. plant thorn synovitis)
- sarcoidosis

Non-inflammatory 'painful joint'
- osteoarthritis
- internal derangement
- osteonecrosis
- stress fracture

Tumours
- pigmented villonodular synovitis

The third pattern is the one in which polyarticular involvement dominates the clinical picture. A variety of inflammatory and non-inflammatory disorders, both common and uncommon, may present as polyarthritis (see Table 33.1).

AETIOLOGY

The accepted aetiology of the common arthropathies is as follows:

- *rheumatoid arthritis*—genetic, microbial and immunological factors play a role in disease susceptibility; autoimmune disease; inflammation drives pathophysiology
- *osteoarthritis*—degenerative condition of articular cartilage with secondary bony changes; environmental factors such as obesity, trauma; genetic factors also contribute

TABLE 33. 1 Distribution of common oligo- and polyarthritides

	Symmetric	Asymmetric
Inflammatory	• Rheumatoid arthritis • Systemic lupus erythematosus • Polymyalgia rheumatica	• Ankylosing spondylitis • Reactive arthritis • Psoriatic arthropathy • Colitic arthritis • Palindromic rheumatism
Degenerative/ crystal-induced	• Osteoarthritis (primary generalised, erosive and nodal types) • CPPD (pseudo-RA type) • Haemochromatosis arthropathy	• Gout (especially oligoarthritis) • CPPD (pseudogout)
Infectious	• Viral arthritis	• Bacterial arthritis, esp *Neisserial* • Bacterial endocarditis

- *crystal arthropathies*:
  - *gout*—inflammatory reaction due to monosodium urate crystals; environmental factors
  - *calcium pyrophosphate disease*—inflammatory reaction to calcium pyrophosphate dihydrate (CPPD) crystal deposition within fibro cartilage or articular cartilage
- *systemic lupus erythematosus (SLE)*—autoimmune disease with environmental factors such as stress, UV exposure, drugs; genetic factors also contribute
- *soft tissue rheumatic syndromes*:
  - *carpal tunnel syndrome*—genetic, environmental (occupational), metabolic (hypothyroidism)
  - *rotator cuff pathology*—ageing, environmental, genetic factors, environmental (occupational).

DIAGNOSIS

As noted above, the history and physical examination are the two most important aspects of the diagnostic process in patients complaining of musculoskeletal systems. However, laboratory tests and imaging may help in confirming a suspected diagnosis or excluding certain conditions.

IMAGING PROCEDURES

X-rays

Plain X-rays often provide useful diagnostic information in patients with inflammatory or degenerative arthritis (see Table 33.2).

CT scanning

Computed tomography (CT) has become widely established as a tool for evaluating bone and soft tissue disorders. In many situations, CT scanning can provide additional information to that provided by plain X-rays because of its increase in dynamic range. It is generally more useful than plain X-rays for imaging of the spine. Subtle cortical and intra-osseous lesions can be visualised by CT. Multiplanar reconstruction helps to better image three-dimensional structures.

TABLE 33.2 Typical X-ray findings in osteoarthritis vs rheumatoid arthritis

	Osteoarthritis	Rheumatoid arthritis
Joint space narrowing	Yes	Yes
Erosions	No	Yes
Periarticular osteoporosis	No	Yes
Subchondral sclerosis	Yes	No

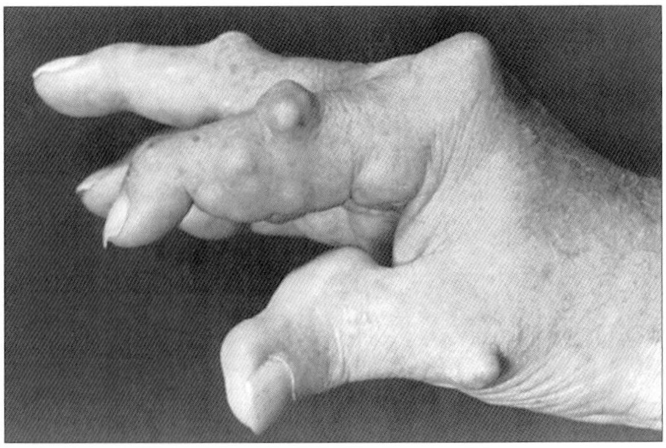

FIGURE 33.7 Rheumatoid arthritis

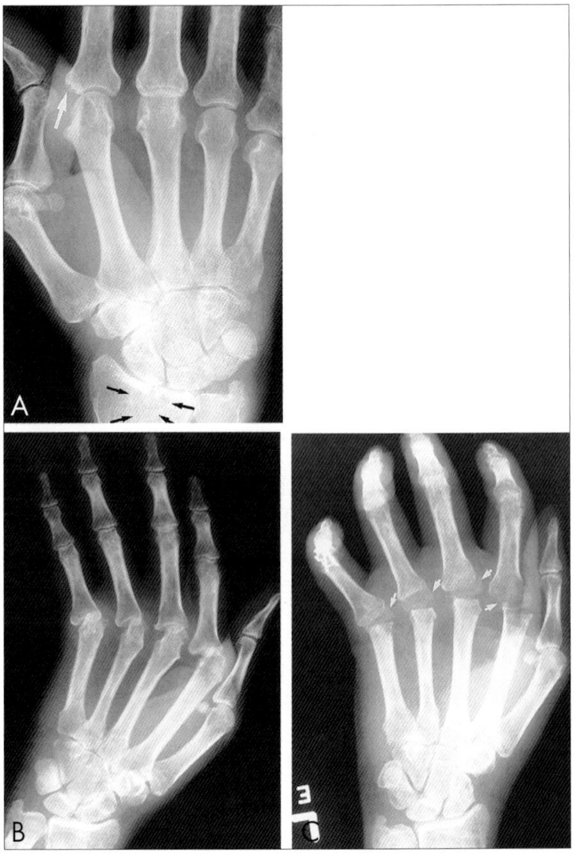

FIGURE 33.8 X-ray of rheumatoid arthritis. **A** Seen typically is narrowing of the carpal joint with subchondrial cyst formation (dark arrows) and periarticular erosions (white arrow). **B** Late changes include subluxation and ulnar derivation at the metacarpophalageal joint. **C** Silicone joint replacements (arrows) in a patient with rapidly progressing disease

Ultrasound

Ultrasound is a more expensive imaging modality used for a wide range of arthritic conditions. Tendon and muscle abnormalities such as rotator cuff tears can be diagnosed using the technique. Synovial effusions, synovial hypertrophy and inflammation can be evaluated using ultrasound. Power Doppler can be used for assessing synovial membrane inflammation. It is important to note that the effectiveness of ultrasound is very much dependent on the experience of the operator.

Magnetic resonance imaging

Magnetic resonance imaging (MRI) offers high-contrast sensitivity for soft tissue and the advantage of a lack of ionising radiation. It can be particularly useful for imaging disc and nerve lesions in the spine as well as soft tissues in sites such as the shoulder and ruptured tendons. However, it is expensive.

LABORATORY TESTS

Acute phase reactants such as C-reactive protein (CRP) and erythrocyte sedimentation rate (ESR) are often useful for excluding or confirming an inflammatory process or assessing whether there is ongoing disease activity. For many diseases, however, more specific laboratory testing is needed.

Antinuclear antibodies

The presence of high concentrations of antinuclear antibodies (ANA) (titre > 1:160) increases suspicion that an autoimmune disorder is present. However, its positivity alone is not diagnostic of disease. The combination of low titres (< 1:80) and few signs or symptoms of musculoskeletal origin suggest a low likelihood of autoimmune disease. A positive ANA in low titre (e.g. 1:40) is commonly found in the normal population. The tests should be performed in an accredited laboratory.

Extractable nuclear antigens

Extractable nuclear antigens (ENAs) may provide further information about the diagnostic subgroup in patients with a positive ANA (see Table 33.3).

Rheumatoid factor

Rheumatoid factors are antibodies directed against the Fc portion of immunoglobulin G (IgG). Patients may have detectable serum rheumatoid factor in a variety of rheumatic disorders, including:

- rheumatoid arthritis
- Sjögren's syndrome
- SLE
- polymyositis.

Rheumatoid factors may be found in up to 5% of young healthy individuals; the higher the titre, the greater the likelihood that the patient has rheumatic disease. Rheumatoid-factor-positive patients with rheumatoid arthritis generally experience more aggressive and

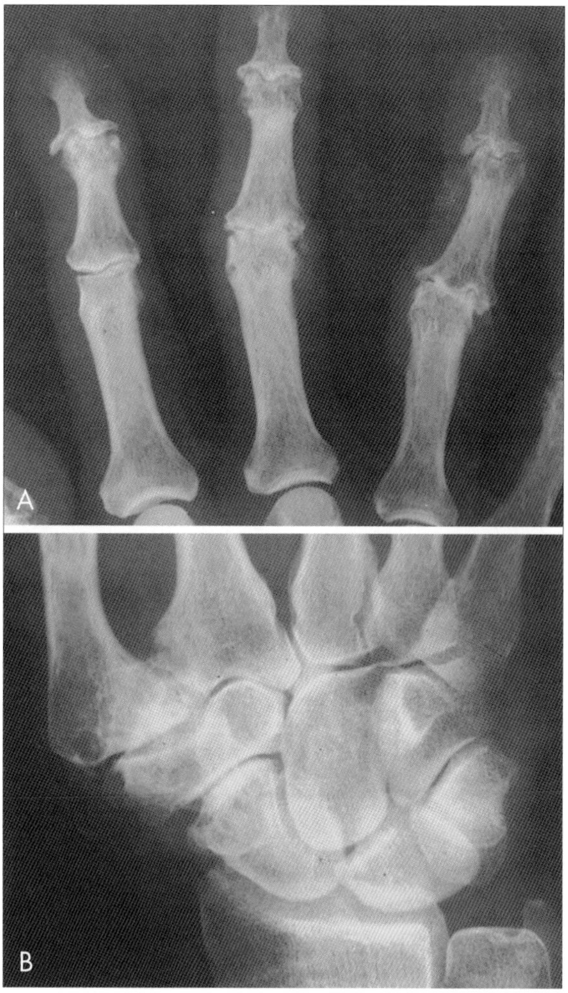

FIGURE 33.9 Osteoarthritis X-ray of **A** fingers and **B** the carpus, showing cartilage loss deviations, sclerosis and spur formation

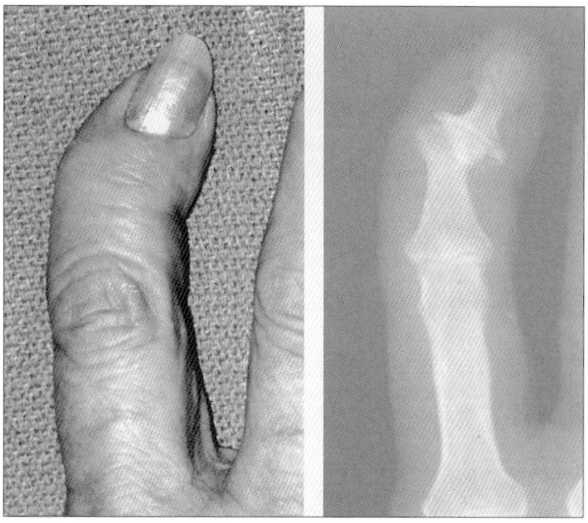

FIGURE 33.10 Osteoarthritis of the finger

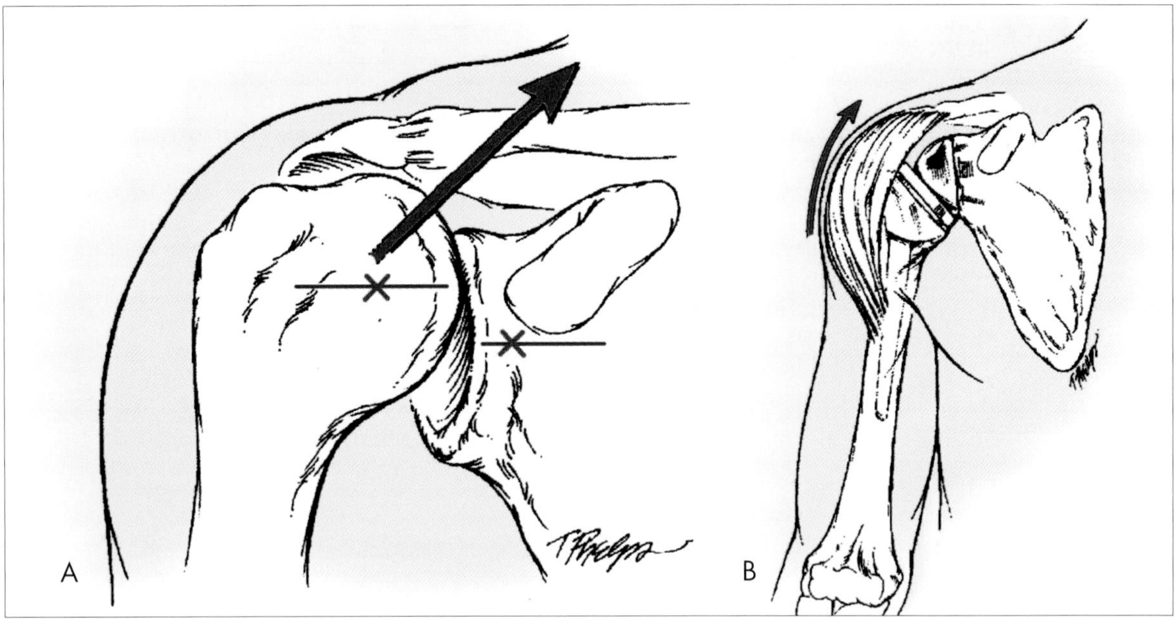

FIGURE 33.11 No rotator cuff tendons **A**—there are few restraints to anterosuperior sublaxation when attempt is made to raise the arm. The pull of the deltoid muscle worsens this by pulling superiorly and medially (arrow). **B** With reverse arthroplasty, the deltoid muscle lever is restored, allowing it to pull the humerous upward and outward (arrow)

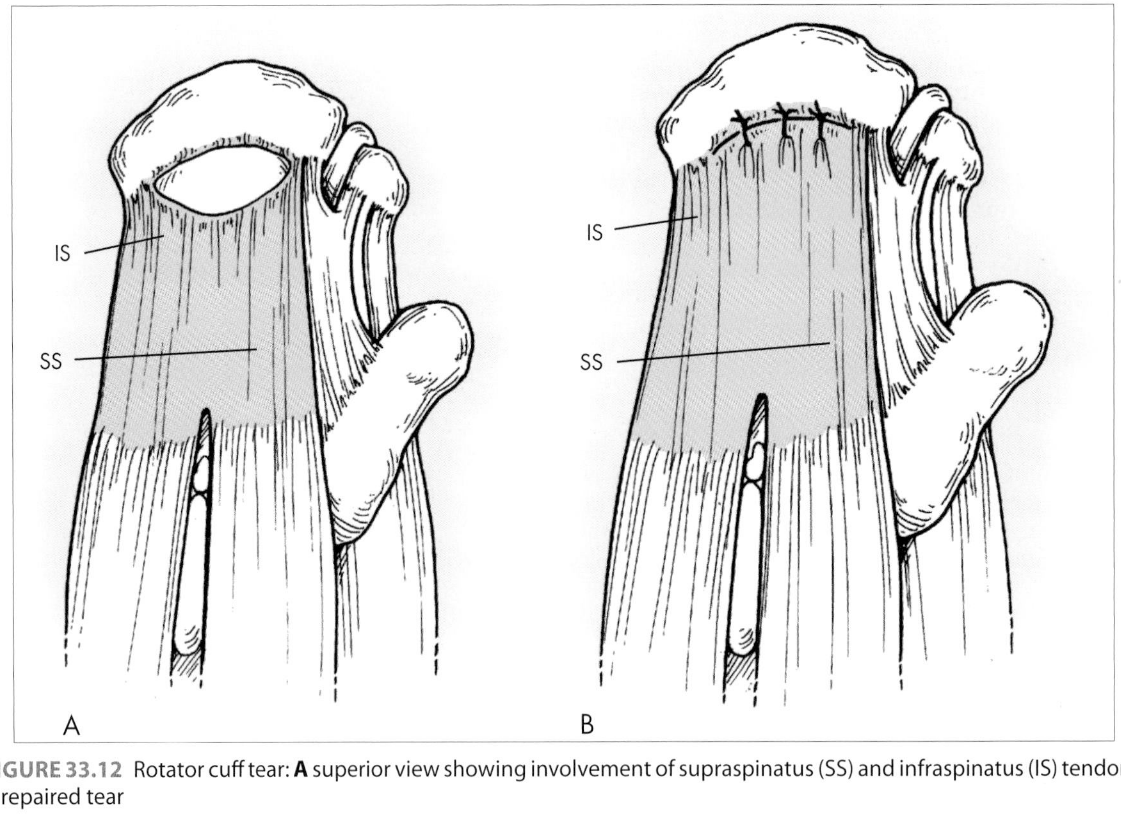

FIGURE 33.12 Rotator cuff tear: **A** superior view showing involvement of supraspinatus (SS) and infraspinatus (IS) tendons; **B** repaired tear

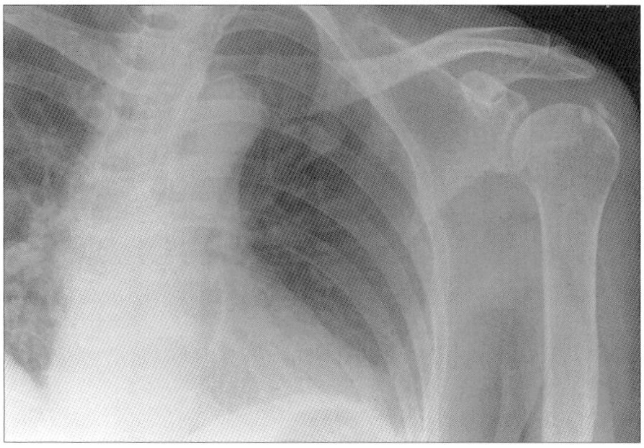

FIGURE 33.13 Rotator cuff calcific tendonitis

TABLE 33.3 ENA subtypes and associations

Subtype	Associations
Sm	SLE
SS-A	Sjögren's syndrome, SLE
SS-B	Sjögren's syndrome, SLE
RNP	Mixed connective tissue disease
Anti-centromere	CREST (limited scleroderma)
Jo-1	Dermatomyositis
Scl-70	Diffuse scleroderma

severe erosive joint disease as well as more extraarticular manifestations than those who are rheumatoid factor negative. However, there is wide inter-patient variability.

Antineutrophil cytoplasmic antibody

The antineutrophil cytoplasmic antibody (ANCA) test is useful in diagnosing certain connective tissue disorders and vasculitis. Two different immunofluorescent patterns can be seen. The cANCA is usually directed against a serum protease called proteinase 3 and found primarily in patients with Wegener's granulomatosis. The pANCA is usually directed again myeloperoxidase and more commonly associated with microscopic polyarteritis, Churg-Strauss syndrome and idiopathic necrotising glomerulonephritis.

Serum uric acid

Measurement of serum uric acid may be helpful in certain clinic situations, particularly in suspected gout or when monitoring urate-lowering therapy. Most patients with asymptomatic hyperuricaemia will never develop gout, so screening patients for hyperuricaemia is not generally recommended. Measurement of 24-hour uric acid may be useful in the evaluation of nephrolithiasis or to classify the patient as an over-producer or under-excreter of uric acid.

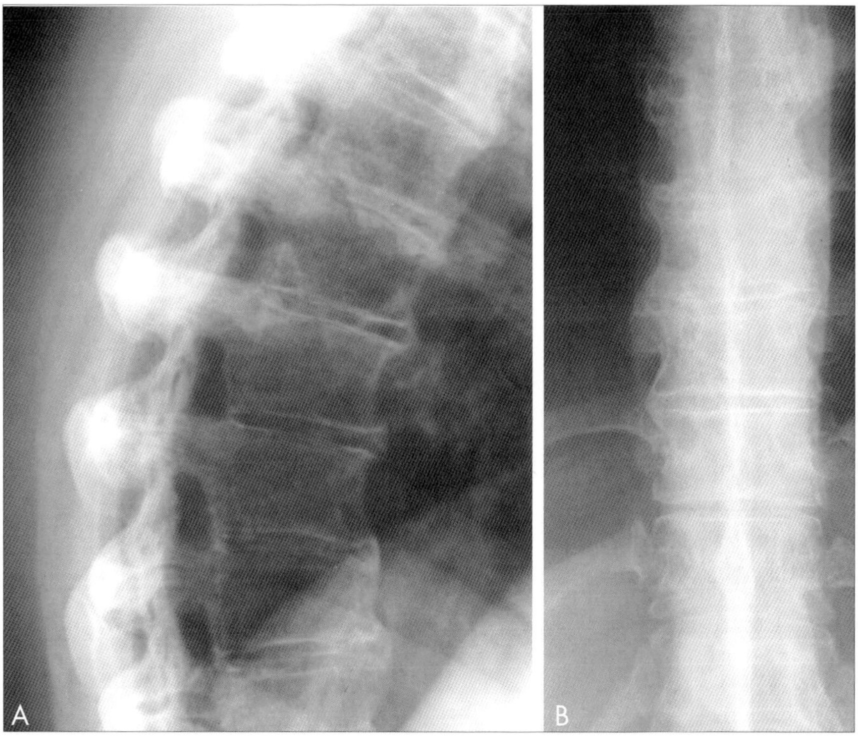

FIGURE 33.14 Hyperostosis X-rays: **A** lateral and **B** anteroposterior views showing bridging osteophytes at multiple levels, out of proportion to the degree of underlying degenerative change

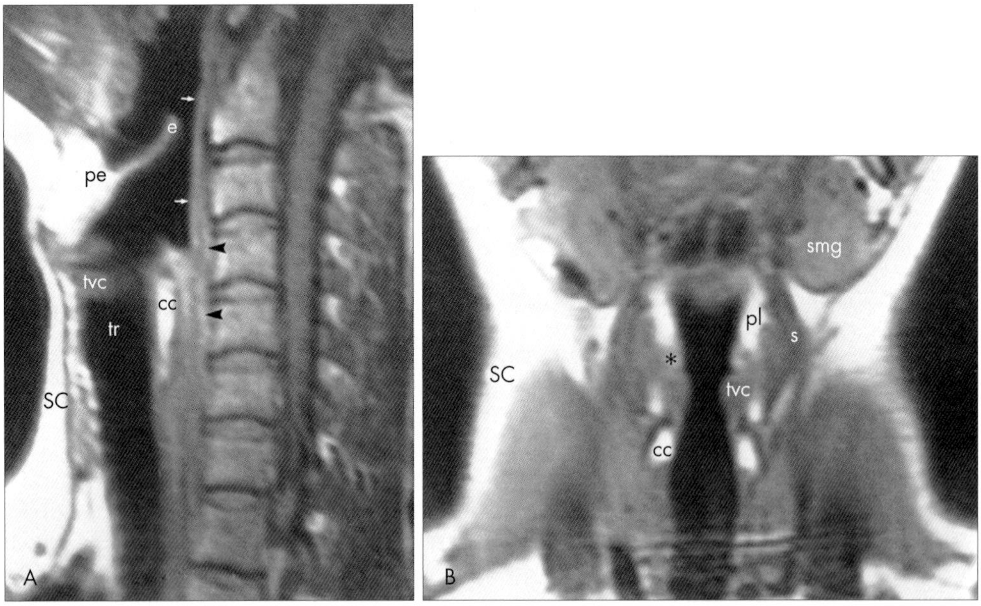

FIGURE 33.15 Infrahyoid neck X-ray: **A** sagittal and **B** coronal images. cc: cricoid cartilage; e: epiglottis; *: false vocal cord; small arrows: pharyngeal mucosal space; pe: pre-epiglottic fat; pl: paralaryngeal fat; arrowheads: retropharyngeal space; s: strap muscle; SC: superficial cervical space; smg: submandibular gland; tr: trachea; tvc: true vocal cord

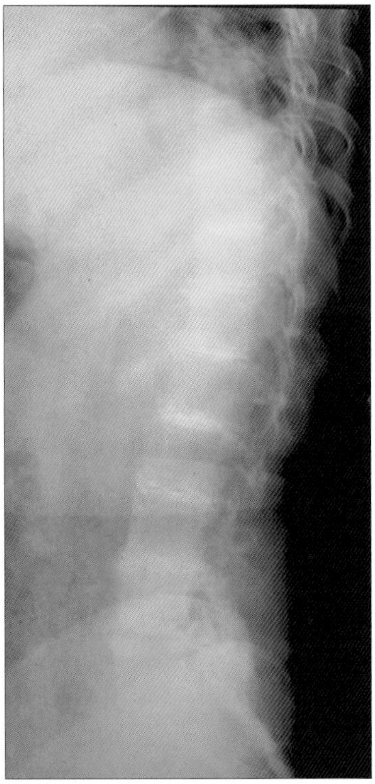

FIGURE 33.16 Alkaptonuria X-ray: spinal abnormalities include widespread disc narrowing, disc calcification and osteoporosis

Synovial fluid analysis

Synovial fluid analysis is very useful in diagnosing bacterial infections, crystal-induced arthritis and haemarthrosis. Its other main value is in allowing classification into inflammatory, non-inflammatory or haemorrhagic categories. It is a safe bedside procedure when using a 'sterile non-touch' technique. The white cell count, culture and polarised light microscopy to determine the presence of crystals are the most valuable studies on synovial fluid.

MANAGEMENT OF DISORDERS

The general practitioner is most often where the initial diagnosis and investigations occur, and plays a central role in coordinating care with other healthcare professionals—this requires good communication between all professionals involved. Other healthcare professionals who may be involved include:

- rheumatologist
- physiotherapist
- occupational therapist
- podiatrist
- pharmacist
- appropriate complementary practitioner
- orthopaedic surgeon.

EDUCATION

With an acute self-limiting form of musculoskeletal problem or arthritis, treatment can be self-limiting and education is not required. With chronic forms of musculoskeletal disease, such as rheumatoid arthritis, education is important and the healthcare professional acts as informed adviser to the patient. Management plans must be mutually agreed.

The primary aim of treatment of rheumatoid arthritis is to prevent joint damage. This helps to improve quality of life and minimise effects on mobility and the need for surgery. When devising a management plan, consideration needs to be given to the patient's level of education, preferences and financial resources.

PHYSIOTHERAPY AND EXERCISE

Exercise and weight loss may be useful for osteoarthritis of the knee. Exercise therapy may also be useful in rheumatoid arthritis, to limit the adverse effects of the disease on muscle strength, endurance and aerobic capacity. An exercise physiologist may be a useful referral for an individualised and supervised exercise program in a person with joint disease.

Hydrotherapy and occupational therapy may improve strength and physical functioning, and help relieve symptoms. Site-specific physiotherapy may be useful in a number of soft-tissue rheumatic disorders (e.g. rotator cuff pathology) and in helping to improve the recovery rate from acute low back pain.

THERAPEUTIC STRATEGIES

Therapeutic strategies in musculoskeletal conditions can be considered non-pharmacological, pharmacological or surgical (see Box 33.4).

INTEGRATIVE APPROACH TO THERAPY

Acupuncture

A large body of evidence exists for the underlying physiological basis of acupuncture in the treatment of pain. Evidence for the efficacy of acupuncture in the treatment of rheumatic and musculoskeletal disorders varies, but its safety is well documented.

Osteopathy

Osteopathy consists of a range of soft tissue stretching, massaging and relaxation techniques, as well as manipulative therapy for specific spinal and soft tissue disorders. Its efficacy remains unproven.

Chiropractic

Beneficial results are reported in some patients from experienced chiropractors. Manipulation is a commonly used technique for the treatment of mechanical and degenerative spinal disorders.

BOX 33.4 Therapeutic approaches in joint disease

Non-pharmacological
- rehabilitation
- education
- knowledge
- general
- specific
- behaviour modification
- relaxation techniques
- stress management
- physiotherapy
- exercise
- general preventive
- specific therapeutic
- rest
- heat/cold
- hydrotherapy
- transcutaneous nerve stimulation
- ultrasound
- mobilisation/manipulation
- devices
- splints
- orthoses
- household modifications
- home/work/walking devices
- complementary medicine
- glucosamine/chondroitin
- fish oil
- acupuncture

Pharmacological
- analgesics
- non-steroidal anti-inflammatory drugs
- antirheumatic drugs
- corticosteroids (systemic, intraarticular)
- immunosuppressive agents
- biological agents
- specific anti-gout therapies
- viscosupplementation

Surgery
- reconstruction
- tendon
- ligament
- arthroplasty
- arthrodesis
- synovectomy
- osteotomy

Herbal

A number of herbal mixtures have been used for arthritis, including devil's claw, St John's wort, evening primrose oil, Ayurvedic medicines and green-lipped mussel.

- Devil's claw (*Harpagophytum procumbens*) is a plant widely used in South African traditional medicine. Extracts of devil's claw roots are widely

used in Europe for rheumatic pain. Two of the active components of devil's claw are harpagoside and harpagide. The potential mechanism of action of devil's claw is still unclear.
- St John's wort (*Hypericum perforatum*) is an aromatic perennial herb that produces golden-yellow flowers that seem to be particularly abundant on 24 June (in the northern hemisphere), the day traditionally celebrated as the birthday of John the Baptist—hence its common name, St John's wort. It has been used to treat arthritis and gout as well as numerous other complaints. In general, the clinical evidence supporting its benefit in inflammatory arthritis is considered weak, and a Cochrane review of its use in depression was inconsistent.[1] There continues to be a need for more high-quality research into, and properly designed randomised trials of, the efficacy and safety of complementary therapies in rheumatoid arthritis.
- Green-lipped mussel (*Perna canaliculus*) is a New Zealand shellfish, of which an extract containing omega-3 polyunsaturated fatty acids has been shown to have anti-inflammatory properties. Commercially this is available as Liprinol®, which has been shown to have anti-inflammatory activity in vitro in inhibiting leukotriene synthesis.

Supplements

Fish oil

Traditional NSAIDs provide symptomatic relief of arthritis by inhibiting the COX enzyme but have significant side effects, particularly in the elderly. Fish oils contain a natural inhibitor of COX, and can reduce reliance on NSAIDs, and reduce cardiovascular risk.

The dietary essential fatty acids are polyunsaturated fatty acids (PUFA) that contain the omega-6 with or without the omega-3 double bond, neither of which can be synthesised endogenously. This is important because the ratios of these fatty acids in the tissues are largely determined by their ratios in the diet. In seeking to alter the balance of omega-3 and omega-6 PUFAs for therapeutic purposes, it is necessary to understand which foods are rich in these fatty acids.

Omega-3 PUFA are found in the flesh of all marine fish, including crustaceans and shellfish. In fish and fish oils, omega-3 PUFA are present as long-chain PUFA. In certain vegetable oils, such as flaxseed, perilla and canola oil, omega-3 PUFA are present as the C18 PUFA, linolenic acid. In sunflower, cottonseed, safflower and soy oils, and the spreads manufactured from them, the main fatty acid is the omega-6 C18 PUFA. Olive oil and canola oil are rich sources of oleic acid, which is a monounsaturated fatty acid containing a single double bond.

Because Western diets are typically low in long-chain omega-3 PUFA, substantial increases in tissue long-chain omega-3 can be achieved by taking a fish oil supplement without additional dietary modification. However, a choice of spreads that are rich in omega-3 PUFA or rich in monounsaturated fatty acids and low in omega-6 PUFA allow higher tissue omega-3 levels to be reached with a given dose of fish oil. To achieve anti-inflammatory doses of long-chain omega-3 PUFA by simply eating fish, a substantial dietary intake is required—greater than would be practical for most people. A daily intake of 2.7 g of long-chain omega-3 fatty acids is the threshold amount that has been shown consistently to deliver an anti-inflammatory effect in groups of patients in randomised trials[2] and is found in 10 mL of standard fish oil (from a bottle of fish oil) daily or nine standard 1000 mg capsules daily. People taking one or two capsules daily will generally have an insufficient dose for any anti-inflammatory effect in conditions like rheumatoid arthritis.

Recommendation: 15 mL fish oil daily to get well within the anti-inflammatory range or 10 capsules per day. A meal of oily fish is equivalent to only one or two capsules. In practice it is better to regard fish eaten as a desirable bonus rather than as a basis for achieving an anti-inflammatory action or making adjustments to capsules or oil.

Glucosamine and chondroitin

Numerous studies indicate that glucosamine alone or combined with chondroitin provides symptomatic benefit for the treatment of osteoarthritis of the knee. However, a lack of standardisation in glucosamine preparations has contributed to inconsistency in study results across trials. A recent updated Cochrane review of glucosamine therapy in osteoarthritis found that pain and function improved by 28% and 21% respectively, compared with placebo.[3] A large NIH-sponsored study found that the combination of glucosamine hydrochloride and chondroitin sulfate was more effective than placebo only in the subgroup with moderate to severe osteoarthritis.[4]

There may also be some effect on 'disease modification'—that is, not just symptoms. In a landmark trial assessing the disease modifying potential of glucosamine sulfate, patients were randomly assigned 1500 mg daily of glucosamine with placebo for 3 years. Patients on placebo had progressive joint space narrowing, whereas no significant joint space loss was seen in patients taking glucosamine.[5] The results have since been questioned because of the radiographic technique used to measure joint space width,[6] and further studies using MRI are needed.

Recommended dose: glucosamine 1500 mg per day; chondroitin 1200 mg per day.

PHARMACOLOGICAL

Simple analgesics

Analgesics, including paracetamol/acetaminophen, have no anti-inflammatory effects. They can be used every 4–6 hours for pain relief if necessary. They seldom produce side effects and are well tolerated.

Non-steroidal anti-inflammatory drugs

Non-steroidal anti-inflammatory drugs (NSAIDs) inhibit the cyclo-oxygenase (COX) enzyme. Two classes of COX enzymes are described: COX-1 and COX-2. Traditional NSAIDs inhibit both COX-1 and COX-2 enzymes. However, selective COX-2 inhibitors have minimal effects on the COX-1 enzyme. As a class of drugs, their use has been limited by adverse effects, mainly upper gastrointestinal. COX-2 specific agents appear to provide anti-inflammatory effects with lesser upper gastrointestinal toxicity but an increase in cardiac events.

NSAIDs act quickly (within hours to a few days) and reduce joint inflammation by inhibiting the production of inflammatory cyclo-oxygenase products, particularly the prostaglandins—small lipid molecules with potent effects on many steps in the inflammatory process. These drugs, of which there are a large number, are potent anti-inflammatory agents. Commonly used agents include diclofenac, naproxen, ketoprofen, sulindac, piroxicam, indomethacin, ibuprofen. Examples with COX-2-specific actions include celecoxib and meloxicam. NSAIDs are usually administered by the oral route, usually in conjunction with food.

In susceptible individuals, NSAIDs are nephrotoxic, by inhibiting prostaglandin-dependent compensatory renal blood flow. Recent studies have also identified an increased risk of cardiovascular events with these agents,[7] suggesting that natural inhibition of COX by fish oils may have certain advantages (see below).

Corticosteroids

Corticosteroids (or glucocorticoids) are hormones produced by the adrenal glands. They have potent anti-inflammatory and immunosuppressive properties. By far the most commonly used compound is prednisone, which is 4–5 times as potent as cortisol and has less mineralocorticoid activity, resulting in less fluid retention. Prednisone is administered orally and acts rapidly to reduce inflammation, resulting in a lessening of joint swelling, pain and stiffness in inflammatory arthritis.

Despite their clinical efficacy, corticosteroids are toxic if used at high doses for prolonged periods. Corticosteroids have important effects on bone metabolism, resulting in osteoporosis and eventual non-traumatic fractures. They interfere with glucose metabolism and are diabetogenic. Corticosteroids cause salt and water retention and may precipitate or exacerbate hypertension. They interfere with ocular lens metabolism, resulting in cataract formation.

Disease-modifying antirheumatic drugs

Disease-modifying antirheumatic drugs (DMARDs) are a group of disparate compounds that share one important feature—they retard the development of bony erosions in rheumatoid arthritis. Drugs in this category include gold compounds, d-penicillamine, sulfasalazine and the antimalarial drug hydroxychloroquine. Immunosuppressive drugs are also sometimes considered in this group. These include the folic acid antagonist methotrexate, the antimetabolite azathioprine, the alkylating agent cyclophosphamide, cyclosporin, which inhibits the production of interleukin-2 by T-lymphocytes, and recently the pyrimidine antagonist leflunomide. Methotrexate is the most widely prescribed drug in this group.

A new era has emerged with the use of biological agents in the treatment of rheumatoid arthritis. These include monoclonal antibodies directed against T-cells (such as infliximab and adalimumab), or proteins (such as etanercept) that block receptors for inflammatory cytokines such as tumour necrosis factor (TNF).

In osteoarthritis, structure-modifying drugs that prevent cartilage degradation remain an area of active research, although claims have been made in this regard for glucosamine and chondroitin via enhancement of proteoglycan synthesis by chondrocytes. (This is discussed in more detail below.)

Opioid analgesia

Opioids have an important role in the management of patients with chronic, intractable pain for whom surgery is not an option and where other modalities have failed. Both oxycodone and tramadol, a weak opioid antagonist, have been used. Their side-effect profile is well described and there are important drug interactions to watch for, notably serotonergic syndrome with tramadol.

Intraarticular and local injection therapy

Pain and inflammation can be effectively relieved by intraarticular corticosteroid injections. Soft-tissue rheumatic syndromes also respond well in many cases to local corticosteroid therapy. Injection techniques that selectively and specifically target the lumbar zygapophyseal joints may be useful in some patients with low back pain.

Viscosupplementation with hyaluronic acid injections has also been used in osteoarthritis. Although no direct comparison between specific products has been performed, viscosupplementation was more efficacious from 5 to 13 weeks with regard to pain, range of motion and Western Ontario and McMaster Universities Index of Osteoarthritis (WOMAC) and Lesquene scores, than placebo.[8] In Australia, the only compound available is hylan G-F 20 (SYNVISC®). It does not attract PBS reimbursement and is only approved for knee osteoarthritis.

RESOURCES

Arthritis Australia, http://www.arthritisaustralia.com.au
Cleland LG, James MJ, Proudman SM. Fish oil: what the prescriber needs to know. Arthritis Res Ther 2006; 8:202.
Hochberg M, Silman A, Smolen J et al. Rheumatology. 3rd edn. London: Mosby; 2003.
March L, Ananda A. Management of osteoarthritis: part 2. Medical Observer 2007; 20 April:27–30.
Sambrook P, Schrieber L, Taylor T et al. The musculoskeletal system. London: Churchill Livingstone; 2001.

REFERENCES

1 Linde K, Berner MM, Kriston L. St John's wort for major depression. Cochrane Database Syst Rev 2008; 3:CD000448.
2 Proudman SM, Cleland LG, James MJ. Dietary omega-3 fats for treatment of inflammatory joint disease: efficacy and utility. Rheum Dis Clin North Am 2008; 34(2): 469–479.
3 Towheed T, Maxwell L, Anastassiades TP et al. Glucosamine therapy for treating osteoarthritis. Cochrane Database Syst Rev 2008; 4:CD002946.
4 Clegg DO, Reda DJ, Harris CL et al. Glucosamine, chondroitin sulfate and the two in combination for painful knee osteoarthritis. N Engl J Med 2006; 354:795–808, 858–860.
5 Reginster JY, Deroisy R, Rovati LC et al. Long-term effects of glucosamine sulphate on osteoarthritis progression: a randomised, placebo-controlled clinical trial. Lancet 2001; 357:247–248.
6 McAlindon T. Glucosamine for osteoarthritis: dawn of a new era? Lancet 2001; 357:247–248.
7 Mukherjee D, Nissen SE, Topol EJ. Risk of cardiovascular events associated with selective COX-2 inhibitors. JAMA 2001; 286(8):954–959.
8 Bellamy N, Campbell J, Robinson V et al. Viscosupplementation for the treatment of osteoarthritis of the knee. Cochrane Database Syst Rev 2005; 2:CD005321.

chapter 34

Musculoskeletal medicine

INTRODUCTION AND OVERVIEW

Musculoskeletal medicine (MSM) is that branch of medicine dealing with the conservative management of disorders of the musculoskeletal system, including the muscles, aponeuroses, joints and bones of the axial and appendicular skeletons, and those parts of the nervous system associated with them. These disorders represent the most common cause of disability in most countries across all age groups[1] and are the third most common reason for presentation to general practice.[2] The direct and indirect costs of this burden are in the $15 billions per annum.[3]

Yet, paradoxically, undergraduate and postgraduate education in MSM is at best elementary. The need for MSM training in medical schools and hospitals has been well established.[4] Currently in Australia there is no public MSM outpatients department (OPD) hospital clinic, which differs from our European and American colleagues, who have vibrant systems in place. For instance, osteopathy and musculoskeletal medicine special-interest doctors are recognised in the United Kingdom, musculoskeletal physicians are recognised in Europe and the United States has osteopathic MDs. Historically in Australia it has been left to the allied healthcare professionals and alternative healthcare practitioners to absorb much of the demand for musculoskeletal (MS) management. The medical profession has been slow to embrace MSM, but has a vital role to play. The optimal management of MSM conditions epitomises the need for an integrated approach from practitioners knowledgeable in the biopsychosocial approach to management. General practitioners with postgraduate MS training can work collaboratively with other healthcare providers to minimise pain and optimise function for patients.

One of the most common MS disorders seen by healthcare practitioners in Australia is spinal pain. Persistent back pain is by far the most common reason for chronic MS patient encounter in Australian general practice, followed by knee, shoulder and neck.[5]

This chapter focuses on the optimal management of spinal pain, although the general principles espoused may be used for all areas of the body.

LOW BACK PAIN

The issue of low back pain (LBP) pervades Western society. Be it through lost work, missed recreation and sporting activities or money spent on prevention or cure, there are few people who have not had dealings with it. Healthcare practitioners have been both blamed for exacerbating its prevalence and given credit for reducing it. It is abundantly covered in the media, and myths circulate swiftly through the populace. This section outlines the evidence on low back pain in a functional fashion.

DEFINITIONS

- *Low back pain* is pain perceived to be arising from lumbar and/or sacral regions of the spine. It has been defined by the IASP[6] as per Figure 34.1. Importantly, low back pain is not perceived to arise from the gluteal, thoracic, loin or groin region, although it may refer into these regions.
- *Acute pain* is pain that has been present for less than 12 weeks, *subacute* pain has been present for longer than 5–7 weeks but less than 12 weeks, and *chronic (persistent) pain* longer than 12 weeks. These terms are common in the research literature and management strategies differ significantly between them.
- *Somatic pain* is pain arising from noxious stimuli to any of the musculoskeletal components of the body. Studies have shown that the sensitivities of these components are: periosteum > ligament

> joint capsule > tendon > fascia > muscle.[7,8] *Somatic referred pain* is pain perceived in a region innervated by nerves other than those that innervate the actual source of pain.[6] Common examples include buttock and posterior thigh pain referred from the lumbar spine, and knee pain referred from the hip.

- *Radicular pain* is pain that arises from irritation of a spinal nerve or its roots. Radiculopathy involves conduction block to a spinal nerve or its root, resulting in numbness and/or weakness.[6] Table 34.1 outlines the differing features of somatic referred pain and radicular pain. Figures 34.2–34.6 show some patterns of referred pain from different vertebral structures. They illustrate the potential of somatic vertebral structures to refer pain to remote areas and thus mimic other pains, such as 'sciatica' and visceral pains.
- *Hyperalgesia* is an increased response to a stimulus that is normally painful. In clinical practice this is commonly seen with persistent pain. It often results in an increase in the referred pain in intensity and area due to central nervous sensitisation.[15] Knowledge of this phenomenon is important in providing patients with a reason for changes in their pain. It is also important for doctors involved in writing reports or assessments, as it invalidates the term 'non-anatomical' in describing distribution of pain. This term is often used in medico-legal reports to suggest that an individual's pain is imaginary or of dubious significance. The use of 'non-anatomical' in describing pain should be obsolete in the twenty-first century.

TABLE 34.1 Somatic versus radicular pain

Somatic referred pain	Radicular pain
Due to spread of pain from deep spinal tissues (including muscles)	Due to chemical or mechanical irritation of nerves
Back pain worse than leg pain, which may be bilateral	Unilateral leg pain worse than back pain
Pain concentrates proximally in buttock and thigh, but may spread below knee	Pain concentrates distally, running into the lower limb, usually extending below the knee
Deep, dull aching, expanding pressure-like quality	Sharp, shooting, electric quality, often deep and superficial
Vague location, varies over time, ill-defined distribution	Pain runs along defined narrow band in dermatome distribution
Poorly defined paraesthesia may be present	Numbness and paraesthesia in dermatomal distribution
Normal reflexes and power (if abnormal, further assessment is needed)	Reflexes may be reduced or absent; motor weakness may be present

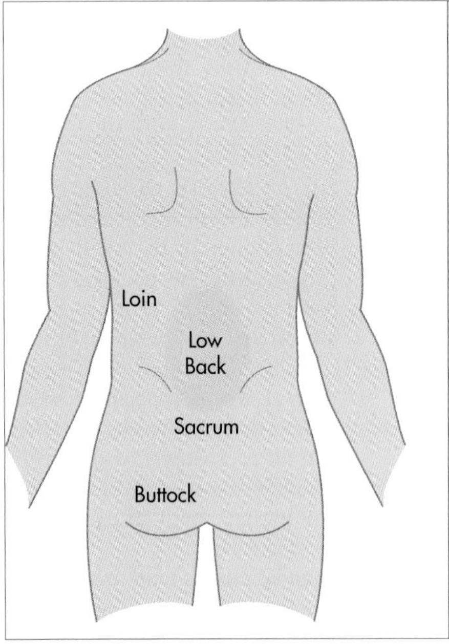

Sacral and gluteal (buttock) pain are commonly sites of referred pain from the lumbar spine. However, in the absence of back pain, look for local causes.

Loin pain may be referred from the thoracic spine, but is less likely to be due to lumbar pathology. Exclude renal problems in the first instance.

Somatic referred pain is pain that arises from somatic tissues in the spine (muscles, ligaments, bones and joints), and spreads distally into the buttocks and legs. It is analogous to arm pain arising from cardiac causes.

Source: RAGGP Guidelines

FIGURE 34.1 Pain sites

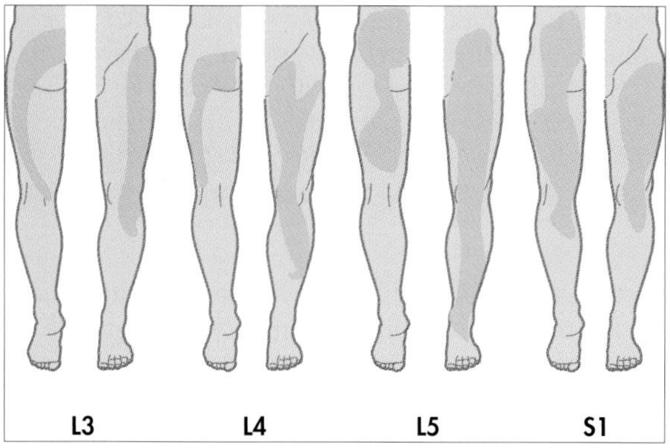

FIGURE 34.2 Patterns of referred pain evoked in normal volunteers by noxious stimulation of interspinous ligaments at the segmental levels indicated (based on Kellgren 1939[9])

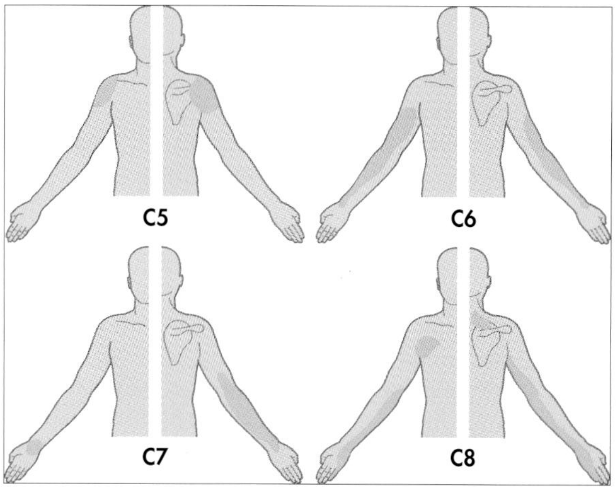

FIGURE 34.3 Patterns of referred pain evoked in normal volunteers by noxious stimulation of interspinous ligaments at the segmental levels indicated (based on Kellgren 1939[9])

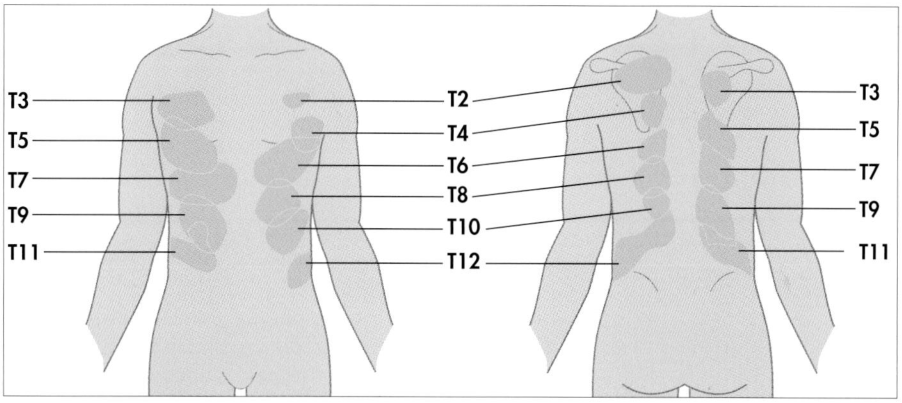

FIGURE 34.4 Patterns of referred pain evoked in normal volunteers by noxious stimulation of interspinous ligaments at the segmental levels indicated (based on Kellgren 1939[9])

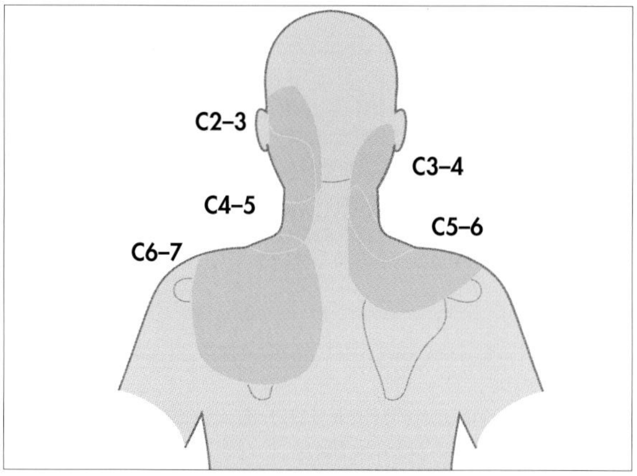

FIGURE 34.5 Patterns of referred pain evoked in normal volunteers and in patients by noxious stimulation of the cervical zygapophyseal joints or intervertebral discs at the segments indicated[10–12]

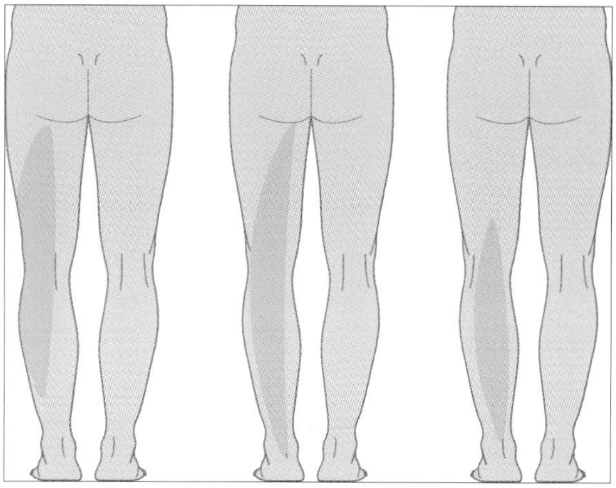

FIGURE 34.6 Various patterns of referred pain produced in normal volunteers or patients by noxious stimulation of lumbar zygapophyseal joints or intervertebral discs[13,14]

EPIDEMIOLOGY

The lifetime prevalence of acute LBP is about 70%,[16] with the cumulative lifetime prevalence of episodes lasting more than 2 weeks being 14%.[17] In Australia, back complaint is the sixth most common reason for presentation to a general practitioner.[2]

Data on the natural history of LBP are variable but instructive when closely analysed. A commonly quoted statement is that, with treatment, '90% of patients recover within 2 months'.[18] This may be true when follow-up is only for 4 weeks.[18] More-rigorous studies with 12-month follow-up reveal a different picture.[19,20] Around 80% of patients remain disabled to some extent at 12 months, with 10–15% highly disabled. These studies paint a picture of recovery followed by relapse. In general, a patient's status at 2 months post presentation reflects their status at 12 months.

An Australian study of acute LBP patients without a compensation claim managed with evidence-based guidelines revealed that 70% can expect to recover and stay recovered at 12 months, with a low risk of recurrence.[21]

BOX 34.2 Red flag indicators

Presence of:
- trauma
- night sweats
- recent surgery
- catheterisation
- venipuncture
- occupational exposure
- hobby exposure
- sporting exposure
- (overseas) travel
- illicit drug use
- weight loss
- history of cancer

Cardiovascular:
- risk factors

Respiratory:
- cough

Urinary:
- UTI
- haematuria
- retention
- stream problems

Reproductive:
- menstrual problems

Haematopoietic:
- problems

Endocrine:
- corticosteroids

Musculoskeletal:
- pain elsewhere

Neurological:
- symptoms/signs

Skin:
- infections
- rashes

GIT:
- diarrhoea

(Source: Bogduk 2003[22])

HISTORY

History-taking primarily allows formulation of a diagnostic framework and assessment of prognosis. It should also be used as a way to gain the patient's trust and begin the process of education and assurance. A reasonable framework is:

- pain history—use pain chart, VAS, disability, recovergram (see also Ch 38, Pain management)
- red flag check—see Box 34.2
- yellow flag check—see Box 34.3.

BOX 34.3 Yellow flag indicators

Work:
- belief that pain is harmful, resulting in fear-avoidance behaviour
- belief that all pain must be abolished before attempting to return to work or normal activity
- expectation of increased pain with activity or work
- fear of increased pain with activity or work
- belief that work is harmful
- poor work history
- unsupportive work environment

Beliefs:
- catastrophising, thinking the worst
- misinterpreting bodily symptoms
- belief that pain is uncontrollable
- poor compliance with exercise
- expectation of 'techno-fix' for pain
- low educational background

Behaviours:
- passive attitude to rehabilitation
- use of extended rest
- reduced activity with significant withdrawal from activities of daily living
- avoidance of normal activity
- impaired sleep because of pain
- increased intake of alcohol or similar substances since the onset of pain

Affective:
- depression
- feeling useless and not needed
- irritability
- anxiety about heightened body sensations
- disinterest in social activity
- over-protective partner/spouse
- socially punitive partner/spouse
- lack of support to talk about problems

(Source: Bogduk 2003[22])

EXAMINATION

Although physical examination of LBP patients will rarely allow a patho-anatomic diagnosis to be made, it remains an extremely valuable tool. Its strength lies in the opportunities it opens (Box 34.4). A confidently performed physical examination in association with meaningful dialogue is an important step in the overall management.

Following the orthopaedic model of 'look, move and feel' is the standard approach. Initial inspection allows a record of asymmetry, pain behaviour, gait and skin lesions. A knowledge of surface landmarks (Fig 34.7) adds more meaning to the descriptions. The physician should be alert for pain behaviour from the patient and its interpretation. Importantly, pain behaviour needs to be recognised as the patient's way of communicating distress. Overt or exaggerated pain behaviour is *not* a sign of malingering but, rather, a signal for the doctor to explore pain management issues in more depth. This would include psychosocial factors as well as biological.

The patient can be moved in all six planes—flexion, extension, lateral flexion left and right, and rotation left and right. Rotation is best performed sitting, to stabilise the pelvis. While the patient is seated, straight leg raising (SLR) and slump testing may be performed (Fig 34.8). With the patient in the supine position, SLR can be assessed as well as leg length. Hip range of movement (ROM) can be assessed, noting that if back pain is reproduced, this is most likely to be from the effects on lumbar/pelvic structures than the hip joint

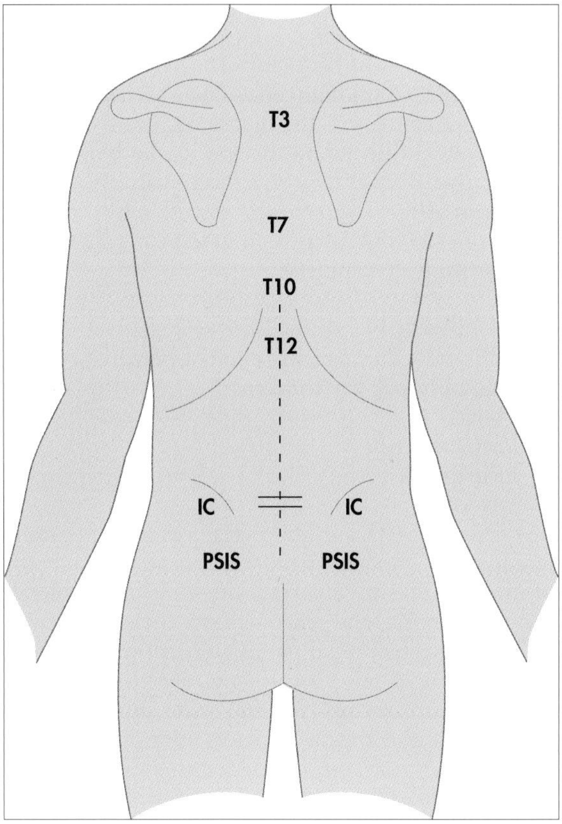

FIGURE 34.7 Surface anatomy landmarks: iliac crests (IC), posterior superior iliac spines (PSIS). Spinous process of L4 lumbar vertebra lies at or just below the level of the iliac crest. Lumbosacral junction (=) lies 10–15° superiorly and towards the midline from the PSISs. T12 can be located by counting spinous processes back from the lumbosacral junction. T10 is at a line drawn along the 12th rib and continued to the midline to meet its contralateral fellow.

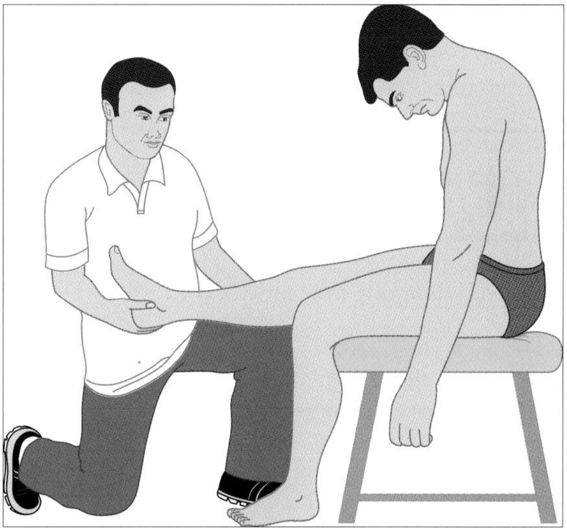

FIGURE 34.8 Slump test. The patient sits on the edge of the couch, then in a stepwise fashion, increased stretch is introduced as follows: i) the patient slumps forward, ii) then flexes the neck, iii) then straightens the leg, iv) then dorsiflexes the foot. Purportedly, if any back or leg pain reproduced so far is eased when the neck is then extended, and/or the ankle plantar flexed, then neuromeningeal irritation, rather than hamstring pain, is invoked (adopted from Kenna & Murtagh[23]).

BOX 34.4 Physical examination opportunities

- Meet patient's expectations
- Enhance doctor–patient relationship, gain trust, increase ability to discuss psychosocial issues
- Reproduce patient's pain
- Reassure patient, positively reinforce normal findings, continue patient education
- Observe pain behaviour
- Detect red flag lesions
- Record impairment and disability
- Detect somatic dysfunction, determine manual therapy options
- Follow patient's progress

(groin/anterolateral thigh pain). In the prone position, hip extension and hip rotation can be assessed.

Palpation should be performed systematically through the paravertebral tissues, sacroiliac and gluteal area. Attention should be paid to insertional areas such as the posterior greater trochanter, parasacrally and the posterior superior iliac spine (PSIS). To assess the sacrotuberous and sacrospinous ligament, levator ani and other paracoccygeal structures, per rectum examination will be needed. Note should be made of hyperalgesia, allodynia and abnormal tissue texture.

Special tests of spinal dysfunction have been described for the lumbar and pelvic region, including many labelled as sacroiliac tests. A combination of tests shows best utility regarding sacro-iliac joints (SIJ) dysfunction.[24]

Examination of the visceral, vascular and neurological systems is determined by the presenting symptoms and history. Neurological examination is only necessary if there is radicular leg pain or neurological symptoms. A quick check of the L5 and S1 myotomes can be performed by asking the patient to stand on their heels, then their toes. The L1–S2 dermatomes are easily checked by touching the centre of the respective zones.

INVESTIGATION

Careful thought is needed before investigating a patient. Concern regarding increasing levels of radiological intervention, especially CT scanning, has become topical.[25,26] The risk of exposure to significant ionising radiation, for questionable clinical benefit along with wasting of limited healthcare resources, should be of concern to the healthcare practitioner and consumer alike. By asking: 'How will this investigation influence my management, what are the chances of a significant finding and will this test detect it?', unnecessary tests are likely to be avoided.

Red flag conditions and their appropriate investigations are shown in Table 34.2. Plain films have a reasonable pick-up rate (Table 34.3) but will miss early disease. CT scans have no role in the investigation of somatic low back pain, except in confirmation of pathology indicated by other investigations or the history/examination. MRI scan is the investigation of choice for red flag conditions of the spine and gives the best information about the status of the intervertebral disc (i.e. presence or absence of modic lesions and high-intensity zones).

Providing the patient with a proper explanation of the role of the investigation is paramount. This is especially so with radiological investigation, where reported abnormalities are, in most cases, not significant (Table 34.4). However, patients risk being alarmed by being referred for unnecessary investigations and misinterpretation of asymptomatic anatomical abnormalities.[29]

DIAGNOSIS

A specific patho-anatomic diagnosis will not be forthcoming for the overwhelming majority of LBP patients. In essence, the initial consultation(s) are primarily to exclude red flag diagnosis and estimate the influence of yellow flags on prognosis. The probability diagnosis will be somatic LBP, and in the acute pain situation no further clarification is necessary. Evidence-informed practice has no value from any further subclassification, even though this is common practice in primary care.[34] Primary practitioners can reasonably use a benign label (ligament or muscle strain) to help reassure their patients that they have a good prognosis.

In the case of persisting pain, precision diagnosis may be sought. Two structures can be relatively easily blocked by guided anaesthetic blocks: the zygapophyseal joints and the sacroiliac joints. Both have validated protocols that must be followed correctly for accurate diagnosis.[35,36] Radiofrequency neurotomy may be used as a treatment if the blocks are positive.[37,38] The intervertebral disc cannot be specifically blocked, but provocative discography has been used to identify a painful disc. The role of discography has been controversial,[39] but it has been used primarily to select patients for fusion surgery.

MANAGEMENT

From the individual patient's point of view, management must address four key concerns:[40]

- 'I hurt'
- 'I can't move'
- 'I can't work'
- 'I'm scared'.

The research data are quite clear on the importance of educating low-back-pain sufferers about the nature of their problem, assuring them of the generally good prognosis and encouraging them to stay as active as possible. What is less clear is the best overall combination of other treatments, such as supervised therapeutic exercise, manual therapy, injections, behavioural therapy, workplace intervention a and myriad other interventions. Few studies have tested combinations of treatments or integrative management, most studies comparing monotherapies against standard/minimal care or another monotherapy. The Australian National Musculoskeletal Medicine Initiative[21] and Blomberg's pragmatic trials[41–44] are significant trials that have compared algorithms involving multiple treatments versus standard care. They are informative for an approach to the four concerns above.

TABLE 34.2 Appropriate investigations for possible serious causes of acute musculoskeletal pain

Suspected condition (and alerting clinical features)		Region of pain				
		Lumbar spinal	**Cervical spinal**	**Thoracic spinal**	**Shoulder**	**Knee**
Fracture History of significant trauma History of minor trauma in association with corticosteroid use, age > 50, history of osteoporosis History of previous fracture or metabolic disease Positive for Canadian C-spine rule Positive for Ottawa Knee rule	All cases	Plain radiography				
	Stress of pars interarticularis	Bone scan				
Infection Fever Sweating Risk factors for infection (invasive medical procedure, indwelling device, injection, injecting drug use, trauma to skin or mucous membrane, immunosuppressive disease or treatment, diabetes mellitus, alcoholism)	All cases	ESR, FBC, CRP				
	Spinal	MRI				
	Osteomyelitis				MRI	
	Joint				Aspiration, culture and microscopy	
Tumour Palpable mass Past history of malignancy Age > 50 years Failure to improve with treatment Unexplained weight loss Pain not relieved by rest	Myeloma	IEPG, serum protein electrophoresis				
	Prostate	PSA				
	All cases	First line: ESR, CRP Second line: MRI				
Crystal arthritis Joint effusion					Aspiration, microscopy	

(continues)

TABLE 34.2 Appropriate investigations for possible serious causes of acute musculoskeletal pain (continued)

Suspected condition (and alerting clinical features)		Region of pain				
		Lumbar spinal	**Cervical spinal**	**Thoracic spinal**	**Shoulder**	**Knee**
Aneurysm Cardiovascular risk factors Anticoagulants Transient ischaemic attacks Bruits Recent history of torsion to neck Absence of musculoskeletal signs	Vertebral, carotid		MRA			
	Aortic	Ultrasound				
Osteonecrosis Immunosuppression Renal dialysis Use of corticosteroids Diabetes, alcoholism					MRI	

CPP: C-reactive protein; ESR: erythrocyte sedimentation rate; FBC: full blood count; IEPG: immunoelectrophoretogram; MRA: magnetic resonance angiography; MRI: magnetic resonance imaging.

Source: Australian Acute Musculoskeletal Pain Guidelines Group (AAMPGG) 2003[27]

TABLE 34.3 Sensitivity* and specificity** of plain films in the evaluation of some pathological causes of back pain

Condition	Sensitivity	Specificity
Malignancy	70%	90%
Osteomyelitis	80–90%	70–90%
Spondylitis	50%	90%

*100% false negative %

**100% minus false positive %

Source: Mazanec 1991[28]

- *'I hurt'*—quick control of pain is paramount. Pain is the fifth vital sign and is an independent risk factor for chronicity. At the first consultation, the patient requires a credible, convincing explanation of the cause of their pain. This should be performed after thorough history-taking and examination, which should be thought of by the practitioner as therapeutic. It needs to be couched in language understandable to the lay person. In most cases, when performed confidently this step will allay patients' concerns regarding their pain and facilitate the other necessary steps in pain management (analgesics, manual therapy, exercises and focal injections).
- *'I can't move'*—the disability associated with acute low back pain can quickly impair a person's ability to work, socialise and perform leisure activities. Patients often become too frightened to move, in case they further 'damage' their spine. Assurance of the benefits of early mobilisation and the dangers of prolonged rest[45] should be incorporated into the explanation of the nature of the patient's condition. Before leaving the first consultation, the patient should have a sound knowledge of appropriate activity and have a program for pacing activities, maintaining movement and controlling any resultant flare of pain or stiffness. This may involve manual therapy, be it manipulation or an exercise regimen or both.
- *'I can't work'*—the work domain and low back pain have been the subject of much debate for years. The experience could be summarised thus: 'If the workplace has a toxic environment, the injured patient is unlikely to return no matter what physical rehabilitation occurs'. Thus the importance of the yellow flag concept as first comprehensively set out in the New Zealand government guidelines.[46]

TABLE 34.4 Spinal disease linked to back pain: prevalence in a primary care population,[30–33] key historical features and their respective positive likelihood ratios[31]

Spinal disease	Primary care prevalence	Key historical feature	Positive likelihood ratio
Compression fracture	4%[31]	Patient aged > 70 years	5.5
		Trauma	2.0
		Corticosteroid use	12.0
Cancer	0.66% (lumbar spine)[32]	Patient aged > 50 years	2.7
	0.63% (thoracic spine)[32]	Previous history of cancer	15.5
		Failure to improve within a month of therapy	3.1
		Unexplained weight loss (>4.5 kg in 6 months)	2.5
		No relief with bed rest	>1.7
		Duration of pain >1 month	2.6
		Age 50+ years, cancer history, unexplained weight loss, failure of conservative therapy	2.5
Ankylosing spondylitis	0.3%[33]	Out of bed at night because of pain	3.1
		Pain not relieved supine	1.6
		Pain duration 3+ months	1.6
		Back pain at night	1.6
		Morning stiffness, 0.5 hours or more	1.6
Spinal osteomyelitis	0.01%[30]	Intravenous drug use, urinary tract infection or skin infection	NA

*Positive likelihood ratios: likelihood, given the presence of the feature(s)[31]

RECOVERGRAM

Name:
Age:

Diagnosis:
Date of onset:

VAS: NUMERICAL RATING SCALE FOR PAIN (X) AND DISABILITY (O)

Pain: 0 = no pain → 10 = worst imaginable pain
Disability: 0 = no limitation of activities → 10 = complete limitation of activities

Date																					
Week number	0	1	2	3	4	5	6	7	8	9	10	11	12	13	14	15	16	17	18	19	20
Visit number																					
10																					
9																					
8																					
7																					
6																					
5																					
4																					
3																					
2																					
1																					
0																					
Global assessment of progress from first visit: 1 = very much worse 2 = much worse 3 = minimally worse 4 = no change 5 = minimally improved 6 = much improved 7 = very much improved																					
Global assessment																					

FIGURE 34.9 Recovergram

(See Box 34.3 for yellow flag indicators.) Returning the worker to his or her occupation in some role as soon as practical with acceptance by their supervisors goes a long way to resolving work issues. The worker must be educated in suitable duties and have a non-adversarial environment to return to, for optimal outcomes.
- *'I'm scared'*—the fear associated with low back pain is a leading cause of disability, even though the fears are most often grounded in myth and mistaken beliefs. Open discussion with the patient about their understanding of the cause of the pain, their expectations regarding recovery and their motivation to actively become involve in the recovery process usually help to overcome their apprehension. Rectifying their fears, educating them in coping skills and reassuring them of the good prognosis are all helpful steps. Formal psychological intervention should be sought if this does not occur within the first few visits.

The above musculoskeletal quartet overview gives a useful framework to address all musculoskeletal patients. It may also be used at each presentation.

Initial presentation

- Take a full pain history and record pain and disability (e.g. recovergram, see Fig 34.9).
- Record red and yellow flags.
- Perform an examination as required from the above information. If spinal dysfunctions are present, then manual therapy should be considered.
- Order investigations deemed necessary from red flags.
- Explain the nature of the patient's condition to them in detail.
- Assure them of the importance of staying active, returning to work and their usual activities, and having a positive outlook regarding recovery. Reassure them that you are available to address any concerns and will review them again soon (this will vary depending on presentation, but is usually a few days to a few weeks).
- Advise them on pain management options (Box 34.5).
- Advise them on ways to maintain movement (Box 34.6).
- Review as necessary. Generally, patients should be followed up until they have recovered (i.e. pain score < 2 visual analogue scale (VAS) and return to full or near full activity).

COMPLEMENTARY THERAPIES

Acupuncture

For low back pain

A 2005 Cochrane review[50] looked at acupuncture for non-specific low back pain and dry-needling for myofascial pain in the lower back. Thirty-five trials were included in the review. The authors concluded that acupuncture relieves pain and improves function in patients with chronic low back pain, compared with no treatment or sham treatment, and this effect was sustained at short-term, but not long-term, follow-up. Acupuncture as an adjunct to conventional treatments is more effective than conventional treatments alone, although the effects are small. Dry-needling can also be a useful adjunct. However, neither acupuncture nor dry-needling are more effective than other treatments, conventional or 'alternative'. These findings were confirmed by an independent 2005 meta-analysis of acupuncture for low back pain, which concluded that acupuncture provides short-term pain relief of chronic low back pain.[51] There was insufficient evidence on acupuncture for acute low back pain.

For neck pain

A 2006 Cochrane review[52] found 10 trials on acupuncture for chronic neck pain, and none for acute or sub-acute neck pain. The authors concluded that there was moderate evidence that acupuncture is more effective than sham treatments in relieving pain both immediately post-treatment and at short-term follow-up. Limited evidence suggests that acupuncture is more effective than massage in the short term. There is moderate evidence that acupuncture is more effective than waitlist control for neck pain with radicular symptoms, at short-term follow-up.

For lateral elbow pain

A 2002 Cochrane review[53] found four small trials of acupuncture for lateral elbow pain of more than

BOX 34.5 Pain management options

1. Give a full explanation of the nature of the pain, and assurance regarding the good chance of full recovery.
2. Encourage the patient to stay active, to minimise pain and disability.
3. Time-contingent use of analgesics to control pain, to allow activity and avoid sleep disruption.
4. Use the safest medication at the lowest effective dose. Opioids may be considered in appropriate patients with careful monitoring.
5. Manual therapies should be considered for a trial to relieve somatic dysfunction.
6. Consider neuropathic pain medication if the pain is predominantly neuropathic in origin.
7. Devil's claw, white willow bark and topical cayeme may all be useful for short-term management.
8. Needling interventions, both dry and wet, may be useful.
9. Guided blocks with a view to radiofrequency neurotomy can be considered in persistent spinal pain.

BOX 34.6 Recommendations for activity and exercise

- Give general advice to stay active, keep flexible and walk without limping.
- The worst thing the patient can do for their back is be too careful.
- Mobilise the spine by gentle activity.
- Build on the patient's personal preferences for exercise; encourage them to set goals.
- Encourage directional preference—i.e. moving in a direction that either reduces pain or doesn't cause pain.
- Make every effort to remove fear about low back pain and avoid sickness behaviour.
- Discourage activities involving static work for the back muscles.
- Treat acute attacks of back pain as an acute muscle spasm, with stretching and light activity.
- With respect to lifting, instruct patients:
  - to avoid twisting with bending
  - to use the thighs with a vertical back for heavy objects
  - to use the back and flex it at other times
  - not to be afraid to lift.
- Explain:
  - that increased tension in muscles, for whatever reason, would increase the pain and thereby add to the problem
  - that longstanding pain could create a vicious circle, with chronic pain as a result.
- Stipulate that all patients must mobilise their lumbar spine through light activity.
- It is not necessary to set exercise goals, but provide the patient with guidelines and encourage them to set their own goals.
- Enquire about and redress any misunderstandings about back pain.
- Encourage and help the patient to try to walk as flexibly as possible.
- Prescribe exercise while a significant other is in attendance at the consultation.
- Reinforce instructions at three months and at one year as a minimum.
- There is evidence for the effectiveness of core stability exercises and Alexander technique programs, but selecting appropriate patients can be problematic.[48,49]
- Remain available to see the patient at their request.

3 weeks duration, and not due to trauma or systemic inflammation. Two trials, with a total of 130 patients, compared needle acupuncture with sham acupuncture. Acupuncture was found to result in greater relief of pain than sham acupuncture (mean difference 18.8 hours), and was more likely to result in 50% more reduction in pain and overall improvement after 10 treatments. However, these changes were not sustained at medium/long-term follow-up (3–12 months).

The other two trials looked at laser acupuncture versus placebo laser, and needle acupuncture plus B_{12} injection versus B_{12} injection alone, and found no differences between acupuncture and control.

The authors concluded that because of the small number of trials, the results should be interpreted with caution, and that there was not enough evidence to determine the role of acupuncture in treating lateral elbow pain.

Since then, two more trials have been published. Tsui and Leung[54] in a small uncontrolled trial ($n = 20$) found that electroacupuncture was superior to manual acupuncture after 2 weeks, and Fink and colleagues[55] found in a small trial ($n = 45$) that both true and sham acupuncture resulted in a decrease in pain and improvement in function after 2 weeks, the difference being significantly greater in the true acupuncture group. At 2-month follow-up the true acupuncture group maintained the improvement in function but pain scores had returned to baseline.

These trials suggest that needle acupuncture may have a short-term benefit in lateral elbow pain, but more trials are needed.

Glucosamine and chondroitin

Glucosamine and chondroitin have anti-inflammatory and chondroprotective effects. They can help rebuild damaged cartilage, and may slow the progression of osteoarthritis following joint injury.

Dose: 1500 mg glucosamine and 1200 mg chondroitin daily. They are more effective in combination than either substance alone for the management of osteoarthritis.

Nutrition

The integrity and functionality of muscles, bones, tendons and joints depends on key nutrients such as magnesium, zinc, selenium, vitamin E, boron and the essential fatty acids. Vitamin C is integral to the formation and maintenance of cartilage and tendons.

As the Western diet is often low in any or all of these nutrients, supplementation and the consumption of nutrient-dense foods should be considered. In cattle and other livestock, the term 'grass tetany' is given to animals when tetanic spasms and eclampsia result from animals consuming pastures low in magnesium.

Bromelian and curcumin have anti-inflammatory and therefore analgesic properties.

Herbal treatments

Anti-inflammatory herbs used in musculoskeletal applications:

- Devil's claw (*Harpagophytum procumbens*)—orally has been shown in several double-blind studies

to be beneficial for longstanding injuries such as chronic low back pain.[56,57] It has been approved for relief of low back pain by ESCOP.[58] It reduces pain and inflammation and has a chondroprotective effect. It compares favourably with medication such as rofecoxib.[6,59] Use cautiously in patients with peptic ulcer, gallstones or pregnancy. Suspend 1 week before major surgery, to avoid increased risk of bleeding.
- Willow bark (*Salix alba*)—used orally for chronic joint or muscle injuries. A Cochrane review in 2006[60] showed moderate evidence that 240 mg salicin daily reduces pain more than placebo in the short term for acute exacerbations of chronic non-specific low back pain. One RCT[61] found that 39% of those treated with willowbark became pain-free after 4 weeks compared with 6% in the placebo group. Response was achieved after 1 week.

  Dose: for acute episodes of non-specific chronic low back pain—willowbark preparations standardised to total salicin content providing 240 mg daily in divided doses.
- *Adaptogens* are a group of herbs used to boost the body's response to stress after injury.
  - Korean ginseng (*Panax ginseng*)—used by many athletes to reduce fatigue, improve strength during convalescence, and facilitate rapid recovery from injury. Used mostly in the short term combined with other herbs, and not during acute infections.
  - Siberian ginseng (*Eleutherococcus senticosus*)—more suitable to long-term use. Not for use in acute infections.
  - *Withania somnifera*—suited to recovery period and reducing fatigue associated with overtraining. Has anti-inflammatory activity exerting selective COX-2 enzyme inhibition.[62]

Topical herbs

- Wintergreen (*Gaultheria procumbens*)—used topically to increase blood flow to chronic joint and muscle injuries. Its essential oil is methyl salicylate.
- *Arnica montana*—used topically to help resolve bruising and swelling of acute injuries.
- Comfrey (*Symphytum officinale*)—used topically for sprains and joint injuries.

INITIAL FOLLOW-UP

1 Record pain/disability.
2 Record red/yellow flags.
3 Repeat examination.
4 Investigate as informed by any changes in red flag status.
5 Repeat education and assurance advice, manage yellow flag issues. This may be done through personal counselling or referring to a psychologist trained in pain management.
6 Consider manual therapy if dysfunctions are present.
7 If dysfunctions are not present and pain management is an issue, consider injections of either corticosteroid or proliferant into tender points.
8 Review as necessary. If steroid injections are performed, review is normally at 2–3 weeks. Proliferant regimens are usually a course of 4–6 injections, 1–2 weeks apart.

FURTHER FOLLOW-UP

- Repeat the first 4 steps above.
- Continue management of yellow flag issues.
- Continue education as to the nature of the problem, and address all the patient's concerns regarding prognosis, lifestyle and work issues, and management options.
- The first 6–8 weeks of management should result in dramatic improvements in pain and disability. If not, then full reassessment of the patient should be undertaken. This will necessarily involve re-evaluation of the diagnosis and treatment strategies in partnership with the patient.

Algorithms can also provide guidance in management. See the appendix for two useful algorithms and associated outcome studies.

Management of chronic persistent low back pain is beyond the scope of this chapter.

SPONDYLOLYSIS/LISTHESIS

The teenage athlete with LBP presents a special dilemma to the health practitioner—that of potential stress fracture of the pars interarticularis. Practitioners should have a high index of suspicion for this condition, to allow early detection and full bony healing.

EPIDEMIOLOGY

The fetal incidence of spondylolysis has conclusively been shown to be zero. It is only on walking that we see spondylolysis occurring. In a study of 32,600 asymptomatic adults, the prevalence of a pars defect was 7.2%.[63] The prevalence has not been shown to be any different in patients suffering from low back pain. There is no significant change in that rate from age 20 to age 80. It is therefore the teenage years that we must be vigilant about, as practitioners.

Most spondylolysis occurs at L5 (85–95%), with most of the rest occurring at the neighbouring L4 (5–15%). There is a strong association with spina bifida occulta.[64] The young athletic populations are at most risk, with gymnasts, cricketers (fast bowlers), footballers, rowers, weight lifters and throwing track and field athletes at highest risk of symptomatic spondylolysis.

PATHOPHYSIOLOGY AND NATURAL HISTORY

The pars interarticularis is the thinnest part of the vertebra. Repetitive mechanical stress from flexion/extension activity of the lumbar spine is the usual cause of fracture to the pars.

In a 45-year follow-up evaluation of first-grade children with a spondylolytic defect, whether symptomatic or not, subjects with bilateral pars defect had a virtually identical course to that of the general population in terms of disability and pain.[65] There appeared to be a marked slowing of slip progression with time, and no subject had reached a 40% slip. Importantly, the authors agreed that there was no justification for advising children and adolescents with spondylolysis and low-grade spondylolisthesis not to participate in sport.

A 7–11-year follow-up of symptomatic young athletes with early-detected spondylolysis recorded similar reassuring findings.[66] Most young athletes conservatively treated will have good functional outcomes at 11-year follow-up. If the pars defect is unilateral, there is a good chance of bony union, but it can take over 3 months.

CLINICAL FEATURES

Pain aggravated by physical activity is the usual presentation of symptomatic spondylolysis. It is usually in the low back and may radiate into the buttocks or proximal thighs. Unfortunately there is no discriminatory symptom or sign for spondylolysis to distinguish it from other causes of mechanical back pain. Reproduction of pain by asking the patient to stand on one leg and hyperextend the lumbar spine is said to be pathognomonic, but no reliability or validity studies have been published.

Most spondylolysis and spondylolisthesis will be asymptomatic. In children, only 13% of individuals with a pars defect have symptoms, and then they usually occur at growth spurts.[67]

IMAGING

To avoid unnecessary radiation, careful thought must be given to ordering radiology. The first rule is not to rush into radiology at the first visit, if there has been no trial of conservative therapy. Most patients suspected of stress fracture are negative to bone scan and X-ray.[68] If, at the 4–6-week mark, there are no signs of the patient settling, then the first step would be a simple lateral of the spine. If spondylolisthesis is present, then no further radiology is necessary. Once there is a slip present, a bone scan is unnecessary as it means there is no possible chance of bony repair of a spondylolysis. The presence of spondylolisthesis does not imply that it is the cause of the back pain, but it does rule out any need for bracing the spine.

If the lateral is normal, then bypass doing oblique radiographs, as they require a great deal of radiation into the gonadal region for no benefit in decision-making. Either treat the patient on suspicion of spondylolysis or do a bone scan/MRI.

If the bone scan is positive, then CT scan through the particular segment will reveal whether a fracture is present and whether it is complete. This will give an indication of the chance of bony healing. It must be pointed out, however, that bony healing is not necessary to achieve an excellent clinical outcome with full return to activities. With this in mind, a strong case can be made for minimal radiological intervention in these patients.

MANAGEMENT

There are no high-quality controlled trials on treatment for spondylolysis. Most studies are uncontrolled case series involving the use of supervised exercise programs, braces and analgesia. Two studies have shown that specific exercise interventions, alone or in combination with other treatments, have a positive effect on low back pain due to spondylolysis and spondylolisthesis; however, the type of exercise was different in both studies.[52]

Factors to consider are:

- *pain management*—this is usually achieved through analgesics, anti-inflammatory agents and avoiding flexion/extension activities; bracing may be considered if pain control proves difficult. Non-pharmacological methods[69] are preferable to pharmacological approaches where possible. An integrative interdisciplinary approach to rehabilitation is usually required, particularly in chronic cases.
- *mind–body techniques*—to assist with pain management
- *stability strengthening*—biomechanical correction, mobilisation, exercises for flexibility and stability and strengthening, soft tissue massage. There are good theoretical reasons for and some clinical evidence to recommend strengthening lumbar stability exercises for patients[70]
- *massage*
- *surgery*—this is rarely needed and usually only considered if there is neurological compromise.

RESOURCES

Australian Association of Musculoskeletal Medicine, http://www.musmed.com

Australasian Faculty of Musculoskeletal Medicine, http://www.afmm.com.au

Australian Family Physician—back pain (June 2004 issue), http://www.racgp.org.au/afp/200406/20040601masters.pdf

Australian Family Physician—musculoskeletal medicine (June 2007 issue), http://www.racgp.org.au/afp/200706

Australasian Musculoskeletal Medicine—journal published biannually by AAMM, http://www.musmed.com/journal.html

REFERENCES

1 Giles LC, Cameron ID, Crotty M. Disability in older Australians: projections for 2006–2031. Med J Aust 2003; 179:130–133.

2 Australian Institute of Health and Welfare. General practice activity in Australia 2006–07. Online. Available: http://www.aihw.gov.au/publications/gep/gpaa06-07/

3 Access Economics. The prevalence, cost and disease burden of arthritis in Australia, Canberra: Arthritis Foundation of Australia; 2001.

4 Woolf AD, Walsh NE, Akesson K. Global care recommendations for musculoskeletal undergraduate curriculum. Ann Rheum Dis 2004; 63:517–524.

5 Charles J, Britt H, Fahridin S. Chronic musculoskeletal problems managed in general practice. Aust Fam Physician 2007; 36:392–393.

6 Merskey H, Bogduk N (eds). Classification of chronic pain. Seattle, WA: IASP Press; 1994.

7 Weddell G, Harpman JA. The neurohistological basis for the sensation of pain provoked from deep fascia, tendon, and periosteum. J Neurol Psychiatry 1940; 3:319–328.

8 Inman VT, Saunders JBD. Referred pain from skeletal structure. J Nerv Ment Dis 1944; 99:660–667.

9 Kellgren JH. On the distribution of pain arising from deep somatic structures with charts of segmental pain areas. Clin Sci 1939; 4:35–46.

10 Dwyer A, Aprill C, Bogduk N. Cervical zygapophyseal joint pain patterns I: a study in normal volunteers. Spine 1990; 15:453–457.

11 Aprill C, Dwyer A, Bogduk N. Cervical zygapophyseal joint pain patterns II: a clinical evaluation. Spine 1990; 15:458–461.

12 Fukui S, Ohseto K, Shiotani M et al. Referred pain distribution of the cervical zygapophyseal joints and cervical dorsal rami. Pain 1996; 68:79–83.

13 McCall IW, Park WM, O'Brien JP. Induced pain referred from posterior lumbar elements in normal subjects. Spine 1979; 4:441–446.

14 Fukui S, Ohseto K, Shiotani M et al. Distribution of referred pain from the lumbar zygapophyseal joints and dorsal rami. Clin J 1997; 13:303–307.

15 Deyo RA, Rainville J, Kent DL. What can the history and physical examination tell us about low back pain? JAMA 1992; 268:760–765.

16 Bogduk N. Mechanisms of musculoskeletal pain. Australasian Musculoskeletal Medicine 2006; 11:6–18.

17 Deyo RA, Tsui-Wu YJ. Descriptive epidemiology of low back pain and its related medical care in the United States. Spine 1987; 12:264–268.

18 Coste J, Delecoeuillerie G, Cohen de Lara A et al. Clinical course and prognostic factors in acute low back pain: an inception cohort study in primary care setting. Br Med J 1994; 308:577–580.

19 Von Korff M, Deyo RA, Cherkin D et al. Back pain in primary care: outcomes at 1 year. Spine 1993; 18: 855–862.

20 Croft PR, Macfarlane GJ, Papageorgiou AC et al. Outcome of low back pain in general practice: a prospective study. Br Med J 1998; 316:1356–1359.

21 McGuirk B, King W, Govind J et al. The safety, efficacy and cost-effectiveness of evidence-based guidelines for the management of acute low back pain in primary care. Spine 2001; 26:2615–2622.

22 Bogduk N. National musculoskeletal medicine initiative. Evidence-based clinical practice guidelines for the management of acute low back pain. CD-ROM Medseed Compass; 2003.

23 Kenna C, Murtagh J. Back pain and spinal manipulation. Sydney: Elsevier; 1997.

24 Hancock MJ, Maher CG, Latimer J et al. Systematic review of tests to identify the disc, SIJ or facet joint as the source of low back pain. Eur Spine J 2007; 16(10):1539–1550.

25 Mendelson R, Conor P. Towards the appropriate use of diagnostic imaging. Med J Aust 2007; 187:5–6.

26 Birnbaum S. CT scanning: too much of a good thing. Br Med J 2007; 334:1006.

27 Australian Acute Musculoskeletal Pain Guidelines Group. Appendix C; 2003. Online. Available: http://www.nhmrc.gov.au

28 Mazanec DJ. Low back pain syndromes. In: Panzer RJ, Black ER, Griner PF, eds. Diagnostic strategies for common medical problems. American College of Physicians; 1991.

29 Borenstein DG, O'Mara JW, Boden SD et al. The value of magnetic resonance imaging of the lumbar spine to predict low-back pain in asymptomatic subjects. J Bone Joint Surg 2001; 83:1306–1311.

30 Liang M, Komaroff AL. Roentgenograms in primary care patients with acute low back pain: a cost effectiveness analysis. Arch Intern Med 1982; 142: 1108–1112.

31 Deyo RA, Rainville J, Kent DL. What can history and physical examination tell us about low back pain? JAMA 1992; 268:760–765.

32 Deyo RA, Diehl AK. Cancer as a cause of back pain: Frequency, clinical presentation, and diagnostic strategies. J Gen Intern Med 1988; 3:230–238.

33 Carter ET, McKenna CH, Brian DD et al. Epidemiology of ankylosing spondylitis in Rochester, Minnesota, 1935–1973. Arthritis Rheum 1979; 22: 365–370.
34 Kent P, Keating JL. Classification in nonspecific low back pain: what methods do primary care clinicians currently use? Spine 2005; 30(12):1433–1440.
35 Bogduk N. International Spinal Injection Society guidelines for the performance of spinal injection procedures. Part1: Zygapophyseal joint blocks. Clin J Pain 1997; 13:285–302.
36 Schwarzer AC, April CN, Bogduk N. The sacroiliac joint in chronic low back pain. Spine 1995; 20:31–37.
37 Binder D, Nampiaparampil D. The provocative lumbar facet joint. Curr Rev Musculoskelet Med 2009; 2(1):15–24.
38 Mulner S. Review article: radiofrequency neurotomy for the treatment of sacroiliac joint syndrome. Curr Rev Musculoskelet Med 2009; 2(1):10–14.
39 Carragee EJ, Alamin TF. Discography: a review. The Spine Journal 2001; 1:364–372.
40 Watson PN. The MSM Quartet. Letter to the editor. Australasian Musculoskeletal Medicine 1999; 2:8–9.
41 Blomberg S. A pragmatic approach to low back pain including manual therapy and steroid injections. A multicenter study in primary health care. 1993; PhD Thesis, Uppsala University, Sweden.
42 Blomberg S, Hallin G, Grann K et al. Manual therapy with steroid injections—a new approach to treatment of low back pain. A controlled multicenter trial with an evaluation by orthopedic surgeons. Spine 1994; 19(5):569–577.
43 Grunnesjo MI, Bogefeldt JP, Svardsudd KF et al. A randomized controlled clinical trial of stay-active care versus manual therapy in addition to stay-active care: functional variables and pain. J Manipulative Physiol Ther 2004; 27(7):431–441.
44 Blomberg S. A pragmatic strategy for low back pain—an integrated multimodal programme based on antidysfunctional medicine. In: Hutson M, ed. Textbook of musculoskeletal medicine. Oxford University Press; 2005:1–20.
45 Hagen KB, Hilde G, Jamtvedt G et al. Bed rest for acute low-back pain and sciatica. Cochrane Database Syst Rev 2004; 4:CD001254.
46 Kendall NAS, Linton SJ, Main CJ. Guide to assessing psychosocial yellow flags in acute low back pain: risk factors for long-term disability and work loss. Wellington, New Zealand: Accident Rehabilitation and Compensation Insurance Corporation of New Zealand and the National Health Committee; 1997. Online. Available: http://www.nhc.govt.nz.
47 Watson P. The recovergram. Australasian Musculoskeletal Medicine 2000; 5(2):24–28.
48 Hammill R, Beazell J, Hart J. Neuromuscular consequences of low back pain and core dysfunction. Clin Sports Med 2008; 27:449–462.
49 Little P, Lewith G, Webley F et al. Randomised controlled trial of Alexander technique lessons, exercise, and massage (ATEAM) for chronic and recurrent back pain. Br Med J 2008; 337:a884.
50 Furlan AD, van Tulder MW, Cherkin DC et al. Acupuncture and dry-needling for low back pain. Cochrane Database Syst Rev 2005; CD001351.
51 Mainheimer E, White A, Berman B et al. Meta-analysis: acupuncture for low back pain. Ann Intern Med 2005; 142:651–663.
52 Trinh KV, Graham N, Gross AR et al. Acupuncture for neck disorders. Cochrane Database Syst Rev 2006; 3:CD004870.
53 Green S, Buchbiner R, Barnsley L et al. Acupuncture for lateral elbow pain. Cochrane Database Syst Rev 2002; CD003527.
54 Tsui P, Leung MCP. Comparison of the effectiveness between manual acupuncture and electro-acupuncture on patients with tennis elbow. Acupunct Electrother Res 2002; 27:107–117.
55 Fink M, Wolkenstein E, Lunnemann M et al. Chronic epicondylitis: effects of real and sham acupuncture treatment: a randomised controlled patient- and examiner-blinded long-term trial. Forsch Komplementarmed 2002; 9:210–215.
56 Laudahn D, Walper A. Efficacy and tolerance of *Harpagyphytum* extract LI 174 in patients with chronic non-radicular back pain. Phytother Res 2001; 15(7):621–624.
57 Chrubasik S, Junck H, Breitschwerdt H et al. Effectiveness of *Harpagophytum* extract WS 1531 in the treatment of exacerbation of low back pain: a randomized, placebo-controlled, double-blind study. Eur J Anaesthesiol 1999; 16(2):118–129.
58 European Scientific Co-operative on Phytomedicine (ESCOP), 2nd edn. Stuttgart: Thieme; 2003.
59 Chrubasik S, Model A, Black et al. A randomised double-blind pilot study comparing Doloteffin® and Vioxx® in the treatment of low back pain. Rheumatology 2003; 42(1):141–148.
60 Gagnier JJ, van Tulder M, Berman B et al. Herbal medicine for low back pain. Cochrane Database Syst Rev 2006; 2:CD004504.
61 Chrubasik S, Eisenberg E, Balan E et al. Treatment of low back pain exacerbations with willowbark extract: a randomised double-blind study. Am J Med 2000; 109(1):9–14.
62 Jayaprakasam B, Nair NG. Cyclooxygenase 2 enzyme inhibitory withanolides from Withania somnifera leaves. Tetrahedron 2003; 59(6):125–132.

63 Moreton RD. Spondylolysis. JAMA 1966; 195: 671–674.

64 Standaert CJ, Herring SA. Spondylosis: a critical review. Br J Sports Med 2000; 34(6):415–422.

65 Beutler WJ, Fredrickson BE, Murtland A et al. The natural history of spondylolysis. Spine 2003; 28:1027–1035.

66 Miller SF, Congeni J, Swanson K. Long-term functional and anatomical follow-up of early detected spondylolysis in young athletes. Am J Sports Med 2004; 32:928–933.

67 Hessinger RN. Spondylolysis and spondylolisthesis in children and adolescents. J Bone Joint Surg 1989; 14:1342–1355.

68 Elliot S, Hutson MA, Wastie ML et al. Bone scintigraphy in the assessment of spondylolysis in patients attending a sports injury clinic. Clin Radiol 1988; 39:269–272.

69 Chou R, Huffman LH. American Pain Society, American College of Physicians. Nonpharmacologic therapies for acute and chronic low back pain: a review of the evidence for an American Pain Society/American College of Physicians clinical practice guideline. Ann Intern Med 2007; 147(7):492–504.

70 O'Sullivan PB, Phyty GD, Twomey LT et al. Evaluation of specific stabilizing exercise in the treatment of chronic low back pain with radiologic diagnosis of spondylolysis or spondylolisthesis. Spine 1997; 22(24):2959–2967.

APPENDIX: ALGORITHMS

ALGORITHM FOR MANAGEMENT OF ACUTE LOW BACK PAIN

ACUTE LOW BACK PAIN ALGORITHM

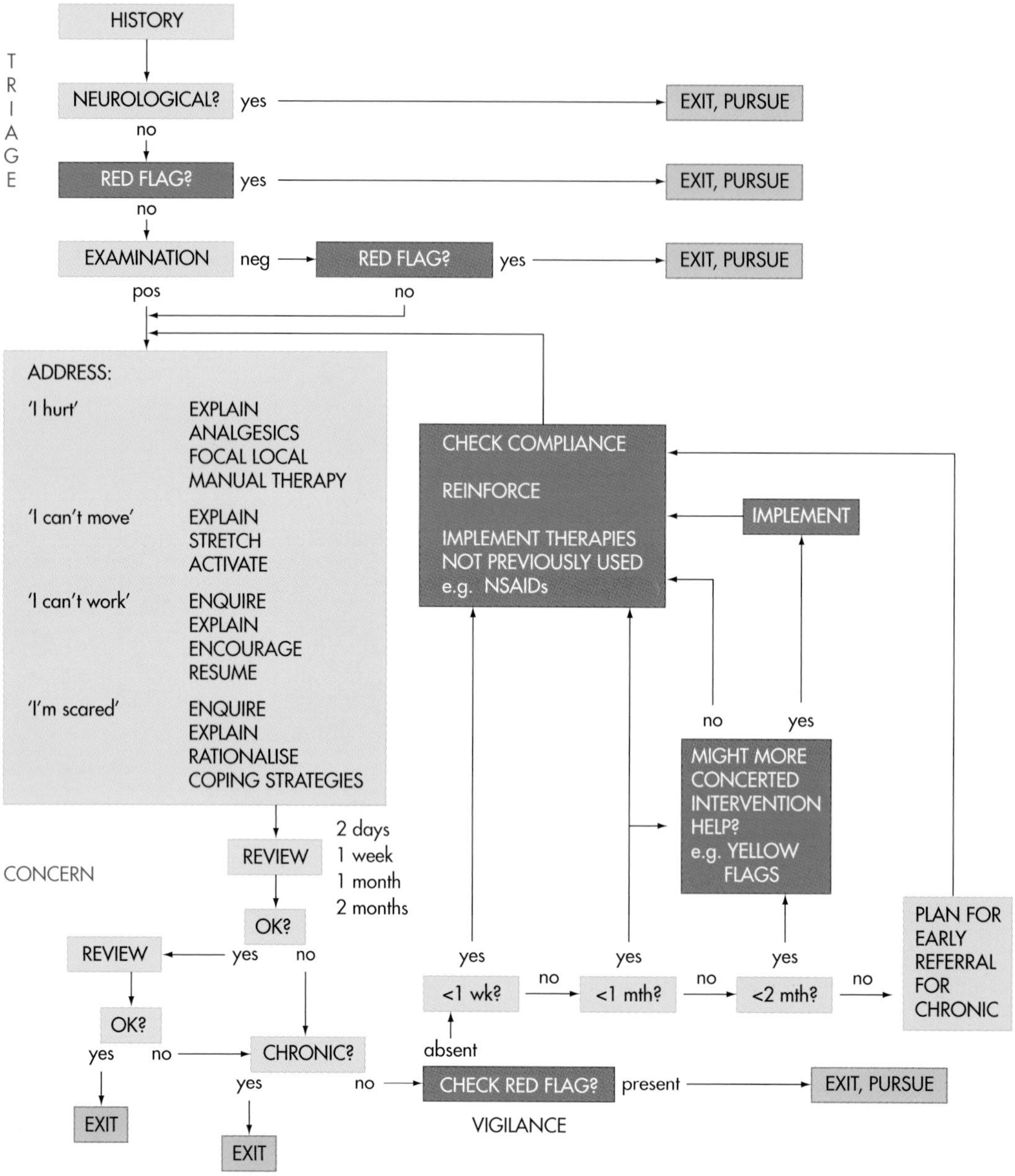

CRITERIA FOR IMAGING IN PRIMARY CARE

1. History of cancer
2. Significant trauma
3. Temperature >37.8°C
4. Body penetration
5. Weight loss
6. Use of corticosteroids
7. No improvement over 1 month
8. Neurological deficit
9. Age > 50 years

After Deyo RA and Diehl AK, J Gen Intern Med 1986; 1:20–25

(Source: McGuirk B, King W, Govind J et al. The safety, efficacy and cost-effectiveness of evidence-based guidelines for the management of acute low back pain in primary care. Spine 2001; 26:2615–2622)

STAYAC ALGORITHM

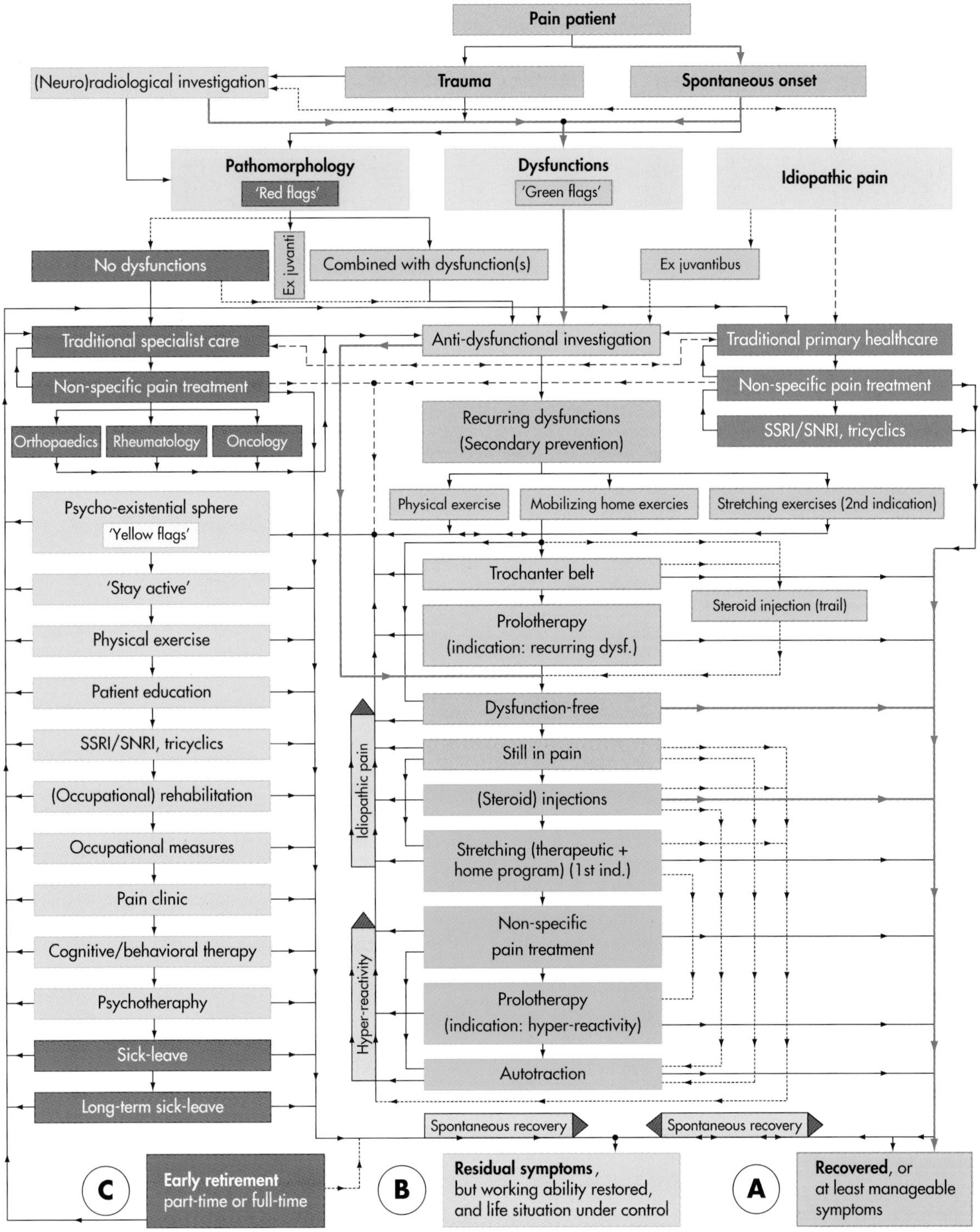

(Source: Blomberg S. A pragmatic strategy for low back pain—an integrated multimodal programme based on antidysfunctional medicine. In: Hutson M, ed. Textbook of musculoskeletal medicine. Oxford University Press; 2005:1–20)

chapter 35

Nails

INTRODUCTION AND OVERVIEW

Nails are important for adornment. Smooth, lustrous nails are considered a sign of health and beauty. The rapid growth of nail salons demonstrates the value that women in particular assign to their nails. Fingernails are also important for fine touch and manipulation. Toenails are protective, especially the large toenails, which bear the brunt of force from jogging, footballing and many other sports.

The nail sits right on the bone of the terminal phalanx, and is closely associated with the distal interphalangeal joint. Toenails especially are prone to repeated microtrauma over the years from footwear, sporting injuries and changes due to arthritis. Fingernails suffer from whatever traumas we put our hands through—chemicals, soaps and detergents and, for some, the added insults of nail salons cutting and dissolving cuticles, using harsh chemicals to apply and remove polishes, false nails, acrylics and so on.

NORMAL NAIL STRUCTURE

The normal nail structure consists of the nail matrix, the nail bed, the proximal and lateral nail folds, the cuticle and the nail plate (Fig 35.1). The nail matrix is made up of the germinative epithelium, and is protected from the environment by the waterproof seal created by the cuticle.

The integrity of the nail depends on the close adhesion of the nail bed and the nail plate, as well as an intact cuticle. The nail bed is closely apposed to the distal phalanx, so changes in the bone and joint will affect the nail.

COMMON NAIL PROBLEMS

HYPERTROPHY AND SUBUNGUAL HYPERKERATOSIS

A number of conditions can cause this problem. Fungal infection, psoriasis and trauma are the most common causes, and may coexist. Fungal infection and trauma are most often seen in toenails; it is rare to have fungal disease in fingernails unless all the toenails are involved too.

Onychomycosis (fungal infection)

Onychomycosis is a relatively common nail disease. A recent European study (Achilles) of 90,000 people aged over 60 years in 16 countries estimated that half had a 'fungal foot infection' and that one-quarter of these had onychomycosis.[1,2] An Australian study of the general population stated the prevalence as 2–8%, but this figure increases with age.[3] An Australian nursing home study put the rate at 22%.[4]

Causes

Most cases of onychomycosis are due to dermatophytes, with *Trichophyton rubrum* and *T. mentagrophytes* var. interdigitale being the most common. They usually affect nails by the distal and lateral subungual route. Repeated microtrauma is a common predisposing factor, and tinea between the toes is often present too.

White superficial onychomycosis and proximal subungual onychomycosis may also occur but are less common.

Diagnosis

A diagnosis of onychomycosis should be made before embarking on treatment. Many diseases mimic onychomycosis. Unfortunately, using fungal microscopy and culture, a negative result is obtained in about 40% of cases where infection is truly present. Ideally, when sending a specimen for micro and culture, plenty of the subungual material should be collected and ground up before plating. Distal nail biopsy gives a much higher yield of positive results. Basically this involves cutting off as large a specimen as possible of distal nail (in fact the patient often

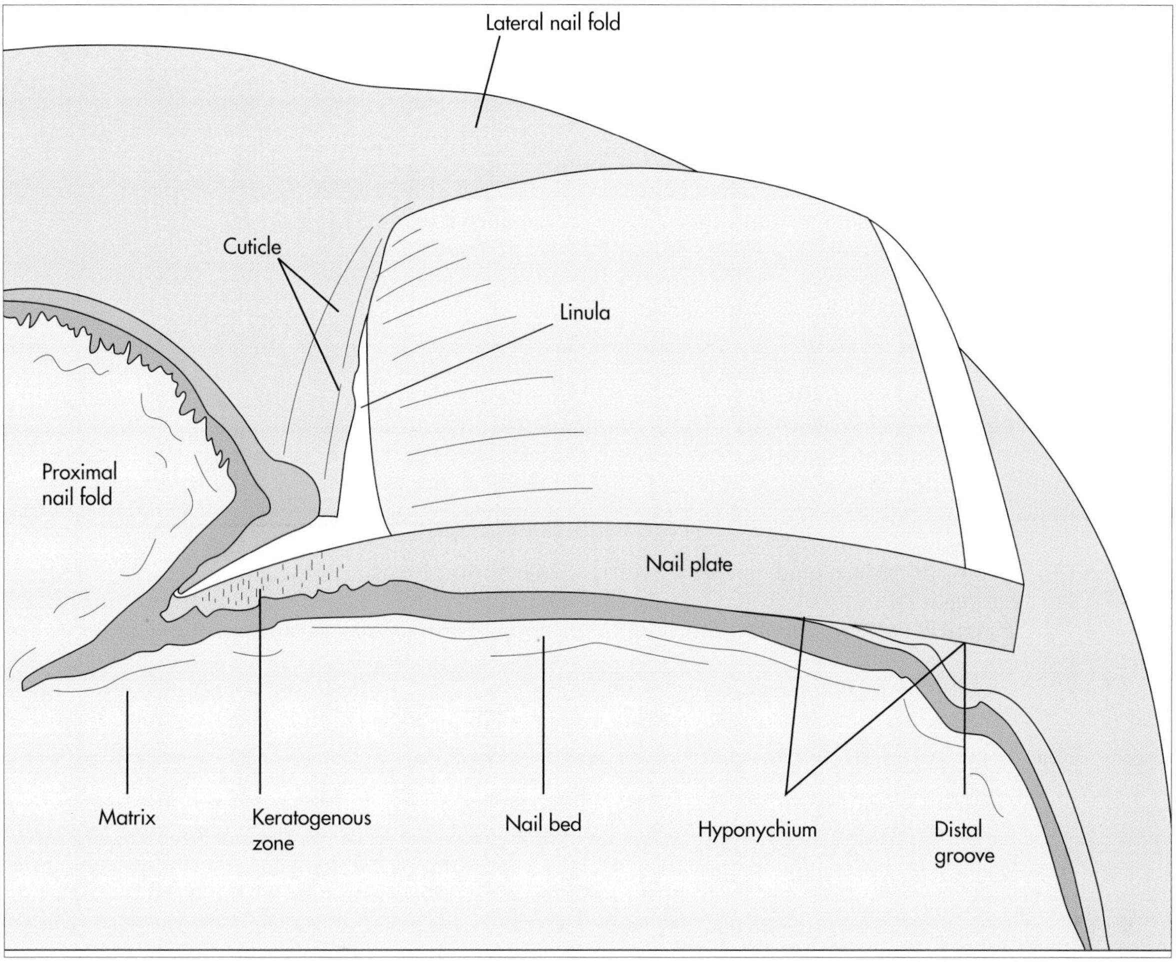

FIGURE 35.1 Diagrammatic drawing of an adult fingertip, showing nail structures through a longitudinal midline plane.

does this best, and you must stop the nail clipping being lost over on the other side of the room). The piece is sent for histopathology as well as micro and culture, and the pathologist looks for hyphae in the nail plate.

Treatment

One option is to have no treatment apart from regular nail clipping. Oral therapy is usually necessary to cure infections in the nail plate. Other treatment options are:

1 *Terbinafine* (*Lamisil®*)—at present the treatment of choice for onychomycosis due to dermatophytes.

   The usual dose is 250 mg daily. It comes as 42 tablets and one repeat. In nail clinics patients are often asked to take the second 42 tablets twice a week; this prolongs the therapy and still gives a reasonable dose in the nail plate.

   It is important to stress to patients that the infected toenails will need to grow out, and this can take up to a year.

   Side effects are normally minimal, but there are some worrying reports of agranulocytosis occurring after a month of therapy. Liver function abnormalities have been reported too. A white cell count and liver function test after a month of treatment are recommended.

2 *Itraconazole* (*Sporanox®*)—also highly effective, often given as 'pulse therapy'. Two tablets twice daily (400 mg) are given for the first week of the month, each month, for 3 months of therapy.

3 *Fluconazole*—weekly oral fluconazole 150 mg for 3 months is used extensively in many countries.

4 *Griseofulvin*—500 mg, two tablets per day is usually required to achieve sufficient dosage in the nail. As this drug is only fungistatic, prolonged treatment of up to 2 years may be needed for toenails, especially in the elderly. Even so, the cure rate is around 50% and relapse is common.

Nausea and headaches may occur, and liver function tests should be monitored with long-term therapy.

5 *Ketoconazole*—can be effective but is inadvisable because of potential liver toxicity.
6 *Topical therapy*—for white superficial onychomycosis or limited disease, topical treatment can be useful, especially in conjunction with removal of diseased nail. Amorolfine (Loceryl®) is the most effective agent currently available in Australia. It is a paint applied weekly after rubbing the nail plate with a file.
7 *Physical treatment*—nail removal, surgically or with 40% urea paste, can be helpful, especially in single nail disease. It is usually advisable to use topical or oral antifungal treatment as well, or the disease may re-occur.

Psoriasis

Involvement of the fingernails and toenails with psoriasis has been reported in up to 50% of psoriasis sufferers.[5] The fingernails are more commonly involved than the toenails.

Pitting and onycholysis are common presentations of nail psoriasis, but the more disfiguring abnormality of hypertrophy and subungual hyperkeratosis is the most distressing. Often all the nails eventually become involved, whereas this is less common in onychomycosis. Fingernails are frequently involved and this appearance upsets patients more than that of their toenails, which can be hidden.

Another difference between onychomycosis and psoriasis is that the nails affected by psoriasis often change; some may recover spontaneously but this does not occur in onychomycosis.

Diagnosis

Distal nail biopsy, as described above, is useful. The pathologist looks for parakeratosis on the nail plate.

Treatment

No treatment is fully effective in all people, and often the patient opts for no treatment.

The following can be used.

1 *Topical calcipitriol.*
2 *Intralesional steroids*—Kenacort®-A10 (triamcinolone acetonide), diluted in Xylocaine® (lignocaine), injected into the proximal nail fold and/or nail bed can give several months of remission.
3 *PUVA* (psoralen plus exposure to ultraviolet A)—topical or oral psoralens with UVA sometimes helps.
4 *Oral methotrexate*—seldom used for nails alone, but if there is widespread skin involvement or arthritis as well, it can be useful.
5 *Oral acitretin*—again, seldom used for nails alone, but can be useful for severe hyperkeratosis.

An alternative approach is of a cosmetic nature. Preformed artificial nails or sculptured artificial nails may be applied if there is enough keratin for adherence. Nail abrasion, usually done by podiatrists, can also help with appearance, and in reducing discomfort from footwear.

Trauma

Trauma, especially to the toenails, is one of the most common causes of nail dystrophy. Repeated microtrauma is particularly common, from shoes and sports, especially jogging, netball and football. Changes to underlying bones and joints with arthritis and ageing can exaggerate the effects of trauma.

Onychogryphosis

Onychogryphosis is most common in the big toenails. The nail plate is thickened and opaque and the nail bed is hyperplastic. In the extreme form the nail looks like a ram's horn. In older patients this is due to biomechanical factors and footwear, and secondary foot anomalies such as hallux valgus are commonly associated.

Pincer nails

Pincer nail deformity is characterised by transverse overcurvature of the nail plate, especially at the distal free edge. The constriction of the distal pulp may be painful, especially in the severe form when the distal phalanx is enclosed. The deformity may lead to ingrown toenails.

The dystrophy is most likely a developmental abnormality for which there may be a hereditary tendency. There seems to be an enlarging of the dorsal bony phalanx with juxtaarticular osteophytes causing widening of the base of the nail, therefore leading to a conical-shaped nail plate.

Treatment with lateral matrix ablation is often necessary, although less invasive treatments have been described.

Habit tic deformity

Habit tic deformity is a deformity usually of the thumb nails, caused by habitual picking and manicuring of the proximal nail fold causing repeated trauma to the nail matrix and resulting in a central depression with transverse grooves at the same angle as the cuticle, giving a washboard or fir tree appearance. Often the cuticle is damaged or absent. This deformity is particularly noticeable in people with large cuticles (Heller's median canaliform dystrophy).

Nail biting (onychophagia)

Nail biting is common in children—up to 50% of children are affected at some stage. Usually it is self-limiting, but it may persist into adulthood with less likelihood of recovery. It may be associated with anxiety or obsessive-compulsive traits, but a primary psychiatric disorder is unlikely.

Treatment requires a highly motivated patient and includes unpleasant-tasting nail preparations, occlusive dressings, behavioural therapy or bribery!

Ingrown toenails

Patients with an ingrown toenail are frequently encountered in general practice. It is a painful condition, due to the penetration and irritation of the soft tissues of the lateral nail fold by an irregular spicule of the lateral nail plate.

Predisposing factors include poorly fitting shoes, incorrect nail trimming, hereditary imbalance between the width of the nail matrix and nail bed, and oral retinoids.

In mild early disease (stage 1), conservative measures such as soaking the foot in warm water, use of topical or oral antibiotics, proper nail-trimming technique and elevation of the corner of the nail can be enough.

Stage 2 disease is characterised by worsening of symptoms, drainage and infection, and can be managed conservatively or surgically. Stage 3 disease is characterised by lateral wall hypertrophy and is best treated with partial nail avulsion, lateral matricectomy and destruction of the lateral wall granulation tissue. Chemical matricectomy with phenol is effective, but surgical matricectomy may offer more controlled tissue destruction and less postoperative drainage.

Trauma is a factor in many other nail conditions discussed here, including onycholysis, chronic paronychia, onychomycosis and brittle nails.

CHRONIC PARONYCHIA

Chronic paronychia is a chronic inflammatory condition of the proximal nail fold and is most common in those who have their hands in and out of water and detergents. The nail cuticle is lost and there is a space between the nail fold and the nail plate. *Candida* species and gram-negative bacteria are commonly cultured here and seem to aggravate the condition. Skin disease affecting nail folds, such as psoriasis, eczema and perniosis, may also contribute.

Treatment

1. General measures include keeping the hands away from soaps and detergents, and wearing gloves where possible. Any contributing skin disease should be treated.
2. Miconazole tincture may be applied twice daily to the space between the nail fold and the nail plate.
3. Nystatin ointment, when hands have to be in water.
4. Topical steroid ointment applied to the proximal nail folds has been shown to be the most effective treatment for this condition.

With treatment the prognosis is good.

ONYCHOLYSIS

Onycholysis—the separation of the nail from its bed—is one of the most common nail conditions. It is found in psoriasis, thyroid disease, yellow nail syndrome and many other conditions, but in a large number of cases no specific cause is found. It is possible that acute trauma initiates it, and once the nail is loosened, repeated minor traumas and secondary infection perpetuate the problem.

Secondary infection may be by yeasts or bacteria. *Pseudomonas aeruginosa* is common and produces green, blue and black discolouration. The exposed nail bed can become covered in keratin, making reattachment unlikely.

Candida albicans is very common as a secondary agent. With time it can grow into the nail plate, preventing reattachment.

Treatment

1. The nail bed should be dried by blowing the area with a hot hair dryer several times a day.
2. Anti-infective agents such as miconazole lotion or 15% sulfacetamide lotion may be applied under the nail plate.
3. If *Pseudomonas* is present, white vinegar soaks for 10–20 minutes twice a day are recommended (10% white vinegar in water).
4. If *C. albicans* is grown from the nail plate, oral treatment with ketoconazole, fluconazole or itraconazole can be very helpful. Three to six months of treatment is often needed, so monitoring of liver function, especially for ketoconazole, is recommended. Terbinafine (Lamisil®) is of no use for this condition.

BRITTLE NAILS

Brittle nails are a reasonably common problem, primarily of cosmetic significance. Clinically there are two alterations to the nail plate: excessive onychorrhexis (longitudinal ridging) and onychoschizia (horizontal layering of the distal nail plate, like the 'split ends' of hair).

Causes

Many factors are associated with brittleness, but water is probably the most important. Repeated wetting and drying has been shown to lead to the above changes. Other chemicals, cement, detergents and alkalis can also lead to dissolution of intercellular adhesive factors and thus to brittle nails.

There are many systemic causes listed, but these are rare. Most people with brittle nails think they must be low in calcium but there is little calcium in the nail and it does not contribute to nail hardness.

Treatment

1. Moisture and trauma should be avoided by wearing cotton and rubber gloves.
2. Oral biotin has been shown in some studies to help. Use Blackmore's hair and nail vitamins or Tricusil® twice a day, as these contain 2.5 mg of biotin, the required daily amount.
3. Nail moisturisers such as 10% urea creams are probably better for the nails than nail hardeners. Alpha-hydroxy acids may also be effective (e.g. lactic acid, glycolic acid creams).

TRACHYONYCHIA (ROUGH NAILS)

Roughness of the nail surface implies disease of the nail matrix. Lichen planus is probably the most common cause, along with alopecia areata and twenty nail dystrophy. In lichen planus, nail changes occur in about 10% of cases but are usually mild and transient. Longitudinal ridging (onychorrhexis) is common along with the roughening. Severe atrophic disease is less common, but devastating when it happens. Scarring can occur between the proximal nail fold and the nail plate. This scar is called a *pterygium*.

Twenty nail dystrophy of childhood is a benign, self-limiting condition with no scarring. Some believe it to be a variant of lichen planus. The child is born with normal nails; then, at a variable age, roughness and ridging of all the nails develop. There are no hair or skin abnormalities. Complete resolution normally occurs after a number of years. In alopecia areata, nail changes again occur in about 10% of cases. Pitting is the most common abnormality, but trachyonychia is not uncommon. Most severe cases are associated with severe alopecia.

Treatment

Treatment is often unnecessary. In more severe cases, treatment is by fluorinated steroids with or without occlusion. In lichen planus with severe atrophy or early pterygium formation, the diagnosis should be confirmed by biopsy and oral steroids should be used to prevent scarring. This is as close as we come to a nail 'dermatological emergency'.

SINGLE NAIL DEFORMITY

When a single abnormal nail develops in the absence of a history of trauma, one should think of a tumour. Myxoid or mucous cysts (due to collagenous degeneration of the extensor tendon) are the most common cause. There may be a swelling in the proximal nail fold, and a linear depression in the nail plate develops.

Other benign tumours include warts (usually obvious), subungual exostoses and glomus tumours (usually painful). Malignant tumours are less common (Bowen's disease, squamous cell carcinoma, melanoma) and present as slowly progressive lesions with destruction of the nail.

Diagnosis often requires surgical exploration (after X-ray), and treatment is by surgical excision.

PIGMENTED BANDS

Longitudinal brown or black bands are relatively common in darker skinned races, but melanoma of the nail still needs to be excluded. Multiple bands that are light in colour and even are usually not of concern.

Trauma leading to a subungual haematoma can cause black staining of the nail bed. Usually the patient remembers trauma, but sometimes in the big toenails trauma from footwear causes bleeding under the nails of which the patient is unaware.

The main problem, however, is whether a single linear pigmented band is caused by a benign naevus, melanocytic hyperplasia of the nail matrix or malignant melanoma. Certain features favour the last:

- one finger only involved
- periungual spread of pigment
- extension of pigment to the free edge of the nail
- darkening with time
- progressive widening of the band, with blurring of the border
- age over 50 years.

Diagnosis

Any suspicious lesion should be biopsied. The proximal nail fold is reflected and the most proximal part of the pigmented band needs to be biopsied, with either a punch or a shave biopsy.

SYSTEMIC DISEASE

KOILONYCHIA

Koilonychia, or spoon-shaped nail deformity, is relatively common, and is only rarely due to iron deficiency anaemia. Most cases are idiopathic or due to chemical trauma. Paradoxically, it can occur in haemochromatosis. In childhood it is a common physiological variant that usually resolves spontaneously.

HALF-AND-HALF NAILS

In this condition there is pallor of the proximal half of the nail plate and erythema of the distal half. This is characteristically seen in renal failure. It can also occur in cardiac or hepatic failure, or with no obvious cause, and the reason for the changes is not clearly understood.

CLUBBING

The characteristic features of clubbing are increased nail plate curvature in both directions, and soft tissue hypertrophy of the digital pulp and nail bed dermis. It is usually gradual in onset, and painless, except in association with carcinoma of the lung. Schamroth's sign is the loss of the diamond-shaped window between apposing nail plates of the corresponding left and right fingers.

Eighty per cent of cases are associated with pulmonary disease, especially chronic infections and cancers.[4] Other associations include endocarditis, bowel diseases, Graves' disease and systemic lupus erythematosus.

BEAU'S LINES

Joseph Beau first described transverse grooves in the nail plate in 1846 as a manifestation of typhoid and other acute systemic diseases. The classic description refers to transverse grooves appearing in all nails 4–8 weeks after the acute illness, They are due to disruption of matrical activity resulting in focal thinning of the nail plate. As well as systemic illness, Beau's lines can be caused by drugs.

If one nail is involved, there has usually been some traumatic event involving the proximal nail fold and/or cuticle (paronychia). In severe cases the nail may be shed (onychomadesis).

YELLOW NAIL SYNDROME

Yellow nail syndrome is an interesting but rare condition in which slow-growing yellow nails develop in association with lymphoedema and/or chronic infective lung disease. The nail disease may precede the other manifestations by many years.

Treatment is of the underlying disease, if one is found. Otherwise vitamin E 800 units a day for 12–18 months has been reported to help.[4] Oral zinc has been reported to be useful in one case.[4]

NAIL CARE

The aesthetic value of nails is as important today as their functional value. The ratio of the length to the breadth of the nail is considered important to its appeal—this should be about equal for the thumb, slightly more for the other nails. Everyone grooms their nails; this may be cleaning and cutting only. Some, especially women, do much more. There are many products available to enhance the appearance of nails, but little data on the efficacy of the products—only adverse reactions are reported.

Most nail manicurists soak the nails before trimming them in an arc fashion. This is probably acceptable for fingernails, but toenails should be cut straight across, to prevent ingrowing of the side of the nail into the lateral nail fold. Filing rather than cutting is less likely to cause shearing and fracturing of the nail plate. The cuticle should never be removed or traumatised, as this removes the water-tight barrier that protects the nail matrix. Unfortunately, manicurists often seem to want to do this, as the cuticle interferes with application of nail polish!

The nail plate is then groomed. This may be just with a cream containing finely ground pumice, talc or kaolin, with wax to increase the shine.

Nail polish consists of pigments suspended in a volatile solvent to which film-formers have been added. The most popular resin used is toluene sulfonamide formaldehyde, which is a cause of allergic contact dermatitis, often manifesting as eyelid dermatitis. Hypoallergenic nail enamels are available, with alternative resins. Pigments are either dissolved or suspended in the lacquer; dissolved pigment is more likely to cause staining of the nails.

Dibutyl phthalate (DBP), a chemical used to keep nail polish from chipping, has been associated with breast cancer in laboratory animals, as well as long-term fertility issues in newborn boys—leaving the cosmetics industry in a heavy debate over whether to continue use of the ingredient. The European Union banned the use of DBP in 2004 and several manufacturers have removed it, or plan to remove it, from their polishes. Toluene-free and DBP-free nail polishes are available.

Apart from reactions to the polish itself, harmful effects can come from nail polish removers, which can cause trachyonychia.

NAIL HARDENERS

Nail hardeners are basically nail polish with different solvent and resin concentrations to make the nail plate less porous. Paradoxically, their prolonged use can make nails more brittle.

NAIL MOISTURISERS

Nail moisturisers are creams and lotions that contain occlusives such as petrolatum and lanolin, or humectants such as glycerine. They can be very useful for brittle nails.

PRE-FORMED ARTIFICIAL NAILS (FALSE NAILS)

Artificial nails are plastic devices glued onto 'normal' nails to make them look longer and more beautiful. The nail plate is roughened by a file to increase adhesion, and a glue, usually ethyl cyanoacrylate, is used. This may cause allergic contact dermatitis, so these nails should not be worn for more than 48 hours at a time.

SCULPTURED NAILS

Sculptured nails are created with the combination of a liquid monomer and a powder polymer cured at room temperature with an organic accelerator. The paste is moulded onto the nail and held in place until it hardens, then the nail is clipped and filed into shape. As the nail grows out, the gap between the acrylic nail and the proximal nail fold must be filled.

Contact dermatitis can occur due to the monomer, now usually ethyl methacrylate.

GEL NAILS

Gel nails are applied in a semi-liquid form onto the 'normal' nail, then cured with ultraviolet light. Allergic reactions to these compounds are frequently reported, causing onycholysis and paronychia.

One of the problems with having beautiful polished, false or sculptured nails is that the wearer wants to keep them long, making them a repository for bacteria. Medical personnel and those in the food handling areas are discouraged from having long or false nails at work.

Despite the numerous reports of negative outcomes from nail grooming, the industry is booming and there must be more positive than negative stories. Nail adornment can be extremely useful for people with damaged, absent, diseased or ragged nails. It is wrong to dismiss complaints of unattractive nails as too trivial!

RESOURCES

Baran R, Dawber R, de Berker D et al. Baran & Dawber's diseases of the nails and their management, 3rd edn. Oxford: Blackwell Science; 2001.

Baran R, Barth J, Dawber R et al. Nail disorders: common presenting signs, differential diagnosis and treatment. New York: Churchill Livingstone; 1991.

REFERENCES

1 Haneke E. Achilles foot-screening project: background, objectives and design. J Europ Acad Dermatol Venereol 2006; 12(S1):S2–S5.

2 Roseeuw D. Achilles foot-screening project: preliminary results of patients screened by dermatologists. Eur Acad Dermatol Venereol 2006; 12(S1):S6–S9.

3 Gill D, Marks R. A review of the epidemiology of tinea unguium in the community. Aust J Dermatol 2002; 40(1):6–13.

4 Tosti A, Piraccini BM, Mariani R et al. Are local and systemic conditions important for the development of onychomycosis? Eur J Dermatol 1998; 8(1):41–44.

5 Baran R, Dawber R, de Berker D et al. Baran & Dawber's diseases of the nails and their management, 3rd edn. Oxford: Blackwell Science; 2001.

chapter 36

Neurology

INTRODUCTION AND OVERVIEW

This chapter discusses the more common neurological symptoms and disorders encountered in general practice, and some of the less-common classic neurological problems that are rarely seen in general practice. It is far from comprehensive—more detailed information can be found in textbooks of neurology.[1,2]

HEADACHE

Headache is probably one of the most common reasons for a patient to consult a general practitioner (GP). Many patients are fearful that they may have a serious neurological disorder, such as a brain tumour, whereas in reality this is rare. In primary care, the risk of brain tumour with a headache presentation is less than 0.1%.[3] The most common causes of headache seen by a GP are primary headaches such as those associated with fever, tension headache and, less often, migraine. The challenge for the GP is to identify the very rare but more sinister causes of headache, such as subarachnoid haemorrhage (SAH), brain tumour, cranial arteritis, meningitis and so on. There are some clinical features that should increase the suspicion of a secondary cause for headache, such as:

- headache of sudden, instantaneous onset
- headache associated with systemic symptoms such as fever, anorexia or weight loss
- presence of focal neurological symptoms
- headache that awakens the patient from their sleep, when they retired to bed without a headache (although migraine headache often awakens patients from their sleep).

HISTORY

Investigations rarely elucidate the cause of headache; it is the history that is used to determine the aetiology of the headache in the great majority of patients. It has been said that if you only have 30 minutes, spend 29 on the history. Ascertain whether this headache is the first that the patient has experienced or whether it is a recurrent headache; if the latter, ask whether this headache is identical to all the others. If so, it is not unreasonable to treat for that same diagnosis. In patients presenting with new-onset headache, *the single most important question* is, 'From the moment you first noticed the headache, how long did it take to reach its maximum severity?' Headache of sudden onset should be regarded as possible SAH until proved otherwise, although with many of the other causes, sudden-onset headache such as cough, benign sex and exertional headache, there are often other clues to the diagnosis (see below). Ascertain whether there were any associated systemic symptoms such as fever, sweats, anorexia or weight loss, and, in the elderly, the presence of scalp tenderness, jaw claudication of proximal muscle, aches and pains (polymyalgia rheumatica), to alert one to the possibility of infection or cranial arteritis. Headache associated with or exacerbated by particular neck movements may point to a cervicogenic musculoskeletal cause.

In patients with focal neurological symptoms, determine whether these developed suddenly or slowly. If slowly, determine whether there was a cumulative neurological deficit or the focal neurological symptoms evolved gradually, with the latter symptoms appearing after the initial symptoms had either partly or completely resolved—a characteristic of migraine.

EXAMINATION

Every patient presenting with headache should be examined for papilloedema and neck stiffness. In elderly patients, the temporal and occipital arteries should be checked for thrombosis. If the patient has had systemic symptoms, the temperature should be checked and a detailed general examination should be performed.

INVESTIGATIONS

A computerised tomography (CT) scan rarely demonstrates any abnormality in most patients presenting to the GP with headache, and yet it is often difficult not to perform in order to reassure the patient that they do not have a brain tumour. A routine CT scan does not routinely examine the pituitary fossa, cavernous sinus, posterior fossa, region of the foramen magnum or cerebral venous system, and disorders in these sites, although very rare, can be missed by a CT scan. Magnetic resonance imaging (MRI) is the modality of choice in these circumstances. In patients with an SAH, a normal CT in the first few hours largely but not always excludes the diagnosis, and in patients with suspected SAH a lumbar puncture (LP) is necessary. An LP should also be performed in patients with suspected meningitis. Perform a full blood examination (FBE), C-reactive protein (CRP) and erythrocyte sedimentation rate (ESR) if there is a suspicion of an infective illness or a systemic problem, or if the patient is elderly.

MANAGEMENT

Apart from symptomatic relief with analgesia, the management is cause-specific and is discussed below.

Headache of sudden onset

Subarachnoid haemorrhage

The diagnosis should be SAH until proved otherwise, because of the potentially disastrous outcome in patients who suffer a recurrent haemorrhage. The headache is maximum in intensity at onset and in general persists for hours (although the warning or 'sentinel' headache representing a less severe rupture of the aneurysm may be so brief that the patient may not consult a medical practitioner). It is usually generalised but may be predominantly occipital or frontal. There is usually nausea and vomiting and, if severe, depression of the conscious state. A focal deficit may occur if haemorrhage also occurs into the parenchyma. The general practice management consists of immediate referral to hospital for assessment. In hospital, management will consist of stabilisation and resuscitation of the patient if necessary, assessment using investigations such as CT and angiography, analgesia and then, possibly, surgery to prevent re-bleed.

Exertional and benign sex headache

It is important to remember that SAH can also occur under these circumstances. In general, patients with these headaches often have a slight warning before the onset of the explosive headache, and this continues with the activity and may resolve if the patient interrupts the exercise or sexual activity. The headache is usually brief, lasting a matter of minutes, and is not associated with nausea or focal neurological symptoms. Men are often too embarrassed to admit that the headache occurred during masturbation and it may be necessary to ask them directly. These headaches often resolve spontaneously with the passage of time, and simple reassurance is often all that is required. If treatment is requested, indomethacin 25–100 mg per day, other non-steroidal anti-inflammatory drugs or a beta-blocker may be employed.

Cough headache

A sudden brief headache may occur with coughing or straining (valsalva). This headache is brief and not associated with any other symptoms. Cough headache is another of the so-called indomethacin-responsive headaches.

Thunderclap headache

This is a syndrome consisting of shortlived headache, sudden and explosive in onset. The CT scan and LP are normal and the aetiology is unclear.

Ice-cream headache

This is the onset of sudden severe headache while eating something very cold. The headache is brief and not associated with any other symptoms, and typically occurs when the cold substance touches the palate.

Ice-pick headache

Ice-pick headache is another sudden-onset headache. It lasts only a matter of seconds but may recur. The pain is very localised, as if being stabbed with an ice-pick or a nail, most commonly in the temple, and there may be a mirror image focus of pain on the opposite side of the head. It is more common in patients with migraine and is another of the indomethacin-responsive syndromes.

Tension headache and chronic daily headache

This is the most common type of headache encountered by the GP. The headache can be generalised, or focal, unilateral or bilateral. Focal neurological symptoms, nausea and systemic symptoms are absent. The headache typically commences some time after awakening and lasts most of the day, and fluctuation in severity during the day is characteristic. The patient may retire with the headache but usually awakens in the morning free of headache. Chronic daily headache is by definition the presence of headaches on a daily basis for six or more months. Although worsening of daily headache is regarded as a 'red flag' for a possible more sinister secondary cause of headache, in fact worsening in terms of increased duration and intensity of headache is not uncommon in these patients, particularly in the setting of increased use of analgesics, a syndrome referred to as the 'analgesic overuse syndrome'. This is a vicious cycle, where increasing use of analgesics (even aspirin or paracetamol) leads to increasing severe headaches, leading to the use of even more of analgesia. A clue is that the patient often states: 'I am taking all these pain killers and they do not seem to work any more.' Many patients also have neck discomfort and when examined may have tenderness in the trapezius and sternocleidomastoid muscles; this often leads to a diagnosis of cervicogenic headache. Here the headache is assumed to be arising from disease in the cervical spine, and yet most patients do not have any demonstrable pathology on imaging or have osteoarthritis that may be an incidental finding, particularly in older patients where it is often present and asymptomatic. Relief of headache can be seen after massage to the neck muscles, physiotherapy or chiropractic, but the benefit may be short-term only.

A multifaceted approach to the treatment of tension-type headache, employing psychological, physiological and pharmacological therapies is recommended.[4] The treatment for the analgesic overuse syndrome is for the patient to withdraw analgesia, which they often find difficult. The use of a tricyclic antidepressant for a short period has been shown to be beneficial.[5]

Migraine

Migraine is a complex headache disorder that has many manifestations. The aetiology is unknown. Patients experience recurrent headaches occasionally associated with recognisable precipitating factors. The diagnosis is entirely dependent on the history of the headache and associated features if present, as currently there are no tests to confirm the diagnosis. The patient with 'classic migraine' rarely presents a diagnostic problem. The headache is preceded by visual phenomena or neurological symptoms, referred to as the *aura*, that commence in one part of the body or visual field and spread, over a period of minutes (on average lasting approximately 30 minutes). The headache is usually throbbing in nature, and commences after the onset of the aura and increases in severity over minutes to hours. It is almost invariably associated with nausea, vomiting, photophobia and phonophobia. The headache persists for hours to days. The associated visual symptoms can vary from photopsia (positive phenomena such as flashing lights or bright dots) to patches of loss of vision, referred to as *scotomata*, that may or may not be surrounded by positive visual phenomena or fortification spectra. The diagnosis is more difficult in patients with recurrent headaches in which gastrointestinal, visual and neurological symptoms are absent. The diagnosis of probable migraine can be made if the patient experiences recurrent headaches that persist for hours on end and are either present on awakening or awaken the patient from their sleep. Rare forms of migraine include hemiplegic migraine and basilar artery migraine. Some patients can experience the aura of a migraine without the subsequent development of a headache, referred to 'migraine without headache' or 'migraine equivalents'. Migraine headaches that occur only at the time of menstruation are referred to as 'menstrual migraine' and are due to the drop in the oestradiol level just prior to menstruation (see Ch 52, Gynaecology).

Management consists of treatment for the individual episodes and, in patients with recurrent headaches, recognising and avoiding precipitating factors, and prophylactic medications.

Once a headache has started, rest in a quiet, darkened room and ensure adequate fluid intake. A combination of magnesium, feverfew and riboflavin can be helpful at the onset of a headache. Several well-designed trials support the effectiveness of spinal manipulation therapy in the treatment of migraine headaches.

In essence, treatment consists of selecting a drug with a potential side-effect profile the patient is willing to contemplate, commencing with the smallest possible dose and increasing up to the minimal required or maximal tolerated dose. Often it is a matter of trial and error.

Initial standard medical treatment often consists of simple analgesia, including non-steroidal anti-inflammatory drugs (NSAIDs) with an antiemetic drug such as prochlorperazine or metoclopramide. Ergot preparations, oral, rectal and subcutaneous, or the triptans, have all been shown to be effective.[6,7]

Prophylaxis for recurrent migraine includes beta-blockers (propanolol, atenolol), tricyclic antidepressants (amitryptiline, nortryptiline), serotonin receptor blockers (pizotifen, methysergide), anticonvulsants (valproic acid, topirimate) or calcium channel blockers (verapamil, flunarazine). Patients are often reluctant to take medication, but may be willing to try a range of integrative medicine approaches.

INTEGRATIVE MANAGEMENT OF HEADACHE/MIGRAINE

Prevention

The goals of prevention are to reduce the frequency, severity and duration of attacks, and to reduce disability.

Triggers

Ask the patient to keep a headache diary to identify triggers. Include date and time. Record food, events, exercise and amount of sleep in the previous 24 hours, and significant life stressors.

Lifestyle

Diet

An elimination–rechallenge diet may help identify triggers. Dietary triggers include chocolate, cheese, monosodium glutamate, tyramine (in aged cheese, red wine, smoked fish, figs), nuts, citrus, dairy and preserved meats (nitrates).

Avoiding smoking, caffeine and alcohol will reduce headache frequency and severity for many patients.

Ensure adequate fluid intake and maintain regular meal times.

Exercise

Exercise may trigger migraine. However, regular moderate exercise can prevent attacks.

Sleep

Ensure sufficient sleep.

Stress management

Stress is a common trigger or exacerbating factor for many headache varieties, and therefore stress management is a central aspect of management. Helpful therapies can include:

- lifestyle alteration
- meditation
- biofeedback
- relaxation techniques such as progressive muscle relaxation and guided imagery.

Herbs and supplements

Magnesium

Intracellular magnesium levels are often lower in people with migraine headaches and magnesium deficiency is common. Two randomised controlled trials (RCTs)[8,9] found that high-dose magnesium reduced the frequency and duration of migraine headaches. Magnesium can also help prevent migraine in women with cyclic headaches related to periods, and is also used in treatment of conditions involving muscle spasm or tension, fibromyalgia, anxiety states and tension headaches.

Riboflavin (vitamin B_2)

Regular riboflavin may help reduce the frequency and shorten the duration of migraine headaches through anti-nociceptive and anti-inflammatory effects.[10] *Dose*: 400 mg/day for at least 3 months, to assess effect in combination with feverfew and magnesium.

SAMe

In a preliminary study, SAMe reduced the frequency, intensity and duration of migraines for most patients.

Feverfew (*Tanacetum parthenium*)

A systematic review of six RCTs[11] concluded that evidence favours feverfew as an effective preventative treatment against migraine, and that it is well tolerated. Note that there is significant variation in the amount of active ingredient in commercially available feverfew preparations.

Physical therapies

Chiropractic

In one study[12] including 127 people with migraine headaches, 22% of those who received chiropractic manipulation reported more than a 90% reduction of migraines and 49% reported a significant reduction of the intensity of each episode. There is some evidence to suggest that patients with tension headache and headache related to neck pain will benefit from chiropractic, although overall the evidence is less strong that chiropractic is beneficial for migraine.[13]

Physiotherapy

A review article[14] evaluating nine studies that tested spinal manipulative therapy for tension or migraine headaches concluded that this technique is comparable to medications used to try to prevent either of these two types of headaches.

Acupuncture

Acupuncture is well studied as an effective treatment for various types of headache. Results from a study published in 2003[15] suggest that having an acupuncture treatment when migraine symptoms first begin is as effective as sumatriptan. Later in the course of the migraine attack, however, the medication works better than acupuncture. A 2001 Cochrane review[16] found 26 trials on acupuncture for headaches. Of these, 16 trials investigated migraine headaches, six tension-type headaches and four various headaches. The majority, although not all, showed acupuncture to be better than placebo/sham acupuncture for tension/migraine headaches, although the quality of many trials was suboptimal. A more recent literature review by Endres and colleagues[17] discussed 10 trials of acupuncture for migraine and concluded that a 6-week course of acupuncture was at least not inferior to a 6-month course of prophylactic treatments, and had a role in the integrated management of migraine headaches.

Drugs for prevention

- Beta-blockers, e.g. propranolol or timolol.
- Tricyclic antidepressants or SSRIs.
- Anticonvulsant medications, e.g. valproate.
- Calcium channel blockers, e.g. verapamil.

- For some women whose headaches are contributed to by the oral contraceptive pill (OCP) it will be important to cease the OCP and organise alternative contraception. There is also concern about the increased risk of stroke in the following groups:
  - women who take the OCP and have migraine with aura
  - women who have migraine without aura, and one additional risk factor:
    - age 35 years or over
    - diabetes
    - a close family member who has had a stroke, heart attack or similar 'vascular' disease before age 45 years
    - a high lipid (cholesterol) level
    - hypertension
    - obesity
    - smoking.

Trigeminal autonomic cephalalgias

The term 'trigeminal autonomic cephalalgias' refers to cluster headaches, chronic paroxysmal hemicrania and SUNCT syndrome.

Cluster headache

The pain of a cluster headache is strictly unilateral and in or around the eye, the temple, frontal or maxillary regions. The pain is excruciatingly severe and is often referred to as 'suicide headache'. The headaches last from 15 minutes to 3 hours, with a curious periodicity, often occurring at the same time of day.

Ipsilateral reddening and watering of the eye and blockage of the nostril are characteristic. A transient Horner's syndrome during the headache is virtually pathognomonic. It is most often seen in men. The attacks occur in bouts or clusters.

Treatment of the acute episode includes oxygen (100%), with a flow rate of at least 7 L/min over 15 minutes, and triptans such as subcutaneous or intranasal sumatriptan. Verapamil up to 240 mg/day is probably the drug of first choice for prophylaxis (maximum dose depends on efficacy or tolerability). Corticosteroids are considered effective in cluster headache, despite the lack of level I or II evidence. Methylprednisolone 100 mg per day (or equivalent corticosteroid) given orally or at up to 500 mg intravenously per day over 5 days (then tapering down) is recommended. Methysergide, lithium and topiramate are recommended as alternative treatments.

Paroxysmal hemicrania

Paroxysmal hemicrania may be either episodic or chronic, and consists of paroxysmal headache attacks very similar to those observed in cluster headache, but the attacks are more frequent and of shorter duration, and lack the circadian rhythm seen with cluster headache. Complete abolition of the headaches with indomethacin is characteristic.

SUNCT syndrome

SUNCT syndrome consists of **s**hort-lasting, **u**nilateral, **n**euralgiform headaches with **c**onjunctival injection and **t**earing lasting between 5 seconds and 4 minutes and occuring from as few as three times per day to as often as 200 times per day. These headaches are also strictly unilateral and periorbital; they are triggered by touching the periorbital region, talking or chewing food. There is mild conjunctival injection and watering of the eye.

Lamotrigine is the most effective preventive agent, with topiramate and gabapentin also being useful.

Idiopathic or benign intracranial hypertension

Idiopathic intracranial hypertension (IIH) or benign intracranial hypertension (BIH) tends to occur in obese females, but can be seen in patients of either sex who are not obese. The headaches are constant and have usually been present for weeks to months prior to presentation. They tend to be constant in nature, generalised and often worse on awakening. The diagnosis relies on the presence of papilloedema in the setting of a normal MRI scan (including magnetic resonance venography (MRV) to exclude cerebral vein thrombosis) and an elevated cerebrospinal fluid (CSF) pressure of > 20 cm H_2O with normal CSF microbiology and biochemistry. Treatment includes recurrent lumbar punctures, acetazolamide and, in resistant cases, lumbo-peritoneal shunt.

Cranial arteritis

Cranial arteritis should be suspected in older patients, typically 75 years of age and older—it is rarely seen in patients under the age of 50 years. The headache is of insidious onset of days to weeks, often with systemic ill health, fever, polymyalgia rheumatica, scalp tenderness and jaw claudication, with the latter two virtually pathognomonic. The ESR is raised, often as high as 100, but *may be normal* early in the course of the illness, and therefore the ESR should be repeated once or twice per week when the diagnosis is suspected and the initial ESR is not raised. Occasionally the diagnosis can be made at the bedside by detecting thrombosed temporal arteries (see Fig 36.1). If the clinical suspicion is high and despite a normal ESR, the patient should be treated with high-dose corticosteroids and a temporal artery biopsy obtained as a matter of urgency. Delays in treatment can result in blindness and, less frequently, cerebral infarction.

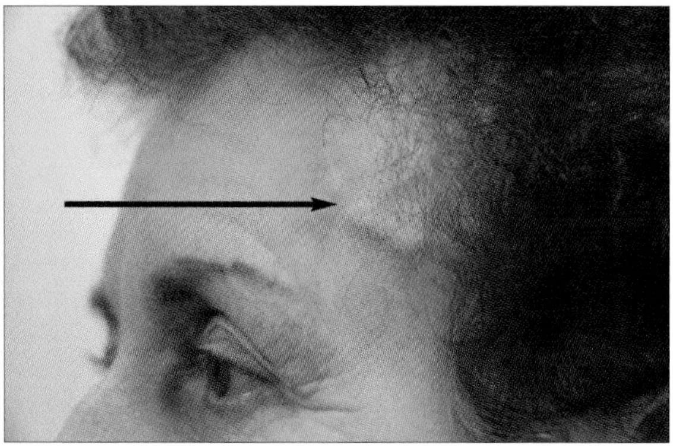

FIGURE 36.1 Thrombosed superficial temporal artery in cranial arteritis (reproduced from Gates 2010[18])

FUNNY TURNS

Intermittent disturbances of neurological function are a very common problem and the list of potential causes is extensive. This section discusses the more common causes encountered by a GP, including syncope, Stokes-Adams attacks, epilepsy, benign positional vertigo and hyperventilation syndrome.

HISTORY

Funny turns consist of intermittent disturbances of function, and therefore the diagnosis is almost entirely dependent upon a very detailed history, as the examination is usually normal and investigations rarely reveal a diagnosis unless they are performed at the time that the patient is having an episode, and even then tests are usually normal.

It is important to obtain a detailed description of not only the circumstances under which the episode occurred, but also the time of the day and the exact nature and distribution of each and every symptom, as well as the timing of each of the individual symptoms in terms of their duration and their relationship to the development of other symptoms.

When obtaining a history, be certain to analyse what was happening immediately *before* the event or 'ictus'. If there is an eyewitness or if the patient does not lose consciousness or memory, ascertain exactly what happened *during* the ictus, and then analyse what happened immediately *after* the ictus, up until the time that the patient regained normal function or behaviour.

EXAMINATION

As already stated, the examination in this situation—measurement of blood pressure lying and standing—may confirm the clinical suspicion of postural hypotension. An irregular pulse may be present in patients with symptoms related to an arrhythmia. A carotid bruit may indicate the presence of a carotid stenosis in a patient with focal cerebral ischaemia. Severe aortic stenosis or the murmur of idiopathic hypertrophic subaortic stenosis may be present in patients with exercise-induced syncope. In patients with posture-induced vertigo, the Hallpike manoeuvre may demonstrate the characteristic delayed onset of vertigo and nystagmus that abates with maintenance with a fixed posture. Hyperventilation—asking the patient to breathe heavily and quickly—can reproduce the symptoms of hyperventilation syndrome, but it is important to remember that hyperventilation will make anyone feel unwell, and therefore the symptoms must be reproduced exactly.

INVESTIGATIONS

The investigations already alluded to rarely, if ever, establish a diagnosis in patients with intermittent disturbances of function. If seizures are frequent or can be precipitated by sleep deprivation or hyperventilation, then video-electroencephalographic monitoring may occasionally detect a seizure (see Fig 36.2). Holter monitoring can on rare occasions detect complete heart block in patients with suspected Stokes-Adams attacks. Symptoms related to hyponatraemia, hypokalaemia or hypocalcaemia are so rare that routine electrolyte estimation is rarely helpful. A full blood examination could detect anaemia or evidence of an infection, but intermittent symptoms related to either of these entities are very rare. Imaging such as CT scan or MRI scan is usually normal, except for patients with focal seizures.

MANAGEMENT

Management is specifically related to the nature of the disturbance, and is discussed in each section below.

Syncope

Syncope is also referred to as *vasovagal syncope* or *neurocardiogenic syncope*. It occurs predominantly in teenagers and young adults. A typical episode consists of prolonged warning symptoms consisting of lightheadedness, clamminess, blurred and then darkening vision, with worsening severity of symptoms and subsequent loss of consciousness (LOC). The patient is limp and, if standing, falls to the ground with eyes closed and no abnormal movements. Pallor is common and bradycardia is present. The period of impaired consciousness is brief—a matter of minutes. An important diagnostic clue is that the patient can prevent LOC if they lie flat immediately. In most instances, reassurance and advice to lie flat immediately is all that is required.

Loss of consciousness is a symptom of a variety of conditions. First episodes of syncope need to be investigated. In older patients particularly, cardiac arrhythmias need to be excluded.

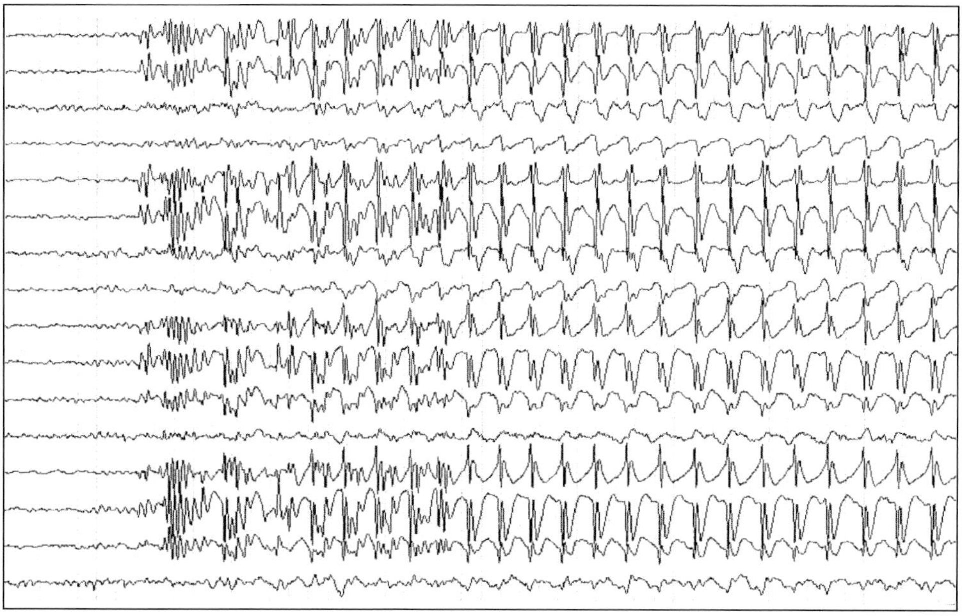

FIGURE 36.2 An EEG showing the classical 3 per second spike and wave characteristic of absence epilepsy (reproduced from Gates 2010[18])

Stokes-Adams attacks

Stokes-Adams syndrome is a disorder of the elderly, although rarely it can occur in younger patients. It consists of sudden LOC without warning, brief and with no 'post-ictal' confusion. It relates to complete heart block, and treatment consists of insertion of a pacemaker.

Epilepsy

Epilepsy is the propensity to recurrent seizures. There are many ways to classify seizures, one common way being to divide them into generalised and partial seizures. *Generalised seizures* include tonic-clonic (previously referred to as grand mal), absence (petit mal), atonic and tonic. *Partial seizures* include simple (no loss of awareness) and complex (loss of awareness) partial seizures. Some patients experience warning symptoms as the initial manifestation of the seizure, referred to as an *aura*, and some patients have a period of drowsiness and confusion after the seizure, referred to as *post-ictal drowsiness* and confusion.

Tonic-clonic seizure

Tonic-clonic seizure may or may not be preceded by an aura. An aura suggests a focal onset. The patient stiffens and may 'cry out'—the so-called 'cri de chat'—the eyes remain open, and this tonic phase, lasting up to 30 seconds, is followed by the clonic phase, with repeated flexing movements of all four limbs. Tongue or cheek biting and incontinence of urine and faeces may also occur. There is a period of post-ictal drowsiness and confusion. Most episodes last less than 2–3 minutes, rarely as long as 20 minutes.[19]

Absence seizure

There is no warning. Suddenly the patient interrupts their behaviour and stares into space. There is often repetitive blinking, but nothing else. After 10 seconds to 1–2 minutes, the patient returns to normal as if nothing has happened. There is normally no post-ictal drowsiness or confusion.

Complex-partial seizure

Often but not invariably there is an aura. There are symptoms such as déjà vu, jamais vu, olfactory or gustatory phenomena, rarely visual or auditory hallucinations. The patient interrupts what they are doing and stares into space. Abnormal movements such as lip smacking, repetitive swallowing or fidgeting are common, and the patient is unresponsive. As opposed to absence seizures, there is a period of post-ictal drowsiness and confusion.

Diagnosis

The diagnosis is essentially a clinical one and based almost entirely on the history of the episode, as only rarely do patients have a seizure while undergoing electro-encephalography (EEG). Current recommendations advocate an EEG, CT or MRI brain scan in all patients presenting with a first unprovoked seizure. The presence of epileptic discharges on an EEG in patients with their first seizure increases the risk of recurrence. Many patients presenting with their first apparent seizure have, on detailed questioning, had unrecognised seizures in the past.[20]

Laboratory tests, such as blood counts, blood glucose and electrolytes, particularly sodium, lumbar puncture and toxicology screening, may be helpful as determined by the specific clinical circumstances based on the history, and physical and neurological examination, but there are insufficient data to support or refute recommending any of these tests for the routine evaluation of adults presenting with an apparent first unprovoked seizure.

Treatment of seizures and epilepsy

Most seizures last only a matter of 1–2, rarely 5, minutes, and the initial management is simply to prevent the patient from harming themselves and to lie them on their side when the seizure is finished. Prolonged seizures and status epilepsy require prompt intervention. Intravenous (IV) lorazepam is the drug of choice in both adults and children.[21]

The principles of management of recurrent seizures are to identify potential precipitating factors, prescribe an appropriate anticonvulsant, monitor the response to treatment, and adjust the dose if appropriate or choose an alternative anticonvulsant. Lifestyle advice is crucial in order to prevent the patient harming themselves or others if they suffer recurrent seizures. Such advice should include not swimming or having a bath if alone, not walking near cliffs or scaling heights, and not driving a motor vehicle or industrial machinery. Each country, and often each state, has different regulations and these should be consulted when advising patients of their inability to drive.

Precipitating factors are uncommon but, when they occur, include flashing lights in patients with photosensitive epilepsy, sleep deprivation, excessive alcohol, forgetting medications and an intercurrent illness.

Choosing the correct drug for the individual patient can be complex, and is determined by the type of epilepsy and the side effect profile the patient is willing to contemplate.

Carbamazepine is the drug of choice for partial or focal seizures, and valproic acid for generalised seizures.[22] However, carbamazepine interferes with the oral contraceptive pill and causes drowsiness; valproic acid can result in hair loss and obesity, side effects that young women are often not willing to contemplate. There are many guidelines[23] and these are frequently evolving and should be consulted on a regular basis.

Integrative management of epilepsy

The adverse effects of antiepileptic pharmaceuticals make it difficult to attain optimal dosage levels in order to prevent seizures in many cases.[24] Current evidence suggests that 25–50% of individuals with epilepsy have tried some form of CAM therapy.[25–27] It is important to note that these therapies are not a substitute for medication; however, depending on the effectiveness of the intervention(s), dosage reductions under medical supervision may be possible.[28]

Mind–body medicine

A systematic review assessing several different meditative practices (meditation, meditative prayer, yoga, relaxation) has revealed some evidence for the efficacy of meditation in the treatment of epilepsy.[29] In particular, studies have demonstrated that transcendental meditation (TM) may be a potential antiepileptic treatment. However, further trials are required, as many of the EEG recordings during TM (increased alpha, theta, gamma frequencies with increased coherence and synchrony) are similar to the neuronal activity that occurs during seizures.[30]

Sleep

It has long been known that there is a close relationship between the physiological state of sleep and the pathological process underlying epileptic seizures, but the connection is still not well understood.[31] Sufferers of epilepsy often demonstrate multiple sleep abnormalities, such as increased sleep latency, fragmented sleep, increased awakenings and stage shifts and an increase in stages 1 and 2 of non-REM sleep.[32] It is important that any sleep disorders are identified and managed as soon as possible, as sleep deprivation has been shown to increase the frequency of epileptiform discharges and seizures.[33–35] Sleep quality, as well as daytime alertness and neurocognitive function, can be improved by anticonvulsant medications, ketogenic dietary principles and vagus nerve stimulation.[33] However, it should be noted that poor sleep can also be an adverse effect of some anticonvulsant drugs.[24,36]

Sunshine

Individuals with epilepsy who have been on long-term treatment with various anticonvulsants may develop hypocalcaemia, osteomalacia and osteopenia that is independent of vitamin D metabolism. It has been demonstrated that there are regional variances in the incidence of drug-induced bone disease and this has been attributed to variances in sunlight exposure, with the majority of reports coming from areas of low sunshine or from institutionalised patients.[37,38]

Exercise

In times past, exercise was restricted for those with epilepsy, rather than encouraged, as it is today. As many people with epilepsy still fear suffering an exercise-induced seizure, they often lead a sedentary life and have poor physical fitness.[39] Although there have been rare cases of exercise-induced seizures, both clinical and experimental data have shown that exercise can reduce the frequency of seizures as well as improving cardiovascular and psychological health.[40,41] Indeed, current evidence demonstrates that regular exercise may have a moderate seizure-preventative effect in 30–40% of this population.[39] Most sporting activities, including contact sports, are safe to participate in, according to current medical recommendations. Supervised water sports and swimming are also considered safe, provided seizures are well controlled. However, sports such as hang-gliding and scuba diving are not recommended, as there is a high risk of severe injury or death if a seizure were to occur.[40] It is imperative that medical advice regarding exercise is individualised for each patient, taking into account their seizure type and frequency.[40]

Yoga

Recent studies have shown that yoga can reduce seizure index and increase quality of life in people with epilepsy.[42] Yoga has also been shown to significantly improve parasympathetic parameters, suggesting that it may have a role in the treatment of autonomic dysfunction in patients with refractory epilepsy.[43]

Diet

Maintaining good blood sugar balance, identifying and eliminating allergenic foods and avoiding suspected triggers such as alcohol, artificial sweeteners, diet soft-drinks, energy drinks and MSG are important in the management of epilepsy.[28,44,45] Growth retardation is common among children with epilepsy and this appears to be secondary to poor dietary intake. Dietary intake of vitamins D, E and K, folate, calcium, linoleic acid and alpha-linolenic acid has been found to be below the recommended daily allowance (RDA) in approximately 30% of children with intractable epilepsy.[46]

Studies of dietary treatments for epilepsy suggest that approximately 50% of children have a 50% reduction in seizures after 6 months. Approximately one-third will achieve more than 90% reduction in their seizures. Such diets maintain their efficacy when provided continuously for several years. Furthermore, long-term benefits may be seen even when the diet is ceased after only a few months, indicating neuroprotective effects.[47] Other dietary guidelines for the management of epilepsy are given below. Recommending such diets in the management of epilepsy needs to be balanced with the overall nutritional needs and health of the patient.

Ketogenic diet

The ketogenic diet is a high-fat, low-carbohydrate, high-protein diet used to treat medically refractory epilepsy.[48] At least 15–20% of patients on the ketogenic diet experience more than 50% reduction in seizure frequency. For this reason, the ketogenic diet should be considered an early treatment for drug-resistant epilepsy, not a 'last resort'.[49–51] The ketogenic diet may also be a valuable therapeutic option for children with drug-resistant focal epilepsy, particularly those with recent deterioration of seizure control.[52,53]

Modified Atkins diet

The modified Atkins diet is a less-restrictive ketogenic diet. It has no restrictions on calories, fluids or protein, and does not involve fasting. As for the ketogenic diet, high-fat foods are encouraged, with 10 g/day of carbohydrate allowed in children and 15 g/day in adults. Approximately 45% of patients have 50–90% seizure reduction, with 28% having more than 90% seizure reduction.[54] The ketogenic diet appears to exert its effects more quickly, although by 6 months the difference is no longer considered significant.[50]

Low glycaemic index diet

A study in 2009 reported on the efficacy, safety and tolerability of the low glycaemic index diet in paediatric intractable epilepsy. More than 50% reduction from baseline seizure frequency was seen in 42%, 50%, 54%, 64% and 66% children at 1, 3, 6, 9 and 12 months respectively.[55]

Nutritional supplementation

Polyunsaturated fatty acids

Increased concentrations of both ketone bodies and polyunsaturated fatty acids (PUFAs) have been found in the cerebrospinal fluid and plasma of patients on the ketogenic diet, and it is thought that a high dietary intake of PUFAs may be one mechanism responsible for the potent anticonvulsant effects of the ketogenic diet.[56,57] Supplementation with omega-3 fatty acids has also been shown to prevent status epilepticus-associated neuropathological changes in animal studies.[58] Although PUFAs have been shown to reduce seizures in several animal models, available data regarding the effects of supplementation in epileptic patients (1–3 g EPA/DHA daily) reveal mixed results with respect to seizure frequency.[59–61] More research is therefore required before PUFAs can be definitively recommended as a treatment option for epilepsy.[56]

Amino acids

Current research suggests that serotonin has an anti-epileptic effect, and serotonin receptors are expressed in almost all networks involved in epilepsies. Some SSRIs, such as fluoxetine, have been found to improve seizure control, and some antiepileptic drugs have recently been found to increase endogenous serotonin levels.[62–64]

Tryptophan

Tryptophan is an essential amino acid and the only brain precursor of serotonin. It has been estimated that patients with epilepsy have approximately 30% lower brain intake of tryptophan compared with controls. Whey proteins that are high in tryptophan but lower in other large neutral amino acids are currently being trialled in combination with antiepileptic medications.[62]

Taurine

Taurine is one of the most abundant free amino acids found mainly in excitable tissues. Taurine is necessary for the production of GABA, one of the major inhibitory neurotransmitters in the limbic system.[65] For this reason, drugs that target GABA receptors are the mainstay of treatment of seizures, with the recent transplantation of GABA-producing cells effectively reducing seizures in several well-established models.[66,67]

There have been multiple animal studies demonstrating that taurine-fed animals have increased levels of GABA and a higher threshold for seizure onset compared to controls.[65] Furthermore, increased taurine levels in the hippocampus improve membrane stabilisation, significantly reducing neuronal cell death and favouring recovery after neuronal hyperactivity.[68,69]

Carnosine

Carnosine is an amino acid with many of the features of a neurotransmitter. It has the ability to act as both a neuromodulator and a neuroprotective agent, and it may indirectly influence neuronal excitability by modulating the effects of zinc and copper.[70–72] Carnosine may have a significant anticonvulsant effect and, as such, it may prove to be a potential anticonvulsant treatment for epilepsy in the future.[73]

Antioxidants

Excessive production of free radicals with neuronal hyperexcitability have been strongly implicated in the pathogenesis of idiopathic epilepsy. There is therefore a possible role of antioxidants in combination with antiepileptic drugs for better seizure control,[74–76] although, as with other chronic illnesses, it is likely that a nutritious diet rich in antioxidants such as vitamins A, C and E is likely to be far more effective than a poor diet supplemented by antioxidants. Results have thus far been mixed for vitamin E supplementation, and more studies are required before definitive recommendations can be made.[77]

Selenium deficiency has been implicated in the pathogenesis of epilepsy.[78] Anticonvulsants may further deplete total body selenium stores, and failure to advise appropriate selenium supplementation, especially to pregnant women taking sodium valproate, may increase the risk of neural tube defects or other free radical mediated damage.[79]

Zinc

Altered zinc homeostasis appears to be associated with epilepsy; however, the definitive role of zinc as a neuromodulator in synapses is still uncertain.[80,81]

Other vitamins and minerals

Many anticonvulsant medications are known to reduce folic acid levels, subsequently raising homocysteine levels. Homocysteine, however, is known to be a convulsing agent that can result in increased seizure recurrence and intractability to medications. In addition, anticonvulsant medications can disturb lipid metabolism, creating hypercholesterolaemia, dyslipidaemia and altered uric acid metabolism. As such, routine supplementation with folic acid, vitamin B_{12}, B_6, C, E and beta-carotene for all those on anticonvulsant medications is important.[82]

A Cochrane review has found that vitamin B_1 improves both neuropsychological and cognitive functions in patients with epilepsy. In the same review, vitamin D was also found to improve bone mineral density in those taking anticonvulsant medications.[28,77]

Manganese deficiency has also been associated with seizures in both animals and humans, according to a systematic review. More research is needed, as it is currently unclear as to whether this is a cause or an effect of the convulsions.[83]

Herbs

Herbal medicine has been used for centuries in many cultures for the treatment of epilepsy and some patients may be self-medicating with herbal medicines. It is therefore important for the GP to ask about the patient's use of herbal preparations, as many herbs can increase the risk of seizures by affecting cytochrome-P450 enzymes and P-glycoproteins, or through possible contamination by heavy metals.[84,85]

Well-designed clinical trials of herbal therapies for epilepsy are scarce. However, based on animal studies and numerous anecdotal observations of clinical benefits in humans, further research is certainly warranted.[84,85]

The flavonoid derivatives from *Scutellaria baicalensis* Georgi, *Artemesia herba-alba*, *Melissa officinalis* and *Salvia triloba* have all been found to exert anticonvulsant effects by exhibiting significant affinity for the GABA(A) receptor benzodiazepine binding site.[86,87] *Ginkgo biloba* appears to have the capacity to both induce and inhibit seizures.[88]

Interestingly, *Curcumin* has also recently been shown to significantly prevent generalisation of electroclinical seizure activity as well as the pathogenesis of iron-induced epileptogenesis.[89,90] Further studies are required.

Various Chinese herbs, such as Chaihu-longu-muli-tang, appear to have antiepileptic properties, and it also appears that the reduction in seizure frequency may be related to the antioxidant effects of the herbs.[91] Shitei-To is another TCM formulation that may have therapeutic effects in the prevention of secondarily generalised seizures. It is made from three medicinal herbs: Shitei (calyx of *Diospyros kaki* L.f), Shokyu (rhizome of *Zingiber officinale* Roscoe) and Choji (flower bud of *Syzygium aromaticum*).[92]

Acupuncture

A 2008 Cochrane review investigated the use of acupuncture in epilepsy. Although there have been some positive trials, as many of the studies were of poor methodological quality it was concluded that current evidence does not support acupuncture as a treatment for epilepsy.[93]

Prevention

Lifestyle measures that may be important in the management of epilepsy have been discussed previously. Furthermore, living as 'cleanly' as possible is important for individuals with epilepsy, as there are numerous documented toxic causes of seizures. These include substance abuse (alcohol and recreational drugs), exposure to various industrial and household products, occupational nickel and other heavy metals.[94] Animal studies have demonstrated that blood lead levels similar to those found in humans living in urban areas with high pollution levels can lower seizure threshold.[95]

Research on hospital admissions of patients in status epilepticus reveals several environmental factors that are either protective or precipitative. It appears that there is a significant diurnal pattern, with the majority of admissions occurring between 4 pm and 5 pm, and least admissions in the early morning hours. Admissions also vary significantly throughout the lunar cycle, with the peak at day 3 after the new moon and trough at 3 days before the new moon. Admissions have been noted to be highest on bright, sunny days, whereas dark days, high humidity and high temperature appear to be significantly protective factors.[96]

Benign positional vertigo

Benign positional vertigo is a not-uncommon condition that can produce disabling attacks of shortlived vertigo precipitated by movement of the head, such as looking up, bending over, turning the head, lying down, getting out of bed or rolling over in bed. Each of these movements stimulates the semicircular canals; in this condition, there are free-moving pathological densities or crystals from the otolith that break off and enter the endolymph, producing abnormal stimulation of the delicate hair cells floating in the fluid. The diagnosis is confirmed by the Hallpike manoeuvre and treatment is by the Epley manoeuvre. Descriptions of how to perform these can be readily obtained from the internet.

Hyperventilation syndrome

Hyperventilation syndrome is a disorder that is frequently missed by the GP. Patients present with lightheadedness (not vertigo) that fluctuates in severity and can persist for minutes to hours. There is often dryness of the mouth and an inability to take a big breath (rather than shortness of breath) and a sense of tightness in the chest. When severe, there can be peri-oral and peripheral paraesthesia in the hands and feet, which occurs without loss of function and at times may be unilateral. The condition can be diagnosed by asking the patient to take deep breaths, in and out, for several minutes—this will reproduce their symptoms. Traditionally, patients have been advised to breath in and out of a paper bag, but this is impractical. The problem is simply resolved by the patient holding their breath in expiration for 20 seconds, taking a breath, breathing out and holding it for another 20 seconds—this is repeated until the symptoms resolve.

MOTOR WEAKNESS

HISTORY

The presence of weakness indicates a lesion somewhere between the motor cortex in the frontal lobe and the relevant muscle group on the contralateral side, with the motor pathways crossing at the level of the foramen magnum. The rapidity of onset of weakness, the pattern of weakness and the presence or absence of significant wasting and/or fasciculations should be elucidated in the history. An enquiry should be made as to the presence of a family history of any disorder causing weakness, as a number of disorders of muscle are familial. The presence of sensory symptoms excludes the anterior horn cell, the motor nerve root, the neuromuscular junction and muscle as the site of the pathology.

EXAMINATION

Central nervous system (CNS) causes of weakness produce a classic 'upper motor neuron' pattern of weakness with finger extension, shoulder abduction and elbow extension in the upper limbs and hip flexion, weakness of dorsiflexion of the feet and knee flexion in the lower limbs. This pattern of weakness would most often be associated with increased tone (with or without clonus), increased reflexes and up-going plantar responses. If the facial muscles are affected with CNS, then the forehead is not affected. In disorders of the peripheral nervous system (PNS), the pattern of weakness will indicate whether the problem is in the anterior horn cell (usually associated with significant wasting and fasciculations), motor nerve root (usually associated with significant radicular pain), plexus, peripheral nerve, neuromuscular junction (fluctuating weakness with exercise) or muscle. The presence of sensory signs excludes disorders of the anterior horn cell, motor nerve root, neuromuscular junction or muscle. In disorders of the PNS, the tone may be normal or decreased, the reflexes are often absent, plantar responses are down-going and, if present, sensory signs will reflect the site of the problem in the PNS. Disorders of muscle are usually associated with preserved reflexes (rare exceptions to this include myotonic dystrophy and inclusion body myositis). If the weakness affects the face, it is important to see whether the muscles that wrinkle the forehead (frontalis muscle) are affected; if so, this points to a lower motor neuron facial palsy. If the forehead is not affected but there is weakness around the mouth, this is an upper motor neuron facial weakness.

INVESTIGATIONS

Magnetic resonance imaging, with its ability to image the spinal cord, brainstem and cerebral hemispheres, has revolutionised the assessment of patients with weakness related to the CNS. It is also superior to computerised tomography at imaging the nerve roots and plexuses. Other tests inlcude creatine kinase (CK), nerve conduction studies (NCS), electromyography (EMG) and muscle biopsy for disorders of muscle. It is also useful to conduct nerve conduction studies for disorders of nerves, in particular individual nerves involved in entrapment syndromes (carpal tunnel syndrome at the wrist, tardy ulnar palsy at the elbow or common peroneal nerve compression at the neck of the fibula), peripheral neuropathy and disorders at the neuromuscular junction where single-fibre EMG (SFEMG) is useful. The cerebrospinal fluid (CSF) may provide vital clues in both CNS and PNS disorders.

MANAGEMENT

Management is disease specific and is discussed below.

Paraplegia

The term *paraplegia* refers to bilateral leg weakness. The most likely causes include spinal cord pathology (resulting in upper motor neuron signs) such as transverse myelitis (sometimes the presenting symptom of multiple sclerosis) or spinal cord compression secondary to spinal cord trauma, malignant vertebral metastases or benign intraspinal tumours. A useful clinical point is that a thoracic cord lesion in a middle-aged to elderly female is a meningioma until proved otherwise. Bilateral leg weakness may also result from PNS problems such as a peripheral neuropathy or even disorders of muscle. Diabetic amyotrophy and lumbosacral neuritis can result in severe pain in the thighs and hip region, and proximal weakness with absent knee reflexes in one or both thighs, evolving over days to weeks.

Monoplegia

Weakness confined to one limb, if it affects the entire limb, is more likely to be central in origin, particularly if it has evolved rapidly. Focal weakness in a limb is more likely to be related to a nerve root or individual nerve, but can also occur with CNS problems. A not-uncommon presentation in general practice is hand weakness, related to either an ulnar nerve lesion or a C8-T1 radiculopathy. In the latter, both the medial and lateral heads of flexor digitorum profundus (FDP) are affected, causing weakness of flexion of the distal phalanges of all four fingers, whereas in an ulnar nerve lesion the lateral two digits are spared (this part of FDP is supplied by the median nerve). The sensory loss will involve the medial two digits and medial aspect of the palm in both conditions, but will be more extensive and up the medial aspect of the forearm in a radiculopathy. Another common presentation is the wrist drop or 'Saturday night palsy', with radial nerve compression in the radial groove causing weakness of wrist and finger extension, weakness of elbow flexion in semi-supination (brachioradialis) but sparing of the triceps. There is often a small area of altered sensation at the base of the thumb. This is a self-limiting condition.

Hemiparesis/hemiplegia

Hemiparesis refers to partial weakness down one side of the body, whereas *hemiplegia* refers to a total loss of strength down one side of the body. Weakness affecting the arm and leg on one side is most likely related to a lesion on the opposite side of the brain, above the level of the foramen magnum where the motor pathway crosses, although a lesion in the upper cervical spinal cord on the same side as the weakness cannot be excluded. Weakness affecting the face, arm and leg on one side clearly points to a lesion affecting the motor pathway above the facial nerve nucleus situated in the pons.

Facial weakness

The most common cause of an upper motor neuron facial weakness would be cerebral ischaemia on the contralateral side. Bell's palsy is the most common cause of a lower motor neuron weakness.

Bell's palsy

Bell's palsy is an acute, idiopathic, unilateral, lower-motor-neuron facial-nerve paralysis of uncertain aetiology. It is one of the most common 'urgent' referrals to a neurologist, because most patients fear that they have suffered a stroke. Patients may often complain of paraesthesia on the face; more often they present with the gradual onset of weakness afflicting one side of the face (bilateral cases are rare but do occur) that develops over hours to days. The inability to wrinkle the forehead on the same side confirms that the weakness relates to a lower motor neuron problem. The presence of hyperacusis in the ipsilateral ear and altered taste on the ipsilateral side of the tongue (related to involvement of the chorda tympani) when present are pathognomonic for Bell's palsy. Facial and corneal sensation are not affected. The condition resolves spontaneously in more than 80–90% of patients.

Corticosteroids and aciclovir have been recommended in the belief that functional outcome is improved.[97] However, a 2009 Cochrane review concluded that corticosteroids and aciclovir have not been proved to be beneficial.[98] Subsequent to this review, a large randomised controlled trial[99] demonstrated complete recovery at 3 months in 83% of patients treated with prednisolone (50 mg per day for 10 days), as opposed to 63.6% for patients treated with placebo. At 9 months, 94.4% of the prednisolone-treated group had completely resolved, compared to 81.6% for the placebo. No benefit was found from aciclovir.

Other therapies that may be useful for some individuals include relaxation techniques, acupuncture, electrical stimulation, biofeedback training and vitamin therapy (including vitamins B_{12} and B_6, and zinc).

Acute and chronic inflammatory demyelinating neuropathy

The term *acute inflammatory demyelinating neuropathy* (AIDP) has replaced the term *(Landry) Guillain-Barré (Strohl) syndrome*. This presents with the rapid onset of weakness usually affecting the limbs, with proximal weakness in the lower limbs and distal weakness in the upper limbs initially, subsequently becoming generalised weakness of the limbs. There is almost invariably neck flexion and occasionally neck extension weakness. The cranial nerves may also be affected, resulting in bilateral facial weakness, palatal weakness or weakness of the extra ocular muscles, resulting in variable patterns including a pseudo-internuclear ophthalmoplegia (INO). The reflexes are absent and there may or may not be peripheral sensory loss. Some patients develop involvement of the autonomic nervous system, resulting in arrythmias, periods of hypertension and hypotension and disturbances of bladder and bowel function. The respiratory muscles are involved in severe cases, and patients will often require long-term ventilation. In addition to supportive measures, either intravenous immunoglobulin (IVIG) or plasma exchange is used in the acute phase.[100–102] IVIG is probably the treatment modality of choice, for ease of use. The prognosis is variable, with approximately 75% of patients making an excellent recovery; the remainder have mild or moderate impairment, with severe disability occurring in less than 5% of patients.

Chronic inflammatory demyelinating neuropathy (CIDP) can cause the same patterns of weakness as AIDP but evolves more slowly (by definition over more than 6 weeks). IVIG or corticosteroids should be considered in sensory and motor CIDP. IVIG should be considered as the initial treatment in pure motor CIDP.[103]

Motor neuron disease

Motor neuron disease (MND), also referred to as amyotrophic lateral sclerosis (ALS), presents with weakness and fatigue associated with significant muscle wasting and fasciculations in the absence of any sensory symptoms. Muscle cramps can occur. Four distinct clinical phenotypes have been identified, with different rates of progression and survival. Patients presenting with global involvement have the worst prognosis, while patients presenting with a flail arm survive longer.[104] When MND affects the bulbar musculature, patients present with a characteristic dysarthria, with wasting and fasciculations of the tongue. At present there is no specific treatment, but these patients should be cared for in specialised centres with expertise in MND.

Myasthenia gravis

Myasthenia gravis is a very rare autoimmune disease and most GPs are not likely to see a case. The characteristic feature is a weakness that is exacerbated by use of the muscle and reduced in intensity by rest. Myasthenia gravis can remain confined to the extra ocular muscles, where it presents with intermittent ptosis and variable horizontal and vertical diplopia—for example, when reading or watching television. Myasthenia affecting muscles in the rest of the body is referred to as *generalised myasthenia*. Myasthenia affecting the bulbar musculature (the lower four cranial nerves) will present with dysarthria exacerbated by talking, dysphagia and difficulty chewing, exacerbated by eating. When it affects the muscles of the arms and legs, patients will complain of increasing weakness when they are trying to do activities such as hanging the washing on the line or washing their hair, or they may complain of increased difficulty walking, and of having to rest. The diagnosis can be made at the bedside by asking the patient to repeatedly exercise and by demonstrating increased weakness; or, if it affects the extra ocular muscles, by asking the patient to look up, and observing increased ptosis and the development of increasing diplopia, the longer the patient is looking up. Applying ice to the ptosed eyelid can lead to a dramatic resolution of the ptosis.[105] Another bedside test is the Tensilon test, where edrophonium hydrochloride is injected and a transient improvement or resolution of symptoms can be observed. The ice test and the Tensilon test both have a high sensitivity (92–95%) and specificity (97%). Antibodies directed against the acetylcholine receptor (ACHR) are highly specific (98%) but the sensitivity varies from one report to another, from as low as 54% to as high as 88%.[106] Electrodiagnostic studies include repetitive nerve stimulation, where a decremental response is observed and the variability of stimulation of the acetylcholine receptor by acetylcholine can be observed with single fibre electromyography (SFEMG)—this is referred to as *increased jitter*. All patients with myasthenia gravis should have a CT scan of the chest to look for thymic hyperplasia (usually seen in younger patients) or a thymoma (in older patients); these can be either benign or locally malignant. Ocular myasthenia gravis sometimes responds to the cholinesterase inhibitor pyridostigmine.[107] Thymectomy is recommended for patients with thymic hyperplasia[108] or thymoma.[109] IVIG is very effective in the treatment of myasthenic crisis and can be used preoperatively prior to thymectomy or prior to any surgery in patients with generalised myasthenia gravis.[101] Corticosteroids, other immunosuppressive agents and plasma exchange are used in patients who fail to respond to thymectomy.[110,111]

Polymyositis and dermatomyositis

Polymyositis and dermatomyositis are very rare inflammatory disorders of muscle. *Dermatomyositis* is more common in younger patients but may also occur in patients with malignancy. Patients present with proximal weakness in their arms and legs, with normal reflexes. Neck flexion weakness is common; rarely the bulbar or respiratory muscles may be affected. The characteristic skin changes seen to imitate myositis include a violaceous discolouration of the eyelids, scaly erythema over the joints on the dorsal aspect of the hands, macular erythema on the posterior neck and shoulders or on the anterior neck and chest, or a violaceous erythema associated with increased pigment and telangiectasia on the anterior neck, chest, posterior shoulders, back and buttocks. Electromyography demonstrates myopathic changes with brief small amplitude polyphasic potentials (BSAPPs) and full recruitment with minimal effort, but also demonstrates fibrillation potentials and positive sharp waves. The definitive diagnosis is established by muscle biopsy. There are few randomised controlled trials regarding treatment; it is largely empirical. Corticosteroids remain the agent of first choice, with other immunosuppressive agents such as azathioprine, cyclophosphamide and cyclosporin used in patients who fail to respond to 3 months of corticosteroids. Prednisolone is commenced at a dose of 1–2 mg per kilogram of body weight and is continued for 2–4 weeks, and then the dose is slowly reduced to a maintenance level over the next 6 months.[112]

PARAESTHESIA AND NUMBNESS

HISTORY

Sensory symptoms affecting various parts of the body are probably one of the most common causes of patients seeking a neurological opinion. In the neurological history it is important to establish whether the symptoms are intermittent or persistent, and, if they are persistent, to determine the time taken from the initial symptom until the symptoms have reached their maximum intensity or maximum extent in terms of which parts of the body are affected. In patients with intermittent symptoms, it is important to establish the duration of the symptoms. In either case, determining the exact distribution of the sensory symptoms, and consulting illustrations that show the sensory pathways and the areas of the body supplied by individual sensory nerve roots or peripheral nerves, will help establish the likely location of the pathological process. The other important aspect to determine from the neurological history is the presence or absence of loss of function as a result of these sensory symptoms. Terms such as 'tingling' and 'numbness' are non-specific, whereas the inability to appreciate pain or the temperature of objects would occur in patients with a peripheral nerve lesion (including a peripheral neuropathy) or involvement of the spinothalamic pathway. Symptoms such as instability in the dark or with the eyes closed, and inability to appreciate what object is in the hand without looking at it, or symptoms such as a sense of swelling in a limb in the absence of objective swelling, or a feeling of tightness as if wearing a tight stocking or glove, indicate problems affecting the pathways for vibration and proprioception.

EXAMINATION

Proprioception is tested in the index finger and big toe. Younger patients can appreciate minute changes; older patients can also detect even small movements of a finger or target. Marked impairment of proprioception in the lower limbs can also be tested by asking the patient to put their feet together and close their eyes—this is referred to as Rhomberg's test. An abnormal test is where the patient becomes unstable with their eyes closed. Vibration is also initially tested on the index finger or big toe using a 128 Hz tuning fork. It is important to remember that vibration sense diminishes in the feet with advancing age, and may even be absent in older patients. Temperature sensation can be tested with either the cold tuning fork or, in patients whose limbs are cold, a warm object such as the examiner's hands. Pain sensation is tested using a sharp object, but a hypodermic needle should not be used. A simple drawing pin or the specific things referred to as 'sharps' can be used. In patients who have objective sensory loss, it is important to test sensation in 360 degrees until the exact distribution of sensory loss is established, and then one can consult a sensory chart to see which part of the nervous system is likely to be affected.

INVESTIGATIONS

Patients are often referred for nerve conduction studies when they have intermittent sensory symptoms affecting their limbs, and it is important to remember that normal nerve conduction studies do not exclude a peripheral nerve lesion in such patients. MRI is the modality of choice when investigating patients with suspected involvement of the spinothalamic pathway or the pathway conveying vibration and proprioception in the CNS.

MANAGEMENT

Management is disease specific. A detailed discussion of all conditions producing sensory symptoms is beyond the scope of this chapter. The most common conditions seen in clinical practice—carpal tunnel syndrome, tardy ulnar palsy, meralgia paraesthetica and hyperventilation syndrome—are discussed, as is the rare entity of transverse myelitis.

Carpal tunnel syndrome

Carpal tunnel syndrome is almost certainly the most common cause of intermittent sensory symptoms. Although in theory these sensory symptoms should be confined to the distribution of the median nerve distal to the wrist, it is not uncommon for patients to complain of altered sensation affecting more proximal parts of the limb. Carpal tunnel syndrome should be suspected in patients who have numbness or tingling precipitated by holding objects, driving, mowing the lawn but in particular in patients who awaken in the middle of the night with numbness in one or both hands that is relieved by either moving the hands and arms or hanging the arms out of the side of the bed. Two simple bedside tests are *Phalen's sign*, where sensory symptoms are precipitated with forced reflection of the wrist, and *Tinel's sign*, where a transient electric shock-like sensation or paraesthesia is precipitated by tapping the median nerve in the carpal tunnel using a tendon hammer. Nerve conduction studies may be normal if symptoms have been present for only a short period of time. On the other hand, in older patients, nerve conduction studies are often very abnormal, even in patients who have only recently noticed symptoms. Nerve conduction studies can also assess the severity of the carpal tunnel syndrome. Symptoms occurring during pregnancy or in the setting of obesity may result following the pregnancy or after weight loss. Patients with mild symptoms may elect to simply tolerate the symptoms; some will use splints of their wrists at night to reduce the intensity of the symptoms. Some patients with mild carpal tunnel syndrome may respond to a corticosteroid injection into the carpal tunnel.[113] Surgical decompression is the definitive treatment in patients with more severe carpal tunnel.[114]

Tardy ulnar palsy

Tardy ulnar palsy is compression of the ulnar nerve at the elbow. The initial symptoms may be either intermittent tingling or numbness affecting the medial 1½ digits and the medial aspect of the palm of the hand, or, alternatively, the insidious onset of sensory loss affecting the medial 1½ digits and the medial aspect of the palm and the back of the hand, together with weakness of the small muscles of the hand. The complaint of weakness is not common, because grip strength is preserved. It would be more common for patients to present having noticed wasting of the small muscles of the hand. This condition is most often unilateral. Patients will have weakness of finger abduction, weakness opposing the thumb to the little finger and a weakness of reflection of the distal phalanx of the fourth and fifth digits but not of the second and third digits (the medial half of the flexor digitorum profundus that flexes the distal phalanges of the fourth and fifth digits is supplied by the arm and nerve, whereas the latter half that flexes the distal phalanges of the second and third digits is supplied by the median nerve). The condition can be confirmed and the site of compression can be defined by nerve conduction studies. Surgical decompression is the treatment of choice.

Meralgia paraesthetica

Numbness, paraesthesia or dysaesthesia (unpleasant sensory symptoms) affecting the lateral aspect of the thigh (see Fig 36.3) is typical of the condition referred to as *meralgia paraesthetica*, and relates to compression of the lateral cutaneous nerve of the thigh beneath the inguinal ligament. Most patients do not seek treatment once the benign nature of the problem is explained to them. Patients with dysaesthesia, on the other hand, can be offered a corticosteroid injection into the site of compression, formal decompression of the nerve, or avulsion of the nerve that results in a resolution of the dysaesthesia, but this is replaced by permanent numbness.

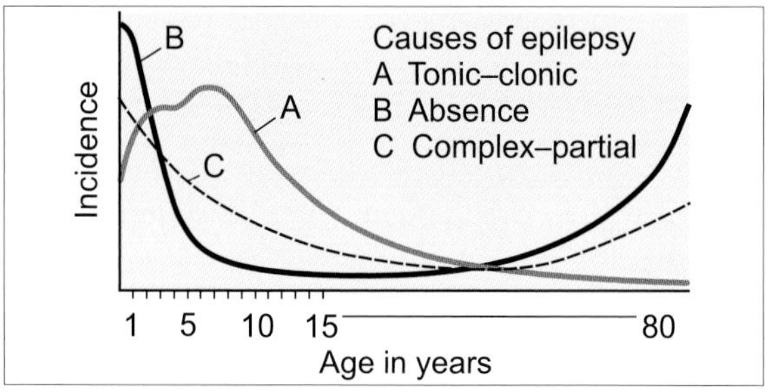

FIGURE 36.3 The area of altered sensation seen in meralgia paraesthetica (reproduced from Gates 2010[18])

Hyperventilation syndrome

A not-uncommon cause of intermittent subjective sensory symptoms in the absence of any objective functional loss is hyperventilation syndrome. Paraesthesia can affect the face, and cause tingling around the mouth, hands and feet. Sometimes only one part of the body may be affected, and occasional patients will have unilateral symptoms. Symptoms can be present for hours on end, waxing and waning in intensity. There is no functional loss when the subject's sensory symptoms are present. The presence of associated non-specific lightheadedness that also waxes and wanes in intensity, and the complaint of an inability to get enough air in (rather than actual shortness of breath) are other typical symptoms of hyperventilation syndrome. In very severe cases the hands and fingers may forcibly flex, an entity referred to as *carpopedal spasm*. The symptoms relate to altered carbon dioxide levels in the blood. Management has been discussed previously.

Transverse myelitis

Transverse myelitis is an inflammatory condition of the spinal cord. Persistent sensory symptoms and sensory loss develop over hours to days and gradually ascend from the feet, up the legs and on to the trunk to just below the level of the myelitis. Weakness in the lower limbs and sphincter disturbance may also occur. Although this can be the presenting symptom of multiple sclerosis, it is more likely to be related to other causes. Patients develop a distinctive sensory level where sensation below that level is impaired.

DISTURBANCES OF VISION

The great majority of patients with blurred vision will have a refractive error that can be corrected by asking them to read the Snellen chart through a small hole in a piece of paper. The more common 'neurological' causes of altered vision relate to abnormalities in the optic nerve, visual field defects due to problems in the visual pathways, or diplopia related to disorders of the third, fourth or sixth cranial nerves or within the brainstem.

HISTORY

Some patients will say they have double vision when what they mean is that there is a loss of vision, and therefore when taking the history it is important to clarify the exact nature of the visual disturbance. Patients will also occasionally confuse a hemi-anopic visual field disturbance with a monocular visual loss and therefore it is important to clarify whether the patient can see all or only half of the object they are looking at. If they can only see half, it is a field disturbance. Diplopia that occurs when the patient is very tired could be due to a problem at the neuromuscular junction, but it is more likely to be related to the breakdown of longstanding strabismus ('lazy eye').

EXAMINATION

The visual acuity in each eye should be tested with the glasses or contact lenses on, to remove any refractive error. Using the index finger in each hand and in each of the upper and lower visual fields will detect a marked hemianopia/quadrantanopia, but a 4 mm red pin is needed to detect more subtle visual field defects, and even this can miss minor abnormalities that can be demonstrated with a Goldman perimeter or a Bjerum screen. Ophthalmoscopic examination of the fundi is difficult but made easier if once or twice a week the non-neurologist practises by examining a 'normal' fundus. The ocular movement should be tested initially by asking the patient to look up to see if there is a gaze palsy on looking up (a 'normal' finding in older patients). Then the ocular movements should be tested in the primary direction action of the extraocular muscles: lateral rectus (lateral gaze); medial rectus (medial gaze); superior rectus (looking up with the eye deviated laterally); and inferior oblique (looking up with the eye deviated medially). The inferior rectus is tested by asking the patient to look down while the eye is deviated laterally, and superior oblique while the eye is deviated medially. If diplopia occurs, cover each eye in succession (cover testing) and ask the patient whether the medial or lateral image disappears. The image furthest from the midline is the abnormal image. This can be difficult, and using red-green glasses is much easier.

INVESTIGATIONS

Investigations will depend on whether the problem is diplopia, monocular visual symptoms or visual disturbance in one field.

MANAGEMENT

Management is disease specific.

Monocular impairment of vision

Amaurosis fugax

Transient loss of vision, as if a blind has descended down over the eye, is typical of amaurosis fugax, indicative of retinal artery ischaemia. This can be associated with internal carotid artery stenosis, but more often it is related to anterior ischaemic optic neuropathy (AION). Rarely, AION may occur in the setting of cranial arteritis. Transient visual loss, referred to as *obscurations*, can also occur with papilloedema.

Optic and retrobulbar neuritis

Optic neuritis and *retrobulbar neuritis* both result in the gradual onset, over hours to days, of severe visual loss, often associated with pain on movement of the eye. There is an afferent pupillary defect (Marcus-Gunn) in the affected eye in both, but the optic disc is swollen with optic but not retrobulbar neuritis. While the most common cause is multiple sclerosis, it can also be a manifestation of connective tissue disease.[115]

Visual loss in one visual field

Although a hemianopia can occur with occipital and parietal lobe lesions, in the former, other manifestations often dominate. When a patient presents with a loss of vision in one visual field, it more likely represents occipital lobe pathology, almost invariably ischaemic in origin and due to an embolus to the posterior cerebral artery.

Diplopia and ptosis

Horizontal diplopia occurs with sixth nerve palsies (which very rarely may be a false localising sign in patients with raised intracranial pressure) or a lesion of the median longitudinal fasciculus (the pathway between the third, fourth and sixth cranial nerves). In the latter, the eye fails to adduct towards the nose on the affected side, and there is leading eye nystagmus on the opposite eye. *Vertical diplopia* occurs with midbrain lesions or affecting the third or fourth cranial nerves, which also produce marked *ptosis*, and impairment of the medial, superior, inferior rectus muscles as well as the inferior oblique. A dilated pupil is a feature of compressive lesions such as aneurysms on the posterior communicating artery, while 'pupil-sparing' third nerve palsies are a feature of lesions with the third nerve (e.g. diabetes).

Fatiguable ptosis becoming worse with, for example, reading, associated with variable vertical and horizontal diplopia, are a feature of myasthenia gravis (see above).

CEREBRAL VASCULAR DISEASE

The term *cerebral vascular disease* refers to the development of a focal neurological deficit as a result of infarction or haemorrhage. The management of patients with cerebral vascular disease is very complex because of the very large number of conditions that can result in either cerebral infarction or intracerebral haemorrhage.

The challenge for the clinician is to:

- determine that the patient is actually suffering from a 'stroke'
- differentiate between infarction and haemorrhage
- elucidate the underlying pathogenesis

and then choose the appropriate treatment in a particular patient, taking into account their past history, social history and listed medications, all of which can influence the choice of therapy. The diagnosis of stroke presents little difficulty when an elderly patient presents with the sudden onset of a focal neurological deficit in the setting of multiple recognised risk factors for stroke. On the other hand, many patients awaken with the neurological deficit and therefore one cannot be certain that the onset was sudden. And stroke can occur in young patients and in patients without recognised risk factors. Some symptoms, such as diplopia or vertigo, will always develop suddenly and may not represent cerebral vascular disease. Obtaining a history from patients is not always possible, because of the presence of speech disturbance or cognitive problems related to the stroke.

Cerebral infarction (CI) rather than intracerebral haemorrhage (ICH) is more common in the era of better management of hypertension. The main causes of CI are atherosclerotic vascular disease with or without stenosis of the major extracranial and, to a lesser extent, intracranial vessels, small vessels (lacunar) infarction related to hypertension and diabetes, and AF. In younger patients (< 45 years of age), alternative causes of stroke need to be considered, such as extracranial artery dissection (see Fig 36.4), a patent foramen ovale, or lupus anticoagulant anticardiolipin antibody syndrome.

PRIMARY PREVENTION

Hippocrates commented that, 'It is difficult to cure a mild case of apoplexy and impossible to cure a severe case'. This holds true even today, and so the focus should be on primary and secondary prevention.

Optimal management of treatable risk factors such as hypertension, smoking, hypercholesterolaemia, obesity and diabetes is the cornerstone of both primary[116] and secondary prevention.

The old adage that a normal blood pressure is 100 plus the patient's age has clearly been shown to be incorrect. The Progress Study[117] demonstrated that the blood pressure should be as close to 120/80 as possible although, in reality, most elderly patients cannot achieve this level of blood pressure due to side effects of medication.

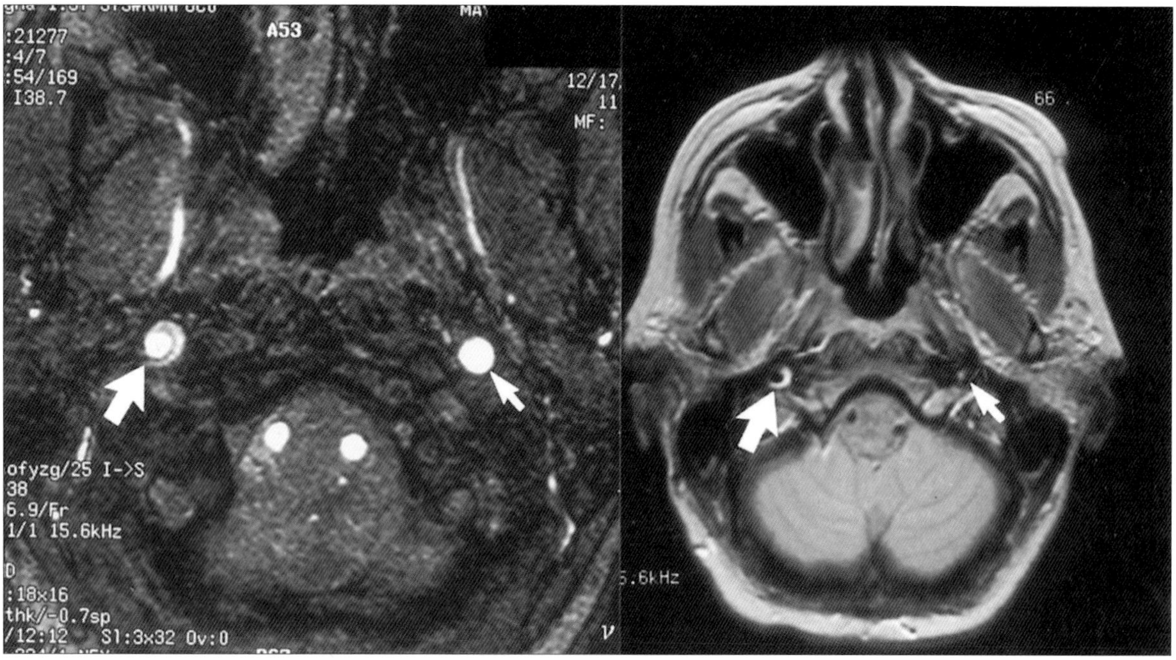

FIGURE 36.4 Internal carotid artery dissection, a rare but important cause of stroke in young patients

Anticoagulation with warfarin (PT INR 2-3) for patients in AF with a CHADS score[118] of two or more significantly reduces the risk of sudden stroke. There is a 70% relative risk reduction with less than 1% mortality and a 1–2% major bleeding risk.[119] Absolute contraindications include bleeding peptic ulcer or other pathology that would predispose to bleeding. A risk of falls and cognitive impairment are *relative* contraindications, and the slightly increased risk of warfarin in these patients needs to be balanced with the risk of stroke using the CHADS score (Table 36.1).

The absolute risk reduction with carotid endarterectomy for patients with asymptomatic carotid stenosis of greater than 50% is 1% per annum.[120]

TABLE 36.1 CHADS score and annual risk of stroke

Score	Annual risk of stroke	95% CI
1	2.8	2.0–3.8
2	4.0	3.1–5.0
3	5.9	4.6–7.3
4	8.5	6.3–11.0
5	12.5	8.2–17.5
6	18.2	10.5–29.4

The CHADS score is calculated as 1 point each for recent (< 3 months) congestive cardiac failure (C), history of hypertension (H), age > 75 (A) and diabetes (D), and 2 points for prior TIA or stroke (S).

HISTORY

In patients with cerebral vascular disease, the history is used to help differentiate between cerebral infarction and intracerebral haemorrhage. The only clues that the stroke may relate to intracerebral haemorrhage are early depression of the conscious state and vomiting, in a cerebral hemisphere lesion, and this may not occur in elderly patients with significant cerebral atrophy.

The history is also used to help determine whether the stroke is in the distribution of the anterior circulation (carotid, middle cerebral and anterior cerebral arteries) or the posterior circulation (vertebral, basilar or post cerebral arteries). The presence of vertigo and diplopia associated with a focal neurological deficit clearly indicate involvement of the brainstem and therefore the most serious circulation. An isolated hemianopia is most likely related to infarction of the occipital lobe, also in the posterior circulation. Dysphasia would point to a dominant hemisphere anterior circulation problem. Although a hemiparesis affecting the face, arm and leg is most likely related to a hemisphere problem, it can relate to an upper pontine or midbrain stroke.

The neurological history should also elicit the presence of risk factors for stroke, which will influence the choice of secondary prevention measures. It will also need to examine the social history, which can have a significant impact on the subsequent management of patients with cerebral vascular disease. Many patients with cerebral vascular disease have multiple other medical problems and are taking a large number of drugs, which will also influence subsequent choice of therapy. Details of past medical problems should be obtained, as many of these will also influence the subsequent choice of therapy—for example, a history of peptic ulcer disease or epistaxis.

In patients with transient ischaemic attacks (defined arbitrarily as an episode of cerebral ischaemia lasting less than 24 hours) the neurological signs have often resolved by the time the patient seeks medical care, and the history is crucial for determining the site of the problem within the nervous system.

EXAMINATION

The neurological examination may be completely normal in patients with transient ischaemic attacks. When neurological signs are present, examination is used to help determine whether the stroke is in the interior or posterior circulation. The pulse should be palpated, looking for possible AF, the blood pressure should be recorded, and the neck should be auscultated to look for a bruit related to carotid artery stenosis, although it is important to remember that the absence of a bruit does not exclude carotid stenosis. The heart should be examined to look for cardiomegaly or the presence of cardiac valve abnormalities, potential sources of cerebral emboli, and if a cardiac murmur is present, the patient should be examined for the possibility of bacterial endocarditis, a rare cause of stroke. The respiratory system should be examined, as many patients have coexistent chronic obstructive airways disease. More importantly, a number of patients with dysphagia will develop aspiration pneumonia. The abdomen should be examined for the possibility of an abdominal aortic aneurysm, and all peripheral pulses should be palpated, as coexistent peripheral vascular disease is not uncommon.

INVESTIGATIONS

Initial investigations that should be performed as a matter of urgency include:

- full blood examination (FBE) and erythrocyte sedimentation rate (ESR)—to exclude anaemia, but also to look for the presence of possible sepsis
- blood sugar—many patients have diabetes; more importantly, hypoglycaemia can rarely present with a focal neurological deficit mimicking a stroke
- urea and creatinine—many patients may have impaired renal function
- liver function tests (LFTs)
- electrocardiogram (ECG)—to look not only for AF but also for the rare instance of a silent myocardial infarct that could be the source of a cerebral embolus.

CT of the brain will differentiate between intracerebral haemorrhage and cerebral infarction. It will also detect the occasional patient with a cerebral tumour, which may mimic a stroke, or the subdural haematoma, which may cause a hemiparesis in the absence of any depression of the conscious state and therefore mimic a stroke.

In patients with either a TIA or a minor stroke in the anterior circulation, ischaemia should have an urgent Doppler carotid ultrasound, as 50% of subsequent strokes after a TIA will occur within the first 24 hours.[121] It is important to remember that a normal CT of the brain does not exclude cerebral ischaemia, particularly in the first 6 hours after onset, but also in patients with ischaemia related to small vessel disease or in the brainstem.

Subsequent investigations

MRI, particularly *diffusion weighted MRI* (dwMRI), can detect cerebral infarction in some patients with transient ischaemic attacks, and can detect cerebral ischaemia as early as 1.5 hours after the onset of symptoms.[122] dwMRI has a sensitivity of more than 90–95% for detecting early (within the first 6 hours after onset) ischaemic changes.[122] It must be performed within the first week, as these changes are transient. It can also detect very small (lacunar) infarcts in both cerebral hemispheres and the brainstem. *Magnetic resonance angiography* (MRA) and *magnetic resonance venography* (MRV) enable imaging of the cerebral circulation. Very rarely, a stroke can relate to cerebral venous thrombosis.

Fasting lipids should be performed, as many patients have hypercholesterolaemia.

Transthoracic and/or trans-oesophageal echocardiography is indicated in patients with a cardiac source for cerebral embolism (in essence, patients with ischaemia in the distribution of the major vessels in the absence of demonstrable vascular disease in those vessels). Patients admitted to stroke units should have cardiac monitoring, in order to detect intermittent AF.[123]

MANAGEMENT

Subsequent management of patients with cerebral vascular disease is very complex and is discussed in each of the individual sections below. This chapter will deal with the management of ischaemic stroke and only briefly touch on intracranial haemorrhage.

Management of ischaemic TIA and stroke

Acute treatment of ischaemic stroke

Ideally, patients should be referred to centres of expertise, as the development of stroke units has led to a reduction in mortality and morbidity. Aspirin in the first 24 hours reduces mortality in the first few weeks after stroke.[124] All patients should have a dysphagia screen and placed on nil orally if they fail, until a detailed speech therapist assessment. Cardiac monitoring is essential, not only to detect AF but also to monitor for other arrhythmias that may occur in the setting of acute myocardial infarction, which occurs in a small percentage of patients with stroke in the early days after stroke. Intravenous fluids are essential to maintain hydration, but 5% glucose should be avoided. Deep vein thrombosis (DVT) prophylaxis with antithrombotic stockings and either unfractionated heparin or low molecular weight heparin should be instituted from day one. Patients should be checked daily for possible aspiration pneumonia.

Thrombolysis

Thrombolysis with tissue plasminogen activator (t-PA) is now a well-established treatment for patients with ischaemic stroke of less than 4.5 hours' duration and a NIHSS score of > 4, provided there are no contraindications.[125] Exclusion criteria include the following:[125]

- intracranial haemorrhage
- time of symptom onset unknown
- symptoms rapidly improving or only minor before onset of infusion
- severe stroke (clinically or on imaging)
- seizure at onset of stroke
- stroke or serious head trauma within the previous 3 months
- combination of stroke and diabetes mellitus
- administration of heparin in the preceding 48 hours
- platelet count < 100,000/mm3
- systolic pressure > 185 mmHg or diastolic pressure > 110 mmHg, or aggressive medication required to reduce the blood pressure to these limits
- blood glucose < 50 mg/dL or > 400 mg/dL
- symptoms suggestive of subarachnoid haemorrhage even if CT scan normal
- oral anticoagulant treatment
- major surgery or severe trauma in preceding 3 months
- other major bleeding disorders.

Secondary prevention

Antiplatelet therapy

In addition to the management of risk factors as discussed above, antiplatelet therapy in the form of aspirin, aspirin and persantin,[126] or clopidogrel[127] is recommended for patients with ischaemic stroke not related to AF or another cardiac source for embolism.

Anticoagulation

Anticoagulation with warfarin (optimal PT INR 2.0–2.5[128]) is recommended for patients with AF or other potential cardiac sources for embolism, such as a cardiomyopathy or artificial heart valve.[129] Recently, dabigatran, a direct thrombin inhibitor, was found at a dose of 110 mg twice a day to be as effective as warfarin[130] although some concerns have been expressed about the methodology of the trial. Despite numerous trials confirming the effectiveness of warfarin, many practitioners are reluctant to prescribe, because of perceived risks. Each area of medicine associated with AF and warfarin has its own perspective. Neurologists see the strokes that could have been prevented by warfarin, neurosurgeons see the complications of warfarin therapy and cardiologists see hundreds of patients with AF who have a very low risk of stroke. As discussed above, the CHADS score allows stratification of risk.

Carotid endarterectomy

Carotid endarterectomy is probably the most potent therapy available for secondary prevention in patients with a symptomatic stenosis of 70% or greater (Fig 36.6). It is associated with a 17% *absolute* risk reduction over 2 years, with numbers needed to treat (NNT) of only 15.[131] As 50% of strokes after TIA occur in the first 24 hours[121] urgent assessment for carotid stenosis with a Doppler carotid ultrasound is essential, although most of these recurrent events may well relate to small vessel disease—the so-called *capsular warning syndrome*.[132]

Carotid stenting

It is hoped that stenting may one day replace endarterectomy for carotid stenosis. A 2010 metanalysis[133] concluded that this stage has not yet been reached.

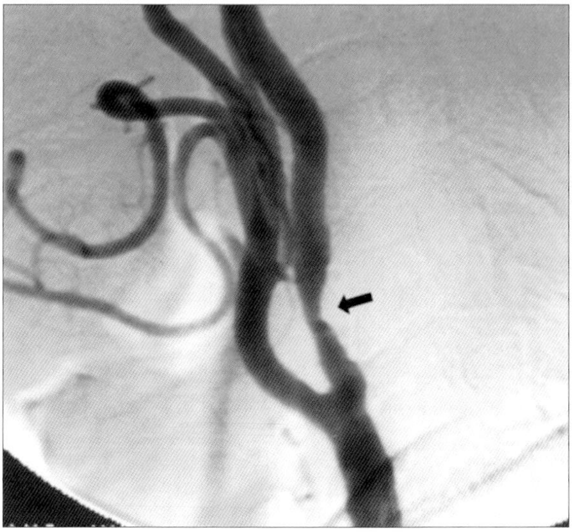

FIGURE 36.5 Severe carotid stenosis, the most important preventable cause of severe stroke after TIA or minor stroke

Integrated management

The integrated management of cardiovascular disease is dealt with extensively in the cardiovascular disease chapter (Ch 25).

ABNORMAL MOVEMENTS AND DIFFICULTY WITH MOVEMENT

Although there are many problems that produce difficulty with walking, probably two of the most common are Parkinson's disease and the frontal lobe apraxia of gait that is often confused with Parkinson's. There are also many 'abnormal movements' in clinical neurology, but only five are discussed in this chapter: benign (essential or familial) tremor, the tremor of Parkinson's, chorea, hemiballismus and the abnormal movements around the mouth referred to as tardive dyskinesia.

HISTORY

Many abnormal movements such as Parkinson's, benign familial tremor and Huntington's chorea are familial, and so it is important to obtain a detailed family history. A detailed list of drugs and medications currently used and those used in the past should be obtained, as a number of abnormal movements are drug induced (e.g tardive dyskinesia, tremor and Parkinsonism, including MPTP-induced Parkinson's). Elicit the circumstances under which the abnormal movements occur, as some occur at rest and others with movement. And finally, determine whether the abnormal movement is still present in sleep—most resolve during sleep, but hemiballismus persists.

EXAMINATION

The various examination findings that differentiate one condition from another are discussed below.

INVESTIGATIONS

At present there are very few investigations that help in the differential diagnosis of most movement disorders. Where applicable they are discussed.

MANAGEMENT

Management is disease specific and is discussed below.

Abnormal movements

Tremor (benign essential, benign familial, resting tremor of Parkinson's)

Benign essential and *benign familial* tremors are identical except that, in the latter, there is a positive family history. This is the patient who complains that the cup rattles in the saucer. This is not a tremor at rest; it occurs with action. The severity of the tremor may be reduced by alcohol, and this can be a diagnostic clue. There is no alteration in tone, nor is there any bradykinesia. Walking is not affected. Hyperthyroidism should be excluded. If the trend is mild, no treatment is required. Primidone and propanolol are the drugs of choice. Alprazolam, atenolol, gabapentin (monotherapy), sotalol and topiramate are probably effective.[134]

The *tremor of Parkinson's*, on the other hand, is present at rest and not when a patient holds an object. In resistant cases, chronic deep brain stimulation or thalamotomy is effective.[134] The tremor may also be noticed when the patient is walking and the arm is hanging down by their side. The tremor is not influenced by alcohol, and in the early stages may be the only manifestation of Parkinson's disease. There are some patients who may only experience tremor, and this is referred to as the *benign tremulous* form of Parkinson's disease. Treatment of the tremor in Parkinson's disease can be very difficult, and it does not always respond as well as the other manifestations to the various levodopa preparations.

Hemiballismus

Hemiballismus is a relatively rare movement disorder characterised by uncontrolled, random, large-amplitude movements of the limbs, likened to a large-amplitude chorea. It is usually caused by a vascular lesion that involves the contralateral subthalamic nucleus (STN) and its afferent and efferent pathways. Occasionally it can occur with infarction at other sites, and it can be a manifestation of multiple sclerosis. It is usually self-limiting and responsive to conservative treatment to prevent injury and dehydration, and the use of drugs to reduce the intensity of the abnormal movements. Tetrabenazine, haloperidol, propanolol, clonazepam, phenytoin and baclofen have all been used, with variable success. Sterotactic pallidotomy has been recommended in refractory cases.[135]

Tardive dyskinesia

Tardive dyskinesia (TD) results from chronic exposure to levodopa, dopamine agonists and dopamine receptor blockers. It is characterised by involuntary, repetitive, purposeless movements of the tongue, jaw, lips, face, trunk, upper extremities, lower extremities and respiratory system. Initially the mouth, lips and tongue are involved, and later the trunk and limbs may be involved. The movements are choreiform in nature. The diagnosis is a clinical one and Wilson's disease needs to be excluded. Approximately one-third of patients will remit upon cessation of the causative agent. Persistent symptoms can occur, particularly in the elderly, those without dentures or those with underlying organic cerebral dysfunction. The incidence may be less with the newer atypical antipsychotic drugs, and these drugs may be useful in treatment, and therefore replacing typical antipsychotic drugs with atypical antipsychotic drugs may be useful. Central anticholinergic drugs that can exacerbate TD should be discontinued. Reserpine, tetrabenazine, clonazepam, baclofen and botulinum toxin injections are recommended in refractory cases.[136]

Chorea: Huntington's and Sydenham's

Chorea is the ceaseless, irregular, rapid, uncontrolled complex body movements that look well coordinated and purposeful but are in fact involuntary. Chorea can affect the face, arms or legs. The abnormal movements are almost continuous.

Huntington's chorea is an autosomal-dominant disorder in middle age with the characteristic chorea, with the subsequent development of abnormal behaviour and dementia. It relates to an expanded and unstable trinucleotide repeat on chromosome 4. The length of the trinucleotide repeats correlates inversely with the age of onset. Genetic testing can confirm the diagnosis. Treatment is symptomatic, with the use of dopamine-depleting agents such as tetrabenazine, reserpine, dopamine agonists such as haloperidol and benzodiazepines such as clonazepam or diazepam.[137]

Sydenham's chorea is a major complication of rheumatic fever due to group A beta-haemolytic streptococcal infection. It is an immune-mediated disorder, with the antibodies triggered by beta-haemolytic streptococcus cross-reacting with antigens in the brain by a molecular mimicry mechanism. Systemic lupus erythematosus (SLE), drug reactions and Wilson's disease should be excluded. Serum antistreptococcal antibodies are also raised in Sydenham's chorea. MRI may show an increase in basal ganglia volume and also evidence of neuronal damage in the ganglia, especially the caudate nuclei and putamina. Single proton emission computed tomography (SPECT) studies can detect both hypo- and hyper-perfusion pattern abnormalities. Valproic acid, haloperidol, carbamazepine or pimozide can be used to treat the chorea.[138]

Difficulty walking: Parkinson's and apraxia of gait

The gait of Parkinson's disease and the apraxic gait seen in frontal lobe disease can at times be very difficult to differentiate. In both entities, patients are 'bradykinetic' and have 'rigidity', although there are subtle differences that enable diagnosis at the bedside. The presence of a resting tremor occurs with Parkinson's disease but not with an apraxic gait.

Parkinson's disease

The most common presentation of Parkinson's disease is a resting tremor, the so-called typical 'pill-rolling' tremor. When Parkinson's disease affects both lower limbs, patients present with difficulty walking, and they walk with small, shuffling steps and do not swing their arms. When there is an associated resting tremor, the diagnosis presents little difficulty. There is a characteristic 'cogwheel' rigidity best tested at rest by slowly flexing and dorsi-flexing the wrist. Occasionally, patients present with unilateral involvement mimicking a hemiparesis. The characteristic pathology of Parkinson's disease is a loss of pigmentation in the substantia nigra and the presence of Lewy bodies, which leads to a deficiency in dopamine. The mainstay of treatment is levodopa replacement therapy; and to reduce side effects from the levodopa, this is combined with a decarboxylase inhibitor such as carbidopa or benserazide. Increasing duration of treatment is associated with great efficacy initially, a shorter duration of action leading to end-of-dose failure, and subsequently the 'on–off' phenomenon whereby periods of bradykinesia alternate with periods of dyskinesia regardless of the timing of the levodopa. *Dyskinesia* refers to the involuntary movements that can occur in patients with longstanding Parkinson's on levodopa, initially as a peak dose phenomenon and subsequently the on–off phenomenon.[139] Dopamine agonists such as cabergoline or pergolide have been used to manage the on–off phenomenon, but in recent years there have been concerns regarding significant side effects of cardiac valve abnormalities and pathological gambling. COMT inhibitors such as entacapone can reduce the dose when one tablet is taken with each dose of levodopa. More recently, pramipexole, a dopamine receptor agonist, has been shown to be very effective in patients with Parkinson's—although less effective than levodopa, it has fewer motor complications. Stereotactic surgery[140] and deep brain stimulation[141] are other treatment modalities in drug-resistant cases.

Apraxia of gait

Apraxia of gait is a perseveration of posture and an inability to perform the serial movements necessary for ambulation, in the absence of weakness, sensory deficit, instability or incoordination. Patients walk with small steps, referred to as the *marche à petit pas* ('walks with little steps'). Patients have a curious alteration in tone, referred to as *gegenhalten* (involuntary resistance), where the rigidity is initially minimal or absent, and increases in severity with more prolonged testing. Palmo-mental and grasp reflexes are usually present. This gait disturbance occurs with frontal lobe problems predominantly on a degenerative or vascular basis, but reversible causes include normal-pressure hydrocephalus, bilateral subdural haematomas or benign frontal lobe tumours. There is no specific pharmacological or surgical therapy. Patients may benefit from supervised physiotherapy.

Integrative management of Parkinson's disease

Recent studies have placed an increasing focus on the role of environmental factors in Parkinson's disease aetiology.[142] For example, there have been many studies concerning the relationship of the neurotoxic effects of certain heavy metals to the risk of developing Parkinson's.[142] In particular, these include chronic exposure to manganese, copper and lead.[143–147] Parkinson's has also recently been characterised by high tissue iron (not currently connected to haemachromatosis) and miscompartmentalisation of zinc and copper.[148,149]

Epidemiological evidence indicates that exposure to pesticides (particularly organophosphates, carbamates, pyrethroids and organochlorides) may also play a significant role in the aetiology of idiopathic Parkinson's disease.[150–155] There is evidence that exposure to the common pesticides, such as maneb, paraquat and rotenone, especially at an early age, increases the risk of Parkinson's.[156,157,152] Despite this evidence, however, ethical challenges in exposure assessment make it impossible to conduct formal studies for further evaluation. Even exposure to pesticides, heavy metals and/or an iron-enriched diet while in the womb may directly reduce the number of dopaminergic neurons or cause increased susceptibility to loss of these neurons, with subsequent environmental insults or ageing.[158,159]

More than 1 year of antidepressant, anxiolytic or hypnotic drugs combined with a family history of Parkinson's have been shown to be associated with significantly increased odds ratios for developing Parkinson's.[156]

Previous work in electronic plants and exposure to fluorides and chlorpyrifos products have also been associated with a significantly increased risk of Parkinson's, as has repeated traumatic episodes of consciousness loss.[150,156] Conversely, cigarette smoking and alcohol intake may be associated with a reduced risk of Parkinson's, although this could not be taken as an argument for taking up smoking.[142,150]

Allied healthcare referrals

Although there is growing evidence that specific allied healthcare interventions are beneficial when integrated into rehabilitation programs, recent Cochrane reviews indicate that there is not enough evidence to support or refute the use of occupational therapy, physiotherapy and speech therapy in Parkinson's disease.[160–162]

Exercise

Several meta-analyses have shown that exercise is beneficial for physical functioning, quality of life, strength, balance and speed of gait for those suffering from Parkinson's.[163–165] A further systematic review has shown that these positive effects decrease when exercise is ceased.[166] In particular, dancing and aerobic exercise have both demonstrated positive effects.[167,168]

Acupuncture

A number of studies, including meta-analyses, have demonstrated possible benefits of acupuncture in the treatment of Parkinson's.[169–171] The symptoms of tremor, rigidity and bradykinesia have especially responded with similar effects from electro-scalp acupuncture.[172,173] The use of acupuncture combined with anti-Parkinson's disease medications has also been found to be synergistic, with reduction of medication dose and reduced adverse drug effects.[174,175]

Herbal therapies

Ayurvedic medicine

Mucuna pruriens (MP) naturally contains levodopa and is the traditional herb used in Ayurveda to treat Parkinson's.[176,177] The pharmaceutical preparation HP-200, which contains MP combined with coenzyme Q10 and nicotine adenine dinucleotide, has been shown to be more effective than conventional levodopa in treating Parkinson's in animal models. Unlike synthetic levodopa, HP-200 was found to significantly restore endogenous levodopa, dopamine, noradrenaline and serotonin in the substantia nigra, suggesting that it has both neurorestorative and neuroprotective effects.[178,179] MP appears to be safe in the treatment of patients with Parkinson's, although more studies are required to confirm its efficacy.[180]

Traditional Chinese medicine

Although there are several preliminary studies showing that moxibustion combined with routine Western medical therapy is more effective than if either is given alone, larger RCTs are required to assess this further.[181]

Nutritional therapies

It has been postulated that imbalances in body metal levels may be a significant risk factor for the development of Parkinson's as well as other neurological diseases.[182] Studies have demonstrated low zinc and high iron and selenium levels in the cerebrospinal fluid of Parkinson's patients who are taking levodopa, which may be correlated with lowered dopamine levels and increased oxidative stress.[183]

Low plasma, platelet and cerebral cortex levels of the antioxidant coenzyme Q10 in patients with Parkinson's has been shown in several studies.[184] A large phase III clinical trial was undertaken in 2008 to determine whether coenzyme Q10 supplementation slowed the progression of Parkinson's.[185]

A meta-analysis of antioxidants has revealed that dietary intake of vitamin E may have a neuroprotective effect, attenuating the risk of Parkinson's.[186] Adequate dietary intake of vitamin B_6 has also been shown to reduce the risk of developing Parkinson's.[187]

Individuals with Parkinson's treated with levodopa have been found to have significantly lower serum levels of folate and vitamin B_{12}.[188] Interestingly, those patients with Parkinson's and depression have significantly lower folate levels, whereas those with Parkinson's and cognitive impairment have lower levels of vitamin B_{12}.[189] Supplementation with these nutrients can lower homocysteine, which can be of particular importance to those Parkinson's individuals at risk of vascular diseases, cognitive impairment or dementia.[188]

Patients with Parkinson's have been found to have significantly lower levels of vitamin D than controls, and therefore vitamin D deficiency may be a significant risk factor in the pathogenesis of Parkinson's.[190] Animal studies have shown that supplementation with vitamin D may help to prevent dopaminergic neuron damage, but further studies on humans are needed.[191]

Diets high in creatine may be beneficial for those individuals with Parkinson's who are on levodopa, to reduce the levodopa-induced dyskinesia that may occur after long-term use of the medication.[192]

Patients with Parkinson's show a significantly reduced zinc status compared with controls.[193] Zinc is required to synthesise superoxide dismutase (SOD), a powerful antioxidant that is normally found in high concentrations in the substantia nigra, where it protects neurons from oxidative stress. Supplementation with zinc significantly increases SOD in in vitro studies.[193] Copper has also been implicated in Parkinson's, as low copper may result in incomplete CNS development and high copper may be involved in the production of free radicals, which can result in mitochondrial damage, DNA breakage and neuronal injury.[194] Magnesium deficiency has also recently been associated with neuronal degeneration in the substantia nigra and, hence, may contribute to the pathogenesis of Parkinson's.[142,195] Animal studies have shown that magnesium might protect against this, but further clinical trials are needed.[196]

A large-scale study of the dietary patterns of 130,000 individuals was conducted over 16 years. Results show that a diet high in fruits, vegetables, legumes, whole grains, nuts, fish and poultry combined with low saturated fat and moderate alcohol consumption was protective against Parkinson's. In contrast, a typical Western diet high in animal and saturated fats was directly associated with an increased risk of Parkinson's.[197,198] In particular, the polyphenols in fruits such as blueberries have been shown to improve neuronal signal conduction and communication.[199]

The correct levels of protein intake in order to prevent Parkinson's are currently debatable, with studies showing mixed results for both ketogenic and low-protein diets.[200–202] Similarly, the consumption of dairy products has been positively associated with increased risk of Parkinson's (especially in men); however, more studies are required to confirm this.[203] The intake of caffeine is controversial; however, recent studies have shown that it may be ingredients in black tea other than caffeine that are responsible for a possible inverse associative risk with Parkinson's.[201–204]

It should be noted that dietary exposure to food contaminants such as polychlorinated biphenyls (PCBs) and methylmercury (MeHg) have been positively associated with Parkinson's, and therefore avoidance of these contaminants where possible is recommended.[205]

Mind–body medicine

Depression is commonly associated with Parkinson's and it has been shown that Parkinson's patients who are suffering from depression may experience faster deterioration in their neurological symptoms, greater cognitive decline and poorer quality of life. There have been several studies showing that therapies such as cognitive behaviour therapy may benefit these patients (and their carers); however, further larger-scale trials are warranted.[206,207] A systematic review of RCTs has shown that the Alexander technique (a process of psychophysical re-education) is effective in reducing disability in those with Parkinson's, and earlier trials have shown that it may be beneficial in reducing depression when combined with drug therapy.[208] Music therapy has also been shown to be effective on both motor and behavioural functioning in those with Parkinson's.[209,210]

MULTIPLE SCLEROSIS

Multiple sclerosis (MS) is the most common neurodegenerative condition affecting young people. It is currently thought to be an immune-mediated disorder of unknown aetiology, due primarily to $CD4^+$ T-cell-mediated immune responses to the major myelin proteins, myelin basic protein (MBP) and proteolipid protein (PLP). As with most other autoimmune conditions, MS is more common among women. In genetically susceptible individuals, factors such as Epstein-Barr virus[211,212] and chlamydia infection[213] have been implicated, as have vitamin D, diet, smoking and stress.[214–218] The complex interplay of vulnerability, causative factors and triggers is far from fully elucidated, but they do point to potential therapies in the integrated management of MS, which will be discussed later. Humoral immune responses are also believed to contribute to the immunopathology. It results in inflammation, demyelination and subsequent gliosis in the central nervous system. MS is rare, with an incidence of approximately 0.1%. The average age of onset is 18–35 years but it may develop in patients at any age and is more common in women. There is a 30–50% increased incidence in children of parents with MS. In younger patients it may present with a clinically isolated syndrome such as optic neuritis or transverse myelitis. A relapsing–remitting course is also characteristic of MS in younger patients, which sometimes transforms to secondary progressive MS. A primary progressive form is characteristic of later-onset (40–55 years of age) MS.

HISTORY

Although intermittent symptoms lasting seconds to minutes may occur with MS, such as the L'hermitte phenomenon (an electric shock-like sensation radiating into the arms and down the back that occurs with neck flexion), trigeminal neuralgia or paroxysmal tonic seizures in general patients present with the gradual onset of a focal neurological deficit evolving over hours to days, and persisting for days to weeks or even months.

The history obtained depends on the part of the nervous system affected. In younger patients, presentations include optic or retrobulbar neuritis (vide supra), transverse myelitis (vide supra) or diplopia, the latter almost invariably related to involvement of the median longitudinal fasciculus within the brainstem producing either a unilateral or a bilateral internuclear ophthalmoplegia. Less commonly, patients may present with the gradual onset of vertigo and dysarthria, reflecting involvement of the cerebellar pathways. Urinary sphincter disturbance related to involvement of the spinal cord is another presentation in young women, although urinary sphincter dysfunction is far more likely to have a non-neurological cause. In patients presenting with the primary progressive form of MS, the history is one of gradual onset, over months to years, of weakness in the lower limb(s) with or without sphincter disturbance and often little in the way of subjective sensory symptoms. Difficulty walking on uneven surfaces, or up and down stairs, is characteristic of patients with spasticity in the lower limbs, also reflecting involvement of the spinal cord.

EXAMINATION

The examination findings will reflect the part of the nervous system involved. An internuclear ophthalmoplegia results in failure of adduction of the ipsilateral (to the side of the lesion) eye towards the nose, associated with leading eye nystagmus in the contralateral eye. The neurological findings associated with optic and retrobulbar neuritis have already been discussed. Neurologists would frequently check the visual acuity, colour vision, pupil reflexes and fundoscopic examination of the optic disc, looking for subtle evidence of asymptomatic involvement of the optic nerve. In this situation, the visual acuity may be mildly impaired in one eye and not corrected with a pinhole or refraction, and there may be an afferent pupillary defect referred to as the Marcus-Gunn phenomena, mild pallor of the optic disc and defects of colour vision. In patients with involvement of the spinal cord, there will be an upper motor neuron pattern of weakness in one or both legs and, in addition, one or both arms even if the latter have been symptomatic (symptoms in one limb with findings in several limbs is often a characteristic feature of MS). The tone will be increased, as will the reflexes, and both plantar reflexes may be extensor. Although mild impairment of sensation is common, a distinct sensory level is most atypical, and the diagnosis of MS should be one of exclusion in this setting.

INVESTIGATIONS

Investigations need to exclude other disorders that can produce multifocal involvement of the CNS, such as acute disseminated encephalomyelitis, antiphospholipid antibody syndrome, Wilson's disease, sarcoidosis, paraneoplastic syndromes, SLE and CNS vasculitis or lymphoma. The diagnosis is currently based on the revised MRI criteria of McDonald.[219] If a patient presents with two or more attacks with objective evidence of two or more lesions, no additional information is required for the diagnosis. On the other hand, if a patient presents with two or more attacks and objective clinical evidence of only one lesion, or one attack with objective evidence of one or more lesions, the MRI scan and CSF analysis can be used to support the clinical diagnosis of MS. The MRI scan demonstrates characteristic abnormalities such as lesions arising from the corpus callosum—the so-called 'Dawson's fingers' (Fig 36.6). Visual evoked responses (VER) can identify subclinical optic nerve lesions, with a

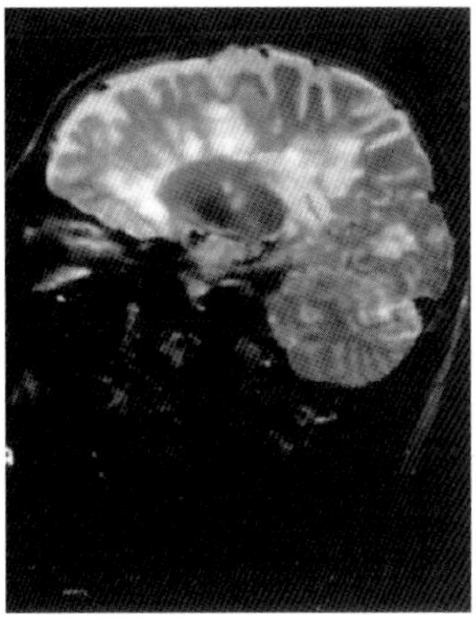

FIGURE 36.6 An MRI scan showing the characteristic 'Dawson's fingers' of multiple sclerosis

prolonged P100 latency and a normal waveform typical of a demyelinating optic neuropathy.[220]

The finding of oligoclonal bands (OCBs) in the CSF and not the serum can improve overall diagnostic accuracy by increasing specificity and negative predictive value.[221] OCBs are also found in, for example, paraneoplastic disorders and CNS infections. Most of these alternative diagnoses can be excluded on clinical grounds and analysis of the CSF. Oligoclonal bands can have a predictive value, as patients presenting with a clinically isolated syndrome (CIS) and a negative MRI are at very low risk of developing MS if their CSF examination is also normal—less than 5% after a median follow-up of 50 months.[222]

MEDICAL MANAGEMENT

Corticosteroids, oral or intravenous, are used in the acute relapse and have been shown to shorten the duration of relapses, but they do not alter the degree of recovery or the long-term prognosis. In recent years, disease-modifying drugs[223] have been developed so rapidly that the management of MS has become very complex and should, ideally, be done in centres with expertise in this area. Drugs such as interferon-alpha, interferon-beta and glatiramer acetate have all been demonstrated to reduce the relapse rate, but their effect on long-term prognosis is uncertain. Immune suppression with azathioprine, cyclophosphamide, cladribine, methotrexate, IVIG or mitoxantrone is often employed, although the evidence of efficacy is limited.[223] Natalizumab is a selective adhesion-molecule inhibitor and has been shown to reduce the risk of sustained progression and disability, and also the rate of clinical relapse in patients with relapsing–remitting MS.[224] Progressive multifocal leucoencephalopathy occurs in less than 1% of patients and appears to be related to the number of infusions.

There is a delicate balance between efficacy and safety. Serious safety issues, including death, have been identified with many of the newer agents, with potential for increased efficacy. Concerns have been identified for natalizumab, rituximab, alemtuzumab, daclizumab, cladribine and fingolimod.[225]

In more advanced MS with increasing disability, other management issues arise, such as recurrent urinary tract infections or, less often, chest infections, pressure sores, depression, appropriate support resources, family relief and appropriate accommodation.

INTEGRATIVE MANAGEMENT

As the causative factors in MS are so varied, it suggests that there are a number of potential points of intervention therapeutically. These interventions have the potential to not only influence quality of life but also to have an impact upon disease progression and outcome. Unfortunately, many people living with MS are not informed about these possible interventions. A person living with MS will need to make informed choices about which therapies to use (or not use), weighing up current evidence along with the potential for positive and negative side effects of integrative medicine and conventional medical options. The GP, in conjunction with the medical specialist, is ideally placed to help patients to decide on a management strategy, foster healthy lifestyle change and monitor progress.

Smoking

There are many studies linking smoking and passive smoking to MS. Those who begin smoking at an early age have an increased risk of developing progressive MS.[226,227]

Environmental exposure

Although no direct links have been made, there appear to be clusters of MS, in various countries, around lead smelters, oil refineries and environments high in air pollution.[228–231] Iron overload and the up-regulation of iron-binding proteins in the brain have been implicated in the pathogenesis of MS, with MRIs revealing significant and pathological iron deposition.[232,233] Similarly, significantly higher urinary concentrations of aluminium have been documented in individuals with MS. Correspondingly, urinary excretions of silicon, a natural antagonist of aluminium, are lower in MS. Aluminium may therefore be another environmental factor associated with the pathogenesis of MS.[233]

Mind–body medicine

Excessive stress is known to exacerbate the course of neurodegenerative diseases.[234] Individuals with MS have been shown to have hypothalamic–pituitary–adrenal (HPA) axis hyperactivity, and therefore any stress-relieving activity or exercise may be of benefit.[235] A 2006 Cochrane review demonstrated a range of psychological interventions that may potentially help those with MS. In particular, CBT has been shown to assist those with MS and depression.[236] This has been confirmed by an Australian longitudinal assessment study of depression, anxiety and fatigue in patients with MS.[237] Interest in the role of mindfulness-based interventions in MS is also growing because of their stress-relieving and potentially neuroprotective neurogenic effects.

Sleep

Sleep problems are more common in those with MS (especially women) compared with the general population.[238] Identifying and managing sleep disorders is an important part of an MS work-up, as fatigue is such a prevalent symptom of MS[239] and sleep has such a significant effect upon mental health. Restless legs syndrome (RLS) is also significantly associated with MS, particularly in those with severe pyramidal and sensory disabilities.[240] Magnesium may assist with RLS.

Sunshine

MS has always been found to be more common in areas further away from the equator. However, over the past five decades, the latitude gradient has been decreasing.[241] It has been well documented that the prevalence of MS is higher in those living at higher latitudes.[242] This observation has been closely associated with the insufficient vitamin D levels that are frequently found in individuals with MS.[243] Lack of sun exposure has also been associated with an increased risk of developing and relapsing from MS.[244,245] It has been discovered that vitamin D deficiency is endemic throughout many countries in the world, including across a wide latitude in Australia.[246] In Australia, this appears to be partly related to excessive sunlight avoidance and sunscreen use.[247] The emphasis should be on responsible sun exposure, not sun avoidance.

Exercise

Current evidence demonstrates that physical activity in individuals with MS counteracts depression and fatigue, and may improve mobility and quality of life.[248–251] Although it is difficult to prescribe a generalised regular exercise program, activities that encourage 'listening to your body' and 'perceived control over fatigue' are recommended.[252,253] Aerobic activity has been shown to improve early anomalies of posture and gait in MS patients and moderate exercise (acute cycling) has been shown to improve anxiety and other mood disturbances. Exercise therapy has been noted to be beneficial for patients with MS not experiencing a relapse, in a 2005 Cochrane review. Studies of yoga have also shown evidence of some benefit to those with MS.

Dietary modification

Despite some clinical evidence of certain dietary regimens being beneficial for individuals with MS, a 2007 Cochrane review stated that more research is necessary.[254] One such regimen involves caloric restriction (under medical supervision), as this has been shown to induce anti-inflammatory, antioxidant and neuroprotective effects.[255,256]

Increased dietary intake of saturated fatty acids has been associated with increased risk of developing MS.[257] Research on a 34-year prospective cohort study of patients with MS published in the *Lancet*[258] gave very promising findings but received relatively little notice in the wider medical community. Swank and Dugan found that over a 34-year follow-up, only 31% of MS patients adhering to a low saturated fat diet (less than 20 g/day) died, compared with approximately 80% of patients not sticking to the diet. Further, in the group who started with a lower level of disability, only 5% died. The rates of disease progression and disability were also vastly different in the two groups, and when those who died from non-MS-related illnesses were excluded from the analysis, 95% survived and remained physically active.

Diets rich in salmon (3–4 times weekly) may provide some protection against demyelination. This is thought to be due to the high content of both omega-3 essential fatty acids and vitamin D.[259]

There is current controversy regarding the possible adverse effects of artificial sweeteners such as aspartame, saccharin and acesulfame-K (ASK) as contributory factors to the development of MS.[260,261]

There is some evidence that individuals with MS have highly significant IgA and IgG antibodies against gliadin and gluten (wheat), as well as significant antibody increases against casein (cow's milk dairy) compared with controls.[262–264] However, recent studies have shown conflicting data, and therefore no specific dietary recommendations on these dietary factors can be made at this time.[265,266]

Nutritional supplementation

Vitamin D

Evidence associates low levels of vitamin D with increased risk of MS and other immune-mediated disorders.[267–271] As such, it is an important modifiable environmental and nutritional factor that has a potential role in both prevention and treatment of MS.[243,267,272] Studies demonstrate lower levels of serum vitamin D_3 in relapsing–remitting MS compared with progressive MS and controls. Furthermore, lower levels have been significantly associated with MS-related disability in women.[270,273] A meta-analysis has shown that vitamin D supplementation significantly reduces all-cause mortality, and therefore it is very important to identify and promptly treat any evidence of deficiency. Those with MS may need more aggressive treatment so that levels are at least 55–70 ng/mL.[271,274] It is important to note, however, that with increasing knowledge of the significance of vitamin D to health maintenance, these reference ranges are likely to be increased in the future. Long-term supplementation with both vitamin D and cod-liver oil in humans has been associated with a reduced risk of developing MS.

Antioxidants

Antioxidants may potentially benefit those with MS, as reactive oxygen species (ROS) have been demonstrated to play major roles in several events in the pathogenesis of MS.[257–277] As yet, there is limited research on the beneficial effects of antioxidants on humans with MS, although studies on animal models demonstrate beneficial effect of vitamins C and E.[276]

PUFAs

Omega-3 essential fatty acids play a major role in the activity of the nervous system, cognitive development, memory-related learning, neuroplasticity of neural membranes, synaptogenesis and synaptic transformation.[278] The human brain has the highest lipid concentration in the body after adipose tissue, and therefore dysregulated lipid metabolism is of prime importance.[279] Both omega-3 and omega-6 deficiencies as well as high levels of monosaturated and saturated fatty acids have been found in individuals with MS. Conversely, both omega-3 and omega-6 supplementation have been shown to reduce clinical signs of disease.[257,280] There is accumulating evidence that both fatty acids can reduce immune-cell activation and result in marked positive clinical effects by various pathways. They may therefore be indicated for the wellbeing of all individuals with MS.[259,281,282] It should be noted, however, that larger clinical trials, preferably with MRI investigations, are required.

B vitamins and iron

For myelin to be continually regenerated in the human body, adequate iron, folate and vitamin B_{12} to enact methylation pathways are required.[283] Elevated homocysteine levels are common and are associated with cognitive impairment and depression in those with MS.[284,285] In Caucasian females, both serum iron and ferritin have been found to be low compared with controls. A small study of patients with relapsing–remitting MS supplemented with myelination-activating nutrients has shown a significant neurological improvement compared with those simply taking multivitamins.[283]

RESOURCES

American Academy of Neurology, http://www.aan.com

Jelinek G. Overcoming multiple sclerosis. An evidence-based guide to recovery. Sydney: Allen & Unwin; 2010.

Neurology, http://www.neurology.org/

Overcoming multiple sclerosis, http://www.overcomingmultiplesclerosis.org/

Therapeutic Guidelines, Neurology, http://www.tg.org.au/index.php?sectionid=46

REFERENCES

1 Rowland L, ed. Merrill's neurology. 11th edn. New York: Lippincott, Williams & Wilkins; 2005.

2 Gates P. Clinical neurology: a primer. Sydney: Elsevier; 2010. Online slideshare: http://www.slideshare.net/AnnekeElsevier/clinical-neurology-a-primer-by-peter-gates-4433610

3 Rasmussen BK. Migraine and tension-type headache in a general population: psychosocial factors. Int J Epidemiol 1992; 21(6):1138–1143.

4 Lance JW. Headache and face pain. Med J Aust 2000; 172(9):450–455.

5 Kudrow L. Cluster headache. Clinical, mechanistic, and treatment aspects. Panminerva Med 1982; 24(1):45–54.

6 Pryse-Phillips WE, Dodick DW, Edmeads JG et al. Guidelines for the diagnosis and management of migraine in clinical practice. Canadian Headache Society. CMAJ 1997; 156(9):1273–1287.

7 Evers S, Afra J, Frese A et al. EFNS guideline on the drug treatment of migraine—revised report of an EFNS taskforce. European Federation of Neurological Societies. Eur J Neurol 2009; 16(9):968–981.

8 Taubert K. Magnesium in migraine. Results of a multicentre pilot study. Fortschr Med 1994; 112(24):328–330.

9 Peikert A, Wilimzig C, Kohne-Völland R. Prophylaxis of migraine with oral magnesium: results from a prospective multi-center, placebo-controlled and double-blind randomized study. Cephalalgia 1996; 16(4):257–263.

10 Schoenen J. The pathophysiology of migraine: a review based on the literature and on personal contributions. Funct Neurol 1998; 13(1):7–15.

11 Ernst E, Pittler MH. The efficacy and safety of feverfew (*Tanacetum parthenium*): an update of a systematic review. Public Health Nutr 2000; 3(4A):509–514.

12 Tuchin PJ, Pollard H, Bonello R. A randomized controlled trial of chiropractic spinal manipulative therapy for Migraine. J Manipulative Physiol Ther 2000; 23(2):91–95.

13 Biondi DM. Physical treatments for headache: a structured review. Headache 2005; 45(6):738–746.

14 Bronfort G, Assendelft WJ, Evans R et al. Efficacy of spinal manipulation for chronic headache: a systematic review. J Manipulative Physiol Ther 2001; 24(7):457–466.

15 Melchart D, Thormaehlen J, Hager S et al. Acupuncture versus placebo versus sumatriptan for early treatment of migraine attacks: a randomized controlled trial. J Intern Med 2003; 253(2):181–188.

16 Melchart D, Linde K, Fischer P et al. Acupuncture for idiopathic headache. Cochrane Database Syst Rev 2001; 1:CD001218.

17 Endres HG, Diener H-C, Molsberger A. Role of acupuncture in the treatment of migraine. Expert Rev Neurother 2007; 7:1121–1134.

18 Gates P. Clinical neurology: a primer. Sydney: Elsevier; 2010.

19 Jenssen S, Gracely EJ, Sperling MR. How long do most seizures last? A systematic comparison of seizures recorded in the epilepsy monitoring unit. Epilepsia 2006; 47(9):1499–1503.

20 King MA, Newton MR, Jackson GD et al. Epileptology of the first-seizure presentation: a clinical, electroencephalographic and magnetic resonance imaging study of 300 consecutive patients. Lancet 1998; 352(9133):1007–1011.

21 Sofou K, Kristjánsdóttir R, Papachatzakis NE et al. Management of prolonged seizures and status epilepticus in childhood: a systematic review. J Child Neurol 2009; 24(8):918–926.

22 Marson AG, Al-Kharusi AM, Alwaidh M et al. The SANAD study of effectiveness of valproate, lamotrigine, or topiramate for generalised and unclassifiable epilepsy: an unblinded randomised controlled trial. SANAD Study group. Lancet 2007; 369(9566):1016–1026.

23 Aylward RL. Epilepsy: a review of reports, guidelines, recommendations and models for the provision of care for patients with epilepsy. Clin Med 2008; 8(4):433–438.

24 Perucca P, Carter J, Vahle V et al. Adverse antiepileptic drug effects: towards a clinically and neurobiologically relevant taxonomy. Neurology 2009; 72(14):1223–1229.

25 Schachter SC. CAM therapies. Curr Opin Neurol 2008; 21(2):184–189.

26 Ricotti V, Delanty N. Use of CAM in epilepsy. Curr Neurol Neurosci Rep 2006; 6(4):347–353.

27 Gross-Tsur V, Lahad A, Shalev RS. Use of complementary medicine in children with ADHD and epilepsy. Paediatr Neurol 2003; 29(1):53–55.

28 Gaby AR. Natural approaches to epilepsy. Altern Med Rev 2007; 12(1):9–24.

29 Arias AJ, Steinberg K, Banga A et al. Systematic review of the efficacy of meditation techniques as treatments for mental illness. J Altern Complement Med 2006; 12(8):817–832.

30 Lansky EP, St Louis EK. Transcendental meditation: a double-edged sword in epilepsy? Epilepsy Behav 2006; 9(3):394–400.

31 Rocamora R, Sanchez-Alvarez JC, Salas-Puig J. The relationship between sleep and epilepsy. Neurologist 2008; 14(6 Suppl 1):S35–S43.

32 Mendez M, Radtke RA. Interactions between sleep and epilepsy. J Clin Neurophysiol 2001; 18(2):106–127.

33 Kotagal P, Yardi N. The relationship between sleep and epilepsy. Semin Pediatr Neurol 2008; 15(2):42–49.

34 deRoos ST, Chillag KL, Keeler M et al. Effects of sleep deprivation on the paediatric EEG. Pediatrics 2009; 123(2):703–708.

35 Sebit MB, Mielke J. Epilepsy in sub-Saharan Africa: its socio-demography, aetilogy, diagnosis and EEG characteristics in Harare, Zimbabwe. East Afr Med J 2005; 82(3):128–137.

36 Kwan P, Yu E, Leung H et al. Association of subjective anxiety, depression and sleep disturbance with quality-of-life ratings in adults with epilepsy. Epilepsia 2009; 15(2):196–201.

37 Weinstein RS, Bryce GF, Sappington LJ et al. Decreased serum ionised calcium and normal vitamin D metabolite levels with anticonvulsant drug treatment. J Clin Endocrin Metab 1984; 58(6):1003–1009.

38 Williams C, Netzloff M, Folkerts L et al. Vitamin D metabolism and anticonvulsant therapy: effect of sunshine on incidence of osteomalacia. South Med J 1984; 77(7):834–836, 842.

39 Nakken KO. Should people with epilepsy exercise? Tidsskr Nor Laegeforen 2000; 120(25):3051–3053.

40 Howard GM, Radloff M, Sevier TL. Epilepsy and sports participation. Curr Sports Med Rep 2004; 3(1):15–19.

41 Arida RM, Cavalheiro EA, da Silva AC et al. Physical activity and epilepsy: proven and predicted benefits. Sports Med 2008; 38(7):607–615.

42 Lundgren T, Dahl J, Yardi N et al. Acceptance and commitment therapy and yoga for drug-refractory epilepsy: a randomised controlled trial. Epilepsy Behav 2008; 13(1):102–108.

43 Sathyaprabha TN, Satishchandra P, Pradhan C et al. Modulation of cardiac autonomic balance with adjuvant yoga therapy in patients with refractory epilepsy. Epilepsy Behav 2008; 12(2):245–252.

44 Mortelmans LJ, van Loo M, de Cauwer HG et al. Seizures and hyponatremia after excessive intake of diet coke. Eur J Emerg Med 2008; 15(1):51.

45 Iyadurai SJ, Chung SS. New-onset seizures in adults: possible association with consumption of popular energy drinks. Epilepsy Behav 2007; 10(3):504–508.

46 Volpe SL, Schall JI, Gallagher PR et al. Nutrient intake of children with intractable epilepsy compared with healthy children. J Am Diet Assoc 2007; 107(6):1014–1018.

47 Kossoff EH, Rho JM. Ketogenic diets: evidence for short- and long-term efficacy. Neurotherapeutics 2009; 6(2):406–414.

48 Weinshenker D. The contribution of noradrenaline and orexigenic neuropeptides to the anticonvulsant effect of the ketogenic diet. Epilepsia 2008; 49(Suppl 8):104–107.

49 Nordli Jr DR. The ketogenic diet, four score and seven years later. Nat Clin Pract Neurol 2009; 5(1):12–13.

50 Porta N, Vallee L, Boutry E et al. Comparison of seizure reduction and serum folic acid levels after receiving the ketogenic and modified Atkins diet. Seizure 2009; 18(5):359–364.

51 Kozak N, Csiba L. Dietary aspects of epilepsy. Ideggyogy Sz 2007; 60(5/6):234–238.
52 Villeneuve N, Pinton F, Bahi-Buisson N et al. The ketogenic diet improves recently worsened focal epilepsy. Dev Med Child Neurol 2009; 51(4):276–281.
53 Hartman AL. Does the effectiveness of the ketogenic diet in different epilepsies yield insights into its mechanisms? Epilepsia 2008; 49(Suppl 8):53–56.
54 Kossoff EH, Dorward JL. The Modified Atkins Diet. Epilepsia 2008; 49(Suppl 8):37–41.
55 Muzykewicz DA, Lyczkowski DA, Memon N et al. Efficacy, safety and tolerability of the low glycaemic index diet in paediatric epilepsy. Epilepsia 2009; 50(5):1118–1126.
56 Farman AH, Lossius MI, Nakken KO. Polyunsaturated fatty acids and epilepsy. Tidsskr Nor Laegeforen 2009; 129(1):26–28.
57 Xu XP, Erichsen D, Börjesson SI et al. Polyunsaturated fatty acids and cerebrospinal fluid from children on the ketogenic diet open a voltage-gated potassium channel: a putative mechanism of antiseizure action. Epilepsy Res 2008; 80(1):57–66.
58 Ferrari D, Cysneiros RM, Scorza CA et al. Neuroprotective activity of n-3 fatty acids against epilepsy-induced hippocampal damage: quantification with immunohistochemical for calcium-binding proteins. Epilepsy Behav 2008; 13(1):36–42.
59 Taha AY, Huot PS, Reza-Lopez S et al. Seizure resistance in fat-1 transgenic mice endogenously synthesising high levels of n-3 polyunsaturated fatty acids. J Neurochem 2008; 105(2):380–388.
60 Pifferi F, Tremblay S, Plourde M et al. Ketones and brain function: possible link to polyunsaturated fatty acids and availability of a new brain PET tracer, 11C-acetoacetate. Epilepsia 2008; 49(Suppl 8):76–79.
61 Bromfield E, Dworetsky B, Hurwitz S et al. A randomised trial of polyunsaturated fatty acids for refractory epilepsy. Epilepsy Behav 2008; 12(1):187–190.
62 Mainardi P, Leonardi A, Albano C. Potentiation of brain serotonin activity may exhibit seizures, especially in drug-resistant epilepsy. Med Hypotheses 2008; 70(4):876–879.
63 Bagdy G, Kecskemeti V, Riba P et al. Serotonin and epilepsy. J Neurochem 2007; 100(4):857–873.
64 Isaac M. Serotonergic 5-HT2C receptors as a potential therapeutic target for the design of antiepileptic drugs. Curr Top Med Chem 2005; 5(1):59–67.
65 El Idrissi A, L'Amoreaux WJ. Selective resistance of taurine-fed mice to isoniazide-potentiated seizures: in vivo functional test for the activity of glutamic acid decarboxylase. Neuroscience 2008; 156(3):693–699.
66 Galanopoulou AS. GABAA receptors in normal development and seizures: friends or foes? Curr Neuropharmacol 2008; 6(1):1–20.
67 Thompson K.Transplantation of GABA-producing cells for seizure control in models of temporal lobe epilepsy. Neurotherapeutics 2009; 6(2):284–294.
68 Baran H. Alterations of taurine in the brain of chronic kainic acid epilepsy model. Amino Acids 2006; 31(3):303–307.
69 Junyent F, Utrera J, Romera R et al. Prevention of epilepsy by taurine treatments in mice experimental model. J Neurosci Res 2009; 87(6):1500–1508.
70 Trombley PQ, Horning MS, Blakemore LJ. Carnosine modulates zinc and copper effects on amino acid receptors and synaptic transmission. Neuroreport 1998; 9(15):3503–3507.
71 Trombley PQ, Horning MS, Blakemore LJ. Interactions between carnosine and zinc and copper: implications for neuromodulation and neuroprotection. Biochemistry (Mosc) 2000; 65(7):807–816.
72 Horning MS, Blakemore LJ, Trombley PQ. Endogenous mechanisms of neuroprotection: role of zinc, copper and carnosine. Brain Res 2000;852(1):56-61.
73 Kozan R, Sefil F, Bagirici F. Anticonvulsant effect of carnosine on penicillin-induced epileptiform activity in rats. Brain Res 2008; 1239:249–255.
74 Devi PU, Manocha A, Vohora D. Seizures, antiepileptics, antioxidants and ox stress: an insight for researchers. Expert Opin Pharmacother 2008; 9(18):3169–3177.
75 Hayashi M. Oxidative stress in developmental brain disorders. Neuropathology 2009; 29(1):1–8.
76 Gupta RC, Milatovic D, Dettbarn WD. Depletion of energy metabolites following acetylcholinesterase inhibitor-induced status epilepticus: protection by antioxidants. Neurotoxicogy 2001; 22(2):271–282.
77 Ranganathan LN, Ramaratnam S. Vitamins for epilepsy. Cochrane Database Syst Rev 2005; 2:CD004304.
78 Kutluhan S, Naziroglu M, Celik O et al. Effects of selenium and topiramate on lipid peroxidation and antioxidant vitamin levels in blood of PTZ-induced epileptic rats. Biol Trace Elem Res 2009; 129:181–189.
79 Gutierrez-Alvarez AM, Moreno CB, Gonzalez-Reyes RE. Changes in selenium levels in epilepsy. Rev Neurol 2005; 40(2):111–116.
80 Moreno CB, Gutierrez-Alvarez AM, Gonzalez-Reyes RE. Zinc and epilepsy: is there a causal relation between them? Rev Neurol 2008; 42(12):754–759.
81 Dominguez MI, Blasco-Ibanez JM, Crespo C et al. Neural overexcitation and implications of NMDA and AMPA receptors in a mouse model of temporal lobe epilepsy implying zinc chelation. Epilepsia 2006; 47(5):887–899.
82 Hamed SA, Nabeshima T. The high atherosclerotic risk among epileptics: the atheroprotective role of multivitamins. J Pharmacol Sci 2005; 98(4):340–353.

83 Gonzalez-Reyes RE, Gutierrez-Alvarez AM, Moreno CB. Manganese and epilepsy: a systematic review of the literature. Brain Res Rev 2007; 53(2):332–336.
84 Schacter SC. Botanics and herbs: a traditional approach to treating epilepsy. Neurotherapeutics 2009; 6(2):415–420.
85 Samuels N, Finkelstein Y, Singer SR et al. Herbal medicine and epilepsy: proconvulsive effects and interactions with antiepileptic drugs. Epilepsia 2008; 49(3):373–380.
86 Huen MS, Leung JW, Ng W et al. 5,7-dihydroxy-6-methoxyflavone, a benzodiazepine site ligand isolated from *Scutellaria baicalensis* Georgi, with selective antagonistic properties. Biochem Pharmacol 2003; 66(1):125–132.
87 Salah SM, Jager AK. Screening of traditionally used Lebanese herbs for neurological activities. J Ethnopharmacol 2005; 97(1):145–149.
88 Harms SL, Garrard J, Schwinghammer P et al. *Gingko biloba* use in nursing home elderly with epilepsy or seizure disorder. Epilepsia 2006; 47(2):323–329.
89 Jyoti A, Sethi P, Sharma D. Curcumin protects against electrobehavioural progression of seizures in the iron-induced experimental model of epileptogenesis. Epilepsy Behav 2009; 14(2):300–308.
90 Sumanont Y, Murakami Y, Tohda M. Effects of manganese complexes of curcumin and diacetylcurcumin on kainic acid-induced neurotoxic responses in the rat hippocampus. Biol Pharm Bull 2007; 30(9):1732–1739.
91 Hung-Ming W, Liu CS, Tsai JJ et al. Antioxidant and anti-convulsant effect of a modified formula of chaihu-longu-muli-tang. Am J Chin Med 2002; 30(2/3):339–346.
92 Minami E, Shibata H, Nomoto M et al. Effect of shitei-to, a traditional Chinese medicine formulation, on pentylenetetrazol-induced kindling in mice. Phytomedicine 2000; 7(1):69–72.
93 Cheuk DK, Wong V. Acupuncture for epilepsy. Cochrane Database Syst Rev 2008; 4:CD005062.
94 Denays R, Kumba C, Lison D et al. First epileptic seizure induced by occupational nickel poisoning. Epilepsia 2005; 46(6):961–962.
95 Arrieta O, Palencia G, Garcia-Arenas G et al. Prolonged exposure to lead lowers the threshold of pentylenetetrazole-induced seizures in rats. Epilepsia 2005; 46(10):1599–1602.
96 Ruegg S, Hunziker P, Marsch S et al. Association of environmental factors with the onset of status epilepticus. Epilepsy Behav 2008; 12(1):66–73.
97 Grogan PM, Gronseth GS. Practice parameter: steroids, acyclovir, and surgery for Bell's palsy (an evidence-based review): report of the Quality Standards Subcommittee of the American Academy of Neurology. Neurology 2001; 56(7):830–836.
98 Salinas RA, Alvarez G, Ferreira J. Corticosteroids for Bell's palsy (idiopathic facial paralysis). Cochrane Database Syst Rev 2009; 2:CD001942.
99 Sullivan FM, Swan IR, Donnan PT et al. A randomised controlled trial of the use of aciclovir and/or prednisolone for the early treatment of Bell's palsy: the BELLS study. Health Technol Assess 2009; 13(47):iii–iv, ix–xi, 1–130.
100 Lehmann HC, Hartung HP, Hetzel GR et al. Plasma exchange in neuroimmunological disorders: part 2. Treatment of neuromuscular disorders. Arch Neurol 2006; 63(8):1066–1071.
101 Lehmann HC, Hartung HP, Hetzel GR et al. Plasma exchange in neuroimmunological disorders: part 1. Rationale and treatment of inflammatory central nervous system disorders. Arch Neurol 2006; 63(7):930–935.
102 Elovaara I, Apostolski S, van Doorn P et al. EFNS guidelines for the use of intravenous immunoglobulin in treatment of neurological diseases: EFNS task force on the use of intravenous immunoglobulin in treatment of neurological diseases. Eur J Neurol 2008; 15(9):893–908.
103 Hughes RA, Raphaël JC, Swan AV et al. Intravenous immunoglobulin for Guillain-Barré syndrome. Cochrane Database Syst Rev 2006; 1:CD002063.
104 Talman P, Forbes A, Mathers S. Clinical phenotypes and natural progression for motor neuron disease: analysis from an Australian database. Amyotroph Lateral Scler 2009; 10(2):79–84.
105 Benatar M, Kaminski H. Medical and surgical treatment for ocular myasthenia. Cochrane Database Syst Rev 2006; 2:CD005081.
106 Sethi KD, Rivner MH, Swift TR. Ice pack test for myasthenia gravis. Neurology 1987; 37(8):1383–1385.
107 Ferreira VF, da Rocha DR, Lima Araújo KG. Advances in drug discovery to assess cholinergic neurotransmission: a systematic review. Curr Drug Discov Technol 2008; 5(3):236–249.
108 Sonett JR, Jaretzki A III. Thymectomy for nonthymomatous myasthenia gravis: a critical analysis. Ann NY Acad Sci 2008; 1132:315–328.
109 Kondo KJ. Optimal therapy for thymoma. Med Invest 2008; 55(1/2):17–28.
110 Chavis PS, Stickler DE, Walker A. Immunosuppressive or surgical treatment for ocular myasthenia gravis. Arch Neurol 2007; 64(12):1792–1794.
111 Hart IK, Sathasivam S, Sharshar T. Immunosuppressive agents for myasthenia gravis. Cochrane Database Syst Rev 2007; 4:CD005224.
112 Wiendl H. Idiopathic inflammatory myopathies: current and future therapeutic options. Neurotherapeutics 2008; 5(4):548–557.
113 Marshall S, Tardif G, Ashworth N. Local corticosteroid injection for carpal tunnel syndrome. Cochrane Database Syst Rev 2007; 2:CD001554.

114 Gautschi OP, Land M, Hoederath P et al. Carpal tunnel syndrome—modern diagnostic and management. Praxis (Bern 1994) 2010; 99(3):163–173.
115 Cikes N, Bosnic D, Sentic M. Non-MS autoimmune demyelination. Clin Neurol Neurosurg 2008; 110(9):905–912.
116 Goldstein LB, Adams R, Alberts MJ et al; American Heart Association; American Stroke Association Stroke Council. Primary prevention of ischemic stroke: a guideline from the American Heart Association/American Stroke Association Stroke Council: cosponsored by the Atherosclerotic Peripheral Vascular Disease Interdisciplinary Working Group; Cardiovascular Nursing Council; Clinical Cardiology Council; Nutrition, Physical Activity, and Metabolism Council; and the Quality of Care and Outcomes Research Interdisciplinary Working Group. Circulation 2006; 113(24):e873–e923.
117 Jackson G. Secondary prevention of stroke: PROGRESS and the evidence for blood pressure reduction. Int J Clin Pract 2001; 55(10):655.
118 Gage BF, Fihn SD, White RH. Warfarin therapy for an octogenarian who has atrial fibrillation. Ann Intern Med 2001; 134(6):465–474.
119 Go AS, Hylek EM, Chang Y et al. Anticoagulation therapy for stroke prevention in atrial fibrillation: how well do randomized trials translate into clinical practice? JAMA 2003; 290(20):2685–2692.
120 MacDougall NJ, Amarasinghe S, Muir KW. Secondary prevention of stroke. Expert Rev Cardiovasc Ther 2009; 7(9):1103–1115.
121 Chandratheva A, Mehta Z, Geraghty OC et al; Oxford Vascular Study. Population-based study of risk and predictors of stroke in the first few hours after a TIA. Neurology 2009; 72(22):1941–1947.
122 Kucinski T, Väterlein O, Glauche V et al. Correlation of apparent diffusion coefficient and computed tomography density in acute ischemic stroke. Stroke 2002; 33(7):1786–1791.
123 Vivanco Hidalgo RM, Rodríguez Campello A, Ois Santiago A et al. Cardiac monitoring in stroke units: importance of diagnosing atrial fibrillation in acute ischemic stroke. Rev Esp Cardiol 2009; 62(5):564–567. [Article in English, Spanish]
124 Ansara AJ, Nisly SA, Arif SA et al. Aspirin dosing for the prevention and treatment of ischemic stroke: an indication-specific review of the literature. Ann Pharmacother 2010; 44(5):851–862.
125 Hacke W, Kaste M, Bluhmki E et al; ECASS Investigators. Thrombolysis with alteplase 3 to 4.5 hours after acute ischemic stroke. N Engl J Med 2008; 359(13):1317–1329.
126 Diener HC. Secondary prevention of ischaemic stroke and TIA. Cardiovasc J Afr 2008; 19(4):229.
127 Simmons BB, Yeo A, Fung K; American Heart Association; American Stroke Association. Current guidelines on antiplatelet agents for secondary prevention of noncardiogenic stroke: an evidence-based review. Postgrad Med 2010; 122(2):49–53.
128 Odén A, Fahlén M, Hart RG. Optimal INR for prevention of stroke and death in atrial fibrillation: a critical appraisal. Throm Res 2006; 117(5):493–499.
129 Saour N, Sieck JO, Mamo LA et al. Trial of different intensities of anticoagulation in patients with prosthetic heart valves. N Engl J Med 1990; 322(7):428–432.
130 Connolly SJ, Ezekowitz MD, Yusuf S et al; RE-LY Steering Committee and Investigators. Dabigatran versus warfarin in patients with atrial fibrillation. N Engl J Med 2009; 361(12):1139–1151.
131 Bakoyiannis C, Economopoulos KP, Georgopoulos S et al. Carotid endarterectomy versus carotid angioplasty with or without stenting for treatment of carotid artery stenosis: an updated meta-analysis of randomized controlled trials. E Int Angiol 2010; 29(3):205–215.
132 Donnan GA, O'Malley HM, Quang L et al. The capsular warning syndrome: pathogenesis and clinical. Neurology 1993; 43(5):957–962.
133 Meier P, Knapp G, Tamhane U et al. Short-term and intermediate-term comparison of endarterectomy versus stenting for carotid artery stenosis: systematic review and meta-analysis of randomised controlled clinical trials. BMJ 2010; 340:c467.
134 Zesiewicz TA, Elble R, Louis ED et al. Practice parameter: therapies for essential tremor: report of the Quality Standards Subcommittee of the American Academy of Neurology. 2005; 64(12):2008–2020.
135 Slavin MJ, Phillips JG, Bradshaw JL et al. Consistency of handwriting movements in dementia of the Alzheimer's type: a comparison with Huntington's and Parkinson's diseases. J Int Neuropsychol Soc 1999; 5(1):20–25.
136 Margolese HC, Chouinard G, Kolivakis TT et al. Tardive dyskinesia in the era of typical and atypical antipsychotics. Part 2: Incidence and management strategies in patients with schizophrenia. Can J Psychiatry 2005; 50(11):703–714.
137 Sharma N, Standaert DG. Inherited movement disorders. Neurol Clin 2002; 20(3):759–778, vii.
138 Gordon N. Sydenham's chorea, and its complications affecting the nervous system. Brain Dev 2009; 31(1):11–14.
139 Miyasaki JM, Martin W, Suchowersky O et al. Practice parameter: initiation of treatment for Parkinson's disease: an evidence-based review: report of the Quality Standards Subcommittee of the American Academy of Neurology. Neurology 2002; 58(1):11–17.
140 Alvarez L, Macias R, Pavón N et al. Therapeutic efficacy of unilateral subthalamotomy in Parkinson's disease:

results in 89 patients followed for up to 36 months. Neurol Neurosurg Psychiatry 2009; 80(9):979–985.

141 Deuschl G, Schade-Brittinger C, Krack P et al. A randomized trial of deep-brain stimulation for Parkinson's disease. German Parkinson Study Group, Neurostimulation Section. N Engl J Med 2006; 355(9):896–908.

142 Guzeva VI, Chukhlovina ML, Chuklovin BA. Environmental factors and Parkinsonian syndrome. Gig Sanit 2008; 2:60–62.

143 Luccini R, Albini E, Benedetti L et al. Neurological and neuropsychological features in Parkinson's disease patients exposed to neurotoxic metals. G Ital Med Lav Ergon 2007; 29(3 Suppl):280–281.

144 Zoni S, Albini E, Luccini R. Neuropsychological testing for the assessment of manganese neurotoxicity: a review and a proposal. Am J Ind Med 2007; 50(11): 812–830.

145 Yokel RA. Blood–brain barrier flux of aluminium, manganese, iron and other metals suspected to contribute to metal-induced neurodegeneration. J Alzheimers Dis 2006; 10(2/3):223–253.

146 Gorell JM, Johnson CC, Rybicki BA et al. Occupational exposure to manganese, copper, lead, iron, mercury and zinc and the risk of Parkinson's disease. Neurotoxicology 1999; 20(2/3):239–247.

147 Coon S, Stark A, Peterson E et al. Whole-body lifetime occupational lead exposure and risk of Parkinson's disease. Environ Health Perpect 2006; 114(12):1872–1876.

148 Barnham KJ, Bush AI. Metals in Alzheimer's and Parkinson's disease. Curr Opin Chem Biol 2008; 12(2):222–228.

149 Squitti R, Gorgone G, Binetti G et al. Metals and oxidative stress in Parkinson's disease from industrial areas with exposition to environmental toxins or metal pollution. G Ital Med Lav Ergon 2007; 29(3 Suppl):294–296.

150 Dhillon AS, Tarbutton GL, Levin JL et al. Pesticide/environmental exposures and Parkinson's disease in East Texas. J Agromedicine 2008; 13(1):37–48.

151 Hancock DB, Martin ER, Mayhew GM et al. Pesticide exposure and risk of Parkinson's disease: a family-based case-control study. BMC Neurol 2008; 8:6.

152 Brown TP, Rumsby PC, Capleton AC et al. Pesticides and Parkinson's disease—is there a link? Environ Health Perspect 2006; 114(2):156–164.

153 Li AA, Mink PJ, McIntosh LJ et al. Evaluation of epidemiologic and animal data associating pesticides with Parkinson's disease. J Occup Environ Med 2005; 47(10):1059–1087.

154 Bjorling-Poulson M, Anderson HR, Grandjean P. Potential developmental neurotoxicity of pesticides in Europe. Environ Health 2008; 7:50.

155 Keifer MC, Firestone J. Neurotoxicity of pesticides 2007; 12(1):17–25.

156 Dick FD, De Palma G, Ahmadi A et al. Environmental risk factors for Parkinson's disease and parkinsonism: the Geoparkinson study. Occup Environ Med 2007; 64(10):666–672.

157 Costello S, Cockburn M, Bronstein J et al. Parkinson's disease and residential exposure to maneb and paraquat from agricultural applications in the central valley of Caifornia. Am J Epidemiol 2009; 169(8):919–926.

158 Barlow BK, Cory-Slechta DA, Richfield EK et al. The gestational environment and Parkinson's disease: evidence for neurodevelopmental origins of a neurodegenerative disorder. Reprod Toxicol 2007; 23(3):457–470.

159 Costa LG, Giordano G, Guizzetti M et al. Neurotoxicity of pesticides: a review. Front Biosci 2008; 13:1240–1249.

160 Dixon L, Duncan D, Johnson P et al. Occupational therapy for patients with Parkinson's disease. Cochrane Database Syst Rev 2007; 3:CD002813.

161 Deane KH, Jones D, Playford ED et al. Physiotherapy for patients with Parkinson's disease: a comparison of techniques. Cochrane Database Syst Rev 2001; 3:CD002817.

162 Deane KH, Whurr R, Playford ED et al. A comparison of speech and language therapy techniques for dysarthria in Parkinson's disease. Cochrane Database Syst Rev 2001; 2:CD002814.

163 Goodwin VA, Richards SH, Taylor RS et al. The effectiveness of exercise interventions for people with Parkinson's disease: systematic review and meta-analysis. Mov Disord 2008; 23(5):631–640.

164 Keus SH, Bloem BR, Hendriks EJ et al. Evidence-based analysis of physical therapy in Parkinson's disease with recommendations for practice and research. Mov Disord 2007; 22(4):451–460.

165 Crizzle AM, Newhouse IJ. Is physical exercise beneficial for persons with Parkinson's disease? Clin J Sport Med 2006; 16(5):422–425.

166 Kwakkel G, de Goede CJ, van Wegen EE. Impact of physical therapy for Parkinson's disease: a critical review of the literature. Parkinsonism Relat Disord 2007; 13 (Suppl 3):S478–S487.

167 Hackney ME, Kantorovich S, Levin R et al. Effects of tango on functional mobility in Parkinson's disease: a preliminary study. J Neurol Phys Ther 2007; 31(4): 173–179.

168 Burini D, Farabollini B, Iacucci S et al. A randomised controlled cross-over trial of aerobic training versus Qigong in advanced Parkinson's disease. Eura Medicophys 2006; 42(3):231–238.

169 Lee MS, Shin BC, Kong JC et al. Effectiveness of acupuncture for Parkinson's disease: a systematic review. Mov Disord 2008; 23(11):1505–1515.

170 Cheng XR, Cheng K. Survey of studies on the mechanism of acupuncture and moxibustion treating diseases abroad. Zhongguo Zhen Jiu 2008; 28(6):463–467.

171 Cristan A, Katz M, Cutrone E et al. Evaluation of acupuncture in the treatment of Parkinson's disease: a double-blind pilot study. Mov Disord 2005; 20(9): 1185–1188.

172 Wang X, Liang XB, Li FQ et al. Therapeutic strategies for Parkinson's disease: the ancient meets the future—traditional Chinese medicine, electroacupuncture, gene therapy and stem cells. Neurochem Res 2008; 33(10):1956–1963.

173 Huang Y, Jiang XM, Li DJ. Effects of ESA on cerebral dopamine transporter in patients with Parkinson's disease. Zhongguo Zhong Xi Yi Jie He Za Zhi 2006; 26(4):303–307.

174 Chang XH, Zhang LZ, Li YJ. Observation on therapeutic effect of acupuncture combined with medicine on Parkinson's disease. Zhongguo Zhen Jiu 2008; 28(9):645–647.

175 Ren XM. Fifty cases of Parkinson's disease treated by acupuncture combined with Madopar. J Trad Chin Med 2008; 28(4):255–277.

176 Manyam BV, Sanchez-Ramos JR. Traditional and complementary therapies in Parkinson's disease. Adv Neurol 1999; 80:565–574.

177 Nader T, Rothenberg S, Averbach R et al. Improvements in chronic diseases with a comprehensive natural medicine approach: a review and case series. Behav Med 2000; 26(1):14–46.

178 Manyam BV, Dhanasekaran M, Hare TA. Effect of antiparkinson drug HP-200 (*Mucuna pruriens*) on the central monoaminergic neurotransmitters. Phytother Res 2004; 18(2):97–101.

179 Manyam BV, Dhanasekaran M, Hare TA. Neuroprotective effects of the anti-parkinson drug *Mucuna puriens*. Phytother Res 2004;18(9): 706–712.

180 Dhanasekaran M, Tharakan B, Manyam BV. Antiparkinson drug *Mucuna puriens* shows antioxidant and metal chelating activity. Phytother Res 2008; 22(1):6–11.

181 Li Q, Zhao D, Bezard E. TCM for Parkinson's disease: a review of Chinese literature. Behav Pharmacol 2006;17(5-6):403–410.

182 Takeda A. Essential trace metals and brain function. Yakugaku Zasshi 2004; 124(9):577–585.

183 Qureshi GA, Qureshi AA, Memon SA et al. Impact of selenium, copper and zinc in on/off Parkinson's disease patients on L-dopa therapy. J Neural Transm Suppl 2006; 71:229–236.

184 Hargreaves IP, Lane A, Sleiman PM. The coenzyme Q10 status of the brain regions of Parkinson's disease patients. Neurosci Lett 2008; 447(1):17–19.

185 Henchcliffe C, Beal MF. Mitochondrial biology and ox stress in Parkinson's disease pathogenesis. Nat Clin Pract Neurol 2008; 4(11):600–609.

186 Etminan M, Gill SS, Samii A. Intake of vitamin E, C and carotenoids and the risk of Parkinson's disease: a meta-analysis. Lancet Neurol 2005; 4(6):362–365.

187 de Lau LM, Koudstaal PJ, Witteman JC et al. Dietary folate, vitamin B_{12} and vitamin B_6 and the risk of Parkinson's disease. Neurology 2006; 67(2):315–318.

188 Triantafyllou NI, Nikolau C, Boufidou F et al. Folate and vitamin B_{12} levels in L-dopa treated Parkinson's disease patients: their relationship to clinical manifestations, mood and cognition. Parkinsonism Relat Disord 2008; 14(4):321–325.

189 Lamberti P, Zoccolella S, Armenise E et al. Hyperhomocysteinaemia in L-dopa treated Parkinson's disease patients: effect of cobalamin and folate administration. Eur J Neurol 2005; 12(5):365–368.

190 Evatt ML, Delong MR, Khazai N et al. Prevalence of vitamin D deficiency in patients with Parkinson's disease and Alzheimers. Arch Neurol 2008; 65(10):1348–1352.

191 Sanchez B, Relova JL, Gallego R et al. 1,25-dihydroxyvitamin D_3 administration to 6-hydroxydopamine-lesioned rats increases glial cell line-derived neurotrophic factor and partially restores tyrosine hydroxylase expression in substantia nigra and striatum. J Neurosci Res 2009; 87(3): 723–732.

192 Valastro B, Dekundy A, Danysz W et al. Oral creatine supplementation attenuates L-dopa induced dyskinesia in 6-hydroxydopamine lesioned rats. Behav Brain Res 2009; 197(1):90–96.

193 Forsleff L, Schauss AG, Bier ID et al. Evidence of functional zinc deficiency in Parkinson's disease. J Altern Comp Med 1999; 5(1):57–64.

194 Desai V, Kaler SG. Role of copper in human neurological disorders. Am J Clin Nutr 2008; 88(3):855S–858S.

195 Oyanagi K, Kawakami E, Kikuchi-Horie K et al. Magnesium deficiency over generations in rats with special references to the pathogenesis of the P-dementia complex and amyotrophic lateral sclerosis of Guam. Neuropathology 2006; 26(2):115–128.

196 Hashimoto T, Nishi K, Nagasao J et al. Magnesium exerts both preventative and ameliorating effects in an in vivo rat Parkinson's disease model involving 1-methyl-4-phenylpyridium (MPP^+) toxicity in dopaminergic neurons. Brain Res 2008; 1197:143–151.

197 Gao X, Chen H, Fung TT et al. Prospective study of dietary pattern and risk of Parkinson's disease. Am J Clin Nutr 2007; 86(5):1486–1494.

198 de Luis Roman D, Aller R, Castano O. Vegetarian diets: effects on health. Rev Clin Esp 2007; 207(3):141–143.

199 Lau FC, Shukitt-Hale B, Joseph JA. Nutritional intervention in brain aging: reducing the effects of inflammation and oxidative stress. Subcell Biochem 2007; 42:299–318.
200 Barichella M, Savardi C, Mauri A et al. Diet with LPP for renal patients increases daily energy expenditure and improves motor function in parkinsonian patients with motor fluctuations. Nutr Neurosci 2007; 10(3/4):129–135.
201 Gasior M, Rogawski MA, Hartman AL. Neuroprotective and disease-modifing effects of the ketogenic diet. Behav Pharmacol 2006; 17(5-6):431–439.
202 Ma L, Zhang L, Gao XH et al. Dietary factors and smoking as risk factors for Parkinson's disease in a rural population in China: a nested case-control study. Acta Neurol Scand 2006; 113(4):278–281.
203 Chen H, O'Reilly E, McCullough ML et al. Consumption of dairy products and risk of Parkinson's disease. Am J Epidemiol 2007; 165(9):998–1006.
204 Tan LC, Koh WP, Yuan JM et al. Differential effects of black vs green tea on risk of Parkinson's disease in the Singapore Chinese Health Study. Am J Epidemiol 2008; 167(5):553–560.
205 Petersen MS, Halling J, Bech S et al. Impact of dietary exposure to food contaminants on the risk of Parkinson's disease. NeuroToxicology 2008; 29(4):584–590.
206 Dobkin RD, Menza M, Bienfait KL. CBT for the treatment of depression in Parkinson's disease: a promising nonpharmacological approach. Expert Rev Neurother 2008; 8(1):27–35.
207 Cole K, Vaughan FL. The feasibility of using CBT for depression associated with Parkinson's disease: a literature review. Parkinsonism Relat Disord 2005; 11(5):269–276.
208 Ernst E, Canter PH. The Alexander technique: a systematic review of controlled clinical trials. Forsch Komplementarmed Klass Nuturheilkd 2003; 10(6):325–329.
209 Paccetti C, Mancini F, Agliera R et al. Active music therapy in Parkinson's disease: an integrative method for motor and emotional rehabilitation. Psychosom Med 2000; 62(3):386–393.
210 Paccetti C, Aglieri R, Mancini F et al. Active music therapy and Parkinson's disease: methods. Funct Neurol 1998; 13(1):57–67.
211 Marrie RA. When one and one make three: HLA and EBV infection in MS. Neurology 2008; 70(13 part 2):1067–1068.
212 Levin LI, Munger KL, Rubertone MV et al. Temporal relationship between elevation of EBV antibody titres and initial onset of neurological symptoms in MS. JAMA 2005; 293(20):2496–2500.
213 Frykholm B. On the question of infectious aetiologies for MS, schizophrenia and chronic fatigue syndrome and their treatment with antibiotics. Med Hypotheses 2009; 72(6):736–739.
214 Ascherio A, Munger K. Epidemiology of MS: from risk factors to prevention. Semin Neurol 2008; 28(1):17–28.
215 Fujihara K. Update on the aetiology and pathogenesis of MS and neuromyelitis optica. Nippon Rinsho 2008; 66(6):1087–1091.
216 Holmey T, Hestvik AL. MS: immunopathogenesis and controversies in defining the cause. Curr Opin Infect Dis 2008; 21(3):271–278.
217 Pugliatti M, Harbo HF, Holmey T et al. Environmental risk factors in MS. Acta Neurol Scand Suppl 2008; 188:34–40.
218 Giovannoni G, Ebers G. MS: the environment and causation. Curr Opin Neurol 2007; 20(3):261–268.
219 Polman CH, Reingold SC, Edan G et al. Diagnostic criteria for multiple sclerosis: 2005 revisions to the 'McDonald Criteria'. Ann Neurol 2005; 58(6):840–846.
220 Chiappa KH. Use of evoked potentials for diagnosis of multiple sclerosis. Neurol Clin. 1988; 6(4):861–880.
221 Zipoli V, Hakiki B, Portaccio E et al. The contribution of cerebrospinal fluid oligoclonal bands to the early diagnosis of multiple sclerosis. Mult Scler 2009; 15(4):472–478.
222 Tintoré M, Sastre-Garriga JJ. New treatment measurements for treatment effects on relapses and progression. Neurol Sci 2008; 274(1/2):80–83.
223 Goodin DS, Frohman EM, Garmany GP Jr et al. Disease-modifying therapies in multiple sclerosis: report of the Therapeutics and Technology Assessment Subcommittee of the American Academy of Neurology and the MS Council for Clinical Practice Guidelines. Neurology 2002; 58(2):169–178.
224 Gold R, Jawad A, Miller DH et al. Expert opinion: guidelines for the use of natalizumab in multiple sclerosis patients previously treated with immunomodulating therapies. J Neuroimmunol 2007; 187(1/2):156–158.
225 Klawiter EC, Cross AH, Naismith RT. The present efficacy of multiple sclerosis therapeutics: is the new 66% just the old 33%? Neurology 2009; 73(12):984–990.
226 Di Pauli F, Reindl M, Ehling R et al. Smoking is a risk factor for early conversion to clinically definite MS. Mult Scler 2008; 14(8):1026–1030.
227 Pittas F, Ponsonby AL, van der Mei IA et al. Smoking is associated with progressive disease course and increased progression in clinical disability in a prospective cohort of people with MS. J Neurol 2009; 256(4):577–585.
228 Williamson DM. Studies of multiple sclerosis in communities concerned about environmental exposures. J Womens Health 2006; 15(7):810–814.
229 Henry JP, Williamson DM, Schiffer DM et al. Investigation of a cluster of multiple sclerosis in two

elementary school cohorts. J Environ Health 2007; 69(10):34–38.
230 Neuberger JS, Lynch SG, Sutton ML et al. Prevalence of multiple sclerosis in a residential area bordering an oil refinery. Neurology 2004; 63(10):1796–1802.
231 Turabelidze G, Schootman M, Zhu BP et al. MS: prevalence and possible lead exposure. J Neurol Sci 2008; 269(1/2):158–162.
232 Abo-Krysha N, Rashed L. The role of iron dysregulation in the pathogenesis of multiple sclerosis: an Egyptian study. Mult Scler 2008; 14(5):602–608.
233 Exley C, Mamutse G, Korchazhkina O et al. Elevated urinary excretion of aluminium and iron in multiple sclerosis. Mult Scler 2006; 12(5):533–540.
234 Esch T, Stafano GB, Fricchione GL et al. The role of stress in neurodegenerative diseases and mental disorders. Neuro Endocrinol Lett 2002; 23(3):199–208.
235 Ysrraelit MC, Gaitan MI, Lopez AS et al. Impaired hypothalamic-pituitary-adrenal axis activity in patients with multiple sclerosis. Neurology 2008; 71(24):1948–1954.
236 Thomas PW, Thomas S, Hillier C et al. Psychological interventions for multiple sclerosis. Cochrane Database Syst Rev 2006; 1:CD004431.
237 Brown RF, Valpiani EM, Tennant CC et al. Longitudinal assessment study of anxiety, depression and fatigue with multiple sclerosis. Psycholog Psychother 2009; 82(Pt 1):41–56.
238 Bamer AM, Johnson KL, Amtmann D et al. Prevalence of sleep problems in individuals with multiple sclerosis. Mult Scler 2008; 14(8):1127–1130.
239 Merlino G, Frattici L, Lenchig C et al. Prevalence of poor sleep among patients with multiple sclerosis: an independent predictor of mental and physical status. Sleep Med 2009; 10(1):26–34.
240 Moreira NC, Damasceno RS, Medieras CA et al. Restless leg syndrome, sleep quality and fatigue in multiple sclerosis. Braz J Med Biol Res 2008; 41(10):932–937.
241 Alonso A, Hernan MA. Temporal trends in the incidence of multiple sclerosis: a systematic review. Neurology 2008; 71(2):129–135.
242 Ascherio A, Munger KL. Environmental risk factors for multiple sclerosis. Part II: Non-infectious factors. Ann Neurol 2007; 6196:504–513.
243 Niino M, Fukazawa T, Kikuchi S et al. Therapeutic potential of vitamin D for multiple sclerosis. Curr Med Chem 2008; 15(5):499–505.
244 Tremiett H, van der Mei IA, Pittas F et al. Monthly ambient sunlight, infections and relapse rates in multiple sclerosis. Neuroepidemiology 2008; 31(4):271–279.
245 Dwyer T, van der Mei I, Ponsonby AL et al. MC1R genotype, past environmental sun exposure and risk of multiple sclerosis. Neurology 2008; 71(8):583–589.
246 Huotari A, Herzig KH. Vitamin D and living in the northern latitudes—an endemic risk area for vitamin D deficiency. Int J Circumpolar Health 2008; 67(2/3):164–178.
247 van der Mei IA, Ponsonby AL, Engelson O et al. The high prevalence of vitamin D insufficiency across Australian populations is only partly explained by season and latitude. Environ Health Perspect 2007; 115(8):1132–1139.
248 Motl RW, Snook EM, Wynn DR et al. Physical activity correlates with neurological impairment and disability in multiple sclerosis. J Nerv Ment Dis 2008; 196(6): 492–495.
249 Waschbisch A, Tallner A, Pfeifer K et al. Multiple sclerosis and exercise: effects of physical activity on the immune system. Der Nervenartz 2009; 80(6): 688–692.
250 Fragaso YD, Santana DL, Pinto RC. The positive effects of a physical activity program for multiple sclerosis patients with fatigue. NeuroRehabilitation 2008; 23(2):153–157.
251 Motl RW, McAuley E, Snook EM et al. Physical activity and quality of life in multiple sclerosis: intermediary roles of disability, fatigue, mood, pain, self-efficacy and social support. Psychol Health Med 2009; 14(1): 111–124.
252 Smith C, Hale L, Olson K et al. How does exercise influence fatigue in people with multiple sclerosis? Disabil Rehabil 2009; 31(9):685–692.
253 Alsano M, Dawes DJ, Arafah A et. What does a structured review of the effectiveness of exercise interventions for persons with multiple sclerosis tell us about the challenges of designing trials? Mult Scler 2009; 15(4):412–421.
254 Farinotti M, Simi S, Di Pietrantonj C et al. Dietary interventions for multiple sclerosis. Cochrane Database Syst Rev 2007; 1:CD004192.
255 Piccio L, Stark JL, Cross AH. Chronic caloric restriction attenuates experimental autoimmune encephalomyelitis. J Leukoc Biol 2008; 84(4):940–948.
256 Fernandes G. Progress in nutritional immunology. Immunol Res 2008; 40(3):244–261.
257 van Meeteren ME, Teunissen CE, Dijkstra CD et al. Antioxidants and polyunsaturated fatty acids in multiple sclerosis. Eur J Clin Nutr 2005; 59(12):1347–1361.
258 Swank RL, Dugan BB. Effect of low saturated fat diet in early and late cases of multiple sclerosis. Lancet 1990; 336(8706):37–39.
259 Liuzzi GM, Latronico T, Rossano R et al. Inhibitory effect of polyunsaturated fatty acids on MMP-9 from microglial cells: implications for complementary multiple sclerosis treatment. Neurochem Res 2007; 32(12):2184–2193.

260 Whitehouse CR, Boullata J, McCauley LA. The potential toxicity of artificial sweeteners. AAOHN J; 56(6):251–259.

261 Bandyopadhyay A, Ghoshal S, Mukherjee A. Genotoxicity testing of low-calorie sweeteners: aspartame, ASK and saccharin. Drug Chem Toxicol 2008; 31(4):447–457.

262 Frisullo G, Nociti V, Iorio R et al. Increased expression of T-bet in circulating B cells from a patient with multiple sclerosis and celiac disease. Hum Immunol 2008; 69(12):837–839.

263 Reichelt KL, Jensen D. IgA antibodies against gliadin and gluten in multiple sclerosis. Acta Neurol Scand 2004; 110(4):239–241.

264 Pengiran Tengah CD, Lock RJ, Unsworth DJ et al. Multiple sclerosis and occult gluten sensitivity. Neurology 2004; 62(12):2326–2327.

265 Borhani Haghighi A, Ansari N, Mokhtari M et al. Multiple sclerosis and gluten sensitivity. Clin Neurol Neurosurg 2007; 109(8):651–653.

266 Nicoletti A, Patti F, Lo Fermo S et al. Frequency of coeliac disease is not increased among multiple sclerosis patients. Mult Scler 2008; 14(5):698–700.

267 Raghuwanshi A, Joshi SS, Christakos S. Vitamin D and multiple sclerosis. J Cell Biochem 2008; 105(2):338–343.

268 Szodoray P, Nakken B, Gaal J et al. The complex role of vitamin D in autoimmune diseases. Scand J Immunol 2008; 68(3):261–269.

269 Smolders J, Damoiseaux J, Menheere P et al. Vitamin D as an immune modulator in multiple sclerosis: a review. Neuroimmunol 2008; 194(1/2):7–17.

270 Correale J, Ysrraelit MC, Gaitan MI. Immunomodulatory effects of vitamin D in multiple sclerosis. Brain 2009; 132(Part 5):1146–1160.

271 van der Mei IA, Ponsonby AL, Dwyer T et al. Vitamin D levels in people with multiple sclerosis and community controls in Tasmania, Australia. J Neurol 2007; 254(5):581–590.

272 Cantorna MT. Vitamin D and multiple sclerosis: an update. Nutr Rev 2008; 66(10 Suppl 2):S135–S138.

273 Kragt J, van Amerongen B, Killestein J et al. Higher levels of 25(OH)D are associated with a lower incidence of multiple sclerosis only in women. Mult Scler 2009; 15(1):9–15.

274 Cannell JJ, Hollis BW. Use of vitamin D in clinical practice. Altern Med Rev 2008; 13(1):6–20.

275 Carlson NG, Rose JW. Antioxidants in multiple sclerosis: do they have a role in therapy? CNS Drugs 2006; 20(6):433–441.

276 Mirshafiey A, Mohsenzadegan M. Antioxidant therapy in multiple sclerosis. Immunopharmacol Immunotoxicol 2009; 31(1):13–29.

277 Schreibeit G, van Horssen J, van Rossum S et al. Therapeutic potential and biological role of endogenous antioxidant enzymes in multiple sclerosis pathology. Brain Res Rev 2007; 56(2):322–330.

278 Mazza M, Pomponi M, Janiri L et al. Omega-3 fatty acids and antioxidants in neurological and psychiatric diseases: an overview. Prog Neuropsychopharmacol Biol Psychiatry 2007; 31(1):12–26.

279 Adibhatia RM, Hatcher JF. Altered lipid metabolism in brain injury and disorders. Subcell Biocem 2008; 49:241–268.

280 Aupperle RP, Denney DR, Lynch SG et al. Omega-3 fatty acids and multiple sclerosis: relationship to depression. J Behav Med 2008; 31(2):127–135.

281 Mehta LR, Dworkin RH, Schwid SR. Polyunsaturated fatty acids and their potential therapeutic role in multiple sclerosis. Nat Clin Pract Neurol 2009; 5(2):82–92.

282 Harbige LS, Sharief MK. Polyunsaturated fatty acids in the pathogenesis and treatment of multiple sclerosis. Br J Nutr 2007; 98(Suppl 1):S46–S53.

283 van Rensburg SJ, Kotze MJ, Hon D et al. Iron and the folate/vitamin B_{12} methylation pathway in multiple sclerosis. Metab Brain Dis 2006; 21(2/3):121–137.

284 Russo C, Morabito F, Luise F et al. Hyperhomocysteinaemia is associated with cognitive impairment in multiple sclerosis. J Neurol 2008; 255(1):64–69.

285 Triantafyllou N, Evangelopoulos ME, Kimiskidis VK et al. Increased plasma homocysteine levels in patients with multiple sclerosis and depression. Ann Gen Psychiatry 2008; 7:17.

chapter 37

Obesity

INTRODUCTION AND OVERVIEW

Practitioners in primary care are uniquely placed to help in the management of patients in all stages of overweight and obesity, and are able to maintain a therapeutic relationship with patients over many years. General practitioners should take a long-term view of weight problems, which can mean avoiding goals for weight management that are unlikely to be achieved. Introducing the stigma of failure through attempting unachievable weight loss may affect this relationship, and therefore knowledge of evidence-based treatments and their outcomes is very important. Weight management should not be equated with weight loss, as many parameters of ill health are substantially improved following minimal changes in weight, and these are more to do with taking on healthier eating and exercise habits than shedding kilograms.

There is little evidence to suggest that complex weight interventions are particularly effective, and so in order to promote sustainability for both practitioners and their patients, management programs should avoid being resource- and time-intensive. The formation of a 'contract' between doctor and patient can help set achievable goals for weight control, and the focus of the intervention can be tailored to their short- and long-term needs and resources. Prevention of weight gain especially in patients rendered vulnerable by health problems or circumstances, management and prevention of potentially irreversible or progressive weight-related comorbidities, and appropriately targeted weight loss, are important and achievable goals for primary care physicians. This chapter aims to discuss weight management in a way that should be applicable to most general practitioners.

BACKGROUND

Increased prevalence of obesity is an issue confounding health policy makers across the developed and developing world (Fig 37.1). In medicine, disciplines that have not had to deal with obesity-related illness are having to change management practices to counter it, and the role of cigarette smoking as our leading preventable cause of illness is rapidly being supplanted by overweight. Population surveys in Australia and internationally, while varying depending on the populations studied,[1,2] show that starting from the paediatric age group, the prevalence of obesity increases in all age groups up to about the sixth decade.

In the United States in 2007–2008, the age-adjusted prevalence of obesity was 33.8% overall, 32.2% among

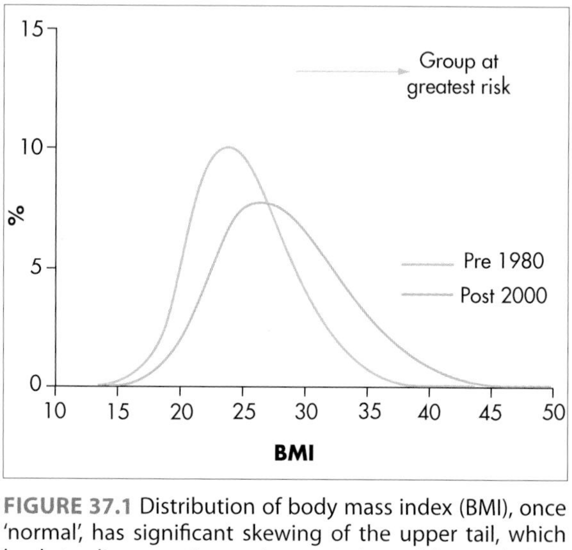

FIGURE 37.1 Distribution of body mass index (BMI), once 'normal', has significant skewing of the upper tail, which leads to disproportionate increases in at-risk populations without a similar change in the population mean BMI (adapted from Ogden et al 2007[3])

men and 35.5% among women. The corresponding prevalence estimates for overweight and obesity combined (BMI ≥ 25) were 68.0%, 72.3% and 64.1%.[4] A review of prevalence estimates in European countries found that the prevalence of obesity based on measured weights and heights varies widely from country to country, with higher prevalences in central, eastern and southern Europe.[5]

The Ausdiab Study showed a prevalence of overweight and obesity in Australia of over 50%.[6] Data for children and adolescents are incomplete but from a demographic point of view at least, the progression from normal weight to overweight and obesity seems to be progressive rather than reversible, so that patients who develop weight problems are more likely to develop further weight problems than undergo substantial improvement. A significant percentage of obese adolescents will be expected to become obese adults.[7]

According to the UK Counterweight Trial, obese patients are more frequent presenters to general practitioner (GP) clinics[8] and more likely to be actively treated with medications[9,10] than the average patient, so the population prevalence of obesity will usually under-represent the number of obese patients that a practitioner will actually see. Normalisation of obesity in the community allows it to be chronically under-recognised, and many patients who could benefit from intervention by a GP will miss out if active screening and action are not part of practice policy.[11,12] Table 37.1 shows BMI and waist circumference values for the Caucasian population. Risk stratification by BMI for non-Caucasian populations is more difficult, and because they may be at risk of adverse metabolic problems at a lower weight, any evidence of excess abdominal adiposity may warrant formal assessment for the metabolic syndrome (Box 37.1). Estimation of childhood and adolescent weight disorders relies on using growth charts created by the American Centers for Disease Control and Prevention, with patients classified as overweight when above the 85th percentile, and obese when above the 95th percentile.

TABLE 37.1 Classification of obesity and overweight in Caucasians[13]

Classification	BMI (kg/m²)	Waist circumference (cm)
Normal range	18.5–24.9	
Overweight	25–29.9	> 94 (male) > 80 (female)
Obese	> 30	> 102 (male) > 88 (female)
Class I	30–34.9	
Class II	35–39.9	
Class III	> 40	

BOX 37.1 Diagnosis of the metabolic syndrome[14,15]

2005 International Diabetes Federation definition of the metabolic syndrome:

- central obesity (waist circumference ≥ 94 cm for Europid men, ≥ 80 cm for Europid women, with ethnicity-specific values for other groups*)

and any two of the following:

- raised serum triglyceride level (≥ 1.7 mmol/L)
- reduced serum HDL-cholesterol level (< 1.03 mmol/L for males, < 1.29 mmol/L for females)
- raised blood pressure (systolic blood pressure ≥ 130 mmHg or diastolic blood pressure ≥ 85 mmHg), or treatment of previously diagnosed hypertension
- impaired fasting glycaemia (fasting plasma glucose (FPG) ≥ 5.6 mmol/L) or previously diagnosed type 2 diabetes

*South Asian and South-East Asian men ≥ 90 cm, women ≥ 80 cm; Japanese men ≥ 85 cm, women ≥ 90 cm.

WHAT CAUSES OBESITY?

While the underlying force driving weight gain in an individual is chronic energy imbalance, the seeming simplicity of weight maintenance hides multiple layers of complexity that relate as much to genetic and environmental factors[16–19] as to voluntary food and exercise choices. Evolution has given us physiological systems that work to maintain 'current weight' without voluntary control and offer significant resistance to weight change (Fig 37.2). In both overfeeding and underfeeding studies there is resistance to changes in body composition, so that diets of energy surplus or restriction, while changing weight in the short term, will usually have little long-term effect on weight. Long-term positive energy imbalance gradually wears down the relatively weak metabolic defences against weight gain and this leads to creation of extra fat stores. These extra stores are rigorously defended when they are threatened by attempts at voluntary weight loss (Box 37.2), and thus chronic weight gain is encouraged and weight loss seemingly unobtainable. Environmental changes leading to increasing availability of energy-dense food, combined with a decline in opportunities to expend calories in everyday activities, have disengaged the 'brakes' that have previously allowed most people to remain weight stable.[20] Failing societal cues for eating and exercise are yet to be replaced by effective public health policy, and lessons learned from successful public health campaigns relying on legislative changes to bolster education (i.e. tobacco smoking) have yet to be applied in obesity prevention. Studies looking at preventing weight gain in 'at-risk' populations are plagued by compliance and methodological problems, but patients who are frequent users of healthcare, such as pregnant women[21] and patients with depressive illness,[22] can benefit from weight management programs, and therefore these patients and others who are regular attendees at GP clinics are ideal candidates for intervention.

OBESITY-RELATED ILLNESS

Weight-related comorbidities are often a mixture of both metabolic and 'mass-related' physical changes (Table 37.2). An overweight patient's expanded adipocyte mass functions as an active endocrine organ, with production

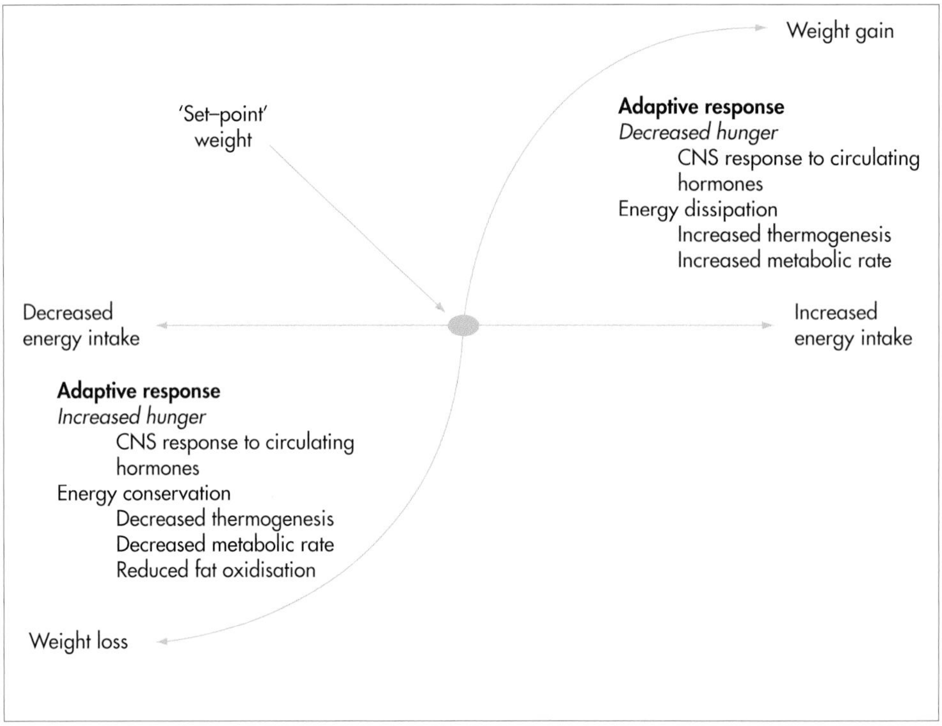

FIGURE 37.2 (and Box 37.2) The relationship between energy intake and weight is not linear.[17,23–26] Most people's weight varies within a 3–5 kg range, and once they leave this range a number of mechanisms are triggered,[27,28] which return that person to their previous range, or, if the energy changes are long-lasting, act to reduce weight change by either increasing (energy excess) or decreasing (energy deficit) metabolic rate[29–32] and altering hunger signals[33,34] to help return the individual to their earlier range.[35] Weight loss triggers a complex array of metabolic and behavioural changes. Patients losing weight often find that they manage early weight loss without great difficulty, then reach a plateau beyond which they cannot go without great effort. They become progressively psychologically distressed the longer the diet persists,[36] and when they cease dieting they recover their lost kilos at a rapid rate, often overshooting their start weight.[37]

TABLE 37.2 Detrimental effects of weight gain*

Metabolic	Physical	Psychosocial	Other
Lipid abnormalities	Obstructive sleep apnoea	Eating disorders	Increased cancer risk
Hypertension	Arthritis	Depression	Asthma
Diabetes	Back pain and non-arthritic soft-tissue disorders	Social isolation	
Steatohepatitis and cirrhosis	Intertrigo	Reduced employment opportunities	
Gallstones	Heart failure	Medical stigma	
Asthma	Reflux		
Polycystic ovarian syndrome (PCOS)	Stress incontinence		

*Some of the disorders fall into multiple categories.

BOX 37.2 Measured physiological responses to weight loss

- Increased hunger and decreased sensation of satiety.
  - During a 'diet', patients record less satiety from standardised meals than before dieting. This tendency increases rather than decreases as duration of diet increases.
  - A number of centrally acting peptides lead to changes in hunger and amplify the enjoyment of eating.
- More recovery of lost fat tissue than other body tissues after starvation.
- After weight loss, 'hyperphagia' (desire to overeat) persists and promotes overshooting of previously lost weight.
  - People on an ad libitum diet following a period of calorie restriction (1500 calories) record above-normal hunger sensations that persist after they have recovered all their previously lost fat mass.
- Increased measurement of parameters of depression.
  - Patients who are 'dieting' but not losing further weight exhibit many features consistent with a depressive illness.
- Decreased metabolic rate.
  - As a result of decreased fat mass, thermogenesis in fat tissue decreases.
  - Sympathetic tone decreases.
- Changing respiratory quotient.
  - Due to a reduction in utilisation of fatty acids as an energy substrate

of endocrine and paracrine substances as well as cytokines, which affect the systemic and portal circulations, leading to the metabolic effects of insulin resistance, including lipid and glucose abnormalities, reproductive hormone changes and hypertension. The physical manifestations of obesity, such as gastro-oesophageal reflux, sleep apnoea and arthritis, probably have metabolic associations also, but these are not well understood, and although obesity is significantly associated with cancers of the uterus, breast, colon and oesophagus, the mechanisms behind this are also not well understood.

SCREENING AND DIAGNOSIS

Routine BMI and waist measurement is a vitally important and often under-utilised screening tool that can lead clinicians towards the diagnosis of early metabolic and cardiovascular disease.

Practices with electronic systems can schedule reminders about BMI checks in the same way that they manage recalls for mammography and Pap smears. Patients diagnosed with an early manifestation of the metabolic syndrome, such as hypercholesterolaemia, can be tagged as being at risk for progression, and management of their problem should also include discussion of weight management. Most clinicians will follow up the diagnosis of any manifestations of the metabolic syndrome with a glucose tolerance test, but other manifestations of obesity-related disease, such as steatohepatitis and cirrhosis, sleep apnoea and increased risk of common cancers, are more difficult to diagnose. Patients presenting with significant obesity or recent weight gain should also be screened for endocrine disorders such as hypothyroidism.

INTEGRATIVE MANAGEMENT

DEFINING GOALS

Despite the diversity in patients needing weight management, and regardless of the resources available to the GP and the patient, the goals need to be health based. Some patients will be seeking weight loss, some will be undergoing treatment for metabolic or physical conditions, and some will be unaware of, or resistant to, linking their weight with their health. When devising a weight control strategy, weight loss itself needs to be viewed as the least effective measure of success and is the least likely outcome. Obtaining and maintaining a reduced-calorie diet combined with any degree of exercise will prevent weight gain, help control cholesterol and blood pressure problems, reduce abdominal girth, prevent progression of impaired glucose tolerance to type 2 diabetes, and potentially reduce mortality risk.[38] Discussing weight issues in terms of health will significantly reduce the risk that the patient will treat your advice in the same manner that they treat the varied, conflicting and erroneous advice they receive from various forms of the dieting 'industry'. Most diet-induced weight loss is invariably followed by weight regain, as the dietary process creates an artificial and unsustainable approach to food and exercise, rather than teaching the skills necessary to manage weight and maintain health in the long term.

When treating weight issues it is important to understand that it is hard for patients to achieve long-term weight loss, and that inadvertent weight gain may lead to physical and metabolic disturbances that promote the tendency to gain even more weight. There is an expectation among many that limiting energy intake will result in weight loss proportional to caloric restriction, whereas in reality this does not appear to be the case. A patient who fails to meet an unrealisable goal should not be allowed to attach the failure to your advice, and if care is taken to focus on non-weight-related targets, this will probably be avoided. It is important not to jeopardise the long-term nature of the relationship between the overweight patient and their GP.

MANAGEMENT OPTIONS

A range of weight management tools is available to the GP and can be used depending on the circumstances of the patient. Some obesity treatments may not be freely available, but most of those used in hospital-based obesity clinics are available in the community (Box 37.3). Guiding patients towards healthy eating habits and sustainable exercise patterns is the ultimate goal, but there will be times when weight loss itself is viewed as important, and if this is the case it is useful to know the nature and effects of obesity therapies. While occasional patients will have dramatic results from non-lifestyle treatments, it is unusual for these to persist, and weight regain usually leaves the patient in worse mental and physical health.

BOX 37.3 Nature and effects of readily available obesity treatments[13,39–45]

Reduced-energy diet

- Dietician-supervised; aims for an energy deficit of 500–1000 calories per day, or 1500 calories intake for women and 1800 calories for men.
- Composition of the diet is probably unimportant, and an average of 3–5 kg weight loss maintained at 2–3 years is expected.

Very-low-energy diet

- Uses meal replacement with commercially available drinks or bars. Used alone provides 600–800 calories per day, or in combination with a normal meal provides 1200 calories per day.
- Used frequently by specialist weight-loss clinics, but requires supervision. For long-term results, best given as part of a diet plan that has the patient moving onto a supervised reduced-energy diet with exercise. One of the easiest and most reliable methods of rapid weight loss available if patients can be compliant, and is associated with some of the best long-term results.

Exercise therapy

- Three to four hours of walking per week will provide 2–3 kg of weight loss, and addition of a significant calorie reduction to this will give only 2–3 kg more. This degree of exercise causes a 1000–1500 calorie deficit *per week*, which is less than a take-away meal, but the beneficial effect on health will far outweigh the minimal effect on weight.
- About 30 minutes most days of moderate-intensity exercise (able to raise heart rate) will confer significant protection from cardiovascular and other diseases, so this should be the *stated goal* for all weight-management patients. More prolonged or intensive exercise should only be encouraged in patients who have managed this amount of exercise over a significant time period.
- About 5 hours a week of moderate-intensity exercise is required to prevent progression of overweight to obesity, and 7–10 hours per week to maintain the 'reduced obese' state—i.e. to prevent weight gain after a diet.

SUCCESSFUL WEIGHT LOSS

Box 37.4 shows data obtained from groups of patients who have not only lost weight, but kept it off in the long term. The medical data are primarily from the National Weight Control Registry,[61] which is an observational study of patients who have maintained > 13.6 kg of weight loss for more than 12 months, and is the largest non-surgical weight-loss cohort in the world. Regardless of the route taken to weight loss, the destination is the same. Patients who lose large amounts of weight consume a diet that is significantly reduced in calories, food choice and spontaneity. They undertake about an hour of aerobic exercise a day, and if they ever regain weight they struggle to lose it again. As patients with

BOX 37.4 Attributes of successful weight-loss patients

In both surgical and non-surgical groups, the key to success is prolonged caloric restriction.[62–74]

Dietary weight loss

- Can arise from virtually any form of diet.
- Conscious weight regulation managed by weighing > once per week.
- Significant caloric reduction maintained over long term (1300 kcal/day women, 1700 kcal/day men).
- Most meals prepared and eaten at home.
- Patients reported meal/snack episodes of 4.5 per day, but ate a significantly reduced range of foods.
- Patients exhibit significant restraint when making dietary choices; disinhibition of dietary restraint from internal cues (emotional) predicts weight relapse.
- Patients who regained weight were unlikely to lose it again; however, the effort of weight maintenance decreases after 2 years.
- One hour or more per day of moderate-intensity exercise (up to 10,000 calorie deficit per week).

Surgical weight loss

- From > 2500 kcal energy intake per day pre-op, patients fall to about 800 kcal per day during significant weight loss, increasing to 1000 kcal per day after this, and levelling out at about 1300 kcal when weight is stable at 18–24 months.
- Surgical patients recorded lower exercise when matched against similar weight-loss patients from the National Weight Control Register, but still more than those who were still obese. They also recorded lower levels of cognitive restraint while eating.
- Weight loss in surgical cohorts appears to relate to effective use of appetite suppression, and this seems to be the key difference between surgical and non-surgical patients, who can develop compensatory hyperphagia in response to weight loss.
- Ability to become physically active (rather than doing set amounts of exercise) increases success.
- Post-surgical patients who gain weight struggle to lose it again.

'Natural' remedies for obesity

by Kerryn Phelps

Reduced caloric intake and increased activity are the most 'natural' remedies for obesity. However, many patients request supplementary assistance with their weight-loss efforts. It is important that the GP is able to have an informed conversation with patients about their options.

Medication review

Some medications increase weight. Review all medications and supplements the patient is taking, and assess for potential to cause increased appetite or weight gain. These might include corticosteroids, antidepressants, antipsychotic agents and antihypertensives. A supervised change or reduction of medication may be possible.

Water

Some patients sense hunger when they are thirsty. Increasing water consumption before a meal may help reduce hunger.[46]

Psyllium

Soluble fibre such as psyllium may help lower insulin levels,[47] reduce hunger,[48] delay gastric emptying and increase the subjective sensation of satiety.

Green tea

Animal studies have shown that green tea consumption reduces food intake, decreases leptin levels and body weight and increases thermogenesis. These results have not been confirmed in human trials.

Gymnema sylvestre

Gymnema sylvestre reduces sweet taste sensation and therefore craving for simple carbohydrates.[49] It can be used to help control blood sugar levels in diabetes.

Zinc

Zinc (15–20 mg per day) may increase lean body mass, and decrease the amount of fat or keep it stable. Zinc increases levels of leptin, a hormone in the body that helps satiety. Perform zinc taste test and supplement as necessary.

Vitamin D

Obesity is associated with vitamin D deficiency. There is an inverse association between BMI and serum levels of 25-hydroxy vitamin D and 1,25 vitamin D. Cross-sectional studies have shown that low 25-hydroxy vitamin D levels are related to glucose intolerance, diabetes, insulin resistance and metabolic syndrome. Assess vitamin D_3 levels and supplement as necessary.

Citrus aurantium

Citrus aurantium is a popular ingredient in weight-loss products, substituting for the banned ephedra in the United States. The main ingredient, synephrine, produces effects on human metabolism that could be useful for reducing fat mass in obese humans because it stimulates lipolysis and raises metabolic rate and fat oxidation through increased thermogenesis.[50] Two small clinical studies suggest possible weight reduction.[51] More research is needed.

Mind–body issues and weight management

by Craig Hassed

For a range of reasons, no integrated approach to weight management should ignore the role of the mind. First, it is well documented that stress and psychological factors often compound poor eating patterns, leading to under- or over-nutrition. Food is often used as compensation for emotional disturbances. Secondly, the mind's effect on allostasis contributes to the development of metabolic syndrome. Thirdly, mind–body therapies have an important role to play in the management of this condition as well as in reducing cardiovascular risk.[52] A range of psychological and mind–body therapies have been trialled with success for weight management and eating disorders.[53] These include mindfulness-based therapies[54,55] and hypnosis,[56] although any psychological strategy that is effective in improving mental health or stress management could also be helpful in weight management. Cognitive behaviour therapy is effective for children, adolescents[57] and adults.[58] Behaviour change strategies also play an important adjunctive role.

It is important to be reminded that the role of psychological therapies is not only to aim for weight loss but also to help improve the quality of a person's life, regardless of their weight. A healthier psychological approach to eating should be seen as a mandatory part of sustainable and healthy weight loss. Dr Rick Kausman's program on weight management is a good example of such an approach that is easy to implement in the primary care setting.[59,60] The following are some of the key points in this program.

- *Achievable and sustainable goals*—as mentioned above, most rapid weight-loss programs do not sustain weight loss by 1–2 years, and in the meantime can reinforce unhealthy attitudes towards food, eating and body image. Smaller changes to food intake, supported by increased physical activity, are gentler, more enjoyable and more likely to be sustained.
- *Positive attitude towards food*—it is natural to enjoy food, but for most people concerned about their weight, guilt, depression, fear or shame are the prime motivators for dietary change. Common language related to food and food advertising—such as being 'good', 'bad', 'guilty' or 'wicked'—confirms such unhelpful attitudes. Breaks in rigid dietary routines often lead to intense guilt and self-loathing as the pendulum swings forcefully from self-deprivation to over-indulgence. Rather than value-laden words like those above, it is better to use terms such as 'everyday foods' and 'sometimes foods'. This gives permission to indulge occasionally, with more enjoyment but less likelihood of overdoing it.
- *Non-hungry eating*—eating patterns are driven by many factors aside from hunger or nutritional need, such as boredom, obligation, habit, celebration and culture. Over time we can lose touch with our bodies and the sensation of real hunger, as opposed

(continued overleaf)

to a desire for food devoid of hunger. We can also become disconnected from our body's messages about when to stop eating. Recognising, respecting and/or re-establishing our body's inbuilt intelligence about what and when to eat is a vital part of eating healthily and maintaining a healthy weight.

- *Body image*—a modern youth culture has evolved in film, advertising and fashion, and revolves around an unhealthily thin body image. In anorexia nervosa there is an inability to experience the normal bodily messages associated with hunger, and a neurological inability to perceive the body's thinness. As such, the rising prevalence of eating disorders is as much a reflection of a societal problem as it is an individual one.
- *Slowing down*—one effect of the busy lives we lead is that we also eat quickly and don't properly taste and chew the food we eat. This significantly reduces enjoyment, impairs the digestive process and doesn't give us time to register when the body has had enough. Eating with attention and slowing down can help to remedy such a problem and is one of the reasons that mindfulness-based activities are helpful.

weight problems are used to eating more and exercising less than their weight-normal peers, it is no surprise that so few can manage the self-imposed deprivation that this entails.

CLINICAL SCENARIOS

Although there are many ways to present with weight problems, patients tend to fall into patterns of presentation, which can help direct advice and treatment along a particular pathway:

- patients at risk of rapid weight gain
- patients with 'reversible' weight-related medical conditions
- patients with established obesity-related disease and disability
- overweight children, especially those with overweight parents.

RAPID WEIGHT GAIN

Most GPs will be familiar with the tendency of some high-risk individuals to gain weight rapidly as a result of lifestyle change or illness. As these weight changes are likely to become permanent unless tackled early, a 'rescue' plan to identify and treat vulnerable patients is worth considering. Patients in the postpartum period, especially if suffering from depression or with a history of weight problems, are a clear example of this, as are patients undergoing treatment for severe depression, or after suffering an injury or disabling musculoskeletal complaint, hysterectomy or diagnosis of an endocrine disorder such as PCOS, thyroid problem or diabetes. Many patients may miss the opportunity to start a weight management plan because of the focus on their mental or physical disorder. Setting aside time to discuss weight management during a separate consultation will be required in many cases, and for patients with depression,[22,75–78] and probably also those in the postpartum period, an exercise program, even if unsustainable in the long term, may be enough to offer significant help.

The diagnosis of diabetes can be followed by weight gain, with some medications, especially insulin, contributing to this.[79] In this group also, regular exercise is

TABLE 37.3 Drug therapy

Drug	Action	Weight loss > placebo
Phentermine, diethylpropion	Non-adrenergic agonists Appetite suppression Serious potential side effects include pulmonary hypertension and heart valve defects. Contraindicated in patients with hypertension, heart disease, glaucoma, or those taking antidepressant medications	3.5 kg
Orlistat	Inhibitor of fat absorption Increases compliance with low-fat diet Side effects include oily stools, flatulence and diarrhoea	2.1 kg
Sibutramine	Inhibits serotonin and noradrenaline reuptake Appetite suppression Serious concerns have been expressed about its safety and it has been suspended from use in the UK and the EU. It is also under review by the FDA and the European Medicines Agency. Concerns involve cardiovascular events and seizures as well as significant side effects	3.5 kg
Fluoxetine	Serotonin reuptake inhibitor Appetite suppression Side effects include anxiety, tremor, sweating and insomnia	3.3 kg

important as a way of increasing insulin sensitivity as well as increasing energy expenditure.

PATIENTS WITH TREATED MEDICAL CONDITIONS

This is the largest group of patients for most GPs. They may have been diagnosed with a manifestation of the metabolic syndrome and will often be in the normal weight range, or may be only a little overweight. The relationship between their medical condition and their lifestyle is likely to be apparent to them, but the importance of preventing weight gain may not be. These patients can have a metabolic disturbance that leads them to develop worsening medical problems with minimal changes in weight, so the key to their management is early identification and attempts to establish healthy eating and exercise patterns.

PATIENTS WITH SIGNIFICANT OBESITY AND OBESITY-RELATED DISEASE

This group of patients is the smallest in number but the most difficult to deal with, and will often consume time and resources without any obvious gains being made. The GP's role in caring for this group is again directed towards achieving health goals that can be maintained. Focusing on weight loss as a primary measure of the success of your relationship with these patients is more likely to lead to detachment of the patient from your practice than actually achieving weight loss. Successful weight management can only come as a result of sustainable healthy eating and exercise habits, but these patients will often require significant rehabilitation of their lifestyle to achieve this.[80] Delegation of some of these tasks to a trusted dietician and an exercise physiologist is important, but these support staff need to be briefed to provide a plan that will not over-stretch the patient and lead to non-compliance. A suggested algorithm for GP-based weight management is given in Fig 37.3, but some of the easiest methods, combining a very-low-energy diet with dietician and exercise program, preferably avoiding pharmacotherapy as 'standalone' treatment,[81] are also some of the most effective,[39,82] and these can be recommended as a core management tool that most practices will be able to access.

These patients often need significant revision of their eating and exercise habits, and detailed instruction about managing the complex task of substituting high-calorie, often packaged or takeaway foods, with similar lower-calorie forms. Patients with a high 'food IQ' will not need this level of structure, and will be just as well served by the formulation of a diet that plans to give them a 500–600 calorie per day deficit to encourage a few months of gentle weight loss.

Exercise for patients with significant obesity and obesity-related disease

Most patients with significant obesity will be unable to manage the enthusiastic exercise challenges recommended by gyms, but will still need to include exercise in their routine. Significantly obese individuals find it difficult to engage in strenuous, and sometimes almost any, exercise. Regular aerobic exercise is difficult to sustain for obese individuals, and its effects on weight loss have been overstated.[62,83–88] The benefits of regular exercise on health, however, cannot be emphasised enough, and it is also useful in reducing the risk of further weight gain.[89] Enlisting the help of an exercise physiologist, or someone with similar interests, is worthwhile in formulating an exercise plan for these patients, as many have physical limitations that make regular exercise difficult. Setting goals for exercise should include goals for incidental exercise such as walking at home and at work, and while using a pedometer is a useful approach to aid this, the aim should be to achieve and sustain minimum rather than 'ideal' targets.

There will be occasions when patients need referral to specialist weight management clinics, or referral for consideration of surgery. One advantage that hospital-based weight management clinics or multidisciplinary integrative clinics may have over general practice is the ready access to experienced support staff with special interest in obese patients, and this makes them ideally placed when caring for patients who can be resource intensive when attempting to correct their substantial lifestyle barriers to weight control. Patients referred to hospital-based clinics will continue to attend their general practice for ongoing care, and when this occurs it is very useful to encourage contact between your own support staff and those in the clinic. Specialist dieticians and exercise physiologists are usually passionate about their work and are an excellent and often under-utilised resource for community practitioners. There is little in the way of published data on weight-loss outcomes from such referrals, but while greater than single-digit (in kilograms) weight loss is unlikely,[90,91] the focused treatment of medical and lifestyle problems will usually justify the intervention.

Psychology referral for patients with significant obesity

Whether to include a psychologist in the care of these patients is a complex issue. While the rate of eating disorders is high in the significantly obese,[92,93] obesity itself is a condition of disordered physiology, and therefore eating disorders are more likely to be a result than a cause of their obesity. Referral to a psychologist with a special interest in weight problems is unlikely to cause weight loss in itself, but it can assist

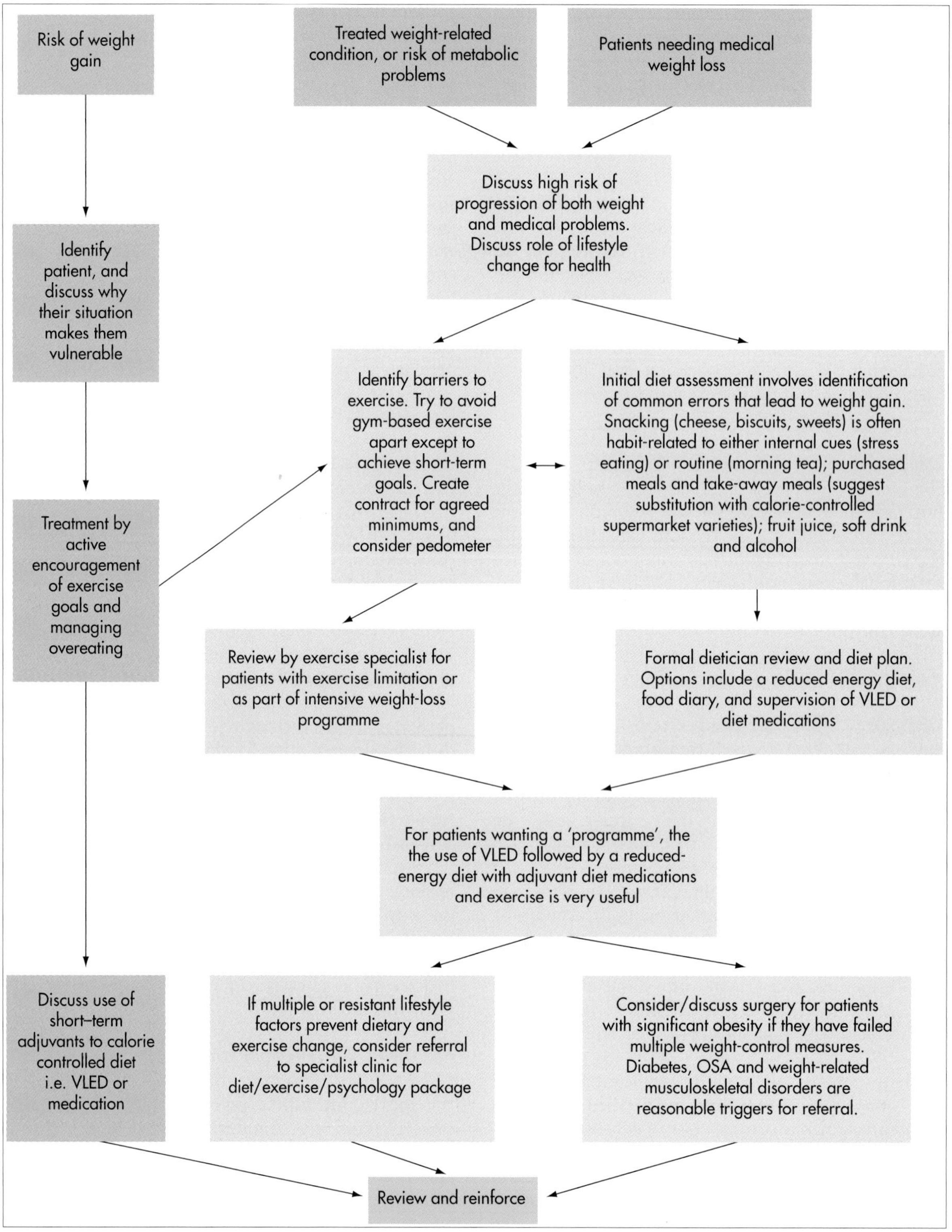

FIGURE 37.3 Suggested algorithm for weight management in general practice. Early identification, focus on healthy sustainable habits and regular review are the important features.

in future weight management if patients are receptive to considering changing their relationship to food and lifestyle. Suggesting referral to a psychologist takes some tact, and needs to be done when the patient is able to understand the reasoning behind the referral.

Surgical intervention for significant obesity

Most GPs will see significantly obese patients who require or seek long-term weight loss. When this is the case it is reasonable to discuss surgical intervention, but obviously there are access and equity issues that will make this impractical for many.[94] In all published comparisons of surgical versus medical treatments for obesity, the magnitude of weight loss achieved and maintained by surgery is 5–10 times greater than any and all medical treatments.[40–42,95] Although the idea of weight-loss surgery appears strange at first glance, it is rapidly being embraced by patients in Australia and overseas. Several types of procedures are available (Fig 37.4), but most work by encouraging patients to embrace low-calorie eating and increased physical activity. These operations significantly reduce hunger and the speed at which patients can eat, and this leads to weight loss

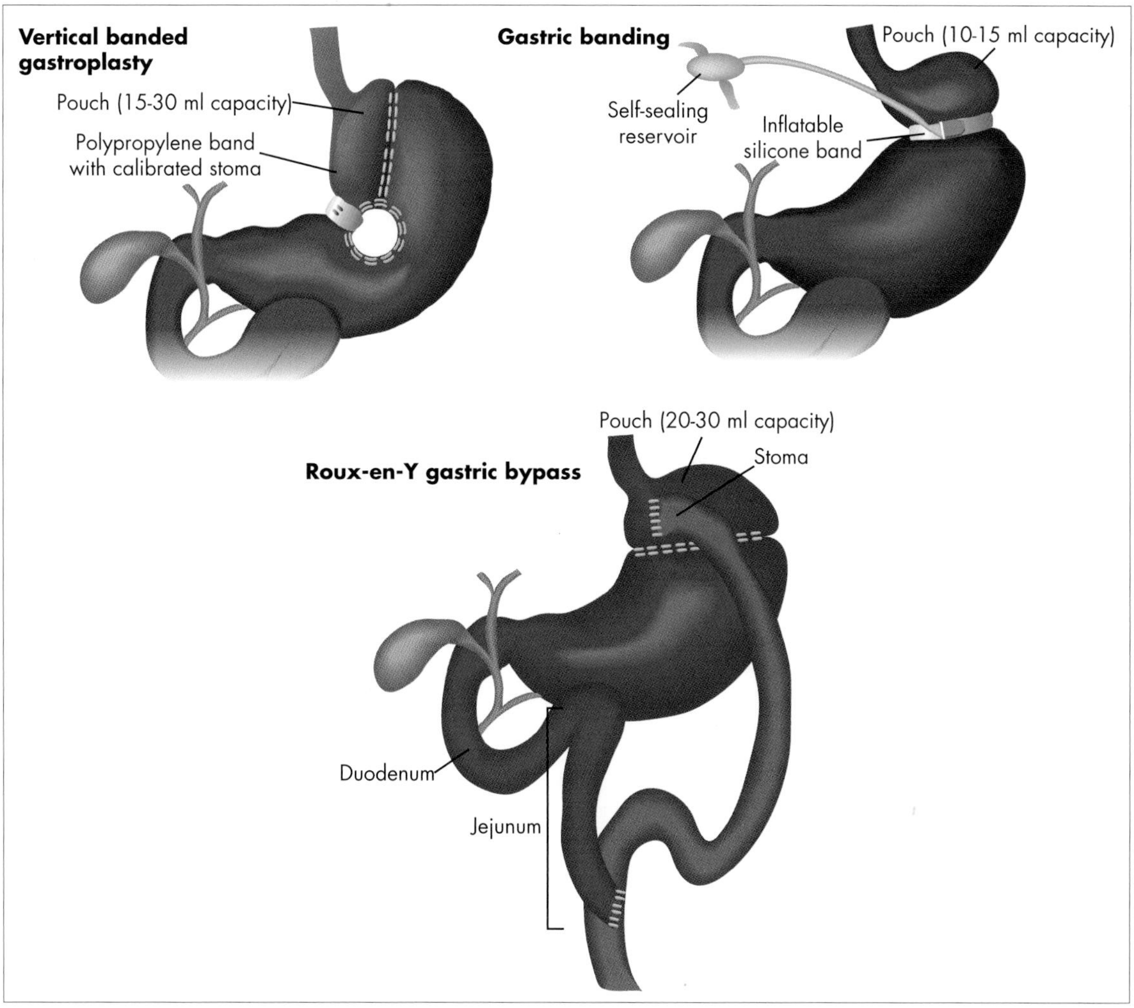

FIGURE 37.4 More than 95% of weight loss procedures are designed to encourage caloric restriction by a number of mechanisms. Appetite suppression and limiting the speed of eating are central to all these operations, but in general the operations are insufficient to cause weight loss without voluntary behaviour change by the recipients. Various forms of laparoscopic gastric banding operations create a 'virtual' pouch of stomach that slows the progress of food into the stomach proper. Pressure from the band leads to prolonged appetite suppression between meals. The laparoscopic gastric bypass creates a small (20 cc) stomach that empties rapidly, leading to neuro-hormonal changes that suppress appetite rapidly during eating, and produce aversion to fatty and high-calorie foods.

through reduced calorie intake. If patients desire to overeat or eat high-calorie foods, they will manage to do this but will not lose weight, and so an important part of preoperative selection of patients is choosing those who wish to change their lifestyle but have been unable to do so (Fig 37.3). The risks of surgery are similar in magnitude to those of laparoscopic cholecystectomy or joint replacement, and while Australia has some of the best results in the world, a lot of this is attributed to the follow-up team, and patients who are unable or unwilling to come to regular review usually fail to embrace the lifestyle changes required and will not lose weight. Obvious candidates for surgical intervention are those with type 2 diabetes (of whom 40–80% can be expected to cease diabetes treatments[44]), severe sleep apnoea and mobility problems who have failed well-supported conservative weight loss efforts.

THE OVERWEIGHT CHILD

Management of weight problems in the young is hampered by under-recognition and by the resistance that many feel about giving and receiving advice on parenting issues, but these barriers should not be allowed to deter clinicians from dealing with what can become a serious and intractable condition.[96] Liberal use of growth charts during routine assessment of children will help de-stigmatise discussions and improve early pick-up, but determining when and how to intervene can be very difficult. There is increasing awareness that childhood obesity increases illness risk, significantly reduces self-esteem[97,98] and quality of life, and usually progresses into adult obesity.

As children have limited ability to control their environment, changing the factors that contribute to obesity requires enlisting the parents or guardians of the child to create an environment where excess calorie consumption and sedentary behaviour are discouraged. As overweight children often live with overweight families, they can have a combination of both genetics and environment working against them from a young age, and this needs to be brought into the discussion whenever possible. Overweight parents can be very unhappy about their own weight, and so this can be used as a factor to drive the 'whole of family' approach to weight management that will be required. While it is known that watching a lot of television,[3] reduced energy expenditure through exercise and disordered parental eating can predispose to weight problems, it is not known whether correcting these problems will reduce weight. Despite the lack of evidence, these factors are potentially the most readily modifiable and so they can form the basis of your interaction with the patient and family. The aim of such an intervention is to promote healthy, reduced-calorie intake and increased exercise, which hopefully will allow the child to decrease their body fat percentage as they grow. Very overweight children may require referral to an accredited practising dietician with a special interest in pediatrics, or to specialist clinics, and as a significant number of eating disorders develop in adolescents, an awareness of the need for psychological help for some patients is also warranted.

CONCLUSION

General practitioners have 'pole position' in weight management due to the long-term relationship they have with patients. This relationship can be used to promote the healthy habits that are the core of successful weight management.[7] A large number of significant health benefits occur very early in the process of weight loss and are related more to a reduction in calorie excess and avoidance of sedentary behaviour than to any particular change in weight. Picking up on these positives, and pointing out that they occur as a result of health improvement rather than weight loss, can set the tone for further consultations in future. When patients understand the difficulties of weight control, and become comfortable with the idea that diets work through calorie restriction rather than through magical alteration in their body's functioning, they can view the weight management tools available and use them appropriately to achieve improved long-term health.

RESOURCES

National Weight Control Registry, http://www.nwcr.ws/

NIH Obesity Information, http://health.nih.gov/topic/Obesity

Zimmet PZ, Alberti KG, Shaw JE. Mainstreaming the metabolic syndrome: a definitive definition. Med J Aust 2005; 183(4):175–176 (this new definition should assist both researchers and clinicians)

REFERENCES

1 Haslam DW, James WP. Obesity. Lancet 2005; 366(9492):1197–1209.

2 Stewart S, Stewart S, Tikellis G et al. Australia's future 'Fat Bomb': a report on the long-term consequences of Australia's expanding waistline on cardiovascular disease. Melbourne, Australia: Baker IDI Heart and Diabetes Institute; 2008.

3 Ogden CL, Carroll MD, McDowell MA et al. Obesity among adults in the United States—no change since 2003–2004. NCHS data brief no 1. Hyattsville, MD: National Center for Health Statistics; 2007.

4 Flegal KM, Carroll MD, Ogden CL et al. Prevalence and trends in obesity among US Adults, 1999–2008. JAMA 2010; 303(3):235–241.

5 Berghöfer A, Pischon T, Reinhold T et al. Obesity prevalence from a European perspective: a systematic review. BMC Public Health 2008;8:200.

6 Cameron AJ, Welborn TA, Zimmet PZ et al. Overweight and obesity in Australia: the 1999–2000 Australian Diabetes, Obesity and Lifestyle Study (AusDiab). Med J Aust 2003; 178(9):427–432.
7 Guo SS, Wu W, Chumlea WC et al. Predicting overweight and obesity in adulthood from body mass index values in childhood and adolescence. Am J Clin Nutr 2002; 76(3):653–658.
8 Frost GS, Lyons GF. Obesity impacts on general practice appointments. Obes Res 2005; 13(8):1442–1429.
9 Counterweight Project Team. The impact of obesity on drug prescribing in primary care. Br J Gen Pract 2005; 55(519):743–749.
10 Ross HM, Laws R, Reckless J et al. Evaluation of the Counterweight Programme for obesity management in primary care: a starting point for continuous improvement. Br J Gen Pract 2008; 58(553):548–554.
11 Laws R. Current approaches to obesity management in UK primary care: the Counterweight Programme. J Hum Nutr Diet 2004; 17(3):183–190.
12 Tan D, Zwar NA, Dennis SM et al. Weight management in general practice: what do patients want? Med J Aust 2006; 185(2):73–75.
13 Proietto J, Baur LA. 10: Management of obesity. Med J Aust 2004; 180(9):474–480.
14 Zimmet PZ, Alberti KG, Shaw JE. Mainstreaming the metabolic syndrome: a definitive definition. Med J Aust 2005; 183(4):175–176.
15 Chew GT, Gan SK, Watts GF. Revisiting the metabolic syndrome. Med J Aust 2006; 185(8):445–449.
16 Cornier MA, Grunwald GK, Johnson SL et al. Effects of short-term overfeeding on hunger, satiety, and energy intake in thin and reduced-obese individuals. Appetite 2004; 43(3):253–259.
17 Morton GJ, Cummings DE, Baskin DG et al. Central nervous system control of food intake and body weight. Nature 2006; 443(7109):289–295.
18 Wisse BE, Kim F, Schwartz MW. Physiology. An integrative view of obesity. Science 2007; 318(5852):928–929.
19 Chung WK, Leibel RL. Considerations regarding the genetics of obesity. Obesity (Silver Spring) 2008; 16(Suppl 3):S33–S39.
20 Swinburn B, Egger G. The runaway weight gain train: too many accelerators, not enough brakes. BMJ 2004; 329(7468):736–739.
21 Guelinckx I, Devlieger R, Beckers K et al. Maternal obesity: pregnancy complications, gestational weight gain and nutrition. Obes Rev 2008; 9(2): 140–150.
22 Blouin M, Tremblay A, Jalbert ME et al. Adiposity and eating behaviors in patients under second generation antipsychotics. Obesity (Silver Spring) 2008; 16: 1780–1797.
23 Bessard T, Schutz Y, Jéquier E et al. Energy expenditure and postprandial thermogenesis in obese women before and after weight loss. Am J Clin Nutr 1983; 38(5):680–693.
24 Schutz Y. Macronutrients and energy balance in obesity. Metabolism 1995; 44(9)(Suppl 3):7–11.
25 Spiegelman BM, Flier JS. Obesity and the regulation of energy balance. Cell 2001; 104(4):531–543.
26 Schutz Y. Dietary fat, lipogenesis and energy balance. Physiol Behav 2004; 83(4):557–564.
27 Weyer C, Pratley RE, Salbe AD et al. Energy expenditure, fat oxidation, and body weight regulation: a study of metabolic adaptation to long-term weight change. J Clin Endocrinol Metab 2000; 85(3):1087–1094.
28 Doucet E, Cameron J. Appetite control after weight loss: what is the role of bloodborne peptides? Appl Physiol Nutr Metab 2007; 32(3):523–532.
29 Leibel RL, Rosenbaum M, Hirsch J et al. Changes in energy expenditure resulting from altered body weight. N Engl J Med 1995; 332(10):621–628.
30 Ranneries C, Bulow J, Buemann B et al. Fat metabolism in formerly obese women. Am J Physiol 1998; 274(1 Pt 1):E155–E161.
31 Crescenzo R, Samec S, Antic V et al. A role for suppressed thermogenesis favoring catch-up fat in the pathophysiology of catch-up growth. Diabetes 2003; 52(5):1090–1097.
32 Major GC, Doucet E, Trayhurn P et al. Clinical significance of adaptive thermogenesis. Int J Obes (Lond) 2007; 31(2):204–212.
33 Doucet E, Imbeault P, St Pierre S et al. Appetite after weight loss by energy restriction and a low-fat diet-exercise follow-up. Int J Obes Relat Metab Disord 2000 24(7):906–914.
34 Drapeau V, King N, Hetherington M et al. Appetite sensations and satiety quotient: predictors of energy intake and weight loss. Appetite 2007; 48(2):159–166.
35 Schwartz MW, Woods SC, Porte DJ et al. Is the energy homeostasis system inherently biased toward weight gain? Diabetes 2003; 52(2):232–238.
36 Chaput JP, Arguin H, Gagnon C et al. Increase in depression symptoms with weight loss: association with glucose homeostasis and thyroid function. Appl Physiol Nutr Metab 2008; 33(1):86–92.
37 Dulloo AG, Jacquet J, Girardier L et al. Poststarvation hyperphagia and body fat overshooting in humans: a role for feedback signals from lean and fat tissues. Am J Clin Nutr 1997; 65(3):717–723.
38 Gregg EW, Gerzoff RB, Thompson TJ et al. Intentional weight loss and death in overweight and obese US adults 35 years of age and older. Ann Intern Med 2003; 138(5):383–389.

39 Egger GJ. Are meal replacements an effective clinical tool for weight loss? A clarification. Med J Aust 2006; 184(11):591.

40 Anderson JW, Konz EC, Frederich RC et al. Long-term weight-loss maintenance: a meta-analysis of US studies. Am J Clin Nutr 2001; 74(5):579–584.

41 Norris SL, Zhang X, Avenelli A et al. Long-term effectiveness of lifestyle and behavioral weight loss interventions in adults with type 2 diabetes: a meta-analysis. Am J Med 2004; 117(10):762–774.

42 Wadden TA, Butryn ML, Wilson C et al. Lifestyle modification for the management of obesity. Gastroenterology 2007; 132(6):2226–2238.

43 Wadden TA, Berkowitz RI, Vogt RA et al. Lifestyle modification in the pharmacologic treatment of obesity: a pilot investigation of a potential primary care approach. Obes Res 1997; 5(3):218–226.

44 Haddock CK, Poston WS, Foreyt JP et al. Effectiveness of Medifast supplements combined with obesity pharmacotherapy: a clinical program evaluation. Eat Weight Disord 2008; 13(2):95–101.

45 Wadden TA, McGuckin BG, Rothman RA et al. Lifestyle modification in the management of obesity. J Gastrointest Surg 2003; 7(4):452–463.

46 van Walleghen EL, Orr JS, Gentile CL et al. Under acute test meal conditions, pre-meal water consumption reduces meal energy intake in older but not younger adults. Obesity 2007; 15:93–99.

47 Sierra M, Garcia JJ, Fernandez N et al. Therapeutic effects of psyllium in type 2 diabetic patients. Eur J Clin Nutr 2002; 56:830–842.

48 Turnbull WH, Thomas HG. The effect of a *Plantago ovata* seed containing preparation on appetite variables, nutrient and energy intake. Int J Obes Relat Metab Disord 1995; 19:338–342.

49 Brala PM, Hagen RL. Effects of sweetness perception and calorie value of a preload on short-term intake. Physiol Behav 1983; 30(1):1–9.

50 Braun L, Cohen M. Herbs and natural supplements. An evidence-based guide. 2nd edn. Sydney: Elsevier; 2007.

51 Preuss HG, DiFerdinando D, Bagchi M et al. *Citrus aurantium* as a thermogenic, weight reduction replacement for ephedra: an overview. J Med 2002; 33:247–264.

52 Innes KE, Vincent HK, Taylor AG. Chronic stress and insulin resistance-related indices of cardiovascular disease risk, part 2: a potential role for mind-body therapies. Altern Ther Health Med 2007; 13(5):44–51.

53 Chrubasik S, Chrubasik C, Torda T. Early impact of a combined dietary and psychological intervention on BMI, blood pressure, and quality of life. Fam Med 2006; 38(3):160.

54 Kristeller J, Hallett C. An exploratory study of a meditation-based intervention for binge eating disorder. J Health Psychol 1999;4:357–363.

55 Singh NN, Lancioni GE, Singh AN et al. A mindfulness-based health wellness program for an adolescent with Prader-Willi syndrome. Behav Modif 2008; 32(2):167–181.

56 Pittler MH, Ernst E. Complementary therapies for reducing body weight: a systematic review. Int J Obes (Lond) 2005; 29(9):1030–1038.

57 Tsiros MD, Sinn N, Brennan L et al. Cognitive behavioral therapy improves diet and body composition in overweight and obese adolescents. Am J Clin Nutr 2008; 87(5):1134–1140.

58 Cochrane G. Role for a sense of self-worth in weight-loss treatments: helping patients develop self-efficacy. Can Fam Phys 200; 54(4):543–547.

59 Kausman R. Tips for long-term weight management. Aus Fam Phys 2000; 29(4):310–313.

60 Kausman R. If not dieting then what? Melbourne: Allen & Unwin; 2004.

61 National Weight Control Registry. Online. Available: http://www.nwcr.ws/

62 Catenacci VA, Ogden LG, Stuht J et al. Physical activity patterns in the National Weight Control Registry. Obesity (Silver Spring) 2008; 16(1):153–161.

63 Flancbaum L, Choban PS, Bradley LR et al. Changes in measured resting energy expenditure after Roux-en-Y gastric bypass for clinically severe obesity. Surgery 1997; 122(5):943–949.

64 Klem ML, Wing RR, McGuire MT et al. A descriptive study of individuals successful at long-term maintenance of substantial weight loss. Am J Clin Nutr 1997; 66(2):239–246.

65 Klem ML, Wing RR, McGuire MT et al. Psychological symptoms in individuals successful at long-term maintenance of weight loss. Health Psychol 1998; 17(4):336–345.

66 McGuire MT, Wing RR, Klem ML et al. Long-term maintenance of weight loss: do people who lose weight through various weight loss methods use different behaviors to maintain their weight? Int J Obes Relat Metab Disord 1998; 22(6):572–577.

67 Shick SM, Wing RR, Klem ML et al. Persons successful at long-term weight loss and maintenance continue to consume a low-energy, low-fat diet. J Am Diet Assoc 1998; 98(4):408–413.

68 McGuire MT, Wing RR, Klem ML et al. What predicts weight regain in a group of successful weight losers? J Consult Clin Psychol 1999; 67(2):177–185.

69 Klem ML. Successful losers. The habits of individuals who have maintained long-term weight loss. Minn Med 2000; 83(11):43–45.

70 Klem ML, Wing RR, Lang W et al. Does weight loss maintenance become easier over time? Obes Res 2000; 8(6):438–444.

71 Klem ML, Wing RR, Chang CC et al. A case-control study of successful maintenance of a substantial weight

loss: individuals who lost weight through surgery versus those who lost weight through non-surgical means. Int J Obes Relat Metab Disord 2000; 24(5):573–579.
72 Raynor HA, Jeffery RW, Phelan S et al. Amount of food group variety consumed in the diet and long-term weight loss maintenance. Obes Res 2005; 13(5):883–890.
73 Raynor DA, Phelan S, Hill JO et al. Television viewing and long-term weight maintenance: results from the National Weight Control Registry. Obesity (Silver Spring) 2006; 14(10):1816–1824.
74 Colles SL, Dixon JB, O'Brien PE. Hunger control and regular physical activity facilitate weight loss after laparoscopic adjustable gastric banding. Obes Surg 2008; 18(7):833–840.
75 Daley AJ, Copeland RJ, Wright NP et al. Exercise therapy as a treatment for psychopathologic conditions in obese and morbidly obese adolescents: a randomized, controlled trial. Pediatrics 2006; 118(5):2126–2134.
76 Diehl JJ, Choi H. Exercise: the data on its role in health, mental health, disease prevention, and productivity. Prim Care 2008; 35(4):803–816.
77 Mead GE, Morley W, Campbell P et al. Exercise for depression. Cochrane Database Syst Rev 2008; 4:CD004366.
78 Weinstein AA, Deuster PA, Francis JL et al. The role of depression in short-term mood and fatigue responses to acute exercise. Int J Behav Med 2010; 17(1):51–57.
79 Russell-Jones D, Khan R. Insulin-associated weight gain in diabetes—causes, effects and coping strategies. Diabetes Obes Metab 2007; 9(6):799–812.
80 Stanton RA. Nutrition problems in an obesogenic environment. Med J Aust 2006; 184(2):76–79.
81 Haddock CK, Poston WS, Dill PL et al. Pharmacotherapy for obesity: a quantitative analysis of four decades of published randomized clinical trials. Int J Obes Relat Metab Disord 2002; 26(2):262–273.
82 Anderson JW, Vichitbandra S, Qian W et al. Long-term weight maintenance after an intensive weight-loss program. J Am Coll Nutr 1999; 18(6):620–627.
83 Miller WC, Koceja DM, Hamilton EJ et al. A meta-analysis of the past 25 years of weight loss research using diet, exercise or diet plus exercise intervention. Int J Obes Relat Metab Disord 1997; 21(10):941–947.
84 Miller WC. How effective are traditional dietary and exercise interventions for weight loss? Med Sci Sports Exerc 1999; 31(8):1129–1134.
85 Neuhouser ML, Miller DL, Kristal AR et al. Diet and exercise habits of patients with diabetes, dyslipidemia, cardiovascular disease or hypertension. J Am Coll Nutr 2002; 21(5):394–401.
86 Saris WH, Blair SN, van Baak MA et al. How much physical activity is enough to prevent unhealthy weight gain? Outcome of the IASO 1st Stock Conference and consensus statement. Obes Rev 2003; 4(2):101–114.
87 Green JS, Stanforth PR, Rankinen T et al. The effects of exercise training on abdominal visceral fat, body composition, and indicators of the metabolic syndrome in postmenopausal women with and without estrogen replacement therapy: the HERITAGE family study. Metab 2004; 53(9):1192–1196.
88 Sevick MA, Miller GD, Loeser RF et al. Cost-effectiveness of exercise and diet in overweight and obese adults with knee osteoarthritis. Med Sci Sports Exerc 2009; 41(6):1167–1174.
89 Weinsier RL, Hunter GR, Desmond RA et al. Free-living activity energy expenditure in women successful and unsuccessful at maintaining a normal body weight. Am J Clin Nutr 2002; 75(3):499–504.
90 Douglas JG, Ford MJ, Munro JF. Patient motivation and predicting outcome in a hospital obesity clinic. Int J Obes 1981; 5(1):33–38.
91 Vasconcelos MP, Jorge Z, Noble EL et al. Assessment of an obesity clinic in a center hospital. Acta Med Port 2004; 17(5):359–366.
92 de Zwaan M. Binge eating disorder and obesity. Int J Obes Relat Metab Disord 2001; 25(Suppl 1):S51–S55.
93 Darby A, Hay P, Mond J et al. The rising prevalence of comorbid obesity and eating disorder behaviors from 1995 to 2005. Int J Eat Disord 2009; 42(2):104–108.
94 Talbot ML, Jorgensen JO, Loi KW. Difficulties in provision of bariatric surgical services to the morbidly obese. Med J Aust 2005; 182(7):344–347.
95 Buchwald H, Avidor Y, Braunwald E et al. Bariatric surgery: a systematic review and meta-analysis. JAMA 2004; 292(14):1724–1737.
96 Cretikos MA, Valenti L, Britt HC et al. General practice management of overweight and obesity in children and adolescents in Australia. Med Care 2008; 46(11):1163–1169.
97 Wang F, Veugelers PJ. Self-esteem and cognitive development in the era of the childhood obesity epidemic. Obes Rev 2008; 9(6):615–623.
98 McCullough N, Muldoon O, Dempster M. Self-perception in overweight and obese children: a cross-sectional study. Child Care Health Dev 2009; 35(3):357–364.

chapter 38

Pain management

INTRODUCTION AND OVERVIEW

One of the most common reasons for people presenting to a healthcare practitioner is the presence of pain. Many people in our community also experience persistent pain, with most studies showing that around 20% of the population suffer from some type of chronic pain problem.[1] In the past 25 years, there have been some major shifts in our thinking regarding the treatment of pain. One is an increased understanding of the biological changes that occur in the presence of pain. These include neuroplastic changes within the central nervous system that need to be addressed as part of successful pain management. The other has been the increasing prominence of a holistic approach to assessment and treatment. This has come from two directions. Pain practitioners have increasingly recognised the limitations of a purely biomedical approach to pain management. Many patients have also demonstrated dissatisfaction with this type of approach. The large number of people using complementary and alternative treatments as part of their pain management indicates the limitations of currently available treatments as well as a desire for a more holistic approach.

Taking an integrative approach to pain management is more, however, than adding in alternative or complementary treatments that merely provide another symptomatic approach to the patient's treatment. Rather, integrative medicine means taking a holistic approach to the person's experience of pain, assessing the relative contribution of all aspects of their pain, whether physical, psychological or spiritual, and applying the most appropriate treatment that evidence has demonstrated to be effective in the management of that aspect. Integrative pain management may therefore involve the judicious use of medications, stress reduction techniques, behavioural modification and re-examination of purpose and meaning. Any or all of these approaches may need to be considered as part of the prescription that best addresses the needs as well as the desires of the person in pain.

TYPES OF PAIN

Pain is often divided clinically into acute, cancer and chronic non-cancer pain. This division reflects differences in treatment approach, although to some extent each of these aims applies to any type of pain (Fig 38.1). For *acute pain*, the emphasis is generally on removing the pain by identifying the cause and providing pain relief until healing occurs. In *cancer pain*, there is a stronger focus on pain relief, as removal of the cause of pain may be difficult. The emphasis in *chronic non-cancer pain* is generally on pain relief, with a stronger focus on pain management. In many chronic pain conditions, the specific cause of the pain cannot be identified with certainty, or may not be treatable. Using an acute pain approach in people with chronic non-cancer pain, with its ongoing search for a cause

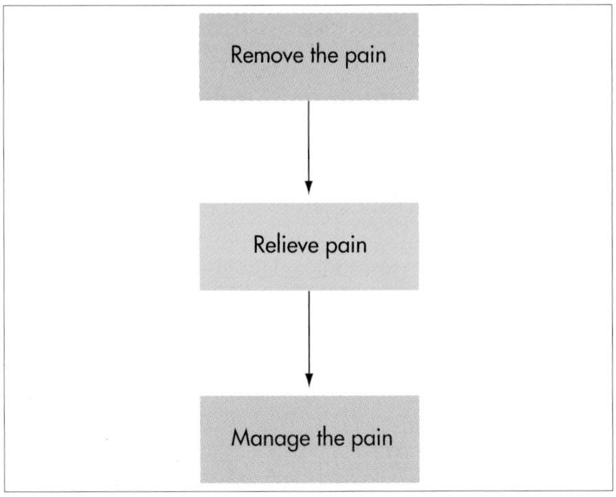

FIGURE 38.1 Aims of pain management

and removal of the pain, can be counter-productive, preventing people from accepting and dealing with their pain, and prolonging and even exacerbating their disability.

PAIN PATHOLOGY

BIOLOGICAL

Pain is a primary indicator of tissue pathology. From a biological perspective, pain can be divided into two pain types, based on underlying mechanisms (Box 38.1). *Nociceptive pain* is pain arising from pathology in somatic and visceral structures, such as bone fractures, appendicitis and renal calculi. *Neuropathic pain* is pain arising from pathology in neural structures, including the peripheral nervous system (e.g. diabetic neuropathic pain and postherpetic neuralgia) and the central nervous system (e.g. spinal cord injury pain and central post-stroke pain). Pain is initiated by damage or potential damage to somatic, visceral or neural tissues. However, a number of secondary changes including sensitisation at the periphery (peripheral sensitisation) and in the central nervous system (central sensitisation) are associated with trauma and the transmission of pain signals.[2] These secondary processes further amplify the pain experience. This means that the treatment of pain often needs to address these secondary changes as well as the underlying cause or generator of the pain.

PSYCHOLOGICAL

Psychological processes are also extremely important in the experience of pain.[3] Although many texts refer to psychogenic pain, pain *caused* by psychological factors is rare and the term may be unhelpful. On the other hand, psychological factors invariably contribute to pain and are a large determinant of the intensity and quality of the pain experience as well as the behaviours that arise as a result of nociceptive and neuropathic stimuli. Mood dysfunction is also a very common *consequence* of pain. Therefore psychological factors need to be considered and assessed in any person who presents with pain.

Psychological factors fall into two main categories. Alterations in *mood*, such as depression, anger, fear and anxiety, may contribute to the pain problem. Our emotional state is strongly linked to activation of descending pathways from the brain to the spinal cord that control the level of amplification of pain signals coming in from the periphery. Both depression and stress-induced anxiety result in increased levels of neurochemicals that result in amplification of incoming pain signals. This results in an increase in the levels of pain that we experience. Therefore, reducing anxiety by providing reassurance and support as well as appropriate management of depression helps to relieve pain by decreasing the level of amplification of pain signals. Unhelpful *cognitions* such as expectation of pain, catastrophising and fear avoidance may also contribute to and exacerbate both pain and pain-related disability.

Brain imaging studies demonstrate that the perception of pain is not localised to any one brain structure or region, but involves the interaction of many regions that register and modify pain signals, including those involved with attention, mood, emotion, fear and cognition. It is therefore extremely difficult to separate the physical aspect of the pain experience from the suffering that accompanies it. 'Pain' can also be experienced vicariously. Empathy, or experiencing another's pain, has been shown to produce changes in brain activity in the observer that are similar to those in the loved one who is actually experiencing the physical pain—apart from the localisation of any pain inputs.[4]

Concluding that mind and emotion affect the experience of pain does not imply that the pain is 'imagined' but that the relationship between pain perception and the extent of physical tissue damage is very variable. There is strong evidence indicating that the central nervous system is sensitised in many chronic pain states, and it is hypothesised that this sensitisation may be maintained by 'sustained attention and arousal'.[5,6] This means that a person with chronic pain can have accentuated pain in the presence of hypervigilance, preoccupation and neuronal hyperactivity, and may go some way to explaining why emotional state has such a major effect on symptomatology for people with chronic pain syndromes. These physiological and psychological changes provide a link between mind and body and a connection between mood, cognitions and the sensation of pain. From a therapeutic perspective, helping to

BOX 38.1 Pain contributors

Biological:
- nociceptive—damage and disease in somatic and visceral structures
- neuropathic—damage or disease in neural structures

Psychological:
- mood—e.g. depression, anxiety, anger
- cognitions—e.g. catastrophising, fear avoidance, self-efficacy

Spiritual:
- loss of purpose, identity and connectedness through disruption of important relationships and activities
- despair and loss of hope
- anger or guilt associated with view of 'higher power' and 'reasons' for pain

Environmental:
- physical—e.g. work, home situation
- social—e.g. relationships with family, friends, colleagues, supervisor
- spiritual—e.g. relationship with 'higher power'

diminish hypervigilance and reactivity to the experience of pain may explain on a clinical and neurological level the better outcomes of people with chronic pain syndromes who include psychological strategies such as stress management or mindfulness as part of their therapeutic approach. Other reasons why the relaxation response or improving emotional state and mental health may help with chronic pain include reduction in muscle tension, the anti-inflammatory effect of stress reduction, improved responsiveness to endorphins and effects on gamma aminobutyric acid (GABA).[7,8]

SPIRITUAL

There is very little information regarding the contribution of spiritual factors to the experience of pain. Even the concept of spirituality is poorly defined. Spirituality is not limited to the religious dimension, and many see spirituality in broad terms involving meaning, purpose and connectedness with no religious connotations. Most people would identify certain activities and relationships that give them a sense of purpose and that enrich and energise them at a deep level. From this perspective, pain can have a significant impact on a person through the disruption of these important and meaningful activities and relationships. This in turn can contribute to the physical experience of pain and add further to depression and loss of hope. However, the relationship between pain and spirituality is not all negative. For many people, the experience of pain can be an opportunity for growth as they re-evaluate their priorities, relationships and direction and find new sources of strength, meaning and hope.

ENVIRONMENTAL INFLUENCES

Pain does not occur in isolation but instead within a context that has a direct bearing on the experience of pain and the person's response to pain. Environmental influences can be divided into three broad categories: physical, social and spiritual (Fig 38.2). *Physical* factors that arise from a person's working or living situation and recreational activities may directly influence or cause pain. For example, for someone in a sedentary occupation with chronic pain, seating posture may have a large bearing on the presence of pain. *Social* factors such as relationships with family, friends, colleagues, employer or supervisor and cultural background can also strongly influence a person's experience of pain and their pain behaviour. For example, the way a spouse or partner responds to a person's pain is a major determinant of the way in which a person with pain will behave. *Spiritual* factors refer to non-physical, non-personal factors that may influence a person's experience of pain. From a religious perspective, it is known that a person's view of God affects their pain.

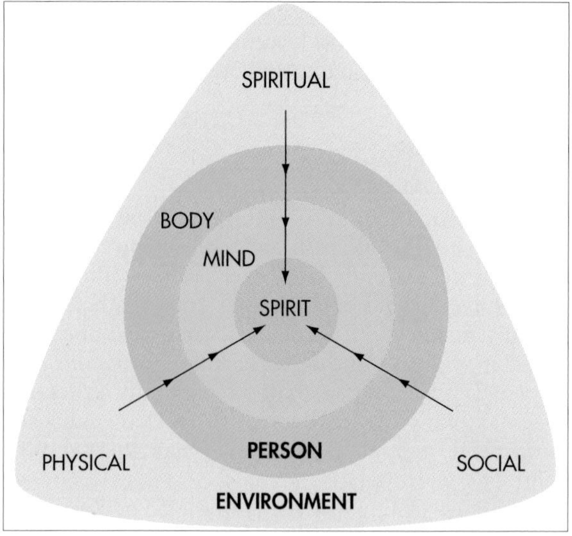

FIGURE 38.2 Interaction between the person and their environment

For example, those who view God as punishing or cruel have worse pain outcomes than those who see God as forgiving.[9] Many people without any religious affiliation also attribute improvement in their pain to an inherent, 'supernatural' ability of certain objects, people or a 'higher power'. Whether these improvements are real or imagined and whether they are simply due to the physical or psychological properties of the intervention is a matter of ongoing debate and study. Nevertheless, it is difficult to consider a person's pain from a holistic perspective without recognising and assessing the possible contribution of these factors to their pain experience.

ASSESSMENT OF PAIN

AIMS OF ASSESSMENT

One aim of pain assessment is first to identify the contribution of biological factors to pain, whether nociceptive or neuropathic. The distinction between nociceptive and neuropathic pain is made because the underlying mechanisms giving rise to pain appear to be different, with different pain characteristics and response to treatment (Table 38.1). Nociceptive pain is often dull or aching and, in the case of musculoskeletal pain, related to activity or position. Although not diagnostic, neuropathic pain is suggested by descriptors such as burning, electric and shock-like with pain present in a region of sensory disturbance. Neuropathic pain often occurs in the absence of stimulation, and minor stimulation such as light touch can lead to exaggerated pain (allodynia).

It is also important to assess the contribution of psychological, spiritual and environmental factors.

TABLE 38.1 Distinguishing nociceptive from neuropathic pain

	Nociceptive	Neuropathic
Symptoms	Dull, aching, worse with movement, positional Relieved by heat, rest, anti-inflammatories	Electric, shock-like, burning, unrelated to activities, associated with paraesthesia, dysaesthesia*, numbness
Signs	Tenderness to palpation and/or on movement Restriction of movement	Disturbance of sensory, motor, reflex function, autonomic changes
Investigations	Somatic or visceral pathology on imaging	Neural pathology on imaging

*Dysaesthesia: unpleasant abnormal sensations, e.g. ants crawling under the skin.

Assessment of *psychological* function includes determining disturbances in mood such as anxiety or depression. It also includes assessing the patient's cognitions, such as their beliefs regarding the cause of their pain, their expectations and preferences for pain management, fear avoidance behaviours, lack of belief in their ability to function normally (self-efficacy), the level of relief they need in order to return to previous activities and the strategies they use to cope with their pain. Assessment of *spiritual* factors may be as simple as finding out what activities and relationships are important to the person and how these have been affected by the pain. This may help understand what gives them strength, purpose and meaning in their life. Further enquiries about a person's beliefs and spiritual practices and how they influence or have been influenced by their experience of pain may also be helpful. Obtaining an *environmental* history focuses on elucidating any factors in their environment that may be contributing to the pain problem. It includes determining the social context of the patient, such as significant relationships, work, hobbies and activities and how these may be acting to reinforce the pain or hinder recovery.

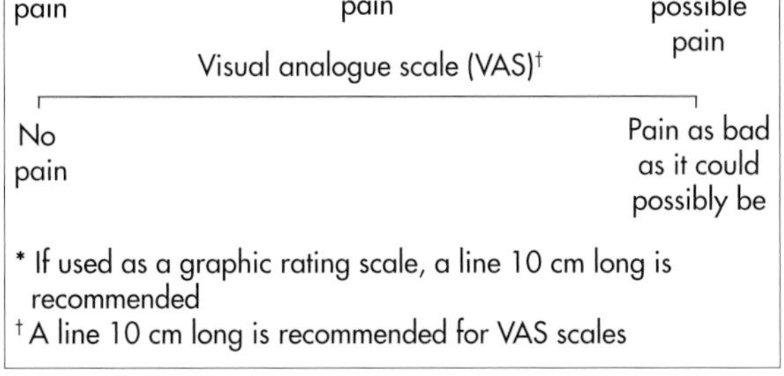

FIGURE 38.3 Pain intensity scales

As well as the contributors to pain, assessment aims to identify the *functional consequences* of pain. This will almost certainly involve the whole person and include physical, psychological and spiritual consequences. For example, acute pain is often associated with physical changes such as an increase in heart rate and blood pressure, pupil dilation and mood changes such as anxiety. Cancer pain may be associated with loss of appetite, anxiety about the diagnosis, and fears and re-evaluation of hopes for the future. A person with chronic non-cancer pain may have postural changes associated with an abnormal gait, sleep disturbance, depression, fear avoidance of activities, interference with social and recreational activities, and loss of identity and meaning in their relationships and work. Although these changes may not be directly contributing to pain, they are important components of the pain problem that need to be addressed. While some may resolve or improve if the pain can be relieved, others may be persistent or severe and require separate attention.

PAIN HISTORY

Taking a patient history is usually the first step towards identifying the main contributors and consequences associated with a person's pain problem. A history provides information that allows some direction as to whether the pain is primarily somatic, visceral or neuropathic, as well as identifying contributing psychosocial factors. For example, lumbar spinal pain precipitated by a lifting incident, that is related to movement, eased by rest, with no radiation to the legs, no numbness or paraesthesiae and a positive response to simple analgesics, including anti-inflammatory drugs, all suggest a primarily somatic nociceptive pain. In addition, sleep disturbance, loss of appetite and loss of enjoyment of activities suggest an accompanying mood disturbance.

A clear history will then provide the basis for further examination and investigations that further refine these preliminary observations. In addition, the history will provide clues regarding other aspects of the person's presentation. The patient's manner, tone, emphasis of certain facts, expressions and language will all help to convey important aspects of their expectations, understanding of their problem and emotional state. Although there are many variations on taking pain history, the basic elements consist of:

- history of the presenting pain problem
- previous pain management
- effect of the pain on the person (associated consequences and effect on function)
- general history (past medical, family, developmental, psychological, social, educational and vocational history) (Box 38.2).

EXAMINATION

As mentioned above, biological pain generators can be broadly divided into nociceptive or neuropathic. Therefore the physical examination can be broadly divided along these same lines into musculoskeletal (or visceral) and neurological (Box 38.3). Other body systems (e.g. cardiovascular, respiratory and gastrointestinal) may also require examination, depending on the individual's presentation. For example, a poor cardiovascular history in a person with low back pain should alert the clinician to the possibility of an underlying vascular cause. This would then warrant careful examination of the vascular system and, potentially, further investigation.

The aim of a physical examination is to identify, where possible, the nature and location of the pathology that may be giving rise to the pain. In addition, any secondary physical consequences or features of the pain, such as muscle deconditioning, allodynia or hyperalgesia, may be a focus of treatment in themselves.

BOX 38.2 Pain history

Pain description
- Location and radiation
- Onset—mechanism of initiating event
- Character/descriptors (aching, sharp, electric etc)
- Temporal characteristics (constant, episodic or intermittent)
- Duration (overall, and of episodes)
- Intensity (verbal—mild, moderate, severe; or numerical rating from 0 to 10)
- Aggravating factors
- Relieving factors

Previous intervention for pain
- Other pain treatments (present and past, and response)
- Pain medications and substances (present and past, and response)

Pain-associated contributors and functional consequences
- Biological (nausea, fatigue, sleep, sexual activity etc)
- Psychological (mood—anxiety, depression, anger etc; cognitions—pain beliefs, concentration, memory, fear avoidance, catastrophising etc)
- Spiritual—source of strength, effect on purpose and meaning, connectedness, beliefs etc
- Environmental (impact on and contribution of physical, social, spiritual environment)

General history
- Medical/psychological problems past and present, and family history
- Other medications including non-prescription, alcohol use and supplements, herbs etc
- Social context and important relationships
- Educational and vocational history, including worker's compensation issues

BOX 38.3 Physical examination

Examination of pain behaviours
- Verbal cues—crying, moaning
- Facial cues—grimacing
- Movement cues—posture, guarding, limping

Examination of the painful region
- Inspection—swelling, skin colour etc
- Palpation—sensitivity to touch (allodynia), palpation of deep structures

Musculoskeletal examination
- Inspection—posture including spinal curvature, guarding, stiffness and gait
- Palpation—generalised, regional or localised tenderness over specific structures
- Movement—active and passive range of joint motion and other features such as crepitus

Neurological examination
- *Sensory*—assessment of large- and small-fibre function in the region of pain compared with non-painful regions using light brushing and pin prick. Consideration should also be given to the use of other modalities such as proprioception, cool (e.g. applying a metal tuning fork) and heat. Record mode (thermal, mechanical), loss or reduction (hypoaesthesia) or increased sensitivity (hyperaesthesia) and level of increase (allodynia or hyperalgesia)*
- *Motor*—determine the impact of pain upon motor function and identify any possible neurological lesion. Includes muscle power (usually 5-point scale), wasting (muscle circumference), increased tone, spasm, clonus or tremor
- *Reflexes*—deep tendon reflexes and Babinski 's sign
- *Autonomic function*—location and nature of changes in temperature, sweating, skin colour, nail and hair growth and oedema (indicative of complex regional pain syndrome; see Box 38.4).

*Allodynia: pain in response to a stimulus which is not normally painful, such as light touch or brushing. Hyperalgesia: heightened response to a stimulus which is normally painful, such as a pin prick.

BOX 38.4 Complex regional pain syndrome

- Complex regional pain syndrome (CRPS) refers to regional pain usually affecting a limb. The person typically complains of generalised burning or aching pain affecting the whole limb.
- The initiating injury can often seem fairly minor and the pain out of proportion to the injury or apparent pathology.
- They may have hypersensitivity to touch (allodynia), and the distinguishing characteristics are autonomic changes including mottling, pallor, reduction in skin temperature, changes in sweating, and swelling.
- If prolonged or severe, CRPS may be associated with bone demineralisation.
- In early stages (generally < 6 months), the patient may respond to sympathetic blocks. However, often the response is poor or of short duration, and other approaches are required, including anticonvulsants, tricyclic antidepressants, spinal cord stimulation and cognitive behavioural approaches with desensitisation and a graduated exposure and exercise program.
- Referral to a multidisciplinary pain clinic is suggested.

INVESTIGATIONS

A wide range of investigations may be indicated to complete an assessment of a patient presenting with persistent pain (Box 38.5). Unfortunately, while most investigations can demonstrate sinister pathology (e.g. fracture, infection, cancer and progressive neurological problems), they are less helpful in identifying the specific mechanisms that may be contributing to persistent pain. For example, in patients with spinal pain, it has been demonstrated that there is a poor correlation between pain report and the presence of pathology on anatomical imaging, even using sophisticated techniques such as magnetic resonance (MR) imaging of the spine.[10,11] In patients with sciatica, imaging is recommended in the acute stage only if there are 'red flags' such as possible infection or malignancy rather than disc herniation, or in the person with severe symptoms who does not respond to 6–8 weeks of conservative management.[12]

Therefore, in ordering further investigations, the clinician needs to be clear as to what information they will provide and whether this information is likely to be of benefit in formulating a diagnosis. In patients with persistent pain who have been adequately investigated, continuing to seek a cause for the pain may make the patient and clinician feel that something is being done. However, a non-specific investigative approach tends to yield less information over time, adds considerably to medical costs and may delay pain management and functional improvement.

BOX 38.5 Investigations

Imaging

The diagnosis of pain relies heavily on imaging techniques. These include:

- X-rays (although of limited value in the diagnosis of back pain and sciatica)
- CT scan
- MRI (± gadolinium)
- bone scan (technetium).

Clinical neurophysiology

May be useful in further characterising any neurological deficit. Useful tests include:

- electromyography (EMG)
- nerve conduction studies (NCS)
- somatosensory evoked potentials (SEP).

Thermography

Significant controversy surrounds the use of this technique in the assessment of persistent pain.[13] Differences in skin temperature can be detected by using an infrared thermometer or thermal imaging.

Thermography does not indicate the presence or magnitude of pain, but reveals alterations in skin temperature that may be due to changes in vascular or neurological function.

However, measurement of temperature differences may be useful in conditions such as complex regional pain syndrome (CRPS) to detect autonomic dysfunction.[14]

MANAGEMENT OF PAIN

There are a large number of options available for the treatment of persistent pain. Sadly, however, many of these options have only limited success and many have substantial side effects. These factors have contributed to the frequent use of psychological and complementary approaches in pain management. Many of the commonly used treatments for pain are listed in the boxes and tables below. Evidence for specific treatments is discussed in the text. Rather than provide an exhaustive review of all the evidence (positive and negative) for each treatment, this text focuses on treatments that have strong (consistent positive findings among multiple high-quality randomised controlled trials (RCTs)) or moderate (consistent findings among multiple low-quality RCTs and/or one high-quality RCT) evidence to support their use.

MINIMAL INTERVENTION: IS THIS A VALID OPTION?

Before examining available treatments, it is worth considering whether it is valid to 'do nothing' for the person with pain. A great danger for the practitioner facing the person in pain is feeling the need to do *something* to relieve the person's suffering. While this is entirely appropriate in the acute pain setting, it may actually contribute to disability in those with persistent

BOX 38.6 Treatment of acute low back pain and sciatica[12,15]

1 History and examination, noting any 'red flags' (such as risk factors for or symptoms and signs of infection, past history of malignancy, osteoporotic fractures, cauda equina syndrome).
2 Identify psychosocial and occupational 'yellow flags' associated with increased risk of progression from acute to chronic.
3 If 'red flags' present, arrange appropriate investigations.
4 If cauda equina syndrome, or acute severe paresis or progressive paresis, refer to neurosurgeon.
5 If 'yellow flags' present, consider behavioural or psychosocial intervention.
6 If no 'red flags' identified, reassure, advise to stay active, use heat and analgesics if necessary.
7 If continuing pain and disability at 6–8 weeks, consider surgery.

pain. In the semi-acute phase of low back pain, it has been demonstrated that long periods of rest have little benefit. Current guidelines indicate that the best approach is analgesia, short-term rest (up to 5 days) and encouragement to return to work (see Box 38.6). Over-medicalisation of chronic pain can lead to increased dependency on pharmacological approaches, increased healthcare practitioner visits, increased passivity and little gain in either pain relief or function.

HERBAL AND HOMEOPATHIC REMEDIES, VITAMINS AND SUPPLEMENTS

Complementary and alternative therapies are widely used in the management of chronic pain, and studies indicate that more than half the population use complementary approaches for the treatment of pain.[16] However, many of the studies that have been done have low subject numbers, are not adequately controlled and have variability in design and outcome measures. Although there are a large number of remedies used, stronger evidence exists for:

- willow bark (*Salix alba*), devil's claw (*Harpagophytum procumbens*) and cayenne (*Capsicum frutescens*) for the relief of low back pain[17,18]
- willow bark (*S. alba*), Phytodolor® (a standardised herbal preparation of aspen, ash and golden rod), S-adenosylmethionine (SAMe), devil's claw (*H. procumbens*), chondroitin sulfate and glucosamine (in moderate to severe pain),[19] ginger extract,[20] capsaicin and avocado–soybean unsaponifiables for osteoarthritis[21,22]
- fish oil and gamma-linolenic acid for pain associated with rheumatoid arthritis[22,23]
- peppermint oil for irritable bowel syndrome[24]
- vitamin B_1 for the treatment of dysmenorrhoea.[25,26]

PHARMACOLOGICAL

Although pharmacological approaches remain the mainstay of pain management (see Table 38.2), it is important to remember the holistic perspective on the management of pain. For example, where the experience of pain is being amplified by emotional, spiritual or existential concerns, the solution is to confront those issues as much as they can be and not merely to mask the problem with ever-escalating doses of medication while leaving the underlying issues unaddressed. Alternatively, providing sensitive and empathic emotional support is adjunctive to, but not a substitute for, the appropriate prescription of analgesics.

Most people with pain rely on prescription, over-the-counter or non-prescription medications for pain relief. As mentioned previously, pain is broadly divided into nociceptive (musculoskeletal and visceral) and neuropathic. The main drugs used for the treatment of *musculoskeletal pain* are non-steroidal anti-inflammatory drugs (NSAIDs), paracetamol and opioids.

- These are generally effective for acute and chronic musculoskeletal pain.
- Best results are achieved with 'around the clock' dosing rather than 'as needed'.
- Pain is usually managed in a stepwise approach using simple analgesics for mild pain, compound analgesics and 'weak' opioids such as tramadol for moderate pain, and 'strong' opioids such as morphine, oxycodone, buprenorphine, hydromorphone, methadone and fentanyl for severe pain.

There has been a swing to increased use of strong opioids for the treatment of chronic non-cancer pain over the past 20 years based on published evidence of the low rate of addiction following short-term use of opioids. Several points are relevant to clinical practice:

- Oral morphine, oxycodone and methadone are regarded as first-line agents for the treatment of moderate to severe chronic non-cancer pain.[27]
- Parenteral administration of strong opioids is best avoided in the management of persistent pain.
- Pethidine should be avoided because of the availability of other effective opioids, the high risk of dependence and the possibility of convulsions from the metabolite norpethidine.
- Long-acting formulations of opioids are preferable to short-acting formulations.

The development of long-acting formulations such as slow- or controlled-release agents and transdermal patches has been an advance in providing more stable levels of analgesia. However, there are an increasing number of people now maintained on strong opioids who still report ongoing pain, with few gains in function

TABLE 38.2 Medications used in pain management

Drug	Indications	Side effects
Paracetamol and NSAIDs		
Paracetamol	Mild to moderate pain (particularly soft tissue and musculoskeletal) Headache Dental pain Dysmenorrhoea Mild procedural pain Supplementation of opioids in moderate to severe pain	Liver toxicity in high doses (> 4 g/day)
NSAIDs (including non-selective and selective COX-1 and COX-2 inhibitors)	Mild to moderate pain associated with inflammation and trauma Back pain and arthralgias with an inflammatory component Metastatic bone pain Headache Toothache Postoperative pain Dysmenorrhoea Acute gout	GI upset including nausea, dyspepsia, bleeding and ulceration, headache, dizziness, drowsiness; pruritis, rash, skin reactions; tinnitus; oedema, hypertension, haematological, renal, hepatic, central nervous, respiratory system effects, hearing, visual disturbances; increased risk of thrombotic events including myocardial infarction and stroke; female infertility Reye's syndrome with aspirin
Opioids		
Morphine Fentanyl Hydromorphone Oxycodone	Unless indicated otherwise, opioids are used for severe acute traumatic, postoperative, cancer and chronic non-cancer pain	All opioids may produce constipation, respiratory depression, hypotension, urinary retention, sedation, nausea, vomiting, sweating, pruritis, hypogonadism, antidiuretic effect, biliary spasm, miosis, increased muscle tone, tolerance, dependence, decreased libido
Codeine	Moderate to severe pain	Approximately 10% of population may be poor metabolisers of codeine; high incidence of constipation
Dextropropoxyphene	Moderate to severe pain	Low-potency opioid with long and variable half-life. Major metabolite is cardiotoxic, and chronic high dosing may result in convulsions and psychosis.
Tramadol	Moderate to severe pain, possible advantage in neuropathic pain because of serotonergic, noradrenergic effects	Serotonergic and noradrenergic actions. Lowers seizure threshold and possibility of serotonin syndrome when mixed with other serotonergic drugs such as MAOIs.
Methadone		NMDA antagonist effect. May be more effective in neuropathic pain conditions. Care required with dose adjustment because of long and variable half-life.
Buprenorphine		Mixed agonist/antagonist. Ceiling effect and may antagonise effects of other opioids.
Pethidine	Some acute pain conditions where a short duration of action is preferable Not indicated for the management of chronic pain	Short duration of action. Metabolite (norpethidine) accumulation and toxicity may occur. Possibility of serotonin syndrome when administered with some drugs, e.g. MAOIs. High addictive potential.

(continued overleaf)

TABLE 38.2 Medications used in pain management (continued)

Drug	Indications	Side effects
Antidepressants		
Tricyclic antidepressants, e.g. amitriptyline, nortriptyline	Neuropathic pain, fibromyalgia	Contraindicated in patients with ischaemic heart disease, heart failure, cardiac conduction disturbances or a history of seizures. Sedation, weight gain and anticholinergic side effects such as constipation, blurred vision, postural hypotension, dry mouth and urinary retention.
Anticonvulsants		
Valproate	Neuropathic pain	Skin reactions, gastrointestinal upset, weight gain, tremor, hair loss, liver dysfunction, haematological and teratogenic effects
Carbamazepine	Neuropathic pain, especially trigeminal neuralgia	CNS toxicity, sedation, nausea, ataxia, diplopia, rash, bone marrow toxicity, hepatotoxicity, hyponatraemia
Gabapentin, pregabalin	Neuropathic pain, fibromyalgia	Dizziness, sedation, ataxia, constipation, dryness of the mouth, peripheral oedema
Other adjuvants		
Ketamine	Neuropathic pain (acute or chronic episodes)	Parenteral administration, narrow therapeutic window, hallucinations
Antiarrhythmics, e.g. lignocaine, mexiletine	Neuropathic pain	Proarrhythmic effects. Drowsiness, GI upset, dizziness with mexiletine.
Corticosteroids, e.g. dexamethasone, prednisone	Reduction of inflammation and oedema	Adverse effects with prolonged use. Local osteoporosis and joint damage with repeated intraarticular use.
Benzodiazepines, e.g. diazepam	Short-term relief of muscle spasm	Drowsiness, memory impairment, ataxia, confusion, dependence with long-term use
Clonazepam	Neuropathic pain	

MAOIs: monamine oxidase inhibitors; NMDA: N-methyl-D-aspartate; NSAIDs: non-steroidal anti-inflammatory drugs.

and other effects such as alterations in endocrine function. This has led to increasing concerns and debate about the wisdom of this approach and has raised several issues.

- Patients need to be warned about the risks of dependence, tolerance and driving while using opioids.
- Side effects such as nausea and constipation require appropriate treatment.
- Opioids should generally not be prescribed in those who have a history of substance abuse.
- A questionnaire (CAGE) is available which may help to identify those at risk of substance abuse (available from the Australian Government Department of Health and Ageing website[27]).

In contrast to musculoskeletal pain, *neuropathic pain* generally responds poorly to anti-inflammatory medications, and opioids have reduced efficacy. Pharmacological treatment of neuropathic pain relies on a number of other adjunctive medications.[28] The two main classes are tricyclic antidepressants and anticonvulsants.

- Tricyclic antidepressants are generally used in lower doses (10–75 mg) than for the treatment of depression and have an analgesic action quite apart from their mood-altering effect. They may also help with sleeplessness and comorbid depression.
- Despite the widespread use of specific reuptake inhibitors and their improved side effect profile, evidence from pain studies still indicates that tricyclic antidepressants have greater efficacy.
- Anticonvulsants have a variety of actions but broadly reduce the abnormal firing of sensory nerves that occurs with neuropathic pain. These include the older anticonvulsants such as valproate and carbamazepine and newer anticonvulsants such as gabapentin and pregabalin.

- Although cost is often an issue, use of the newer anticonvulsants with their better side effect profile is gradually replacing the use of older anticonvulsants. The possible exception to this is carbamazepine, which still is regarded as the first-line agent in the treatment of trigeminal neuralgia.

TABLE 38.3 Biological treatments

Nociceptive	Neuropathic
Pharmacological	
Simple analgesics, e.g. paracetamol, NSAIDs, opioids Antispasmodics (if spasm present) Glucosamine, herbal medicines, traditional Chinese medicine, traditional Indian medicine (Ayurveda), homeopathic remedies, naturopathic preparations, aromatherapy, vitamins and supplements, diet	Antidepressants, anticonvulsants, opioids, other adjuvants
Physical	
Physiotherapy, chiropractic, osteopathy, craniosacral therapy, massage Specific techniques, e.g. Alexander, Pilates, t'ai chi, qi gong, yoga, Rolfing, therapeutic touch, reiki	Little benefit
Stimulation techniques	
TENS, acupuncture, magnets, low-level laser therapy	TENS, acupuncture, spinal cord stimulation, deep brain stimulation, motor cortex stimulation
Nerve blocks	
Skeletal blocks, e.g. facet joint blocks Epidural blockade Nerve root blocks	
Surgical	
Nerve, spinal cord section (indicated only in cancer pain)	Dorsal root entry zone (DREZ) lesions (brachial plexus avulsion) Other procedures provide short-term relief with high likelihood of pain returning
Spinal drug delivery	
Intrathecal opioids	Intrathecal opioids, clonidine

- As well as the tricyclic antidepressants and the anticonvulsants, a number of other medications and topical local anaesthetics are used but with more limited evidence of efficacy.

STIMULATION TECHNIQUES

A variety of stimulation techniques such as acupuncture, transcutaneous electrical nerve stimulation (TENS), low-level laser therapy, electromagnetic fields, spinal cord stimulation, deep brain stimulation and motor cortex stimulation are used, with varying levels of invasiveness and support. Although many studies do not provide long-term outcomes, there is positive support from at least one well-controlled trial for:

- high-frequency TENS for primary dysmenorrhoea[29] and osteoarthritic knee pain[30]
- low-level laser therapy for treatment of chronic neck pain and osteoarthritic knee pain[30,31]
- electroacupuncture for labour pain,[32] 'idiopathic' headache,[33] acute dental pain and postoperative pain, fibromyalgia,[34] shoulder pain,[35] lateral epicondylitis (short-term relief),[36] chronic neck pain (short-term relief),[37] chronic low back pain (short-term relief)[38] and osteoarthritic knee pain.[30]

PHYSICAL AND MANUAL THERAPIES

Although physical and manual therapies are widely used in the treatment of musculoskeletal pain problems (Table 38.3), there is continuing debate about their

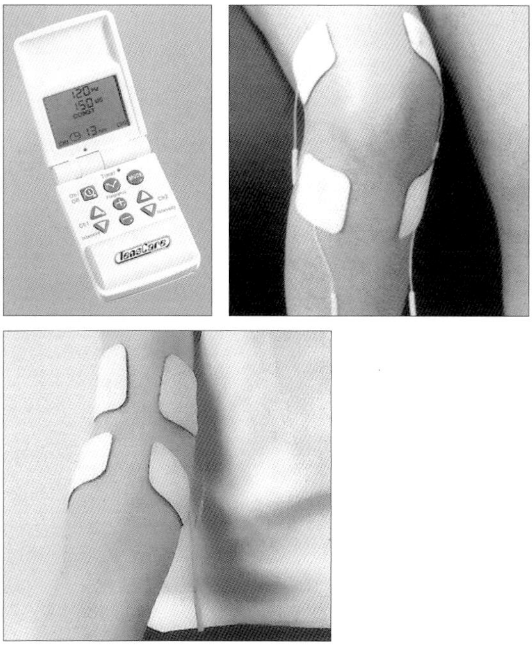

FIGURE 38.4 TENS machine/ treatment

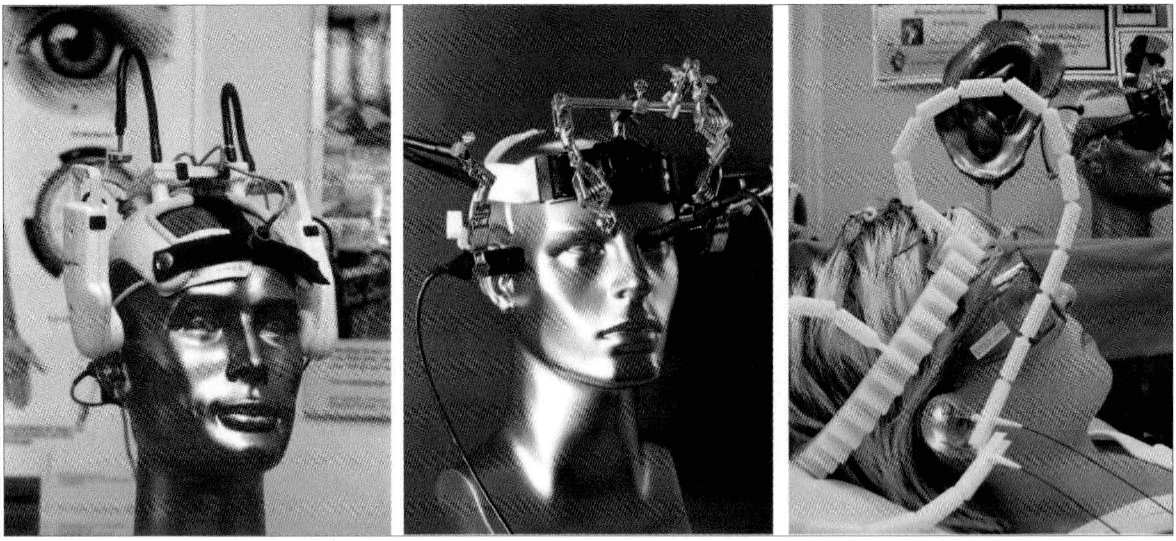

FIGURE 38.5 Electro acupuncture

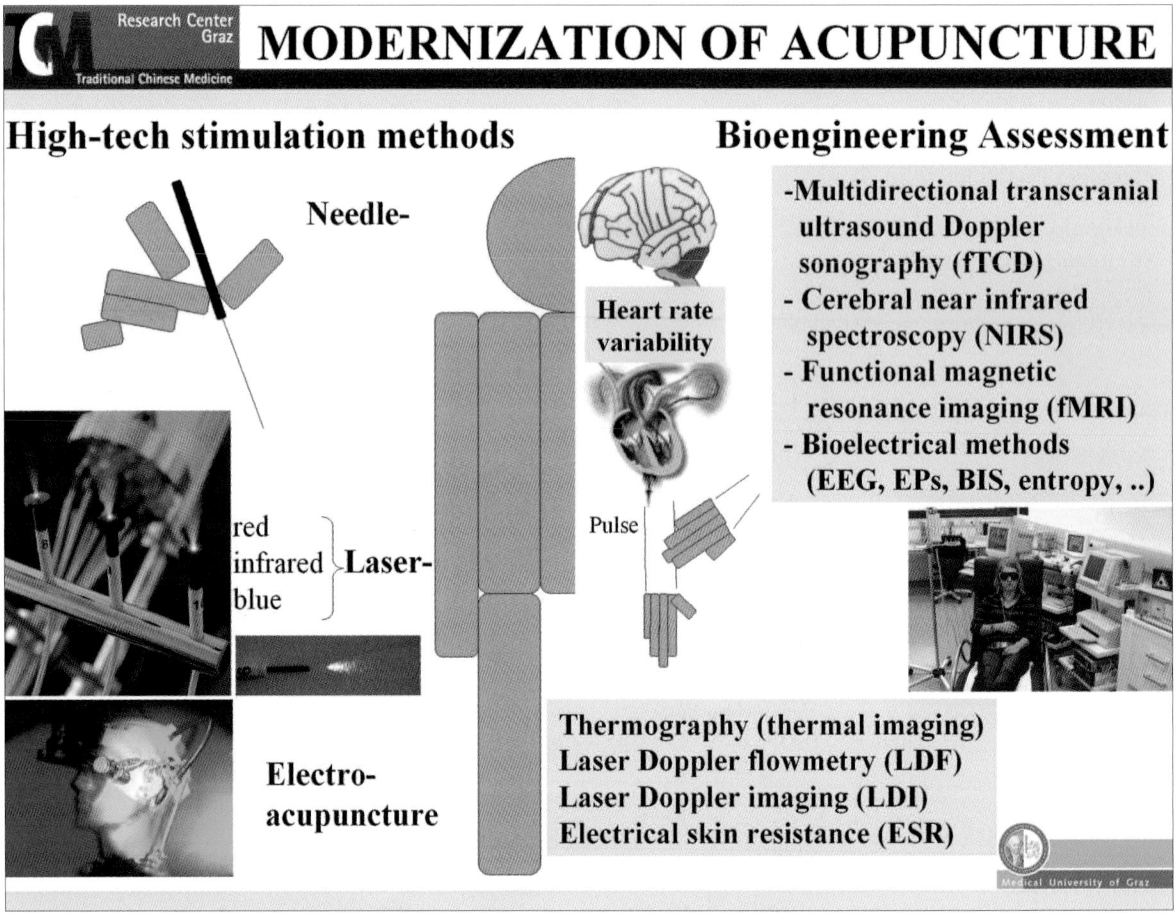

FIGURE 38.6 Laser acupuncture

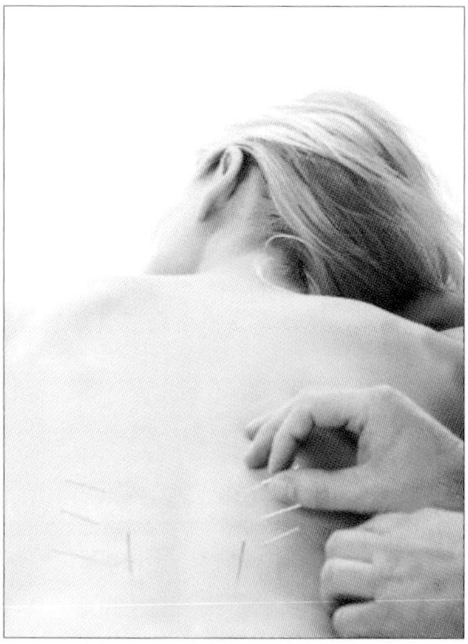

FIGURE 38.7 Needle acupuncture

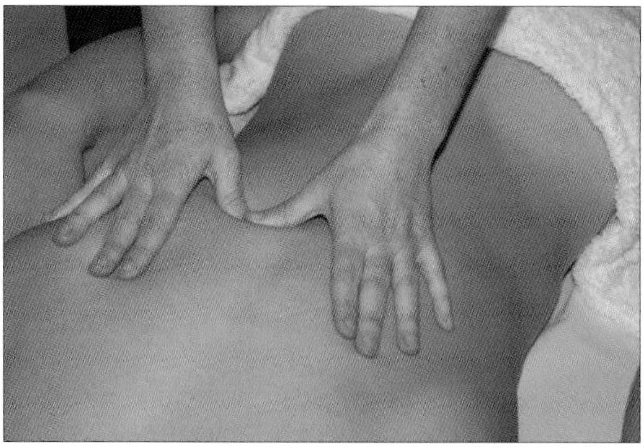

FIGURE 38.8 Massage therapy for back pain

long-term effectiveness. There is stronger evidence for some approaches as indicated below:

- Spinal manipulation and neck exercises have a positive effect on cervicogenic headache.[39]
- Physiotherapist-directed exercise and advice have significant beneficial effects on pain and function in people with subacute low back pain at 6 weeks but with only a small effect on function at 12 months.[40]
- Massage has a positive effect in low back pain that is maintained for at least 12 months.[41]
- Heat is effective for the relief of acute low back pain.[42]
- Exercise, spinal manipulation and interdisciplinary rehabilitation are effective for chronic and subacute low back pain.[43]
- Physical conditioning programs that include a cognitive behavioural approach plus intensive physical training are effective in reducing disability associated with chronic back pain.[44]
- Yoga has been demonstrated to be superior to exercise and a self-care book in the treatment of low back pain.[44]
- One study demonstrated a positive short-term effect of therapeutic touch on tension-type headache.[45]

Chiropractic and osteopathy are widely used treatments in the management of spinal pain. However, there is very little research that compares the two techniques or other forms of spinal manipulation.

- As indicated above, there is evidence that spinal manipulation may be beneficial in the treatment of cervicogenic headache and chronic and subacute low back pain.
- There are reports of worsening disc protrusion or cauda equina syndrome following low back manipulation, but these are extremely rare and serious adverse events have been reported to be as low as 1 per 1 million visits.[42]
- Rotational cervical manipulation may be associated with vertebral artery dissection. Although the incidence is very low, it may be associated with serious and permanent disability and the potential benefit does not appear to justify the risk.

As mentioned previously, the experience of pain is 'holistic' in that every part of our mental, emotional and physical make-up is affected when we experience chronic pain. Therefore the management of chronic pain needs to address the mind as well as the body. For this reason, mind–body practices such as mindfulness, hypnosis and relaxation therapies (see Box 38.7) can reduce hypervigilance, arousal and reactivity, and reduce anxiety or depression by helping to gently shift the focus of attention. Such adjunctive techniques have excellent long-term effects in the management of chronic pain and related symptoms for those who are motivated to use them.[46–48]

Mood is often affected by the presence of persistent pain and may need to be addressed by use of anti-depressant or anxiolytic medications and cognitive behavioural approaches. Several cognitive, behavioural or mind–body approaches, including those listed below, have been demonstrated to be effective in reducing pain.

- Cognitive behavioural interventions that focus on building coping strategies such as reducing fear avoidance or catastrophising, and may take the form of individual counselling or intensive group interventions, generally have a significant impact on functional outcomes such as medication use, mood, activity levels and sleep, with less impact on pain levels,[49] and there is good evidence of

BOX 38.7 Psychological treatments

- Relaxation techniques, e.g. progressive muscle relaxation, breathing techniques
- Attentional techniques, e.g. imagery, music
- Meditation, e.g. mindfulness meditation, transcendental meditation
- Hypnosis, self-hypnosis
- Humour
- Distraction, desensitisation
- Cognitive behaviour therapy—group or individual
- Education—therapist-directed education, self-education and self-management
- Psychotherapy
- Biofeedback

moderate efficacy in chronic and subacute low back pain.[42]

- Education regarding surgical procedures, including the nature of the procedure and the likely experience of pain, may be helpful.[50]
- Relaxation techniques such as progressive muscle relaxation and self-hypnosis may be effective in reducing pain.[51]
- Meditation, including techniques such as mindfulness meditation, may be useful in helping patients to cope with chronic pain.[46] Its mode of action may be by reducing the preoccupation/hypervigilance and hyperreactivity that often accompany chronic pain.
- Hypnosis may reduce acute pain and labour pain.[38]
- Attentional techniques such as imagery or focusing on the sensory rather than emotional aspects of the pain.[52]
- Music reduces pain intensity in acute pain.[53]

SPIRITUAL

There is wide variation in understanding as to what constitutes a spiritual approach to treatment (see Box 38.8), and very little evidence regarding the effectiveness of most treatments. Some people use the term to refer to treatments such as reiki, therapeutic touch or prayer that are believed to have a spiritual quality even when they are used simply with the aim of producing physical healing and symptomatic relief. On the other hand, spiritual approaches may refer to treatments or activities that are engaged in with the aim of addressing a person at a deeper, 'spiritual' level and trying to build qualities such as meaning, courage, gratitude and hope. For example, some people may find that music, art or a relationship with a higher power develops these qualities and gives them strength. People in pain can feel that they no longer have a meaningful purpose if activities and relationships they valued as important are lost or affected. It may be helpful to work with the person to develop a purpose beyond their pain which they recognise as meaningful. Using a spiritual approach then may include the process of identifying and fostering relationships and activities which strengthen a person's spirit and provide the person with a purpose that again brings meaning and hope to their life. As mentioned previously, pain and suffering can actually be positive things by providing the person with the catalyst for change, and many people can emerge from pain and suffering with a deeper sense of meaning, strength and purpose.

BOX 38.8 Spiritual approaches to pain management

- Spiritual healing practices (e.g. therapeutic touch, prayer)
- Activities that a person finds spiritually moving (e.g. music, art therapy)
- Looking to a 'higher power' for spiritual strength
- Developing 'spiritual' qualities (e.g. gratitude, forgiveness, courage)
- Re-evaluation of meaning and purpose

SURGERY

Surgery has a major role in the treatment of pain, although results are usually poorer when the primary criterion for surgery is pain relief. Outcomes studies indicate that at 12 months there is little advantage of surgery over conservative management in the treatment of low back and sciatica.[54] Therefore, while surgery may be indicated for those with severe pain, continuing neurological compromise and disability despite intensive conservative treatment, these studies suggest that the long-term outcomes between the two groups are similar. In addition, further surgical intervention in people with chronic back pain results in a decreasing likelihood of success with possible complications such as epidural fibrosis. Therefore, the promise of pain relief with re-operation is fraught with danger.

OTHER MEDICAL AND PARAMEDICAL APPROACHES

Because of the multifactorial nature of pain, treatment is often heavily reliant on input from other healthcare professionals. The treatment of pain, and chronic pain in particular, will often benefit from assessment and treatment in an interdisciplinary setting. Pain management centres can provide a comprehensive assessment with input from appropriately qualified practitioners such as rheumatologists, psychiatrists, neurologists, anaesthetists, physiotherapists, occupational therapists, clinical psychologists, social workers, nurses and other specialties that have expertise in the underlying condition that may be giving rise to the pain. A comprehensive assessment may help to provide a holistic treatment plan that addresses the many factors involved in the pain problem. This can help to avoid the expense, frustration and disappointment that sometimes occur when people seek out a long list of various practitioners in the hope of finding the person who is going to take away their pain.

SELF-MANAGEMENT

Chronic pain is increasingly moving towards a self-management approach. Education by the primary care physician should encourage the person with chronic pain to manage the pain by themselves. Resources such as the book *Manage Your Pain*[55] are available which provide the patient with active coping strategies to assist them to manage chronic pain effectively, with reduced reliance on healthcare professionals and medications. Other resources such as patient information sheets on acute low back pain and other acute musculoskeletal pain problems are available and can be downloaded from the National Health and Medical Research Council of Australia website (see the Resources list below).

LIFESTYLE

The management of chronic pain is strongly dependent on lifestyle choices. Although many people with chronic pain limit their activities because of pain, many also make these limitations because of unnecessary fear avoidance, inaccurate advice or unrealistic expectations of pain relief. This inactivity results in increasing deconditioning and associated health problems such as weight gain, depression and hypertension. Once adequate investigations to determine the cause of pain have been done and appropriate treatments trialled, people with chronic pain should be encouraged to commit to a graduated exercise and activity program that is initially set at a reasonable level but with a realistic goal. People should be encouraged to reach their goal despite the presence of pain.

ONGOING REVIEW

Although there is little evidence to support the best approach to the ongoing management of people with persistent pain, best outcomes may be achieved by regular scheduled visits with the primary care practitioner. Having scheduled visits may help to reduce anxiety, reduce the overall number of visits, minimise the number of emergency calls and help to change the focus to self-management rather than dependency on the practitioner to deal with crises. This approach may be more beneficial to the person in managing their pain effectively as well as more satisfying for the practitioner, who becomes more of a partner in dealing with the pain than someone who is called on to get rid of the pain when it reaches intolerable levels.

CANCER PAIN: SPECIFIC ISSUES

Many of the issues raised above are applicable to the person with cancer who has pain, and many of the approaches are used in common. Despite many people's fears, a large number of cancers are not necessarily associated with severe pain. However, there are several distinctive features about the person with cancer pain, including the following:

- Pain may be due to the cancer itself because of direct invasion and organ involvement. However, in about 20% of cases, pain is due to cancer treatment such as surgery-related trauma or nerve injury following irradiation or chemotherapy.
- Pain itself may be associated with different emotions in the person with cancer or previously diagnosed cancer. It may arouse fears of disease recurrence and progression and therefore may hold much stronger overtones.
- Although it is also important that the person with cancer manages and copes with their pain, limited life expectancy usually means a greater emphasis on pain relief rather than pain management. Some people with cancer are still concerned about becoming drug addicts or that they will have nothing left in reserve 'when the pain gets really bad'. People with cancer should be reassured about the almost nonexistent likelihood of psychological dependence, the availability of appropriate medications even when the pain is severe, and the positive aspects of being able to live with low levels of pain even when the outlook is poor.
- In practice this means that people with cancer pain are usually treated more aggressively with much higher doses of opioids if required and possibly more invasive procedures such as parenteral or spinal administration of drugs. Even neuroablative procedures, which have virtually no place in the treatment of the person with chronic non-cancer pain, may be considered in the person with severe pain and limited life expectancy.
- Opioids remain the mainstay of pharmacological treatment for moderate to severe pain. However, as with other types of chronic non-cancer pain, other medications that are appropriate to the underlying pathology, such as NSAIDs and anti-neuropathic medications, should be used where an inflammatory or neuropathic component is believed to be present. A simple analgesic such as paracetamol may still be appropriate even with high doses of opioid because of its complementary mode of action. The WHO ladder[56] remains a standard approach to the use of pharmacological agents.
- Other psychosocial issues that may be specific to cancer need to be considered. For example,

facing the end of life raises many issues such as acceptance, grief, fear of death, unresolved relationship issues and questions of faith. Some of these may also influence the experience of pain. Being aware of issues that are important to the individual who is suffering from pain and dealing with them appropriately may make a huge difference to the quality of a person's last years, months and days.

RESOURCES

Berman BM. Integrative approaches to pain management: how to get the best of both worlds. BMJ 2003; 326(7402):1320–1321.

Handbook for Health Professionals. Ch 17, Managing chronic pain. Department of Health and Ageing. Online. Available: http://www.aodgp.gov.au/internet/aodgp/publishing.nsf/content/pain-1

National Health & Medical Research Council (NHMRC). Evidence-based management of acute musculoskeletal pain. Online. Available: http://www.nhmrc.gov.au/publications/synopses/cp94syn.htm

National Health & Medical Research Council (NHMRC). Acute pain management: scientific evidence. Online. Available: http://www.nhmrc.gov.au/publications/synopses/cp104syn.htm

Nicholas MK, Molloy A, Beeston L et al. *Manage your pain.* Sydney: ABC Books; 2007.

Patel G, Euler D, Audette JF. Complementary and alternative medicine for non-cancer pain. Med Clin North Am 2007; 91(1):141–167.

Therapeutic guidelines: Analgesic. Version 5. Melbourne: Therapeutic Guidelines Ltd; 2007.

REFERENCES

1 Blyth FM, March LM, Brnabic AJM et al. Chronic pain in Australia: a prevalence study. Pain 2001; 89: 127–134.

2 Siddall PJ, Cousins MJ. Persistent pain as a disease entity: implications for clinical management. Anesth Analg 2004; 99(2):510–520.

3 Turk DC. The role of psychological factors in chronic pain. Acta Anaesthesiol Scand 1999; 43:885–888.

4 Singer T, Seymour B, O'Doherty J et al. Empathy for pain involves the affective but not sensory components of pain. Science 2004; 303(5661):1157–1162.

5 Eriksen HR, Ursin H. Subjective health complaints, sensitization, and sustained cognitive activation (stress). J Psychom Res 2004; 56(4):445–448.

6 Ursin H, Eriksen HR. Sensitization, subjective health complaints, and sustained arousal. Ann NY Acad Sci 2001; 933:119–129.

7 Elias AN, Wilson AF. Serum hormonal concentrations following transcendental meditation—potential role of gamma aminobutyric acid. Med Hypotheses 1995; 44(4):287–291.

8 Harte JL, Eifert GH, Smith R. The effects of running and meditation on beta-endorphin, corticotrophin-releasing hormone and cortisol in plasma, and on mood. Biol Psychol 1995; 40(3):251–265.

9 Rippentrop AE, Altmaier EM, Chen JJ et al. The relationship between religion/spirituality and physical health, mental health, and pain in a chronic pain population. Pain 2005; 116(3):311–321.

10 Jensen MC, Brant-Zawadzki MN, Obuchowski N et al. Magnetic resonance imaging of the lumbar spine in people without back pain. N Engl J Med 1994; 331:69–73.

11 Schellhas KP, Smith MD, Gundry CR et al. Cervical discogenic pain: prospective correlation of magnetic resonance imaging and discography in asymptomatic subjects and pain sufferers. Spine 1996; 21:300–312.

12 Koes BW, van Tulder MW, Peul WC. Diagnosis and treatment of sciatica. BMJ 2007; 334(7607): 1313–1317.

13 LaBorde TC. Reimbursement for unproven therapies: the case of thermography. JAMA 1993; 270(21):2558–2559.

14 Rommel O, Habler H-J, Schurmann M. Laboratory tests for complex regional pain syndrome. In: Wilson P, Stanton-Hicks M, Harden RN, eds. CRPS: current diagnosis and therapy, progress in pain research and management, Vol. 32. Seattle: IASP Press; 2005.

15 de Jager JP, Ahern MJ. Improved evidence-based management of acute musculoskeletal pain: guidelines from the National Health and Medical Research Council are now available. Med J Aust 2004; 181(10):527–528.

16 Patel G, Euler D, Audette JF. Complementary and alternative medicine for noncancer pain. Med Clin North Am 2007; 91(1):141–167.

17 Chrubasik S, Eisenberg E, Balan E et al. Treatment of low back pain exacerbations with willow bark extract: a randomized double-blind study. Am J Med 2000; 109(1):9–14.

18 Gagnier JJ, vanTulder M, Berman B et al. Herbal medicine for low back pain. Cochrane Database Syst Rev 2006; 2:CD004504.

19 Clegg DO, Reda DJ, Harris CL et al. Glucosamine, chondroitin sulfate, and the two in combination for painful knee osteoarthritis. N Engl J Med 2006; 354(8):795–808.

20 Altman RD, Marcussen KC. Effects of a ginger extract on knee pain in patients with osteoarthritis. Arthritis Rheum 2001; 44(11):2531–2538.

21 Soeken KL. Selected CAM therapies for arthritis-related pain: the evidence from systematic reviews. Clin J Pain 2004; 20(1):13–18.

22 Little CV, Parsons T, Logan S. Herbal therapy for treating osteoarthritis. Cochrane Database Syst Rev 2001; 1:CD002947.

23 Fortin P, Lew R, Liang M et al. Validation of a meta-analysis: the effects of fish oil in rheumatoid arthritis. J Clin Epidemiol 1995; 48(11):1379–1390.

24 Pittler MH, Ernst E. Peppermint oil for irritable bowel syndrome: a critical review and meta-analysis. Am J Gastroenterol 1998; 93(7):1131–1135.

25 Gokhale L. Curative treatment of primary (spasmodic) dysmenorrhoea. Indian J Med Res 1996; 103:227–231.

26 Proctor ML, Murphy PA. Herbal and dietary therapies for primary and secondary dysmenorrhoea. Cochrane Database Syst Rev 2001; 3:CD002124.

27 Department of Health and Ageing. Substance abuse assessment. A manual of mental health care in general practice; 2003. Online. Available: http://www.health.gov.au/internet/main/publishing.nsf/Content/mental-pubs-m-mangp-toc~mental-pubs-m-mangp-18~mental-pubs-m-mangp-18-as

28 Dworkin RH, O'Connor AB, Backonja M et al. Pharmacologic management of neuropathic pain: evidence-based recommendations. Pain 2007; 132(3):237–251.

29 Proctor ML, Smith CA, Farquhar CM et al. Transcutaneous electrical nerve stimulation and acupuncture for primary dysmenorrhoea. Cochrane Database Syst Rev 2002; 1:CD002123.

30 Bjordal J, Johnson M, Lopes-Martins R et al. Short-term efficacy of physical interventions in osteoarthritic knee pain. A systematic review and meta-analysis of randomised placebo-controlled trials. BMC Musculoskelet Disord 2007; 8(1):51.

31 Chow RT, Heller GZ, Barnsley L. The effect of 300 mW, 830 nm laser on chronic neck pain: a double-blind, randomized, placebo-controlled study. Pain 2006; 124(1/2):201–210.

32 Smith CA, Collins CT, Cyna AM et al. Complementary and alternative therapies for pain management in labour. Cochrane Database Syst Rev 2006; 4:CD003521.

33 Melchart D, Linde K, Fischer P et al. Acupuncture for idiopathic headache. Cochrane Database Syst Rev 2001; 1:CD001218.

34 Berman BM, Ezzo J, Hadhazy V et al. Is acupuncture effective in the treatment of fibromyalgia? J Fam Pract 1999; 48(3):213–218.

35 Guerra de Hoyos JA, Andres Martin MdC, Bassas y Baena de Leon E et al. Randomised trial of long term effect of acupuncture for shoulder pain. Pain 2004; 112(3):289–298.

36 Trinh KV, Phillips SD, Ho E et al. Acupuncture for the alleviation of lateral epicondyle pain: a systematic review. Rheumatology 2004; 43(9):1085–1090.

37 Trinh KV, Graham N, Gross AR et al. Acupuncture for neck disorders. Cochrane Database Syst Rev 2006; 3:CD004870.

38 Furlan AD, van Tulder M, Cherkin D et al. Acupuncture and dry-needling for low back pain: an updated systematic review within the framework of the Cochrane collaboration. Spine 2005; 30(8): 944–963.

39 Jull G, Trott P, Potter H et al. A randomized controlled trial of exercise and manipulative therapy for cervicogenic headache. Spine 2002; 27(17):1835–1843.

40 Pengel LHM, Refshauge KM, Maher CG et al. Physiotherapist-directed exercise, advice, or both for subacute low back pain: a randomized trial. Ann Intern Med 2007; 146(11):787–796.

41 Cherkin DC, Eisenberg D, Sherman KJ et al. Randomized trial comparing traditional Chinese medical acupuncture, therapeutic massage, and self-care education for chronic low back pain. Arch Intern Med 2001; 161(8):1081–1088.

42 Chou R, Huffman LH, American Pain Society et al. Nonpharmacologic therapies for acute and chronic low back pain: a review of the evidence for an American Pain Society/American College of Physicians clinical practice guideline. Ann Intern Med 2007; 147(7): 492–504.

43 Schonstein E, Kenny DT, Keating J et al. Work conditioning, work hardening and functional restoration for workers with back and neck pain. Cochrane Database Syst Rev 2003; 1:CD001822.

44 Sherman KJ, Cherkin DC, Erro J et al. Comparing yoga, exercise, and a self-care book for chronic low back pain: a randomized, controlled trial. Ann Intern Med 2005; 143(12):849–856.

45 Keller E, Bzdek V. Effects of therapeutic touch on tension headache pain. Nurs Res 1986; 35(2):101–106.

46 Kabat-Zinn J, Lipworth L, Burney R. The clinical use of mindfulness meditation for the self-regulation of chronic pain. J Behav Med 1985; 8(2):163–190.

47 Carmody J, Baer RA. Relationships between mindfulness practice and levels of mindfulness, medical and psychological symptoms of well-being in a mindfulness-based stress reduction program. J Behav Med 2008; 31(1):23–33.

48 Gonsalkorale WM, Miller V, Afzal A et al. Long-term benefits of hypnotherapy for irritable bowel sundrome. Gut 2003; 52(11):1623–1629.

49 Morley S, Eccleston C, Williams AC. Systematic review and meta-analysis of randomized controlled trials of cognitive behaviour therapy and behaviour therapy for chronic pain in adults, excluding headache. Pain 1999; 80:1–13.

50 Suls J, Wan C. Effects of sensory and procedural information on coping with stressful medical

procedures and pain: a meta-analysis. J Consult Clin Psychol 1989; 57(3):372–379.
51 Luebbert K, Dahme B, Hasenbring M. The effectiveness of relaxation training in reducing treatment-related symptoms and improving emotional adjustment in acute non-surgical cancer treatment: a meta-analytical review. Psycho-Oncology 2001; 10(6):490–502.
52 Miro J, Raich RM. Effects of a brief and economical intervention in preparing patients for surgery: does coping style matter? Pain 1999; 83(3):471–475.
53 Cepeda MS, Carr DB, Lau J et al. Music for pain r elief. Cochrane Database Syst Rev 2006; 2:CD004843.
54 Peul WC, van Houwelingen HC, van den Hout WB et al. Surgery versus prolonged conservative treatment for sciatica. N Engl J Med 2007; 356(22):2245–2256.
55 Nicholas MK, Molloy A, Beeston L et al. Manage your pain. Sydney: ABC Books; 2007.
56 World Health Organization. Cancer pain relief. Geneva: WHO; 1986.

chapter 39

Palliative medicine

INTRODUCTION AND OVERVIEW

In the mind of the general public, palliative care is commonly equated with terminal care, and many members of the medical community no doubt share this opinion. Traditionally, palliative care has predominantly provided service to cancer patients and their families. However, the role of palliative care is much richer and more varied than this. Palliative care principles can readily be applied to many incurable diseases as they become more severe, and can also be useful in the management of symptoms during the earlier stages of disease.

Palliative care, at its best, is provided by a team of individuals working towards common goals for a particular patient. The team may include doctors, nurses, allied healthcare staff, counsellors and family members. Symptom control, achievement of optimal quality of life and assistance with decision-making are all components of palliative care that can be provided by the general practitioner (GP). The critical role of the GP in the coordination of patient care is particularly pronounced for patients with advanced disease. Furthermore, a GP who has known a patient for much of their life is likely to have worthwhile insight into their values and wishes, and is well placed to assist them in negotiating difficult transitions.

GOALS OF CARE

It is often helpful to establish and focus upon the goals of care for a patient. These will be influenced by the nature and stage of the disease, the age of the patient, their general health and their life philosophy. As cancer progresses, the situation may become more complex and decisions may seem increasingly difficult. It is helpful at these times to return the focus to the goals of care and reflect on the outcome that we are trying to achieve. This will assist in more clearly identifying a pathway that is likely to accomplish these objectives. The GP should take an active role in reviewing the overall situation and incorporating a holistic understanding of their patient.

For example, a 55-year-old woman first confronted with a diagnosis of breast cancer is likely to elect to pursue chemotherapy if this is advised. She will consider the temporary side effects, reduction in quality of life and time taken to attend therapy to be worthwhile in view of the potential benefits. An 83-year-old woman with multiple other medical issues resulting in some frailty will often be more susceptible to adverse effects of routine chemotherapy for breast cancer. She may find the effort required to attend clinics, undergo invasive investigations or procedures and the time taken to recover from each cycle of chemotherapy to be an unacceptable trade-off for the potential benefits, which in all probability will be of a lesser magnitude.

Many important decisions may need to be made by a person confronted with a life-limiting illness. For an excellent and practical guideline on how to approach this, the reader is referred to Clayton & Hancock, 'Clinical practice guidelines for communicating prognosis and end-of-life issues with adults in the advanced stages of a terminal illness, and their caregivers', published as a supplement in the *Medical Journal of Australia*.[1]

CARING FOR THE WHOLE PERSON

Nowhere is integrated and holistic care more important than when dealing with death and dying. Obviously the physical aspects of care need to be attended to, and dealing with various symptoms will be dealt with in detail in this chapter. Obvious also is the impact of emotional, social and spiritual/existential aspects involved in confronting end-of-life issues.

A deep-seated fear of dying, for example, or long-standing and unresolved guilt can have an enormous impact on how a patient deals with physical pain. It is not uncommon for deeper emotional and existential issues to influence and magnify such symptoms. If physical treatments only are administered (e.g. prescribing escalating doses of pain killers) but the underlying emotional and existential issues are not acknowledged or dealt with, then the problem of pain will likely be unsolvable, whereas if these deeper issues are dealt with well, the pain will often be far more manageable.

Most patients confronting life-threatening illnesses wish to speak to their medical team about spiritual and religious issues (see Ch 12, Spirituality). Whether the doctor provides such counselling or helps to link the patient with counsellors, pastoral care and allied healthcare professionals, one way or another this aspect of care needs to take place and not be ignored among the more obvious and apparently more pressing physical needs.

At all times one needs to also bear in mind that it is the whole family who will be experiencing the grief and anxiety associated with the illness—sometimes far more grief and anxiety that the patient, who may already have come to terms with their situation.

THE ROLE OF COMPLEMENTARY THERAPIES

The frequency of complementary therapy use by cancer patients may be as high as 83%[2] (see Ch 24, Cancer). This includes herbal medicines, music therapy and physical therapies such as acupuncture, among others. Patients use these therapies to improve symptoms, in the hope of curing cancer or increasing survival, and as a response to pressure from family or friends.[3] It is certainly reasonable to encourage the use of those therapies that are proving helpful to the patient without causing undue hardship or interfering with conventional treatment. Some incur a considerable cost with little or no benefit, and occasionally there may be a risk of the therapy interfering with conventional medical care or causing harm to the patient. For example, many herbs can interact with drugs such as warfarin. The GP has an important role in discussing the use of such therapies with the patient.

PAIN

Pain is a complex experience involving specific neural pathways that convey nociceptive information to consciousness. Neuronal systems also exist that modify pain—for example, descending inhibitory pathways in the central nervous system. This chapter focuses mainly on cancer pain, but many of the principles can be applied to non-malignant pain in patients with advanced or near end-stage disease. Chronic pain, while sharing some features, requires important differences in approach and is not discussed here (see Ch 38, Pain management).

Pain is common is cancer and more so in advanced malignancy, with 70–90% of patients reporting pain.[4] It is also common in the elderly (28–86% of nursing home residents[5]) and in those with other chronic disease (e.g. 40% of patients with Parkinson's disease). As such, competent assessment and management of pain is a crucial skill for GPs.

The most effective approach to cancer pain requires consideration of the pathophysiology as well as the aetiology of the pain.

PATHOPHYSIOLOGY

Pathophysiology is important, as the different pain types respond differently to specific medications and thus can guide therapy.

- *Somatic pain* is caused by activation of peripheral nociceptors in response to inflammation or injury of surrounding tissues. Examples include bone metastases, arthritic pain and burn injury.
- *Visceral pain* occurs when nociceptors in thoracic or abdominal viscera are activated by infiltration, distension or compression of the organ. Liver metastases or bowel obstruction are examples.
- *Neuropathic pain* results from direct injury to the peripheral or central nervous system, such as peripheral neuropathy, spinal cord compression or cancer infiltration of a neural plexus.

It is common for cancer patients to have mixed somatic and neuropathic pain, for example when a rib metastasis causes bone pain and also has a neuropathic element by involving the intercostal nerve.

In addition, pain can also be classified on the basis of 'timing'. *Incident pain* describes pain that occurs with movement; *breakthrough pain* refers to pain that 'breaks through' otherwise adequate levels of analgesia.

AETIOLOGY

In patients with cancer, pain may be:

- cancer-related—e.g. bone metastasis, infiltration of nerves or organs
- treatment-related—e.g. mucositis secondary to chemotherapy-induced neutropenia
- non-cancer-related—e.g. coexisting osteoarthritis.

HISTORY AND EXAMINATION

Careful history and examination can often assist in determining the likely pathophysiology and aetiology of a patient's pain. The history will focus on the qualities, temporal features and other descriptive features of the pain. Details such as location, duration, onset, offset, relieving and exacerbating features should be elicited, along with a description of pain quality. It is clearly important to enquire about other symptoms such as nausea and vomiting, history of a recent fall, previous treatments and so on.

- Somatic pain descriptors include dull, constant, aching. Pain is usually well localised. This pain responds well to simple analgesics and to opioids.
- Visceral pain may have a gnawing, colicky or cramping character, feels deep and is less well localised. Be aware that visceral pain may be referred to other sites, e.g. shoulder tip pain from liver metastases, central abdominal pain from early appendicitis.
- Neuropathic pain may be described as burning, shooting or constricting, and often has a particularly unpleasant character. It can occur in paroxysms with or without a more constant component. Neuropathic pain may be felt in a dermatomal or peripheral nerve distribution. Features such as anaesthesia or allodynia strongly suggest an element of neuropathic pain.

The focus of the examination will be determined by the specifics of the pain and the patient's previous history, but a general approach should include:

- overview of the patient—are they confused, markedly cachexic, dehydrated?
- a careful examination of the affected area, looking for tenderness, signs of deformity, infection, presence of a mass, loss of function and so on
- neurological examination to elicit any weakness or sensory abnormality, as it is possible that the patient will not have noticed these or recognised their importance.

INVESTIGATIONS

It is not possible to cover the scope of investigations that may be relevant. Some form of radiological imaging is generally useful to accurately determine the cause of the problem, but initiation of good analgesia should not be delayed while waiting for these results. In appropriate clinical circumstances, a variety of other investigations such as a full blood count, urine culture or calcium level will be indicated.

INTEGRATIVE MANAGEMENT

- Prevention—not realistic in the conventional sense, but severe, ongoing problems may potentially be minimised if pain is addressed promptly and effectively. For example, rapid initiation of therapy for shingles can reduce the incidence of postherpetic neuralgia.[6]
- Evaluation—in all cases, pain should be adequately evaluated. Some patients will choose not to pursue intervention but these are a minority, with relatively low levels of pain and greater general wellbeing.
- Self-help, lifestyle, home remedies—some strategies that patients are able to use in order to relieve pain include the use of heat or cold packs, resting the affected area (not always possible) and various relaxation strategies.

Non-pharmacological

- Transcutaneous electrical nerve stimulation (TENS) machines are useful for some patients, often as part of a comprehensive pain management strategy.
- Complementary therapies have a role in pain management, in providing analgesia and in raising the pain threshold.
  - Acupuncture is increasingly being used in pain management, including by GPs. Limited evidence is available regarding its use in advanced cancer, although various reviews of the literature conclude that benefit is likely.[7,8]
  - Massage appears to be of some benefit in reducing pain and the anxiety associated with it. However, in some groups the benefit appears to be short-lived.[9] A recent Cochrane review stated that overall there was insufficient evidence to draw firm conclusions about the benefit of massage.[10] The addition of aromatherapy was not shown to provide any additional benefit.
  - Music therapy is available through various avenues, including community palliative care services. It has been shown to reduce pain in cancer patients.[2,11]
  - Other strategies employed by patients include hypnotherapy, meditation, relaxation and imagery. Trials are not consistent in demonstrating benefit.

Pharmacological

The choice of agent will depend on:

- pain severity
- likely aetiology of the pain
- presumed mechanism of pain (somatic, neuropathic etc)
- analgesics already tried
- patient preferences, fears and allergies.

Generally, analgesia for cancer pain should be given:

- orally
- around the clock rather than 'as required'
- in adequate doses—using a combination of drugs may enable lower doses of each drug to be used, with fewer side effects.

Simple analgesics

- Paracetamol—the precise mechanism of action remains uncertain, although it may act on a cyclo-

oxygenase enzyme (COX-3) only present in the brain. It can provide useful analgesia alone for mild pain or in combination with other agents for more severe pain. Newer preparations enable 8-hourly dosing to provide 24 hours of cover. Maximum doses should not be exceeded.
- NSAIDs—these have a particular role when the possibility of an inflammatory component to the pain exists, for example with bone metastases, cellulitis, thrombophlebitis. The side-effect profile should always be considered when using NSAIDs.
- Tramadol—this agent acts on multiple neurotransmitters, including weak affinity for the opioid receptor.

BOX 39.1 Case study: opioid titration

Mr P is a 72-year-old man with pain due to metastatic colon cancer. In addition to simple analgesics he requires an opioid to adequately manage his pain. He is commenced on slow-release (SR) morphine 15 mg 12-hourly as baseline analgesia with immediate release (IR) morphine mixture 2.5–5 mg as needed for breakthrough pain ($^1/_{12}$ to $^1/_6$ of 24-hour baseline dose). Aperients are prescribed prophylactically.

On review 3 days later he has consistently required 4–5 doses/24 hours of 2.5 mg morphine in order to control his pain, representing ~20 mg additional morphine. His baseline SR morphine is therefore increased to 25 mg 12-hourly with good effect. Thereafter he requires few additional doses.

Opioids

Opioids are the mainstay of cancer pain management. They are particularly useful for somatic and visceral pain, as well as having an important role in neuropathic pain. The reader is referred to other textbooks for more in-depth advice on use of opioids in cancer pain. Some basic principles are listed here.
- In the elderly particularly, start low, go slow.
- Opioids should be used around the clock rather than 'prn'. This has become much easier with the availability of slow-release preparations of morphine, oxycodone, fentanyl and so on.
- Injectable opioids have no advantage over oral where the patient is able to swallow and has a functioning gut.
- Provide 'breakthrough' medications to deal with exacerbations of pain. Ensure that these are rapid-acting rather than slow-acting. The breakthrough dose is approximately one-tenth of the total 24-hour baseline dose (see the example in Box 39.1; see Table 39.1 for conversions). The dose may need to be rounded to, for practical reasons.
- Calibrate the dose (see the example in Box 39.1).
- Avoid constipation. Most patients will experience constipation with opioids (although there is a lower frequency with fentanyl). Prescribe regular laxatives at the same time as the opioids are prescribed.
- Be mindful of other common side effects, such as nausea (~30% initially) and drowsiness. Respiratory depression rarely, if ever, occurs without other signs of excessive dose, such as drowsiness.
- Patients must be warned that when opioids are commenced or increased, their ability to drive safely may be compromised. Once the dose is stable, patients can drive, provided they are not drowsy. They should be warned about additive effects of other sedative drugs, including alcohol, and advised not to drive if they use alcohol or other drugs.

Adjuvant agents

Adjuvant agents are particularly useful in neuropathic pain. The traditional classes of drugs that have efficacy are the anticonvulsants (carbamazepine, sodium valproate, gabapentin etc) and tricyclic antidepressants. Corticosteroids have an important role in spinal cord compression, nerve root compression and so on. There are a number of other drugs that are used to manage neuropathic pain but consultation with a pain or palliative medicine specialist is advised. All these agents have side effects and the potential for drug interactions, and some require monitoring of levels or other blood parameters. Their use should be individualised.

TABLE 39.1 Opioid conversion to morphine equivalent

	Conversion from oral morphine	10 mg oral morphine equivalent	30 mg oral morphine equivalent	100 mg oral morphine equivalent
Morphine oral	1:1	10 mg	30 mg	100 mg
Morphine parenteral	3:1	3.3 mg	10 mg	33 mg
Oxycodone	1.5–2:1	5–7.5 mg	15–20 mg	50–75 mg
Fentanyl topical	100:1	*12.5 µg/h patch	*12.5–25 µg/h patch	*25–50 µg/h patch

*Wide variation is observed between patients. The manufacturer provides quite conservative recommended conversions, with some variation from the above table.

- Radiotherapy, chemotherapy, surgery, antibiotics and so on may all have a role, depending on the cause of the pain. Many of these modalities will take some time to commence or for an effect to be seen, and so it is essential that analgesia is attended to simultaneously.
- Ongoing review is critical. Adequate control of pain requires ongoing efforts. Doses of drugs may need to be titrated to maximise effect and minimise side effects. Referral back to the treating specialist (medical oncologist, radiation oncologist or other) will be appropriate for many patients, but in the very late stages of disease, additional appointments, investigations and aggressive treatments may impose too great a burden on the patient. Advice from a palliative medicine physician or pain specialist may be appropriate.

PITFALLS

- Spinal cord compression—beware radicular pain, back pain or leg pain in a patient with known bone metastases! Approximately 90% of patients treated prior to developing weakness or paraplegia will retain independent mobility but this falls to 10% if they are unable to walk when treatment begins. Preserved continence is not reassuring.
- Continuing to escalate opioid dose without adequate response—this is a complex issue, but important concepts to consider are:
  - Could the pain be neuropathic or visceral in origin and therefore poorly responsive to opioids?
  - Are there psychosocial issues contributing to the distress, that could be dealt with?
  - Could there be an element of opioid toxicity?
  - Has there been diversion of the opioid?

Consultation with a palliative medicine specialist is strongly recommended. It is rare to achieve incremental analgesia with escalation of morphine above 1000 mg/24 h.

- Failure to prescribe aperients with opioids.
- Hypercalcaemia can present with pain as a symptom.

CONSTIPATION

Constipation may be defined in terms of frequency of defecation (< 3 times/week) or the passage of small, hard faeces with some difficulty. It is prevalent in chronic illness, particularly malignancy, affecting up to 63% of elderly inpatients. Many of the standard approaches to this common symptom are less helpful in the setting of advanced disease.

AETIOLOGY/PATHOLOGY

There are many factors that may contribute to the development of constipation in patients with cancer or other life-limiting disease. A common pathophysiological feature is slowed colonic transit time. Constipation may be a feature of the cancer itself, due to the general effects of advanced disease, a result of treatment or unrelated to the primary problem.

Cancer can cause constipation through intestinal obstruction, spinal cord or cauda equina compression and as a result of hypercalcaemia. Patients with advanced disease commonly have reduced food intake, particularly in relation to high-fibre foods, may be chronically dehydrated and suffer from generalised muscle weakness and tend to have reduced activity levels. These can all predispose to constipation.

Many medications cause constipation; most important in this context are the opioids, tricyclic antidepressants, other drugs with anticholinergic effects (e.g. hyoscine), iron supplements, certain chemotherapeutic agents (vinca alkaloids, thalidomide), diuretics, 5-HT_3 antagonists (ondansetron, tropisetron etc) and antacids. Comorbid conditions such as cerebrovascular disease may also contribute.

HISTORY AND EXAMINATION

History should include specific details of the symptoms, including:

- duration of symptoms—is this a long-term or recent complaint?
- onset—was it sudden (potentially implying bowel obstruction)?
- sensation of incomplete evacuation—suggests the presence of a rectal mass
- urge to defecate—absence may reflect damage to perineal nerves
- presence of blood.

Other important information includes:

- associated symptoms such as nausea, abdominal pain, bloating—specifically enquire about back pain, numbness and other symptoms that may suggest spinal cord/cauda equina compression
- medication list, including non-prescription items and complementary therapies—St John's wort, goldenseal, echinacea and shark cartilage are among the herbal remedies that are reported to cause constipation in some patients
- assessment of diet, activity, mood and general wellbeing
- strategies already undertaken by the patient to relieve constipation.

Abdominal and anorectal examination can provide much information, completed by a general examination. Specific features to be alert for are:

- presence of palpable abdominal and pelvic masses, due to either organomegaly, metastatic deposits or faecal loading

- bowel sounds—'tinkling' or absent sounds suggest bowel obstruction
- loss of anal tone, decreased perianal sensation—consider urgent referral for evaluation of spinal cord compression
- faeces or other masses in the rectum, anal fissures—note whether faeces are hard or soft
- general features, dehydration, weakness.

INVESTIGATIONS

Routine investigations are not required. If clinical findings are suggestive of bowel obstruction, plain abdominal X-ray can help to confirm this. Occasionally it may be useful to demonstrate the extent of faecal loading. With a suggestive clinical situation, calcium levels should be checked and, potentially, thyroid function. Suspicion of spinal cord compression should prompt urgent referral and investigation as appropriate.

INTEGRATIVE MANAGEMENT

Preventative measures consist of optimal symptom control, physical activity within the patient's limitations and maintaining adequate oral hydration. Patients with advanced disease are generally unable to consume sufficient fibre to reduce constipation, and use of fibre supplements without sufficient fluid intake can be counter-productive. Perhaps the most important preventative measure is to prescribe regular laxatives at the same time that an opioid is prescribed.

Not treating constipation is only a valid option in the very last days of life, as untreated constipation can cause severe discomfort and distress.

Many patients will be aware of particular foods or strategies that are of benefit. Some examples are licorice, beer or dried fruit. Natural therapies with demonstrated benefit include cascara, senna and pureed rhubarb.[12]

Pharmacological

Most patients, particularly those requiring opioid analgesia, will need laxatives to ease constipation. These should be taken regularly rather than 'as needed', with the dose titrated to maintain comfort. Laxatives can be classed as softening agents or peristaltic agents (Box 39.2), and the initial choice of drug can be guided by the predominant symptom—that is, hard faeces or faeces that are soft but difficult to pass. Bowel obstruction should be excluded prior to commencing laxatives, particularly the stimulants.

More recently available in Australia is methylnaltrexone bromide. This is a selective μ-opioid receptor antagonist, specifically targeted at the treatment of opioid-induced constipation. Because it has very limited capacity to cross the blood–brain barrier it is able to reverse the constipating effect of opioids in the bowel, without compromising analgesia. It is given as a subcutaneous injection and usually has a rapid onset of action, usually within 4 hours.[13]

Suppositories or enemas may be required, particularly when there is evidence of rectal loading or impaction, when oral therapy is not possible, or where a trial of oral laxatives has been unsuccessful. The mechanism of action is similar, with softening agents such as glycerine suppositories and stimulant agents such as bisacodyl Microlax™ (containing sodium citrate, sodium lauryl sulfoacetate and sorbitol) and sodium picosulfate.

BOX 39.2 Laxatives

Softening agents
- docusate
- sorbitol
- lactulose

Stimulants
- senna
- bisacodyl
- sodium picosulfate

Doses

Patients with advanced disease, particularly those requiring opioids for pain management, will require regular laxatives and commonly require higher than average doses. The aim of therapy is to ensure comfortable passage of faeces and relief of associated symptoms.

PITFALLS

- Faecal impaction with overflow presenting as diarrhoea.
- Failure to prescribe laxatives when opioids are commenced.

NAUSEA/VOMITING

Nausea is another symptom frequently encountered in general practice, occurring in a wide range of conditions including pregnancy (up to 80%) and myocardial infarction (50% experience nausea or vomiting). Between 40% and 70% of patients with advanced cancer are troubled by this symptom.

PATHOPHYSIOLOGY AND AETIOLOGY

Vomiting is controlled by the vomiting centre (VC), a number of adjacent, coordinated sites located in the lateral reticular formation of the medulla. The physiology of nausea is not as well understood but it may arise when stimuli excite the VC without sufficient amplification to trigger the vomiting cascade. A variety of neurotransmitters are involved at various sites, and knowledge of these can be exploited in order to target therapy (Table 39.2).

TABLE 39.2 Summary of nausea pathophysiology, aetiology and treatment

Site	Neurotransmitters	Examples of triggers*	Relevant antiemetic agents
CTZ	5-HT_3, D_2	Drugs (opioids, chemotherapy, NSAIDs, antibiotics), metabolic (hypercalcaemia, uraemia, infection)	Haloperidol, prochlorperazine, metoclopramide, domperidone
Vagal & SNS afferents	5-HT_4, D_2	Constipation, bowel obstruction, hepatomegaly, gastric outlet obstruction, gastritis	Haloperidol
Vestibular nucleii	M, H_1	Motion sickness	Cyclizine, promethazine
CNS	H_1	Raised ICP, anxiety, anticipatory nausea (prior to chemotherapy), cerebral lesion	Cyclizine, promethazine, corticosteroid (for raised ICP)
VC	5-HT_3, M, H_1		

*Particularly in advanced cancer.
CNS: central nervous system; CTZ: chemoreceptor trigger zone; ICP: intracranial pressure; SNS: sympathetic nervous system; VC: vomiting centre.

Inputs to the VC include the chemoreceptor trigger zone (CTZ), located in the floor of the fourth ventricle. An effective absence of the blood–brain barrier allows chemosensitive nerve cell endings direct contact with cerebrospinal fluid, which is in chemical equilibrium with blood. The relevant neurotransmitters are serotonin (5-HT_3) and dopamine (D_2). Vagal and sympathetic afferents are activated by gastric irritation, gastric distension, intestinal obstruction, constipation, liver disease and so on. Important neurotransmitters are 5-HT_4 and D_2. Vestibular nuclei activated by labyrinthitis, motion sickness and so on act via muscarinic (M) and histaminergic (H_1) neurotransmitters. Further input comes from the CNS (H_1) and is important in nausea induced by anxiety, fear, raised intracranial pressure, cerebral lesion, meningitis and the senses (taste, smell). Important neurotransmitters of the VC are H_1, M and 5-HT_3.

HISTORY

Obtain details from the patient when possible, in their own words. Consider frequency, volume and colour of vomitus. Does nausea precede vomiting? Have any triggers been identified? Enquire about the presence of other symptoms such as headache, dizziness, abdominal pain, constipation or features of anxiety. A complete list of medications, including non-prescribed and even illicit drugs, should be requested.

Various features can point to a possible cause:

- epigastric pain—gastritis
- small volume—squashed stomach
- very large volume—gastric stasis
- heartburn—reflux
- drowsy and confused—hypercalcaemia or raised ICP (e.g. due to cerebral metastases).

EXAMINATION

General examination needs to include vital signs, conscious state and an assessment of hydration. In the abdomen look for hepatomegaly, ascites, masses and a succussion splash. If the history raises the possibility of a CNS cause, a neurological examination is indicated.

INVESTIGATIONS

These should be tailored to the clinical situation but may reasonably include:

- electrolytes, including corrected or ionised calcium and estimation of renal function
- mid-stream urine examination (MSU).

The role of diagnostic imaging will depend not only on the particular symptoms but also on the overall condition of the patient and the goals of care. Transport to a radiology practice may not be in the best interests of patients who are particularly frail, who have very advanced disease or are confused, and where the clinical picture is unlikely to be clarified by available imaging. In other cases CT scanning of the brain or abdomen could be particularly helpful.

INTEGRATED MANAGEMENT

- Prevention of nausea and vomiting will be possible only in a limited number of circumstances, for example prior to emetogenic chemotherapy. Approximately one-third of patients who are prescribed morphine will experience nausea, often transiently, so routine prophylaxis is not generally recommended. It is reasonable to warn the patient that nausea can occur and even to provide a prescription for antiemetics, to be filled if required.
- Not actively treating nausea is seldom indicated, due to the unpleasant nature of the symptom.
- Self-help strategies can be of use. Some patients benefit from meditation, massage or other forms of

relaxation therapy, particularly in the setting of chemotherapy. Home remedies include the use of ginger preparations, cinnamon tea and peppermint.[12]
- A Cochrane review of acupuncture for chemotherapy-induced nausea and vomiting showed benefit in reducing acute vomiting but not acute or delayed nausea.[14] Acupuncture should be used in conjunction with antiemetics in this situation.
- Lifestyle measures include reducing activity after eating, reducing exposure to food smells, providing small portions of non-greasy food, and cold or warm rather than hot meals.

Pharmacological

Principles

1. Identify the likely cause of nausea and vomiting.
2. Identify the pathway and neurotransmitter involved.
3. Choose the most potent antagonist to the receptor identified. If several mechanisms are identified, choose the most potent for each one rather than one with several weak actions. It is also useful to identify previously helpful drugs.
4. Choose a route of administration that will ensure the drug reaches its site of action, e.g. 5-HT_3 antagonist wafers, rectal or IV administration.
5. Give antiemetics regularly and titrate the dose.
6. If symptoms persist, consider another cause.

Antiemetic drugs

- Dopamine antagonists—butyrophenones (haloperidol, droperidol), phenothiazines (prochlorperazine, chlorpromazine, levomepromazine (methotrimeprazine)). Starting dose of haloperidol may be as low as 0.25 mg b.i.d., titrate to 1.5–2.5 mg t.d.s.
- Prokinetics (metoclopramide and domperidone) act on D_2 and 5-HT_3 receptors.
- Antihistamines (cyclizine, promethazine)
- 5-HT_3 antagonists (ondansetron, tropisetron)
- Corticosteroids to reduce raised ICP.

Other management

Review other medications. If opioids are implicated, switching to another opioid can result in reduced nausea. Discussion with a palliative medicine specialist can be helpful in this situation and is recommended. Alternatives to selective serotonin reuptake inhibitors (SSRIs) may need to be considered. Digoxin doses often need to be reduced in frail patients.

Treat hypercalcaemia in appropriate circumstances. Once again, this may be unwarranted in very end-stage situations.

Treat underlying conditions such as infection or constipation. Referral back to treating specialists will be indicated for some patients, for example if raised ICP is suspected. Once again, the goals of care must be considered.

In refractory cases, such as persistent gastric outlet obstruction, it is sometimes necessary to resort to measures such as a nasogastric tube. Advice should be sought from a palliative medicine specialist.

PITFALLS

- Attempting to manage established vomiting with oral medications. A short course of parenteral therapy to gain control of vomiting is used, followed by oral antiemetics.
- Opioid-induced nausea responds well to D_2 antagonists. Another option is to change opioids, as patients vary in their susceptibility to nausea with different opioids.
- Drugs with prokinetic activity should be avoided when there is suspicion or evidence of bowel obstruction or gastric outlet obstruction.

ANOREXIA/CACHEXIA

Eating, food and meals are clearly much more than a means of sustenance. Joining family or friends at the table for dinner maintains social connections and has emotional benefits. There are also times when meals have particular cultural or religious significance. When a loved one is unable to enjoy specially prepared dishes, it can act as a harsh reminder of the toll taken by the disease. Some families will find this symptom intolerable and request that something be tried.

A cancer anorexia/cachexia syndrome has been described where:

- tissue wasting is out of proportion to anorexia
- fat loss is not preferential (as is the case with starvation) and
- supplemental feeding does not correct the weight loss.

Despite causing great distress to patients and their families, little is known about the pathophysiology of this condition.

Anorexia is common in advanced cancer, affecting up to 85% of patients. There are many contributing factors including (but not limited to) chronic nausea, constipation, dysphagia, infection, circulating cytokines, depression and altered taste. In cancer patients, the aetiology of anorexia is commonly multifactorial.

CLINICAL

A careful history and examination is required, aiming to detect the presence of treatable factors. Specific enquiry should be made about the presence of nausea, constipation, mouth pain, dysphagia and so on. Features indicative of depression or the presence of infection should also be sought (e.g. dysuria, productive cough, rigors) and a list of medications obtained.

Examination needs to be comprehensive. Note the presence and extent of wasting. Examine the mouth for evidence of mucositis or oral candidiasis, palpate for hepatomegaly or other abdominal masses that may be compressing the stomach. Consider any evidence of an infective process, such as fever, signs of pneumonia or cellulitis.

INVESTIGATIONS

There are few 'routine' investigations. The clinical findings will dictate the testing that should be done.

INTEGRATED MANAGEMENT

- Explanation to the patient and family is crucial. This may require a discussion of the possible causes contributing to the symptom in the individual patient, reassurance that the weight loss and reduced intake does not reflect poorly on the carer, and some practical advice. When a patient is in the last stages of their illness, further reassurance should be given that reduced appetite and intake is a normal part of the dying process and that it is rare for patients with advanced cancer to complain of being hungry. In the last stages, the most common symptom associated with inability to eat is a dry mouth. Patients and carers can be reassured that this can be readily managed with simple measures (mouth swabs, lip balm, small sips of water, grapeseed oil).
- Potentially reversible causes should be sought and treated (e.g. oral candidiasis, depression, constipation).
- Practical advice includes:
  - providing small portions of food more frequently
  - avoiding hot meals where the aromas can trigger nausea
  - identifying foods that the patient can manage most easily; for example, many patients find softer food (custard, yoghurt) or soups easier to digest
  - some patients find that a small amount of alcohol improves their appetite
  - sometimes an appropriate exercise program is useful.

Pharmacological measures

Several appetite stimulants have been proposed but few have proven benefit in rigorous trials. The available options are often limited in their utility due to limited efficacy and the presence of side effects.

- Corticosteroids, e.g. dexamethasone 4–8 mg daily:
  - May improve appetite, food intake, strength, performance status and wellbeing.
  - Do not improve survival.
  - There are many side effects (e.g. oral candidiasis, muscle weakness, fluid retention) and therefore if there is no benefit after 4–5 days, cease.
  - Benefits seem to be transient—2–6 weeks in most studies.
- Progestational agents:
  - Megestrol acetate is of benefit in patients with malignancy, although a Cochrane review in 2005 was unable to define the optimal dose.[15] It has many potential side effects, including deep vein thrombosis and fluid retention, and can be expensive for patients.
- Cannabinoids:
  - No benefit has been consistently demonstrated despite popular belief to the contrary. Side effects are troublesome, particularly in the elderly.
- Omega-3 fatty acids, especially eicosapentanoic acids:
  - There are data to suggest that these agents are of benefit. Most studies have focused on pancreatic cancer. However, a recent Cochrane review concluded that the evidence was insufficient to support the use of eicosapentanoic acids to treat cachexia in advanced cancer patients.[16]
  - They are thought to work by down-regulating pro-inflammatory cytokine and eicosanoid pathways.
  - The main difficulty in practice is with the palatability of the products.

Supplemental feeding

Many patients or families will wish to explore the possibility of supplemental feeding. The discussion needs to be handled sensitively but the salient points are as follows:

- Aggressive nutritional therapy does not significantly influence the outcome of patients with advanced cancer.
- No information is available to support or exclude improved quality of life with nutritional support in advanced cancer.
- It can make it more difficult for the patient to be cared for at home, particularly in the case of parenteral nutrition.
- There may be increased risk of infection or aspiration and, potentially, worsening of nausea.

Ongoing review

In the latter stages of disease, weighing the patient frequently is not recommended. Weight loss is often unavoidable, and repeated weighing merely reinforces the distress.

OTHER SYMPTOMS AND CARE IN THE LAST DAYS OF LIFE

Dyspnoea is a particularly difficult symptom to manage and often precipitates admission for inpatient care. A general approach would include assessment for readily reversible components (infection, new pleural effusion etc) and seeking advice from a palliative medicine specialist. Morphine and benzodiazepines are the mainstays of symptomatic management.

LAST DAYS OF LIFE

Many people express a wish to die at home, and support from a GP is a crucial part of assisting them to achieve this aim. Management in the terminal phase is dictated by attention to comfort and dignity, with the cessation of those treatments that no longer provide benefit or are no longer possible. Points to consider include the following:

- Cease unnecessary medications and interventions. Most drugs other than those directly providing symptom relief can be ceased—for example, antihypertensives, iron supplements, aspirin, antibiotics.
- Convert from oral to subcutaneous delivery where appropriate. The most common drugs required are opioid analgesics, benzodiazepines and antiemetics. Syringe drivers are a convenient method of providing continuous subcutaneous infusions, thereby obviating the need for regular injections in many situations. See Box 39.2 for a list of drugs that can be given subcutaneously.
- Provide a supply of medications that can be used if required, often by community nurses. Useful drugs include an injectable opioid, injectable antiemetic and a benzodiazepine, in either injectable or sublingual form (e.g. clonazepam drops).
- Accumulating oropharyngeal secretions occasionally cause noisy breathing or a 'death rattle'. The most important aspects of management are explanation to the family that this is not a painful symptom for the patient and the use of judicious positioning to minimise the noise. If medication is required, glycopyrrolate is preferred over hyoscine or atropine as it does not cross the blood–brain barrier and therefore does not risk precipitating a delirium. None of these agents will significantly reduce respiratory secretions in a patient with respiratory sepsis.
- The use of an indwelling catheter may be appropriate for some patients who find that activity exacerbates pain or who develop urinary retention.

BOX 39.2 Drugs used via the subcutaneous route in palliative care

Analgesics
- morphine
- oxycodone
- hydromorphone
- ketorolac

Antiemetics
- metoclopramide
- haloperidol
- cyclizine
- levomepromazine

Sedatives
- midazolam
- clonazepam

Other
- glycopyrrolate
- hyoscine hydrobromide
- hyoscine butylbromide
- dexamethasone

- Terminal restlessness or agitation represents an emergency situation due to the extremely distressing nature of this symptom for families. Reversible causes (e.g. urinary retention) should be excluded but otherwise pharmacological treatment is required. It may respond to relatively small doses of sedative but occasionally high doses are required, and resistant cases may require the use of agents such as levomepromazine (methotrimeprazine) or phenobarbitone. The aim is to control the distress without necessarily rendering the patient unconscious. Urgent consultation with a palliative care specialist is strongly urged.
- Mouthcare is an important aspect of terminal care. A dry mouth can be uncomfortable and distressing. This symptom can be readily managed with frequent sips of fluid or with drops of grapeseed oil applied as needed. This is cheaper and often more palatable than artificial saliva preparations.
- Supporting the family is a key aspect of care in the last days of life. They should be provided with explanations about common symptoms, what might be expected around the time of death and how to assist children at this time, as well as given opportunities to ask questions.

RESOURCES

CareSearch, palliative care knowledge network—an online resource of palliative care information and evidence, http://www.caresearch.com.au

Memorial Sloan Kettering Cancer Centre, http://www.mskcc.org

Memorial Sloan Kettering Cancer Centre, Integrative Medicine Service, http://www.mskcc.org/mskcc/html/1979.cfm

Palliative Care Australia—includes fact sheets, reports and a resource directory, http://www.pallcare.org.au

Therapeutic Guidelines, Palliative Care—concise, practical information on all aspects of palliative care

Twycross R. Introducing palliative care, 2nd edn. Oxford: Radcliffe Medical Press; c1997—a concise but comprehensive introduction to all aspects of palliative care, including communication, ethics, drug profiles and more

Woodruff R. Palliative medicine: evidence-based symptomatic and supportive care for patients with advanced cancer, 4th edn. Melbourne, Victoria: Oxford University Press; 2004—written by an Australian oncologist/palliative care physician

REFERENCES

1 Clayton JM, Hancock KM, Tattersall MHN et al. Clinical practice guidelines for communicating prognosis and end-of-life issues with adults in the advanced stages of a terminal illness, and their caregivers. Med J Aust 2007; 186(12):S18.

2 Zappa SB, Cassileth BR. Complementary approaches to palliative oncological care. J Nurs Care Qual 2003; 18(1):22–26.

3 Oneschuk D, Hanson J, Bruera E. Complementary therapy use: a survey of community- and hospital-based patients with advanced cancer. Palliat Med 2000; 14(5):432–434.

4 Foley KM. Acute and chronic cancer pain syndromes. In: Doyle D, Hanks G, Cherny N et al, eds. Oxford textbook of palliative medicine, 3rd edn. Oxford: Oxford University Press; 2004:298–316.

5 Pain in residential aged care facilities. Management strategies. Sydney: Australian Pain Society; 2005.

6 Bowsher D. The effects of pre-emptive treatment of postherpetic neuralgia with amitriptyline: a randomized, double-blind, placebo-controlled trial. J Pain Symptom Manage 1997; 13(6):327–331.

7 Bardia A, Barton DL, Prokop LJ et al. Efficacy of complementary and alternative medicine therapies in relieving cancer pain: a systematic review. J Clin Oncol 2006; 24(34):5457–5464.

8 Deng G, Cassileth BR. Integrative oncology: complementary therapies for pain, anxiety, and mood disturbance. CA: Cancer J Clin 2005; 55:109–116.

9 Cassileth BR, Vickers AJ. Massage therapy for symptom control: outcome study at a major cancer center. J Pain Symptom Manage 2004; 28(3):244–249.

10 Fellowes D, Barnes K, Wilkinson S. Aromatherapy and massage for symptom relief in patients with cancer. Cochrane Database Syst Rev 2004; 3:CD002287.

11 Beck SL. The therapeutic use of music for cancer-related pain. Oncol Nurs Forum 1991; 18:1327–1337.

12 Cassileth BR. Complementary and alternative cancer medicine. J Clin Oncol 1999; 17(11 Suppl):44–52.

13 Portenoy RK, Thomas J, Moehl Boatwright ML et al. Subcutaneous methylnaltrexone for the treatment of opioid-induced constipation in patients with advanced illness: a double-blind, randomized, parallel group, dose-ranging study. J Pain Symptom Manage 2008; 35(5):458–468.

14 Ezzo JM, Richardson MA, Vickers A et al. Acupuncture-points stimulation for chemotherapy-induced nausea or vomiting. Cochrane Database Syst Rev 2006; 2:CD002285.

15 Berenstein EG, Ortiz Z. Megestrol acetate for the treatment of anorexia-cachexia syndrome. Cochrane Database Syst Rev 2005; 2:CD004310.

16 Dewey A, Baughan C, Dean T et al. Eicosapentaenoic acid (EPA, an omega-3 fatty acid from fish oils) for the treatment of cancer cachexia. Cochrane Database Syst Rev 2007; 1:CD004597.

chapter 40

Psychiatry and psychological medicine

INTRODUCTION AND OVERVIEW

Psychiatric disorders are highly prevalent. Depressive and anxiety disorders occur in up to 25% of primary care patients.[1] The World Health Organization Global Burden of Disease Project (cited in Davies 2000[2]) identified that psychiatric illnesses in developed economies account for over 20% of years of life lost through premature mortality and years lived with a disability. The economic impact is enormous in direct costs to the healthcare system and indirect costs to the community.

The National Survey of Mental Health and Wellbeing found a one-year prevalence of 20% of adults surveyed with a psychiatric illness and noted that, while only a third of those suffering from a psychiatric disorder sought treatment, most of those presented to their general practitioner (GP). Indeed, of patients who seek help for their psychiatric symptoms, 75–90% see a GP.[4] A GP seeing 40 patients a day could expect that eight would require support or treatment for anxiety or depression.[5]

Given the size of the problem, it is clearly beyond the scope of this chapter to do more than provide a framework for the GP in the assessment and understanding of patients who present with psychiatric disorders, and then to briefly describe the management of some of the conditions that present in general practice, emphasising high-prevalence disorders.

The most common psychiatric disorders presenting to GPs are depression, anxiety, adjustment disorders, and alcohol abuse and dependence (dealt with in Ch 62). The prognoses of anxiety, depression and psychotic disorders are all improved by early detection and intervention, and so the GP's role is pivotal in improving the level of functioning and quality of life of their patients. The GP is uniquely positioned to assess psychiatric symptoms, because they will have often seen a patient over an extended timeframe and so will have access to information about the patient and their premorbid functioning.

OBJECTIVE OF THE CONSULTATION

With every patient there are three questions that the GP is endeavouring to answer:

- What is wrong (or what is the diagnosis)?
- Why did whatever is wrong with the patient go wrong with them?
- What are we going to do about it (treatment approach)?

Like any other branch of medicine, to answer these questions requires an adequate history and examination, followed by the GP using the information and data available to answer the above three questions.

PSYCHIATRIC HISTORY

A standard psychiatric history requires information in a number of categories. Although, obviously, in general practice it is difficult to obtain all the information, much of the history may already be known.

A psychiatric interview includes:

- demographics
- presenting complaint (including current symptoms)
- past history (both medical and psychiatric)
- medication and medication history
- alcohol, cigarette and drug history
- forensic history
- family history
- developmental history and personal history
- premorbid personality
- level of functional impairment.

The interview is described in most psychiatric texts, including *Foundations of Clinical Psychiatry*.[6]

EXAMINATION

Both a mental state examination and a physical examination are indicated.

MENTAL STATE EXAMINATION

Unlike the physical examination, the mental state examination occurs throughout the consultation, as the patient's emotional, behavioural and thinking states are observed by the GP. It helps to make notes about the patient's mental state throughout the interview, particularly in noting affective changes and any thought disorder.

- *Appearance and behaviour*—describe what is observed.
- *Speech*—describe the quality and process of speech, which can range from mute, to the slowed speech of psychomotor-retarded depression, to the very rapid and pressured speech of mania.
- *Affect*—observe the patient's emotional state during the interview, noting fluctuations and whether it is congruent or incongruent with the content of the conversation. For example, the tearfulness of a patient describing the recent death of their parent would be mood congruent.

  In patients with schizophrenia or post-traumatic stress disorder, affect is sometimes blunted, with a reduction in the intensity that would normally be anticipated. For example, a patient may say he or she is being watched by aliens in a rather 'matter of fact' fashion, in contrast to the extreme level of agitation and anxiety you would expect were such a delusional belief to be true.
- *Thought process*—does the history flow in a normal conversational fashion? Manic thoughts are so fast that the conversation appears to take jumps, and there appears to be little connection between sentences. In schizophrenia the conversation may not be understandable. It is difficult to recall such disorganised thought unless you have recorded it at the time.
- *Thought content*—thought content includes the depressed themes of depressive disorders, the nihilistic delusions and descriptions of hopelessness, helplessness and guilt in psychotic depression, and the ruminations of obsessive compulsive disorder. The delusional beliefs of psychosis are described here, as is suicidal or homicidal ideation.
- *Perception*—perception most commonly relates to auditory hallucinations, although all sensory modalities can be involved.
- *Cognitive testing or cognition*—assessment of a patient's cognition is an important aspect of a mental state examination and a number of commonly used instruments are available, such as the mini-mental state examination (MMSE).[7] If a patient has come to the appointment on their own and on time, their cognition is probably intact. The MMSE is particularly important where there is a history of alcohol abuse or when dementia-like disorders are suspected.
- *Insight*—probably the most practical assessment of insight is whether the patient believes they have an illness that is treatable and is amenable to such treatment.
- *Judgment*—judgment is best assessed by asking what the patient plans to do next. For example, a patient with depression who plans to resign because they believe they are hampering their employer's business opportunities probably has impaired judgment.

For further details about mental state examination, see *The psychiatric mental state examination* by Trzepacz and Baker.[8]

HINTS TO ENHANCE A PSYCHIATRIC CONSULTATION

- *Set aside time*—in an often busy consulting day it is sometimes difficult to take the time to elicit psychiatric symptoms, and so if suspicious of psychological symptoms, making arrangements for a longer consultation is a priority. It is important to keep interruptions to an absolute minimum and ensure privacy.
- *Opening the interview*—psychiatric interviews are usually best started with neutral subjects such as details of current circumstances, while listening with an empathic ear and observing the patient's emotional and behavioural responses. Gentle encouragement, such as asking the patient, 'What do you mean?' or perhaps repeating the patient's last phrase as a question, can help to clarify symptoms. For example, if a patient has described feeling very sad, the GP might say, 'You mention that you have been feeling really sad—have you ever thought that life is not worth living?'.
- *Summarise back to the patient*—it is helpful to reflect back to the patient the history that they have given to you and also to clarify whether you have correctly identified relevant features of the history.
- *Concluding the interview*—it is often useful when completing any patient interview to ask if there is anything they believe to be important that has not yet been raised.

COMMON INTERVIEW DIFFICULTIES

Most interactions with patients are relatively straightforward; however, sometimes difficulties arise. Some of these are discussed below.

- *Lack of trust*—trust is essential in any successful interaction. Usually a patient is seeing a GP who they already trust; however, if it is evident that the patient is not being open, tact and reassurance are required, as is the ability to tolerate deficits in the history.

  Possible reasons for a lack of trust are suspiciousness due to developing persecutory ideation, embarrassment about things they have either done or imagined doing, or believing that emotional symptoms reflect a weakness of character.
- *Tearfulness*—in the context of a busy general practice, an emotionally distressed patient presents a challenge. However, such demonstrations of emotional distress can be usefully reflected back to the patient, such as saying, 'I can see this has been very upsetting for you'.
- *Anger and hostility*—aggression and anger can be prejudicial to an effective interview. Management of anger and hostility will be discussed later.
- *Over-familiarity*—some patients, particularly those with maladaptive personality styles, require the GP to be on their guard. It is important not to take compliments at face value—for example, when a patient says that they have finally found someone who understands them.

DIAGNOSIS

(or: *What is wrong with the patient?*)
While patients and healthcare professionals want to know the 'diagnosis', it is important not to be lulled into a false sense of understanding. In psychiatry, a categorical classification diagnostic system is used, most commonly the *Diagnostic and Statistical Manual of Mental Disorders (DSM IV-TR)*.[9] Such a diagnostic system has a number of benefits, including enhanced communication between professionals and facilitating evidence-based research.

However, a categorical classification system does not have a dimensional capacity and patients with symptoms that do not meet the full criteria for the application of a label can often have marked distress and significant functional impairment. In some ways the use of such a labelling system is akin to a patient presenting with a sore throat and, after a thorough examination, being diagnosed with 'sore throat disorder'. Diagnostic labels are useful as long as these limitations are recognised and with an awareness that they often change over time as more becomes known about the patient's symptoms.

FORMULATION

(or: *Why did whatever is wrong with the patient go wrong with them?*)
Why is the patient here with these symptoms at this particular time? It is the formulation that reflects the integrative nature of psychiatry. It reflects the complexities of a biological, psychological and social paradigm.

It may help to conceptualise patients as being like a three-legged kitchen stool. One leg of the stool represents the biological brain, the second leg represents their psychology (the way they think, process and react to things) and the third leg represents the world in which they live. There is no such thing as a patient whose presentation does not reflect the complexity of the abovementioned stool.

The biological perspective includes family history and any genetic vulnerability. Previous episodes increase the risk of subsequent episodes. Medical illnesses, concomitant medication and substance use and abuse can also influence the reason for a patient presenting.

From a psychological perspective, the developmental history may suggest vulnerabilities. Personality style, coping strategies (both adaptive and maladaptive), loss issues and the patient's patterns of thinking and behaviour also help understanding.

Also, patients live in a real world with relationships and concerns that need to be taken into account in understanding them. For example, it is more difficult to treat a depressed woman with antidepressants and psychotherapy if she is in a violent domestic relationship.

TREATMENT

(or: *What are we going to do about it?*)
Treatment is predicated on the abovementioned biological, psychological and social understanding. It requires use of evidence-based interventions targeting the biological brain and the psychological make-up of the patient, and taking into consideration the realities of their environment. The rationale for the three-legged stool metaphor is that a treatment intervention failing to address one or other dimensions is unlikely to be successful.

It is this that makes psychiatric presentations a paradigm of the integrative approach itself, in that the whole of the person, in all their dimensions, needs to be considered in order to treat symptoms, maximise function and enhance quality of life.

PSYCHIATRIC EMERGENCIES: RISK TO SELF AND OTHERS

Before dealing with some of the common conditions in general practice, suicide and violence will be addressed.

SUICIDAL PATIENTS

Managing a suicidal patient is highly stressful. Suicide is not random or pointless but, rather, a way out of a problem or a crisis that is invariably causing intense suffering.

Suicide was the eleventh leading cause of death in the United States in 2006.[10] An estimated 12–25 suicides are attempted, for every suicide death.[11] Recently the suicide rate in Australia has decreased, but it continues to be a significant problem. Since 1990, more male deaths in Australia have been attributed to suicide than to non-intentional motor traffic fatalities. The overall rate has remained relatively stable, at 11 per 100,000 of population per year in the United States and Australia. It is a rare occurrence with a very low base rate, while each of the risk factors is common. This makes prediction and prevention of suicide a difficult task. The majority of patients who suicide have seen their GP in the month before.[12]

Risk factors for suicide

The most significant risk factor for suicide is previous attempts. Other risk factors are:

- sense of hopelessness
- age—risk rises with age; peak in males is between 15 and 24 years
- gender—males are much more likely to suicide than females, in a ratio of about 4:1[13] (young women have an increased risk of self-harm compared with young men)
- marriage/partnered status—risk is increased for those who are separated, divorced, widowed, single or living alone
- unemployment and retirement
- physical illness
- psychiatric disorder—the risk is significantly higher than in the general population in patients with severe major depressive disorder, bipolar affective disorder, schizophrenia or borderline personality disorder
- current relationship difficulties
- history of sexual abuse
- availability of means (e.g. firearms in the home)
- alcohol and other substance abuse
- incarceration.

Suicide assessment

The most important aspect of management is to ask. Initially this can be relatively indirect—for example, 'Does it ever seem that life is not worth living?'. Then ask more directly. There is little evidence that asking about suicide gives the idea to the patient—indeed, current popular culture mentions suicide in both literature and music. But be prepared to follow up the question with a discussion of alternative solutions to the person's problems.

Assess the plans, intention or organisation of the suicide plan. Ask about future activities. Document things they plan to do in the next few weeks. Assess underlying psychiatric disorders.

If the patient is suicidal but wanting help, it may be possible to manage them at home, provided they have social supports. Alternatively, they may agree voluntarily to be assessed by public or private psychiatry services.

If concerned about the person's safety, use the appropriate local mental health legislation to ensure that the patient is first and foremost given 'asylum' and assessed by a psychiatrist or crisis team.

VIOLENCE AND AGGRESSION

Aggression is a major problem in society today, and dealing with it is certainly one of the most difficult tasks facing GPs. Management begins with treating the aggression first.

Aggression may be adaptive and may be triggered by environmentally appropriate and highly specific stimuli. It may be a normal reaction to a realistic threat, or a maladaptive reaction. It may be out of proportion to the stimuli or aimed at unrealistic or inappropriate stimuli. It may be impulsive or uncontrolled and it may be non-specific.

Violence, like suicide, is very difficult to predict. The most robust risk factor is a history of violence. Fear of violence by psychiatric patients probably contributes to societal stigma. Patients with depression and anxiety are probably less dangerous than the general community; patients with schizophrenia have a risk of violence approximately equal to that in young men in the general population. Dementia patients also have an increased risk of being violent towards their carers.

While psychiatric disorders alone are a poor predictor of violence, some psychiatric disorders have a higher risk. These are:

- delirium and acute brain syndromes
- psychotic and related disorders
- personality and related disorders
- alcohol and drug intoxication/withdrawal.

Risk factors

Risk factors for violence/aggression are:

- statement of intent
- specific plan
- means
- male
- youth
- history of violence and antisocial acts
- low socioeconomic status
- poor social support
- recent psychosocial stress.

Mental state assessment of aggressive patients

Formal testing is usually not possible. General appearance can be noted, as can the level of behavioural activity. The mainstay of the mental state assessment is to determine whether you can establish adequate communication with the patient.

It may be possible to determine the intellectual level of the patient, their mood state, emotional control, reality orientation, presence or absence of intoxication or withdrawal and potential for insight.

Management of potentially violent patients

- Keep yourself safe.
- Know of past violence.
- Be alert.
- Assume that aggression is possible.
- Keep the environment safe. (Don't have objects that could be used as weapons easily accessible.)
- Keep a safe distance.
- Have an escape route and help at hand.
- Trust your instincts—if you feel afraid, make any excuse to leave the room.

Approaching an aggressive patient

People who are aggressive or angry tend to cause us to feel angry. It is important to control your anger or fear, and demonstrate respectful control of the situation. To that end, try to understand where the patient 'is at', using a non-aggressive stance.

- Recognise the patient's fear and insecurity, but show that you are in calm control.
- Set appropriate limits. For example, accept that the patient may be talking loudly but tell them that you want to listen to them and are unable to do so when they shout.
- Admit that you feel fearful or concerned.
- Be humane and respectful, recognising that the aggression has an underlying meaning. Nevertheless, the patient needs to know that violence is not acceptable.
- Avoid making outright refusals or concrete promises. Rather, establish that decisions may be able to be made once the situation has calmed down.
- If aggression is related to a specific situation or person, try and separate them.
- Restrict access to weapons.
- There is no place for heroics.
- If there are identifiable potential victims, the duty to warn them takes priority over confidentiality.
- Treat mental disorders, possibly using mental health legislation.
- If there is no evidence of a mental disorder, ask the person to leave, and if necessary call the police.

The rest of this chapter briefly discusses some of the more common disorders presenting in general practice.

DEPRESSION

Up to 10% of people who see a GP have depression, often with anxiety. Patients with depressive disorders can present with a range of symptoms that may or may not fulfill the criteria for a label of major depressive disorder, but patients with a severe depressive syndrome always have anhedonia (loss of interest in usually enjoyed activities).

Other neurovegetative symptoms include insomnia, often with early-morning wakening, diminished appetite, diurnal mood variation, impaired energy and motivation, diminished libido, and poor memory and concentration. Patients will often describe a sense of hopelessness, helplessness and guilt. With hopelessness it is important to ask whether the patient has plans for the future. An absence of such plans increases the suicide risk.

General practice patients often present with comorbid physical illness. It is not always easy to identify symptoms of depression in the context of physical illness.

Particular patient groups with an increased risk of depression include:

- chronic illness
- central nervous system illnesses (stroke or Parkinson's disease)
- pain and fatigue syndromes with no clear diagnosis
- the elderly
- people living alone
- comorbid substance abuse, including alcohol and amphetamines
- postpartum women
- recent losses
- transitional changes
- adolescents with behavioural changes.

INVESTIGATION

In the vast majority of patients with depression there is no underlying medical explanation. However, there are a number of neurological and medical causes of depression symptoms. These include thyroid disorders, Parkinson's disease, malignancies, infections such as infectious mononucleosis, rheumatoid arthritis and sleep apnoea. If the history and examination suggest it, then appropriate investigations may be indicated. These can include thyroid function tests, complete blood picture, electrolytes and brain CT scan.

If the depression proves to be treatment refractory, investigations need to be considered.

It is important to review pharmacotherapy, as a number of drugs can cause depression symptoms. There are many of these, including indomethacin, griseofulvin, tetracyclines, beta-blockers and levodopa.

SCREENING INSTRUMENTS (DEPRESSION AND ANXIETY)

General practice is busy, and GPs have substantial time constraints. Patients presenting to GPs with depression will commonly complain of somatic symptoms rather than emotional symptoms. These can include joint pain, headache, fatigue, muscle aches, gastrointestinal upset and dizziness. This probably reflects the fact that patients perceive that doctors are mostly interested in their physical complaints, as well as the reality that it is probably easier to articulate physical symptoms than psychological ones.

The use of screening instruments in these patients can be a helpful way of identifying the level of psychological distress and possibly the need for intervention, and also set a baseline measure.

Questionnaires like the Depression Anxiety Stress Scales (DASS, developed by Lovibond SA and Lovibond PF) or the SPHERE can be helpful. (The DASS and SPHERE instruments can be obtained from the web addresses in the Resources list at the end of this chapter.)

But the GP's clinical impression is still the primary assessment tool. And don't forget that asking, 'Are you feeling depressed?' works.

TREATMENT

As the causes of depression arise from a wide range of biopsychosocial factors, the integrated management of depression needs to attend to all these factors if it is to optimise outcomes. An over-reliance on any one aspect of patient care to the exclusion of the others risks inadequate management or mismanagement of the mental health problem. For example, the management of mental health problems is often overly reliant on pharmacological strategies alone, sometimes marginalising the importance of psychological strategies, other potential therapies and lifestyle factors. Conversely, if a patient with severe mental health problems were to be denied the use of pharmacological therapies because of personal or practitioner preferences, there would be a greater risk of sub-optimal outcome for the patient. Therefore, any holistic management strategy will not be an either/or approach but will use all safe and effective therapies available and tailor them according to the patient's needs and wishes. This section therefore presents a range of possible strategies from which the clinician can draw, starting with general and supportive measures such as lifestyle management and psychological approaches, which should be included in the management of all patients, and then considering the rational and judicious use of pharmacological and other therapies.

Mental healthcare

Lifestyle management: the ESSENCE model

Education

Psychoeducation is essential. It is helpful to explain the physiological basis of symptoms, and to discuss the high prevalence of depression and that it is not a 'personality weakness'.

Stress management

While many theories about the psychological understanding of depression exist, and proponents of different psychological theories claim effectiveness in depression, in general practice the therapy with the widest utility and best evidence for efficacy is *cognitive behaviour therapy* (CBT).

People develop particular ways of thinking about the world that may or may not predispose them to the development of psychological symptoms. CBT endeavours to elucidate the negative thoughts people have when they are evaluating the events that occur in their lives, and helps them to learn more constructive ways of evaluating the event. It also seeks to use behavioural approaches to help improve functioning, develop skills and overcome behaviours such as avoidance, which often reinforce unhelpful thought patterns.

For example, a 'perfectionistic' patient may believe that only doing things perfectly is adequate and that anything less than perfect is a failure. While this thinking style can be adaptive—for example, an accountant needs the books to balance—a patient may find that with a new baby she is unable to control the baby's sleeping, eating and punctuality, and consequently believes that she is a failure as a mother, which may precipitate a depressive episode.

Cognitive therapy is a guided process whereby patients learn to recognise links between their emotions and thoughts, evaluate the evidence supporting their initial thoughts, and then find alternatives.

For example, a depressed patient may expect a telephone call from a friend. When the call doesn't occur, they personalise this, thinking, 'My friend no longer likes me. I must have done something wrong', which exacerbates their depression. Cognitive therapy helps the patient to recognise that the escalation of depression symptoms is related to their thoughts and to find alternative explanations, such as that their friend is forgetful or may have had another appointment or perhaps has a faulty telephone. The intensity of the psychological symptoms is reduced. And the patient develops a sense of power over their emotions.

CBT is available from trained GPs, psychologists and psychiatrists. There are also internet-based programs, including Mood Gym and Climatetv (see Resources list).

Despite its attractiveness, CBT does not suit everybody. Some patients want a therapist who will do the work for them. It can be useful to give a patient some reading homework (such as a rationale of CBT). If, two weeks later, they say they haven't had time to read it, the task can be reset. If at the next appointment they still haven't read it, they probably won't take an active role in therapy and it is likely to be unsuccessful. A more behavioural approach might be indicated in such patients.

Behavioural therapeutic interventions for depression, while easier to recommend than cognitive approaches, are nevertheless not always easy to implement. A range of CBT-based strategies can be used, including structured problem-solving, anger management and assertiveness training, interpersonal therapy and activity scheduling. It is beyond the scope of this textbook to outline these approaches in detail but these strategies can be easily learned by GPs, and can increase the range of options available to suitably trained and motivated GPs in the primary care management of mental health problems.

Managing insomnia is also vital for managing mental health problems, particularly depression. In fact, some patients with depression will find that their depression resolves if they use and maintain effective behavioural strategies for improving sleep.[14]

The other approach to therapy that is gaining particular attention among medical practitioners and psychologists alike is the mindfulness-based approach. Originally pioneered in the health setting by Jon Kabat-Zinn's mindfulness-based stress reduction (MBSR), mindfulness has made a transformation from a complementary to a mainstream approach within a relatively short space of time. This has been driven in large part by recent research particularly in the fields of mental health and neuroscience.

Psychologists Teasdale, Williams and Segal took the work of Kabat-Zinn a step further when they used mindfulness principles to underpin a new approach to cognitive therapy—mindfulness-based cognitive therapy (MBCT). Other variations of mindfulness-based approaches include dialectical behavioural therapy (DBT), acceptance commitment therapy (ACT) and the Stress Release Program (SRP).

MBCT has been shown to significantly reduce depressive relapse.[15,16] Mindfulness, as opposed to conventional cognitive therapy, does not seek to change the content of thought but instead seeks to change the relationship a person has to their thoughts (and emotions and sensations also).[17] When, for example, we experience a thought, emotion or sensation that we dislike, our habitual reaction is to become highly judgmental of it and therefore to try and suppress it or become reactive to it. Experience, however, teaches us that the more reactive we become to an unpleasant experience, the more it monopolises our attention, thereby accentuating its impact. Furthermore, through habitual rumination, particularly about the past and the future, we create or replay stressors and negative situations, often without realising that we are doing it. Therefore, through cultivating a greater capacity to focus on present-moment reality, and by fostering metacognitive awareness (the capacity to objectively stand back from one's thoughts and just see them as events, rather than facts), people with anxiety and depression can more fully engage with life (through greater focus on the present moment), undo the tendency to amplify the impact of unpleasant experiences and minimise the unconscious tendency to ruminate.

The various approaches to mindfulness-based therapies are based on mindfulness meditation. It is important to recognise that mindfulness meditation is not a distraction; quite the opposite. It is a mental discipline used to help train the capacities and cognitive insights that will help the person to undo the processes driving their depression or anxiety for the vast majority of the day when they are not meditating.

Another area where mindfulness is proving important is in the training of healthcare professionals. It has been found not only to reduce burnout and improve general wellbeing, coping and mental health among medical students and doctors,[18,19] but also to assist in the development of communication, empathy and emotional intelligence.[20] Overall, mindfulness-based approaches seem to be extremely safe.[21] Caution should be exercised when using mindfulness with patients with a history of psychosis. It should only be used in remission, if at all, and only by experienced practitioners. It may also be better not to try to commence mindfulness therapy for people with acute and severe depression and anxiety. Generally it is better to wait until the person has stabilised to some extent before commencing mindfulness therapy. People should also be cautious in doing intensive or prolonged practice when new to the approach.

Spirituality

Having an active search for meaning, including having a religious or spiritual dimension to one's life, appears to be protective against mental health problems.[22,23] It can also help a person to recover more quickly or to cope better if mental health problems do arise.

Exercise

Regular exercise has antidepressant benefits and should be recommended to all patients with depression.[24]

A strategy is to write a prescription for a 30-minute walk, five days per week. Being written on a prescription pad can increase the patient's perception of the treatment's validity, and encouraging them to walk with a friend can help them commit to the activity.

In order for exercise to be a successful intervention for mental health problems it needs to be done regularly. Unfortunately, finding and maintaining motivation to undertake a regular exercise program is a major challenge for many people with depression and anxiety. For these people, encouragement, structured programs, regular guidance and exercising with the support of others is very important and can be instrumental to the success of any exercise-based interventions. Exercise is a powerful, accessible and attractive approach that is ideal for adolescent depression, and it can be effective at any age. Physical exercise also provides help for a range of symptoms associated with depression, including lack of vitality and concentration, as well as improved physical health outcomes.[25]

Elevation of mood is universally seen with various exercise programs, independent of disease; however, aerobic exercise appears to be most effective in improving mental health. A number of studies have demonstrated that regular physical exercise results in mood elevation in both healthy and clinically depressed people. A large proportion of these studies have reported antidepressant and anxiolytic (anxiety-relieving) effects of exercise.[26] Higher-intensity exercise seems to be more effective than low-intensity exercise. Exercise has also been useful in the management of alcohol and substance abuse, which commonly accompany mental health problems. The mechanism of action in depression and anxiety is not completely clear, but some of the likely mechanisms include:

- increased cerebral neurotransmitters, such as serotonin[27]
- improvement in sleep and help with insomnia[28]
- increase in self-esteem by giving a sense of achievement and mastery
- acting as a therapeutic distraction to reduce rumination about worries and concerns
- improvement in general health, vitality and physical fitness
- release of pent-up anger, frustration and hostility
- increase in social engagement, particularly in team sports
- reduced need for medications associated with depression (e.g. beta-blockers, sedatives).

Nutrition

Nutrition has not generally been thought of as a core element in the management of mental health issues, but it should be. Poor nutrition can play a causative role in some patients' mood changes, or may exacerbate symptoms if left unaddressed. For example, adolescents in the lowest quintile of diet quality have an odds ratio of 1.79 for developing depression, compared to those in the highest quintile for diet quality (e.g. whole food, balanced, adequate fruits and vegetables, not calorie dense).[29] Unfortunately, for many people food is a source of loathing and guilt, especially when one is dealing with eating addiction or eating disorders, or is locked in a pitched battle to control weight. Before considering the particular foods that might be useful for mental health, it is important to remember the following:

- Food is to be enjoyed.
- The foods found to be beneficial for depression or anxiety may be helpful for other mental health problems including bipolar disorder and schizophrenia.
- Some foods have a therapeutic effect on depression and anxiety, but others will also be important in offsetting some of the symptoms and physical health-related problems associated with poor mental health.
- Mental health is a complex, multifactorial area of health, and diet is one piece of the jigsaw.

The *Medical Journal of Australia* reviewed the evidence regarding the direct effects of food on mood and drew the following conclusions:[30]

- Eating breakfast regularly leads to improved mood, better memory, more energy and feelings of calmness.
- Eating regular meals and nutritious afternoon snacks may improve cognitive performance.
- Slow weight reduction in overweight women can help to elevate mood.
- High levels of refined sugar consumption were found to be linked to a greater prevalence of depression.

Food and depression

The role of nutrition in the management of depression is currently far from mainstream, but the GP needs to consider its use on the back of a growing body of research and an increasing interest among patients wishing to self-manage mental health problems. A few examples of the role of food for the management of mental health problems are given below, with the caution that this is still a relatively new field and should not replace the use of other psychological and pharmacological therapies when they are indicated.

One key study[31] conclusively showed that low dietary intake of fish and seafood is associated with higher incidence of depression. Omega-3 fatty acid supplementation reduces symptoms of depression in unipolar and bipolar mood disorders.[32] Regular omega-3 fatty acid consumption is associated with a 30% reduction in risk of mental health problems.[33]

Chocolate has now been confirmed as a food that improves mood, but probably only in the short term.[34] It does not seem to be so useful when consumed in excess as a comfort food rather than in moderation. Dark chocolate is preferable.

High levels of saturated fat consumption may be linked to a greater prevalence of depression.[35]

Supplements

Some specific nutritional supplements show promise as therapeutic agents that should be considered in depression, although, as with other categories of illness, a nutritionally rich diet is far more beneficial than a poor diet boosted with nutritional supplements.

- *Folate*—it has been estimated that 15–38% of depressed people also have a folate deficiency.[36] Dietary folate below median,[37] low folate and a MTHFR C677T genotype are all independently associated with increased risk of depression.[38] There is evidence of a reduced response to fluoxetine with declining folate levels.[39] Preliminary studies have also shown it to be useful in the treatment of major depressive disorders.[40] Food sources include tomato juice, green beans, broccoli, spinach, asparagus, okra, black-eyed peas, lentils, navy, pinto and garbanzo beans. *Dose*: 500 µg/day.
- *SAMe (s-adenosyl-L-methionine)*—400–1600 mg daily may raise levels of the brain chemical dopamine. Meta-analyses have concluded that SAMe is superior to placebo, as effective as tricyclic antidepressants, and better tolerated in the treatment of depressive disorders, but may have significant side effects.[41,42] SAMe is not to be taken without medical supervision. The body usually manufactures all the SAMe it needs from the amino acid methionine, which is found in ordinary dietary sources such as meats, soybeans, eggs, seeds and lentils.
- Foods high in *B vitamins*, particularly B_6, have long been thought to help with prevention of depression. Foods rich in a range of B vitamins include potatoes, bananas, lentils, chilli peppers, tempeh, liver, turkey, spinach, broccoli, mushrooms and tuna.
- *5-HTP (5-hydroxytryptophan)*[43] is an amino acid that is used to make serotonin and melatonin, and can enhance mood and sleep. Foods that contain the amino acid tryptophan can help raise levels of 5-HTP. Such foods include red meats (beef, pork, lamb and wild game), poultry (chicken and turkey) and seafood (tuna, salmon, halibut and shrimp), as well as cottage cheese, Swiss cheese, peanuts, cashews and avocados. Vitamin C assists in the production of 5-HTP and is an excellent antioxidant. 5-HTP, 100 mg three times per day, may also help. Caution must be exercised, as combination with antidepressant medication may cause serotonin syndrome.

Food and anxiety

Much of the nutritional information on depression applies for anxiety also. During times of anxiety and increased stress (high allostatic load), there are greater demands on the body's nutrients. They are used more rapidly to meet the increased biochemical needs of metabolism, and so there is an increased need for many nutrients.

One particular aspect of the stress placed on the body is an increase in oxidation and free-radical production, and so antioxidants are an extra important part of the diet. Licorice also provides adrenal support and can help as an antioxidant.[44] There is some evidence to suggest that omega-3 fatty acids may also reduce symptoms of anxiety.[45]

Magnesium[46] is a mineral with many uses in the body, including relaxing tense muscles, maintaining normal nerve function and cardiac rhythm, and helping to maintain stable blood sugar levels and immune function.

As in depression, the B vitamins[47] are considered helpful in general, but B_6 seems to be particularly important. Vitamin B_6 can be found in potato, banana, chicken breast, sunflower seeds, trout, spinach and avocado.

Hypoglycaemia can make an anxious person feel more anxious, because there are similarities between some of the symptoms associated with each. This can be avoided by eating regularly (possibly every 3 hours) and snacking on healthy low-GI foods. Ensure adequate fluid intake.

Removing stimulants from the diet is important for many patients, as these can add to the level of anxiety. Typical stimulants include coffee, tea, chocolate and caffeine-based soft drinks. Coffee and other caffeine-containing foods increase alertness but can increase heart rate and aggravate agitation and depression, which is particularly important to note in relation to the increasing numbers of adolescents attempting to use caffeine as a mood-enhancing drug.[48]

Connectedness

Relationships, upbringing and social circumstances profoundly influence the way we think and cope, and this can sensitise a person to the development of depression or anxiety disorders later in life. Social isolation, relationship break-up, educational status, disadvantage, unemployment and socioeconomic conditions can all influence one's susceptibility and response to mental health problems.

The sub-cultures we identify with in society and the music we listen to can create an atmosphere that is therapeutic or reinforces depression and anxiety.

The importance of supportive and stable relationships (e.g. marriage, family and friends) cannot be over-emphasised. Consciously seeking and nurturing such relationships has a flip-side in that patients may need to be prepared to leave behind those relationships that consistently undermine their efforts at growth.

Connectedness is also nurtured through community engagement and involvement with groups such as clubs and interest groups. Attending these can be therapeutic in itself, apart from any other benefits. Connectedness and support can be fostered in other ways as well, including via healthcare professionals, support groups and group therapy, and via information technology (IT). There are increasing numbers of IT-based mental health interventions that provide information, self-help strategies and links to healthcare interventions. Connectedness and support will not only have a beneficial effect on mood and self-esteem but, depending on the group, can also help to support us in making other healthy changes such as improving diet or exercise.

Developing a regular, structured activity schedule with regular pleasurable activities is a most useful strategy for patients with depression. Explaining to patients with symptoms of depression that developing a structured day has significant antidepressant benefits can be significantly empowering to a patient. Listed websites and books such as the *Management of Mental Disorders* (WHO; see Resources list) have easy-to-follow instructions on how to do this.

Patients often have difficulty being motivated. In mild to moderate depression, it is helpful to encourage the patient by explaining that feeling like doing something will often come after doing it, and that this is preferable to waiting until we feel like doing something before doing it.

Environment

Environment can have a range of beneficial or deleterious effects on emotional state. It is not hard to observe the effect of a sports crowd on mood, or the effect of a beautiful garden or park. It is hard to maintain good mental health if one lives in a war zone, and living in an overcrowded or noisy environment can be a significant stressor for many people. Positive and safe environments can foster health behaviours, such as exercise, that can be important for good mental health.

Environment influences a person at every stage of the life cycle. For example, the intrauterine environment during pregnancy can influence development in later life in profound ways. A mother who is smoking during pregnancy increases the risk of mental health problems in her offspring later in life.[49] Extreme stress, particularly in the first semester of pregnancy, can significantly increase the incidence of schizophrenia in the offspring. Elderly people who are living in a non-stimulating environment will have declining mental health as a result. Environment can foster and support social interaction, opportunities and learning, and influence safety, particularly in the workplace.

Environment can also have an impact in other ways. Air pollution, for example, may be another factor in exacerbating depression.[50] Climate change and drought affect economies and communities, and these can have secondary effects on the mental health of the farmers and communities involved.

Sunlight is an important modulator of mood. There is a natural rise and fall in mood with the seasons, but for some the fall is enough to lead to depression. Regular, moderate sun exposure has been found to be beneficial for mental health, particularly those with seasonal affective disorder (SAD), which is a type of depression.[51] Light stimulates brain chemicals and mood, which is probably a hangover from evolution, when we would have gone into a relative hibernation when food was scarce. Exposure to sunlight may also have a beneficial effect on schizophrenia.[52]

Pharmacological

Antidepressant medications represent the most established treatment for major depressive disorder and few would argue with their use, particularly for severe depression, but there is some controversy over their effectiveness and widespread use particularly for mild to moderate depression and in children and adolescents. Meta-analyses have questioned whether they have a therapeutic effect greater than placebo for patients with less severe depression.[53] Despite their popularity, a meta-analysis found that the magnitude of benefit of antidepressant medication compared with placebo may be minimal or nonexistent, on average, in patients with mild or moderate symptoms, but increasing with severity of depression symptoms; that is, for patients with very severe depression, the benefit of medications over placebo is clear.

It is likely that patients with a strong preference for an integrative approach will be less inclined towards a pharmacological solution, but any patient with moderate to severe depression, whether they are sympathetic to integrative medicine or not, should certainly think very carefully before declining the use of antidepressants as at least a part of their total management approach.

In general, the first-line pharmacological antidepressant is a selective serotonin reuptake inhibitor (SSRI).

However, if the patient has a depressive disorder with loss of interest in almost all activities, and melancholic features such as early morning wakening, marked diurnal mood variation, significant psychomotor retardation, marked anorexia or weight loss and marked excessive/inappropriate guilt, a dual-action antidepressant such as a selective serotonin and norepinephrine reuptake inhibitor (SNRI) can also be considered as a first-line biological treatment. If the first drug is not effective after an adequate trial (with dose optimisation as described below), an alternative SSRI or an SNRI can be used. Ensure that the first agent is slowly ceased and that the appropriate washout time is observed. The *Therapeutic Guidelines: Psychotropic version 5* (2003) provides an excellent guide to choosing an antidepressant.[54]

The GP should become familiar with a couple of antidepressants in each class, with knowledge of side effects and possible drug interactions. If a patient has previously responded to a particular antidepressant, unless some new contraindication has arisen it is sensible to use that agent again, although it will not necessarily have the same efficacy in a separate episode.

The most important goal of pharmacotherapy is ensuring dose optimisation. Wait 4–6 weeks at each dose before increasing. A drug has not failed until a 6-week trial at maximum recommended dose, balanced against the incidence and acceptability of side effects. The *MIMS* and the *Australian Medicines Handbook* provide advice on maximum doses.[55,56]

For a first episode of depression, when in remission treat for a minimum of 12 months. For a second episode treat for 2–5 years, and after a third episode treat indefinitely.

The use of antidepressant drugs in children and adolescents is controversial. Because of ethical considerations in research there is very little high-quality evidence on efficacy and tolerability in this patient group. Nevertheless, depression can occur and can have a substantially deleterious effect on the social and academic function of the young person. Anecdotally, careful treatment with SSRIs can be effective in remitting symptoms and improving function. Such prescribing needs careful discussion and informed consent from the young person and their parents.

The younger the child, the more caution should be applied, and seeking a second opinion from a child and adolescent psychiatrist early is preferable.

There has been some recent controversy about antidepressants increasing the risk of suicide in young people. The reliability of the evidence for this is being debated but it is prudent for a doctor prescribing antidepressant drugs for all age groups, and particularly the young, to be vigilant about suicidal risk.

Herbal (St John's wort)

A Cochrane review[57] found that the available evidence suggests that the *Hypericum* extracts tested in the included trials:

- are superior to placebo in patients with major depression
- are similarly effective as standard antidepressants, and
- have fewer side effects than standard antidepressants.

The association of country of origin and precision with size of effects complicates the interpretation, however. Because of its low incidence of side effects, it is not unreasonable to begin with a therapeutic trial of St John's wort, particularly in patients who are resistant to taking pharmaceutical antidepressant medications. St John's wort is a well-tolerated medicine with few side effects; however, drug interactions are possible. For a patient already taking antidepressant medication or other medicines in general, check to make sure that no untoward drug interactions will occur with the introduction of this medicine.

ANXIETY DISORDERS

Anxiety disorders are the most common psychiatric illnesses, with a one-year prevalence of 9.7%,[3] and can cause significant distress for large numbers of patients.

Fear is the response to a realistic and immediate danger, whereas in anxiety the fearful response, with the same physiological arousal, occurs in the absence of any specific danger or in the anticipation of problems or challenges. The behavioural response to anxiety is a modification of the fight-or-flight response, but in the absence of something that is easily fought, patients respond with avoidant behaviour, withdrawal from functional activities and self-medication with drugs or alcohol. Patients also present with a range of physical symptoms including fatigue, headache and nausea. Different anxiety disorders share significant similarities in both understanding and management.

SOME OF THE ANXIETY DISORDERS

- *Panic and related disorders*—the first panic attack often occurs in the late teens. While 20% of adults will experience one panic attack in their lives, in any one year only about 2% of the population experience significant panic attacks. The fear is of either dying or losing control. Agoraphobia, where the anxiety is of being in a situation or place from which escape might be difficult, affects about 2% of the population per year, with an onset in the mid to late twenties.
- *Social phobia*—fear of scrutiny is as common as the combined prevalence of panic disorder and

agoraphobia, and occurs equally commonly in men and women.

- *Specific phobia*—at least 8% of the population have a diagnosable specific phobia, although only about 10% of these people seek treatment.
- *Generalised anxiety disorder*—persistent, generalised and excessive feelings of anxiety are relatively common, affecting 2–8% of the population, with age of onset between 20 and 40 years of age.
- *Obsessive–compulsive disorder*—this disorder presents with obsessive, intrusive, unwanted thoughts that the individual finds difficult to control, and/or persistent and uncontrollable compulsions or urges to perform certain behaviours. It affects approximately 0.6% of the population. It generally first occurs in childhood or early adolescence in a fluctuating pattern.
- *Post-traumatic stress disorder*—this disorder presents with a range of specific symptoms, most notably featuring re-experiencing and avoidant behaviours developing after exposure to a significant traumatic event.

INVESTIGATIONS

In patients presenting with anxiety disorders in middle and late age, similarly to patients with depression, organic aetiologies need to be searched for more aggressively than in patients who present with their first episodes in late teenage or early adulthood.

Cardiac arrhythmias may produce symptoms of anxiety, and hyperthyroidism and hypoglycaemia can present with anxiety. Substance abuse and intoxication must be considered, and caffeine use not uncommonly can produce a chronic anxiety pattern or may precipitate a panic attack.

The use of investigations is determined by the findings in the history and physical examination.

MANAGEMENT

Check for symptoms of depression and risk of suicide.

Certain strategies are applicable to all anxiety disorders. The provision of reassurance, explanation and education is imperative. Remove physical factors contributing to the symptoms, and manage caffeine, cigarette smoking and alcohol use.

For most anxiety disorders seen in general practice, psychological interventions are probably sufficient. These include assisting patients to recognise the normal adaptiveness of anxiety and the negative consequences of avoidance (physical or pharmacological, including alcohol) in exacerbating anxiety. There are many resources teaching relaxation training, structured problem solving as for depression and cognitive and behavioural therapy. Resources on the internet can be helpful.

Often the most helpful treatment is a behavioural therapeutic exposure intervention. Patients are fearful of situations that provoke their anxiety. Use the analogy of the person who wants to ride a horse but who has fallen off. If you ask a patient to tell you the best way to help a person who has fallen off a horse but who wants to ride again to bring about that outcome, most will tell you that they need to get back on the horse. Obviously, if one has fallen off a horse, the thought of riding is extremely anxiety provoking. However, if they want to ride again, a graded exposure is required. Using blinkers, having somebody sit with them, tethering the horse or even using a Shetland pony are strategies that are still likely cause to anxiety and have no guarantee of safety; however, such a strategy has the best likelihood of getting them riding again.

Alternatively, seeing someone regularly to talk about the original fall and about how anxious they feel might seem caring to the patient because 'somebody understands', but such an approach risks perpetuating the avoidance. With this rationale, patients are far more receptive to the development and implementation of exposure-based behavioural therapeutic interventions. Books such as *Management of Mental Disorders* by the WHO[58] or websites such as Climatetv (see Resources list) help patients develop exposure-based interventions.

Biological

Pharmacotherapy has a role in disabling anxiety. In a crisis, benzodiazepines are extremely useful but have a high risk of dependency; therefore, they are reserved for short-term use. Ongoing benzodiazepine use is an avoidance strategy and risks dependency.

Most anxiety disorders respond to the newer SSRIs, although anxiety may be exacerbated by these medications in some patients. The therapeutic drug guidelines provide details of doses and indications.

The same maxim applies as in the use of these drugs for patients with depression, in that dose optimisation is an imperative, with doses being increased according to tolerability and efficacy until the maximum therapeutic dose necessary is reached.

Lifestyle: the ESSENCE approach

All the key points mentioned above in the ESSENCE section on depression are relevant in the management of anxiety. For patients with anxiety it is also advisable to avoid abuse of alcohol, tobacco and caffeine.

Herbal

Patients with anxiety and depression commonly self-prescribe herbal medicines. It is advisable for a health practitioner to have training in the use of any herbs and formulas before prescribing them, and to have a reliable source of information available when concerns about interactions with medications arise.

In patients suffering from anxiety and sleep disturbances, phytomedicines may have a valid place alongside synthetics, and GPs will at least need to be equipped for conversations with patients about the potential benefits and risks.

Many herbs have anxiolytic effects and a broad mechanism of action.

One review[59] reported that commonly used traditional herbs with varying levels of evidence for alleviating anxiety include the following:

- kava (*Piper methysticum*)[60]
- chamomile (*Matricaria recutita*)
- valerian (*Valeriana officinalis*), often combined with lemon balm (*Melissa officinalis*) or with St John's wort (*Hypericum perforatum*)
- passionflower (*Passiflora incarnata*)[61]
- rhodiola (*Rhodiola rosea*)
- *Bacopa monnieri*
- *Centella asiatica*
- *Withania somnifera*
- *Ziziphus jujuba* var. spinosa.

Acupuncture

There is some evidence that acupuncture can help reduce the symptoms of anxiety, especially when combined with behavioural desensitisation (including psychotherapy).[62] One study showed that benefits continued for as long as one year after treatment. Treatment is based on an individualised assessment of the excesses and deficiencies of *qi* located in various meridians. In traditional Chinese medicine, it is considered that a qi deficiency is often detected in the kidney or spleen meridians in anxiety states.

Social

Functional impairment is significant because often the anxiety and its associated avoidance has resulted in a patient withdrawing from the workplace or from their social network. The rationale of an exposure-based intervention to facilitate the patient returning, in a graded fashion, to the workplace and to a social role is an important aspect of therapy.

It needs to be constantly remembered that patients with anxiety disorders will often self-medicate and, unless asked, the use of agents, particularly alcohol and benzodiazepines, can be under-appreciated.

PSYCHIATRIC DISORDERS IN THE ELDERLY

The number of people aged over 65 years is likely to double by 2040. While most elderly people are fit, active and healthy, old age is often a time of loss and disability, where many are widowed and alone and where serious physical, sensory and mental conditions can have a significant impact on independence and autonomy. The elderly therefore require increasing levels of support and extensively use primary care and specialist medical services.

Allow for deafness, poor vision and frailty, and in elderly patients with confusion keep questions brief and simple. Do not shout or patronise.

Collateral history is also essential where there is confusion or memory deficit.

GENERAL PRINCIPLES OF MANAGEMENT

Symptoms have often evolved over time and there is generally no need to rush. Quickly resorting to pharmacological interventions can be inappropriate; the importance of a biological, psychological and social approach is paramount.

When using psycho-pharmacotherapy, consider the reduction in body water, renal clearance and plasma albumin in the elderly that can heighten bioavailability, increase the time of storage and also delay excretion of drugs with the potential for side effects. Many elderly people take other medications and have concomitant physical illnesses that can interact with psycho-pharmacotherapy.

DEMENTIA

Dementia is a syndrome involving changes in memory, intellect, behaviour and personality, often noted by others. Its prevalence is 1% of the population at age 65 years, doubling every 5 years until at age 85 years, 25% of elderly people have dementia. The common dementias are Alzheimer's dementia (50%), cerebrovascular dementia (15%) and Lewy body dementia (15%).

The time of onset of cognitive impairment and the pattern of progression is crucial.

Delirium versus dementia

Differences between the symptoms of dementia and those of delirium are listed in Table 40.1. Delirium can occur at any age and is a medical emergency, with the primary objective being to identify the cause. It is more common in older people and can superimpose on a developing dementia.

When assessing cognitive impairment there can sometimes be a mismatch between symptoms as presented and observed cognitive function. For example, a loyal spouse may minimise symptoms in order to keep

TABLE 40.1 Differential diagnosis of delirium and dementia

Clinical feature	Delirium	Dementia
Onset	Abrupt, possibly with a precise date	Gradual (unless vascular)
Duration	Acute (days to weeks)	Chronic (months to years)
Reversible?	Usually	Generally irreversible; decline may be progressive
Disorientation	Early and pronounced in most cases	Later in illness (months to years)
Consistency	Varies from moment to moment, hour to hour	More stable day to day
Consciousness	Clouded, fluctuating	Not usually affected
Attention span	Strikingly short	Not particularly affected
Psychomotor changes	Striking: hyperactive or hypoactive	Usually only occur in late dementia

Source: Gauthier, Burns & Pettit 1997[63]

a patient at home, or a child may exaggerate the degree of cognitive impairment in order to get assistance. Patients suspected of having dementia can often blame lack of knowledge of what day it is and other pertinent observations or orientation on retirement, poor vision or hearing and social isolation, but most cognitively intact people are aware of these things.

Not uncommonly, patients developing dementia suddenly reach a time where the demand on them exceeds their coping capacity, leading to marked anxiety or agitation—the so-called 'catastrophic reaction'.

Cognitive testing needs to take into account issues such as poor vision, hearing, comorbid depression, educational level, language and lack of cooperation. Short, structured questionnaires such as the Mini-Mental State Examination are useful, but often it is the tone of the answers that reveals much. For example, when asking an elderly patient about what day it is, a bland response such as 'one day seems much like another' or, in a person who has previously described an interest in world affairs who is asked about recent events, the remark 'I don't follow the news any more' is revealing.

Tact and sensitivity are essential.

Investigations

Having determined that a patient has dementia, it is imperative to exclude treatable causes. Differential diagnosis of dementia includes:

- urinary tract infection
- adverse effects of prescribed medication
- alcohol excess
- depression
- eyesight or hearing problems
- diabetes
- thyroid disease
- renal disease
- hyponatraemia
- poor nutrition
- brain tumour
- head injury
- infection.

After the history and a thorough physical examination, including neurological assessment (gait etc), a number of investigations may be appropriate, depending on the clinical context. These could include:

- full blood count
- B_{12}, and folate and iron studies
- biochemistry
- thyroid function tests
- urinalysis
- CT scan
- ECG
- chest X-ray
- sexually transmitted disease screen
- brain MRI.

Management

Do not be nihilistic: advice, education and carer support are essential.

Acetyl cholinesterase inhibitors can delay cognitive decline, but most psychotropic drugs can worsen confusion. Atypical antipsychotic drugs can help behavioural symptoms of dementia.

One of the important aspects of managing patients with cognitive deficits is involving families and carers, and clarifying legal issues such as Power of Attorney, Will and Enduring Power of Guardianship. Careful assessment of testamentary capacity is important. Essentially the question is whether the patient can comprehend in adequate detail the nature of a decision and its consequences. It is not essential that the doctor agrees with the decision, but it is important that the GP documents their opinion and, if asked to provide an opinion of a patient's testamentary capacity, provides a caveat that any such determination, in the absence of any significant medical event, is valid only for a limited period.

Medication

There is no known cure for senile dementia but some medications have a small effect in slowing progression of the disease or providing some relief of symptoms.

- Cholinesterase inhibitors (donepezil (Aricept®), rivastigmine (Excelon®), galantamine (Razadyne®)) may offer symptom relief for a short time in patients with mild to moderate depression.
- Memantine (Ebixa®/Namenda®) is currently indicated for use for people with moderately severe to severe Alzheimer's disease, but the effect is likely to be small.
- Antipsychotics (haloperidol (Serenace®)) are used to control agitation, aggression, delusions and hallucinations.

An integrated approach has been shown to slow cognitive decline.[64]

Lifestyle: the ESSENCE model

- *Education*—having an education and an engaged mind actively involved with stimulating pastimes has been found to be protective against dementia. Even engaging in these activities when elderly is protective and can slow the progression. Having inadequate stimulation and unstimulating pastimes such as excessive television watching increases risk and accelerates dementia.
- *Stress management*—poor mental health is a risk factor in itself for dementia. Evidence is also accumulating that a range of psychological strategies, and in particular mindfulness, not only have the capacity to enhance mental health but also improve focus and memory, and stimulate neurogenesis in the hippocampus and prefrontal cortex.[65]
- *Spirituality*—any improvements in mental health or coping related to meaning and spirituality are likely to be important for preventing, managing or coping with dementia, for the patient and their family.
- *Nutrition*—nutritional deficiencies should be corrected. Healthy nutrition, omega-3 fatty acids, reduced saturated fat intake and avoidance of excessive alcohol are all preventive for dementia and look to slow the progression of it.
- *Exercise*—regular exercise as tolerated can both prevent and slow the rate of progression of dementia. Exercise, among other things, helps to stimulate neurogenesis (including in the hippocampus), improve memory and concentration and improve mental health.
- *Connectedness*—relationships and social interaction significantly protect against dementia, and can assist in slowing progression and in coping.
- *Environment*—the importance of a stimulating and engaging physical and social environment cannot be overstated.

Herbal

Ginkgo biloba and brahmi (*Bacopa monnieri*) are popular herbs that have long been used for improving cognitive impairment, but the evidence is inconsistent.

PSYCHOTIC DISORDERS

The main psychotic disorders are schizophrenia and bipolar affective disorder I. These are low-prevalence disorders, schizophrenia occurring in 1% and bipolar affective disorder I in 1.2% of the population. Both have a significant genetic vulnerability.

In psychotic illnesses there is often a significant delay of over 12 months between first symptoms and treatment, and at least 75% of these patients will have seen a GP during that period. The longer the time to treat, the worse the prognosis. It is conceptualised that the psychotic illness itself is neurotoxic, similarly to the way in which prolonged coma or lengthy post-traumatic amnesia worsens the prognosis.

The hallmark of psychotic disorders are delusions (false ideas about reality), perceptual abnormalities and disorganised thinking. There is often a history of prodromal deterioration in patients diagnosed with schizophrenia in the 2–5 years before presentation. Nevertheless, 25–40% of patients with DSM IV-TR schizophrenia will only have one episode. Good prognostic indicators are a rapid onset of symptoms, rapid recovery, presence of affective symptoms and stable premorbid personality.

Schizophrenia begins in late adolescence or early adulthood in men, and in the early to mid twenties in women. If a patient presents with unusual thinking or changes in mood or behaviour, it is useful to at least consider the possibility that it is a prodrome, to use structured problem-solving techniques, to enlist supports such as drug and alcohol agencies if there is a substance problem, and to elicit family education and support.

The presence of one manic episode is sufficient to diagnose bipolar disorder I. Manic patients have elevated or irritable mood for a period of one week, with decreased sleep, increased self-esteem, increased energy, and rapid and jumping thoughts (flight of ideas). They are distractible and impulsive, and often risk damaging their reputation or incurring financial loss or legal problems.

INVESTIGATIONS FOR PATIENTS WITH A FIRST EPISODE OF PSYCHOSIS

The recommendations of clinical guidelines on the management of psychosis are that a number of investigations to exclude treatable pathology, as indicated by the history and physical examination, are indicated. These can include:

- an EEG if temporal lobe epilepsy is considered
- CT scan of the brain
- thyroid function test
- syphilis serology
- HIV serology
- B_{12} and folate
- ESR, complete blood picture, electrolytes
- fasting blood sugar
- serum calcium and phosphate
- urine and blood drug screens.

ROLE OF ILLICIT SUBSTANCES

It is worth briefly noting the contribution of illicit substances, most notably cannabis, to schizophrenia. There is controversy as to the role of cannabis in the development of psychotic disorders; however, it is probably best to consider that cannabis, while not causative of psychosis, can unmask symptoms in a vulnerable brain. This conceptualisation tends to reduce the risk of both patients and their families blaming the patient for causing the psychosis. It can also help in encouraging the patient to avoid illicit substances. The concept that, for the person with a predisposition to psychosis, the patient is 'allergic' to cannabis and needs to avoid it and other drugs in a similar fashion to the person with an allergy to penicillin having to avoid that drug, enables the doctor to advise the patient strongly to avoid the substance, without having to adopt a moralistic view.

MANAGEMENT

Schizophrenia-type psychosis

If a patient with a psychotic illness can be managed at home, the maxim is to go slowly and start with a low dose of atypical antipsychotic. The dose can be increased in the first week to the initial target dose (for example: risperidone 2 mg, olanzapine 10 mg, quetiapine 300 mg). After 3 weeks, if there has been response, the dose can be increased slowly over the next month to 4 mg, 20 mg and 800 mg respectively.[15,16]

Agitation can settle in hours or days but the positive symptoms of schizophrenia can sometimes take weeks or even months. Once first-episode symptoms are in remission, it is reasonable to try and stop medication, with vigilant observation of the mental state after 1 or 2 years.

After a second episode of psychosis, treatment needs to continue for at least 5 years after remission; after a third episode, treatment should be considered lifelong.

Manic-type psychosis

For mania, the treatment of choice is mood stabilisers. (Seek advice in patients during the reproductive years due to the problems of both teratogenicity and effects on the newborn of drugs like sodium valproate and lithium.)

A major part of managing psychotic illnesses is to help the patient and their family identify warning signs of and triggers that may precipitate an illness relapse. For example, sleep deprivation (from, for instance, a patient doing excessive overtime or night shifts) may be a trigger for an episode of illness. However, reduction in sleep requirement may be the first indicator of an evolving manic episode.

Encourage the patient to keep a mood and sleep diary, to identify both triggers and warning signs. Try to involve the family. The relapse signature varies from individual to individual and can be used to assist the GP to develop a management plan. GPs can help provide continuity of care and to monitor mental state. Strategies such as going for walks, exercising, talking and watching television can help manage symptoms such as hallucinations.

The GP can monitor side effects of both the illness and its treatment, including weight gain and emergent diabetes. Patients with schizophrenia and bipolar disorder have increased morbidity and mortality from general medical conditions compared to the normal population, even in the absence of treatment with atypical antipsychotics and other drugs.

PATIENTS WITH CHRONIC PHYSICAL SYMPTOMS FOR WHICH NO ORGANIC CAUSE IS IDENTIFIED

This includes patients with chronic pain. These patients challenge both GPs and psychiatrists. The principles of management are described below.

MEDICAL EXAMINATION AND NECESSARY INVESTIGATIONS

Explain the results of investigations and examination carefully and then, importantly, explain how emotional states can modulate pain perception. To avoid excessive and unnecessary procedures and investigations, it helps to set regular, time-limited appointments. Encourage the patient not to see multiple doctors. Only refer the patient if there is a clear reason, but ensure that all reasonable measures have been undertaken to diagnose treatable underlying pathology.

DIAGNOSING CONCOMITANT PSYCHIATRIC ILLNESS

In acknowledging ongoing pain symptoms, the focus is on the management of the pain. For example, it is helpful to explain to the patient that any reduction in tension can lead to a reduction in pain and that the focus is on rehabilitation rather than cure.

It is important to identify psychosocial precipitants and to help the patient to problem-solve these. Often it is important to involve the family where previously there has been a focus on the symptoms, instead switching the focus to the need to reinforce appropriate coping strategies.

Such patients cause significant frustration for doctors. It is important to be aware of that frustration and to have a clear plan, which, in the absence of any abnormal findings and investigations, can sometimes best be viewed as palliative, albeit for the long term. Sometimes it helps to refer the patient for a psychiatric assessment, but always tell the patient that you are doing so.

PERSONALITY DISORDERS

The personality and coping style of the patient can have an impact, both positive and negative, on the assessment, treatment efficacy and prognosis. It can also have an impact on the health of the doctor.

A person with a healthy personality copes with the environment and interpersonal relationships by first trying to manipulate the factors to best suit themselves. They then have the capacity to recognise when this is no longer feasible, and the flexibility to adapt to inflexible external demands. In order to do this, a person needs an innate ability to take responsibility for their own cognitions, emotions and behaviour. They need to be of sufficient maturity and to demonstrate adequate intelligence.

Personality disorder diagnoses are purely descriptive and do not eliminate the need to understand the entirety that is the person. For that reason, such patients often have significant comorbid anxiety, depression and substance abuse problems.

Personality disorders are not in themselves inherently untreatable; however, they often cause significant frustration for GPs. They can lead to diagnostic difficulties such as the 'diagnosis' being incorrect or missed, or comorbid conditions also being missed. In general, patients with personality disorders are not 'good' patients, and it is not uncommon for patients with maladaptive personality styles to cause interpersonal problems between the clinician and the patient. These then become the focus of attention.

MANAGEMENT

The most important initial task in managing patients with disordered personalities is to engage them in a therapeutic relationship. You cannot assume that the patient has the capacity to be engaged; even if the GP wishes it, engagement requires active collaboration between both the GP and the patient. A lack of adequate engagement can lead to major diagnostic and treatment difficulties.

Common obstacles to engagement include unrealistic expectations of the patient and the clinician, basic mistrust of the professionals by the patient, and ambivalence from the patient about both seeking out and receiving help.

Correctable reasons for treatment failure in patients with personality disorders include:

- inadequate engagement in treatment
- unrealistic treatment expectations
- unrealistic timeframe for treatment
- inconsistent delivery of treatment
- unresolved covert staff disagreements
- inadequate inter-staff communication
- undue delay in response to a deterioration or improvement in the patient's clinical status.

Patients with maladaptive personalities often precipitate 'splitting' of staff, for which the most important pre-emptive strike is education of the staff. It is important to be clear with the patient, possibly using treatment contracts that specify what particular staff are able to provide and/or tolerate. Regular meetings of all the relevant clinicians to identify and resolve differing attitudes to treatment can be helpful. Not infrequently, patients with significant personality disorders will tell the GP a different version of events to that given to the psychiatrist or mental health teams, and communication between the members of the treating team is essential.

Patients with the diagnostic label *borderline personality disorder* can be difficult to manage and are often treated rather dismissively. Nevertheless, these patients have a significant mortality rate by suicide of approximately 10%.

Borderline personality disorder patients have difficulties with 'here and now' and generally the focus of therapy is on current problems and stressors rather than past problems. The GP can have problems with counter-transference, and such patients often demonstrate idealised transference versus devalued transference, in that one moment the doctor is the 'best in the world' and the next they are being denigrated for being the worst. Such patients are frequently those with whom doctors have boundary transgressions.

The strategy for managing displays of over-familiarity and idealisation is to be objective and careful, and unambiguous in your response. It is important with these patients to set clear limits of both what you can and cannot do, and your availability and accessibility. Be open and discuss these issues with the patient.

Acknowledge the individual's responsibility for their behaviour, but also acknowledge the need for such behaviour and to assist the patient to find alternative behaviours and responses using structured problem-solving techniques.

It can be useful to ask for a second opinion with patients who have difficult personality styles. Usually the outcome of such opinions is that the GP is doing an excellent job and that it is reasonable to continue to see a dependent patient on a regular basis, and that it is acceptable to set limits with the patient with a borderline personality style.

GET TO KNOW YOUR LOCAL PSYCHIATRIC RESOURCES

As is the case in all specialities, it is helpful for the GP to develop a working relationship with a psychiatrist or two who, at the very least, are available to give telephone advice. Get to know private psychiatrists and their billing practices.

The public mental health sector varies from state to state and area to area, but GPs who clarify local referral protocols and systems will often find that a little effort pre-emptively can save a great deal of time when dealing with an acute or complex patient.

RESOURCES

Australian Centre for Posttraumatic Mental Health, http://www.acpmh.unimelb.edu.au/

Australian Medicines Handbook, http://www.amh.net.au/

Beyondblue, http://www.beyondblue.org.au

Black Dog Institute (mood disorders and depression resource), http://www.blackdoginstitute.org.au/

BluePages (depression resource), http://bluepages.anu.edu.au/home/

Climate GP (CBT for anxiety and depression), http://www.climate.tv/

Depression Anxiety Stress Scales, http://www2.psy.unsw.edu.au/groups/dass/

Mental Health First Aid, http://www.mhfa.com.au/program_overview.shtml

MoodGYM (online CBT for depression), http://www.moodgym.anu.edu.au/

Organization of Teratology Information Specialists (information on drugs in pregnancy), http://www.otispregnancy.org/

RANZCP (clinical practice guidelines), http://www.ranzcp.org/

Reach Out (for younger people), http://www.reachout.com.au

Reach Out Central, http://www.reachoutcentral.com.au/

SPHERE, http://www.spheregp.com.au/ (can also be accessed from the Beyondblue website)

University of Adelaide Library, Treatment Guidelines for Mental Health, http://www.adelaide.edu.au/library/guide/med/menthealth/guidelines.html

WHO Treatment Protocol Project. Management of mental disorders, 4th edn. Vols 1 & 2. Sydney: WHO Collaborating Centre for Evidence in Mental Health Policy; 2004

REFERENCES

1 Sartorius, N, Ustun TB, Lecrubier Y et al. Depression comorbid with anxiety: Results from the WHO study on psychological disorders in primary health care. Br J Psychol 1996; 168(Suppl 30):S38–S43.

2 Davies J. A manual of mental health care in general practice. Commonwealth Department of Health and Aged Care; 2000. Online. Available: http://www.health.gov.au/internet/wcms/publishing.nsf/Content/mental-pubs-m-mangp

3 Andrews G, Hall W, Teesson M et al. The mental health of Australians. Canberra: Commonwealth Department of Health and Aged Care; 1999.

4 Casey PR. A guide to psychiatry in primary care. Petersfield, UK: Wrightson Biomedical Publishing; 1997.

5 Ellen SR, Norman TR, Burrows GD. Assessing anxiety and depression in primary care. Practice essentials: mental health. Sydney: Australian Medical Publishing; 1998.

6 Bloch S, Singh BS, eds. Foundations of clinical psychiatry. 2nd edn. Melbourne: Melbourne University Press; 2001.

7 Folstein MF, Folstein SE, McHugh PR. 'Mini-mental state'. A practical method for grading the cognitive state of patients for the clinician. J Psychiatr Res 1975; 12(3):189–198.

8 Trzepacz PT, Baker RW. The psychiatric mental state examination. New York: Oxford University Press; 1993.

9 American Psychiatric Association. Diagnostic and statistical manual of mental disorders. 4th edn, text rev. Washington DC: APA; 2000.

10 National Institute of Mental Health. Suicide in the US: statistics and prevention; 2009. Online. Available: http://www.nimh.nih.gov/health/publications/suicide-in-the-us-statistics-and-prevention/index.shtml

11 Centers for Disease Control and Prevention, National Center for Injury Prevention and Control. Web-based Injury Statistics Query and Reporting System (WISQARS). Online. Available: http://www.cdc.gov/ncipc/wisqars

12 Jason B. Luoma MA, Catherine E et al. Contact with mental health and primary care providers before suicide: a review of the evidence. Am J Psychiatry 2002; 159:909–916.

13 World Health Organization. Suicide rates (per 100,000), by country, year, and gender. Most recent year available; May 2003. Online. Available: http://www.who.int/mental_health/prevention/suicide/suiciderates/en/
14 Morawetz D. Insomnia and depression: which comes first? Sleep Res Online 2003; 5(2):77–81.
15 Teasdale J, Segal Z, Williams J et al. Prevention of relapse/recurrence in major depression by mindfulness-based cognitive therapy. J Consul Clin Psychol 2000; 68(4):615–623.
16 Ma SH, Teasdale JD. Mindfulness-based cognitive therapy for depression: replication and exploration of differential relapse prevention effects. J Consult Clin Psychol 2004; 72(1):31–40.
17 Teasdale J, Segal Z, Williams J. How does cognitive therapy prevent depressive relapse and why should attention control (mindfulness) training help? Behav Res Ther 1995; 33:25–39.
18 Shapiro S, Schwartz G, Bonner G. Effects of mindfulness-based stress reduction on medical and pre-medical students. J Behav Med 1998; 21(6):581–599.
19 Hassed C, de Lisle S, Sullivan G et al. Enhancing the health of medical students: outcomes of an integrated mindfulness and lifestyle program. Adv Health Sci Educ Theory Pract 2009; 14(3):387–398.
20 Krasner MS, Epstein RM, Beckman H et al. Association of an educational program in mindful communication with burnout, empathy, and attitudes among primary care physicians. JAMA 2009; 302(12):1338–1340.
21 Melbourne Academic Mindfulness Interest Group. Mindfulness-based psychotherapies: a review of conceptual foundations, empirical evidence and practical considerations. Aust NZ J Psych 2006; 40:285–294.
22 McCullough M, Larson D. Religion and depression: a review of the literature. Twin Research 1999; 2(2):126–136.
23 Koenig H, George L, Peterson B. Religiosity and remission of depression in medically ill older patients. Am J Psychiatry 1998; 155:536–542.
24 Sjösten N, Kivelä SL. The effects of physical exercise on depressive symptoms among the aged: a systematic review. Int J Geriatr Psychiatry 2006; 21(5):410–418.
25 Warburton DE, Nicol CW, Bredin SS. Health benefits of physical activity: the evidence. CMAJ 2006; 174(6):801–809.
26 Byrne A, Byrne DG. The effect of exercise on depression, anxiety and other mood states: a review. J Psychosom Res 1993;13(3):160–170.
27 Chaouloff F. Effects of acute physical exercise on central serotonergic systems. Med Sci Sports Exerc 1997; 29(1):58–62.
28 King AC, Oman RF, Brassington GS et al. Moderate-intensity exercise and self-rated quality of sleep in older adults. JAMA 1997; 277(1):32–37.
29 Jacka FN, Kremer PJ, Leslie ER et al. Associations between diet quality and depressed mood in adolescents: results from the Australian Healthy Neighbourhoods Study. Aust NZ J Psychiatry 2010; 44(5):435–442.
30 Jorm AF, Christensen H, Griffiths KM et al. Effectiveness of complementary and self-help treatments for depression. Med J Aust 2002; 176(Suppl):S84–S96.
31 Peet M. International variations in the outcome of schizophrenia and the prevalence of depression in relation to national dietary practices: an ecological analysis. Br J Psychiatry 2004; 184:404–408.
32 Ross BM, Seguin J, Sieswerda LE. Omega-3 fatty acids as treatments for mental illness: which disorder and which fatty acid? Lipids Health Dis 2007; 6(1):21.
33 Sanchez-Villegas A, Henriquez P, Figueiras A et al. Long chain omega-3 fatty acids intake, fish consumption and mental disorders in the SUN cohort study. Eur J Nutr 2007; 46(6):337–346.
34 Parker G, Crawford J. Chocolate craving when depressed: a personality marker. Br J Psychiatry 2007; 191:351–352.
35 Akbaraly TN, Brunner EJ, Ferrie JE et al. Dietary pattern and depressive symptoms in middle age. Br J Psychiatry 2009; 195(5):408–413.
36 Alpert JF, Fava M. Nutrition and depression. The role of folate. Nutr Rev 1997; 55(5):145–149.
37 Tolmunen T, Hintikka J, Ruusunen A et al. Dietary folate and the risk of depression in Finnish middle-aged men: a prospective follow-up study. Psychother Psychosom 2004; 73(6):334–339.
38 Kelly C, McDonnell AP, Johnston TG et al. The MTHFR C677T polymorphism is associated with depressive episodes in patients from Northern Ireland. J Psychopharmacol 2004; 18(4):567–571.
39 Papakostas G, Petersen T, Lebowitz BD et al. The relationship between serum folate, vitamin B_{12} and homocysteine levels in major depressive disorder and the timing of improvement with fluoxetine. Int J Neuropsychopharmacol 2005; 8(4):523–528.
40 Taylor MJ, Carney SM, Goodwin GM et al. Folate for depressive disorders: systematic review and meta-analysis of randomized controlled trials. J Psychopharmacol 2004; 18:251–256.
41 Fetrow CW, Avila JR. Efficacy of the dietary supplement S-adenosyl-L-methionine. Ann Pharmacother 2001; 35(11):1414–1425.
42 Bressa GM. S-adenosyl-L-methionine (SAMe) as antidepressant: meta-analysis of clinical studies. Acta Neurologica Scandinavica 1994; 154(Suppl):7–14.
43 Birdsall T. 5-hydroxytryptophan: a clinically effective serotonin precursor. Alt Med Rev 1998; 3(4):271–280.

44 Haraguchi H, Yoshida N, Ishikawa H et al. Protection of mitochondrial functions against oxidative stresses by isoflavans from *Glycyrrhiza glabra*. J Pharm Pharmacol 2000; 52(2):219–223.

45 Ross BM, Seguin J, Sieswerda LE. Omega-3 fatty acids as treatments for mental illness: which disorder and which fatty acid? Lipids Health Dis 2007; 6(1):21.

46 de Souza MC, Walker AF, Robinson P et al. A synergistic effect of a daily supplement for 1 month of 200 mg magnesium plus 50 mg vitamin B6 for the relief of anxiety-related premenstrual symptoms: a randomized, double-blind, crossover study. J Women's Health Gend-based Med 2000; 9(2):131–139.

47 Carroll D, Ring C, Suter M et al. The effects of an oral multivitamin combination with calcium, magnesium, and zinc on psychological well-being in healthy young male volunteers: a double-blind placebo-controlled trial. Psychopharmacology 2000; 150:220–225.

48 Whalen DJ, Silk JS, Semel M et al. Caffeine consumption, sleep, and affect in the natural environments of depressed youth and healthy controls. J Pediatr Psychol 2008; 33(4):358–367.

49 Cornelius MD, Goldschmidt L, DeGenna N et al. Smoking during teenage pregnancies: effects on behavioral problems in offspring. Nicotine Tob Res 2007; 9(7):739–750.

50 Szyszkowicz M. Air pollution and emergency department visits for depression in Edmonton, Canada. Int J Occup Med Environ Health 2007; 20(3):241–245.

51 Levitan RD. The chronobiology and neurobiology of winter seasonal affective disorder. Dialogues Clin Neurosci 2007; 9(3):315–324.

52 McGrath J, Selten JP, Chant D. Long-term trends in sunshine duration and its association with schizophrenia birth rates and age at first registration—data from Australia and the Netherlands. Schizophr Res 2002; 54(3):199–212.

53 Jay C, Fournier MA, de Rubeis RJ et al. Antidepressant drug effects and depression severity: a patient-level meta-analysis. JAMA 2010; 303(1):47–53.

54 Therapeutic Guidelines: Psychotropic 5. Therapeutic Guidelines Ltd; 2003. Online. Available: http://www.tg.com.au

55 MIMS Online. MIMS Australia Pty Ltd. Online. Available: http://www.mims.com.au/index.php?option=com_frontpage&Itemid=1

56 Australian Medicines Handbook. Australian Medicines Handbook Pty Ltd; 2009. Online. Available: http://www.amh.net.au/

57 Linde K, Berner MM, Kriston L. St John's wort for major depression. Cochrane Database Syst Rev 2008; 4:CD000448.

58 World Health Organization, Treatment Protocol Project. Management of mental disorders. 4th edn. Vols 1 & 2. Sydney: WHO Collaborating Centre for Evidence in Mental Health Policy; 2004.

59 Saeed SA, Bloch RM, Antonacci DJ. Herbal and dietary supplements for treatment of anxiety disorders. Am Fam Physician 2007; 76(4):549–556. Review.

60 Bilia AR, Gallon S, Vincieri FF. Kava-kava and anxiety: growing knowledge about the efficacy and safety. Life Sci 2002; 70:2581–2597.

61 Akhondzadeh S, Naghavi HR, Vazirian M et al. Passionflower in the treatment of generalised anxiety: a pilot double-blind randomized controlled trial with oxazepam. J Clin Pharm Ther 2001; 26:362–367.

62 Guizhen L, Yunjun Z, Linxiang G et al. Comparative study on acupuncture combined with behavioral desensitization for treatment of anxiety neuroses. Am J Acupunct 1998; 26:117–120.

63 Gauthier S, Burns A, Pettit W. Alzheimer's disease in primary care. London: Martin Dunitz; 1997.

64 Bragin, V Chemodanova M, Dzhafarova N et al. Integrated treatment approach improves cognitive function in demented and clinically depressed patients. Am J Alzheimers Dis Other Demen 2005; 20(1):21–26.

65 Luders E, Toga AW, Lepore N et al. The underlying anatomical correlates of long-term meditation: larger hippocampal and frontal volumes of gray matter. Neuroimage 2009; 45(3):672–678.

chapter 41

Respiratory medicine

INTRODUCTION AND OVERVIEW

The human respiratory system is complex and finely tuned. Fortunately, two factors are of enormous benefit to us. First, there is a large reserve of function, greater than many of us are ever going to call upon; and secondly, the respiratory system can tolerate quite a degree of insult before symptoms appear. The predominant symptoms of respiratory problems that present to GPs are breathlessness, cough, sputum, wheeze and chest pain.

Diagnosis is the important first step in medical practice, and the classic method of adequate history, appropriate physical examination, thinking about the clinical problem and then considering special investigations will clarify most situations.

IMPORTANT CONDITIONS

The four diagnoses that are most prominent and/or important in general practice are:

- asthma
- chronic obstructive pulmonary disease (COPD)
- lung cancer
- infections.

The Bettering the Evaluation And Care of Health (BEACH) data show the distribution of respiratory problems managed in general practice (Table 41.1).[1]

Infections of particular importance are best considered as:

- bacterial—community-acquired pneumonia
- viral—viral upper respiratory tract infection (URTI)
- other—including opportunistic infections (PCP) and tuberculosis (TB).

ASTHMA

BACKGROUND AND PREVALENCE

It is estimated that worldwide as many as 300 million people of all ages have currently diagnosed asthma. The prevalence of asthma in Australia is quite high, with one in six children (14–16%) and one in nine adults (10–12%) having the disease.[2] There is variation between

TABLE 41.1 Important respiratory conditions managed in general practice

Problem managed	Number	% total problems	Rate per 100 encounters	95% CI
Respiratory (total)	20,112	13.5	20.8	20.2–21.4
URTI	5,914	4.0	6.1	5.7–6.6
Immunisation (respiratory)*	2,726	1.8	2.8	2.4–3.2
Asthma	2,117	1.4	2.2	2.1–2.3
Acute bronchitits/bronchiolitis	2,550	1.7	2.6	2.4–2.8
Sinusitus	1,312	0.9	1.4	1.2–1.5
Tonsillitis	852	0.6	0.9	0.8–1.0
COPD	790	0.5	0.8	0.7–0.9

URTI: upper respiratory tract infection. *Immunisation against respiratory illnesses (influenza, pneumonia)

Source: Britt et al. 2009[1]

countries in the incidence of asthma (this is detailed in the document *Global burden of asthma* (see Resources list at the end of this chapter)).

The condition we call asthma involves a number of pathological processes including inflammation, smooth muscle spasm and increased airways secretions. In essence it is a chronic inflammatory disorder affecting the airways. Many types of cells play a role in this inflammatory process, including mast cells, eosinophils, T-lymphocytes, macrophages, neutrophils and epithelial cells. Individuals who experience asthma generally have a genetic susceptibility that can also be affected by lifestyle and environmental factors. Airway inflammation causes recurrent episodes of asthma associated with the symptoms of wheezing, shortness of breath, chest tightness, and also coughing, most commonly at night or in the early morning or in response to exercise. These episodes of wheezing and dyspnoea brought on by widespread airflow obstruction will reverse spontaneously or with treatment.[2] In those disposed to airway hypersensitivity, the inflammation is usually triggered by environmental factors such as allergens, irritants and temperature change. Psychological and emotional factors can also trigger or aggravate episodes of asthma.

AETIOLOGY

Asthma manifests as a combination of atopy, bronchial hyper-reactivity and IgE- and non-IgE-mediated acute and chronic immune responses. Most authorities accept that it occurs as a result of the action of a variety of environmental stimuli on genetically predisposed people.[3]

PATHOLOGY

The description of asthma given above, based on the National Asthma Council of Australia's definition, covers the pathology of asthma quite succinctly.

DIAGNOSTIC APPROACH

It is important that a careful clinical history is taken (see below). An examination is done (in order to assist in excluding other differential diagnoses) and objective lung function testing, preferably spirometry, is performed.

HISTORY

As asthma is most often an intermittent disease, the history is of symptoms that wax and wane—there are episodes of symptoms. The most sensitive symptom of uncontrolled or destabilising asthma is awakening during the night with asthma symptoms such as chest tightness, breathlessness and wheeze. If the patient (or witness) reports hearing a wheeze with expiration, this is very suggestive, but not diagnostic, of asthma. Other information that supports the diagnosis of asthma include:

- a personal history of previous recurrent episodes of asthma (or symptoms suggestive of asthma if the diagnosis has not yet been made)
- normal respiratory and functional performance in the intervals between episodes
- a personal history of atopic (especially flexoral) eczema
- a family history of asthma.

If there are clearly identifiable triggers that precipitate episodes of cough, breathlessness or wheeze, this is strongly suggestive of asthma. The more common asthma triggers are viral URTI, change in ambient air temperature, house dust mite and exercise.

EXAMINATION

Physical examination is, on most occasions, normal unless the patient is in the midst of an asthma attack (i.e. an episode of bronchospasm). In the past, the chronic untreated asthma sufferer sometimes had a deformed thoracic area with a barrel chest and spreading of the

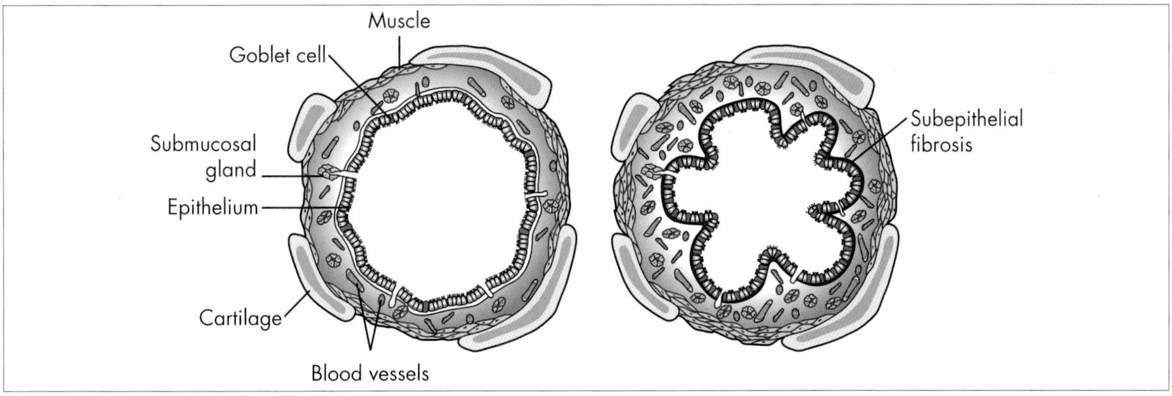

FIGURE 41.1 Airway affected by asthma (right); a healthy airway is shown on the left

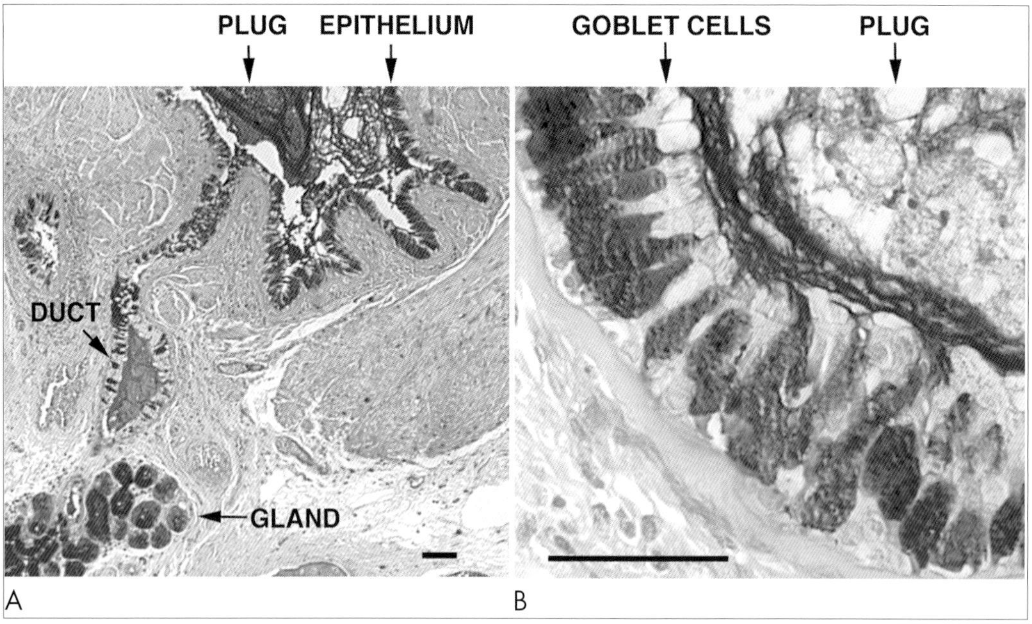

FIGURE 41.2 Mucus hypersecretion in asthma: **A** The airway lumen is plugged with mucus released from the submucosal gland via a gland duct; **B** (higher magnification) Mucus can be seen streaming from the luminal tips of the goblet cells into the lumen

ribs, but this is now only seen, in developed countries, in historical textbooks of medicine.

INVESTIGATIONS

- *In the consulting room*—spirometry is the 'gold standard' for objective lung function testing.
- *Away from the surgery*—encouraging self-monitoring by the measurement of peak expiratory flow rate (PEFR) is worthwhile. This is particularly important where the history suggests occupational or hobby-associated asthma. PEFR is also an important way for some patients to self-monitor their asthma, so they know when control of their asthma is slipping.
- *Pathology*—if one is looking for an allergic cause of asthma, sometimes radioallergosorbent testing (RAST) or skin prick testing is useful in helping to identify specific triggers. However, careful history taking will often narrow the allergens to a manageable number so that specific investigations are not needed.
- *Special tests*—these are rarely needed unless one is attempting to exclude differential diagnoses that have not been excluded by clinical methods.

INTEGRATED MANAGEMENT

Prevention

The 'hygiene hypothesis'[4] is a theory, still being debated,[5] that links an increased risk of atopic disease with reduced microbial exposure from a variety of sources during childhood. Epidemiological studies are providing increasingly strong evidence that protection from atopic disorders including asthma is afforded by early-life exposure to environmental microbes. For example, children who are raised on farms, who drink unpasteurised milk, have more older siblings or attend day care at an earlier age are protected to some extent against asthma. This may explain to some extent the 'asthma epidemic that has been occurring, especially in developed nations, over the past several decades'.[6]

If the 'hygiene hypothesis' is correct, letting children 'get down and dirty' may become a preventive activity!

Respiratory hygiene and minimising spread of infection is important in preventing exacerbations. Ensure routine immunisation against *Haemophilus influenzae*, seasonal influenza and pertussis (whooping cough).

Active surveillance

If we look back to when there were no effective treatments for asthma, the consequences of providing no active intervention are well described. Although patients can sometimes learn to ride out mild asthma attacks using self-help techniques such as breathing exercises, thereby reducing the need for reliever medication, doing nothing for moderate to severe asthma, or not taking preventer medications where asthma episodes are frequent, would not be considered a valid option. A worst-case scenario is that it is life-threatening. This is especially so for those with a history of brittle asthma and severe attacks.

Self-help

Many self-help strategies or home remedies are suggested but robust evidence of their efficacy is often lacking. Self-help strategies or home remedies that have been subjected to scrutiny and are listed in the medical literature are described below.

Tobacco avoidance

Cease smoking and avoid exposure to other people's smoke. Exposure to cigarette smoke can trigger asthma attacks, increase the frequency of asthma attacks, cause the need for higher doses of preventer and reliever medication, increase the need for asthma medication and reduce lung function. Children exposed to cigarette smoke are more likely to develop asthma and have more severe symptoms and more frequent attacks.

House dust mite control

The major allergen in house dust comes from mites. Although methods of reducing dust mite exposure, such as adequate ventilation, keeping a dust-free environment and having regular fresh bed linen, are intended to reduce asthma symptoms, these methods have not been as successful as expected.[7]

Ion generator

Although marketed for use in homes to reduce asthma by removing dust and smoke particles, and although some studies show that ion generators can alter airways function, 'the few studies which have been conducted in the homes of people with asthma, demonstrate no significant benefit in improving lung function or symptoms'.[8]

Pets

Some people with asthma are allergic to their own and others' pets. The solution for many is the removal of the pets, to reduce exposure to the allergens in their hair and skin, but other methods such as pet washing, sprays and air filtration units can help reduce the amount of allergen in the air and on the floor of the home. The evidence is not at present conclusive.[9]

Caffeine

Caffeine (a methylxanthine drug) is related to the theophyllines that used to be commonly prescribed for asthma. These have an effect on the airway musculature. Caffeine is commonly found in coffee, tea, cola drinks and cocoa, and it has been found that even small amounts of caffeine can improve lung function for up to 4 hours, but for some the amount required to improve symptoms may be offset by the other side effects of caffeine.[10]

Fish oil

Many people with asthma who change their diets to include more fish oil do not improve their asthma,[11] but other evidence has suggested that others do. There has been some work published on taking fish oil supplements (rather than just increasing fish in the diet). In one study,[12] some benefit was shown in people with predominately exercise-induced bronchospasm (EIB) but the authors have given the guarded advice that 'fish oil supplementation may represent a potentially beneficial non-pharmacological intervention in asthmatic patients with EIB'.

Vitamin C, vitamin E and beta-carotenes

There is a great deal of research under way into whether specific dietary supplementation is of benefit in asthma. Consensus on the importance of eating enough fresh fruit is yet to emerge, but one review found that:

> Longitudinal data support the hypothesis that fresh fruit consumption has a beneficial effect on the lung. Among children, consumption of fresh fruit, particularly fruit high in Vitamin C, has been related to a lower prevalence of asthma symptoms and higher lung function.[13]

The message is therefore that a healthy diet is far more likely to be beneficial in asthma than supplements, particularly in the presence of a poor diet.[13]

Tartrazine exclusion

Tartrazine is one of the most commonly used food and medication additives or colourants. The evidence that tartrazine makes asthma worse, or that avoiding it makes asthma patients better, is questionable.[14]

Pharmacological

The cornerstone of asthma management is the use of inhaled corticosteroids. The greatest challenge is in deciding when they are required and in what dose. The recommendation of the National Asthma Council Australia is summarised in Figure 41.3.[2a]

Surgical

There has been some very early work on destroying the muscle layer in the airways as a means of minimising asthma symptoms, but this is still experimental.

Breathing exercises

The way in which 'breathing exercise' or 're-training' is understood varies depending on the form of the therapy, the therapist providing the therapy and the cultural

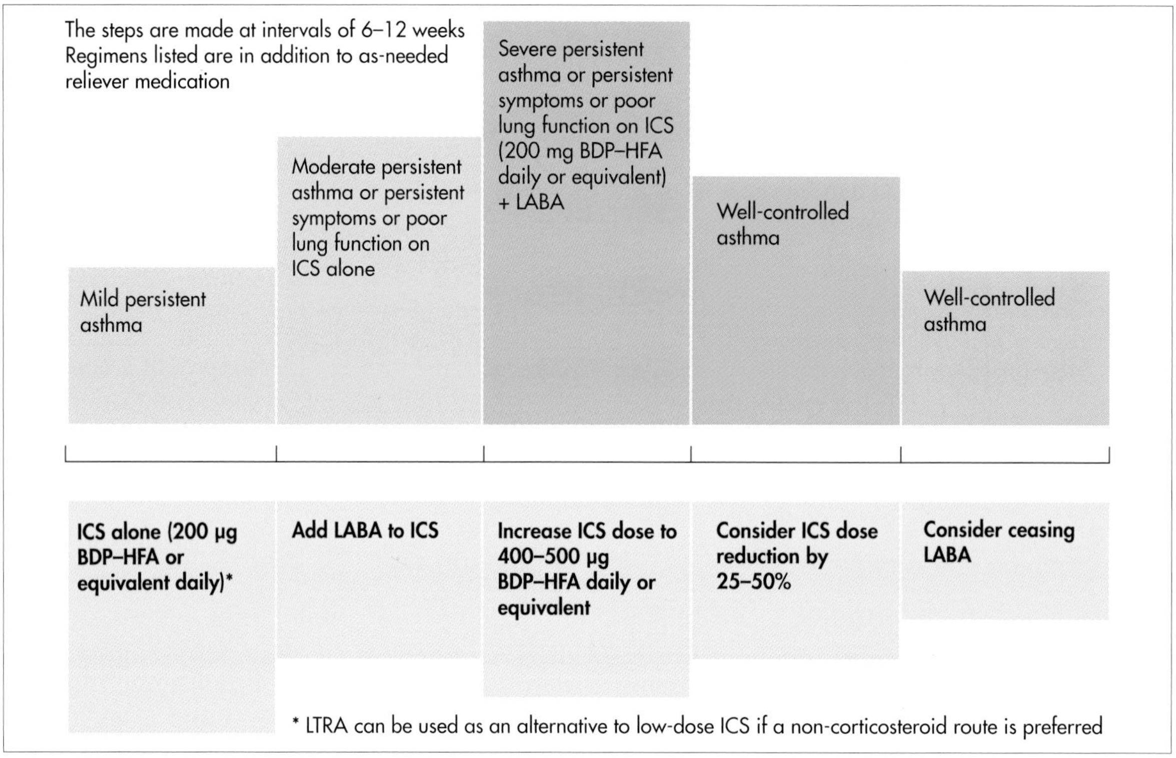
The steps are made at intervals of 6–12 weeks
Regimens listed are in addition to as-needed reliever medication
Mild persistent asthma
Moderate persistent asthma or persistent symptoms or poor lung function on ICS alone
Severe persistent asthma or persistent symptoms or poor lung function on ICS (200 mg BDP–HFA daily or equivalent) + LABA
Well-controlled asthma
Well-controlled asthma
ICS alone (200 μg BDP–HFA or equivalent daily)*
Add LABA to ICS
Increase ICS dose to 400–500 μg BDP–HFA daily or equivalent
Consider ICS dose reduction by 25–50%
Consider ceasing LABA
* LTRA can be used as an alternative to low-dose ICS if a non-corticosteroid route is preferred

FIGURE 41.3 Management of mild, moderate and severe persistent asthma (from NACA 2006[2]). BDP-HFA: beclomethasone dipropionate; ICS: inhaled corticosteroid; LABA: long-acting beta-2 agonist; LTRA: leukotriene receptor antagonist

background of the person having the therapy. Some of the earlier studies of breathing exercises were small or had methodological flaws, but more recent studies demonstrate a trend for improvement.[15] Evidence on breathing exercises, including yoga-based breathing exercises[16], in asthma suggests that they can provide objective and subjective benefit and can be useful in reducing the need for reliever and preventer use.[17] The Buteyko method is also widely used in asthma. Evidence suggests that it provides subjective benefit, although results indicating whether it also provides objective benefit have been inconsistent. It is best to learn breathing exercises from health professionals trained in their use.

Complementary therapies

Dietary supplements

There has been much interest in whether specific dietary supplementation can influence the clinical course of asthma. Many entities and results have been examined but the authors of the studies are careful in making claims. One study showed that the lipid extract of New Zealand green-lipped mussel had a beneficial effect in patients with atopic asthma.[18]

Adolescents with a less nutritious diet, with a lower intake of antioxidants and anti-inflammatory micronutrients, have poorer pulmonary function and increased respiratory symptoms, especially among smokers. The likely explanation is that these nutrients promote respiratory health and lessen the effects of oxidative stress.[19] Dietary supplementation or adequate intake of lycopene and foods rich in vitamin A may also be beneficial in asthma.[20]

Acupuncture

The evidence is not clear and consistent enough to make firm recommendations about the value of acupuncture in asthma.[21] It may be that some forms of acupuncture are more beneficial than others, or that acupuncture is beneficial for some variants of asthma but not others.

Alexander Technique

The Alexander Technique is a form of movement-based physical therapy. It is commonly used to correct posture and bring the body into natural alignment, and also as an aid to relaxation and greater body awareness. Although there are some positive findings, a review of trials found that there was not enough evidence to show a benefit of the Alexander Technique in reducing the need to use medication for asthma.[22]

Herbal treatments

Evidence from 27 trials covering 21 different herbal treatments for both adults and children, and from both inpatient and outpatient settings, was inconclusive generally because of methodological limitations of the trials. Although further trials of high quality are needed to assess the use of herbal treatments in asthma, there is enough positive preliminary evidence to suggest that some of these compounds will prove to be of benefit.[23]

Homeopathy

Different types of homeopathy are used for asthma, such as classical homeopathy (tailored to an individual's bodily and psychological constitution and their symptoms) or isopathy (e.g. using a dilution of an agent that causes an allergy, such as pollen). In the existing studies on homeopathy and asthma, the type of homeopathy used varies and study designs are sometimes poor. Consequently, there is no strong evidence that homeopathy is effective for asthma.[24]

Speleotherapy

Speleotherapy, or staying in an underground environment such as a cave or mine, is believed by some to be of benefit for people with asthma. If benefits are there, it is believed that they come from air quality, underground climate (cool and humid), air pressure or radiation. Evidence is more anecdotal than derived from high-quality randomised controlled trials.[25]

ONGOING REVIEW AND/OR MONITORING

Asthma is a chronic disease and, as such, is worthy of regular planned medical review. However, it is the experience of many clinicians that people with asthma tend to view their asthma as an intermittent disease and so take medications and seek treatment only when they are particularly troubled by symptoms.

IMPORTANT PITFALLS

Making an accurate diagnosis of asthma can be particularly difficult in the paediatric age group, when the history and response to empirical treatment are the only guides. In the older patient, it is important to differentiate asthma from COPD (see below) but, at the same time, to be aware that some people have a mixed picture. If there is significant reversibility on spirometry (post-bronchodilator FEV_1 increases by 200 mL and 12%), treat as asthma.

PROGNOSIS

More children than adults manifest asthma and so the assumption is that, as a problem, asthma 'weakens' with age. It is probably better to accept the view of the National Asthma Council Australia that:[2]

> education, together with self-monitoring, appropriate drug therapy, regular medical review and a written asthma action plan, reduces morbidity and mortality.

Most people with asthma lead normal lives and can participate competitively in sport.

PATIENT EDUCATION

There is a wealth of useful material available at the National Asthma Council Australia website (see Resources list).

CHRONIC OBSTRUCTIVE PULMONARY DISEASE

BACKGROUND AND PREVALENCE

Chronic obstructive pulmonary disease (COPD) is a major cause of disability, hospital admission and premature death. It is commonly associated with other diseases including heart disease, lung cancer, stroke, pneumonia and depression.[26] In a community-based survey that included lung function testing, doctor-diagnosed chronic bronchitis or emphysema was reported by 4.3% of the population. When clinical diagnosis is combined with complex lung function testing and an FEV_1/FVC of less than 75%, around 12% of the population have some evidence of emphysema.[27] This figure will be considerably higher in countries where anti-smoking legislation and campaigns are less prominent.

Definition

According to the Australian and New Zealand guidelines on COPD,[26] COPD is:

> characterised by airway inflammation and airflow limitation that is not fully reversible. It is a progressive, disabling disease with serious complications and exacerbations that are major burdens for healthcare systems.

AETIOLOGY

COPD is really a group of diseases that are clustered together—the more common sub-types are emphysema, chronic bronchitis and fixed airflow obstruction due to asthma.

COPD is the end result of chronic insults to the lungs. 70% of COPD is related to cigarette smoking[28] but it can result from any particulate matter insult (in low-income countries this is often the indoor burning of biomass for cooking and heating) or air pollution.

PATHOLOGY

As the term 'COPD' covers a number of discrete entities (emphysema, chronic bronchitis, fixed airflow obstruction with chronic asthma), the pathology of each is different and is beyond the scope of this chapter.

DIAGNOSTIC APPROACH

The tried and true pattern of adequate history, appropriate physical examination, thinking about the clinical problem and then considering special investigations will clarify most situations.

HISTORY

The cardinal symptoms are:

- breathlessness
- cough
- sputum.

How these symptoms combine gives an indication of the underlying cause of the COPD. There is usually a past or present history of cigarette smoking.

- emphysema—predominant breathlessness, especially on (often minimal) exertion
- chronic bronchitis—the formal definition is: 'the production of sputum on most days for 3 months over 2 successive years'. In milder cases this is often discounted by the patient as being a 'smoker's cough'.

EXAMINATION

The physical examination gives an indication of the predominant pathology:

- emphysema—signs of hyperinflation (barrel-chested with increase in anterioposterior (AP) diameter, pursed-lip breathing, use of accessory muscles of respiration)
- chronic bronchitis—prolonged expiratory phase of respiration.

INVESTIGATIONS

- Consulting room—spirometry and pulse oximetry
- Pathology—FBC demonstrating polycythaemia
- Special tests—chest X-ray will give a suggestion of hyperinflation, flattening of the diaphragm. CT scanning, especially high-resolution CT, gives a view of the lung parenchyma and is most helpful for diagnosing emphysema and bronchiectasis.

INTEGRATIVE MANAGEMENT

One of the problems with COPD is the acute exacerbations that occur. They are diagnosed when there is an increase in any (or all) of the common COPD symptoms, especially increased shortness of breath, increase in cough, and/or increase in amount or purulence of sputum. It seems that the earlier symptoms of an exacerbation are increase in dyspnoea and cough, and the increase in purulence of the sputum comes later.

Exacerbations cause both physical and psychological distress to the patient and are a substantial burden on the health system.

Of exacerbations, approximately 80% are infectious (40–50% bacterial, 30–40% viral and 5–10% atypical) and 20% are non-infectious (due to either an increase in the environmental load of irritants or non-compliance with management strategies including medications). The viral exacerbations correlate with viral epidemics

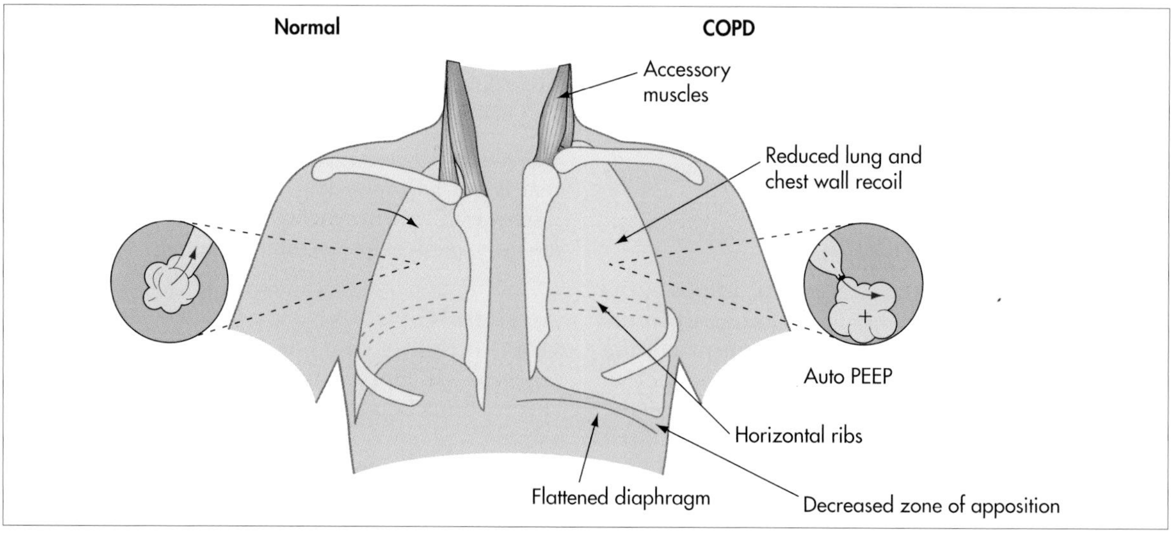

FIGURE 41.4 Clinical features of COPD

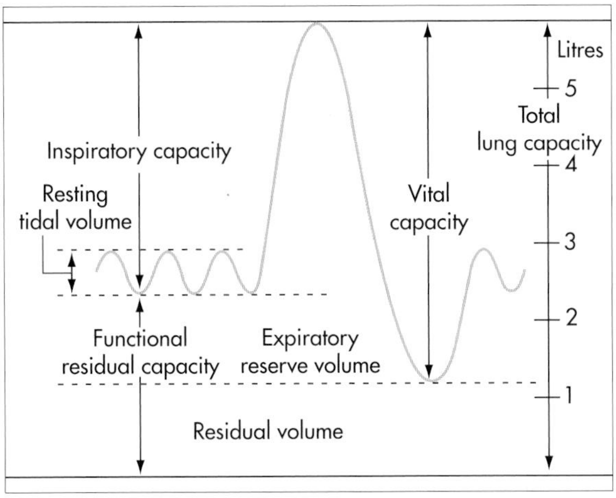

FIGURE 41.5 Spirometry tests

among children. COPD sufferers who are still smoking get more viral infections than non-smokers and so get more exacerbations.

Prevention

As COPD in industrialised countries is commonly due to cigarette smoking, all healthcare providers should be aware of the need to identify and then try to assist smoking cessation in those who smoke cigarettes.

It is worth noting that, in terms of particulate insult to the lungs, one marijuana 'bong' is considered to be equivalent to five cigarettes and so, in those who use marijuana, this needs to be added in to the particulate load when calculating 'pack years'.

At present the only thing known to reduce the rate of decline in lung function in COPD due to cigarette smoking is to encourage the patient to stop smoking.

In countries where the indoor burning of biomass fuels is used for cooking and heating, enabling extraction of the smoke and particulate matter with chimneys and flues should be encouraged, in order to reduce the incidence of COPD.

Respiratory hygiene and minimising spread of infection is important. Ensure routine immunisation against *Haemophilus influenzae*, seasonal influenza and pertussis (whooping cough).

Self-help

As most smokers quit without any particular medical intervention, simply identifying and advising current cigarette smokers to quit is of benefit (see Ch 62, Substance misuse).

Pharmacological

The stages of COPD are defined using spirometry. The definition depends on having a post-bronchodilator FEV_1/FVC ratio ≤ 0.7. The severity of the COPD is graded on the degree of airflow obstruction compared with the population (in Fig 41.6 this is stated as '% predicted'). Therefore, mild COPD is a FEV_1/FVC ratio ≤ 0.7 with $FEV_1 \geq 80\%$ predicted for a person of the same age, gender, height and ethnicity. Modern electronic spirometers calculate the '% predicted' for the practitioner.

Surgical

Lung volume reduction surgery is a major operation sometimes offered to people with severe emphysema. The assessment of patients being considered for operation is complex and is usually reserved for specialised multidisciplinary units. There is significant perioperative mortality with this surgery. The outcomes of surgery suggest that, in patients who survive up to 3 months post surgery, there is significantly better health status and lung function in those who have the surgery than in those who have the usual medical care alone.[29]

Paramedical

Pulmonary rehabilitation programs have been shown to improve the physical functioning, symptoms and mental health of people with COPD. It reduces hospitalisations and has been shown to be cost effective.

Complementary therapies

Herbal medicines

The effectiveness of herbal medicines for treating COPD is not well established and so more high-quality trials are needed.[30]

Nutritional supplementation

Low body weight is common in people with COPD, which impairs heart and lung function enough to reduce the person's ability to exercise as an aid to recovery. A degree of malnutrition is common in people with COPD and can signify a lack of self-care or other comorbidity, but it is unclear whether this is the cause of their deterioration, or just a sign of disease progression. It is questionable whether nutritional supplementation makes a significant difference to the course of COPD itself, but it will nevertheless be useful for general wellbeing.[31]

With emphysema in particular, the work of breathing is increased so much that the sufferer cannot take in sufficient calories to avoid weight and lean muscle loss. Pulmonary rehabilitation programs often attend to this but these people will often benefit from a review by a dietician, and consideration of protein and caloric supplementation and of whether multivitamin supplements are necessary.

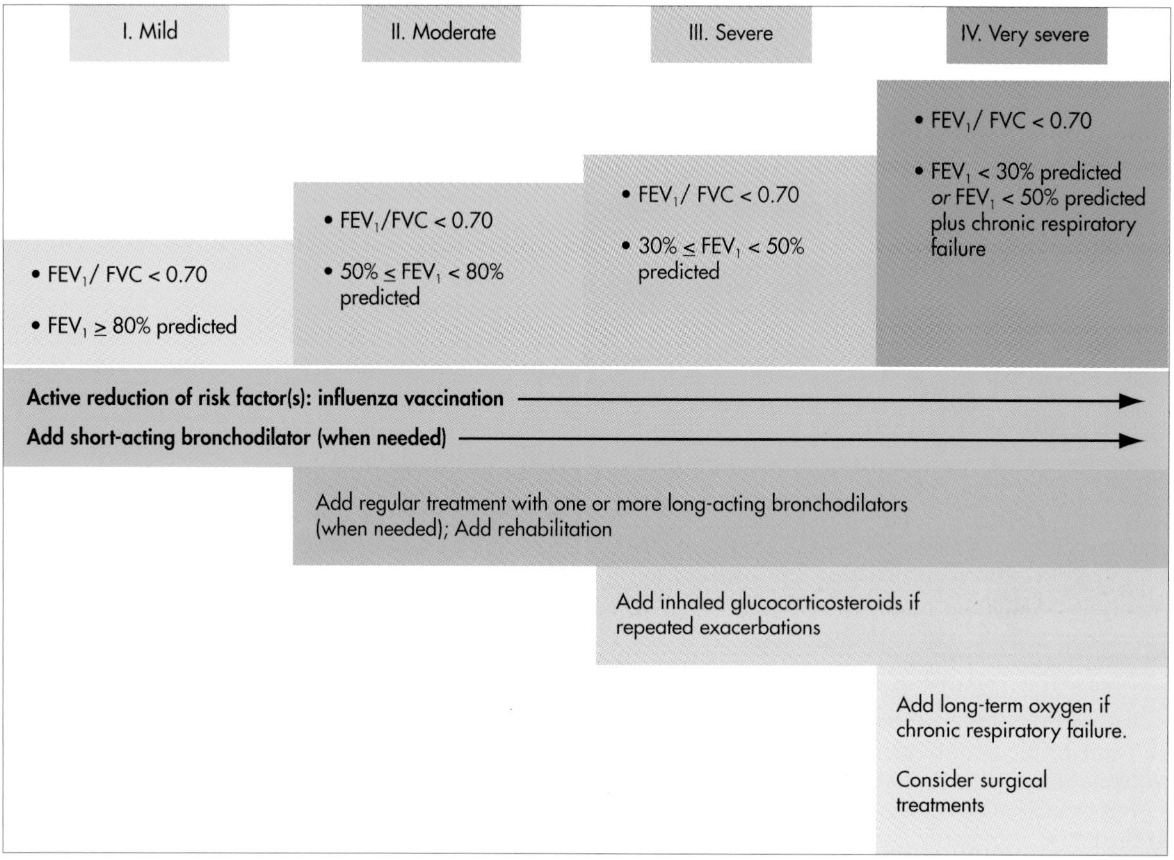

FIGURE 41.6 Therapy at each stage of COPD (Source: Global Initiative for Chronic Obstructive Lung Disease www.goldcopd.org)

ONGOING REVIEW AND/OR MONITORING

Unfortunately, COPD is a progressive disease. The rate of progression is affected by whether:

- the lung irritation is removed (be it cigarette smoking or exposure to wood smoke from indoor cooking and heating)
- the patient has acute infective exacerbations of their disease. In addition, these people often have significant comorbidities such as cardiovascular disease, due to the same factor—cigarette smoking.

Because of these matters, these patients are often frequent attenders in the primary healthcare system. Because of this they are seen often but only occasionally have a formal review or ongoing monitoring of their COPD—the healthcare system is often reacting to an acute problem rather than planning ongoing care of their chronic disease.

A planned review visit for COPD should include:

- review of symptoms
- enquiry regarding smoking status
- review of medication and inhaler device use
- lung function testing
- immunisation status
- review of the written COPD action plan for exacerbations.

IMPORTANT PITFALLS

Asthma and COPD share some features and treatment modalities. It is important to attempt to differentiate between the two, as the finer points of management and the prognoses of the two diseases are different.

PROGNOSIS

COPD is a relentlessly progressive disease and the best that can be hoped for is to slow the rate of progression and minimise symptoms. It is possible to predict the longer-term progression of COPD by using the BODE index.[32] The BODE parameters, measurable in general practice, are:

- B—body mass index
- O—degree of obstruction
- D—level of dyspnoea
- E—exercise distance.

The prognosis of COPD depends on disease severity and, as earlier diagnosis and smoking cessation influence this, all healthcare providers should aim to assess and provide advice on smoking to the people they see in consultation.

PATIENT EDUCATION

A wealth of patient information is available (see the Resources list).

LUNG CANCER

According to the World Health Organization, cancer is a leading cause of death worldwide: it accounted for 7.9 million deaths (around 13% of all deaths) in 2007. Most cancer deaths are caused by cancer of the lung, stomach, liver, colon and breast cancer. Tobacco use is the single most important risk factor for cancer.[33]

In a general practice caring for approximately 10,000 patients, there may be four new lung cancer diagnoses per year.[34]

Small-cell lung cancer has usually spread into the bloodstream by the time it is diagnosed. However, it is sensitive to both chemotherapy and radiotherapy, which are usually administered as the first line of treatment, rather than surgery.

Non-small-cell lung cancer represents approximately 80% of lung cancers.[35] Non-small-cell lung cancers are broadly divided by their main cell type into squamous cell, adenocarcinoma and large cell. If detected early it can initially be managed with local treatments such as surgery and/or radiotherapy.

AETIOLOGY

Insults to the respiratory tract are the most common cause of cancer. The most common insult to the lung is that caused by cigarette smoking, but other risk factors include:

- increasing age
- exposure to lung irritants—asbestos; occupational dusts and chemicals, most notably silica, cadmium, arsenic, nickel, chromium and beryllium.

DIAGNOSTIC APPROACH

Adequate clinical history, appropriate physical examination, thinking about the clinical problem and then considering special investigations will clarify most situations.

HISTORY

Chronic cough is probably the most common symptom of lung cancer. Unfortunately, those with COPD also have a chronic cough and, as there is a shared causative factor (cigarette smoking), the doctor needs to consider lung cancer developing in someone with COPD.

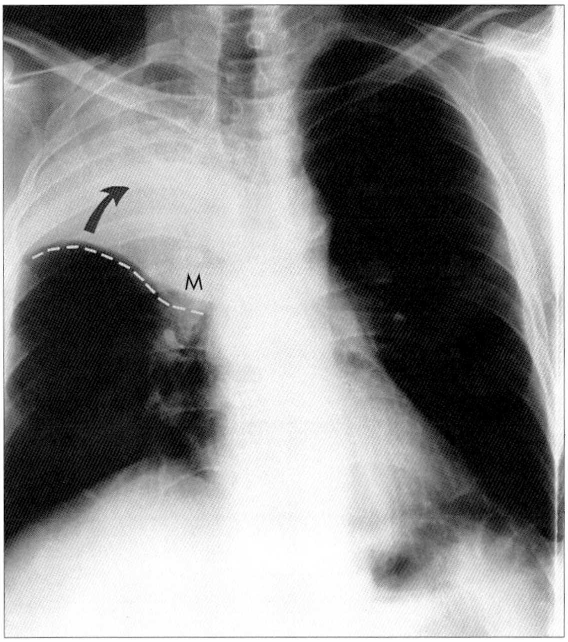

FIGURE 41.7 Chest X-ray of lung cancer: the 'golden S' sign—with a mass near the hilum, the inferior margin of the upper lobe takes on an S shape as it goes around the mass

Haemoptysis and undesired weight loss can alert the clinician to the presence of a malignancy. In a person who has an infection such as pneumonia in the upper zones, be aware that there may be an obstructing lesion.

EXAMINATION

There may be clinical evidence of COPD or regional lymphadenopathy.

INVESTIGATIONS

- In the consulting room, spirometry may demonstrate COPD (which often has the same aetiology as lung cancer).
- Pathology:
  - sputum cytology—has a low sensitivity but the specimen must be properly collected, not just saliva
  - special tests—chest X-ray and CT scanning may demonstrate the mass, and bronchoscopy is recommended to get tissue for pathological examination.

INTEGRATIVE MANAGEMENT

Prevention

As cigarette smoking and working with dusts and chemicals are known to cause lung cancer, preventive strategies based on encouraging and supporting smoking cessation and mandating protective programs for those who are exposed to noxious dusts and chemicals are critical in preventing lung cancers.

Surveillance

Surveillance alone is not a valid option unless the malignancy is so far advanced that palliation is all that can be offered (see Ch 39, Palliative medicine).

Self-help

Smoking cessation, even after diagnosis, may improve the efficacy of the various treatment modalities.

Pharmacological

Each type of lung cancer has a preferred treatment and this is specialised work. The oncology team will determine which regimen is most likely to have maximal effect.

Surgical

Surgical treatment of lung cancer depends on the type of lung cancer and its anatomical distribution. Again, these decisions need to be made by experts in this specialised area.

Complementary therapies

There are many therapies that can make the person with cancer feel better—massage, relaxation and meditation are examples (see Ch 24, Cancer).

IMPORTANT PITFALLS

Making a diagnosis is important, and appropriate investigation of patients at risk of lung cancer is crucial.

PROGNOSIS

Small-cell lung cancer

Small-cell lung cancer is an aggressive disease. The median survival time for limited disease is 18–24 months, with only 25% of patients alive after 5 years. More extensive disease is treated with chemotherapy and, even with this treatment, median survival is in the order of 12 months, with only 10% of patients surviving for 2 years.[36]

Non-small-cell lung cancer

Of patients with operable non-small-cell lung cancers that have not metastasised, up to 80% can expect to be alive at 5 years. For tumours that have spread to the lymph nodes, the 5-year survival rate drops to 25–30%. For patients with more widespread metastatic spread but who are still fit enough to receive chemotherapy, the 5-year survival rate is in the order of 15–35%.[37]

PATIENT EDUCATION

Providing education about not taking up smoking or cessation if it has already commenced is a crucial role for the GP.

INFECTIONS

Respiratory infections can be classified as viral, bacterial, atypical or tuberculosis.

VIRAL UPPER RESPIRATORY TRACT INFECTIONS

The prevalence of upper respiratory tract infections (URTI) is shown in Table 41.2.

Aetiology

General practitioners can become 'local' epidemiologists in that they often become aware quite quickly that 'something is around'. The common cold, coryza or URTI presents with a constellation of symptoms familiar to all. One needs to differentiate the common URTI from a 'true' influenza. With an influenza infection there are more systemic symptoms, with a significant fever (> 38.5°C), myalgia, arthralgia and headache.

Diagnosis

The common cold is so familiar to GPs that diagnosis is not a problem.

Treatment

- *Self-help*—usually common, simple, symptomatic measures are recommended (paracetamol, bed rest and oral fluids).

  Most of the respiratory infections seen in primary care are self-limiting viral URTIs. Even though it is almost impossible for people to avoid coming into contact with these viruses, it is important to keep the defences in the best possible condition and so minimise the number of URTIs contracted. How to maintain the healthiest possible immune system is discussed elsewhere (see Ch 32, Principles of the immune system).

TABLE 41.2 Respiratory problems managed in primary care

Problem managed	Number	% total problems	Rate per 100 encounters	95% CI
All respiratory problems	20,112	13.5	20.8	20.2–21.4
URTI	5,914	4.0	6.1	5.7–6.6

Source: Britt et al 2009[1]

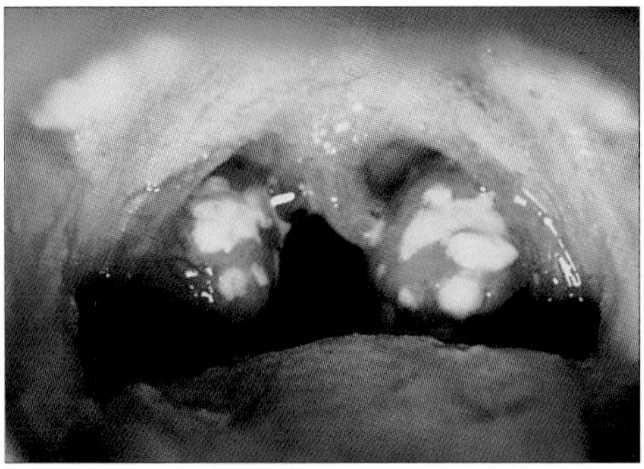

FIGURE 41.8 Pharyngitis

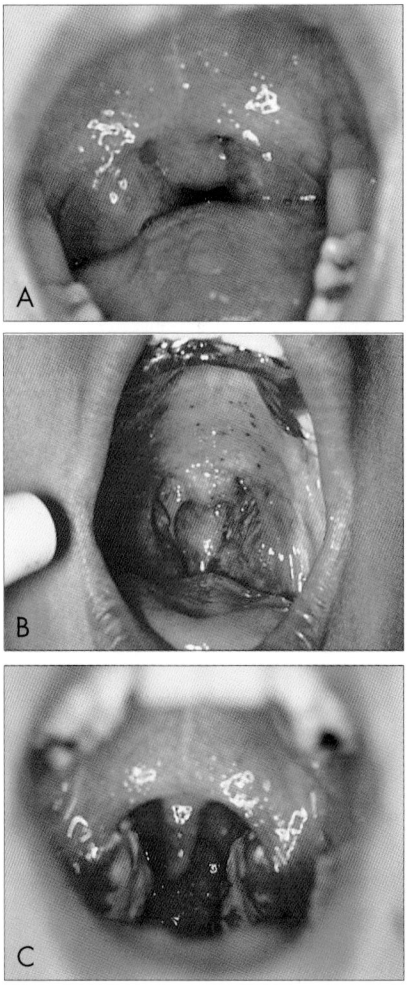

FIGURE 41.9 Bacterial tonsillitis: **A** Diffuse tonsillar and pharyngeal erythema can be produced by a variety of pathogens; **B** Intense erythema with acute tonsillar enlargement and palatal petechiae is highly suggestive of group A beta-streptococcal infection; **C** Exudative tonsillitis is most commonly seen with either group A streptococcal or Epstein-Barr virus infection

- *Steam inhalation*—although this has been used for generations, evidence as to whether it improves nasal congestion for a person with a cold is insufficient. Some studies found that inhaling steam helped symptoms, but others did not; and there were some adverse effects, such as discomfort or irritation of the nose or lips.[37]
- *Pharmacological*—for the simple URTI, paracetamol is usually all that is required.

Complementary therapies

- *Echinacea*—this has been widely used for preventing and treating the common cold. Echinacea preparations available on the market differ greatly, as different species, plant parts (e.g. herb, root or both) and manufacturing methods (drying, alcoholic extraction or pressing) are used. A review of 16 controlled clinical trials on different *Echinacea* preparations for preventing and treating common colds suggests that the evidence that it can help to shorten the duration of the cold and related symptoms is stronger than evidence that it can prevent colds.[38]
- *Andrographis paniculata*—has been shown to have antiviral properties and to shorten the duration and severity of symptoms of the common cold.[39] Typical dose: 500 mg t.d.s.
- *Astragalus*—has antiviral properties and stimulates the immune system, suggesting that it may be effective at preventing colds. Standardised extract: 250–500 mg, 3–4 times a day.
- Vitamin C—a 2007 Cochrane review[40] found that vitamin C reduced the duration and severity of common cold symptoms slightly. However, with regard to prevention, 'The failure of vitamin C supplementation to reduce the incidence of colds in the normal population indicates that routine mega-dose prophylaxis is not rationally justified for community use. But evidence suggests that it could be justified in people exposed to brief periods of severe physical exercise or cold environments'.
- Zinc—deficiency should be corrected. Clinical trial data support the value of zinc in reducing the duration and severity of symptoms of the common cold when administered within 24 hours of the onset of common cold symptoms. However, overall data studying the use of various forms of zinc for treatment of colds are inconclusive.[41]
- Homoeopathic oscillococcinum—research suggests that this does not seem to prevent influenza but it may shorten the duration of the illness.[42]

Ongoing review and/or monitoring

Most URTIs are self-limiting. It is prudent to warn the patient to contact their GP if the URTI does not follow the expected pattern, as there is always the possibility of bacterial super-infection or exacerbation of an underlying comorbidity.

Prognosis is excellent unless there are significant co-morbidities that can render the patient vulnerable to complications. A common cause of destabilisation of asthma is a viral URTI. Many acute exacerbations of COPD are precipitated by viral infections. If the patient is immunocompromised (e.g. HIV/AIDS, malignancy and iatrogenic immunosuppression), an URTI is capable of causing many problems.

Patient education

Rest, simple symptomatic treatments, cough hygiene and some degree of 'isolation' to minimise spread of the virus are important messages to give to the patient.

TUBERCULOSIS

Tuberculosis (TB) remains a global problem. In 2008, there were an estimated 9.4 million incident cases worldwide—this is equivalent to 139 cases per 100,000 population. Most of the estimated number of cases in 2008 occurred in Asia (55%) and Africa (30%).[43]

Tuberculosis is a notifiable disease, as it is quite contagious. As such, cases should be notified promptly to the relevant public health authorities. Both the World Health Organization and the International Union against Tuberculosis and Lung Disease run international programs for TB prevention and management.

The symptoms of TB are vague (cough, sputum, breathlessness, haemoptysis, weight loss, fever, malaise and anorexia).[44] Think of it in the person with a chronic cough, particularly if it is productive. There are also extra-pulmonary manifestations of TB, including lymph nodes, genitourinary tract, pleura, pericardium, bones and joints, meninges, eye, skin, adrenal glands and gut.

Immigrant populations from areas of high background incidence—Indian subcontinent, Africa, South-East Asia and the former Eastern Bloc countries—are a high-risk group as reactivation can occur in the presence of immunosuppression.

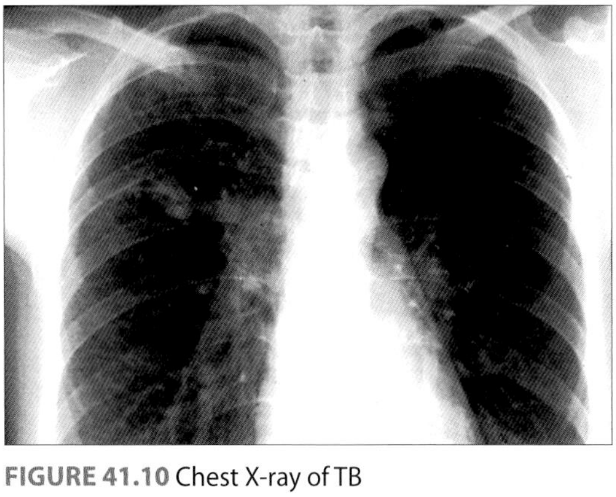

FIGURE 41.10 Chest X-ray of TB

Tuberculosis should also be considered in those at risk of a reactivation of quiescent TB—the immunosuppressed. Consider the large number of people in your practice who are on immunosuppressive therapy (e.g. post-transplant patients, rheumatoid disease, systemic lupus erythematosus (SLE), polymyalgia rheumatica, recurrent rescue prednisolone for acute exacerbations of COPD). Also consider diseases that are inherently immunosuppressive—HIV/AIDS and many cancers. There are a large number of people in these categories and this heightens their risk of reactivation of TB.

Diagnosis

Diagnosis is made on the basis of the chest X-ray and sputum microscopy and culture.[44] Polymerase chain reaction (PCR) rapid diagnostic tests are available in some places but the more important thing is that the possibility of TB is considered and acted upon.

A Mantoux test may be a useful guide.

Biopsy of accessible extra-pulmonary lesions such as lymph nodes may be performed.

Consider HIV testing.

Treatment

According to *Australian Therapeutic Guidelines: Respiratory*,[45] patients with TB should:

- be managed only by specialists with appropriate training and experience
- be notified promptly to the relevant state public health authorities
- have contact tracing performed by public health nurses liaising closely with the treating doctors.

Because of concerns about drug resistance, bacterial confirmation of the diagnosis, and drug susceptibility testing, should be strenuously pursued.

Adequate adherence to anti-tuberculous therapy is vital in order to:

- achieve a satisfactory treatment outcome
- reduce the risk of transmission to contacts
- reduce the risk of relapse
- prevent the emergence of drug resistance.

Measures to improve adherence include:

- comprehensive patient and family education (in the form of verbal and written information)
- close and consistent follow-up
- provision of directly observed therapy (DOT).

The most common drugs used to treat TB are isoniazid, rifampin, pyrazinamide, ethambutol and streptomycin, usually in combinations of four. If problems with supply of anti-tuberculous drugs arise, the state health department should be contacted.

- Probiotics will be a necessary adjunct.
- Avoid alcohol during treatment because of potential hepatotoxicity.
- Avoid tobacco smoke.
- There are significant public health issues with TB and so expert assistance is usually required when the diagnosis has been made.

Nutrition

Many patients with active TB experience severe weight loss and some show signs of vitamin and mineral deficiencies. Patients with TB/HIV co-infection are even worse off nutritionally. Nutritional advice and support are important elements in recovery.

Frequent (six times a day) meals with a high-energy and high-protein diet are helpful in the acute stages of the illness.

Multivitamin and mineral supplementation:

- zinc
- vitamin C
- *Astragalus*
- protein and calorie supplementation—may be necessary where appetite is lacking.

Prevention

- BCG vaccination should be considered in some at-risk populations.
- Maintain immune system function (see Ch 32, Principles of the immune system)
- Sufficient sleep and rest.
- Exercise 30 minutes per day.
- Fresh whole foods including fruit and vegetables.
- Maintain respiratory hygiene.

COMMUNITY-ACQUIRED PNEUMONIA AND THE ATYPICAL INFECTIONS

In general practice, when dealing with community-acquired pneumonia and the atypical infections, the most important thing is to consider them in the differential diagnosis.

In community-acquired pneumonia (CAP), the patient is unwell, with high fever. It is more than a simple URTI. The disease is more common in the very young and the very old. The most common organism is *Streptococcus pneumoniae* but, in one study, in 22% of cases of CAP where an organism was identified, it was an atypical organism (*Mycoplasma pneumoniae*, *Chlamydia pneumoniae* and *Legionella* spp).[46]

Think of atypical respiratory infections especially in the context of the person with an impaired immune system. A prominent example is *Pneumocystis jiroveci* (*carinii*) (formerly PCP) infection in those with HIV infection.

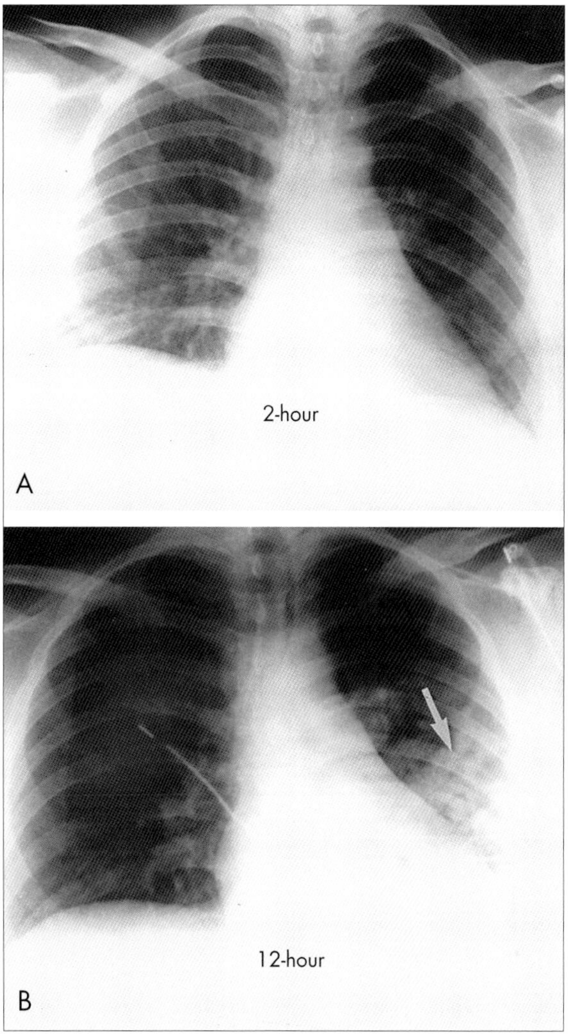

FIGURE 41.11 Chest X-ray of pneumonia obtained soon after aspiration may appear normal (**A**); it takes 6–12 hours for an alveolar infiltrate to develop (arrow, **B**)

Diagnostic approach

- *History*—the patient has a chest infection, often productive of purulent sputum, and is systemically unwell.
- *Examination*—there may be some localising signs on respiratory examination.

Investigations

- *Consulting room*—there may be a reduction in oxygen saturation (if you have access to a pulse oximeter).
- *Pathology*—sputum (a properly collected sample) for microscopy, culture and sensitivity (MCS) is important but, if the patient is very unwell, commencing treatment should not be delayed while these samples are being tested.
- *Special tests*—a chest X-ray will assist diagnosis.

Integrated management

Prevention

Respiratory hygiene and minimising spread of infection is important. Ensure routine immunisations against *Haemophilus influenzae*, influenza and pertussis (whooping cough).

Some children with specific medical problems require vaccination against invasive pneumococcal disease (IPD) separately from the usual immunisation program. These conditions are listed in Box 41.1.

Self-help

Maintaining adequate nutrition is important in preventing infection in susceptible children.

Pharmacological

If CAP is suspected, consultation with the local infectious disease physician or microbiology service will guide the GP as to the most appropriate antibiotic to be used.

BOX 41.1 Underlying medical conditions predisposing children aged 9 years or younger to IPD[47]

- Diseases compromising immune response to pneumococcal infection:
  - congenital immune deficiency including symptomatic IgG subclass or isolated IgA deficiency (but children who require monthly immunoglobulin infusion are unlikely to benefit from vaccination)
  - immunosuppressive therapy (including corticosteroid therapy ≥ 2 mg/kg per day of prednisolone or equivalent for more than 2 weeks) or radiation therapy, where there is sufficient immune reconstitution for vaccine response to be expected
  - compromised splenic fuanction due to sickle haemoglobinopathies, or congenital or acquired asplenia
  - haematological malignancies
  - HIV infection, before and after development of AIDS
  - renal failure, or relapsing or persistent nephrotic syndrome
  - Down syndrome.
- Anatomical or metabolic abnormalities associated with higher rates or severity of IPD:
  - cardiac disease associated with cyanosis or cardiac failure
  - all premature infants with chronic lung disease
  - all infants born at less than 28 weeks' gestation
  - cystic fibrosis
  - insulin-dependent diabetes mellitus
  - proven or presumptive cerebrospinal fluid (CSF) leak
  - intracranial shunts and cochlear implants.

Ongoing review and/or monitoring

These patients are often very unwell, and hospital admission will need to be considered. There are validated severity scales (e.g. CURB-65) that guide diagnosis, but how to proceed remains a clinical decision.[46]

Important pitfalls

Perhaps the greatest risk for the GP is of underestimating the severity of the patient's condition.

Prognosis

The mortality from CAP has altered little since antibiotics became readily available—it is still a significant cause of mortality. In Australia, pneumonia and influenza cause 2% of male deaths and 2.7% of female deaths.[48]

RESOURCES

Australian Lung Foundation, http://www.lungnet.com.au
Cancer Council of Australia, http://www.cancer.org.au
Global Initiative for Asthma (GINA), Global Burden of Asthma, http://www.ginasthma.com
International Primary Care Respiratory Group (IPCRG), http://www.theipcrg.org
National Asthma Council Australia, http://www.NationalAsthma.org.au
World Health Organization, http://www.who.int

REFERENCES

1 Britt H, Miller GC, Charles J et al. General practice activity in Australia 2008–09. Canberra: Australian Institute of Health and Welfare; December 2009. Cat. GEP 25; Table 7.2.
2 National Asthma Council Australia (NACA). Asthma management handbook 2006. Melbourne: NACA; 2006. a p 3.
3 Holgate ST, Boushey HA, Fabbri LM, eds. Difficult asthma. London: Martin Dunitz; 1999:183.
4 Strachan DP. Hay fever, hygiene, and household size. BMJ 1989; 299:1259–1260.
5 Goldberg S, Israeli E, Schwartz S et al. Asthma prevalence, family size, and birth order. Chest 2007; 131(6):1747–1752.
6 Kline JN. Eat dirt. CpG DNA and immunomodulation of asthma. Proc Am Thorac Soc 2007; 4:283–288.
7 Gøtzsche PC, Johansen HK. House dust mite control measures for asthma. Cochrane Database Syst Rev 2008; 2:CD001187.
8 Blackhall K, Appleton S, Cates CJ. Ionisers for chronic asthma. Cochrane Database Syst Rev 2003; 2:CD002986.
9 Kilburn S, Lasserson TJ, McKean M. Pet allergen control measures for allergic asthma in children and adults. Cochrane Database Syst Rev 2003; 1:CD002989.
10 Welsh EJ, Bara AI, Barley EA et al. Caffeine for asthma. Cochrane Database Syst Rev 2010; 1:CD001112.

11 Thien FCK, De Luca S, Woods R et al. Dietary marine fatty acids (fish oil) for asthma in adults and children. Cochrane Database Syst Rev 2002; 2:CD001283.
12 Mickelborough TD, Lindley MR, Ionescu AA et al. Protective effect of fish oil supplementation on exercise-induced bronchoconstriction in asthma. Chest 2006; 129:39–49.
13 Romieu I, Trenga C. Diet and obstructive lung diseases. (Review) Epidemiol Rev 2001; 23(2):268–287.
14 Ram FS, Ardern KD. Tartrazine exclusion for allergic asthma. Cochrane Database Syst Rev 2001; 4:CD000460.
15 Holloway E, Ram FSF. Breathing exercises for asthma. Cochrane Database Syst Rev 2004; 1:CD001277.
16 Nagendra H, Nagarathna R. An integrated approach of yoga therapy for bronchial asthma: a 3–54 month prospective study. J Asthma 1986; 23(3):123–137.
17 Slader CA, Reddel HK, Spencer LM et al. Double blind randomized controlled trial of two different breathing techniques in the management of asthma. Thorax 2006; 61:651–656.
18 Emelyanov A, Fedoseev G, Krasnoschekova O et al. Treatment of asthma with lipid extract of New Zealand green-lipped mussel: a randomised clinical trial. Eur Respir J 2002; 20:596–600.
19 Burns JS, Dockery DW, Neas LM et al. Low dietary nutrient intakes and respiratory health in adolescents. Chest 2007; 132(1):238–245.
20 Riccioni G, Bucciarelli T, Mancini B et al. Plasma lycopene and antioxidant vitamins in asthma: the PLAVA study. J Asthma 2007; 44(6):429–432.
21 McCarney RW, Brinkhaus B, Lasserson TJ et al. Acupuncture for chronic asthma. Cochrane Database Syst Rev 2003; 3:CD000008.
22 Dennis J, Cates CJ. Alexander technique for chronic asthma. Cochrane Database Syst Rev 2000; 2:CD000995.
23 Arnold E, Clark CE, Lasserson TJ et al. Herbal interventions for chronic asthma in adults and children. Cochrane Database Syst Rev 2008; 1:CD005989.
24 McCarney RW, Linde K, Lasserson TJ. Homeopathy for chronic asthma. Cochrane Database Syst Rev 2004; 1:CD000353.
25 Beamon S, Falkenbach A, Fainburg G et al. Speleotherapy for asthma. Cochrane Database Syst Rev 2001; 2:CD001741.
26 McKenzie DK, Abramson M, Crockett AJ et al. The COPD-X Plan: Australian and New Zealand guidelines for the management of chronic obstructive pulmonary disease, 2009. Online. Available: http://www.copdx.org.au/guidelines/
27 Abramson M, Raven J, Skoric B, et al. Prevalence of COPD amongst middle aged and older adults. Respirology 2003; 8(Suppl 2):A59.
28 Wilson D, Adams R, Appleton S et al. Difficulties identifying and targeting COPD and population-attributable risk of smoking for COPD. A population study. Chest 2005; 128:2035–2042.
29 Tiong LU, Gibson PG, Hensley MJ et al. Lung volume reduction surgery for diffuse emphysema. Cochrane Database Syst Rev 2006; 4:CD001001.
30 Guo R, Pittler MH, Ernst E. Herbal medicines for the treatment of COPD: a systematic review. Eur Respir J 2006; 28:330–338.
31 Ferreira IM, Brooks D, Lacasse Y et al. Nutritional supplementation for stable chronic obstructive pulmonary disease. Cochrane Database Syst Rev 2005; 2:CD000998.
32 Celli BR, Cote CG, Marin JM et al. The body-mass index, airflow obstruction, dyspnea, and exercise capacity index in chronic obstructive pulmonary disease. N Engl J Med 2004; 350:1005–1012.
33 World Health Organization. Cancer. Online. Available: www.who.int/cancer/en/index.html 2 April 2010.
34 McAvoy B, Elwood M, Staples M. Cancer in Australia. An update for GPs. Aust Family Physician 2005; 34(1/2):41–45.
35 Cancer Council Australia. Lung cancer—non small cell. Online. Available: http://www.cancer.org.au/Healthprofessionals/cancertypes/lungcancernonsmallcell.htm. Last updated 2003.
36 Cancer Council Australia. Lung cancer—small cell. Online. Available: www.cancer.org.au/Healthprofessionals/cancertypes/lungcancersmallcell.htm. Last updated 2003.
37 Singh M. Heated, humidified air for the common cold. Cochrane Database Syst Rev 2006; 3:CD001728.
38 Linde K, Barrett B, Wölkart K et al. Echinacea for preventing and treating the common cold. Cochrane Database Syst Rev 2006; 1:CD000530.
39 Saxena RC, Singh R, Kumar P et al. A randomized double blind placebo controlled clinical evaluation of extract of *Andrographis paniculata* (KalmCold) in patients with uncomplicated upper respiratory tract infection. Phytomedicine 2010; 17(3/4):178–185.
40 Hemilä H, Chalker E, Treacy B et al. Vitamin C for preventing and treating the common cold. Cochrane Database Syst Rev 2007; 3:CD000980.
41 Hulisz D. Efficacy of zinc against common cold viruses: an overview. J Am Pharm Assoc 2004; 44:594–603.
42 Vickers AJ, Smith C. Homoeopathic Oscillococcinum for preventing and treating influenza and influenza-like syndromes. Cochrane Database Syst Rev 2006; 3:CD001957.
43 World Health Organization. WHO Library Cataloguing-in-Publication Data. Global tuberculosis control: a short update to the 2009 report. WHO/HTM/TB/2009.426, pp. 4–5.
44 Campbell IA, Bah-Sow O. Pulmonary tuberculosis: diagnosis and treatment. BMJ 2006; 332:1194–1197.

45 Therapeutic Guidelines. Respiratory. North Melbourne: Therapeutic Guidelines Ltd; 2006.

46 Durrington HJ, Summers C. Recent changes in the management of community acquired pneumonia in adults. BMJ 2008; 336:1429–1433.

47 Australian Government. Australian immunisation handbook, 9th edn. 2008: 246.

48 Australian Institute of Health and Welfare. Australia's health no. 9. Cat. No. AUS 44. Canberra: AIHW; 2004.

chapter 42

Skin

The skin, the skin
'Tis a wonderful thing.
Keeps the outside out
And the inside in.

INTRODUCTION AND OVERVIEW

The skin is the most obvious organ in the body and every practitioner sees lots of it—about two square metres of it walks through the door with each adult patient. Skin is our interface with the environment and it always tells us things about the patient.

Every primary practitioner sees a wide variety of skin diseases in patients of all age groups, including eczema, psoriasis, infections, acne, urticaria, various pigmented lesions and solar damage including skin cancer. Up to 15% of general practice presentations are for skin conditions.

The skin can itch, burn, swell and appear unsightly, and this can frequently lead to anxiety or psychological reactions. The skin presents to the world and even an apparently trivial skin blemish may be considered a major problem by the patient. Many skin conditions can also cause such persistent discomfort and inconvenience in day-to-day living that patients feel restricted, even in the most basic of activities, resulting in loss of confidence, low self-esteem and diminished quality of life.

The more skin conditions can be understood and managed in relation to the patient's general health, the more likely there is to be a cure, sustained relief or benefit to the patient as a whole.

This chapter is too brief to give a comprehensive coverage of skin disease. Instead, it provides a framework to enable a clinician to approach skin conditions from an integrative perspective, using some common conditions as examples. Some skin conditions are covered at greater length, with integrative approaches, while others have been included only briefly, to represent what is common in primary care practice.

As in other areas of medicine it is important to ensure that both diagnosis and treatment of skin conditions address causes, rather than suppressing symptoms alone. Skin conditions often have multiple contributing causes, including topical influences, autoimmune or genetic susceptibility, food factors and numerous ancillary triggers.

AETIOLOGY

Many people have a predisposition to skin disease before triggers or precipitating events cause the condition to appear. Allergic or autoimmune predisposition, dry skin, excessive sun exposure, stress or nutritional deficiencies can all set the scene. The triggers may include infection (bacteria, fungi, yeasts, viruses, parasites) or trauma, leading to inflammation or neoplastic change. There are also systemic diseases that have skin manifestations, such as diabetes, thyroid disease, high lipids, and deficiencies including fatty acids, zinc, iron and B vitamins.

DIAGNOSIS

While diagnosis of many skin conditions relies on pattern recognition, sometimes it is elusive. A well-honed systematic approach is essential for diagnosis.

Systematic steps:

1 History
2 Examination
3 Accurate description of lesions or skin
4 Differential diagnosis
5 Special tests
6 Diagnosis
7 Treatment plan.

- *History*—in addition to the history of the condition, questions relating to general health are also needed. Past medical history, family history,

TABLE 42.1 Terminology of lesions

Term	Small (< 5 mm)	Large (> 5 mm)	
Flat colour change	Macule	Patch	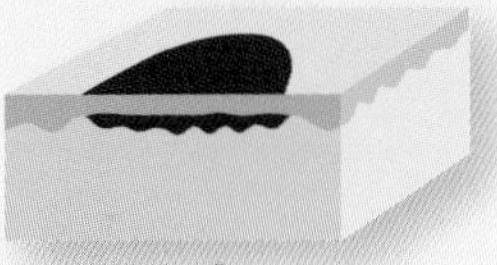 Macule
Elevated lump	Papule	Nodule: > 5 mm in width & depth Plaque: > 2 cm with little depth	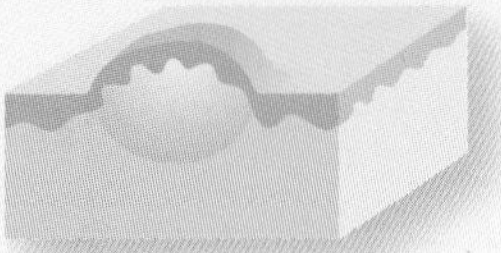 Plaque 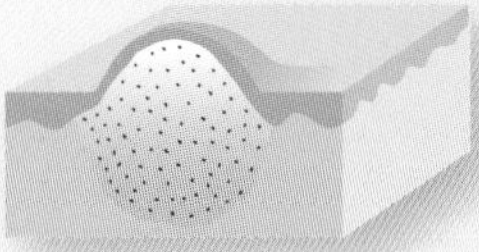 Nodule
Pus-filled lesion	Pustule	Abscess	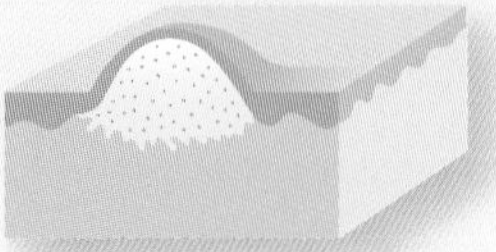 Pustule
Fluid-filled blister	Vesicle	Bulla	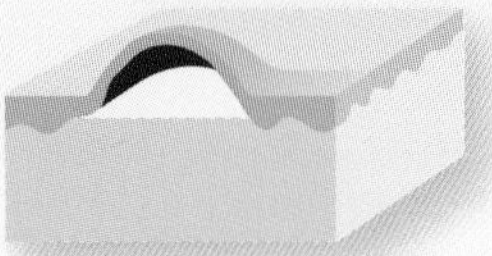 Vesicle (subepidermal)
Extravasated blood	Petechia (pinhead) Purpura (< 2 mm)	Ecchymosis Haematoma: swelling, gross bleed	
Dermal oedema	Wheal (any size)	Angio-oedema	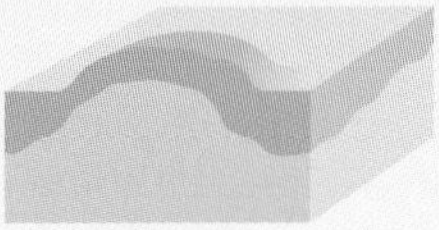 Wheal

Adapted from Hunter et al. 1995[1] and Gawkrodger 1992[2]

allergic history, a nutritional assessment, including supplements, and medications are all important. Listen to patients, as they often have perceptions about their skin and ideas that provide clues to the causes or triggers for the condition.

- *Examination*
  - Dermatology is a visual branch of medicine, and in order to ensure accurate diagnosis, examination requires a bright light and good magnification.
  - Dermoscopy is a valuable examination tool for pigmented lesions. An ultraviolet Wood's lamp can cause fungal infections and erythrasma to fluoresce.
  - Examine the whole skin in addition to the specific lesion. Have a good look—touch, stretch and feel the texture and thickness.
- *Accurate description of lesions or skin*—an accurate description (Table 42.1) requires careful observation and often leads directly to the

diagnosis. A dermatology atlas and comprehensive text are helpful.
- *Special tests*—take the time and make the effort to do the tests. Investigations are:
  - swabs, skin scrapings or nail clippings
  - punch, shave or incisional biopsy. These are simple procedures that take little extra time and often make or confirm a diagnosis. It is important to provide a brief clinical outline, a description of the lesion and, if possible, a differential diagnosis for the histopathologist, as microscopic appearances can be equivocal.
- *Diagnosis* will arise from the above systematic approach. Remember that the skin is a reflector of systemic conditions.

TREATMENT PLAN

Each skin condition requires specific treatment measures. In general, however, integrated management could include the following:

- *Prevention*—where triggers are identifiable; for example, avoidance of arginine-rich foods (peanuts, almonds and chocolate) with herpetic infections; management of sun exposure to minimise solar sun damage while ensuring adequate sun exposure to manufacture vitamin D in the skin.
- *Surveillance*—Hippocrates said to 'Make a habit of two things—to help or at least to do no harm'. The positive diagnosis of benign or self-limiting conditions such as pityriasis rosea, keratosis pilaris, granuloma annulare or toxic viral rashes is important, as they often require no intervention.
- *Self-help and general remedies* that aim to improve the patient's general health and benefit the condition. For example:
  - Reduce exposure to heat, spices or alcohol with rosacea.
  - Reducing immune stressors can reduce the threshold to autoimmune disease that affects or reflects in the skin. These diseases include vitiligo, melanoma, halo naevus, idiopathic thrombocytopenic purpura, Hashimoto's thyroiditis, systemic lupus erythematosus, scleroderma and diabetic skin disease. Stressors that reduce a patient's adaptive capacity include emotional stress (including anxiety and depression), chemical load, allergic load, hormonal imbalance, fatigue, endocrine disease, chronic viral infections and nutritional deficiencies (zinc, iron, vitamin D, vitamin B_{12} or folic acid). These stressors are common and need to be addressed.
- *Pharmacological relief* is important—a teenager with severe acne can try multiple nutritional and topical measures but needs treatment with a high probability of a rapid response. This will often include topical as well as oral treatments.
- *Surgical excision* is still the treatment of choice for the majority of skin cancers. Excision provides a specimen, which is always sent to pathology. The dermatopathologist will confirm or make the diagnosis and establish the presence of a margin of safety around the malignant lesion.

IMPORTANT PITFALLS IN SKIN MANAGEMENT

- Remember to take skin conditions seriously. Most are not fatal but many cause angst and suffering, or low mortality with high morbidity. Take the trouble to assess the impact of the condition on the patient. For example, most young people with moderate acne experience significant loss of confidence, depression or even difficulty gaining employment.
- Work for a positive diagnosis before committing to long-term treatment. For example, is it psoriasis, eczema or fungal?
- Do not use fluorinated steroids on the face, especially around the mouth.
- Do not use steroids on rashes where there could be fungal infections as this can lead to extension of the infection, known as tinea incognito.

SPECIFIC SKIN CONDITIONS

In order to see how a well-honed systematic approach can be applied in practice, we will look at the management of some specific skin conditions. Some of these conditions are well managed using an integrative approach and are discussed more fully. Others require standard medical treatment alone, and many of these are covered only briefly, in order to provide a more representative picture of skin presentations.

ECZEMA

Eczema is the most common skin reaction. It is an inflammatory disorder and the term is interchangeable with *dermatitis*, although sometimes 'dermatitis' is used when the cause is external or exogenous (Box 42.1).

Contact or exogenous eczema

- *Irritant contact*—occurs whenever irritant materials are in prolonged contact with the skin. This is not an allergy and does not reflect individual sensitivity. It is a direct irritant effect of substances such as detergent, petrol or solvents. Irritant contact dermatitis of the hands is the most common occupational disease.

BOX 42.1 Classification of eczema

Contact or exogenous eczema
- irritant contact eczema (90%)
- allergic contact eczema
- photosensitive

Constitutional or endogenous eczema
- atopic
- pompholyx (dyshidrotic)
- hyperkeratotic
  - discoid or nummular
  - asteatotic or eczema craquelé
  - seborrhoeic eczema of adults or infants

BOX 42.2 Common contact allergens

- adhesives
- antibiotic
- cement, leather, matches
- chromates
- cosmetic preservatives, laboratories, white shoes, deodorants
- cosmetics, creams containing lanolin
- cosmetics, soaps
- epoxy resin
- formaldehyde
- fragrances/perfume mix
- gloves, shoes, elastic straps, tyres
- jewellery, watch straps, jean studs, coins, tools
- lignocaine
- neomycin
- nickel
- parabens
- preservative
- rubber chemicals
- topical local anaesthetic
- wool alcohols

- *Allergic contact*—occurs when there is an allergic reaction to an agent in contact with the skin (Box 42.2). There are many causes. These may be suspected from the history and confirmed by patch testing if necessary.
- *Photosensitive dermatitis* is eczema in light-exposed areas, often as a side effect of a drug.
- *Napkin dermatitis* is a specific form of irritant contact dermatitis following prolonged contact with urine and faeces.
- Plant contact dermatitis.

Constitutional or endogenous eczema

- *Atopic eczema* (see next section)
- *Pompholyx or dyshidrotic eczema*—this is a common hand or foot eczema characterised by small blisters on the palms or soles, especially at the margins, that burst and heal with peeling. Because the skin is thick, inflammatory fluid is trapped in the skin, leading to this characteristic appearance. A potent topical steroid ointment is required.
- *Hyperkeratotic eczema*
- *Discoid or nummular eczema*—the pattern of one or more oval or coin-shaped plaques of eczema is characteristic. The cause is unknown but lesions may occur on any part of the body, particularly on the legs.
- *Asteatotic eczema* or *eczema craquelé*—a dry and itchy form of eczema on the legs that produces a 'crazy paving' type of appearance. It is related to dry skin (xerosis) and is common later in life.
- *Seborrhoeic eczema*—a red, itchy, scaling rash that commonly affects the scalp and midline areas of the face, including around the nose and between the eyebrows. The ears may also be involved, and occasionally areas on the central chest and axillae are affected. It is thought to be caused by sensitivity to a yeast, *Malassezia*. The eyelids often have scales and redness (blepharitis).

  Patients often notice that seborrhoeic eczema is worse when they are tired, run-down or eating excessive sugar or refined carbohydrates. Yeasts feed on sugar.

  Management is most effective when anti-yeast shampoos or creams are combined with a diet that avoids sugar and refined or high-GI carbohydrates.
- *Infantile seborrhoeic eczema*—affects newborns up to 6 months of age, manifesting as cradle cap, napkin dermatitis or sometimes spreading over the whole trunk.

Atopic eczema

Atopic eczema is dealt with in detail here, as it is a good example of how a practitioner can make a great contribution to the wellbeing of the patient and their family, by employing integrative principles. This discussion emphasises management in children, where atopic eczema is most common, but the principles can be adapted to all age groups.

Atopic eczema is common, often very itchy and usually begins in young children from allergic families. Atopic patients have an allergic predisposition to asthma, eczema, hay fever, urticaria and other allergies. It is important to spend time with the patient, collecting information and piecing together the puzzle. Patients or parents will tell you the answers if you ask and listen. Avoid reflex prescriptions for medications, including nutritional supplements.

Atopic eczema can be likened to a slow-burning scrub fire. It is much more than a steroid-responsive dermatosis. Each patient needs to be managed with an appreciation of the causes, triggers and individual patterns of their disease.

The prevalence of atopic eczema and allergic disease has increased dramatically over the past three decades. One theory put forward to explain this is the 'hygiene hypothesis', which argues that early childhood exposure to infections inhibits the tendency to develop allergic disease. The idea behind this hypothesis is that bacterial and viral infections during childhood somehow 'tone up' the immune system and thereby reduce the tendency to develop allergic disease. Children in Western societies have a more hygienic and 'sanitised' lifestyle and a greater risk of developing allergic illness. The increasing prevalence of autoimmune disease may be related.

The cause of atopic eczema is probably multifactorial: genetic, immunological and environmental.

Other predisposing factors to be considered may include a family history of allergies, early introduction of cow's milk or wheat, and of antibiotics (beta-lactam), vaccinations (pertussis, influenza), dust mite or cockroach exposure, a smoking parent and stress.

Atopic eczema will resolve in at least half of children by the age of five, but a significant number will go on to develop asthma. Atopic eczema is a T helper 2 (Th2) dominant disease.

Clinical presentation

Commencing around 3 months of age, atopic eczema is characterised by dryness, itching and scaling. The rash is usually symmetrical and commences on the cheeks and flexures. There is often subsequent excoriation and lichenification from scratching.

Assessment

A detailed history should be taken, including suspected allergies, details of the diet and preparations used to treat the skin. The family will usually have suspicions about factors thaat may be contributing, and clues will emerge about foods or general triggers. These families have a child with a chronic disease that requires ongoing monitoring, considerable thought and a lot of care each day. The impact on the family as a whole needs to be appreciated.

Food sensitivity is more likely to be a factor in childhood eczema than in adults, and parents will often ask about this. Features in the history that suggest food intolerance as more probable than inhalant allergy include: early age of onset; past history of atopic disease; infective pattern to asthma; sinusitis, otitis media, glue ear or grommets; associated symptoms relating to other systems, such as irritable bowel syndrome, migraine, fatigue, behaviour problems in children; recurrent croup; positive family history of food problems; negative skin tests for inhalants; and a poor response to drug therapy.

Children tend to react to foods that they eat frequently or crave. Wheat, potato, tomato, cows' milk and citrus are common food sensitivities that may contribute to eczema.

Sometimes skin testing for inhalant allergens, and particularly for those that can be avoided, such as house dust mite, cat or dog, can be useful. Radioallergosorbent test (RAST) is an alternative technique with blood testing to test for IgE-mediated allergies.

Most food sensitivity is not IgE mediated, and skin or blood testing (IgE or IgG) is not reliable in excluding food problems. The most accurate way of diagnosing food sensitivities is through food elimination and challenge dietary testing.

Prevention

(See also Ch 55, Child health and development.)

- Pregnant mothers with a family history of atopy or allergies should have their diet discussed. Avoidance of specific foods such as egg white or shellfish in pregnancy may reduce the risk of atopic disease in the baby, but there should also be discussion of the patient's food intake to ensure that there is a good variety of foods and moderation of intake of foods where there has been a family problem.
- A good level of antioxidant intake during pregnancy reduces allergic disease in the first 2 years of life.
- Breastfeeding should be encouraged, as this is protective of the infant's immunological health.

And for all age groups:

- Avoid known or suspected allergens, to reduce the allergic load on the individual.
- Minimise exposure to potentially toxic or sensitising chemicals in the environment. These include petrochemicals, pesticides, deodorisers, aldehydes, solvents and other volatile organic chemicals.

Treatment

These approaches are directed towards young children, but are adaptable to all age groups.

- Once a young child has atopic eczema, reducing dust in the bedroom and removing pets and feathers are precautionary measures.
- Reduce trigger factors, including woollen clothes in contact with the skin.
- Avoiding contact with skin infections, especially cold sores or herpetic infections, helps to prevent infections that cause more severe eruptions in eczematous skin.
- Treat dry skin—like dry leather, dry skin does not respond well to soaps or detergents, and needs oil or moisturising preparations to keep it soft and

healthy. How well would leather shoes respond to regular washing with soap and hot water? Similarly, eczematous skin is best cleansed with cooler water and minimal use of a soap substitute or cream.

- Emollients or moisturisers are useful for greasing dry skin (xerosis). Although many commercial brands have petrochemical bases, they usually work well in practice. Often these base preparations have added ingredients such as oils or colloidal oatmeal. Plant oils can also be useful topically, and include evening primrose, vitamin E, rosehip and coconut oils. Emollients soak into the skin within 2 hours and need to be used frequently to moisturise the skin effectively. These oils can also be applied as ointments or creams. Creams contain water and therefore also preservatives, which have the potential for sensitisation. The more greasy the emollient the more effective, but often also the less cosmetically acceptable.
- Ensure there are adequate oils in the diet. Fish oil (adult dose 1000 mg caps, four daily) or flaxseed oil (especially for vegetarians), which is a comparable omega-3 fatty acid. Omega-6 fatty acids such as evening primrose oil can be used in smaller doses and also applied topically as an emollient. Dietary olive oil can be used for dressings, salads and cooking.
- Infection is important in atopic eczema. Up to 80% of eczema is colonised by pathogenic bacteria, especially *Staphylococcus aureus*. The more severe the dermatitis, the denser the infection. *S. aureus* causes direct irritation or exotoxin immunological sensitisation. Bacteria belong on the outside of the skin but in eczema they readily penetrate the skin, causing inflammation and itching. Scratching then ploughs in more bacteria. Antiseptic measures or topical antibiotics can help eradicate infection and aid repair of the barrier function of the skin.

  Infection control measures in atopic eczema:
  - Condy's crystals ($KMnO_4$)—1:8000 solution gives a light-pink solution in the bath and is a safe and effective antiseptic
  - other antiseptics in the bath water—these include triclosan and benzalkonium chloride in oil
  - calendula cream[3]—has antiseptic properties for topical use
  - topical antibiotic—(e.g. mupirocin ointment) for established localised bacterial infection
  - oral antibiotics—for more widespread or severe local infection.
- Anti-inflammatory agents such as topical corticosteroid ointments or pimecrolimus cream (for the face) reduce inflammation and restore the barrier function of the skin, moisture and normal texture.
- Know the forms and doses of topical medications. Common forms: ointments are oil in oil, creams are oil in water, and lotions contain still more water.
- Different potencies of topical corticosteroids are used for different areas and age groups. Use only hydrocortisone on the face, and only the more potent fluorinated topical corticosteroids on the hands and feet where the skin is thick. Hydrocortisone can be effective on the trunk and limbs in children.
- Non-steroidal pimecrolimus cream can be useful, especially on the face.
- How much ointment will be needed? To work out the dose needed, use the 'rule of hand' (Fig 42.1).[4] Four hand areas (using the area under the flat of the hand) requires one gram of ointment per treatment. For example, if ointment is being used daily over eight hand areas, this is 2 grams daily,

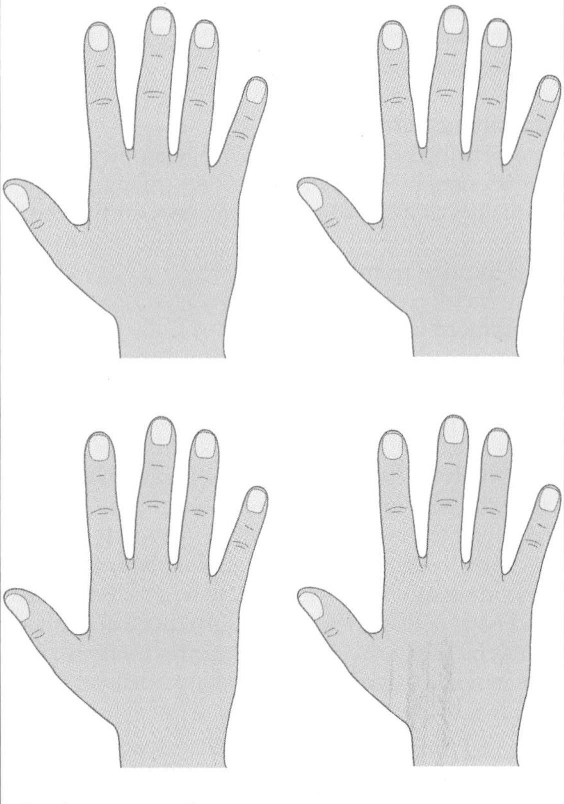

4 hand areas = 1 g of ointment.
30 g will cover a single application over the whole body

FIGURE 42.1 Rule of hand for estimating dosage of topical therapy[3]

and a 15-gram tube will last 1 week. It is important to prescribe an adequate quantity to last until the next review.
- Put out the fire. Cool down the inflammation of eczema. Eat, drink, dress, sleep, bathe, shower and think *cool*. Inflammatory conditions are like a grass fire—easier to prevent than to put out. Turning down the central heating, avoiding heating foods such as spices, sleeping and dressing cool, bathing or showering cool and keeping a cool head, all help. Traditional Chinese medicine incorporates concepts of heat in diagnosis and treatment.
- Nutritional supplements:
  - *omega-3 fatty acids*—replace arachidonic acid and lead to reduced levels of inflammatory mediators and IgE. Sources are:
    - deep-sea cold water fish such as salmon, sardines, herrings, mackerel or fish oil capsules 1000 mg (adult dose: four daily)
    - flaxseed (linseed) oil, LSA (linseed, sunflower, almond mix). Fish oil may have more anti-inflammatory action than flaxseed oil.
  - *evening primrose oil*—can be used and absorbed as a topical emollient in children
  - *olive oil*—can be used in dressings, salads and cooking
  - *probiotics*—helpful to ensure normal bowel flora, which has a role in immune system regulation. With the number of antibiotics and antiseptics in foods and the environment, probiotics should probably be used intermittently by most people. Probiotics benefit atopic eczema in both children and adults. Children have different bacterial populations in the gut and need preparations containing bifidobacteria; *acidophilus in yoghurt* provides fewer beneficial bacteria
  - adequate *glutathionone peroxidase*—provided by selenium supplementation (50–200 μg daily adult dose) if necessary
  - *antioxidants*—vitamin C, vitamin E, beta-carotene, selenium
  - increase fresh vegetables, fruits and foods rich in naturally occurring dietary antioxidants
  - thiamin B_6 and folate
  - *zinc*—adequate levels enhance immunity
  - *traditional Chinese medicine*—especially Chinese herbs, including *Panax ginseng*[5] (Korean ginseng), which increases Th1 cells.

Eczema causes significant morbidity for the patient and their family.[6] Treat the patient and the family as a whole. Remember the total load on the system.

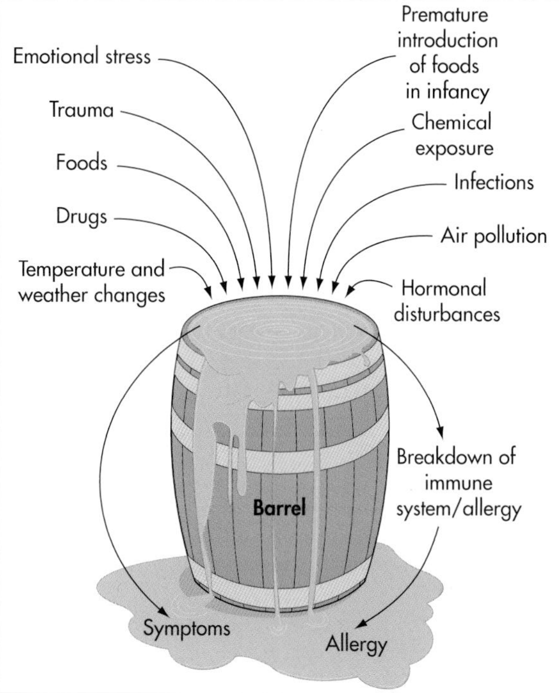

FIGURE 42.2 The barrel effect

Remember that the body as a whole (including the nervous system and the mind) is always trying to heal itself, always trying to maintain balance in a life of constant 'wear and tear'. Many factors contribute to this wearing down of the system, and the total load on the individual is always important. When the stressors on the body are too much for it to manage, the 'barrel' overflows and symptoms result (Fig 42.2). Stress or anxiety, therefore, having a pro-inflammatory effect, is commonly associated with exacerbations of eczema, whereas stress reduction techniques are associated with improved control and reduced exacerbations.[7]

PSORIASIS

Psoriasis is a chronic condition commonly characterised by symmetrical, well-defined red plaques with silvery white scale. Psoriasis can affect many parts of the body, with varying appearances. The nails, joints and eyes may also be affected.

Causes and triggers

- *Genetic*—there is usually a family history.
- *Infections* (especially streptococcal throat) may precipitate guttate (small spot) psoriasis.
- *Drugs*—beta-blockers, lithium, chloroquin or quinine and steroid withdrawal (quinine is used to provide the bitter flavour in tonic water and bitter lemon drinks).

- *Injury* to the skin (Koebner phenomenon)—includes sunburn, trauma and surgery.
- *Sunlight*—10% of patients develop more severe psoriasis with exposure to sunlight.
- *Stress* often has a significant role at least in aggravating psoriasis.
- *Cigarette smoking* and *excessive alcohol intake.*

Pathophysiology

Psoriasis is characterised by epidermal hyperproliferation, with epidermal cells dividing and moving to the surface of the skin. This normally takes 28 days but in psoriasis it is accelerated to 4 days. Psoriasis is a T helper 1 (Th1) dominant disease.

Treatment

Aims of therapy:

- reduce inflammation
- promote growth of healthy skin
- reduce stress and the stress resulting from the condition.

Medical treatment depends on the location:

- extensor surfaces
  - calcipitriol
  - dithranol
  - topical corticosteroids
- scalp
  - tar preparations
  - steroid lotion or cream
- flexures
  - topical corticosteroid creams rather than ointments.

Lifestyle factors including exercise, nutrition and stress management can all influence psoriasis.

Dietary guidelines

Many patients report improvement with diets that include large quantities of fresh fruits and vegetables, small amounts of protein from fish and fowl, fibre supplements, olive oil and minimisation of red meat, processed foods and highly refined carbohydrates.

Foods to eat:

- a diet rich in fresh fruits and vegetables, especially carrots, garlic, turmeric/curcumin, nuts and seeds
- fish, especially oily fish, flaxseed oil and olive oil for cooking.

Foods to avoid or restrict:

- foods to which sensitivity has been demonstrated; gluten sensitivity needs to be excluded[8]
- chemical additives, colourings, flavourings and preservatives, including processed meats such as bacon, ham, corned beef and sausages
- 'spicy' foods, including spices, chillies, peppers and the deadly nightshade family (potato, tomato, capsicum, chilli)
- alcohol, sugar, sweets, coffee, soft drinks and fruit juices—minimise intake.

Nutritional supplements

- *Fish oil*—4000 mg daily or vitamin A 10,000 IU; other omega-3 oils including flaxseed oil also reduce Th1
- *Vitamin D* (sunlight or vitamin D_3, 2000 IU orally daily)—down-regulates Th1, which may explain summer improvement
- *Omega-6 oils*—modulate Th1/Th2 balance
- *Folic acid* 1–5 mg (especially for patients requiring methotrexate)
- *B vitamins* (especially B_6, B_{12} and folic acid)—reduce homocysteine and may improve psoriasis; betaine also decreases homocysteine and dampens down the Th1 immune response. Dose of vitamin B_{12} varies according to level of deficiency. Current recommendation is 2000 μg of oral B_{12} daily, followed by 1000 μg daily and then 1000 μg weekly and, finally, monthly
- *Zinc* 30 mg daily (depending on testing) with copper 2 mg
- *Vitamin C*
- *Probiotics* such as *Lactobacillus acidophilus*, *L. plantarum*, *L. rhamnosus*, *L. fermentans* or bifidobacteria
- *Beta-sitosterol*, found in the cells and membranes of all oil-producing plants, fruit, vegetables, grains, seeds and trees, ideally in a balanced diet or supplemented
- *Selenium* 50–200 μg daily
- Multivitamin B and multimineral supplement.

Lifestyle

- Exercise decreases Th1 and helps psoriasis.
- Cigarette (or marijuana) smoking should be avoided.
- Minimise chemical exposure—chlorine, hairsprays, perfumes, household cleaning agents, insecticides, aerosol sprays, paints and thinners, plasticisers and printing chemicals.
- Because psoriasis can affect the patient's self-image and confidence, psychological management may be beneficial. Anxiety and stress often contribute to flares in psoriasis. Mind–body therapies such as mindfulness-based interventions have been found to improve the clearing rate for patients with severe psoriasis when used as an adjunct with other medical therapies.

Herbal treatments

Phytomedicines can assist in the management of symptoms of chronic autoimmune, inflammatory skin conditions such as psoriasis. Topical (and internal) use of plant oils high in omega-3 and -6 fatty acids are also of benefit. Saponin-rich herbs have a beneficial effect on the symptoms of persistent psoriasis. They must be used under expert professional supervision.

Common herbs used are:

- evening primrose oil[9] (*Oenothera biennis*)—anti-inflammatory
- sarsaparilla[10] (*Smilax officinalis*)—anti-inflammatory, antipruritic, alterative (saponin rich)
- turmeric[11] (*Curcuma longa*)—anti-inflammatory, antioxidant, hepatoprotective.

Topically:

- celandine (*Cheladonium majus*)—inhibits keratinocyte proliferation
- aloe vera 0.5% cream[12]—may be effective.

Other herbal treatments for psoriasis include:

- Western herbs—yellow saffron,[13] ginseng[14] and polypodium[15]
- ayurvedic herb *Coleus forskohlii*[16] (traditional use but no evidence of efficacy)
- traditional Chinese herbs—including *Rehmania glutinosa*, *Angelica sinesis*, *Salvia miltorrhiza*, *Dictamnus dasycarpus*, *Smilax glabra*, *Oldenlandia diffusa*, *Lithospermum erythrorhizon*, *Paeonia lactiflora*.[17]

INFECTIONS

Host factors are important and infection is more common with impaired immunity. When infections thrive, spread more rapidly than usual or recur despite appropriate therapy, it is important to ask why this may be happening. Causes of impaired host immunity or reduced threshold to infection can include:

- eczema
- nutritional deficiencies such as iron, vitamin B_{12}, vitamin C, vitamin D, zinc or low protein intake
- diabetes or hyperglycaemia
- physical or emotional stress
- food sensitivity.

Therefore, in the prevention or management of infectious diseases, particularly those that have a chronic and relapsing course, attention should be given to lifestyle and psychological factors.

Viral infections

Warts

Warts are a very common infection of the skin and mucous membranes caused by papillomavirus. As with other infections, the viability of a wart depends on the immunity of the host. Warts are very susceptible to lifestyle and psychological influences that increase immunity.

Other treatments include:

- salicylic acid preparations, sometimes in combination with lactic acid
- liquid nitrogen cryotherapy, repeated if necessary every 2–3 weeks
- salicylic acid 70% in linseed oil plasters (pare down after 5 days)
- curettage and cautery under local anaesthetic—rarely used now
- immunotherapy with DCP (diphencyprone), which is a potent topical sensitiser.

General measures to enhance immunity and general wellbeing can be important, and include: nutrition, antioxidants and immunostimulant herbs.

Check for zinc deficiency. Recalcitrant warts may respond to zinc supplementation.[18]

Because warts can be painful and potentially infectious, some treatment should be offered. First-line physical treatments such as curettage with diathermy or excision are rarely indicated and can lead to scarring. It should be remembered that in the presence of normal immunity, warts will nearly always resolve over time without active therapy.

Herpes simplex

Herpes simplex virus 1 and 2 infections cause primary and recurrent oral and genital infections. Genital herpes and oral cold sores are frequently painful and emotionally distressing. It is important to recognise the emotional stigma that patients with herpes often feel. Treatment measures can include:

- avoidance (by all patients with herpetic infections) of arginine-rich foods (chocolate, peanuts, almonds)
- antioxidants, including vitamins C, A, D and selenium
- echinacea and immunostimulant herbs[19]
- lysine
- avoidance of trigger foods or physical factors such as excessive sunlight or wind
- probiotics supplementation.

Herpes zoster

Patients with shingles will feel unwell for days or weeks, but the greatest morbidity is from post-herpetic neuralgia. Early intervention with antiviral agents, antioxidants and especially vitamin C (oral or intravenous), immunostimulant herbs, optimal nutrition and topical vitamin E oil will reduce the morbidity. It should be remembered that, with a debilitating systemic condition like shingles, there is no substitute for rest.

Molluscum contagiosum

Molluscum contagiosum is a common benign skin infection, with dome-shaped papules that have central umbilication. Lesions eventually resolve spontaneously. Most children will only tolerate treatment of a limited number of lesions at a time.

Treatment options:

- 5% benzoyl peroxide
- tape stripping (duct/Leukosilk®/Micropore® tape)—change daily after bath or shower for 4–8 weeks
- Duofilm® lotion (17% salicylic acid, 17% lactic acid) or gel (27% salicylic acid) used twice weekly
- Imiquimod cream thrice weekly for 3 weeks.

Fungal and yeast infections

Tinea of the body, feet, hands, scalp, flexures or incognito are common. The characteristic appearance of tinea on the body is an asymmetrical annular erythematous rash with a slightly raised margin and peripheral scale. Ringworm or tinea spreads outwards.

- Confirm the diagnosis when treating tinea. Take scrapings, nail clippings or plucked hairs rather than guess. Confident treatment based on a positive diagnosis will provide a better outcome.
- Beware of tinea incognito or fungal infection treated and modified with topical corticosteroids.
- Check the toenails, as recurrent fungal infections in the skin can come from unrecognised toenail tinea (onychomycosis).

Thrush or *Candida albicans* is a common commensal infection in warm, moist environments. Yeast and fungal infections thrive in 'tropical' (warm and moist) environments such as on the feet or in the groin or flexures.

Pityriasis versicolor is a benign skin reaction to *Malassezia furfur* yeast infection. It causes small patches of altered skin colour, especially on the trunk. It is more common in people who sweat heavily and in hot, humid climates.

Bacterial infections

Bacterial infections include impetigo, folliculitis, boils, cellulitis and erysipelas. Remember that appropriate antibiotics will treat bacterial infection but pus needs to drain. When bacterial infections persist, remember host factors including diabetes or deficiencies of iron, zinc or vitamin D.

INSECT BITES

Insect bites are common and often present with a secondary allergy rash. This may take the form of papular urticaria, where there may be a small number of primary bites with numerous itchy papules spread over many parts of the body.

Scabies

A common example of insect bites is scabies. Scabies is an intensely itchy mite infestation usually affecting the forearms and web spaces of the fingers, together with the cooler areas of the areolae in women and the scrotum in men (papulonodules). It has an incubation period of 3–4 weeks with 10–15 mites. Itch is increased by warmth.

Diagnosis

Diagnosis is made on the clinical picture and confirmed with skin scrapes or shave of the entire burrow to enable microscopic visualisation of the mite.

Treatment

- Topical permethrin cream 5%, from the neck down. This should be left on overnight and washed off in the morning. Clothes should be tumble dried after a hot wash. Re-treat symptomatic cases after 1 week.
- Treat eczema after scabies with a fluorinated topical corticosteroid ointment and emollients.
- Scabetic nodules may need intralesional steroid injection.
- Pregnancy alternative—10% sulfur in soft white paraffin daily for 3 days.
- Infants under 6 months—as for pregnancy (need the scalp to be treated as well), or daily crotamiton cream for 3 days.
- Resistant cases—oral ivermectin 12 mg stat and repeat after 10 days.

ACNE

Most people have at least some acne during their teenage years. Acne is redness, swelling and inflammation of the hair and oil gland unit (pilosebaceous follicle) of the skin. In acne there are blackheads and whiteheads (comedones) or pimples, abscesses and inflammation (redness and soreness), and eventually there may be scars. Changing levels of androgen and heredity set the stage, but all the causes are not known.

Most young people with acne (as with eczema and psoriasis) experience degrees of shame, embarrassment, anxiety, depression, loss of self-confidence or significant difficulty with employment. It is important that practitioners take acne seriously, treat it enthusiastically and encourage regular review.[20] Patients need to be reassured that acne is not infectious, is not caused by poor hygiene, and can be controlled.

What produces acne?

Acne is produced by pores blocked with plugs of oily secretions and skin material, increased sebum (oil) from the sebaceous glands, bacteria thriving in the oily secretions, and inflammation from oil and bacteria bursting out of the comedones (Fig 42.3).

Treatment

The aim of treatment is to control these steps and prevent or minimise the development of scars that may be permanent.

- Retinoids (adapalene or retinoic acid) unblock pores.
- Benzoyl peroxide reduces bacteria and unblocks pores.
- Azelaic acid reduces bacteria and unblocks pores.
- Antibiotics (topical such as erythromycin or clindamycin, or oral such as minocycline) reduce bacteria and inflammation.
- Isotretinoin can be curative for severe acne.

Patients need to be reminded to:

- use water-based rather than oil-based make-up
- use oil-free sunscreens
- eat good food, including plenty of fruit, vegetables and fish
- avoid squeezing pimples, as this causes the infection and inflammation to spread
- avoid thick, oily moisturisers that block the pores of the skin
- wash the skin gently without excessive scrubbing
- follow through the treatment and discuss problems with their practitioner.

Other points:

- Most treatments take at least 4 weeks to work, and longer to achieve full effect. Reassurance is needed that all acne can be controlled.
- It is normal for lotions or gels to irritate or burn at the start of treatment.
- Acne often has to get worse before it gets better!
- Antibiotics by mouth can potentially interfere with the efficacy of the oral contraceptive pill.
- 10% picolinic acid gel can be used.[21]

General management

- Wash once or twice a day only, with low-residue soap or soap substitute in lukewarm water.
- Topical therapy
- Dietary measures:
  - Minimise sugar intake—sugar ingestion causes increased insulin levels, which may trigger the release of androgens and activate pro-inflammatory cytokines, including leptin.
  - Restrict refined carbohydrates, especially wheat.
  - Avoid caffeine-containing foods or drinks.
  - While it is unwise to generalise about the effect on acne of foods such as chocolate and fats, individual patients may notice specific triggers.
- Supplements:
  - zinc 30 mg daily
  - vitamins A, C and E
  - vitamin A or beta-carotene 10 mg daily
  - fish oil capsules 4000 IU daily
  - vitamin D—ensure adequate sun exposure in winter, or check blood levels and supplement
- Herbal treatment:
  - *Vitex*[22] (chaste tree) tablets—2 tablets on rising
  - *Arctium*[23] (burdock root)

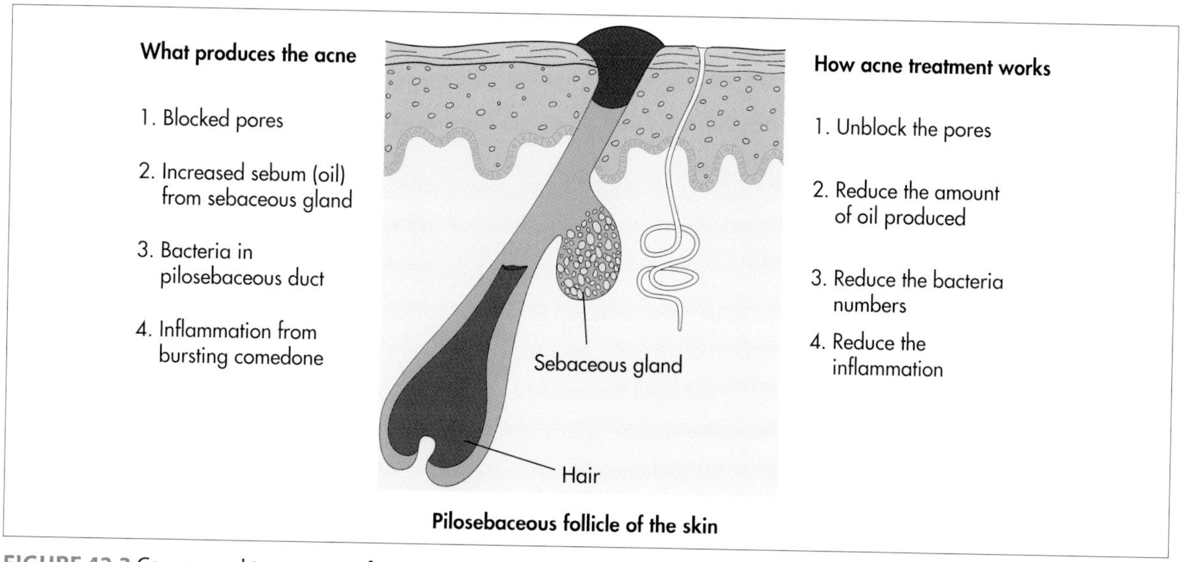

What produces the acne
1. Blocked pores
2. Increased sebum (oil) from sebaceous gland
3. Bacteria in pilosebaceous duct
4. Inflammation from bursting comedone
Sebaceous gland
Hair
How acne treatment works
1. Unblock the pores
2. Reduce the amount of oil produced
3. Reduce the bacteria numbers
4. Reduce the inflammation
Pilosebaceous follicle of the skin

FIGURE 42.3 Causes and treatment of acne

ROSACEA

Rosacea is a chronic inflammatory disorder of the skin of the face characterised by persistent redness and dilated blood vessels of the cheeks, nose, chin and forehead. It is more common with fair skin. It is a blushing disorder. Acute episodes occur with papules, swelling and pustules (Ace of clubs distribution, the curse of the Celts). The cause is unknown but exposure to sunlight and UV light damage play a role. *Demodex* mites have been found in the skin of affected individuals.

The following can be aggravants:

- alcohol, hot drinks or hot spicy foods, which cause facial vessels to dilate
- temperature fluctuations and hot weather—there may be impairment in the vasomotor tone of facial blood vessels
- topical corticosteroids—these have a profoundly deleterious effect and should always be avoided.

Treatment

Rosacea usually responds within a few days to oral antibiotic therapy and although treatment may need to be maintained for about 10 weeks, often only low doses are required. The initial course can be repeated if or when there is a flare. If oral maintenance therapy is required, low doses on alternate days may be sufficient. Oral antibiotic therapy should be followed by probiotic supplementation to replace gut flora. Topical therapy will usually be adequate for milder cases and for longer-term maintenance.

Acute rosacea (with erythema and papules):

- topical metronidazole 0.75% (up to 1.5%) gel applied sparingly twice daily, with second-line topical treatment of clindamycin 1% lotion
- oral minocycline 50 mg b.i.d. or doxycycline 100 mg daily, reducing after several weeks and continuing for 6–12 weeks
- erythromycin 250 mg q.i.d. as second-line oral therapy

Chronic rosacea with erythema and telangiectasia—treatment is more difficult.

- Avoid factors that cause flushing.
- Avoid UV exposure and use sunscreens.
- Apply soothing emollients.
- Zinc supplementation may be beneficial for rosacea.

Complications

- Conjunctivitis, blepharitis, styes and rosacea keratitis (rare)
- Rhinophyma (sebaceous gland hyperplasia)—surgery, dermabrasion or isotretinoin
- Lymphoedema around eyes or forehead.

URTICARIA, ANGIO-OEDEMA AND ALLERGIC RASHES

Urticaria (hives, wheals) is a common eruption characterised by transient dermal oedema. *Angio-oedema* is the same reaction as urticaria, but in the deep dermis and subcutaneous tissues, with oedema spreading more diffusely. Angio-oedema often affects the face and neck.

There are many manifestations of allergic rashes in response to antigenic exposure through contact, ingestion or exposure to infections such as viruses.

Urticaria is an example of a skin condition that is easy to recognise but for which a cause is often difficult to discover.

Questions to ask:

- Is it urticaria? Could it be scabies, tinea, contact dermatitis, dermatitis herpetiformis or pruritus related to lymphoma, biliary obstruction or cancer?
- Is it simple urticaria? A residual bruise or stain points to vasculitis. Systemic upset points to systemic disease.
- Is the eruption acute or chronic? Acute is often allergic, but chronic is less likely to be allergic.
- Can trigger factors be identified?

Management

- Emergency treatment for severe urticaria is adrenaline with the possible addition of steroids. Urticaria becomes a medical emergency when it is widespread or affecting the airway or breathing.
- An antihistamine such as cetirizine is first-line treatment for the majority of urticarial eruptions.

General measures include the following:

- Avoid non-specific precipitants, including unnecessary allergenic foods, food additives, temperature stress, exertion and alcohol.
- Eat, drink, dress, bathe, sleep and think *cool*. All these measures cool the fire.
- Vitamin C (sodium ascorbate) 1000 mg × 2–5 doses daily (for food reactions, take enough ascorbate until the stools become loose. This will 'flush' the food through the digestive tract).
- For food allergies, take an alkalinising agent such as sodium bicarbonate, one teaspoon in water followed by another glass of water up to three times daily, or 'Tri-Salts' (3 parts $NaHCO_3$, 2 parts $KHCO_3$ and 1 part $CaCO_3$).
- Drink copious water.
- See Table 42.2.

ENVIRONMENTAL INJURY AND SKIN CANCER

Skin cancer is the most common cancer in the body, and Australia has the highest incidence in the world.

TABLE 42.2 Management of urticaria

Type	Causes & diagnosis	Treatment
Acute (week): likely to be allergic	*Drugs*: aspirin, antibiotics (beef, chicken), NSAIDs, quinine, morphine, codeine	AH
	Insect stings: bee, wasp	
	Foods: salicylates, amines, benzoates, preservatives, colourings, peanut, shellfish, egg white	Avoidance
	Infection: focal sepsis, viral, worms, parasites, e.g. *Candida*, protozoa	Empirical metronidazole
	Idiopathic	
Physical	*Cold*: icy water	Self-limiting, AH
	Pressure (delayed): weights for 8 hours	Self-limiting, AH
	Solar: sunlight or solar stimulation	
	Aquagenic: water	Bicarbonate in water
	Cholinergic/heat: heat, exercise or stress. Five minutes of exercise will evoke < 2 mm diameter wheals	± AH
	Dermographism: 2% population, most common	
Chronic (years): non-allergic	History of implants, silicon, rubber, prosthesis, nickel, iodine *Diagnosis*: FBE, ESR, LFTs, stool & urine micro & culture, X-ray chest & sinus, complement, auto antibodies, HepBsAg	AH, e.g. cetirizine (empirical metronidazole)

AH: antihistamines; FBE: full blood examination; HepBsAg: hepatitis B virus surface antigen; LFT: liver function test.

Currently 280,000 skin cancers are diagnosed each year, including 8000 melanomas. Around 1200 Australians die each year of skin cancer and the incidence continues to rise. The highest incidence of melanoma in Australia extends from Sydney up the coast to Far North Queensland. Melanomas are more likely to occur with intermittent sun exposure, such as in weekend beachgoers. Non-melanoma skin cancer is more common inland and appears to be more closely related to total sun exposure.

What causes skin cancer?

Exposure to excessive ultraviolet (UV) rays from the sun is the major cause. UVA rays penetrate more deeply than UVB and are the most carcinogenic wave band. Other traumatic or damaging agents include:

- petrochemicals—e.g. a ship's engineer exposed to heat and petrochemical vapours
- chemicals, such as chlorinated pools in combination with sunshine
- trauma or heat damage to the skin, including dryness
- poor general health, especially problems of the immune system
- immunosuppressive drug therapy
- clear, hot, sunny days in summer—risk is greatest on these days, as they have the highest UV index
- geography—areas where the risk is greater include at altitude in mountains or with aviation and where there is increased reflection of UV rays from reflective surfaces such as snow, water, sand or granite
- pale skin—more vulnerable to solar damage and skin cancer.

Classification

Non-melanoma skin cancer

Basal cell carcinoma (BCC) is the most common skin cancer and can be superficial, nodular or tough (pigmented, recurrent, infiltrating, morphoeic, desmoplastic).[24] Spread is local. BCC appears as a red papule or plaque, which may have a pearly edge. The pearly edge becomes more obvious when the skin is stretched under good light.

Squamous cell carcinoma (SCC)—there can be a continuum from solar or actinic keratosis to intraepidermal cancer (IEC or Bowen's disease) to SCC. SCC grows locally but can later spread to regional nodes and beyond. High-risk locations include the lip, ear and scalp. Recurrent tumours also carry a higher risk.

Melanoma

Melanoma is the most malignant of common skin cancers. Melanomas are usually pigmented and many arise from normal skin. Melanomas tend to be irregular, and initially grow laterally before later deep spread with increase in thickness and increased risk of metastatic spread.

Other

Other forms of skin cancer include Merkel cell carcinoma and other less common skin tumours.

Prevention

- Avoiding, and protecting the skin from, excessive UV exposure is the main preventative approach. This has been reinforced through the national 'Slip Slop Slap' campaign in Australia, which encourages people to 'slip on a shirt, slop on sunscreen, slap on a hat and sunglasses'.
- Correcting predisposing factors in general health includes moisturising dry skin, and improving general nutrition where there may be low levels of iron or antioxidants, vitamin D, vitamin C, zinc, vitamin B_6 or low protein intake.
- Keep the skin healthy—skin cancers generally become more common as people age. With age and time there is a progressive loss of functions in the skin. Dry skin or xerosis needs to be managed as it leaves the skin more vulnerable to disease, including infections and malignant change.
  - Use external moisturisers or emollients—these oils, ointments or creams soften the skin, rather like polishing and preserving leather in shoes.
  - Avoid hot water, detergents and soap, which wash out natural oils.
  - A diet rich in healthy oils will also prevent dryness—these dietary oils include fish oil or flaxseed oil (omega-3 fatty acids), some omega-6 fatty acids from vegetable sources and olive oil.
  - Drink plenty of fresh water.
  - Avoid excessive heat—'Dress, bathe, sleep and think cool'.
- Many people are vitamin D deficient, especially at the end of winter. This can be checked with a simple blood test, 25-OH vitamin D. Vitamin D has a role in preventing cancer and it acts to tan and possibly repair solar skin damage. Ironically, many Australians need less sun exposure in summer than they currently get, but many in the southern states need more sun exposure in winter than they currently receive. Outdoor exercise could help give multiple benefits compared with being indoors or exercising only in gyms during winter. Vitamin D_3 (cholecalciferol) can be taken as a supplement where blood levels are inadequate.

Checking the skin:

- Examination includes checking the skin all over to identify general abnormalities, and specific examination of pigmented lesions and moles.

BOX 42.3 Risk features in pigmented lesions

Edinburgh system

- Major symptoms:
  - Change in size
  - Change in shape
  - Change in colour
- Minor symptoms:
  - Inflammation
  - Crusting or bleeding
  - Sensory change, e.g. itch
  - Diameter > 7 mm

US system

- A—Asymmetry
- B—Border irregularity
- C—Colour variability
- D—Difference/diameter > 6 mm
- E—Enlarging/elevation

Dermoscopy is a useful skill to improve the diagnosis of pigmented lesions.

- Most patients with melanoma have noticed a change in the skin in the previous few months. There are two systems for assessing features suspicious of melanoma in pigmented lesions (Box 42.3).

Treatment of premalignant lesions

- Observation of solar or actinic keratoses (SK) is often appropriate, especially in low-risk areas of the body or in the frail or elderly patient. SKs may resolve spontaneously.
- Liquid nitrogen cryotherapy destroys abnormal cells by freezing and thawing abnormal tissue. Using a spray gun or cotton wool stick dipped in nitrogen, the SK and a surrounding millimetre of normal skin is frozen for a predetermined 'freeze time' of around 10 seconds.
- Immunostimulant therapy with imiquimod cream stimulates the body's immune system to heal SKs.
- Diclofenac sodium 3% gel can likewise be used over weeks to eradicate SKs.
- Therapy with imiquimod cream, diclofenac gel or 5-fluorouracil cream is particularly useful where there is a more extensive area of solar damage, such as the face and scalp.
- Shave, punch or excision biopsy for lesions that do not resolve or that appear more substantial, or where the diagnosis is in doubt. Be prepared to biopsy lesions that are atypical in any way, or that persist after ablative therapy, especially in high-risk parts of the body.
- Send all excised or biopsy specimens to pathology.

Treatment of malignant skin cancer

- Surgical excision of non-melanoma skin cancer is sometimes preceded by biopsy: punch, shave, incisional or excisional. Surgical excision has the advantage of providing a specimen for histopathological confirmation of the diagnosis, as well as establishing that there is a margin of safety around the excised tumour. Surgical excision remains the gold standard for treating skin cancer.
- Other treatments for superficial BCCs are curettage, imiquimod cream, diathermy or photodynamic therapy. These are not suitable for tough BCCs, which require surgical excision.
- Mohs surgery is a specialised surgical technique for excising high-risk BCCs, especially on the face near vital structures.
- SCCs require surgical excision, especially from high-risk areas of the lip, ear or scalp, or recurrent tumours.
- Surgical excision with an adequate margin is the only curative treatment for melanoma. The width of the surgical margin depends on the thickness of the melanoma measured by the histopathologist at the initial excision. Melanomas are usually re-excised with a margin of safety, which increases with the increasing tumour depth.
- Non-surgical treatments such as liquid nitrogen cryotherapy, laser or imiquimod cream do not provide confirmation of histology or evidence of adequate clearance. These should only be used for superficial, straightforward, non-melanoma tumours in low-risk areas where the diagnosis is clear.

Examine the rest of the skin after a malignant skin cancer has been diagnosed.

AGEING SKIN, DRY SKIN AND WOUND HEALING

With many chronic skin diseases and in the elderly, the skin tends to be dry. The functions of the skin deteriorate with age. Oil glands don't work as well and, like old leather, the skin dries out and cracks. Oils can be used externally and internally. Essential fatty acids and oils in the diet make a difference to the health of the skin. Some oils such as fish oil also have anti-inflammatory functions. Topical evening primrose oil may benefit eczema and there are many oils that can be used topically, including vitamin E, rosemary, coconut or evening primrose oil.

It should be remembered that keeping the skin healthy with moisturisers and oils is more than a cosmetic exercise. Healthy skin is less likely to break down or undergo malignant change.

Wound healing depends on multiple general and local factors. Healing is aided by:

- good circulation
- adequate exercise levels
- avoidance of smoking
- normal weight
- normal blood sugar levels
- local factors including good circulation and tissue vitality
- adequate levels of vitamin B_6, vitamin C, iron, zinc and protein.

SYSTEMIC DISEASES AND THE SKIN

The skin frequently reflects underlying health or disease and can provide vital windows or clues to assist the practitioner in identifying systemic conditions.

- Autoimmune conditions of the skin—halo naevus, vitiligo, alopecia areata, Addison's disease and melanoma—should alert the practitioner to the possibility of coexisting systemic autoimmune conditions.
- Skin can be an early reflector of systemic illness in diabetes, Graves' disease, Hashimoto's thyroiditis, pernicious anaemia, rheumatoid arthritis (RA), systemic lupus erythematosus (SLE), morphea and lichen sclerosis.
- Skin infections that persist may be associated with low levels of ferritin, vitamin B_{12} or vitamin D, or with early diabetes.
- Dermatitis herpetiformis is linked with coeliac disease.
- Acquired ichthyosis can be associated with Hodgkin's disease.
- Erythema gyratum repens may reflect underlying malignancy.
- Nail fold abnormalities occur in Raynaud's phenomenon, SLE, RA, dermatomyositis, systemic sclerosis and CREST syndrome.
- Cutaneous xanthomas may be associated with hyperlipidaemia.

Although skin presentations are often simple and can be summarily treated, almost all skin diseases can be considered from an integrative perspective. A comprehensive integrative approach to the management of skin conditions will usually have a positive, and sometimes dramatic, impact on a patient's general health. It is important to have well-informed patients by being a caring practitioner who educates and who constantly learns.

RESOURCES

American Academy of Dermatology, http://www.aad.org/

Australian College of Dermatologists, http://www.dermcoll.asn.au/public/default.asp

Burns T, Breathnach S, Cox N et al. eds. Textbook of dermatology. 7th edn. Oxford: Blackwell Science; 2004.

du Vivier A. Dermatology in practice. London: Mosby-Wolfe; 1995.

emedicine, dermatology articles. A useful website covering a wide range of dermatological conditions, http://emedicine.medscape.com/dermatology

Gawkrodger DJ. Dermatology: an illustrated colour text. Edinburgh: Churchill Livingstone; 1992. A useful and illustrated textbook of dermatology.

Hunter JAA, Savin JA, Dahl MV. Clinical dermatology. 3rd edn. Oxford: Blackwell Science; 2002.

Marks R. Roxburgh's common skin diseases. 16th edn. London: Chapman & Hall Medical; 1993.

REFERENCES

1 Hunter JC, Savin J, Dahl M. Clinical dermatology. 2nd edn. Oxford: Blackwell Science; 1995:36.

2 Gawkrodger DJ. Dermatology: an illustrated colour text. Edinburgh: Churchill Livingstone; 1992:13.

3 Pommier P, Gomez F, Sunyach MP et al. Phase III randomized trial of *Calendula officinalis* compared with trolamine for the prevention of acute dermatitis during irradiation for breast cancer. J Clin Oncol 2004; 22(8):1447–1453.

4 Long CC, Findlay AY. The rule of hand. Arch Dermatol 1992; 128:1129–1130.

5 Surh Y, Lee J, Choi K et al. Effects of selected ginsenosides on phorbol ester-induced expression of cyclooxygenase-2 and activation of NF-kappaB and ERK1/2 in mouse skin. Ann NY Acad Sci 2002; 973:396–401.

6 Holm EA, Wulf HC, Stegmann H et al. Life quality assessment among patients with atopic eczema. Br J Dermatol 2006; 154(4):719–725.

7 Hoare C, Li Wan Po A, Williams H. Systematic review of treatments for atopic eczema. Health Technol Assess 2000; 4(37):1–191.

8 Michaelsson G, Kristjansson G, Pihl Lundin I et al. Palmoplantar pustulosis and gluten sensitivity. Br J Dermatol 2007; 156(4):659–666.

9 Berbis P, Hesse S, Privat Y. Essential fatty acids and the skin. Allerg Immunol (Paris) 1990; 22(6): 225–231.

10 Weiss R, Fintelmann V. Herbal medicine. 2nd edn. Stuttgart: Thieme; 2000.

11 Strimpakos A, Sharma R. *Curcumin*: preventive and therapeutic properties in laboratory studies and clinical trials. Antiox Redox Signal 2008; 10(3):511–545.

12 Choonhakarn C, Busaracome P, Sripanidkulchai et al. A prospective, randomized clinical trial comparing topical aloe vera with 0.1% triamcinolone acetonide in mild to moderate plaque psoriasis. J Eur Acad Dermatol Venereol 2010; 24(2):168–172.

13 Brown AC, Hairfield M, Richards D et al. Medical nutrition therapy as a potential complementary treatment for psoriasis—five case reports. Altern Med Rev 2004; 9(3):297–307.

14 Shin Y-W, Bae E-A, Kim D-H. Inhibitory effect of ginsenoside Rg5 and its metabolite ginsenoside Rh3 in an oxazolone-induced mouse chronic dermatitis model. Arch Pharm Res 2006; 29(8):685–690.

15 Vasange-Tuominen M, Perera-Ivarsson P, Shen J et al. The fern *Polypodium decumanum*, used in the treatment of psoriasis, and its fatty acid constituents as inhibitors of leukotriene B4 formation. Prostaglandins Leukot Essent Fatty Acids 1994; 50(5):279–284.

16 Anon. *Coleus forskohlii*. A monograph. Altern Med Rev 2006; 11(1):47–51.

17 Tse W. Use of common Chinese herbs in the treatment of psoriasis. Clin Exp Dermatol 2003; 28(5):469–475.

18 Al-Gurairi FT, Al-Waiz M, Sharquie KE. Oral zinc sulphate in the treatment of recalcitrant viral warts: randomized placebo-controlled clinical trial. Br J Dermatol 2002; 146(3):423–431.

19 Schneider S, Reichling J, Stintzing F et al. Anti-herpetic properties of hydroalcoholic extracts and pressed juice from *Echinacea pallida*. Plant Med 2010; 76(3):265–272.

20 Basra MKA, Sue-Ho R, Finlay AY. The Family Dermatology Life Quality Index: measuring the secondary impact of skin disease. Br J Dermatol 2007; 156(3):528–538.

21 Heffernan MP, Nelson MM, Anadkat MJ. A pilot study of the safety and efficacy of picolinic acid gel in the treatment of acne vulgaris. Br J Dermatol 2007; 156(3):548–552.

22 Amman W. Acne vulgaris and *Agnus castus* (Agnolyt). Z Allgemeinmed 1975; 51(35):1645–1648.

23 Mills S, Bone K. Principles and practice of phytotherapy. Modern Herbal Medicine. London: Churchill Livingstone; 2000.

24 Dixon AJ, Hall SH. Managing skin cancer. Aust Fam Physician 2005; 34(8):669–671.

chapter 43

Sleep disorders

INTRODUCTION AND OVERVIEW

As the quantity and quality of our sleep influences how we feel and function during the day, there is increasing awareness of the significant impact that disorders of sleep have on patients and society as a whole. Sleep disorders affect not only our day-to-day functioning, but also have medical morbidity and mortality consequences, as well as societal and economic costs. For example, both obstructive sleep apnoea and periodic limb movements with concomitant sleep disruption lead to excessive daytime sleepiness which in turn is associated with driving and industrial accidents. The most common sleep disorder, insomnia, is associated with daytime fatigue and impaired memory, alertness, motor performance and mood. Furthermore, recent research has found that sleep loss may have significant effects on mental health and the cardiovascular, immune and endocrine systems, contributing to hypertension, increased risk of cerebrovascular accident, obesity and diabetes.

There are many types of sleep disorders, with different aetiologies, presentations and treatments. Generally, sleep disorders can be classified into one of four groups: hypersomnias, parasomnias, insomnia and sleep–wake schedule disorders. Some sleep disorders need to be referred to a specialised sleep disorders clinic for diagnosis and treatment. Other sleep problems can be diagnosed and managed within general practice and will be emphasised in this chapter.

In the first part of this chapter we provide a brief introduction to the sleep process. In the second part, we outline sleep disorders such as obstructive sleep apnoea, narcolepsy and sleep-related movement disorders, bruxism and the parasomnias, which require referral to a specialised sleep centre. In the final part we describe the diagnosis and management of the more common but heterogenous sleep disorders of insomnia and sleep–wake schedule disorders. More detailed accounts of all these areas are available.[1]

THE NATURE OF SLEEP

It seems that the general public, as well as those with sleep disorders, believe that normal sleep is a long, continuous period of unconsciousness/inactivity. When asked to draw a graph to represent normal sleep, most people draw a U-shaped curve, with many hours of continuous deep sleep in the middle of the sleep period. This belief not only is incorrect, but will be worrisome when the person experiences awakenings in the middle of the night, and may lead to the development of insomnia.

Sleep research over the past 50 years has confirmed some interesting and very important facts about the nature of the sleep process. A state of sleep was discovered during which the sympathetic nervous system ('fight-or-flight' mechanism) was activated. It has variously been called activated, paradoxical and dreaming sleep, but now officially is termed *rapid eye movement* or *REM sleep*. One of its interesting characteristics is that it occurs in about four or five discrete episodes (only a few minutes long initially, up to 30–40 minutes in duration later) spaced about 90 minutes apart during a normal sleep period. But most of our sleep (80%) occurs between these REM sleep episodes. This non-REM state of sleep has been subdivided into different stages based on the variety of EEG cortical activity, from light (easily awoken, sleep not perceived) Stage 1 sleep to the deepest or behaviourally non-responsive Stage 4 sleep. The 90-minute non-REM/REM sleep cycles repeat four or five times during the nocturnal sleep period in a roller-coaster type pattern, as illustrated in Fig 43.1.

An intriguing aspect of this typical sleep pattern is the spontaneous lightening of sleep at the end of each deep sleep phase. As a result of this 90-minute cycle of lighter sleep throughout the sleep period, awakenings

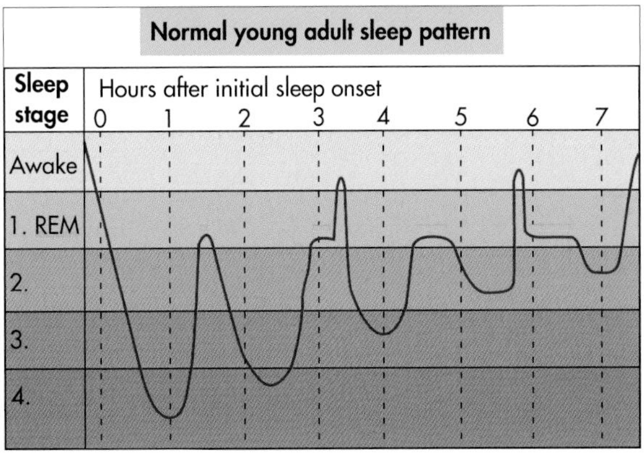

FIGURE 43.1 A typical journey through the stages of sleep, as indicated by the solid red line, in the sleep period of a healthy young adult. Note that stages 3 and 4 are more prominent early, and REM sleep and brief awakenings later in the period.

out of this lighter sleep are normal events. Even children and adolescents who normally sleep 'soundly' have these awakenings but they are usually brief and not recalled. Normal ageing results in sleep becoming lighter, with more awakenings that are more likely to be remembered. Therefore, awakenings are a normal part of the sleep period, particularly in more mature individuals, but need not have any detrimental impact on daytime functioning.

Another curious aspect of sleep is that we cannot directly perceive our own sleep. Therefore, judgments about time spent sleeping are often incorrect. Our minds are usually active, with some fleeting images and thoughts, during sleep. When we awaken we may be aware of only the last vestiges of this activity because earlier thoughts are not stored in long-term memory. People with chronic insomnia are more likely to attribute these thoughts, incorrectly, to the state of being awake.[2] Therefore two awakenings—for example, an hour apart—may seem to be a continuous hour of wakefulness rather than two brief, separate awakenings, thus leading to an underestimation of total sleep time. Because multiple awakenings become more common with age, there is an increased vulnerability to underestimating sleep time, concern about sleep and the likelihood of developing insomnia.

BIOLOGICAL DETERMINERS OF SLEEP PROPENSITY

Sleep homeostasis

Sleep acts like other basic biological drives regulating such processes as nutritional balance (hunger/eating), in that sleep drive or pressure builds steadily the longer we are awake (go without sleep) and decreases or is satisfied by sleeping. Young adult humans strike a balance of sleep and wakefulness in a ratio of about one to two, or about 8 hours asleep to 16 hours awake on average. Some individuals naturally require less sleep (6–7 hours), while others show signs of insufficient sleep if they do not get at least 8–9 hours.

Circadian rhythms

Independent of the sleep homeostasis mechanism, another major influence on sleepiness/alertness arises from our circadian (*circa* = about, *dia* = a day) or 24-hour rhythms.[3] Virtually all our physiological, biochemical and hormonal measures show circadian variation—that is, variation from peak to trough (minimum) and back to peak, taking about 24 hours to complete a full cycle. To some extent they are influenced directly by the 24-hour external environment (night/day) and our behaviour. However, free of all these influences they are shown to be endogenous. The circadian timing of these rhythms is controlled by a small nucleus in the hypothalamus of the brain, the suprachiasmatic nucleus (SCN). For example, the SCN signals the peripheral vasculature to vasodilate at about 8 pm, starting the process of decreasing core body temperature to its trough at about 4–5 am. The SCN signals the pineal gland to start manufacturing and secreting the hormone melatonin at about 9 pm and to stop its activity at about 4 am. Likewise, many other biological rhythms are kept in synchrony, a main function of which is to maximise sleepiness at night and alertness during the day, for us diurnal-adapted humans.

Maximum circadian alertness occurs at about the time of core temperature peak (6–9 pm for most individuals) and maximum circadian sleepiness is at the trough of core temperature (about 4–5 am). A few hours later (9–11 am), alertness increases again. Thus most individuals would have a circadian sleep-conducive zone from about 11 pm to about 7 am. The variation of circadian temperature, melatonin and sleepiness for a normal sleeper is illustrated in Fig 43.2.

However, this 'sleepy' zone is bracketed by 'alert' zones (one normally in the early evening and one in the later morning), which can be problematic if the timing of the circadian system comes adrift. For example, if the circadian timing is delayed by 2–3 hours, the evening alert zone may span the time when sleep is intended (e.g. 11 pm) and thus inhibit sleep. Alternatively, an early-timed circadian rhythm may wake an individual prematurely before sufficient sleep is obtained.[4]

The SCN, serving as the central body clock, receives its main sensory input from the optic nerve, arising from retinal ganglion cells. Retinal light stimulation, particularly at the blue end of the spectrum, is capable of re-timing the SCN clock. Considerable research has shown that light stimulation before the core body

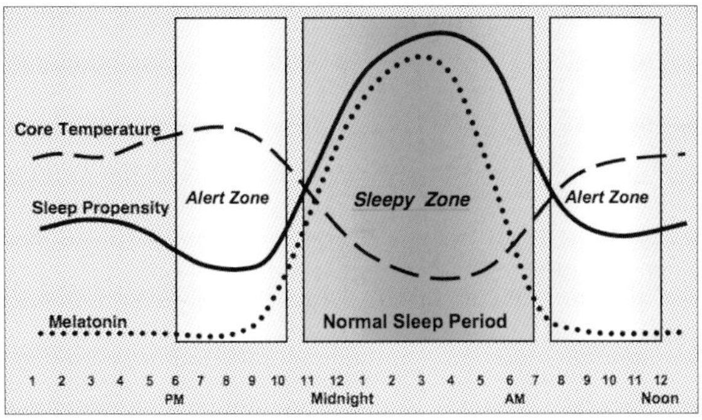

FIGURE 43.2 For a normally good sleep between 11 pm and 7 am, the figure shows the associated circadian variation of core body temperature (dashed line), melatonin (dotted line), and sleep propensity (solid line).

temperature minimum produces a delay of the circadian timing and, conversely, light stimulation after the core temperature minimum results in a shift of the clock to earlier times. Therefore, a sleep difficulty resulting from circadian timing gone astray may be treated with appropriately timed light stimulation. For example, sleep-onset insomnia arising from a circadian delay can be treated with morning bright light, and the opposite timing problem, early morning awakening insomnia arising from an abnormally early timed circadian rhythm, can be treated with evening bright light.

Although the SCN signals the pineal gland to secrete melatonin during the night, the SCN is also sensitive to melatonin feedback and can be influenced in its timing if melatonin is administered exogenously outside the normal sleep period. Melatonin administered several hours before typical sleep onset (e.g. 5–7 pm) can advance the circadian rhythm (reset to an earlier time). Conversely, melatonin administered late in the typical sleep period (e.g. 5–8 am) can delay circadian rhythms along with the circadian sleep-conducive period. Thus both bright light and exogenous melatonin can be used in a 'push–pull' manner to readjust circadian timing. (These sleep disorders and treatments are elaborated upon later, in the sections on insomnia and circadian rhythm sleep disorders.)

NORMAL PSYCHOLOGICAL AND BEHAVIOURAL DETERMINERS OF SLEEP PROPENSITY

Sleep propensity can also be influenced by a myriad normal psychological and behavioural variables, including learned responses, perceptions of danger/safety, ingestion of stimulants/sedatives and physical activity/inactivity. For example, if the tendency to fall asleep while watching a favourite television program happens frequently, it can become a learned or conditioned sleeping response. The opposite tendency, for people with insomnia to become alert when attempting to fall asleep despite being sleepy before bedtime, is also a conditioned response. An awakening at night may be perceived as a potential threat for its negative impact on meeting obligations the following day. The brain's threat response or 'fight-or-flight' system will be activated, resulting in increased physiological activation and alertness inhibitory to sleep. Furthermore, if this perceived threat and subsequent fight-or-flight response occurs frequently enough in the same circumstances, it can become a conditioned response to that occasion of awakening and, therefore, occur automatically regardless of any subsequent daytime obligations. This process describes the putative conditioned or learned basis of 'psychophysiological insomnia' assumed to be present in most cases of chronic insomnia.

THE IMPACT OF SLEEP UPON HEALTH

An adequate amount of good-quality sleep on a regular basis is crucial to physical and mental wellbeing. It should be considered one of the 'big three' health promoters, in addition to nutrition and exercise. However, unlike eating and exercise, over which we have direct control, sleep cannot be forced. In fact, trying hard to sleep can be counter-productive. Providing the right behavioural and mental conditions for sleep is the best approach to prevent the development of sleep disorders.

Chronic sleep problems can have a negative impact on health but, equally, chronic health problems can affect sleep. For example, factors predicting the later development of insomnia include being overweight (35% more likely than average), physical inactivity (42%), alcohol dependence (75%) and having a joint or lower back disorder (195%).[5] Having a major psychiatric disorder increases the risk eight-fold. Managing the sleep problem in such situations therefore requires attention to the underlying health problem.

The mismanagement of sleep problems and the overuse of sedatives can also have a negative impact upon health.[6,7] Only a small proportion of patients taking sleeping pills regularly will note improvement in their insomnia in the long term. A higher proportion will report that their insomnia is worsened by them, despite the fact that the person soon finds themselves unable to sleep without them. Sleep medications can also be associated with a worsening of depression and reduced energy. Using pharmacological methods alone for management of long-term insomnia is an inadequate and incomplete solution.[8] Sleeping tablets also accumulate in the body, particularly in the elderly for whom the half-life of the drugs is far longer, and are associated with other problems such as falls, drowsiness and lowered life expectancy.

LIFESTYLE FACTORS AND SLEEP

Education

As the problems associated with poorer sleep become more recognised, educating people from an early age as to what constitutes healthy sleep (as illustrated in Fig 43.1), and helping a person with sleep problems to understand the ways in which they can improve sleep, is an increasingly important role for the general practitioner.

Stress management

The two-way links between poor sleep and poor mental health are now well established. Depression and anxiety produce effects on various stress hormones including cortisol and catechols, which also have a negative impact on sleep patterns.[9] The vicious circle of stress leading to poor sleep, lowered mood and more stress is a common one in our community.

It has been a common assumption in medical circles that sleep disturbance is secondary to depression, which is true, but evidence also suggests that it goes the other way as well. If a detailed chronological history is taken from a patient with depression, it is often found that sleep disturbance precedes the onset of lowered mood.[10–12] Because a patient may present with concerns about the mood, the underlying role of sleep may be undervalued. Chronic insomnia nearly trebles the risk of depression, and in one study was found to be second only to recent bereavement as a risk factor and was a more significant risk factor than having had a previous episode of depression.[13] Another study put the risk for depression at four times greater for women and twice as great for men if they suffered from long-term insomnia.[14]

Some studies suggest that, if people with depression undertake effective behavioural strategies for improving sleep, the depression will resolve in 57% of people and be improved by more than 40% in another 13%.[15] These kinds of findings have been replicated in other studies on other behavioural interventions for insomnia in those with depression.[16]

Therefore, the management of sleep problems always needs to take mental health into account, and the holistic management of mental health problems always needs to include sleep.

Exercise

Being active during the day and exercising regularly will tend to improve sleep at night and wakefulness in the day.[17,18] Some people find that vigorous exercise close to bedtime has a negative effect on sleep, because of sympathetic nervous system (SNS) activation. A solution can be to exercise earlier or to have a period of quiet activity between exercising and going to bed.

In the absence of chronic fatigue syndrome or other significant medical conditions, there are many people who oversleep and yet feel chronically tired. It would be easy to believe that the solution is to get more sleep, whereas it is likely that a better solution would be to include more activity in one's daily life and not to sleep past what the body and mind need. (This will be explored in more detail later.)

Nutrition

An increasing number of people these days try to boost their available energy with stimulants such as caffeine and 'energy drinks'. Unfortunately, these can exacerbate the original problem. Quality sleep is the optimal and natural way to replenish energy and is of central importance to our mental and physical health. Minimising caffeine and avoiding it entirely for up to 6 hours before bedtime, and avoiding alcohol abuse, are two of the simplest steps to help many people improve their sleep.

Tryptophan is a precursor to melatonin, so tryptophan-rich foods such as seaweed products or milk can boost melatonin levels, as can calorie restriction and foods rich in calcium, magnesium, vitamin B_6 and niacinamide.

Connectedness

A number of potential sources of distress (e.g. loss of job, marital difficulties, bereavement) will normally trigger the 'flight-or-flight' mechanism and lead to shortened sleep and more awakenings. Rather than ruminating about the sleep problem, it may be more effective to resolve the underlying issue with problem-solving behaviour or counselling. The sleep problem, if of short duration, is likely to resolve in response to this approach.

However, a sleep problem can remain long after the precipitating problem has gone. This suggests the presence of conditioned insomnia, which can be addressed by the non-drug techniques discussed later.

Environment

Obviously, a noisy, light or unsettled environment is not conducive to good sleep patterns. For example, living on a main road or near an industrial area or major building works, or having a noisy dog next door, can be problematic for some people. Ear plugs and eye shades can be useful in these conditions. Most important is to avoid becoming angry or distressed about the noise, as this is more likely to disturb sleep than the noise itself.

Having adequate sunlight during the day and avoiding bright light close to bedtime or if you happen to wake during the night is important for having adequate melatonin levels at night.[19,20]

SLEEP DISORDERS

A large range of sleep disorders will be evident in general practice. It is important to be attentive to the clinical signs of these various disorders in order to provide appropriate diagnosis and treatment. Some sleep disorders are diagnosed and managed better at specialist sleep disorders units, and others can be managed within general practice using a range of behavioural and cognitive techniques.

SLEEP DISORDERS REQUIRING REFERRAL

In this section we outline a range of sleep disorders that are best referred to a specialist unit for confirmation of diagnosis and initial treatment. Table 43.1 summarises the most common clinical symptoms and how they relate to the different sleep disorders outlined below.

Sleep disorders such as obstructive sleep apnoea, periodic limb movements in sleep, restless legs syndrome, narcolepsy, parasomnias and REM sleep behaviour disorder are diagnosed by clinical symptoms and overnight polysomnography (PSG) and should be referred to a sleep disorders unit for diagnosis and initial management. Overnight PSG involves an appointment to sleep in a motel-like room in a sleep disorders unit, usually associated with a hospital. Various sensors are attached to the skin of the head to measure brain waves (EEG), eye movements (EOG) and muscle tension (EMG), the finger or earlobe for blood oxygen saturation; a nasal cannula is used to measure nasal pressure during respiration, chest and abdominal pressure transducers measure breathing, and a sleep position sensor is used. These sensors are connected by thin wires to a box at the bed head and recorded on computer for subsequent analysis. Although this procedure appears intrusive, most patients obtain close to their usual sleep. (Contacts for these services can be found in the Resources list.)

Obstructive sleep apnoea

Obstructive sleep apnoea (OSA) is characterised by repetitive episodes of upper airway collapse and obstruction of airflow during sleep. These events can result in reductions in blood oxygen saturation and are usually terminated by brief arousals from sleep.[21]

Prevalence

OSA can occur in any age group, but in adults the prevalence rate for mild OSA has been estimated at 24%

TABLE 43.1 Clinical symptoms, possible diagnosis and clinical management decisions

Initial clinical symptoms	Hypothesised diagnosis	Confirmatory symptoms	Management decision
Daytime sleepiness	Narcolepsy	Overwhelming daytime sleepiness, sleep attacks, insomnia	Sleep disorders unit
Loud snoring Gasping Stop breathing	Obstructive sleep apnoea (OSA)	Snoring, gasping, witnessed apnoeas, morning headache, daytime sleepiness, obesity	Sleep disorders unit
Daytime tiredness/ fatigue Sleeping difficulties	Insomnia	Difficulty initiating sleep Night-time awakenings Waking too early Daytime tiredness/fatigue	See Table 43.2
Restless legs	Restless legs syndrome	Aching, itchy, crawly feeling in legs Uncontrollable urge to move legs Symptoms greatest in evening at bedtime	Sleep disorders unit
Kicking at night	Periodic limb movements in sleep	Twitching legs and arms while asleep Daytime sleepiness	Sleep disorders unit
Unusual behaviour during sleep	Sleepwalking Night terrors Bruxism REM behaviour disorder (RBD)	No memory of event, first half of night Screaming, fear response Tooth grinding, morning headache Sleep-related injuries, disruptive behaviour	GP, psychologist Paediatrician Sleep disorders unit

in men and 9% in women, and for moderate to severe OSA, 4% in men and 2% in women.[21,22] The prevalence rate increases with age, with a higher rate in overweight middle-aged males and in women after menopause.

Diagnosis

Clinical symptoms include excessive daytime sleepiness and fatigue despite apparently adequate sleep time. Other clinical symptoms that are usually reported by the bed partner are heavy snoring and/or choking sounds, cessation of breathing for short periods (10–30 seconds) with resumption by gasping for breath. The patient may complain of a dry mouth and headache on awakening in the morning. An overnight PSG will report abnormalities of sleep architecture, the number of respiratory events per hour of sleep time and amount of oxygen desaturation.

Management

Lifestyle changes such as avoiding alcohol in the evening, losing weight, quitting smoking and using special pillows or devices to avoid sleeping on one's back can help in treating OSA. If appropriate, one conservative treatment is an oral appliance to keep the airway open during sleep. If these conservative methods are ineffective in preventing obstruction of airway and decreasing daytime sleepiness, continuous positive airway pressure (CPAP) is usually recommended by the sleep physician. This involves wearing a nasal mask attached to an air pump to produce a mild positive airway pressure and is usually successful at maintaining airway patency and allowing unobstructed breathing during sleep. In some cases surgical procedures are recommended.

Obstructive sleep apnoea in children

OSA is surprisingly common in children (1–10%) and presents some clinical symptoms similar to those of adults (e.g. snoring, choking, daytime sleepiness) with additional daytime symptoms of hyperactivity, difficulty concentrating, excessive irritability, behaviour problems, meal refusals, failure to thrive and enuresis. The overlap of many clinical symptoms with those of attention deficit hyperactivity disorder (ADHD) can lead to an incorrect ADHD diagnosis and potentially inappropriate pharmacotherapy. Overnight PSG can provide a differential diagnosis. The most common aetiology of OSA in children is enlarged tonsils and adenoids. Adeno-tonsillectomy is, therefore, the most common and successful treatment for OSA and its associated symptoms in these children.

Narcolepsy

Narcolepsy, a disorder of excessive daytime sleepiness, is a rare, chronic, neurological disorder with prevalence rates in the United States and Europe of approximately 1 in 2000 people.[23] Age of onset is typically adolescence or young adulthood.

Diagnosis

Narcolepsy is characterised by excessive and overwhelming daytime sleepiness temporarily relieved by a brief sleep. An adequate bed period at night but somewhat disrupted sleep is usually reported. Narcolepsy may be accompanied by cataplexy that is characterised by sudden weakening of large skeletal muscles provoked by emotional response, for example, elation, laughter, surprise or anger.[21] The loss of muscle tone may range from a mild sensation of weakness to complete paralysis and collapse. Hypnagogic hallucinations and sleep paralysis are also associated with 'narcolepsy with cataplexy'. An overnight PSG and a daytime multiple sleep latency test are commonly used in the diagnosis of this disorder.

Management

Sleep physicians may use stimulants during the day and hypnotics at night to control excessive daytime sleepiness, and antidepressants to ameliorate cataplexy. Lifestyle changes that may be useful include a regular bedtime schedule, and avoiding caffeine and alcohol within 6 hours before bedtime. Short, regular daytime naps are also recommended to ameliorate the sleepiness symptoms. This may require negotiation with schools and employers to modify class/work schedules, with the added benefit of informing those in the patient's social environment of the presence of a medical, rather than motivational, condition.

Sleep-related movement disorders

Sleep-related movement disorders include the conditions of restless legs syndrome (RLS), periodic limb movements in sleep (PLMS) and sleep-related bruxism, all of which can affect sleep quality and daytime functioning.

Restless legs syndrome

Restless legs syndrome (RLS) is a sensorimotor disorder characterised by uncomfortable sensations in the legs, such as aching or internal itchy or burning feelings, that causes an irresistible urge to move the legs. These unpleasant feelings are most noticeable and problematic in the evening or whenever the person is trying to relax, but then often decline during the early morning period, suggesting a circadian influence. RLS can therefore prolong sleep onset and contribute to insomnia. PSG findings have demonstrated fragmented non-REM and REM sleep in individuals with RLS.[24]

Prevalence

RLS is reported by 5–10% of the population and occurs up to two times more commonly in women than in men.[21] A recent survey found that clinically significant RLS, occurring at least twice a week and causing moderate distress, occurs in almost 3% of the population.[25] RLS is generally idiopathic, and in 40–60% of cases there is a familial association. RLS may also be symptomatic of such associated conditions as peripheral neuropathies, uraemia, iron deficiency, diabetes, Parkinson's disease and pregnancy.[26]

Diagnosis

RLS can be diagnosed by the presence of clinical symptoms and further evaluated using an immobilisation test, which is generally carried out in a sleep disorders unit.

Management

Treatment options include both behavioural and pharmacological approaches. Lifestyle changes of possible benefit include a balanced diet and avoiding caffeine, nicotine and alcohol in the evening. RLS appears to respond to dopaminergic agonists as short-term therapy.[27] Because RLS is strongly associated with periodic limb movements in sleep (see below), the diagnoses and treatment of both would best rely on PSG and sleep physician respectively at a sleep disorders unit.

- Hot baths help some patients.
- Exercise early in the day.
- Magnesium supplementation may reduce symptom severity.[28]
- Assess for and correct iron deficiency (restless legs may be associated with iron deficiency).

Periodic limb movements in sleep

Periodic limb movements in sleep (PLMS) are characterised by periodic episodes of repetitive (every 20–40 seconds) short bursts (0.5–5 seconds) of limb movements that occur during sleep.[21] They arise from dorsiflexion of the ankle and toes and a partial flexion of the knee. PLMS may sometimes occur in the arms. Although typically the individual is unaware of these movements, they can be associated with a cortical arousal or an awakening and hence lead to sleep onset and/or sleep maintenance problems and concomitant daytime sleepiness and fatigue.[21]

Prevalence

The prevalence of PLMS is estimated to be 4–11% in adults, with PLMS occurring in 80–90% of people with RLS.[21,29] A large cross-sectional European study found that factors associated with PLMS are female gender, shift work, caffeine intake and stress.[30]

Diagnosis

Although clinical symptoms may be acutely evident to a bed partner, who may suffer from sleep disturbance from the frequent movements, diagnosis should be confirmed with PSG measured as the number of PLMS per hour of total sleep time.[21]

Management

Lifestyle measures that target the associated factors include reducing caffeine and nicotine intake, and stress management. One study has shown that magnesium supplementation can help. Most treatments use the newer dopaminergic medications that have been found to fully suppress PLMS. However, these potent drugs should be used cautiously as they are not free of side effects, including daytime augmentation of RLS symptoms.[21]

Sleep-related bruxism

Sleep bruxism (SB) is characterised by grinding or clenching of the teeth during sleep and is usually associated with cortical arousals but rarely full awakenings.[21] It is associated with temporomandibular pain, headaches and tooth wear.

Prevalence

Prevalence is highest in childhood (14–17%) and then decreases over the lifespan to about 3% in older adults.[21] A large cross-sectional survey found that risk factors for SB include OSA, loud snoring, heavy alcohol consumption, caffeine consumption (> 6 cups), smoking, anxiety and stress.[31]

Diagnosis

The condition is diagnosed from EMG during a clinical PSG. Bruxism occurs more frequently in the lighter stages (Stages 1 and 2) of sleep.

Management

The management of SB includes pharmacological (clonazepam), psychological and occlusal therapeutic approaches.[32] Occlusal splints, fitted by a dentist, appear to be a more symptomatic treatment option. Psychological therapies have used biofeedback, relaxation, hypnosis, counselling, sleep hygiene and lifestyle changes. A recent study compared the effectiveness of an occlusal splint to cognitive–behavioural treatment (CBT) for sleep bruxism.[32] The CBT comprised progressive muscle relaxation, nocturnal feedback and stress-management training. Both groups experienced significant reductions in SB activity and associated symptoms as well as improved psychological measures.

Parasomnias

Parasomnias are undesirable physical events or experiences that occur during entry into sleep, within sleep or during arousal from sleep. They involve sleep-related behaviours and experiences over which there is no conscious, deliberate control.[21] These events can be injurious to the patient and others and can produce a significant disruption of the sleep–wake pattern. This section discusses the more common parasomnias including NREM disorders such as sleep terrors and sleepwalking, and parasomnias associated with REM sleep such as nightmares and REM sleep behaviour disorder (RBD).

According to the International Classification of Sleep Disorders[21] only RBD requires PSG for a diagnosis, although an overnight sleep study can confirm a clinical diagnosis of other parasomnias and rule out other disorders, such as epilepsy. Diagnosis of other parasomnias requires a clinical interview with the individual and a family member to elucidate the description, timing, frequency and duration of the behavioural event.

Non-REM: sleep terrors and sleepwalking

Sleep terrors and sleepwalking are disorders caused by partial arousal from slow-wave sleep and therefore typically occur 1 to 3 hours after sleep onset, when slow-wave sleep is usually most prominent.[33] Apart from diminished alertness, both are associated with amnesia for the event. They are common in childhood and decrease in incidence during early adolescence, when slow-wave sleep declines.

Sleep terrors are accompanied by a cry or piercing scream and behavioural manifestations of intense fear such as dilated pupils and pallor of the skin.[21] Sleepwalking (somnambulism) consists of a series of complex behaviours such as walking about in a lowered state of consciousness, and impaired judgment.[21]

As both sleep terrors and sleep walking are associated with irregular sleep schedules, sleep deprivation and psychosocial stress, helpful actions include increasing time in bed and a regular sleep pattern.[33] Adults experiencing sleepwalking and sleep terrors may also have a past or current history of depression or anxiety; however, control of these psychiatric disorders does not control the parasomnias.[21] A recent study has found that sleep-disordered breathing is associated with parasomnias, with respiratory effort leading to a number of arousal reactions occurring in slow-wave sleep.[34] Referral to a sleep disorders unit and PSG may be indicated in this instance.

REM: nightmares

Nightmares are characterised by awakening primarily from REM sleep, experienced as disturbing mentations.[35]

Prevalence and diagnosis

Up to 50% of children between 3 and 5 years of age experience nightmares severe enough to disturb their parents.[21] In adults, 50–85% report experiencing at least an occasional nightmare.[21] Because nightmares typically arise during REM sleep, they usually occur in the latter half of the night when REM propensity is high. Numerous studies have indicated that nightmares are associated with increased life stress, anxiety and other psychopathologies. Nightmares can also be associated with alcohol abuse and some medications that initially suppress REM sleep, and when these are stopped, REM rebound may occur, with often bizarre and frightening nightmares.

Management

Stress management techniques and cognitive behaviour therapy for anxiety may be recommended, as well as avoidance of chronic sleep restriction and excessive alcohol consumption before bed.

REM sleep behaviour disorder

REM sleep behaviour disorder seems to be caused by a failure of the normal muscle paralysis of REM sleep and is characterised by abnormal behaviours such as physically active (often violent) episodes, usually associated with dream recall. When aroused to reality, the patient will report that they had a violent dream and reinterpreted the present environment in terms consistent with the dream. RBD is more likely to occur in the latter half of the night when REM sleep is more frequent.

Prevalence

RBD is uncommon but tends to affect mainly men aged 50 years and older, and may be idiopathic or associated with other neurological disorders.[21,36]

Diagnosis

Differential diagnosis of RBD is made from PSG by the presence of abnormal REM sleep behaviours or failure of EMG suppression during REM sleep.

Management

Following diagnosis, medication such as clonazepam may be indicated. Ensure adequate sleep to avoid curtailing REM sleep with its potential subsequent REM rebound, which may exacerbate RBD.

INSOMNIA

In this final section we describe the common sleep disorders that may be managed in general practice.

Insomnia is defined as chronic difficulty with initiation, consolidation or duration of sleep, resulting in daytime impairment.[21] It is the most common sleep disturbance in the general population and is said to be the third-highest complaint seen by the GP. Epidemiological surveys have yielded prevalence rates of 20–40% in the adult population, with 10–20% experiencing severe or frequent insomnia.[37] Insomnia is often comorbid with other disorders (e.g. chronic pain, depression, anxiety) and therefore the GP needs to be alert for sleep problems when treating other physical and psychological disorders. Although insomnia may have been originally secondary to other health problems, if of long duration the insomnia is likely to be self-sustaining and require its own treatment.

Table 43.2 describes the three main types of insomnia complaints seen by the GP—that is, sleep onset, sleep maintenance and/or early morning awakening insomnia. These are illustrated in Fig 43.3, with examples of different sleep patterns from a typical sleep diary. Some patients may have a combination of insomnia diagnoses—for example, they may present with sleep onset insomnia but have a combination of psychophysiological insomnia as well as a delayed circadian rhythm, or they may have sleep maintenance insomnia as well as sleep onset insomnia.

Management

Still the most common medical treatment for insomnia is hypnotics and, more recently, antidepressants. However, these have negative consequences such as tolerance, dependence, withdrawal rebound insomnia and altered sleep physiology, as well as side effects such as amnesia, psychomotor slowing, cognitive impairment and unusual night-time behaviours. Particularly in the older population, hypnotics tend to exacerbate all the normal cognitive/behavioural impairment of ageing as well as potentially interacting with a patient's other medications. Medication may provide temporary symptomatic relief only and does not address the causes of insomnia. In recent studies, cognitive behaviour therapy for chronic insomnia has been shown to be comparable to pharmacotherapy in the short term and more effective in the long term.[38,39] Cognitive/behaviour and light therapies aimed at correcting the underlying aetiologies are suggested to produce greater long-term effectiveness. However, it is important to correctly identify the subtype of insomnia and its likely aetiology in order to provide the most appropriate treatment. Figure 43.3 and Table 43.2 can be used as a guide to this process. Identify the pattern of insomnia in Figure 43.3, then check the treatment suggestions in Table 43.2, which are elaborated in detail below.

In addition, insomnia non-drug treatment programs conducted in most major cities worldwide successfully use evidence-based therapies such as stimulus control, bedtime restriction and cognitive therapy and bright light to treat the different insomnia subtypes. (See the Resources list at the end of this chapter for websites of sleep clinics and practitioners.)

Non-drug, evidence-based insomnia treatments

Good sleep practices (sleep hygiene)

A good bedtime routine includes the following measures:

- Avoid vigorous exercise at least 2 hours before bedtime.
- Avoid caffeine drinks (stimulants) within 6 hours before bedtime.
- Avoid alcohol before bedtime, as it can lead to night-time awakening.
- Nicotine (smoking and patches) increases alertness. Smoking reduction or withdrawal can improve sleep as well as general health.
- Avoid going to bed hungry or after a big meal.
- Have a 'wind down' period (30–60 minutes) for relaxing in dim light before bed.
- Avoid a fixed bedtime or going to bed too early. Use feelings of sleepiness, not fatigue, as your guide for bedtime.
- Get rid of the bedroom clock if checking the time is a habit that is associated with worry about your sleep.
- Have a fixed wake-up time.

Short 'power-naps' (less than 20 minutes) may be rejuvenating when experiencing daytime sleepiness. A longer sleep (longer than 20–30 minutes), where one goes into deep sleep, often results in shorter and broken sleep that night. Furthermore, when we come out of a longer, deep sleep during the day or early evening, we can experience a period of lethargy for up to an hour after awakening, referred to as sleep inertia, which can counteract the rejuvenating purpose of daytime sleep.

Stimulus control therapy

Difficulty falling asleep may be due to an association that has developed between bedtime and difficulties with falling asleep. The process of getting ready for bed and going to bed may become stimuli that trigger negative emotions such as anxiety, frustration, worry—known as 'conditioned insomnia'.

To extinguish these responses:

- Reserve the bedroom for sleep or sexual activity—no TV, computers, eating or arguing.
- Go to bed only when feeling sleepy, as opposed to going to bed because you feel exhausted or tired or believe it should be bedtime.
- If you are unable to fall asleep within a short time (e.g. 15–20 mins) or are feeling anxious or alert, get out of bed and go to another room and read or watch TV under dim lights. Return to bed again only when feeling sleepy.

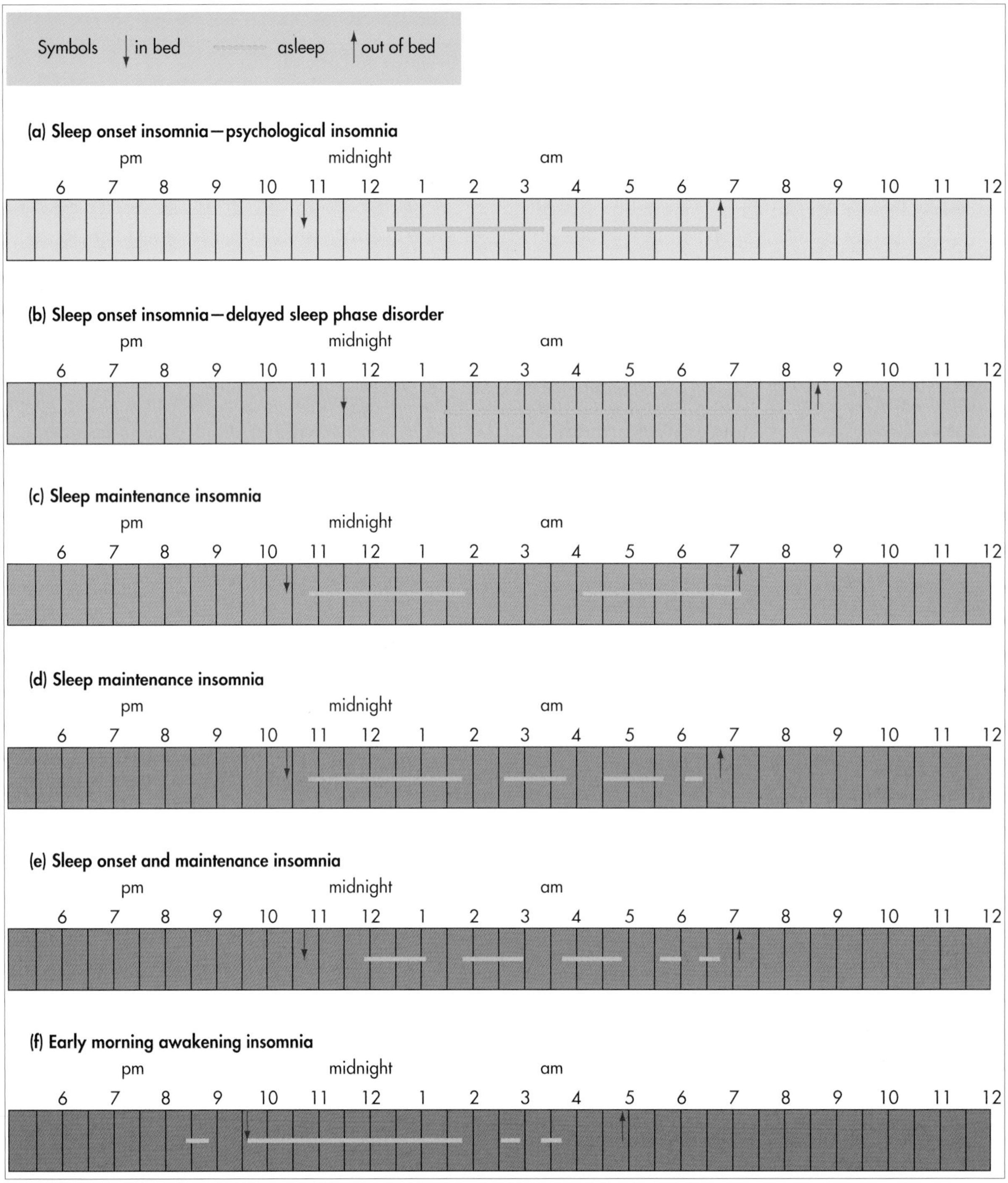

FIGURE 43.3 Examples of typical sleep patterns for different subtypes of insomnia diagnoses: (a, b) sleep onset insomnia, (c, d) sleep maintenance insomnia, (e) sleep onset and sleep maintenance insomnia and (f) early morning awakening insomnia

TABLE 43.2 Clinical symptoms of insomnia subtypes and suggested treatment options

Clinical symptoms of insomnia type	Treatment suggestions
Sleep onset insomnia	
Psychophysiological insomnia (PI) (Fig 43.2a) • Long time taken to fall asleep (> 30 min) at desired bedtime • Sometimes fall asleep when sleep is not intended • May sleep better away from home • Anxious about sleep, mentally/physically aroused after going to bed • Some daytime impairment (tired, fatigued, irritable)	Stimulus control therapy Cognitive therapy Relaxation therapy Good sleep practices
Delayed sleep phase disorder (DPSD) (Fig 43.2b) • Normal sleep duration but later sleep pattern • Long sleep latency at normal bedtime (e.g. 11 pm) but shorter latency at later time (e.g. 2 am) • Able to sleep late in the morning if given opportunity • Difficulty trying to awaken at desired time (e.g. 7 am)	Stimulus control therapy Morning bright light Dim light in evening Good sleep practices
Sleep maintenance insomnia (Fig 43.2c,d) • Usually no difficulty falling asleep at desired time • Waking in middle of the night feeling anxious/alert • Difficulty falling back to sleep • Some daytime impairment (tired, fatigued, irritable)	Bedtime restriction Cognitive therapy Evening bright light Good sleep practices Relaxation therapy
Sleep onset and sleep maintenance (Fig 43.2e) • Long sleep latency (> 30 min) • Waking in the middle of the night, difficulty falling back to sleep • Some daytime impairment (fatigue, distress)	Bedtime restriction Cognitive therapy Good sleep practices Relaxation therapy
Early morning awakening insomnia (Fig 43.2f) • Early evening sleepiness (falling asleep in front of TV) • Able to fall asleep quickly at usual bedtime • Early morning awakening (e.g. before 5 am) and unable to fall back to sleep • Some daytime impairment	Evening bright light Dim light in morning

- Keep repeating the above step until you fall asleep quickly.
- Keep a regular time for arising from bed, even on weekends, and get some light stimulation after arising.

In the first few nights/weeks this is likely to result in many times out of bed before rapid onset of sleep. In winter months it would be helpful to keep another room warm, to encourage you to get up when needed. Gradually, as sleep pressure builds and conditioned insomnia declines, sleep will occur more quickly, with fewer out-of-beds required.

Bedtime restriction

People who experience sleeplessness during the night often stay in bed longer in the hope of 'catching up' on lost sleep. This exacerbates the problem, as it usually increases time spent awake in bed. Spending too long in bed results in shallow and fragmented sleep, anxiety and daytime tiredness, and reinforces the conditioned insomnia.

By restricting the amount of time spent in bed, sleep will become consolidated due to an increase in sleep homeostatic pressure. To do this:

- Estimate the patient's average total sleep time (e.g. 6 hours).
- Set a period in bed for only that amount of time (e.g. 6 hours).
- Choose a regular wake-up time to suit personal circumstances and then set a regular bedtime (e.g. 12 am to 6 am).
- Avoid daytime naps, to help increase sleep pressure.
- Assess the sleep pattern after a week and, if sleep is more consolidated with few awakenings, gradually extend time in bed by 15–30 minutes each week until daytime sleepiness/fatigue abates.

Cognitive therapy

Unhelpful and unrealistic thoughts and beliefs about sleep can lead to anxiety, and emotional and somatic arousal, which all interfere with the sleep process.

Cognitive therapy involves:

- explaining the normal sleep process (e.g. awakenings are normal)
- replacing unhelpful thoughts with more realistic, helpful thoughts and beliefs (e.g. feeling tired after a fragmented sleep is normal, but despite

taking more effort, the following day can still be successful, and recovery sleep the following night is likely).

Relaxation techniques

- Learn a relaxation technique, such as diaphragmatic breathing, visualisation, meditation. All these involve focusing on a non-provocative idea/image in order to keep worrisome thoughts at bay. When extraneous thoughts re-enter consciousness, be mindful of that (don't be discouraged, it will happen) and regain your focus on your relaxation image/idea. Practise this relaxation technique until proficient before using it in bed for sleep.
- Do something relaxing in the hour before bed—no computer work, computer games, business or arguments.
- If you have a lot on your mind, it can be helpful to spend a few minutes (e.g. 15–30 minutes in the early evening) planning the next day or thinking about the day's activities.

Morning bright light

Morning bright light will advance a delayed circadian rhythm and lead to an earlier sleep pattern.[4] For example, if a patient wishes to sleep between 11 pm and 7 am but is unable to fall asleep until 3 am and has difficulty waking earlier than 11 am, they may have delayed sleep phase disorder.[21] To advance the sleep period back to the preferred earlier time, we suggest the following protocol:

1. Establish the patient's ad lib wake-up time (sleep-in time, e.g. 11 am).
2. Commence light therapy sessions. The patient is exposed to 1 hour of bright light, possibly outdoor light, 30 minutes before this time (e.g. 10.30 am). Note: an artificial light device in the morning may be necessary during winter.
3. Gradually advance wake-up time and morning light exposure by 15–30 minutes each day until the preferred wake-up time is reached (e.g. 10 am, 9.30 am, 9 am, 8.30 am …).
4. Avoid bright light in the evenings—no computer or stimulating activity.
5. Keep a regular sleep/wake schedule, to prevent relapse delay of sleep phase.

Evening bright light

The abnormally early timed circadian rhythm and sleep pattern can be delayed by exposure to bright evening light.[4] The patient with an early timed circadian rhythm (advanced sleep phase[21]) will struggle to stay awake until the desired or conventional bedtime and may experience frequently unintentional naps in the evening before retiring to bed. They will also experience early morning awakening. For example, the patient may have overwhelming sleepiness at 8 pm, prolong bedtime until 10 pm but despite this, still wake at 4 am and be unable to fall back to sleep. We suggest the following:

- Develop a habit of spending up to 60 minutes outdoors late in the day or early evening. An artificial light device may be used in winter with light exposure for 1 hour before bedtime.
- Do some light exercise early in the evening (walking, stretching).
- Avoid morning sunlight or other bright light within 1–2 hours after waking (may need to wear dark glasses).

Melatonin

Melatonin may be useful for those with a circadian rhythm sleep disorder. Because melatonin can re-time the circadian rhythm, it can be useful for treating the insomnias with a circadian mistiming component. In severe sleep onset insomnia, low-dose melatonin (0.5–1.0 mg) may be helpful if taken in the early evening (e.g. 6–8 pm). This will shift the underlying circadian rhythm to an earlier time and result in the ability to fall asleep earlier.

When early sleep onset with premature early morning awakenings is the problem, evening bright light and low-dose (0.3–0.5 mg) melatonin taken in the early morning (e.g. 3–5 am) can help to delay the abnormally early rhythms and allow longer sleep in the morning. It should be noted that pure melatonin, which is necessary for this effect, can only be obtained by prescription in Australia. In the United States, it is available in health food stores.

Herbal treatments

Common herbal treatments for insomnia include:

- *Valerian* (*Valeriana officinalis*)—usually used in combination with other herbal treatments. Not all research results are positive, but results from several well-conducted placebo-controlled studies suggest that valerian reduces sleep latency and increases sleep quality in poor sleepers if taken for more than 2 weeks.[40]
- *Lavender*—a number of controlled trials and observational studies suggest that inhalation of ambient lavender oil has a relaxing effect and can reduce anxiety and improve mood, concentration and sleep.[41]
- *Lemon balm*—often prescribed in combination with other herbs such as valerian in the treatment of insomnia.[42]

CONCLUSION

It is important to be alert to the clinical symptoms of sleep disorders in medical practice as these disorders will often not be the presenting problem. Many of these disorders are prevalent and cause significant morbidity. However, the field of sleep disorders has made, and will continue to make, considerable advances in diagnosis and treatment. Many of the suspected disorders would best be managed by referral to a specialist sleep disorders unit, while some of the most prevalent can be managed by the general practitioner using a variety of proven non-drug therapies.

RESOURCES

American Academy of Sleep Medicine, http://www.aasmnet.org

Australasian Sleep Association, http://www.sleep.org.au

Australasian Sleep Association, information on sleep disorders, http://www.sleepaus.on.net/factsheets.html

Australasian Sleep Association, insomnia treatment services (in each Australian state), http://www.sleepaus.on.net/servicesinsomniatreatments.php

British Sleep Society, http://www.sleeping.org.uk/

European Sleep Research Society, http://www.esrs.eu/cms/front_content.php

Lack L, Wright H, Bearpark H. Insomnia: how to sleep easy. Sydney: Media 21; 2003.

Morin CM, Espie CA. Insomnia: a clinical guide to assessment and treatment. New York: Kluwer Academic/Plenum; 2003.

Poceta JS, Mitler MM. Sleep disorders: diagnosis and treatment. New Jersey: Humana Press; 1998.

REFERENCES

1 Poceta JS, Mitler MM. Sleep disorders: diagnosis and treatment. New Jersey: Humana Press; 1998.

2 Mercer JD, Bootzin RR, Lack LC. Insomniacs' perception of wake instead of sleep. Sleep 2002; 25:564–571.

3 Borbely AA. A two-process model of sleep regulation. Human Neurob 1982; 1:195–204.

4 Lack LC, Wright HR. Treating chronobiological components of chronic insomnia. Sleep Med 2007; 8:637–644.

5 Janson C, Lindberg E, Gislason T et al. Insomnia in men—a 10-year prospective population-based study. Sleep 2001; 24(4):425–430.

6 Mant A, Mattick RP, de Burgh S et al. Benzodiazepine prescribing in general practice: dispelling some myths. Fam Pract 1995; 12(1):37–43.

7 Mant A, de Burgh S, Mattick RP et al. Insomnia in general practice. Results from NSW General Practice Survey 1991–1992. Aust Fam Physician 1996; Suppl 1:S15–S18.

8 Hohagen F, Rink K, Kappler C et al. Prevalence and treatment of insomnia in general practice. A longitudinal study. Eur Arch Psychiatry Clin Neurosci 1993; 242(6):329–336.

9 Steiger A. Sleep and endocrinology. J Intern Med 2003; 254(1):13–22.

10 Holsboer-Trachsler E, Seifritz E. Sleep in depression and sleep deprivation: a brief conceptual review. World J Biol Psychiatry 2000; 1(4):180–186.

11 Buysse DJ. Insomnia, depression and aging. Assessing sleep and mood interactions in older adults. Geriatrics 2004; 59(2):47–51; quiz 52.

12 Riemann D, Voderholzer U. Primary insomnia: a risk factor for depression? J Affect Disord 2003; 76(1–3):255–259.

13 Cole MG, Dendukuri N. Risk factors for depression among elderly community subjects: a systematic review and meta-analysis. Am J Psychiatry 2003; 160(6):1147–1156.

14 Mallon L, Broman J, Hetta J. Relationship between insomnia, depression, and mortality: a 12-year follow-up of older adults in the community. Int Psychogeriatr 2000; 12(3):295–306.

15 Morawetz D. Insomnia and depression: which comes first? Sleep Res Online 2003; 5(2):77–81.

16 Germain A, Moul DE, Franzen PL et al. Effects of a brief behavioral treatment for late-life insomnia: preliminary findings. J Clin Sleep Med 2006; 2(4):403–406.

17 Merrill RM, Aldana SG, Greenlaw RL et al. The effects of an intensive lifestyle modification program on sleep and stress disorders. J Nutr Health Aging 2007; 11(3):242–248.

18 Youngstedt SD. Effects of exercise on sleep. Clin Sports Med 2005; 24(2):355–365, xi.

19 Tooley GA, Armstrong SM, Norman TR et al. Acute increases in night-time plasma melatonin levels following a period of meditation. Biol Psychol 2000; 53(1):69–78.

20 Massion AO, Teas J, Hebert JR et al. Meditation, melatonin and breast/prostate cancer: hypothesis and preliminary data. Med Hypotheses 1995; 44(1):39–46.

21 American Academy of Sleep Medicine. International classification of sleep disorders: Diagnostic and coding manual. 2nd edn. Westchester, Illinois: AASM; 2005.

22 Shamsuzzaman ASM, Gersh BJ, Somers VK. Obstructive sleep apnea: implications for cardiac and vascular disease. JAMA 2003; 290:1906–1914.

23 Ohayon MM, Zulley J, Smirne S et al. Prevalence of narcolepsy, symptomatology and diagnosis in the European general population. Neurology 2002; 58:1826–1833.

24 Hornyak M, Feige B, Voderholzer U et al. Polysomnography findings in patients with restless

legs syndrome and in healthy controls: a comparative observational study. Sleep 2007; 30:861–865.
25 Allen RP, Walters AS, Montplaisir J et al. Restless legs syndrome prevalence and impact. Arch Intern Med 2005; 165:1286–1292.
26 Zucconi M, Ferini-Strambi L. Epidemiology and clinical findings of restless legs syndrome. Sleep Med 2004; 5:293–299.
27 Oertel WH, Benes H, Bedenschatz R et al. Efficacy of cabergoline in restless legs syndrome: a placebo-controlled study with polysomnography (CATOR). Neurology 2006; 67:1040–1046.
28 Hornyak M, Voderholzer U, Hohagen F et al. Magnesium therapy for periodic leg movements-related insomnia and restless legs syndrome: an open pilot study. Sleep 1998; 21(5):501–505.
29 Hornyak M, Feige B, Riemann D et al. Periodic leg movements in sleep and periodic limb movement disorder: prevalence, clinical significance and treatment. Sleep Med Rev 2006; 10:169–177.
30 Ohayon MM, Roth T. Prevalence of restless legs syndrome and periodic limb movement disorder in the general population. J Psychosom Res 2002; 53: 547–554.
31 Ohayon MM, Li KL, Guilleminault C. Risk factors for sleep bruxism in the general population. Chest 2001; 119:53–61.
32 Ommerborn MA, Schneider C, Giraki M et al. Effects of an occlusal splint compared with cognitive–behavioral treatment on sleep bruxism activity. Eur J Oral Sci 2007; 115:7–14.
33 D'Cruz OF, Vaughn BV. Parasomnias—an update. Sem Pediatr Neurol 2001; 8:251–257.
34 Espa F, Dauvilliers Y, Ondze B et al. Arousal reactions in sleepwalking and night terrors in adults: the role of respiratory events. Sleep 2002; 25:32–36.
35 Nielsen T, Levin R. Nightmares: a new neurocognitive model. Sleep Med Rev 2007; 11:295–310.
36 Schenck CH, Mahowald MW. REM sleep behavior disorder: clinical, developmental, and neuroscience perspectives 16 years after its formal identification in sleep. Sleep 2002; 25:120–138.
37 Ford DE, Kamerow DB. Epidemiology of sleep disturbance and psychiatric disorders: an opportunity for prevention. JAMA 1989; 262:1479–1484.
38 Smith MT, Perlis ML, Park A et al. Comparative meta-analysis of pharmacotherapy and behavior therapy for persistent insomnia. Am J Psychiatry 2002; 159:5–11.
39 Morin CM, Colecchi C, Stone J et al. Behavioral and pharmacological therapies for late-life insomnia: randomised controlled trial. JAMA 1999; 281:991–999.
40 Donath F, Quispe S, Diefenback K et al. Critical evaluation of the effect of valerian extract on sleep structure and sleep quality. Pharmacopsychiatry 2000; 33(2):1333–1336.
41 Goel N, Kim H, Lao R. An olfactory stimulus modifies night time sleep in young men and women. Chronobiol Int 2005; 22(5):889–904.
42 Cerny A, Schmidt K. Tolerability and efficacy of valerian/lemon balm in healthy volunteers: a double blind, placebo-controlled multicentre study. Fitoterapia 1999; 70(3):221–228.

chapter 44

Sports medicine

INTRODUCTION AND OVERVIEW

Sports medicine encompasses healthcare for the exercising individual. The first associations for sports medicine practitioners appeared in the second half of the twentieth century (for example, the American College of Sports Medicine was founded in 1954 and the Australian Sports Medicine Federation was founded in 1963). For much of the twentieth century there was a perception that the major scope of sports medicine was care for the elite athlete. This perspective has even led to the cynical view that because injuries are common in sports, athletes should be characterised with groups such as smokers as being responsible for their own medical conditions.[1] In recent years, it has become increasingly apparent that the benefits of exercise in general (and most sporting activities) far outweigh the risks in terms of injuries.[2] Lack of physical activity, along with tobacco smoking and poor diet, is one of the three great reversible risk factors for disease in Western societies.[3] While the scope of sports medicine still involves care of high-level athletes, its potential for helping society as a whole is just beginning to be realised.

Most initial presentations for sports injuries will be to a hospital accident and emergency department or to the general practitioner. Referral to a sports medicine practitioner, rheumatologist, physiotherapist, chiropractor, orthopaedic surgeon, sports psychologist, exercise physiologist or other healthcare practitioner may be necessary as part of a management plan for acute care or rehabilitation.

Exercise prescription for the general population is that people should be physically active for more than 30 minutes on at least 5 days per week.[2] (See also Ch 9, Exercise as therapy.) Sports medicine helps people to adhere to this prescription.

Musculoskeletal conditions can tend to be trivialised when viewed alongside other medical conditions that can lead to death and greater disability. However, by successfully managing these so-called 'minor' musculoskeletal injuries, sports medicine can enable ongoing exercise, which is critical for prevention of diabetes, heart disease, cancer and osteoporosis.[4] The sports medicine attitude towards elite athletes of 'keeping them on the field' should also be applied to the rest of the population, in keeping them from becoming physically inactive.

Sports medicine encompasses specialist sports physician practice and is a sub-discipline of other branches of medicine, particularly general practice, emergency medicine, orthopaedic surgery, rehabilitation medicine and rheumatology. Sports medicine has been recognised by most Western countries as a specialist branch of medicine, and further sports medicine education is available (in the form of certificates, diplomas and Masters degrees) for all medical practitioners.

Much of the skill in sports medicine practice involves perspective. It is probably true to assert that most people (particularly those over the age of 30) perceive some musculoskeletal pain or discomfort on a daily basis. Although almost everyone who reports pain would like to reduce it where possible, it is not mandatory to diagnose and treat every symptom arising from the musculoskeletal system. Part of the sports medicine history involves the question of what physical activity the patient wants/needs to do, and whether the symptoms prevent this activity. Once more serious causes of pain have been excluded, being able to reassure a patient that their musculoskeletal pain is not sinister or dangerous is often an important part of sports medicine practice.

Certain symptoms or body parts (e.g. knee pain) in sports medicine are easily amenable to clinical diagnosis and in these situations an attempt at diagnosis should be made. For other symptoms or body parts (e.g. low back pain), clinical diagnosis is notoriously inaccurate.[4] This most certainly does not mean that every patient requires imaging,[5] but instead that a management plan in most instances can be implemented based on a functional (rather than anatomical) diagnosis.

ANKLE SPRAIN

Ankle sprains are one of the most common sports injuries to present to the GP, most commonly affecting the lateral ligament complex.

THERAPEUTICS

Management of the acute joint injury involves management of the injury locally and systemically to enhance the healing process.

- *Acute care* of the injury involves the principles of PRICE[6] for several days after the injury—**p**rotection, **r**est, **i**ce, **c**ompression and **e**levation of the affected area.
- *Ice* (wrapped in a cloth or a towel; do not apply ice directly to the skin)—reduces pain, bleeding and inflammation.
- *Analgesia* may be required, particularly for more severe injuries.
- *Short-term walking cast* immobilisation may be necessary, particularly in severe grades of tears or where there is an associated avulsion fracture[7]; followed by functional bracing.
- *Taping*—the use of an elastic bandage has fewer complications than taping (especially skin irritation), but appears to be associated with a slower return to work and sport, and more reported instability than a semi-rigid ankle support.[8]

Acupuncture

Acupuncture may be effective for pain management in acute ligament/joint injuries.

Massage

Therapeutic massage is effective at increasing circulation and may relieve spasm in surrounding muscle groups.

Nutrition and supplements

- *Vitamin C* (1 g/day) and *beta-carotene* (50,000 IU per day for 5 days) both help connective tissue production and may reduce pain.
- *Vitamin E* (400 IU/day) has antioxidant effects in injured tissue.
- *Bromelain* has anti-inflammatory effects and helps reduce swelling.
- *Turmeric* (*Curcuma longa*) helps reduce swelling and enhances the effect of bromelain. *Dose*: 250–500 mg each of turmeric and bromelain, three times a day between meals.
- *Zinc* (15–30 mg per day) to assist healing.
- *Glucosamine and chondroitin* may assist in healing of joint injuries, although most published studies relate to degenerative knee injuries. Usual doses are: glucosamine 1500 per day; chondroitin 800–1200 mg per day, divided into two to four doses. They are often combined in one supplement.
- *Aescin*, the active ingredient in horse chestnut (*Aesculus hippocastanum*), applied topically, may reduce tenderness and swelling. Apply a gel with 2% aescin to the affected area every 2–3 hours.
- *Arnica* (topical or oral)—for reducing swelling in acute injury. Do not apply topically if the skin has open cuts over the injured area. Traditional use; evidence is lacking.
- *Comfrey root ointment (avoid applying to open wounds)* decreases pain and improves function.[9]

Prevention

- Ankle supports in the form of semi-rigid orthoses or air-cast braces, to prevent ankle sprain during high-risk sporting activities (e.g. soccer, basketball), especially in people with previous ankle injuries.[10]
- Adequate rehabilitation of previous ankle injuries with joint flexibility improvement and muscle strengthening.
- Proprioceptive balance training[11] in pre-season preparation and in-season training programs. This may be taught to individuals by a sports physiotherapist.
- Avoid over-training fatigued muscles.

KNEE INJURIES

Knee injuries are common in many sports, with surgical procedures performed on the knee joint more commonly than on virtually any other structure in the body. The combination of increasing average life expectancy and increasing body mass index means that most of the population will suffer from a knee complaint at some time during their life.

Although knee MRI is more sensitive than clinical examination for certain conditions, because the knee is an accessible peripheral joint it is generally possible for an experienced clinician to make an accurate diagnosis of many knee injuries using history and clinical examination. For a GP assessing a knee injury it is most important to recognise the diagnostic possibilities from the history (Table 44.1) and to be aware of which clinical diagnoses can be made without the need for imaging or specialist assessment.

Clinical diagnosis of some injuries such as those to the anterior cruciate ligament (ACL) can be difficult for examiners who lack regular exposure to managing such injuries. However, a GP with a special interest

TABLE 44.1 Diagnosing the major knee injuries (clinical and imaging)

Diagnosis	Clinical diagnosis	Investigations
Anterior cruciate ligament (ACL) tear	History of suddenly giving way. Experienced examiners can confirm with Lachman's and pivot shift tests in most cases	MRI useful for high-level athletes with haemarthrosis when early diagnosis is required
Posterior cruciate ligament tear	Contact injury to the ground (on a flexed knee) or clash of knees (AFL ruckmen). Positive posterior drawer	Usually not necessary
Medial collateral ligament tear	Contact valgus injury, increased valgus stress	Usually not necessary
Tibio-fibular sprains/ posterolateral complex injuries	Generally hyperextension mechanism (rare injury)	MRI to assess severity and whether surgery may be required (only required in severe cases)
Meniscal tears	Combination of medial or lateral pain and joint-line tenderness, mechanical symptoms, effusion and positive McMurray's test	MRI scanning useful for confirming that surgery is indicated
Articular cartilage injuries	Knee effusion and history of locking or catching may indicate a significant lesion	X-ray to assess overall state of knee degeneration. MRI for pinpointing specific lesions, but X-ray is more likely than MRI to alter management
Knee inflammatory or infective conditions	Knee effusion, pain, fever, no history of trauma (or history of invasive procedure, e.g. injection or arthroscopy)	X-ray and pathology tests indicated (FBC, ESR, C-reactive protein, uric acid)
Patellar tendinopathy (or Osgood-Schlatter syndrome in adolescents)	History of sporting activity, gradual onset of pain, tenderness at either end of the patellar tendon	Ultrasound or MRI may assist with prognosis but do not generally alter management. Use X-ray instead in adolescents
Patellar tendon rupture	Sudden-onset injury, inability to support weight	Investigations indicated before surgery (ultrasound or MRI)
Hamstring insertional tendinopathy	Tenderness on medial side below joint line	Usually not necessary
Iliotibial band syndrome	History of running (or cycling), pain on slow running. Tenderness on lateral side above joint line	Usually not necessary
Patellofemoral pain	Pain with the knee bent (sitting or squatting)	Usually not necessary
Prepatellar bursitis	History of kneeling or landing on kneecap. Swelling cannot be balloted underneath the patella	Usually not necessary
Patellofemoral instability	Patellofemoral apprehension, history of dislocations	X-ray (with skyline view of patellofemoral joint) helpful

in sports injuries and who is confident with using the Lachman (Fig 44.1) and pivot shift tests can often make this diagnosis. It is equally appropriate, when this diagnosis is suspected, to refer for MRI or specialist assessment when the diagnosis is in doubt. Although modern radiological techniques such as MRI can assist in the diagnosis of knee injuries, there is a tendency for overuse of investigations in cases where the diagnosis can be clearly established using clinical examination alone.[5] It is important to remember that a high incidence of abnormality in normal asymptomatic knees is detected on knee MRI.[12] In general the attitude towards investigation of knee injuries should fall somewhere between the potential mismanagement in an emergency department when a normal knee X-ray is used to declare that the injury is 'minor', and the modern (equally inappropriate) tendency to use MRI scanning to confirm every clinical diagnosis.

KNEE MENISCAL TEARS AND ARTICULAR CARTILAGE LESIONS

Meniscal lesions are extremely common and can often be found on MRI in asymptomatic individuals. Although MRI has assisted with greater accuracy in diagnosis, the decision to undergo surgery should be made on clinical grounds. Traditionally these are:

- mechanical symptoms (catching and/or locking)
- restrictions in range of movement (in the extremes of flexion or extension)
- positive McMurray's test, being a feeling of pain and/or catching when the examiner rotates the tibia with the knee close to full flexion
- recurrent knee joint effusions.

These indications should not be altered by the presence of in-substance signal change in the meniscus on an MRI scan. The information gained from MRI can be useful to avoid or delay surgery in a patient with knee pain due to low-grade articular cartilage degeneration. A recent controversial but landmark randomised controlled trial cast serious doubt on the value of knee 'chondroplasty' (smoothing of roughened areas of degenerate chondral surfaces) for mild–moderate degenerative articular cartilage change, showing no improvement with chondroplasty compared with placebo surgery.[13] Although the authors claimed that many thousands of unnecessary arthroscopies are performed each year, there has been no reaction from orthopaedic surgery bodies, or insurance companies, to limit the indications for this potentially lucrative procedure.[14] There is something of a role for arthroscopic management of certain chondral lesions, but the indications should probably be limited to cases in which there are loose bodies, mechanical symptoms of locking, or recurrent large effusions rather than knee pain with evidence of degenerative change on X-ray or MRI.

Where there are degenerative changes in the knee causing pain (but not to a degree that indicates that joint replacement is needed), the best management is to recommend moderate activity, quadriceps strengthening, glucosamine and chondroitin tablets and hyaluronic acid injections. Hyaluronic acid injections are normally given as a series of 3–5 × 2–3 mL injections weekly. While evidence indicates that outcomes are improved in knee osteoarthritis,[15] the patient and their insurer must decide whether the possible benefits are worth the expense of the treatment.

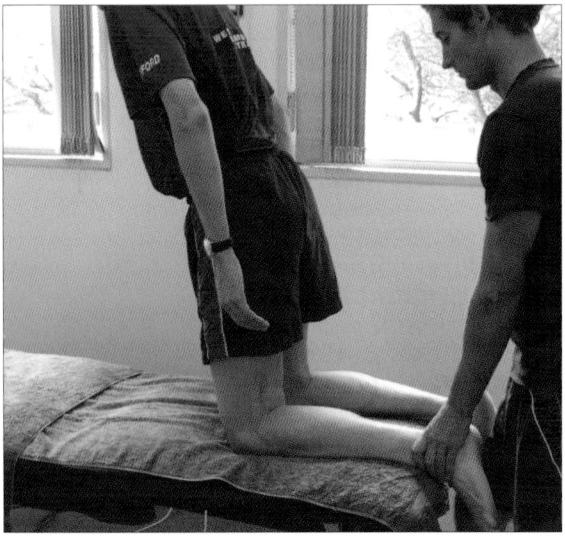
FIGURE 44.1 Lachman test

PATELLOFEMORAL PAIN SYNDROME

The history in this condition usually includes pain on activities that involve prolonged knee bending (such as sitting) and during knee squatting, sometimes with obvious wasting of the vastus medialis (inner quadriceps) muscle. Although patellofemoral pain syndrome is primarily a clinical diagnosis best managed conservatively, investigations using MRI suggest that subtle patellofemoral joint articular cartilage lesions are common. Treatment includes strengthening of the muscle plus taping or bracing the patella (usually into a more medial position) to assist the muscle in holding the patella in its correct alignment.

Non-impact forms of training may be required, to maintain fitness while the symptoms are settling. Ensure quality sports footwear. Orthotics and arch supports may also be advised.

ANTERIOR CRUCIATE LIGAMENT INJURIES

The knee anterior cruciate ligament (ACL) injury is rightly considered the most important acute diagnosis of the sporting knee because of its frequency and devastating impact on athletes. However, it is worth bearing in mind that an unstable ACL is a condition that affects the ability to participate in multidirectional sports and has relatively minimal effect on straight-line sports and everyday activities. Although the absolute number of ACL injuries occurring is greater in males (due to the greater likelihood of them playing at-risk sports),[16] numerous studies have shown that the relative risk for ACL injury in females in much greater when they play the same sports.[17,18]

The most common mechanisms of ACL injury are:

- a non-contact change of direction when the foot becomes 'stuck' to the surface
- a hyperextension on landing from a jump
- a direct valgus force from a blow to the leg from the outside.

The clinical diagnosis of ACL instability can be made in most cases using the Lachman and pivot shift tests. With the Lachman test (Fig 44.1), the amount of anterior drawer at 30° of flexion is relevant, but the 'end point' feel to movement is even more important for determining an intact ACL. When the pivot shift test is performed on a deficient ACL the tibia can be subluxed forward in internal rotation (relative to the femur) with an extended knee, and relocates with passive flexion. Successful use of these tests requires substantial exposure to examining stable and unstable knees, which is normally not part of medical school curriculum. Most sports physicians and orthopaedic surgeons who treat knee injuries can make the diagnosis clinically, particularly in either chronic cases or in the immediate acute scenario (on the sideline). The most difficult time to diagnose an ACL injury is in the days immediately after the injury, when there may be a large, tense haemarthrosis. At this time the accuracy of MRI examination may be greater than that of an experienced examiner. The natural history of an ACL injury is that the ligament generally heals in a suboptimal position, meaning that the knee is prone to instability (and therefore secondary cartilage injuries) during twisting movements.

After a diagnosis of ACL injury has been made, the patient is faced with difficult decisions about surgical reconstruction and whether to return to twisting sport. Younger patients are more likely to fail conservative treatment for ACL injuries. However, even surgical reconstruction cannot promise a completely normal knee. On return to sports such as football after reconstruction, the player has a four- to ten-fold increase in the risk of re-injuring the ACL (on either the graft or the contralateral side),[19] and further surgery for cartilage injuries is not uncommon. The choice of graft for ACL reconstruction is made by the surgeon, but there have been many randomised controlled trials comparing the two most popular choices (patellar tendon graft and four-strand hamstring tendon grafts). A consistent finding has been equivalent levels of function and patient satisfaction for each type of graft, but with trends towards greater stability in the patellar tendon graft groups and less secondary morbidity from the graft site in the hamstring tendon groups.[20] This means certain patients can be recommended to have certain grafts based on their relative needs for stability versus avoiding morbidity, but either graft choice is satisfactory in the hands of an experienced knee surgeon.

Management of the major knee injuries is summarised in Table 44.2.

TENDON INJURIES

Tendon injuries make up a large proportion of musculoskeletal pain in both athletes and the general community. The most common form is 'tendinopathy', which was previously but inaccurately known as 'tendinitis' when it was thought that these were inflammatory conditions.[22,23] It is now best to think of tendinopathies as degenerative conditions although, fortunately, the degenerative change is semi-reversible. Some of the most common forms of tendinopathy are tennis elbow (lateral epicondylitis), rotator cuff tendinopathy, De Quervain's wrist tendinopathy, adductor (groin) tendinopathy, Achilles tendinopathy and patellar tendinopathy ('jumper's knee'). The other common condition related to tendinopathies is plantar fasciitis, which strictly speaking is an enthesopathy, not a tendinopathy, as there is no muscle directly attached to the plantar fascia (and hence it is not a tendon).

The most common variety of tendinopathy is insertional (affecting the bone–tendon interface), although Achilles tendinopathy is an exception as it most commonly affects the mid-tendon substance. Some types of insertional tendinopathy are prone to intra-tendinous calcification. Insertional tendinopathies appear to be a combined 'underuse–overuse' injury, with the weakened under-surface of the tendon not bearing enough load and the normal outer portion of the tendon often overloaded.[23] The key underlying management is to recommend moderate loads that the injured tendon can withstand, rather than continuing with overloads or recommending complete rest. Sudden increases in load are risky for all tendons and hence complete inactivity is risky for tendon injury (as return to 'normal' activity will represent a sudden increase in load). This paradigm explains why tendinopathy is common in middle-aged people who suddenly take up exercise after a period of inactivity.

The middle-ground approach to tendinopathy is moderate loading within pain limits, followed by gradual increases in load as the weakened section of the tendon repairs itself. Some experts recommend exercising through the pain barrier, with complete immobilisation now out of favour and considered overly conservative.[18] Eccentric strengthening (loading as the tendon is lengthening) appears to be the best type of specific rehabilitation exercise.[24]

Because inflammation and impingement are not generally considered significant pathologies in this condition, NSAIDs and cortisone injections are not generally recommended.[25] Other newer treatment options successfully used for patellar or similar tendinopathies include nitrate patches,[25–28] extracorporeal shock-wave therapy[29] and polidocanol injections.[25] Nitrate patches are those used to treat angina, with the lowest dose (5 mg/24 h) cut into quarters (NITRO-DUR® or Minitran™) and applied daily to the affected body part (Fig 44.2).

ROTATOR CUFF TENDINOPATHY AND 'TENNIS ELBOW'

The two most common tendinopathies in the upper limb affect the supraspinatus tendon in the shoulder and the common extensor origin at the elbow. Supraspinatus tendinopathy is a special case as the phenomenon of

TABLE 44.2 Recommended management (conservative versus surgical) for the major knee injuries

Diagnosis	Conservative management	Surgical management
Anterior cruciate ligament (ACL) tear	In patients who do not have symptomatic instability, older athletes and/or those prepared to avoid multidirectional sports	ACL reconstruction is the management of choice for the young athlete who wishes to continue with multidirectional sports
Posterior cruciate ligament tear	Usually rest for 6–8 weeks is sufficient	Rarely indicated (?only when combined with posterolateral instability)
Medial collateral ligament tear	Rest (± knee brace) for 1–12 weeks, depending on severity Low-level laser therapy may improve healing[21]	Rarely indicated (?high-level athletes with complete ruptures at the tibial insertion)
Tibio-fibular sprains/posterolateral complex injuries	Minor lateral ligament sprains can recover with 2–6 weeks' rest	Biceps tendon ruptures and/or combined lateral and posterior cruciate ligament injuries (rare) are managed surgically
Meniscal tears	Degenerative tears in the older athlete that do not give rise to mechanical symptoms can be managed conservatively	Arthroscopic partial meniscectomy is generally the treatment of choice for mensical tears. Meniscal repair can occasionally be successful in acute peripheral tears in younger athletes
Articular cartilage injuries	Almost all mild–moderate articular cartilage injuries (extremely common) should be managed conservatively, even though complete cure is unlikely	Arthroscopic surgery for articular cartilage lesions is probably over-performed (as it also fails to cure), although it is still indicated when there are mechanical symptoms such as locking. Total knee replacement in severe cases
Patellar tendinopathy	Physiotherapy, eccentric strengthening, activity within pain limits and some other therapeutic treatments (although COX-2 inhibitors and cortisone are not recommended)	Rarely indicated
Patellar tendon rupture	Treat surgically	Acute surgical repair is the most appropriate treatment
Osgood-Schlatter syndrome (in adolescents)	Activity within pain limits, calf and gluteal strengthening, reassurance	Rarely indicated (?when impingement caused by excessive ossification)
Hamstring insertional tendinopathy	Anti-inflammatory gel, cortisone injection, eccentric strengthening	Occasionally indicated for chronic cases with bursa formation
Iliotibial band syndrome	Cortisone injection, avoidance of aggravating activities (e.g. downhill jogging)	Indicated for cases resistant to conservative treatment
Patellofemoral pain	Physiotherapy, taping, strengthening	Rarely indicated (?when there is persistent knee joint effusion)
Prepatellar bursitis	Aspiration and cortisone injection (± antibiotics)	Indicated for cases resistant to conservative treatment
Patellofemoral instability	Physiotherapy, bracing, strengthening	Indicated for recurrent dislocations
Knee infections or inflammatory conditions	Cortisone injections for proven inflammatory conditions (e.g. gout)	Hospital admission (antibiotics, lavage) for knee joint infections

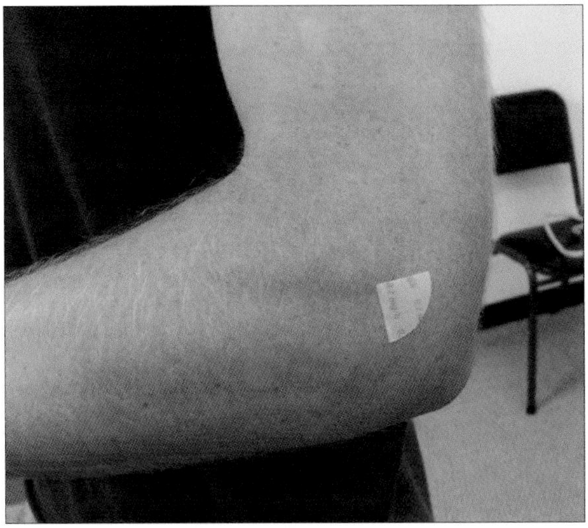

FIGURE 44.2 Nitrate patches used in quarters for 'tennis elbow'

impingement is generally associated with this condition. It is clinically important to assess how much of the patient's pain is due to the intrinsic pathology of tendon, compared with secondary impingement. Weakness on rotator cuff strength testing can suggest tendon damage, but shoulder ultrasound is probably the best way to accurately differentiate this from impingement. If impingement is the predominant cause of pain, NSAIDs and cortisone injections are indicated. For intrinsic tendinopathy, scapular stabilising exercises and nitrate patches are more-specific treatments.

While tennis elbow is common in amateur tennis players, it is such a ubiquitous form of tendinopathy in middle-aged patients that the vast majority of cases are in non-tennis players. The pain on the lateral side of the elbow can radiate down the forearm, but it is wrist and finger extension movements that aggravate the pain.

Therapeutics

- Modalities that may assist recovery include physiotherapy, massage, acupuncture[30] and transcutaneous electrical nerve stimulation (TENS).
- Try a brace centered over the proximal forearm.
- Check sports equipment (e.g. racquet size) for correct fit.

Supplements

- Healing may be assisted by vitamin C (1 g/day)
- Calcium (1500 mg/day) and magnesium (750 mg/day) to aid healing of connective tissues and muscles
- Vitamin E (400–800 mg/day)
- Essential fatty acids from fish oil (1000–1500 IU one to three times a day) to reduce inflammation
- Bromelain (250–750 mg three times a day between meals)
- Curcumin (*Curcuma longa*) / turmeric (200–400 mg three times a day between meals) to reduce inflammation.

Pharmaceutical

- Nitrate patches and eccentric exercises have been shown to help recovery.
- Cortisone injections give short-term pain relief but may damage the tendon in the longer term.[30]
- Botulinum toxin injections into the muscle can relieve the pain of tennis elbow but at a cost of temporary loss of extension of the third finger.

LOWER-LIMB TENDINOPATHIES

Management of lower-limb tendinopathies follows similar principles, although because the tendons bear heavy loads, cortisone injections are riskier and should generally be avoided. The key management principle is graduated loading, including eccentric (lengthening only) strengthening exercises.[24] An example of an eccentric exercise is shown in Fig 44.3 for the hamstring muscle group. For patellar tendinopathy ('jumper's knee') the exercises are best done on a decline board (30° downslope), which encourages loading of the patellar tendon while lengthening only.[31] Other exercises should strengthen or mobilise other deficiencies in the lower limb (e.g. calf and gluteal strengthening and hamstring stretching). Very few patients require total rest from weightbearing or immobilisation. Surgery for many lower-limb tendinopathies has limited success, although it is indicated for tendon rupture.

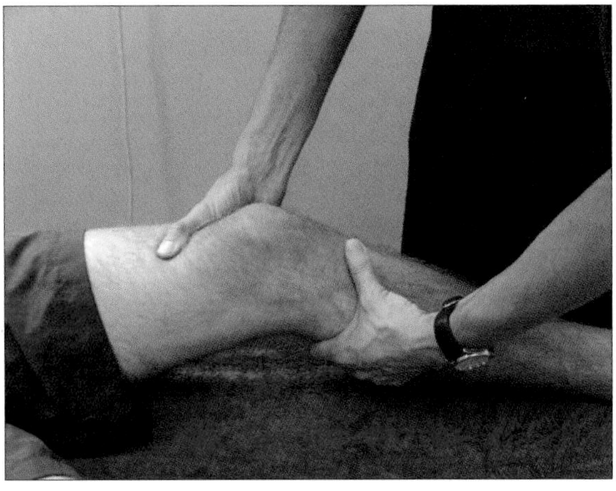

FIGURE 44.3 Hamstring eccentric exercises

In adolescents, similar conditions are common but with more tendency to self-limitation as they are epiphyseal overloads. They are, unfortunately, known by their cumbersome eponymous names such as Osgood-Schlatter disease (at the tibial tubercle just below the knee) and Sever's disease (below the Achilles attachment on the calcaneus).

In most cases (both adults and adolescents) there is little need to investigate; when this is necessary, plain X-ray in adolescents and ultrasound in adults are the modalities of choice. As is the case with many other pathologies, there is a high incidence of tendon imaging abnormalities in asymptomatic athletes.

GROIN INJURIES

Groin injuries are often due to chronic tendinopathy (particularly of the adductor muscle group), although the differential diagnosis of groin pain is extremely complicated.[32] Chronic groin pain is often due to osteitis pubis,[33] which is probably a bony stress overload lesion at the end stage of insertional tendinopathy. The standard treatment of chronic groin overuse injuries is reduction of load (rather than total rest) to a level where the pain is not worsening. Fortunately, many football players can continue to play once a week and limit their training without aggravating a chronic groin injury. In the off-season, jogging is generally encouraged, followed in order by faster running, maximal sprinting, kicking from a standing start, change of direction movements and then kicking on the run. Surgery is sometimes indicated, including hernia repair and adductor tenotomy.[34] In addition to unresolved chronic pain, the indication for adductor tenotomy includes painful reduction of range of passive hip abduction, as surgery can correct this. A hernia repair is indicated if there is pain and clinical or imaging (usually ultrasound) evidence of a hernia or posterior inguinal wall deficit.[35]

TENDON RUPTURES

The other tendon injuries of note are complete ruptures of tendons, which are not uncommon in older individuals and particularly affect the supraspinatus tendon and the Achilles tendon. Other common tendons to rupture in ball-sport players are the finger flexor tendons. The optimal management is acute surgical repair, as this leads to the best functional outcome. This management is problematic in high-level football players, for example, who are likely to wish to return shortly after surgery, which jeopardises the surgical repair. Many professional players elect to continue to play important games and put up with the inevitable fixed flexion deformity. Tendons that rupture and have nearby agonists, such as long head of biceps brachii and distal semitendinosus, are often managed conservatively as the functional deficit is generally acceptable. Full-thickness rotator cuff tendon tears, proximal hamstring, Achilles tendon and patellar tendon ruptures are not common but need to be managed surgically in active individuals.

DRUGS IN SPORT

The topic of drugs in sport is of major interest to those who work in the sports medicine field and the lay public who follow professional sport. However, even GPs who have no interest in sport must now have a basic understanding of the restrictions on drugs in elite sport. The reason for this is that any doctor can potentially treat an elite athlete as a patient and therefore has a responsibility to try to avoid prescribing medications that would be illegal in that sport. Drugs in sport laws follow a principle of strict liability, where, unfortunately, it is not a defence to have been prescribed a banned drug for a medical condition not related to sport. This can put a GP in a difficult position in which he or she can be seen as an accessory to breaking 'drugs in sport' laws for following routine medical practice.

Prohibitions on the use of dangerous performance-enhancing drugs have been introduced to almost all elite-level sports over the past four decades. Anti-doping laws attempt to minimise the number of athletes engaging in doping, although the enforcement of anti-doping laws is, predictably, not 100% successful. However, sport without anti-doping laws would further disadvantage those athletes who want to compete at an elite level without risking their health.

The World Anti-Doping Agency (WADA) is responsible for developing and implementing uniform anti-doping standards worldwide (with respect to lists of banned drugs and penalties for abusing them). The World Anti-Doping Code (WADA Code) was adopted after consultation with governments, sporting bodies, national anti-doping agencies and other relevant parties in 2003 by all Olympic federations, many nations and many elite sports.

Anti-doping laws do not relate just to positive tests for prohibited substances. Refusing to submit to testing procedures, tampering with samples (before or after they are submitted), possession and/or trafficking of illegal substances, and refusal to supply accurate regular whereabouts information to authorities (to allow for regular unannounced out-of-competition testing) can lead to doping infringements. Therefore, medical practitioners may also be subject to doping sanctions and suspended from involvement in elite sport.

WADA enforces the principle of strict liability because there is generally no reasonable doubt that a drug discovered within an athlete's urine or blood sample (taken under a strict protocol) was present within the athlete's system, yet it would be far too difficult, in the majority of cases, to prove intent to cheat beyond reasonable doubt. Strict liability for doping offences is controversial, although the WADA Code does offer the athlete some opportunity to consider the unique circumstances of each case.

THERAPEUTIC USE EXEMPTIONS

The WADA Code has a process for granting exemptions for the legitimate medical use of banned substances. All applications must be prospective and registered (except in emergency situations). Some medications are banned with the proviso that they may be used for certain medical indications, which require notification prior to their use. Prospective approval to take a banned drug via a Therapeutic Use Exemption (TUE) process for a documented medical condition is currently provided (under the WADA Code) if:

- the condition poses significant impairment to health, and
- there is no additional enhancement of performance (other than return to normal state of health following treatment of the legitimate medical condition), and
- no reasonable therapeutic alternative exists to treat the condition.

Drugs with a potential for abuse and performance enhancement must be assessed by an expert panel. Each country has its sports drug agency to assess these claims. TUEs are commonly granted for the use of oral glucocorticosteroids to treat severe asthma or inflammatory bowel disease.

Major controversy also surrounds testing for non-performance-enhancing but illegal drugs, which athletes may take for social (or recreational) purposes. The banning of stimulants, such as cocaine, when competing is universally accepted. The dilemma lies in whether stimulant drugs should be tested out-of-competition (where presumably they convey no performance advantage) and whether drugs such as marijuana, which are illegal but unlikely to confer any performance advantage, should be tested for and potentially lead to disqualification. The argument offered by WADA is that these drugs affect the health of the athlete, and that taking drugs inappropriately is against the spirit of sport.

It may be considered an invasion of privacy to test for non-performance-enhancing drugs out of athletic competition. However, it is hard to argue in defence of athletes who choose to break not only anti-doping but also criminal laws by using illicit social drugs. It may be more appropriate that these athletes receive counselling, and perhaps shorter suspensions, than other athletes found using drugs that would give them an unfair performance advantage.

SPORTS PSYCHOLOGY

Any person who has participated in sport, let alone competed at the elite level, will recognise that sport involves the mind as much as it does the body. Sports psychology is therefore important for two main reasons: in relation to improving performance, and in relation to mental health.

PERFORMANCE

Most serious athletes now dedicate a significant amount of time in their training regimen to training their minds. Understanding, for example, how to train attention, particularly when under pressure, can mean the difference between a higher or lower level of performance when the pressure is greatest. Athletes speak about states like the 'zone' or 'flow states' and we now know that these are trainable states of attention through practices such as mindfulness or visualisation exercises. A crucial aspect of this is being able to train one's attention onto the process and to unhook attention from anxiety about the outcome, which often distracts attention from performing in the moment. Training teams requires particular skills in setting common goals, fostering team spirit and cohesion, and in dealing with conflict between team members.

Another aspect of mental training is learning how to cope with physical discomfort, particularly in endurance sports such as distance running, cycling or swimming, and in playing with injuries, which is increasingly common particularly in professional sports. Deciding how fast to go, when to stop or when not to participate in the first place is an important aspect of being able to perform safely and well, as well as assisting in being able to recover more quickly and to have a sustainable career in the longer term. Athletes are prone not only to injuring their bodies through driving them too hard, but also to over-anxiousness regarding injury, particularly where the stakes associated with being injured are high.

MENTAL HEALTH

Athletes are not only subject to the normal mental health issues prevalent in the community, but they also have a range of particular mental health issues to deal with. For example, competing at a high level is associated with significant self-restraint from activities that others would enjoy as a normal part of life. Rigorous diets and training schedules can be very hard to maintain and this issue can be particularly important for young athletes, especially when being trained and driven overly hard by ambitious parents.

Anxiety and depression are common among high-performing athletes. The unbridled joy often publicly displayed when winning is the other side of the coin of the intense disappointment often borne privately when having lost or performed poorly. Furthermore, ambition or anxiety about performance can lead elite athletes to set extraordinarily high expectations or participate when they possibly should not. Such concerns are also a significant contributor to the risk of taking performance-enhancing drugs and all the health and legal problems that this entails.

Having long-term injuries can lead to intense disappointment and even depression, especially when a long-term and valued goal has been worked towards but is no longer possible. When an athlete's career comes to an end, especially when that end is unexpected and premature, it is not uncommon for there to be a significant and challenging period of adjustment. Often the disappointment and isolation associated with retirement from the sport is compounded by adjusting to a new life and career for which the athlete has not adequately prepared.

CONCLUSION

Knee injuries, tendinopathy and drugs in sport have been chosen as example topics with high current relevance to both specialist sports physicians and GPs. However, sports medicine has a far wider scope that cannot be fully covered in a single book chapter. For further resources, please consult the Resources list below.

Sports medicine is an emerging field that particularly has scope for community (non-hospital) practice, and hence it is very relevant to general practice. GPs are now aware that lack of exercise is a major risk factor for many diseases. There is a move towards treating non-exercisers as the medical profession treats smokers—that doctors must try to convince these patient that their lifestyle choices are unhealthy and require changing. However, doctors who are correctly advising their patients that they must exercise need to be in a position where they can provide basic management of the injuries that may be associated with exercise. For this reason, the past ostracism of sports medicine by much of the mainstream medical community has been misplaced.[36]

Australia has been a world leader in the development of quality sports medicine practice, possibly because of the elevated status of professional sport in this country.[36] However, in prevention of sports injuries and recognition of sports medicine as a specialty area, it has fallen behind other countries, most notably New Zealand.[37,38] In Australia, only 50% of the population is physically active at recommended levels, meaning that physical inactivity may soon surpass cigarette smoking as the number one cause of preventable diseases.[3]

For the sake of preventing illness and disease, the exercise prescription is probably the most important prescription that a GP can write in the twenty-first century. A basic knowledge of sports medicine is essential to assist patients in adhering to this important prescription.

RESOURCES

ASDMAC (Australian Sports Drug Medical Advisory Committee), http://www.asdmac.org.au

Australasian College of Sports Physicians, http://www.acsp.org.au/

Brukner P, Khan K. Clinical sports medicine, 3rd edn. Sydney: McGraw Hill; 2006. One of the world's leading general sports medicine texts. Pitched at a perfect level for medical students, physiotherapists, general practitioners and doctors undertaking postgraduate study in sports medicine. For information: http://www.clinicalsportsmedicine.com/

injuryupdate, an Australian website on sports injuries, http://www.injuryupdate.com.au/

Medical Journal of Australia, sports medicine papers, http://www.mja.com.au/Topics/Sports%20medicine.html

National Sports Information Centre, Australian Institute of Sport, http://www.ausport.gov.au/nsic/index.asp

Sports Medicine Australia, http://www.sma.org.au/

World Anti-Doping Agency, http://www.wada-ama.org/en/

REFERENCES

1 Finer N. Rationing joint replacements: Trust's decision seems to be based on prejudice or attributing blame [letter]. BMJ 2005; 331:1472.

2 Brukner P, Brown W. Is exercise good for you? Med J Aust 2005; 183(10):538–541.

3 Mokdad A, Marks J, Stroup D et al. Actual causes of death in the United States, 2000. JAMA 2004; 291(10):1238–1245.

4 Bigos S, Davis G. Scientific application of sports medicine principles for acute low back problems. J Orthop Sports Phys Ther 1996; 24(4):192–207.

5 Orchard J, Read J, Anderson I. The use of diagnostic imaging in sports medicine. Med J Aust 2005; 183(9):482–486.

6 Ivins D. Acute ankle sprain: an update. Am Fam Physician 2006; 74(10):1714–1720.

7 Haraguchi N, Toga H, Shiba N et al. Avulsion fracture of the lateral ankle ligament complex in severe inversion injury: incidence and clinical outcome. Am J Sports Med 2007; 35(7):1144–1152.

8 Kerkhoffs GM, Struijs PA, Marti RK. Different functional treatment strategies for acute lateral ankle ligament injuries in adults. Cochrane Database Syst Rev 2002; 3:CD002938.

9 Predel HG, Giannetti B, Koll R et al. Efficacy of a comfrey root extract ointment in comparison to a diclofenac gel in the treatment of ankle distortions: results of an observer-blind, randomized, multicenter study. Phytomedicine 2005; 12(10):707–714.

10 Quinn K, Parker P, de Bie R et al. Interventions for preventing ankle ligament injuries. Cochrane Database Syst Rev 2000; 2:CD000018.
11 McGuine TA, Keene JS. The effect of a balance training program on the risk of ankle sprains in high school athletes. Am J Sports Med 2006; 34(7):1103–1111.
12 Beattie K, Boulos P, Pui M et al. Abnormalities identified in the knees of asymptomatic volunteers using peripheral magnetic resonance imaging. Osteoarthritis Cartilage 2005; 13(3):181–186.
13 Moseley J, O'Malley K, Petersen N et al. A controlled trial of arthroscopic surgery for osteoarthritis of the knee. N Engl J Med 2002; 347:81–88.
14 Orchard J. Health insurance rebates in sports medicine should consider scientific evidence [editorial]. J Sci Med Sport 2002; 5(4):v–viii.
15 Strand V, Conaghan P, Lohmander L et al. An integrated analysis of five double-blind, randomized controlled trials evaluating the safety and efficacy of a hyaluronan product for intra-articular injection in osteoarthritis of the knee. Osteoarthritis Cartilage 2006; 14: 859–866.
16 Orchard J, Chivers I, Aldous D. Seasonal and geographical analysis of ACL injury risk in Australia. Sport Health 2005; 23(4):20–27.
17 Arendt E, Agel J, Dick R. Anterior cruciate ligament injury patterns among collegiate men and women. J Athlet Train 1999; 34(2):86–92.
18 Arendt E, Dick R. Knee injury patterns among men and women in collegiate basketball and soccer. NCAA data and review of the literature. Am J Sports Med 1995; 23(6):694–701.
19 Orchard J, Seward H, McGivern J et al. Intrinsic and extrinsic risk factors for anterior cruciate ligament injury in Australian footballers. Am J Sports Med 2001; 29(2):196–200.
20 Anderson A, Snyder R, Lipscomb A. Anterior cruciate ligament reconstruction. A prospective randomized study of three surgical methods. Am J Sports Med 2001; 29(3):272–279.
21 Bayat M, Delbari A, Almaseyeh MA. Low-level laser therapy improves early healing of medial collateral ligament injuries in rats. Photomed Laser Surg 2005; 23(6):556–560.
22 Khan KM, Cook JL, Bonar F et al. Histopathology of common tendinopathies. Update and implications for clinical management. Sports Med 1999; 27:393–408.
23 Orchard J, Cook J, Halpin N. Stress-shielding as a cause of insertional tendinopathy: the operative technique of limited adductor tenotomy supports this theory. J Sci Med Sport 2004; 7(4):424–428.
24 Alfredson H, Pietila T, Jonsson P et al. Heavy-load eccentric calf-muscle training for the treatment of chronic Achilles tendinosis. Am J Sports Med 1998; 26:360–366.
25 Paoloni J, Orchard J. The use of therapeutic medications for soft-tissue injuries in sports medicine. Med J Aust 2005; 183(7):384–388.
26 Paoloni J, Nelson J, Murrell G. Topical glyceryl trinitrate application in the treatment of chronic supraspinatus tendinopathy. A randomized, double-blind, placebo controlled clinical trial. Am J Sports Med 2005; 33(6): 8–16.
27 Paoloni J, Appleyard R, Nelson J et al. Topical glyceryl trinitrate treatment of chronic noninsertional achilles tendinopathy. A randomized, double-blind, placebo-controlled trial. J Bone Joint Surg Am 2004; 86A(5):916–922.
28 Paoloni J, Appleyard R, Nelson J et al. Topical nitric oxide application in the treatment of chronic extensor tendinosis at the elbow: a randomized, double-blinded, placebo-controlled clinical trial. Am J Sports Med 2003; 31(6):915–920.
29 Gerdesmeyer L, Wagenpfeil S, Haake M et al. Extracorporeal shock wave therapy for the treatment of chronic calcifying tendonitis of the rotator cuff: a randomized controlled trial. JAMA 2003; 290(19):2573–2580.
30 Bisset L, Paungmali A, Vicenzino B et al. A systematic review and meta-analysis of clinical trials on physical interventions for lateral epicondylalgia. Br J Sports Med 2005; 39(7):411–422.
31 Cook J, Khan K. What is the most appropriate treatment for patellar tendinopathy? In: MacAuley D, Best T, eds. Evidence-based sports medicine. London: BMJ; 2002:422.
32 Fricker P, Taunton J, Ammann W. Osteitis pubis in athletes: infection, inflammation or injury? Sports Med 1991; 12(4):266–279.
33 Verrall G, Slavotinek J, Fon G. Incidence of pubic bone marrow oedema in Australian rules football players: relation to groin pain. Brit J Sports Med 2001; 35(1):28–33.
34 Orchard J, Read J, Verrall G et al. Pathophysiology of chronic groin pain in the athlete. Intern Sports Med J 2000; 1(1):134–147.
35 Orchard J, Read J, Neophyton J et al. Groin pain associated with ultrasound findings of inguinal canal posterior wall deficiency in Australian Rules footballers. Br J Sports Med 1998; 32(2):134–139.
36 Orchard J, Brukner P. Sport and exercise medicine in Australia. Med J Aust 2005; 183(7):383.
37 Orchard J, Leeder S, Moorhead G et al. Australia urgently needs a federal government body dedicated to monitoring and preventing sports injuries. Med J Aust 2007; 187(9):505–506.
38 Orchard J, Finch C. Australia needs to follow New Zealand's lead on sports injuries. Med J Aust 2002; 177(1):38–39.

chapter 45

Travel medicine

INTRODUCTION AND OVERVIEW

There has been an increasing trend for people to travel internationally.[1] Ease of air transportation has ensured that nearly 1 billion people travel internationally each year to every part of the globe.[2] These travellers are potentially exposed to infectious diseases for which they have no immunity, as well as other serious threats to wellbeing, such as accidents and exacerbation of pre-existing medical and dental conditions. Conservatively, it is estimated that 30–50% of travellers become ill or are injured while travelling.[3,4] Relative estimated monthly incidence rates of various health problems have been compiled elsewhere.[3] The risk of severe injury is thought to be greater for people when travelling abroad.[1,5]

In terms of morbidity, infectious diseases such as respiratory tract infection and traveller's diarrhoea, and injuries, are important concerns for travellers.[1,4,5] The main health complaints of returned travellers vary considerably, depending on the country visited and the duration of the visit. Some studies have reported, based on travel insurance claims, that respiratory, musculoskeletal, gastrointestinal, ear, nose and throat, and dental conditions were the most common presenting problems,[6] whereas others have found that infectious disease (43.5%), accidents involving the extremities (15.3%), psychiatric conditions (8.2%), pulmonary disorders (4.7%) and accidents involving the head (4.7%) were the most common.[3,7] Fortunately, few travellers die abroad, and those who do tend to die of pre-existing conditions, such as myocardial infarction in travellers with known ischaemic heart disease. However, accidents are also a major cause of travel-related mortality.[8] This chapter highlights some of the current issues in travel medicine, but excludes specific discussion concerning migrant health.

DEFINING TRAVEL MEDICINE

Travel medicine is a new multidisciplinary specialty area that has emerged in response to the growing needs of the travelling population worldwide. Nearly all general practitioners (GPs) will need a basic knowledge of travel medicine, some GPs will make it an area of special interest and there are medical specialists whose whole practice is travel medicine.

Travel medicine seeks to prevent illnesses and injuries occurring to travellers going abroad and manages problems arising in travellers coming back or coming from abroad. It is also concerned about the impact of tourism on health and advocates for improved health and safety services for tourists.[9a]

The latter aspect recognises the impact of travel on ecosystems around the world, particularly the introduction and spread of diseases and disease resistance.

The roles of the GP or travel health adviser in the provision of travel health advice can be regarded as a continuum (Fig 45.1) and include:

- providing pre-travel assessment and advice, which may take place in a travel medicine clinic, during a standard general practice consultation, or through giving advice to other practitioners
- advising on other precautions that should be taken against diseases to which the person is likely to be exposed during travel
- immunising travellers for their protection
- immunising travellers to provide the relevant certificates to facilitate travel through epidemiological control posts at sea and air ports
- prescribing appropriate prophylactic and self-treatment medications
- advising on important safety nets for travellers abroad, including travel insurance and finding medical assistance abroad

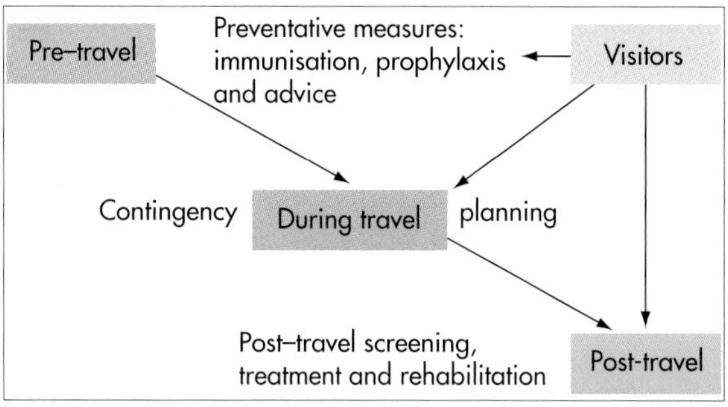

FIGURE 45.1 Relationships in the continuum of travel medicine

- advising on follow-up of travellers returning from overseas
- managing medical problems of travellers from abroad, which may also involve aeromedical evacuation, emergency assistance and even 'good Samaritan' acts on board aircraft or abroad
- providing advice on health, including pre-existing problems while away
- informing public health authorities about travellers presenting with any possible notifiable disease.

PRE-TRAVEL HEALTH CONSULTATION

The pre-travel health consultation involves consideration of and advice about various aspects of travel-related health, including fitness to travel and the health risks of travelling in itself, including exposure to infectious diseases and diseases arising from travel. This may necessitate the provision of malaria and other chemoprophylaxis, and various vaccinations. The areas that may be covered in the pre-travel health consultation with travellers are listed in Table 45.1.

Before the pre-travel consultation, a risk assessment needs to be undertaken, evaluating the risks of both the destination and the individual travelling there. Information on the exact itinerary and special medical problems of the traveller needs to be obtained early, up to 6–8 weeks before travel for most travellers, perhaps longer when travellers are going overseas for long-term employment, placement or holiday touring. In the clinic setting, it is preferable that this information is obtained well before the traveller presents for their first face-to-face consultation. It is necessary to establish:

- where they are travelling
- which areas of those countries they plan to go to
- what they plan to do in that country
- how they are going to get there
- at what time of year they are departing
- how long they will be travelling for.

This information may be obtained by a standardised questionnaire, which may be developed in the context of a travel clinic network or general practice network, or by individual travel health advisers. The World Health Organization (WHO) has provided an example of the types of questions to be asked in international travel and health.[12] Practice or clinic staff can assist by ensuring that this information is obtained before the formal consultation. It is important that the procedure is time efficient for a practice, to improve flow and time management.

In the general practice setting, detailed records may be available to assist in assessing the traveller's medical risks for travel. In any event, these records may need updating if the traveller has not presented to the GP for

TABLE 45.1 Areas that might be covered in pre-travel preparation of patients going aboard

Advise/discuss	
Insects	Repellents, nets, permethrin
Ingestions	Care with food and water
Infections	Skin, environment
Indiscretions	STIs, HIV
Injuries	Accident avoidance, safety
Immersion	Schistosomiasis
Insurance	Health and travel insurance
	Finding medical assistance abroad
	First aid advice
Vaccinate	
Always	National immunisation schedule vaccines
Often	Hepatitis A, influenza
Sometimes	Typhoid
	Japanese encephalitis
	Meningococcal disease
	Polio
	Rabies
	Tetanus–diphtheria
	Yellow fever
Older travellers	Pneumococcus
	Influenza
	Pandemic influenza, e.g. pandemic (H1N1) 2009
Prescribe	
Always	Regular medication
Sometimes	Antimalarial medication
	Diarrhoeal self-treatment
	Condoms
	Traveller's medical kit

Source: modified from Seelan & Leggat 2003[10] and Ingram & Ellis-Pegler 1996[11]

some time. Travel clinics, general practices and those in the travel industry should make it clear to prospective travellers that they should present early before travel, to obtain their travel medicine advice, immunisations and chemoprophylaxis or be referred for specialist advice, such as a pre-travel dental check. This may be best stated in a formal practice policy, so that travellers are aware of these possible requirements, which might be advertised in clinic newsletters, websites or practice updates or reminders.

ESTABLISHING THE RISKS

The risks of travel that need to be assessed for most travellers include the risks of the:

- destination
- mode of travel
- traveller's medical history
- intervention.

It is important in travel medicine to establish the risks of the destination and the mode of travel in terms of the hazards and the potential exposure to these hazards, and to examine the traveller's medical history to establish host risks, which may affect selection and use of interventions in the pre-travel health consultation. These are then weighed against the risks of the intervention.

The risks of the destination and any specific requirements for travel health advice may be obtained from a variety of resources. The WHO publishes a booklet entitled *International Travel and Health*.[12] Several other publications and sources of information relevant to travel medicine are also available. Online computerised databases have long since been mooted as useful aids for providing the most up-to-date and validated information for advising on travel medicine.[13]

POST-TRAVEL CONSULTATION

The traveller should also be advised of the possible need for follow-up and management after travel, particularly if going to a high-risk area (e.g. for malaria) or if they have any illness upon return (e.g. fever; persistent or bloody, mucous diarrhoea).[14] It must be impressed upon the traveller that, in the event of any illness upon return, they should inform the treating physician of their recent travel and that they have travelled, for example, to a malaria area. It is important, if seeing a traveller with a post-travel health problem, that a risk assessment similar to the pre-travel health consultation is undertaken, guided by the presenting features of the illness or injury against a background of the patient's general health. Even travellers who have been seen in the clinic or general practice for pre-travel health advice may need to have the risk assessment re-evaluated if any of the parameters of risk have changed (e.g. the person has travelled to a new destination). The risks of travel may also be modified by:

- having travel insurance and access to an emergency assistance service
- post-travel screening and interventions
- malaria eradication
- empirical eradication treatment (e.g. deworming treatment).

The effective early management of post-travel health problems early can significantly reduce morbidity and mortality, among travellers, from diseases such as malaria, which may still occur post travel as no intervention is necessarily 100% protective. Managing the risk and these travel health problems in a timely manner can also reduce the risk to local populations from this disease, and post travel it may assist in reducing the risks to the traveller's own community (e.g. in dengue recognition and management).

DEVELOPMENTS IN TRAVEL MEDICINE

Several key developments in the past two decades have ensured the continuing emergence of travel medicine as a specialty area. The development of national programs and guidelines in travel health was an important advance, as this recognised the need to develop a consensus strategy for combating commonly encountered infectious diseases and other problems encountered by travellers. Examples of these include the former Australian Government's Travel Safe® Programme, including the publication of Australian guidelines for travel health,[15] and the US Centers for Disease Control and Prevention (CDC) travel health program.[16] These programs and guidelines were directed at the major providers of travel health advice, such as general practices and public health agencies, but also travel clinics and travel agents. Internationally, the World Health Organization has also been producing travel health guidelines. (Examples of major travel health guidelines can be found in the Resources list.)

Three main challenges confront effective travel medicine practice.

- Travellers must recognise the need for travel health advice before travelling abroad, particularly given that a recent airport survey suggested that only 50% of international travellers abroad had sought pre-travel health advice.[17]
- Travellers need to seek travel health advice in a timely manner, preferably 6–8 weeks before travel.
- Travellers should obtain travel health advice from a qualified source. In the survey previously mentioned, only one-third of travellers had sought pre-travel health advice from a healthcare professional.[17]

Many of these challenges can be at least partially addressed through industry and government cooperation, particularly at the level of the travel agent or airline, which have initial contact with travellers. Many countries now have foreign travel advisory services that help keep practitioners advised about things such as important travel warnings and global disease outbreaks.

One of the most important factors influencing whether travellers seek health advice is the perceived risk and severity of tropical diseases,[1] despite their relatively low health and safety risk to travellers compared with accidents and less exotic conditions such as traveller's diarrhoea. In addition to the prevention of potentially lethal diseases and injuries among travellers abroad, the importance of providing travel health services is also increasingly being recognised in relation to early detection and reporting of imported infections.

PROFESSIONAL INITIATIVES

The International Society of Travel Medicine (ISTM), established in 1991, has taken the lead in establishing a global professional base for travel medicine. Some of the important early initiatives of the ISTM were the provision of travel health alerts to subscribers, a journal, biennial conferences, a global listing of travel health practitioners, and a collaborative disease-reporting network (GeoSentinel) with the CDC in the United States.[18] GeoSentinel has played a role regionally in examining post-travel health problems.[19] More recently, the ISTM has developed a certification program based on a detailed body of knowledge in travel medicine leading to a Certificate of Travel Health.[20] GeoSentinel is an excellent example of the contribution of travel medicine to the early detection and reporting of imported infections, to which several sites in Australia and New Zealand contribute.[21]

The Asia Pacific Travel Health Association also conducts biennial conferences in travel medicine in the Asia-Pacific region, in alternate years to the ISTM's annual conference and in parallel with its endorsed regional conference. The two major journals in travel medicine are currently the ISTM's *Journal of Travel Medicine*, published by Wiley-Blackwell, and *Travel Medicine and Infectious Diseases*, published by Elsevier Science. In Australia, the development of a professional body in travel medicine, the first Faculty of Travel Medicine (FTM), has been achieved[22] as part of the Australasian College of Tropical Medicine (ACTM). The FTM works in close association with the New Zealand Society of Travel Medicine, established in 1997. The ACTM produces the *Annals of the ACTM*, which is subtitled 'A journal of tropical and travel medicine', reflecting the major interests of the college and its faculty. The Royal College of Physicians and Surgeons of Glasgow subsequently founded an FTM in 2006.

In addition, there are a number of valuable internet and related resources, which also provide information on disease distribution and prevention (see Resources list). Access to current policy guidelines and up-to-date health intelligence, usually provided in travel medicine from internet-based resources, is essential. Continuing research is essential for a better understanding of the epidemiology of travel-related diseases and injuries, which in turn leads to the development of improved guidelines in travel medicine and more effective preventive measures to combat infectious diseases and prevent injuries associated with travel.

VECTOR-BORNE DISEASES

Vector-borne diseases remain among the great personal concerns for travellers abroad, especially those travelling to more remote tropical areas. Some vector-borne diseases also represent a potential public health problem when returning home. Malaria remains the single most important vector-borne disease problem, although arboviral diseases such as dengue and Japanese encephalitis (JE) are also becoming increasingly important international travel-related health problems. Some vector-borne diseases are important for local travel within a country or region—an example is scrub typhus, which has affected soldiers in northern Queensland, Australia.[23,24]

Personal protective measures remain the first line of defence for vector-borne diseases. Travellers need to be aware of when the vectors bite and the seasonal nature of some of these vectors. Table 45.2 summarises the biting behaviour of mosquitoes that carry major diseases. Other vectors also have peak biting times between dusk and dawn (e.g. phlebotomine sandflies transmitting leishmaniasis). Preventive measures are

TABLE 45.2 Time of peak biting activity of mosquito genus by disease

Mosquito genus	Peak times of activity	Examples of diseases transmitted
Anopheles	Usually night ('dusk to dawn'), mainly rural	Malaria, lymphatic filariasis
Culex	Usually evening/night ('dusk to dawn')	Japanese encephalitis, West Nile virus, lymphatic filariasis
Aedes	Usually day biting, midday	Dengue, yellow fever, lymphatic filariasis
Mansonia	Usually night	Lymphatic filariasis

mostly directed at reducing contact with vectors, such as: staying in screened or air-conditioned accommodation where possible; spraying the accommodation area; using permethrin-impregnated clothing to cover as much of the body as possible; using diethyl methyl toluamide (or DEET) repellents; controlling vermin and stray animals; and using bed nets soaked in permethrin, and fine-mesh bed nets to prevent sandfly bites. Currently available non-DEET repellents do not provide protection for durations similar to those of DEET-based repellents.[25] For example, a number of citronella products have been tested, but these give very short-term protection.[25] Soybean oil (2%) provides some protection, but again of much shorter duration than DEET-based products.[25] More recently, 20% Citrodiol®, a lemon-eucalyptus extract, has been found to be as effective as DEET in preventing mosquito and other insect bites and provides about 7–8 hours protection.[26]

MALARIA

Malaria is a serious disease caused by a protozoan parasite largely confined to the tropics. The WHO estimates that there are more than 500 million cases of malaria infection and 2.5 million deaths due to malaria worldwide annually.[27] Most cases and deaths occur due to infection with *Plasmodium falciparum* species of malaria, although infection due to *P. vivax* also remains important, especially as dormant liver stages of the life cycle can cause relapses, sometimes several, for months after returning home. While Australia is malaria-free, suitable vectors of the *Anopheles* mosquito can be found in many parts of tropical northern Australia, resulting in occasional reports of local transmission from imported cases of malaria.[28,29]

Standard malaria preventive measures are considered part of pre-travel health planning for travellers to malaria areas, based on disease patterns and policy guidelines. Current disease-prevention measures against malaria include the use of malarial chemoprophylaxis, personal protective measures against insect bites, environmental health measures against disease vectors, malaria eradication treatment for liver stages, including hypnozoites, and gametocyes on return from the malaria area, and early detection and treatment of malaria cases in order to avoid serious complications of the infection.

The growing incidence of chloroquine and multiple drug resistance in *P. falciparum* and, more recently, *P. vivax* have limited the antimalarial drug options for malaria chemoprophylaxis. Current recommended malaria chemoprophylaxis options include doxycycline (one 100 mg tablet daily), mefloquine (one tablet weekly), and atovaquone plus proguanil or Malarone® (one tablet daily, consisting of 250 mg of atovaquone and 100 mg of proguanil).[16] Chloroquine continues to be recommended as malaria chemoprophylaxis for malaria in the few areas where there is no chloroquine resistance.

Malaria eradication

Current eradication treatment for malaria is primaquine (two 7.5 mg tablets twice daily for 2 weeks), although tafenoquine was trialled in defence force personnel in East Timor as both an alternative eradication treatment (400 mg daily for 3 days) and a weekly-dose chemoprophylactic agent.[30]

Because of the incidence of neuropsychiatric side effects, such as anxiety and nightmares, it is advisable for travellers taking mefloquine for the first time to take several trial doses, possibly commencing as early as 3 weeks before departure.[31] It is also advisable that travellers are given trial doses of other antimalarials, such as doxycycline and Malarone®, that they might be taking for the first time well before departure. This is to ensure that there is time to consider alternative chemoprophylactic drugs.[31] If travel is commenced at short notice, modification to antimalarial regimens may have to be done abroad, which is less satisfactory. There are varying opinions on how long antimalarial drugs should continue to be taken after leaving an antimalarial area. However, antimalarial drugs that have no pre-erythrocytic effects on the liver stages of the malarial parasite, such as doxycycline and mefloquine, should be continued for up to 4 weeks afterwards. This relates to the time it takes for parasites to develop in the liver and infect the bloodstream. Chemoprophylaxis with Malarone®, which also has some effects on the hepatic stages of *P. falciparum* parasites, may be able to be given for shorter periods (e.g. one week) after return.[32]

For travellers to more remote areas, standby treatment in the event of overt malaria infection while abroad may also be useful. 'Standby treatment consists of a course of antimalarial drugs that travellers to malaria endemic areas can use for self-treatment if they are unable to gain access to medical advice within 24 hours of becoming unwell.'[31a] In these situations, a traveller's medical kit may be supplied with a thermometer, possibly an immunochromatographic test (ICT) malaria diagnostic kit and written instructions, and an appropriate malaria treatment course and written instructions, and the traveller must seek medical advice as soon as possible. Newer antimalarials that may be useful for standby treatment include Malarone® and Riamet®, the latter containing 20 mg artemether and 120 mg lumefantrine.[33]

ARBOVIRAL DISEASES

There are many arboviral diseases that may affect travellers. Apart from yellow fever, which has a widespread distribution in many parts of South America and Africa and is controlled by international health regulations,[34] two of the most important arboviral diseases for travellers are dengue fever and Japanese encephalitis, because in recent years people have been travelling to more remote areas where these diseases are endemic. Both diseases are transmitted by various species of mosquitoes.

Dengue fever is a major global public health problem. The WHO estimates that there are more than 50 million cases per year.[34] Dengue is a viral illness transmitted by *Aedes* mosquito species, classically *Aedes aegypti*. Infection may range from subclinical to fever, arthralgia and rash, or be complicated by haemorrhagic diatheses or shock syndromes. Treatment is supportive, while management of the problem is directed towards early detection of the disease and preventing transmission upon return to receptive countries.[35] Numerous outbreaks of dengue have been attributed to travellers returning with the disease, associated with delays in detecting the condition.[35] With travellers arriving or returning from abroad during the incubation period of the disease, it is vital that there is a collaborative effort made by various civilian public health authorities to contain and prevent the transmission of the disease among the local population.[36] Until a vaccination becomes available, the mainstays of dengue prevention are personal protective measures and environmental health measures against disease vectors.[35]

Japanese encephalitis (JE) is the leading cause of viral encephalitis in Asia. The WHO estimates that there are more than 70,000 cases annually in South-East Asia.[37] Up to a third of clinical cases die and about half of clinical cases of JE have permanent residual neurological sequelae.[37] Despite the availability of a vaccine against JE, the immunogenicity of these vaccines has recently been questioned and concerns have been raised regarding adverse reactions reported with vaccination.[38] The current development of safer and more immunogenic second-generation JE vaccines will be important for travellers in this region in the future.[37]

PREVENTION OF INFECTIOUS DISEASES THROUGH VACCINATION

A number of infectious diseases of travellers can be prevented by immunisation. There are few mandatory vaccines, for which certification is necessary, and these include yellow fever and meningococcal meningitis. Yellow fever vaccination is required for all travellers entering or returning from a yellow fever endemic area, which is prescribed by the WHO.[27,39] Meningococcal vaccination is required for travellers to Mecca.[27]

The travel medicine consultation is also an opportunity to update routine and national schedule vaccinations for diseases that may afflict travellers anywhere. There are also a variety of vaccinations that may be required for travellers to particular destinations. It would seem prudent to vaccinate travellers against diseases that might be acquired through food and water, such as hepatitis A, typhoid and polio,[31] as well as using other measures to combat these diseases. The most common vaccine-preventable diseases of travellers are hepatitis A and influenza[3]; however, typhoid vaccination should also be considered for travel to many developing countries. Polio vaccination is rarely required these days, with a concerted campaign for global eradication; however, it may be required in situations where polio outbreaks have been reported.[31]

There are a number of other infectious diseases, such as hepatitis B, JE and rabies, that may afflict travellers to certain destinations or are a result of the nature of their travel and are vaccine preventable (see Table 45.1).

For older travellers, pneumococcal and influenza vaccinations should also be considered. The development of combination vaccines, such as hepatitis A plus typhoid and hepatitis A plus B, has greatly reduced the number of injections required.[31] The development of rapid schedules for travellers departing at short notice has been useful in providing protection within 4 weeks.[31] Many diseases have no vaccination. For example, some parasitic diseases, such as intestinal and filarial helminths, can only be prevented through personal protective measures against the infective stages of the parasite and/or through periodic treatment or eradication treatment on return.

TRAVELLER'S DIARRHOEA

Traveller's diarrhoea (see Ch 30, Gastroenterology) is a common problem for travellers and emphasises the importance of being able to communicate basic public health advice to the individual. It also highlights the need for a sound knowledge of tropical diseases. In general, reference may need to be made to:

- water sources and water purification, which may involve the use of both filters and compounds such as iodine, or advice on how to boil water
- specific diseases and the consequences of diseases potentially acquired from food and water
- oral rehydration salts and their use
- the need for antibiotic prophylaxis
- selection and use of anti-motility drugs
- selection and use of standby antibiotic drugs
- awareness that some foods, such as some cereals, nuts, seeds and spicy foods containing chilli or ginger, may contain aflatoxins, which may be a non-pathogenic cause of diarrhoea
- the possible role of probiotics in preventing traveller's diarrhoea.

A recent meta-analysis suggested that several probiotics have significant efficacy in preventing traveller's diarrhoea, in particular *Saccharomyces boulardii* and a mixture of *Lactobacillus acidophilus* and *Bifidobacterium bifidum*.[40]

Despite the importance of advice concerning the prevention of traveller's diarrhoea, it is interesting to note that constipation is also of considerable inconvenience for travellers, and may also need attention.

NON-INFECTIOUS HAZARDS OF TRAVEL

Despite the emphasis on infectious disease in travel medicine, the single most common preventable cause of death among travellers is accidental injury.[8,41]

The patterns of mortality among travellers from the United States, Switzerland, Canada and Australia are similar. This is illustrated by research indicating that about 35% of deaths of Australian travellers abroad were the result of ischaemic heart disease, with natural causes overall accounting for some 50% of deaths.[8] Trauma accounted for 25% of deaths abroad.[8] Injuries were the reported cause of 18% of all deaths, with the major group being motor vehicle accidents, accounting for 7% of all deaths, which appeared to be over-represented in developing countries.[8] Infectious disease was reported as the cause of death in only 2.4% of those who died while travelling abroad.[8]

A similar pattern of mortality was observed in Swiss,[41] American[42] and Canadian[43] travellers abroad. Deaths of travellers have also resulted from air crashes, drowning, boating accidents, skiing accidents, bombs and electrocution.[8] Homicides, suicides and executions combined accounted for about 8% of all deaths.[8] Most fatal accidents in American and Swiss travellers were traffic or swimming accidents.[41,42] Deaths of tourists visiting Australia were similarly found to be due mainly to motor vehicle accidents and accidental drowning.[44]

ISSUES IN AVIATION MEDICINE AND ALTITUDE

Travel medicine is also a key component of the activities of many healthcare professionals working in aviation medicine. In addition to undertaking aviation medical examinations and advising their own staff who are travelling, airline medical departments review passengers' clearances to fly and provide advice to travel health advisers. Some travellers need special clearance to fly in cases of aeromedical evacuation (AME) on commercial aircraft and in certain prescribed circumstances of normal travel, such as after recent surgery or with serious physical or mental incapacity,[45] and liaison by travel health advisers with the airline medical departments is usually advisable. Healthcare professionals working in aviation medicine also become involved in developing policies and guidelines for dealing with in-flight emergencies involving travellers as well as training in first aid for flight attendants. Physicians working in aviation medicine have their own national or regional professional organisations.

While some medical practitioners undertake the work of Designated Aviation Medical Examiners,[46] particularly in respect of pilots, air traffic controllers and, in some instances, flight attendants, travel health advisers also need to be aware of the potential health effects of modern airline travel. These include the effects of reduced atmospheric pressure, low humidity, closed environment, inactivity, the effects of crossing several time zones on circadian rhythm, alcohol, and the general effects of aircraft motion and movement.[47] These effects can produce conditions such as barotrauma, dehydration, jet lag, motion sickness, claustrophobia and panic attacks, air rage and spread of infectious disease, and can contribute to the development of deep venous thrombosis (DVT) and venous thromboembolism (VTE).[47] Concerns have also been raised about the transmission of tuberculosis through close proximity to infected travellers on commercial aircraft.[48] The provision of travel health advice and preventive measures for these conditions also largely falls to the travel medicine provider.

While considerable attention has been focused on DVT and VTE, it remains uncertain what the contribution of air travel is to the development of this condition among travellers. What seems to be clear is that the development of DVT and VTE is multifactorial.[49] While the identification of travellers with predisposing risk factors would seem useful, it is only an option where the risks of side effects of the screening procedure do not outweigh the risks of developing DVT after a long-haul flight, which is estimated to be about 1 in 200,000 for travellers on a 12-hour long haul journey.[50] In the meantime, conservative measures should be recommended, such as in-flight exercises, restriction of alcoholic and caffeinated beverages and drinking lots of water. Other preventive measures for some at-risk cases, such as subcutaneous heparin, are worthy of investigation.[31] Current epidemiological research and pathophysiological studies are helping to establish which travellers are at greatest risk, which will in turn lead to appropriate intervention studies.

One of the most interesting problems in travel medicine has been the prevention of altitude illness. It has been difficult to find associations that might be useful in screening for individuals at higher risk; hence the focus has been on early treatment or the use of prophylactic agents such as acetazolamide. Natural compounds have been explored and *Ginkgo biloba* has been widely used; however, a recent trial suggested that *Ginkgo biloba* performed very poorly compared with drugs such as azetazolamide.[51] Further studies are probably needed in human populations at risk.

TRAVEL ADVISORIES

In recent times, travel advisories have assumed great importance in endeavouring to ensure the safety and security of travellers. Travel advisory services include the US State Department,[52] the Australian Department of Foreign Affairs and Trade,[53] and the UK Foreign and Commonwealth Office.[54] Travellers have suffered numerous casualties from recent acts of terrorism, most notably the Bali bombings, and natural disasters, most notably the Asian tsunami, both of which required a rapid multiagency response to rescue travellers from the affected areas.[55–57]

TRAVEL INSURANCE

Because of the potentially high costs of medical and dental treatment abroad, which may not be covered by private health insurance or local national health services, and the potential high costs associated with AME, all travellers should be advised of the need for comprehensive travel insurance. Travel insurance policies normally underwrite travel-related, medical and dental expenses incurred by travellers abroad under conditions specified by the travel insurance policy. In addition, travel insurance companies often provide a direct service, usually through their emergency assistance service contractors, to assist travellers abroad. This may include assistance with accessing or obtaining medical care while overseas, including AME. For example, claims for reimbursement of medical and dental expenses abroad made up more than two-thirds of all travel insurance claims in Australia and Switzerland.[6,7] In the Australian study, almost one in five Australian travellers abroad had been found to have used the travel insurer's emergency assistance service.[6]

Travel insurance is the most important safety net for travellers in the event of illness, injury or unforeseen events, and should be reinforced by GPs and travel health advisers. Studies have shown that about 60% of GPs in New Zealand,[58] 39% of GPs in Australia[10] and 39% of travel clinics worldwide[59] usually advise travellers about travel insurance. Although the majority of GPs also usually advise travellers about ways to find medical assistance abroad,[58] GPs need to ensure that they provide advice on suitable travel insurance companies, especially as a source of medical assistance while travelling. However, it is not known what proportion of travel agents or airlines currently give advice on travel insurance routinely, although most airlines operating internationally now provide more travel health advice in their in-flight magazines.[60]

SUMMARY

Travel medicine is emerging as a new multidisciplinary specialty area catering for an increasing number of travellers worldwide. General practitioners and other travel health advisers are engaged in the provision of pre-travel health advice, chemoprophylaxis against travel-related diseases, traveller's medical kits and post-travel assessments and eradication treatment for various travel-related diseases. They are also in a key position to liaise with public health authorities on possible imported disease risks. In terms of risk assessment and provision of preventive measures, vector-borne diseases, particularly malaria and the arboviral diseases, stand out as major concerns for travellers; however, common problems such as traveller's diarrhoea and respiratory tract infection also need to be addressed. Travel and aviation medicine have many linkages, especially in terms of fitness to fly and dealing with problems that may arise in travellers due to the physiological and psychological stresses of travel. In the face of recent terrorism and conflict, travel advisories have assumed great importance in travellers' planning. Travel insurance remains an important safety net for travellers, and provides coverage for medical and dental treatment abroad as well as an emergency assistance service, which may include aeromedical evacuation.

RESOURCES

Australian Department of Foreign Affairs and Trade, http://www.dfat.gov.au

Canada, Public Health Agency of Canada, Travel Health, http://www.phac-aspc.gc.ca/tmp-pmv/

CDC, Health Information for International Travel, http://wwwn.cdc.gov/travel/default.aspx

CDC, Morbidity and Mortality Weekly Report, http://www.cdc.gov/mmwr

CIA World Factbook, https://www.cia.gov/library/publications/the-world-factbook/

Faculty of Travel Medicine/New Zealand Society of Travel Medicine, Australasian College of Tropical Medicine, http://www.tropmed.org/travel/index.html

Faculty of Travel Medicine, Royal College of Physicians and Surgeons of Glasgow, http://www.rcpsg.ac.uk/Travel%20Medicine/

James Cook University, Travel Medicine Program, http://www.jcu.edu.au

International Association for Medical Assistance to Travellers, http://www.iamat.org

International Society of Travel Medicine, http://www.istm.org

South African Society of Travel Medicine, Travel medicine Program, http://www.sastm.org.za/

UK Fit for Travel, http://www.fitfortravel.nhs.uk/home.aspx

UK Foreign and Commonwealth Office, http://www.fco.gov.uk/en/

University of Otago, Travel medicine program, http://www.otago.ac.nz

US Department of State, Bureau of Consular Affairs, http://travel.state.gov/

WHO, International Travel and Health, http://www.who.int/ith/index.html

WHO, Weekly Epidemiological Record, http://www.who.int/wer

Worldwise Travellers Health Centres of New Zealand, http://www.worldwise.co.nz

REFERENCES

1 Behrens RH. Protecting the health of the international traveller. Trans R Soc Trop Med Hyg 1990; 84:611–612, 629.

2 World Tourism Organisation. Online. Available: http://www.unwto.org/index.php 5 December 2007.

3 Steffen R, de Bernardis C, Banos A. Travel epidemiology—a global perspective. Int J Antimicrobiol Agents 2003; 21:89–95.

4 Cossar JH, Reid D, Fallon RJ et al. A cumulative review of studies on travellers, their experience of illness and the implications of these findings. J Infect 1990; 21:27–42.

5 Bewes PC. Trauma and accidents: practical aspects of the prevention and management of trauma associated with travel. Br Med Bull 1993; 49:454–464.

6 Leggat PA, Leggat FW. Travel insurance claims made by travelers from Australia. J Travel Med 2002; 9: 59–65.

7 Somer Kniestedt RA, Steffen R. Travel health insurance: indicator of serious travel health risks. J Travel Med 2003; 10:185–189.

8 Prociv P. Deaths of Australian travellers overseas. Med J Aust 1995; 163:27–30.

9 Leggat PA, Ross MH, Goldsmid JM. Introduction to travel medicine (Ch 1). In: Leggat PA, Goldsmid JM, eds. Primer of travel medicine. 3rd rev edn. Brisbane: ACTM; 2005:3–21. a p 3.

10 Seelan ST, Leggat PA. Health advice given by general practitioners for travellers from Australia. Travel Med Inf Dis 2003; 1:47–52.

11 Ingram RJH, Ellis-Pegler RB. What's new in travel medicine? NZ Public Health Rep 1996; 3(8):57–59.

12 World Health Organization. International travel and health. Geneva: WHO; 2007. Online. Available: http://www.who.int/ith 5 December 2007.

13 Cossar JH, Walker E, Reid D et al. Computerised advice on malaria prevention and immunisation. BMJ 1988; 296:358.

14 Looke DFM, Robson JMB. Infections in the returned traveller. Med J Aust 2002; 177:212–219.

15 Commonwealth Department of Health. Health information for international travel; 1995. 4th edn. Canberra: AGPS.

16 Centers for Disease Control and Prevention. Health information for international travel 2009–2010. Online. Available: http://wwwn.cdc.gov/travel/default.aspx 25 March 2010.

17 Wilder-Smith A, Khairullah NS, Song JH et al. Travel health knowledge, attitudes and practices among Australasian travelers. J Travel Med 2004; 11:9–15.

18 Freedman DO, Kozarsky PE, Weld LH et al. GeoSentinel: The Global Emerging Infections Sentinel network of the International Society of Travel Medicine. J Travel Med 1999; 6:94–98.

19 International Society of Travel Medicine. GeoSentinel. Online. Available: http://www.istm.org 5 December 2007.

20 Kozarsky PE, Keystone JS. Body of knowledge for the practice of travel medicine. J Travel Med 2002; 9:112–115.

21 Shaw MTM, Leggat PA, Weld LH et al. Illness in returned travellers presenting at GeoSentinel sites in New Zealand. Aust NZ J Pub Health 2003; 27:82–86.

22 Leggat PA, Klein M. The Australasian Faculty of Travel Medicine. Travel Med Inf Dis 2004; 2:47–49.

23 McBride WJH, Taylor CT, Pryor JA et al. Scrub typhus in north Queensland. Med J Aust 1999; 170:318–320.

24 Likeman RK. Scrub typhus: a recent outbreak among military personnel in North Queensland. ADF Health 2006; 7:10–13.

25 Fradin MS, Day JF. Comparative efficacy of insect repellents against mosquito bites. N Engl J Med 2002; 347:13–18.

26 Centers for Disease Control (CDC). Updated information regarding insect repellents. Online. Available: http://www.cdc.gov/ncidod/dvbid/westnile/RepellentUpdates.htm 5 May 2010.

27 World Health Organization. Malaria. Fact sheet. Updated April 2010. Online. Available: http://www.who.int/mediacentre/factsheets/fs094/en/ 5 May 2010.

28 Hanna JN, Ritchie SA, Eisen DP et al. An outbreak of *Plasmodium vivax* malaria in Far North Queensland, 2002. Med J Aust 2004; 180:24–28.

29 Brookes DL, Ritchie SA, van den Hurk AF et al. *Plasmodium vivax* malaria acquired in far north Queensland. Med J Aust 1997; 166:82–83.

30 Edstein MD, Nasveld PE, Rieckmann KH. The challenge of effective chemoprophylaxis against malaria. ADF Health 2001; 2:12–16.

31 Zuckerman JN. Recent developments: travel medicine. BMJ 2002; 325:260–264. a p 262.

32 Looareesuwan S, Chulay JD, Canfield CJ et al. Malarone (atovaquone and proguanil hydrochloride): a review of its clinical development for treatment of malaria.

Malarone Clinical Trials Study Group. Am J Trop Med Hyg 1999; 60:533–541.
33 Omari AA, Preston C, Garner P. Artemether-lumefantrine for treating uncomplicated falciparum malaria. Cochrane Database Syst Rev 2002; 3:CD003125.
34 World Health Organization. Dengue and dengue haemorrhagic fever. Fact sheet no. 117. March 2009. Online. Available: http://www.who.int/mediacentre/factsheets/fs117/en/ 5 May 2010.
35 Malcolm RL, Hanna JN, Phillips DA. The timeliness of notification of clinically suspected cases of dengue imported into north Queensland. Aust NZ J Pub Health 1999; 23:414–417.
36 Kitchener S, Leggat PA, Brennan L et al. The importation of dengue by soldiers returning from East Timor to north Queensland, Australia. J Travel Med 2002; 9:180–183.
37 Kitchener S. Most recent developments in Japanese encephalitis vaccines. Aust Mil Med 2002; 11:88–92.
38 Kurane I, Takasaki T. Immunogenicity and protective efficacy of the current inactivated Japanese encephalitis vaccine against different Japanese encephalitis virus strains. Vaccine 2000; 18(Suppl 2):33–35.
39 World Health Organization. International health regulations. Geneva: WHO; 2005. Online. Available: http://www.who.int/ihr/en/ 5 May 2010.
40 McFarland LV. Meta-analysis of probiotics for the prevention of traveler's diarrhea. Travel Med Inf Dis 2007; 5:97–105.
41 Steffen R. Travel medicine: prevention based on epidemiological data. Trans R Soc Trop Med Hyg 1991; 85:156–162.
42 Baker TD, Hargarten SW, Guptill KS. The uncounted dead—American civilians dying overseas. Pub Health Rep 1992; 107:155–159.
43 MacPherson DW, Gushulak BD, Sandhu J. Death and international travel: the Canadian experience 1996 to 2004. J Travel Med 2007; 14:77–84.
44 Leggat PA, Wilks J. Overseas visitor deaths in Australia, 2001 to 2003. J Travel Med 2009; 16:243–247.
45 Cheng I. Screening of passenger fitness to fly and medical kits on board commercial aircraft. J Aust Soc Ae Space Med 2009; 4:14–18.
46 Civil Aviation Safety Authority. Designated aviation medical examiner handbook. Rev November 2008. Online. Available: http://www.casa.gov.au/scripts/nc.dll?WCMS:STANDARD:1001:pc=PC_91302 5 May 2010.
47 Graham H, Putland J, Leggat P. Air travel for people with special needs (Ch 8). In: Leggat PA, Goldsmid JM eds. Primer of travel medicine. 3rd rev ed. Brisbane: ACTM; 2005:100–112.
48 World Health Organization. Tuberculosis and air travel. Geneva: WHO; 2001.
49 Mendis S, Yach D, Alwan A. Air travel and venous thromboembolism. Bull World Health Org 2002; 80:403–406.
50 Gallus AS, Goghlan DC. Travel and venous thrombosis. Curr Opin Pulm Med 2002; 8:372–378.
51 Chow T, Browne V, Heileson HL et al. *Ginkgo biloba* and acetazolamide prophylaxis for acute mountain sickness. Arch Intern Med 2005; 165:296–301.
52 US Department of State, Bureau of Consular Affairs. Online. Available: http://travel.state.gov/ 6 May 2010.
53 Department of Foreign Affairs and Trade, Australia. Smartraveller. Online. Available: http://www.smartraveller.gov.au 5 May 2010.
54 Foreign and Commonwealth Office. Online. Available: http://www.fco.gov.uk/en/ 5 May 2010.
55 Leggat PA, Leggat FW. Emergency assistance provided abroad to insured travellers from Australia following the Bali bombing. Travel Med Inf Dis 2004; 2:41–45.
56 Hampson GV, Cook SP, Frederiksen SR. The Australian Defence Force response to the Bali bombing, 12 October 2002. Med J Aust 2002; 77:620–623.
57 Leggat PA, Leggat FW. Assistance provided abroad to insured travellers from Australia following the 2004 Asian Tsunami. Travel Med Inf Dis 2007; 5:47–50.
58 Leggat PA, Heydon JL, Menon A. Safety advice for travelers from New Zealand. J Travel Med 1998; 5:61–64.
59 Hill DR, Behrens RH. A survey of travel clinics throughout the world. J Travel Med 1996; 3:46–51.
60 Leggat PA. Travel health advice provided by inflight magazines of international airlines in Australia. J Travel Med 1997; 4:102–103.

chapter 46

Urology

INTRODUCTION AND OVERVIEW

Symptoms suggesting urological pathology are common presentations in primary care. These include recurrent urinary tract infections, frequency and urgency of micturition, nocturia and urinary incontinence.

Acute presentations to general practitioners or hospital emergency departments often involve pain: acute loin pain, testicular pain and the pain of urinary retention. Some signs may be suspicious for malignancy (e.g. haematuria). In addition, lumps in the scrotum and testes are a frequent cause for patient concern. A systematic approach to these presentations is easily followed, and history and examination will provide the diagnosis in the majority of cases.

HISTORY AND EXAMINATION

History and examination of genitourinary presentations will necessarily differ between male and female patients.

ADULT MALE

History

History taking should include the presenting complaint and any associated symptoms that may not be volunteered (e.g. haematuria, haematospermia, urethral discharge). Enquire about erectile function and recent sexual activity.

Smoking and occupational history (increase risk of bladder cancer) should be obtained. It is important to obtain an assessment of both chronicity and severity as this will guide management, particularly in bladder outlet obstruction. Nocturia is a common symptom in middle age, in both men and women.

Current medications and allergies should be noted, as well as past surgical procedures.

Family history of prostate cancer will be potentially relevant to diagnosis and screening.

Various symptoms scores have been defined for assessing the severity of lower urinary tract symptoms (LUTS), the most notable being the International Prostate Symptom Score (IPSS). This can easily be remembered by the acronym FUNWISE: **F**requency, **U**rgency, **N**octuria, **W**eak stream, **I**ntermittency, **S**training, incomplete **E**mptying. It is scored from 0 to 5 based on the number of times the symptom has occurred in the past month, and the score is then totalled from 0 to 35. A score of 0–7 is defined as mildly symptomatic, 8–19 moderately symptomatic and 20–35 severely symptomatic. In addition there is a quality of life score from 0 (delighted) to 6 (terrible). These scores are useful for assessing severity and response to treatment, and are widely used.

Examination

Examination of a male presenting with a genitourinary problem will incorporate a general physical examination including an abdominal examination and examination of the penis, scrotum, testes and hernial orifices. Percuss for a palpable bladder and ballot for a palpable kidney. The examination of the prostate is regarded by some men as invasive and avoided by many doctors, but it is invaluable in the diagnosis and management of prostate diseases. Historical descriptions of the characteristics of benign and malignant prostate glands are largely erroneous (e.g. obliteration of the median sulcus); they are usually soft or hard, large or small. Nodules may be felt, and these are often suspicious for malignancy but may also represent intra-prostatic stones.

ADULT FEMALE

History

History will begin with the presenting complaint. Ask about frequency and urgency of micturition, nocturia and urinary incontinence, haematuria, loin pain and vaginal discharge. Ask about a history of past urinary tract infections, gynaecological conditions and procedures, menstruation pattern and bowel function. If appropriate, enquire about recent sexual activity.

Ask about current medications and allergies.

Examination

Examination of a female presenting with a genitourinary problem will incorporate a general physical examination including an abdominal and gynaecological examination. Specific gynaecological conditions should be sought, such as prolapse, fibroids or vaginal atrophy. Asking the woman to cough with a full bladder can give an indication as to the severity of stress incontinence.

BEDSIDE UROLOGICAL TESTS

Dipstick and/or microbiological examination of the urine is valuable for the diagnosis of urinary tract infection and microscopic haematuria. The collection of urine samples for microbiology should be done aseptically. The GP should instruct the patient in how to collect the sample. The patient should wash their hands and the urethra should be swabbed (from front to back in females) with saline-soaked gauze. In females, the labia should be parted and the initial part of the void should be then made into the toilet, the midstream should be voided into the specimen container and the remainder in the toilet. The specimen should then be labelled and note made of whether the patient is menstruating. The specimen should be placed in a specimen bag for transportation to the laboratory.

Urine examination is carried out at the bedside, usually using urine dipstick analysis or similar cellulose strips. These contain reagents sensitive to various substances in urine such as blood, leucocytes, protein, glucose, nitrite, bilirubin and urobilinogen. A diagnosis of urinary tract infection (UTI) can be made confidently in the presence of leucocytes, nitrites and protein. It is possible to treat on this basis alone but a midstream sample for culture should also be sent, to ensure that the correct antibiotic is used.

Urinary catheters

Urinary catheterisation is usually straightforward in the anatomically normal lower urinary tract. Adult urinary catheters used in urological surgery are sized from 12 French (Charriere or Ch) to 24 French and above. The gauge equates to the circumference in mm and is approximately three times the diameter in mm. Other catheters such as the Coudé tip catheter and the Tiemann's are used to negotiate the prostatic urethra but these are uncommonly used and inhabit the realms of the specialist. For patients with acute retention of urine, a 12 Ch catheter is usually sufficient. Although these were traditionally made of rubber, silicone is now widely used. Silicone catheters have the advantage of softness without the risk of perishing and can be left in the bladder for up to 12 weeks.

Technique

Catheterisation should be carried out using aseptic technique, and consideration given to antibiotic prophylaxis in immunocompromised or unwell patients. Prepare with antiseptic and drape the area. Fenestrated drapes are usually included in catheterisation packs for this purpose. Use 1% lignocaine gel (e.g. Instillagel®) to anaesthetise and lubricate the urethra, and allow 5 minutes to achieve maximum effect. Use the smallest catheter to effect drainage (usually 12 or 14 Ch) and insert until urine is seen to drain. Only then can the balloon be inflated. Usually 10 mL of either normal saline or sterile water is used to fill the balloon. Connect the tubing to a proprietary urinary drainage bag.

If it not possible to perform urethral drainage, suprapubic drainage is sometimes required. A palpable bladder is a prerequisite for this. Seldinger kits are now available to aid avoidance of adjacent organs (bowel and large vessels), but the standard proprietary kits such as Add-a-Cath® are still commonly available. Fine-bore tubes designed for the draining of ascites are best avoided.

UROLITHIASIS

INCIDENCE

Stones are extremely common and have a significant economic impact on a largely working population. The lifetime risk of stone formation has been reported in the range of 12% for men and 5% for women. Approximately 50% of these patients will have a second episode in their lifetime. The peak incidence is 30–45 years of age and men are three times more likely to suffer than women.

AETIOLOGY

Theories of stone formation are by no means complete, partly due to the difficulties of mimicking in vivo disease with an in vitro model. What is clear, however, is that supersaturated urine is a prerequisite to stone formation. The nucleation theory suggests that stones originate from crystals in supersaturated urine, whereas the crystal inhibition theory suggests that it is an absence of urinary inhibitors that differentiates the stone former from the non-stone former. Some work has gone into examination of potential inhibitors, particularly magnesium and citrate. Types of stones are listed in Table 46.1.

TABLE 46.1 Types of stones

Type of stone	Incidence (%)
Calcium oxalate / calcium phosphate	80–85
Urate	5–10
Struvite (magnesium, ammonium, phosphate)	5–10
Cystine	≈1–2
Xanthine	≈1–2

Risk factors for stone disease

- *Genetic*—there is a strong association between family history and incidence of stone disease, more than doubling the risk compared with the general population.
- *Medications*—certain drugs have been implicated in renal stone formation, particularly indinavir, an anti-retroviral drug now very uncommonly used.
- *Chemotherapeutic drugs* can cause hyperuricaemia as a side effect of protein breakdown of tumours.
- *Soft drink consumption* has been examined as a cause but the evidence is poor (relative risk for sucrose is 1.5).
- *High protein/purine diet*—high intake of animal proteins has been shown to change urinary pH, increase uric acid excretion, reduce urinary citrate and increase urinary calcium. Significant levels of purines are found in anchovies, asparagus, cauliflower, legumes, mushrooms, organ meats, poultry, sardines, spinach. By extension, a vegetarian diet appears to have a protective effect, although the effect is small.
- *High sodium/salt intake*—this causes increased urinary calcium excretion and has been shown to increase the risk of stones by approximately 1.3.
- *Low fluid intake.*

SIGNS AND SYMPTOMS

Urinary stone disease presents either acutely as renal colic or more insidiously with renal angle pain, haematuria or recurrent infections. Renal colic is a common emergency presentation, with very severe pain in the loin. The pain has been described as being more severe than labour, by patients who have endured both. Pain relief should be a priority for these patients when seen in an emergency setting. The pain is often described as a 'colic' but can be relentless. It often radiates to the groin or testicle, and testicular pain may be the predominant symptom. The differential diagnosis includes musculoskeletal pain and incipient herpes zoster. In the elderly, ruptured abdominal aortic aneurysm may mimic renal colic. In situations where immediate imaging is not available, this is a diagnosis to consider.

INVESTIGATIONS

Non-contrast CT of the kidneys (CTKUB) is the imaging of choice for kidney stone disease. It has largely replaced the classic intravenous pyelogram (IVP) because it gives better anatomical detail with similar radiation exposure. Measurement of serum creatinine and testing of urine for infection should be carried out.

THERAPEUTICS

Renal colic

The immediate priority is to relieve pain. Non-steroidal anti-inflammatory agents such as indomethacin or diclofenac are often used in this situation. Opiates such as morphine may be required in addition. Pethidine should be avoided as there is no evidence for superior efficacy and it has more potential as a drug of abuse. Many patients will be able to be discharged after a period of observation once a firm diagnosis has been made, as many small stones pass spontaneously.

Management of renal stones

Management of renal stones depends on many factors, including size and position, coexistent infection, renal failure and so on. Mandatory indications for immediate treatment include:

- obstructed infected kidney
- stone unlikely to pass spontaneously (e.g. > 1 cm in size)
- single kidney
- persistent pain.

In addition, social factors sometimes supervene (e.g. incipient long-haul flight). People working in certain professions, such as pilots, are forbidden from working with a renal stone, and that may influence the timing of intervention.

There is good evidence that the use of alpha-blocking drugs and calcium antagonists can assist in the passage of small stones in the lower ureter, and these are often prescribed initially in combination with pain relief.

Methods of stone removal

Ureteric stones can be removed with the assistance of ureteroscopes, which can be either rigid (rod-lens), semi-rigid or flexible (fibre-optic). There have been considerable improvements in the technology of these techniques in recent years. A wide array of baskets is available and these can be used in combination with energy sources such as pneumatic lithotripsy or (holmium) laser. External shock wave lithotripsy (ESWL) is also commonly used, particularly for small stones in the kidney, and these techniques may need to be used in combination.

For larger stones in the kidney, staghorn calculi and so on, percutaneous access may be required to carry out stone surgery. It is unusual for open renal ureteric or renal surgery to be required.

PREVENTION

In order to identify risk of further stone formation, certain investigations are carried out in patients after their first episode of colic. Some authors suggest that metabolic evaluation should be carried out only on those patients with multiple or recurrent stones.

Measurement of serum calcium and urate will identify hypercalcaemic and hyperuricosuric patients. Identification of metabolic abnormalities associated with recurrent stone disease is usually carried out by analysis of 24-hour urine excretion (volume, pH, levels of calcium, phosphate and uric acid, oxalate, citrate, creatinine). Stone analysis may also assist following operative procedure or spontaneous passage.

The most common abnormality found is idiopathic hypercalciuria (with normal serum calcium). This is most easily treated with an increased fluid intake of 1.5–2 L per day.

Chemoprevention is a holy grail for stone disease. Urinary inhibitors such as potassium citrate, alone or in combination with a thiazide diuretic, can be used. Thiazide diuretics decrease hypercalciuria by increasing reabsorption of calcium from the distal tubule. Citric acid (as lemon juice) can be taken but large amounts (100–150 mL of pure lemon juice) are required to produce enough citrate in the urine.

Where possible, avoid medications likely to increase stone risk.

Diet

Dietary fact sheets containing sensible advice are invaluable in reducing further episodes of stone disease. The following points should be included:

- Increase water intake (1.5–2 L of water per day).
- Reduce consumption of soft drinks.
- Reduce high-purine foods in urate stone formers (alcohol, anchovy, asparagus, cauliflower, legumes, mushrooms, organ meats, poultry, sardines, spinach).
- Reduce salt intake.

Dietary restriction of calcium has a counterintuitive effect on the risk of subsequent stones, and is to be discouraged.

Supplements

- Calcium citrate is preferred for postmenopausal women with stone disease. The increase in urinary calcium is counteracted by the concomitant increase in urinary citrate.
- Magnesium reduces calcium oxalate risk.
- Vitamin B_6 decreases oxalate production (foods rich in vitamin B_6 include oily fish, whole grains, poultry, soybean, avocado, bananas, nuts). *Dose*: 50 mg/day.[1]

URINARY TRACT INFECTION

INCIDENCE

Urinary tract infection (UTI) is a common condition of young women, with an estimate of 10% of women aged between 16 and 65 years suffering from one UTI per year. It is predominantly a condition of women, but prostatic hypertrophy causes the incidence to increase in men over the age of 65 years. UTIs are classified as:

- uncomplicated lower UTI (cystitis)
- uncomplicated pyelonephritis
- complicated pyelonephritis
- urosepsis.

AETIOLOGY

UTIs can be acquired haematogenously but the vast majority arrive through ascending infection via the urethra. Bacteria vary in their virulence and this may vary depending on host factors such as obstruction, immunocompromise and so on. Most UTIs are caused by a single bacterial species. *Escherichia coli* is responsible for the vast majority, mostly of the O serotype. Less common pathogens include *Proteus*, *Pseudomonas*, *Klebsiella* and, rarely, *Staphylococcus*. The finding of persistent less common bacteria such as *Proteus* should prompt investigation for underlying pathology such as stone disease.

SIGNS AND SYMPTOMS

Simple cystitis in women usually gives a classic combination of symptoms: pain on micturition (dysuria), frequency, malaise and occasionally haematuria. In addition, patients may notice an odour associated with the urine. Pyelonephritis can cause significant morbidity, and patients may be pyrexial, with fevers, loin pain and potential sepsis. They frequently, but not always, have a preceding or coincident cystitis. Urinalysis will commonly demonstrate evidence of UTI (leucocytes, erythrocytes and nitrites), and culture of blood and urine will confirm infection with the same bacteria that lead to uncomplicated UTI.

INVESTIGATIONS

- *Urinalysis*—simple dipstick analysis of urine in the presence of symptoms will give the diagnosis in the majority of cases. In simple UTI, this may be sufficient, but a significant number of UTIs will not respond to empirical antibiotics, because of either resistance or lack of sensitivity. For this reason, urine culture is recommended. A culture result is usually available within a few days, such that prescribed antibiotics can be amended.

- *Urine culture*—the gold standard for identification of UTI is culture. Add a urine *Chlamydia* PCR if appropriate. Patients with dysuria and frequency may have false negative urine culture if organisms are fastidious or anaerobic.
- *Upper tract investigation* is not required for uncomplicated UTI. In patients with pyelonephritis, some upper tract imaging is required to rule out hydronephrosis and stone. An ultrasound of kidneys is usually sufficient. If there is evidence of complicated pyelonephritis (failure to settle, persistent pain), a contrast-enhanced CT scan may be required. It must be borne in mind that an abdominal CT carries a significant radiation dosage, with its attendant risk of malignancy.
- *Cystoscopy* is reserved for patients with recurrent UTI in whom no cause can be found. In young women, this is almost invariably normal. It is more common to find bladder outlet obstruction in elderly men, and a similar work-up to lower urinary tract symptoms is indicated.

THERAPEUTICS

- *Antibiotics*—the choice and duration of antibiotics is guided by local guidelines and antibiotic sensitivities. Trimethoprim or cephalexin have the advantage of being inexpensive and well tolerated, and are commonly used to treat uncomplicated UTI, although trimethoprim has limited sensitivity in *Enterococcus* and *Pseudomonas* species.
- Complicated UTIs are more commonly treated with quinolones (e.g. ciprofloxacin) or intravenous aminoglycosides. These are highly effective against gram-negative bacteria.
- Encourage fluid intake.
- Alkalinising urine (sodium citrotartrate) may help symptomatic dysuria.

PREVENTION

- *Hygiene measures*—many women will already be familiar with strategies to avoid UTI and these need to be taught to young girls from the age of toilet training. They include wiping from front to back after voiding, and avoidance of bath products, lubricants and synthetic underwear. In sexually active women, there may be a strong association between intercourse and UTI. Various measures such as voiding prior to, and after, intercourse or showering prior to intercourse can reduce the risk. Some authors advocate pre-coital antibiotics if the association is strong. (Often a single dose 4–6 hours beforehand is sufficient, or afterwards if not done so.)
- *Cranberry juice*—as either pure juice or as tablets, has been shown to reduce the incidence of UTI in women with recurrent cystitis by as much as half. Compliance with pure juice can be low but this is overcome by taking one tablet twice daily.
- Encourage *fluids.*
- *Long-term low-dose antibiotics*—this is rarely necessary and has been implicated in the emergence of resistant bacterial strains. Nevertheless, it is sometimes used, if only for a limited period (3–6 months). A prophylactic dose of trimethoprim or cephalexin can reduce the recurrence rate by as much as 95%. Self-start antibiotics can also be used in this way in patients with recurrent UTI, and the duration of antibiotic use may be less if employed in this way. For motivated patients, this is preferable. If antibiotics are used, they should be accompanied by a probiotic such as *Lactobacillus acidophilus.*

UTI IN CHILDREN

Incidence

UTI is a common bacterial infection causing illness in infants and children. It may lead to non-specific illness and the diagnosis is often more difficult to make than in adults. In this age group, a definitive microbiological diagnosis may not always be possible.

Aetiology

UTI in children may have no underlying cause, but the possibility of underlying congenital abnormality must be considered. This is discussed below.

Signs and symptoms

In infants aged 3 months or less, fever and lethargy may predominate, with offensive urine and specific urinary symptoms being less common. In older infants, abdominal pain and tenderness may be more apparent, but failure to thrive and vague abdominal pain may predominate. In children above toddler age, dysuria and frequency may be more apparent than constitutional symptoms.

Investigations

Clean-catch urine is recommended. This takes patience and persistence. Urine collection pads may be used if this is not possible. Suprapubic aspiration may be required in the unwell infant prior to initiation of antibiotic treatment.

Therapeutics

Young children with UTI are mostly managed in hospital. Older children may be managed in the community but should be referred to a paediatrician. A 7–10 day course of antibiotics may be required.

Prevention and management

The investigation and management of UTI in children is a matter of debate and there has been criticism of over-investigation with invasive testing in the past. In general, the younger the infant, the greater the likelihood of underlying anatomical abnormality such as severe vesicoureteric reflux. For this reason, ultrasound is recommended as a first investigation, followed by micturating cyst-urethrography (MCUG). DMSA renography may be carried out under the care of a paediatrician in secondary care.

A diagnosis of reflux nephropathy is usually treated by prophylactic antibiotics, as most reflux will improve spontaneously over time. Circumcision has been shown to reduce the incidence of UTI in young boys with a congenital anomaly and should be considered. Severe reflux may need to be managed surgically with either endoscopic or open anti-reflux surgery.

INCONTINENCE

Urinary incontinence is the involuntary loss of urine. It is both a clinical sign and a symptom. The prevalence of incontinence increases with age and it is more common in women than men. Estimates are that 7–19% of adult women suffer from some form of urinary incontinence, with wide differences seen between different cultures and races.

Incontinence is not only a hygienic issue but it can negatively affect a patient's quality of life, with social, psychological and sexual impairment.

Urinary incontinence may be classified as:

- *stress incontinence* (SUI)—loss of urine associated with abdominal effort, e.g. coughing, laughing, sneezing or straining
- *urge incontinence* (UUI)—urine loss that is preceded by the sudden uncontrollable desire to void
- *mixed incontinence*—a combination of both stress and urge incontinence
- *continuous (total) incontinence*—persistent loss of urine
- *overflow incontinence*—uncontrolled urine loss due to urinary retention
- *nocturnal enuresis*—loss of urine during sleep.

AETIOLOGY

(See Fig 46.1) Stress incontinence is more commonly seen with multiple vaginal deliveries and increasing age. Female continence is dependent on the supports of the bladder neck and urethra as well as the external sphincter located at the mid-urethral level. Tissue laxity and atrophy allow hypermobility with incomplete urethral closure. Male SUI is much less common and is usually due to traumatic sphincteric injury (e.g. prostatectomy for benign or malignant disease or pelvic fracture with urethral rupture).

Patients with UUI have increased urinary frequency and difficulty postponing voiding. They may report large-volume losses on the way to the toilet. Conditions that result in bladder irritation, such as infections, stones and tumours, may be causative and should be excluded. Detrusor overactivity is a common cause of UUI that is diagnosed with urodynamic studies. Detrusor overactivity is frequently idiopathic (overactive bladder) or it may be associated with longstanding bladder outlet obstruction or neurological disease (e.g. diabetic neuropathy, multiple sclerosis and spina bifida).

Continuous incontinence may be non-urethral and can occur with urinary fistulas and ectopic ureteric orifices.

Overflow incontinence is defined by urine leakage from a distended bladder. It results from bladder outlet obstruction or poor bladder contractility.

SIGNS AND SYMPTOMS

A careful history should document the type, onset and severity of the incontinence. Associated urinary symptoms should be assessed as well as background fluid intake and voiding habits. The completion of a bladder diary may be beneficial in this regard. The presence of pain, haematuria or voiding difficulty may indicate complicated cases. Physical examination should include a neurological assessment including perineal sensation, anal sphincter tone and control of pelvic floor muscles.

Elderly patients may develop incontinence secondary to reversible conditions, which should be actively sought. These include: delirium, excess urine output, limited mobility, stool impaction and medications.

INVESTIGATIONS

Urinalysis and urine culture are routine. Imaging, such as with an ultrasound, is commonly done to assess the post-void residual and rule out pathology. Cystourethroscopy may be performed when indicated to evaluate the lower urinary tract anatomy.

Urodynamic studies with cystometry involve pressure/volume monitoring during artificial bladder filling. This is combined with fluoroscopy to define leakage. Information on bladder sensation, capacity, compliance and detrusor overactivity is provided. Urodynamics are indicated for patients with complicated or refractory incontinence, all those with neurological disease and prior to surgical therapy.

THERAPEUTICS

Stress incontinence

Conservative treatment involves fluid management, timed voiding and pelvic floor muscle exercises.

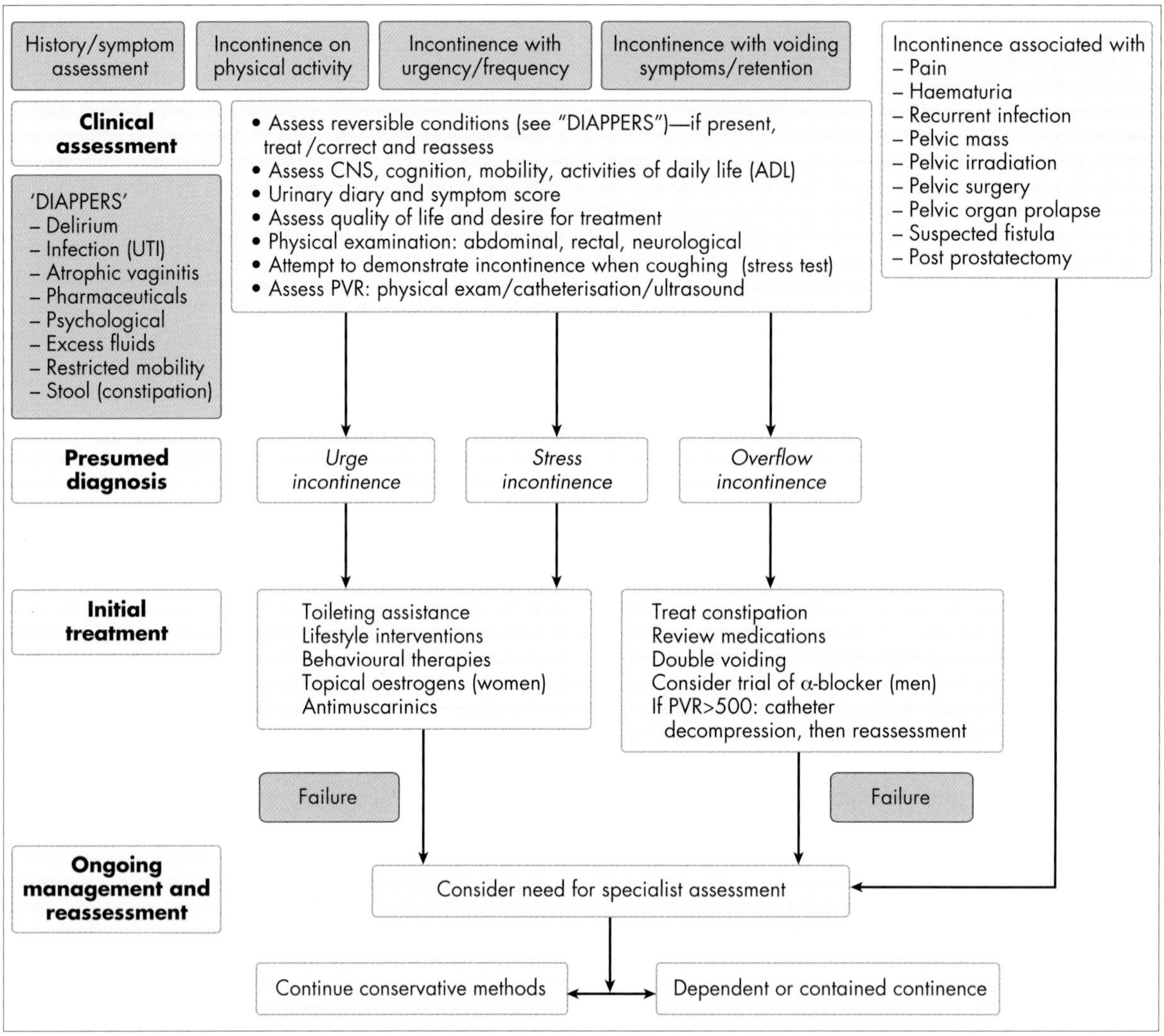

FIGURE 46.1 Main types/causes of incontinence, and their management

Smoking cessation, elimination of constipation, oestrogen replacement and correction of obesity are also appropriate. Surgical therapy for female SUI involves bolstering the mid-urethral complex or bladder neck suspension. Colposuspension surgery involves elevation of the tissues surrounding the bladder neck behind the pubis, thus preventing mobility. Colposuspension has been largely replaced by urethral sling procedures. Autologous or synthetic slings are placed via the obturator foramen or retropubic space around the middle or proximal urethra to form a hammock for urethral support. The outcome data for synthetic slings (trans-vaginal tape, transobturator tape, etc) are now quite mature and they seem to remain effective at long-term follow-up.

Urge incontinence

Elimination of obvious bladder irritants, outlet obstruction and neurological disease will define overactive bladder (OAB). Anticholinergic medications (oxybutinin, toltoredine, solifenacin and darifenacin) are beneficial, along with bladder training. Anticholinergics may have significant side effects and should be used with caution in patients with glaucoma, obstructed voiding or cognitive impairment. Intravesical botulinum toxin injections are useful, but expensive, for refractory cases.

Complicated cases

Complicated cases may require more invasive therapy. Severe sphincteric deficiency such as that seen post prostatectomy or with lower motor neuron disease may be treated with an artificial urinary sphincter. An artificial sphincter involves the placement of a silicone cuff around the urethra, which is connected to a reservoir buried in the retropubic space. Fluid is cycled in and out of the cuff by a pump that is placed in the scrotum or labia. Debilitating UUI may require bladder augmentation surgery or a urinary diversion such as with an ileal conduit.

PREVENTION

Avoidance of exacerbating factors such as constipation, obesity, smoking and the treatment of asthma may prevent or reduce stress incontinence.

BENIGN PROSTATIC HYPERPLASIA

INCIDENCE

Benign prostatic hyperplasia (BPH) is a common clinical condition of the ageing man. Studies suggest that about 30% of men older than 65 years will suffer from clinical BPH. The definition of BPH is not standardised, and it may be used to refer to:

- histological features of stromoglandular proliferation
- benign prostatic enlargement
- clinical BPH—the most commonly used definition indicating the presence of lower urinary tract symptoms (LUTS) from bladder outlet obstruction by a non-cancerous prostate gland.

AETIOLOGY

BPH is an age-related process that is androgen dependent. Histological changes, prostate size and LUTS are all more prevalent with increasing age. BPH does have an inheritable component and severe forms may be hereditary.

SIGNS AND SYMPTOMS

The most common presentation of BPH is with LUTS due to bladder outlet obstruction. These symptoms can be assessed with validated scoring systems (e.g. IPSS, see above) and with a voiding diary. Occasionally, BPH-related complications such as recurrent urinary tract infections, recurrent haematuria, bladder calculi, bladder diverticula or urinary retention may lead to presentation.

History and physical examination aim to determine the impact of BPH and exclude differential diagnoses. Digital rectal examination is important to evaluate prostatic size and for possible cancer.

INVESTIGATIONS

There are a variety of investigations that may be used in the evaluation of patients with BPH. The more common tests are listed below.

- urine microscopy, culture and sensitivity—for *all* patients
- urine cytology, upper tract imaging and cystoscopy—if haematuria is present
- renal tract ultrasound—performed when information regarding renal anatomy and upper tract changes (e.g. hydronephrosis and stones), bladder anatomy, prostate size and post-void residual is sought
- flexible cystoscopy—not routinely indicated but may be done when urethral anatomy is questioned (e.g. stricture disease, previous prostatic surgery) or when bladder pathology needs to be excluded
- voiding flow rate with residual—a useful adjunct in assessing obstructive LUTS that may indicate aetiology by its pattern
- serum creatinine—may be measured when renal function may be compromised (e.g. urinary retention)
- prostate-specific antigen measurement—should be considered where the diagnosis of prostate cancer may alter the treatment plan
- urodynamic studies—indicated where confounding conditions may be responsible for LUTS (e.g. neurological disease or previous failed prostatic surgery).

INTEGRATED THERAPEUTICS

Many men with bladder outlet obstruction due to BPH are not significantly bothered by their symptoms and may be appropriate for watchful waiting. Many men will remain stable or have improvement with long-term observation. For men who are bothered by their symptoms, medical therapy should be considered.

- Regular physical exercise—most of the literature supports a clinically significant, independent and strong inverse relationship between exercise and the development of BPH/LUTS.[2]
- Supplements:
  - quercetin 500 mg b.i.d. combined with bromelain
  - beta sitosterol[3]
  - saw palmetto[4]
  - *Pygeum africanum*[5] (50–100 mg extract daily) may be useful
  - stinging nettle[6]
  - pumpkin seed oil extracts standardised for fatty acid content—have been used in BPH studies in the amount of 160 mg t.i.d. with meals
  - vitamin C 1000 mg daily
  - zinc 60 mg daily
  - omega-3 fatty acids 2000–4000 mg daily as anti-inflammatory.

Pharmaceutical

Alpha-blocking agents (e.g. tamsulosin or prazosin) provide rapid symptomatic improvement and improve urine flow. These are usually first-line pharmaceutical agents for BPH therapy. Inhibitors of 5-alpha reductase (e.g. finasteride and dutasteride) block the conversion of testosterone to dihydrotestosterone, the more potent androgen within the prostate. These agents result in a gradual decrease in prostatic size (20–30%), improve urinary symptoms and prevent disease progression. They are useful in men with significantly enlarged prostates and may be used alone or in combination with alpha-blockers. However, they may reduce PSA, altering the monitoring of prostate cancer.

Surgery

Surgical therapy is indicated for failed medical therapy and for BPH-related complications. Transurethral prostatic resection (TURP) remains the mainstay for surgical management of BPH. Possible complications include: haemorrhage, infection, stricture formation, retrograde ejaculation and, rarely, stress incontinence. The 'TURP syndrome' is a rare and potentially fatal complication that occurs from absorption of hypotonic irrigation solution. Erectile dysfunction has been reported post TURP; however, the rates appear to be similar to those of age-matched cohorts. Men with a very large prostate gland may require open surgical excision. Laser surgery may provide an alternative approach to TURP. Holmium laser enucleation of the prostate (HOLEP) provides similar results to traditional surgery and may be performed for large glands or in anticoagulated patients. Photoselective vaporisation with KTP (greenlight) laser is being increasingly used and may be performed as a day procedure. Less invasive measures such as radiofrequency needle ablation (TUNA) and microwave thermotherapy (TUMT) provide symptomatic benefit that in general is less than that seen with TURP, and are not widely performed.

Prevention

No preventative strategies exist.

PROSTATITIS

Chronic prostatitis is a difficult condition to manage, and has been calculated to be responsible for two million outpatient visits in the United States in 2009. The majority of these patients fulfill the criteria for chronic pelvic pain syndrome and most do not respond to antibiotics. It is characterised by diagnostic uncertainty and unsatisfactory outcomes.

Acute prostatitis is a serious but uncommon infection, often requiring inpatient treatment. Parenteral quinolone and aminoglycoside antibiotics may be required.

BOX 46.1 NIH classification of prostatitis

I Acute bacterial prostatitis
II Chronic bacterial prostatitis
III Chronic abacterial prostatitis—chronic pelvic pain syndrome
- A—Inflammatory chronic pelvic pain syndrome (white cells in semen/expressed prostatic secretions)
- B—Non-inflammatory chronic pelvic pain syndrome (no white cells in semen/expressed prostatic secretions)

IV Asymptomatic inflammatory prostatitis (histological prostatitis)

In less severe cases, long courses of oral quinolones (e.g. 3 weeks) may be sufficient. It may rarely be complicated by prostatic abscesses, which may require surgical intervention.

Bacterial prostatitis is usually divided into acute and chronic, depending on the duration of symptoms. The National Institutes of Health classification is frequently used and is outlined in Box 46.1.

AETIOLOGY

The aetiology of acute and chronic prostatitis is unclear. It is assumed that acute prostatitis begins with a cystitis or a urethritis, which then spreads to involve the gland along the prostatic ducts. There is a strong association between chronic prostatitis and bladder outlet obstruction, but true chronic pelvic pain syndrome may exist without any pre-existing urinary pathology.

SIGNS AND SYMPTOMS

Acute prostatitis is associated with severe urinary symptoms, fever and possible signs of sepsis. Chronic prostatitis/chronic pelvic pain syndrome is a constellation of symptoms. Testicular, perineal, rectal or penile pain may predominate. In addition, frequency of micturition and dysuria are common. The pain may be debilitating, with many of the characteristics associated with chronic pain elsewhere.

INVESTIGATIONS

The investigations for chronic prostatitis should include:

- urinalysis and urine culture
- exclusion of sexually transmitted disease using urine PCR for chlamydia
- assessment of lower urinary tract dysfunction using a flow rate and voiding chart
- an attempt to culture a prostatic pathogen for either urine or expressed prostatic secretions (EPS). This can be achieved by using the 'Stamey three glass test' where the patient voids 15–20 mL of urine into the first glass (voided bladder (VB)

urine 1), then performs an MSU as described above (VB2). The prostate is then massaged by the doctor and the prostatic secretions expressed (expressed prostatic secretions (EPS)). The patient then voids 10–15 mL into a third container (VB3). In essence, bacteria or white cells in VB1 suggests urethritis, in VB2 cystitis and in EPS prostatitis.

THERAPEUTICS

Standard medical treatment for acute prostatitis usually involves antibiotics for 4–12 weeks (with probiotics), combined with anti-inflammatory medication (NSAIDs). Usually, quinolones (e.g. ofloxacin), trimethoprim or tetracyclines are used. Alpha-blockers may help if there is trouble with micturition, and are usually tried in addition. However, there is a lack of proven efficacy for conventional medical treatment of chronic abacterial prostatitis/chronic pelvic pain syndrome.

Where symptoms are chronic or refractory to treatment, the condition may represent non-bacterial prostatitis. Standard medical treatment is usually unhelpful for this condition.

The following combination can be trialled:[7]

- cernilton, a flower pollen extract (500–1000 mg 2–3 times/day)[8]
- quercetin 500 mg b.d. combined with bromelain
- beta sitosterol
- saw palmetto[3] inhibits 5-alpha-reductase, dose 320 mg/day
- stinging nettle
- vitamin C 1000 mg daily
- zinc 60 mg daily
- omega-3 fatty acids 2000–4000 mg daily
- avoid alcohol and caffeine.

URINARY RETENTION

INCIDENCE

Various longitudinal community studies have attempted to measure the risk of acute retention in men with benign prostatic hyperplasia (BPH). A recent study identified men with BPH and randomised them into receiving placebo, or treatment with alpha-blockers and/or 5-alpha reductase inhibitors. The placebo arm represented untreated BPH and 2% of those men developed acute retention in 5 years. A similar study estimated the risk of retention in untreated men with BPH was 23% after 20 years.

AETIOLOGY

Urinary retention can be either acute (commonly) or chronic (rare). Acute retention is often caused by obstruction to the outflow tract in elderly men, due to BPH or, less commonly, malignant disease. Less common causes include urethral stricture disease and spinal cord injury.

Acute urinary retention in hospital commonly follows surgery, particularly to the groin, anus or hip. In these cases, pain and anti-cholinergic side effects of anaesthetic agents often conspire to inhibit voluntary voiding. In the community, alcohol, anticholinergics and tricyclic antidepressants are sometimes implicated.

Chronic retention of urine is an insidious condition seen in elderly men. They often describe a painless swelling of the abdomen associated with nocturia and incontinence, caused by overflow of urine from a distended bladder. Most of these are low pressure, and renal function is preserved, but there may be bilateral hydronephrosis if the pressure within the bladder is high. This is an emergency and has to be relieved by catheterisation. In cases of acute renal failure, catheterisation can lead to a large diuresis and profound fluid shifts, and requires careful management. A regimen of replacing hourly losses with normal saline may be required. Daily weights may assist the fluid management in these cases. Bladder outlet surgery is mandatory in these patients as a removal of the catheter will result in further episodes of renal failure. This should be delayed for at least 6 weeks to allow glomerular and tubular function to recover.

INVESTIGATIONS

The investigation of patients with retention of urine is similar to those with lower urinary tract symptoms (LUTS). At the time of catheterisation, a sample of urine is sent for culture and sensitivity. Blood tests for creatinine and full blood count are checked. PSA measurement at the time of retention is a controversial topic but is probably best avoided. Significant increases in PSA can be seen in cases of retention and this will require at least a further PSA after an interval to ensure that it has returned to normal. In contrast, some authors suggest that a normal PSA is reassuring and a very high PSA associated with metastatic prostate cancer can speed diagnosis. Clinical examination of the prostate is required to assess for size and possible malignancy.

THERAPEUTICS

Simple measures can be tried, to assist voiding. Sitting in a warm bath, pain relief or simply sitting out of bed for the hospitalised patient can be useful manoeuvres. If catheterisation is required, the patient should be catheterised as described above. Some units prefer suprapubic catheterisation as a routine. The ability to carry out a trial of voiding without removing the catheter must be weighed against the additional morbidity associated with suprapubic catheterisation.

There is good evidence that the addition of an alpha-blocker (e.g. tamsulosin 400 mcg OD) can improve the percentage of men who void following removal of the catheter. This is normally started on admission and requires at least two doses. Approximately half of men will void following a first episode of retention. In patients who have an obvious precipitant and minimal LUTS prior, this is more likely to succeed. In men who have had worsening symptoms over a long period culminating in an episode of retention, it is less likely and they are best managed with prostate surgery in the first instance.

RENAL DISEASE

Diseases of the kidney are important in general practice for a range of reasons. First, when severe they cause considerable morbidity and mortality. Secondly, they are common, particularly in some sections of the community, such as the elderly and indigenous peoples, and they are regularly co-managed by GPs. Thirdly, their management can be complex and includes not just managing the illness itself but also the symptoms commonly associated with kidney diseases. Fourthly, many of the symptoms and signs associated with chronic kidney disease can come on slowly and are both ill-defined and common, so as to mimic other illnesses, thereby causing diagnostic problems.

Kidney disease is mentioned in a number of other chapters in the context of its association with other illnesses and risk factors. For example, it is discussed in the chapter on diabetes (Ch 26) in the context of complications and monitoring, and in the chapter on cardiovascular disease (Ch 25) due to its role in hypertension. This section of the chapter will therefore focus on kidney failure.

KIDNEY FAILURE

Kidney failure is defined as acute or chronic, depending on whether the decline in renal function has occurred for days/weeks or longer.

Acute kidney failure

Acute kidney failure (AKF) is a sudden and significant decrease in renal function, which leads to a number of sequelae. These include oliguria (less than 400 mL/day in adults or 0.5–1.0 mL/kg/h in children and infants, or nil in the case of ureteric obstruction) and electrolyte imbalance.

Aetiology

AKF can arise from a variety of causes, including:

- *pre-renal*—causes of kidney hypoperfusion such as severe dehydration, blood loss or major and prolonged drop in blood pressure
- *intrinsic*—causes of kidney diseases such as glomerulonephritis or toxic overload (as with certain drugs, such as chemotherapy)
- *post-renal*—causes such as prostate enlargement or ureteric obstruction due to renal calculi.

Polypharmacy, particularly with commonly prescribed medications for the elderly, such as anti-inflammatory medications, diuretics and ACE inhibitors, is a very common cause of AKF. Other medications can exacerbate complications of kidney failure, such as hyperkalaemia. Drugs that can do this include diuretics such as aldactone and Moduretic®, ACE inhibitors, anti-inflammatory medications and AIIR antagonists. It is also worth bearing in mind that medications that are excreted through the kidney may have a substantially longer half-life in the elderly, due to poorer excretion.

Investigations

Tests for AKF will include :

- estimated glomerular filtration rate (eGFR)
- serum creatinine, and urea and electrolytes
- identifying the underlying cause (e.g. plain abdominal X-ray in the presence of renal colic).

Management

AKF is potentially life-threatening and requires urgent diagnosis and admission to hospital. The underlying cause needs to then be identified and treated, such as restoration of fluids or blood, or passing of the calculus.

Recovery from AKF tends to be good, provided the underlying cause can be alleviated, although there is a risk of chronic kidney failure in the future. Sometimes dialysis may be required in the short term until normal kidney function returns.

Chronic kidney failure

Chronic kidney failure (CKF) is defined as a measured or estimated glomerular filtration rate (eGFR) of < 60 mL/min/1.73 m^2 and/or evidence of kidney damage for three or more months, such as proteinuria (ratio of > 30 mg albumin to 1 g creatinine on untimed (spot) urine testing), abnormal renal function tests or abnormalities in imaging tests (scarring or polycystic kidneys).

The majority of patients will be managed in general practice.

Like other organ systems, the kidney has a significant functional reserve of approximately 75–80%. This means that 75% of renal function can be lost without any significant electrolyte or metabolic results or symptoms. Beyond that point (less than 20% of renal function), the effects of diminishing renal function can be measured and symptoms become noticeable. At less than 10% of renal function, the mortality rate rises sharply without dialysis or kidney transplant.

BOX 46.2 Common causes of chronic kidney failure

- Diabetes mellitus
- Hypertension
- Glomerulonephritis
- Renal artery stenosis
- Polycystic kidney disease
- Toxins and pharmaceuticals—e.g. aspirin, anti-inflammatory medications such as ibuprofen and the COX-2 inhibitors, codeine, antibiotics including gentamicin, vancomicin and tetracyclines, ACE inhibitors and lithium
- Reflux nephropathy
- Outflow obstruction of the bladder
- Connective tissue disorders, e.g. SLE
- Amyloidosis
- Gout

Aetiology

CKF can arise from diseases that primarily originate in the kidney itself, or from other illnesses that affect the kidney (Box 46.2). Many of these illnesses, such as type 2 diabetes, hypertension and vascular disease, are lifestyle related and are therefore preventable.

CKF can be diagnosed on investigating indicative symptoms and signs, but as the early stages are usually asymptomatic, often diagnosis will depend on clinical suspicion resulting in testing of at-risk groups, or on the results of blood tests or screening done for other reasons.

Signs and symptoms

Early CKF is commonly asymptomatic. The most common early symptoms are generally non-specific and related to uraemia, such as malaise, nausea, vomiting, weight loss and anorexia and lethargy. As the kidney disease progresses, further symptoms and signs are caused by the complications.

The symptoms associated with CKF are largely due to effects on fluids and electrolytes, homeostasis and erythropoietin. Symptoms (e.g. pruritis), signs (e.g. unexplained hypertension, fatigue or anaemia) and laboratory findings (e.g. proteinuria, uraemia) should raise the clinical suspicion of CKF. Box 46.3 outlines the main symptoms and signs of CKF.

When confirmed upon measurement of the eGFR, serum creatinine and urea, further tests should also be directed at determining the underlying cause of the CKF, such as diabetes.

Investigations

When a clinical suspicion of CKF is aroused, it needs to be confirmed on investigations and the severity of various complications determined. The following tests should be considered by the GP, although a range of others may also be performed by a renal specialist.

BOX 46.3 Signs and symptoms of chronic kidney failure

Symptoms

- Symptoms associated with uraemia:
  - nausea, vomiting, weight loss, anorexia, diarrhoea, bad taste in mouth and bad breath
- Electrolyte imbalance:
  - phosphate—itching, bone pain
  - potassium—arrhythmias, muscle weakness
  - calcium—muscle cramps
  - acidosis
- Fluid balance:
  - swelling of ankles and legs, shortness of breath and aggravation of heart failure
- Inadequate erythropoetin
  - tiredness, malaise, dizziness, drowsiness
- Skin pigmentation—yellowish
- Easy bruising and epistaxis
- Polyuria and nocturia

Signs

- General appearance—pale, weight loss
- Skin—dry, scratch marks, yellowish pigmentation, bruising, purpura
- Fluid balance—peripheral oedema, signs of congestive cardiac failure (CCF)
- Anaemia—pallor, pale conjunctiva
- Nails—leuconychia
- Urine—haematuria, proteinuria, polyuria
- Cardiovascular—hypertension, signs of CCF
- Neurological—from drowsiness to confusion, seizures and coma in severe cases
- Muscular—weakness and muscle spasm
- Respiratory—tachypnoea
- Prostate—potential prostatic enlargement in cases of obstructed outflow
- Eyes—retinopathy secondary to diabetes or hypertension
- Abdomen—renal enlargement, particularly with polycystic kidneys, or small scarred kidneys with chronic kidney damage
- Signs of underlying illness contributing to CKF, e.g. diabetes

- Urine tests:
  - Test for glucose, blood, protein and albuminuria (initially with a dipstick). The albumin:creatinine ratio (ACR) is now used to help establish the severity of CKF. ACR on a random spot urine sample is carried out to further quantify proteinuria (albuminuria). Where this is abnormal, repeat specimen a few weeks later to determine whether it is persistent. If positive, two further tests for ACR are done in the next 2 months. Albuminuria is stratified according to International Diabetes Federation guidelines[9] as shown in Table 46.2.

TABLE 46.2 International Diabetes Federation guidelines[8] on albuminuria

	Urinary ACR (mg/mmol)	
	Women	**Men**
Normoalbuminuria	< 3.5	< 2.5
Microalbuminuria	3.5–35	2.5–25
Macroalbuminuria	> 35	> 25

  - Haematuria—exclude non-glomerular haematuria such as menstruation, urinary tract infection, urinary neoplasm, calculus, prostatic disease. Glomerular haematuria is related to kidney disease. Persistent haematuria or haematuria with other indicators of kidney damage requires investigation.
- Electrolytes:
  - sodium, chloride, potassium, calcium, phosphate, bicarbonate.
- Renal function tests:
  - urea, creatinine, creatinine clearance
  - eGFR.
- Full blood examination.
- Blood pressure assessment.
- Ultrasound imaging of the kidney and urinary tract
- Further tests as indicated, such as looking for the cause of the CKF or assessing general wellbeing—blood glucose, urate, lipids, ECG, lupus serology, iron studies.
- Further tests generally ordered by a nephrologist—could include kidney biopsy, immunological tests.

Kidney function is measured by the eGFR, measured in mL/min. Creatinine is the most commonly used compound used to calculate the eGFR. The formula used to calculate eGFR is:

$$eGFR = \frac{\text{urine concentration of creatinine} \times \text{urine flow}}{\text{plasma concentration of creatinine}}$$

The eGFR varies with age, gender and size, and so what would be considered normal kidney function needs to be interpreted in light of these parameters.

CKF is divided into five stages according to the eGFR:

1 > 90: normal
2 60–90: mild
3 30–60: moderate
4 15–30: severe
5 < 15: end-stage.

Patients with moderate levels of kidney failure or above should be referred to a renal specialist (Box 46.4) for advice and co-management.

BOX 46.4 Indications for referral to a nephrologist

- eGFR < 30 mL/min/1.73 m^2
- Unexplained decline in renal function (> 15% reduction in eGFR in 3 months)
- Proteinuria > 1 g/24 h
- Glomerular haematuria (particularly if proteinuria is present)
- CKD and hypertension unable to achieve or maintain at target
- Unexplained anaemia (Hb < 100 g/L) with eGFR

Integrative management

The management of CKF can be complex and prolonged, and needs specialist referral, close monitoring and review by a multidisciplinary team. The following are some of the key principles of managing CKF.

- *Treat underlying conditions* that may be contributing to or exacerbating the CKF—these commonly include hypertension, diabetic control or the cessation of some medications.
- *Assess and manage cardiovascular risk factors* such as hypertension, cholesterol, smoking and diabetes. Optimal management of these risk factors slows the progression of CKF (Box 46.5 lists treatment targets).
- *Control blood pressure*—ACE inhibitors are first-line for management of hypertension, and multiple medications may be required to achieve optimal blood pressure control. If hypertension is resistant to medication, consider renal artery stenosis.
- For eGFR 30–59, an ACE inhibitor or ARB agent used singly or in combination reduces proteinuria/albuminuria significantly and is associated with improved outcomes.
- *Electrolyte balance*—particularly phosphate and potassium. Calcium carbonate can be used for patients with high phosphate levels because it binds to phosphate. Avoid potassium-sparing diuretics.
- *Fluid balance* is important, being careful to avoid dehydration, which can further impair kidney

BOX 46.5 Treatment targets

- Maintain blood pressure < 130/80 mmHg. Maintain BP <125/75 if proteinuria > 1 g/24 h or diabetes present.
- Proteinuria will usually halve with blockade of angiotensin and this has a reno-protective effect, so ACE inhibitor or ARB are first-line medications.
- Maintain total cholesterol < 4.0 mmol/L, LDL < 2.5 mmol/L.
- Pre-prandial blood glucose 4.4–6.7 mmol/L, HbA_{1c} < 7.0% with lifestyle management, oral hypoglycaemics, insulin (see Ch 26, Diabetes).

function, and over-hydration, which can exacerbate oedema and CCF.

- *Manage intercurrent illnesses and risk factors*, particularly urinary tract infections, cardiovascular disease and diabetes.
- *Nutrition* can be a significant concern and care should be taken to have a low-protein diet and avoid excess intake of electrolytes such as potassium and sodium—advise low-sodium foods and no added salt. Referral to an accredited practising dietician with experience in renal disease is appropriate.
- *Avoid hydrogenated vegetable oils*, because they are high in trans-fatty acids.
- *Manage anaemia* with adequate iron and erythropoetin.
- *Manage symptoms*, especially nausea.
- *Prescribe medications with caution*, because of the potential for many drugs to exacerbate CKF, such as those mentioned previously, or to accumulate due to a longer half-life. Some examples of drugs that do accumulate in those with CKF are provided below, but it is always advisable to check drug information sheets before prescribing any medications to patients with significant levels of CKF. A lower dose of these medications would generally be recommended if a decision is made to prescribe them, taking care to monitor the patient closely for side effects. Examples:
  - antibiotics—penicillin, co-trimoxazole, flagyl, quinolones
  - cardiovascular drugs—atenolol, sotalol, digoxin
  - diabetic medications—insulin, sufonylureas, metformin
  - lithium
  - codeine
  - methotrexate.
- *General support for the patient and the family*, including psychological support and, commonly, assistance with issues such as finances and employment.
- *A healthy lifestyle* should be encouraged in as much as it is possible. This will assist with maintaining wellbeing as well as slowing decline in kidney function.
- *Dialysis or kidney transplant* are the last resort for patients with end-stage kidney failure. When more conservative measures have failed and kidney function continues to decline, leading to a level of symptoms that is having a significant impact on the patient's life, these options should be discussed and an assessment made by the specialist team as to the appropriateness of the various options available. Although they are not without their complications, risks and expense, when successful they can often lead to a rapid and significant improvement in quality of life.

Prevention

- Cease and avoid smoking.
- Maintain healthy BMI.
- Maintain blood pressure in normal range.
- Prevent diabetes or manage existing diabetes.
- Maintain waist circumference < 94 cm for males, < 80 cm for females.
- Encourage at least 30 minutes exercise daily.
- Limit dietary salt intake.
- Moderate alcohol consumption.
- Immunise against influenza and pneumococcal disease if diabetes or end-stage kidney disease present.
- Avoid NSAIDs and COX-2 inhibitors.

BLADDER CANCER

INCIDENCE

Bladder cancer is the second most common urological cancer. Incidence rates vary worldwide and are highest in Egypt, North America and Western Europe. Bladder tumours are three times more common in men and are most often diagnosed after age 55.

AETIOLOGY

Transitional cell carcinoma (TCC) is the most common type of bladder cancer (> 90%). The most important risk factors associated with bladder cancer are cigarette smoking and occupational exposure to urothelial carcinogens (e.g. aromatic amines, polycyclic hydrocarbons) such as in the textile and dye industries. Other possible causes include analgesic abuse, cyclophosphamide exposure and previous radiation. The bladder is the most common site of TCC occurrence, but it is important to note that the entire urothelium is at risk of neoplastic changes.

Squamous cell carcinomas of the bladder are rare (5%) and are associated with chronic inflammation, such as with stones or schistosomiasis. Adenocarcinomas are even rarer (1%) and may be associated with persistent urachal remnants.

SIGNS AND SYMPTOMS

The most common presentation is painless haematuria, which is typically gross. Other urinary symptoms such as frequency, urgency and dysuria are less common, and if present indicate associated in-situ carcinoma or muscle-invasive disease.

INVESTIGATIONS

Endoscopic examination of the lower urinary tract (cystoscopy) is the diagnostic standard for bladder cancer, and is combined with urinary studies and radiological imaging. Urinary cytology has only moderate sensitivity but good specificity for the detection of urothelial cancers, and is more useful in post-therapy surveillance.

Radiological studies including ultrasound, intravenous urography (IVU) and CT urography may detect the presence of a tumour but cannot replace cystoscopy. Their utility is in the staging of disease extent and assessing for upper urinary tract pathology.

THERAPEUTICS

Transurethral resection of bladder tumour (TURBT) in combination with bimanual palpation provides local disease staging and in many cases is therapeutic. Bladder cancer may be classified according to appearance (papillary or sessile) or whether it is superficial or muscle-invasive.

TURBT is essential in determining the grade (low or high) and local stage of the tumour (TNM classification), which are used in deciding on prognosis and treatment. TNM stages are as follows:

- Ta papillary, urothelial confined
- Tis carcinoma in-situ
- T1 lamina propria invasion
- T2 muscle wall invasion
- T3 extension through bladder wall
- T4 invasion of surrounding organs.

Non-muscle-invasive tumours are treated with complete TURBT. This is followed by periodic surveillance cystoscopy and urinary cytology for life. Tumours that are at higher risk of disease progression (i.e. high tumour grade, T1 or associated with Tis) should be considered for Bacillus Calmette-Guérin (BCG) intravesical therapy. BCG therapy is effective in reducing recurrence rate and disease progression.

Muscle invasive disease is treated by radical cystectomy and urinary diversion with an ileal conduit or a neo-bladder in select patients. Radiation therapy is an option for patients desiring bladder preservation, poor surgical candidates and those with unresectable disease. Patients with unresectable disease or metastases are treated with chemotherapy.

PREVENTION

Smoking cessation reduces the risk of developing bladder cancer, with a greater than 30% risk reduction in 1–4 years, and 60% after 25 years. The risk, however, never decreases to that of non-smokers.

RENAL CELL CANCER

INCIDENCE

Renal cell carcinomas are adenocarcinomas of renal tubular cells. They represent 2–3% of all adult malignancies and are the most lethal urological cancer.

AETIOLOGY

Renal cell carcinomas (RCC) are more common after middle age and in men. There is some association with cigarette smoking. There are a number of familial syndromes associated with increased risk of RCC, most notably Von Hippel Lindau's disease (up to 50% develop RCC).

SIGNS AND SYMPTOMS

The 'classic' presentation of RCC, with flank pain, haematuria and a palpable abdominal mass, is no longer common. These features herald advanced disease. The majority of renal tumours are now incidental discoveries on abdominal imaging carried out for other reasons. Less commonly, patients may present with a paraneoplastic syndrome, such as hypertension, anaemia, pyrexia of unknown origin (PUO), abnormal liver function tests, hypercalcaemia or erythrocytosis. These result from tumour endocrine activity with the production of renin, parathyroid-like peptides, erythropoietin and so on. The plethora of possible presentations has resulted in the coining of the term the 'internist's tumour'.

INVESTIGATIONS

High-quality triple phase CT scan of the abdomen and pelvis is the imaging modality of choice for renal tumours. The presence of a solid enhancing renal parenchymal lesion is considered an RCC until proved otherwise. Imaging should also exclude nodal disease and bony, liver, adrenal or venous involvement. The presence of a normal contralateral kidney without synchronous lesion is also assessed. Chest imaging with X-rays or CT should be done to assess lung metastases. Baseline blood studies including FBC, renal function tests, LFTs and calcium should be drawn. Renal tumour biopsy is rarely indicated but may be used to assess atypical lesions, such as with suspected renal lymphoma.

Cystic lesions are treated according to their level of complexity; this is determined by the presence of septations, calcification and solid components. Simple cysts are uniformly benign and require no therapy unless symptomatic. Complex cysts will require either surveillance with follow-up imaging or resection, depending on the level of complexity.

THERAPEUTICS

Radical nephrectomy is the standard treatment for RCC. Partial nephrectomy is an option for smaller (< 4 cm) exophytic tumours and may be mandatory where radical nephrectomy will result in renal insufficiency, such as in a solitary kidney. Cancer-specific survival rates for partial nephrectomy are equivalent to radical nephrectomy for treating small renal tumours. Both radical and partial nephrectomy can be accomplished open or laparoscopically. Unfortunately, up to a third of patients present with metastatic disease.

Organ-confined tumours of < 7 cm carry a good long-term prognosis. Solitary metastatic deposits can be resected along with nephrectomy, with reasonable outcome. Locally invasive tumours or those with nodal or metastatic deposits are associated with very poor survival rates. In situations where a single metastatic deposit is present, nephrectomy may be combined with resection of the metastasis, with reasonable outcome. Venous extension is not such a poor prognostic factor and even when extensive can be excised at nephrectomy. Renal cell carcinomas are resistant to radiotherapy and chemotherapy. For patients with advanced disease at diagnosis, tyrosine kinase inhibitors (sunitinib and sorafenib) have resulted in disease stabilisation or even regression, but are not curative.

PREVENTION

No preventative measures currently exist.

TESTICULAR CANCER

INCIDENCE

Testicular cancer represents 1–1.5% of male tumours and 5% of urological tumours in general. The vast majority are germ cell tumours (GCTs) and can be classified histologically as pure seminomas or non-seminomas (NSGCT). Presentation is most common in the third or fourth decade of life.

AETIOLOGY

Risk factors for the development of testicular cancer include undescended testes (cryptorchidism), familial history, Klinefelter's syndrome, infertility and the presence of tumour in the contralateral testicle. Testicular cancer is more common in men of Scandinavian descent.

SIGNS AND SYMPTOMS

The most common presentation is the casual discovery of a unilateral testicular mass. Pain is reported in only 20–25% of cases. Occasionally scrotal trauma leads to the detection of a mass. Rarely, diagnosis is made during the work-up of secondary gynaecomastia or abdominal discomfort from retroperitoneal nodal involvement.

Physical examination should aim to characterise the scrotal mass as well as look for distant disease (abdominal masses, supraclavicular nodes).

INVESTIGATIONS

Scrotal ultrasound is invaluable in evaluating a testicular mass. It has excellent diagnostic accuracy for testis tumours and can exclude possible differentials (i.e. epididymitis and hernia).

The tumour markers human chorionic gonadotrophin (HCG), alpha-fetoprotein (aFP) and lactate dehydrogenase (LDH) are useful for the diagnosis, staging and prognosis of testicular GCTs. These markers are also used in post-treatment surveillance and may aid therapeutic decisions.

Imaging is critical in the staging of GCTs. Testicular GCTs spread in an ordered manner to the retroperitoneal nodes adjacent to the great vessels, with distant nodal or haematogenous dissemination occurring thereafter. Contrast CT scan should be done to assess for involvement of the retroperitoneum, mediastinum or visceral organs. PET scans are not indicated for the initial diagnosis but may be useful in assessing treatment response.

THERAPEUTICS

Radical/inguinal orchidectomy, which involves the excision of the testicle within its tunical coverings, is the initial treatment for localised testicular cancer. Surgery provides local staging and histological classification, which determines further treatment.

Post orchidectomy, patients with locally confined (Stage I) seminoma may be managed with single-agent chemotherapy (carboplatin), radiotherapy to the retroperitoneum or surveillance. Surveillance is best suited for those without adverse risk factors on pathological assessment (i.e. tumour size > 4 cm or Rete testis involvement). Seminomas with small-volume retroperitoneal disease can be treated with either combination chemotherapy (bleomycin, etoposide and cisplatin (BEP)) or radiation. Bulky nodes or distant disease is treated with chemotherapy (BEP).

Patients with locally confined NSGCT are usually treated with adjuvant chemotherapy (BEP) or retroperitoneal lymph node dissection (RPLND); those without adverse histological features may be selected for surveillance. Retroperitoneal nodal involvement is treated with chemotherapy and RPLND for residual disease post chemotherapy.

Most patients with GCTs enjoy a favourable prognosis. Non-pulmonary visceral metastases and persistently elevated tumour markers post orchidectomy are poor prognostic factors.

PREVENTION

- Correction of undescended testes in children.
- The excision of undescended testes in post-pubertal men is recommended, to prevent the subsequent development of testicular cancers.

ADRENAL DISEASES

Paired adrenal glands lie adjacent to the upper aspect of each kidney. These glands are composed of an

TABLE 46.3 Causes of adrenal diseases

Non-neoplastic	Neoplastic
Adrenal cyst	Adrenal adenoma
Adrenocortical hyperplasia	Adrenal carcinoma
Haematoma/abscess	Phaeochromocytoma
Myelolipoma	Metastatic deposit

outer cortex (mesodermal origin) and inner medulla (neuroectodermal origin). Adrenal cortical function involves the production of aldosterone, cortisol and adrenal androgens as part of normal homeostasis. The adrenal medulla is composed of chromaffin cells, which produce the catecholamines epinephrine and norepinephrine.

The adrenal gland may be the site of a variety of benign and malignant diseases (Table 46.3).

INCIDENCE

Most adrenal tumours are now discovered incidentally on abdominal imaging. Estimates are that 1–5% of abdominal CT scans will detect an adrenal mass. When an adrenal lesion is detected in a patient with a history of malignancy, 75% of these lesions prove to be metastatic deposits, and two-thirds of lesions found in patients without a cancer history are benign.

AETIOLOGY

While the majority of adrenal lesions are of unknown aetiology, there are a few genetic syndromes associated with the development of adrenal tumours. For example, phaeochromocytomas may be associated with von Hippel Lindau disease, MEN 2 or neurofibromatosis.

SIGNS AND SYMPTOMS

Functional tumours may present with symptoms associated with hormone production. Cortisol excess produces Cushing's syndrome, with obesity, hypertension, muscle weakness, cutaneous striae and glucose intolerance. Conn's syndrome results from aldosterone excess, with hypertension, hypokalaemia, polydipsia and polyuria. Phaeochromocytoma is a rare cause of hypertension that may be paroxysmal and associated with headaches, palpitations, sweating, anxiety and chest pain.

Adrenal carcinomas are rare aggressive tumours commonly presenting with pain and constitutional symptoms. They typically secrete multiple compounds and may present with virilisation or feminisation.

INVESTIGATIONS

Imaging with CT or MRI defines the size and character of the adrenal lesion. Adenomas tend to have low signal intensity due to their high lipid content. Myelolipomas and cysts are usually easily identified on routine imaging. Adrenal carcinomas tend to be heterogenous with calcification and they have high signal intensity on T2-weighted MRI.

Following the diagnosis of an adrenal lesion, functional studies are indicated to detect secretory activity. Cortisol production is assessed with 24-hour urine samples. Elevated urinary levels of the catecholamine metabolites metanephrines and vanillyl mandelic acid (VMA) are found with phaeochromocytoma. Aldosterone excess results in HTN with hypokalaemia and an abnormal renin:aldosterone ratio. Dexamethasone suppression testing may be required to differentiate pituitary pathology (Cushing's disease), adrenal hyperplasia or adenoma.

THERAPEUTICS

All biochemically active lesions require surgical excision. Special attention should be paid to preoperative alpha-adrenergic blockade for phaeochromocytomas, to avoid hypertensive emergencies, and steroid replacement in Cushing's syndrome, to limit adrenal insufficiency.

The majority of asymptomatic non-functional lesions are benign; however, larger adenomas share imaging features with carcinomas. It has been shown that more than 90% of adrenal carcinomas are larger than 6 cm at diagnosis and adrenal tumours less than 4 cm have a 2% chance of being malignant. Tumours that are larger than 5 cm at diagnosis and those with suspicious features on T2-weighted MRI are possibly carcinomas and should be excised. Other tumours may be observed.

Adrenal tumours may be resected via open or laparoscopic approach. Suspected adrenocortical carcinomas are best dealt with open due to their tendency for local invasion, which may require en-bloc resection of surrounding organs.

PREVENTION

No preventative strategies exist.

PENILE DISORDERS

Penile disorders may be classified anatomically and functionally as:

- disorders affecting the prepuce
- disorders affecting the urethral meatus
- disorders affecting the glans
- disorders affecting the penile shaft
- sexually transmitted infections
- sexual and functional disorders.

DISORDERS OF THE PREPUCE

Phimosis is stenosis of the preputial orifice that prevents retraction of the foreskin over the glans. This may be considered primary (childhood) or secondary (previously retractible). Congenital adhesions between the glans and prepuce are present at birth and tend to loosen with age; about 90% of boys have a retractible foreskin by the age of 3 years. Inability to retract the foreskin persists in 1% of pubertal males. Pathological phimosis occurs from trauma or infection, with a resultant fibrotic ring. Recurrent infections of the glans and preputial sac (balanoposthitis) may cause and result from phimosis. Infections may result from poor foreskin hygiene (failure to retract the foreskin and clean underlying smegma daily) and are more common in diabetics.

Treatment may be initially conservative, with the application of steroid creams. Circumcision is indicated where adult phimosis prevents normal hygiene.

Paraphimosis is the inability to replace a retracted foreskin. This may occur after forcible retraction of a phimotic prepuce or where the prepuce has been left retracted (e.g. post catheterisation). The resultant constricting band can result in a vicious cycle of congestion and oedema of the glans and prepuce, with the potential for necrosis when severe. Treatment is by prompt replacement of the foreskin. This usually requires manual decompression of the oedema and occasionally a dorsal slit under local anaesthetic.

A short frenulum results in ventral deviation of the glans when the prepuce is retracted. This may result in tears during cleaning or intercourse. Treatment is usually by circumcision, although frenuloplasty may be sufficient.

Circumcision is the surgical excision of the prepuce. It is most commonly performed on male neonates for social or religious reasons. Circumcision may be medically indicated for recurrent balanoposthitis, recurrent UTIs associated with abnormal anatomy and in secondary phimosis. Although the procedural risks are low, there is an increased risk of meatal stenosis, concealed penis and the potential for excessive skin removal or damage to the glans. Potential benefits include some protection against sexually transmitted diseases and penile cancer as well as cosmetic considerations. Circumcision is contraindicated in the presence of congenital penile anomalies (e.g. hypospadias), as the prepuce may be required for reconstructive surgery.

DISORDERS AFFECTING THE URETHRAL MEATUS

The external urethral meatus is a sagittal slit that is the narrowest point of the urethra. The urethra just proximal to the meatus is dilated and this configuration produces rotational streaming and focuses the issuing urinary stream.

Hypospadias is malpositioning of the urethral meatus to the undersurface of the penis. Congenital hypospadias are most commonly distal (glandular or coronal). More proximal (severe) hypospadias may be penile or perineal. This disorder is associated with an incomplete foreskin and a ventral band connecting the meatus to its normal position, with a resulting ventral chordee.

Epispadias, the reverse disorder, is much less common and is usually associated with gross defects of fusion of the anterior bladder and urethra and of the pelvic girdle (extroversion).

Meatal strictures may be congenital or acquired. A meatal ulcer is a common problem in infancy and is virtually confined to circumcised infants. Meatal strictures can follow ammoniacal dermatitis (nappy rash) in babies. Any urethral discharge should be noted, its character observed and a bacteriological swab taken for smear and culture. Meatal strictures may be treated with simple dilation or meatoplasty.

DISORDERS AFFECTING THE GLANS

Discharge from the prepuce with inflammatory skin changes suggests an underlying disorder. The glans is examined after gently retracting the prepuce fully.

Balanitis and balanoposthitis are often non-specific but may be due to a number of specific venereal infections or secondary to malignant or premalignant conditions. Treatment with antibiotic or antifungal creams may hasten resolution. Recurrent episodes should prompt urological consultation.

Penile carcinoma is an uncommon condition that is largely preventable with adequate penile hygiene.

Premalignant lesions of the glans include:

- leukoplakia—an area of whitish, painless indurated epithelium secondary to chronic balanitis
- erythroplasia of Queyrat (or Paget's disease)—an indurated plaque of epithelium of similar origin with a violaceous hue, which is similar to Bowen's disease of the skin elsewhere and indicates carcinoma-in-situ of the glans, prepuce or shaft.

Penile carcinoma usually starts as a warty or nodular growth on the glans, coronal sulcus or the inner aspect of the prepuce. It may resemble genital warts. Progressive growth is associated with purulent and bloody discharge. The lesion eventually develops the typical appearance of a squamous cell cancer, with elevation, induration and fungative ulceration. Associated groin nodes may be inflammatory or malignant.

Treatment is by surgical excision with an adequate margin, usually a partial penectomy. Palpable nodes may also need excision based on the stage and grade of the primary lesion or their persistence after antibiotic therapy.

DISORDERS AFFECTING THE PENILE SHAFT

Subcutaneous induration of the shaft with a firm, non-tender plaque of fibrous tissue in the fascia surrounding the corpus cavernosum on one or both sides is due to *Peyronie's disease*, a condition of unknown cause akin to Dupuytren's disease and which results in irreversible damage of the tunica albuginea of the corpora cavernosa. Peyronie's disease is one of the causes of chordee during erection. The natural history of the disease is an active and painful phase of plaque development and then a quiescent phase. The active phase is treated symptomatically and no further treatment of the quiescent phase is required unless chordee that limits voiding in the upright position or sexual penetration results from the plaque.

A *fractured penis* defines rupture of the corpora cavernosa due to forcible bending. This occurs exclusively with an erect penis and may involve one or both corpora and in severe cases the urethra as well. It is most commonly the result of intercourse but may occur with self-manipulation. The typical history is that of trauma with an audible 'cracking' sound followed by immediate loss of erection and the onset of penile bruising and swelling. The diagnosis is made clinically. Surgical repair of the corporal rent is undertaken to prevent penile angulation, pain and erectile dysfunction.

SEXUALLY TRANSMITTED INFECTIONS

The management of sexually transmitted infections (STIs) requires up-to-date knowledge of diagnostic and treatment practices, awareness of contact tracing and compassionate, non-judgmental care. An increasing number of patients with STIs have human immunodeficiency virus (HIV) infection, with either overt disease or positive antibody titre. All patients who present with a suspected STI should be screened for HIV and hepatitis B and C.

As a general rule it should be assumed that an ulcer on the glans penis is a syphilitic ulcer until proved otherwise. Care to prevent cross-infection should be taken. Syphilitic ulcers take about 4 weeks to appear from the time of contact. The chancre is usually painless. The lesion first appears as a firm reddened macule, usually in the coronal sulcus which, in most cases, undergoes ulceration and eventually regresses. The inguinal lymph nodes are invariably enlarged and are firm, discrete and mobile. Patients are not toxic at the time of penile ulceration but become so during the secondary stage of the disease (about 6–8 weeks after the appearance of the penile lesion). The causal organism, *Treponema pallidum*, is recognised by dark-field examination of exudate obtained from the lesion. The diagnosis may also be made by positive serology.

Pain during micturition with a purulent discharge is commonly due to gonococcal urethritis. The causative organism is *Neisseria gonorrhoeae*. Infection often also involves the epididymis, seminal vesicles, prostate and bladder. Urethral stricture is a late complication.

Ulceration, particularly if painful, may be due to herpes simplex infection. This viral infection starts as a patch of erythema on the inner surface of the prepuce or on the glans, which develops vesicles and pustules that, on abrasion, form small ulcers. The diagnosis is made cytologically by finding the characteristic 'ground glass' inclusion in giant cells from the involved epithelium. The common venereal viral warts (condylomata acuminata) occasionally ulcerate. Rare causes of ulceration include chancroid (soft chancre). Chancroid is an acute ulcerative lesion with lymphadenopathy caused by *Haemophilus ducreyi*. Other diseases diagnosed by smear and culture are lymphogranuloma venereum (Chlamydia) and granuloma inguinale (Donovan bacillus). These infections are more common in tropical countries. Penile candidiasis presents as an itchy balanitis with white plaques.

Sexually transmitted infections usually respond to antibiotics. Syphilis is treated with penicillin. Azithromycin 1 g orally in a single dose or doxycycline 100 mg orally twice a day for 7 days is the treatment of choice for non-gonococcal urethritis in men or other infection with *Chlamydia trachomatis*. Uncomplicated gonococcal infections are treated with ceftriaxone. Herpes genitalis is treated with aciclovir. Chancroid is treated with sulfonamides, granuloma venereum and inguinale with tetracycline, and venereal warts with topical anti-viral cream or local diathermy excision. Treatment of the patient's partner is important in preventing recurrence.

SEXUAL AND FUNCTIONAL DISORDERS

Impotence is a common problem and is defined as failure to obtain or maintain an erection strong enough for satisfactory sexual activity. Organic causes can be grouped by aetiology and are most commonly:

- vasculogenic—associated with and having the same risk factors as generalised vascular disease
- traumatic—particularly to the pelvic nerves and vasculature (including surgery for prostate cancer)
- neurogenic—including spinal cord injury and multiple sclerosis
- endocrine—including diabetes, where the autonomic neuropathy and vascular insufficiency result in loss of erections
- any debilitating disease (anaemia, carcinoma)
- old age.

Many drugs (alcohol, opiates, hypotensives, phenothiazines and sedatives) are thought to be contributory, although the association is often poorly understood. Functional causes associated with psychogenic factors are not as common as a primary cause; these are usually diagnoses of exclusion once organic causes have been excluded.

Management of impotence has been revolutionised by the development of phosphodiesterase type-5 (PDE5) enzyme inhibitors. These drugs act in the breakdown of cyclic guanosine monophosphate (cGMP), which causes smooth muscle relaxation in the arterioles of the corpora cavernosa, hence increasing intracavernosal blood flow and invoking erection. These drugs (sildenafil, tadalafil and vardenafil) can be taken by most patients, except where there is concomitant nitrate use for the management of angina. There is a small incidence of minor side effects such as headache and facial flushing. Initial management of impotence may therefore take place in the primary care setting where, after careful history and examination to exclude organic pathologies that should otherwise be treated, a trial of PDE5 inhibitors may take place. Local intracavernosal injections of a vasodilator, such as alprostadil or a papaverine-based mixture, can be used in patients who do not respond to PDE5 drugs. Long-term compliance with this treatment is poor. Implanting an inflatable penile prosthetic device, which has high satisfaction and efficacy rates, is suitable for men who want a long-term 'cure' of erectile dysfunction.

Priapism is a persistent erection, not associated with sexual stimulation, lasting more than 4 hours. It may be divided into veno-occlusive (low-flow) and arterial (high-flow) states. The corpora cavernosa are stiff and distended and painful; the corpus spongiosum and glans are flaccid. *Low-flow priapism* occurs where there is venous stasis, which can be due to multiple causes, including persistent spasm of the venous smooth muscle sphincters that maintain erection, after use of intracavernosal injection for impotence, conditions causing hyper-coagulable states such as sickle cell anaemia, multiple myeloma or leukaemia, other malignancy, and other drugs including anticoagulants, phenothiazine, fluoxetine and cocaine. *High-flow priapism* results from an arteriovenous anomaly after pelvic, perineal or penile trauma and, unlike low-flow, is generally not painful early on. If prolonged, priapism of either cause will lead to thrombosis of the veins draining erectile tissue. Subsequently, even though priapism is relieved, there may be permanent impotence.

If initial treatment with cold showers and oral pseudoephedrine fails, then intracavernosal injections with vasoactive agents such as phenylephrine (with cardiac monitoring) should be attempted. If these measures fail, a shunt between one of the corpora cavernosa and the corpus spongiosum or between corpus cavernosum and saphenous vein should be carried out within 6 hours. Prompt therapy is required, to reduce permanent erectile dysfunction.

RESOURCES

emedicine, urology articles (an online resource for patients and doctors), http://emedicine.medscape.com/urology

European Association of Urology, urological guidelines (authoritative and much used), http://www.uroweb.org/guidelines/online-guidelines/

Kidney Health Australia, Chronic kidney disease management in general practice, http://www.kidney.org.au/LinkClick.aspx?fileticket=dSUlcQgPd6o%3d&tabid=635&mid=1584

Society for Chronic Pelvic Pain and Interstitial Cystitis, http://ucpps.org/

REFERENCES

1 Goldfarb DS, Coe FL. Prevention of recurrent nephrolithiasis. American Family Physician 2009; 15 November. Online. Available: http://www.aafp.org/afp/991115ap/2269.html

2 Sea J, Poon KS, McVary KT. Review of exercise and the risk of benign prostatic hyperplasia. Phys Sportsmed 2009; 37(4):75–83.

3 Wilt TJ, MacDonald R, Ishani A. Beta-sitosterol for the treatment of benign prostatic hyperplasia: a systematic review. BJU Int 1999; 83(9):976–983.

4 Kaplan SA, Volpe MA, Te AE. A prospective, 1-year trial using saw palmetto versus finasteride in the treatment of category III prostatitis/chronic pelvic pain syndrome. J Urol 2004; 171:284–288.

5 Wilt T, Ishani A, MacDonald R et al. *Pygeum africanum* for benign prostatic hyperplasia. Cochrane Database Syst Rev 2002; 1:CD001044.

6 Konrad L, Müller HH, Lenz C et al. Antiproliferative effect on human prostate cancer cells by a stinging nettle root (*Urtica dioica*) extract. Planta Med 2000; 66(1):44–47.

7 Shoskes DA, Kannan Manickam AE. Herbal and complementary medicine in chronic prostatitis. World J Urol 2003; 21:109–113.

8 Elist J. Effects of pollen extract preparation Prostat/Poltit on lower urinary tract symptoms in patients with chronic nonbacterial prostatitis/chronic pelvic pain syndrome: a randomized, double-blind, placebo-controlled study. Urology 2006; 67:60–63.

9 International Diabetes Federation. Clinical Guidelines Task Force. Global guideline for type 2 diabetes. Brussels: IDF; 2005.

chapter 47

Weight problems and eating disorders

INTRODUCTION AND OVERVIEW

Eating disorders are characterised by a preoccupation with thoughts about body weight, food, eating or exercise and a need for the person to control their weight or eating or exercise in order to stop intense negative feelings. These thoughts interfere with all aspects of the person's daily life. This description could also include people who are very obese (BMI > 35 kg/m^2) as they cannot tolerate the feeling of energy restriction that would be consistent with gentle weight loss, and it includes the third of obese people who binge eat.

The content of this chapter is limited to anorexia- and bulimia-like disorders. These eating disorders are characterised by the use of inappropriate behaviours to control body weight and feelings, as evidenced by low body weight, high body weight, extreme weight-control behaviours such as vomiting and starvation, excessive exercise and binge eating.

Eating disorders can also be thought of as 'weight disorders' as body weight is the major preoccupation, or 'energy control disorders' as they are associated with inappropriate energy control behaviours that may be associated with high, normal or low body weight. There may be only one eating disorder rather than the three or four cited by the American Psychiatric Association, as the differences are often based on artificial divisions, such as body weight or the frequency of the behaviours employed. It is often easiest to communicate about patients by describing their behaviours and their body weight. For example:

- Patient A has an eating disorder characterised by low body weight, binge eating and self-induced vomiting.
- Patient B has a normal body weight, exercises excessively and compulsively, and restricts her food intake episodically.
- Patient C is overweight, binge eats in the evening but does not eat during the day.

CURRENT AMERICAN PSYCHIATRIC ASSOCIATION CRITERIA

The American Psychiatric Association (APA) criteria are being revised at present, and amenorrhoea will be removed from the criteria for anorexia nervosa. The current official APA diagnoses are anorexia nervosa, bulimia nervosa and eating disorder not otherwise specified (EDNOS), and a binge-eating disorder is proposed. The borders between these diagnoses are blurry and a patient can have all the criteria for more than one of these eating disorders or move from one diagnosis to another. To help overcome this problem, the diagnoses are made by following a hierarchy, with anorexia nervosa taking precedence over bulimia nervosa and EDNOS being the 'leftover' category. Binge-eating disorder can be considered separately or as part of EDNOS.

For communication with healthcare professionals, EDNOS patients may be described as having an anorexia nervosa-like disorder, or a bulimia nervosa-like disorder or a non-specific disorder associated with other behaviours such as chewing and spitting, or a chaotic pattern of any mix of these behaviours. Despite EDNOS patients' failure to fulfill the anorexia or bulimia nervosa diagnoses, they can be extremely unwell, both medically and psychologically.

BACKGROUND

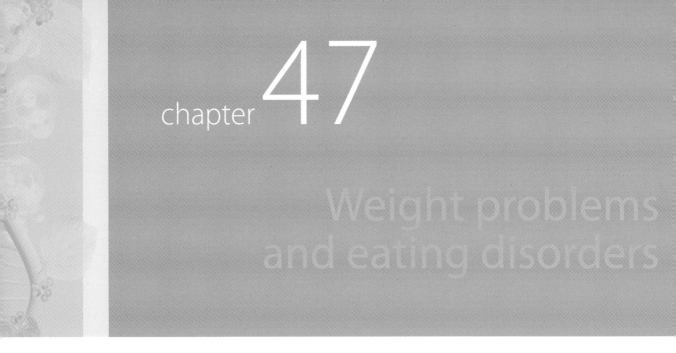

Anorexia nervosa was first described by Sir William Withey Gull in 1873, although he mistakenly assumed that the emaciated woman he discussed had no appetite. Binge eating among anorexia nervosa patients was described in 1979 and the first diagnostic criteria for bulimia nervosa was proposed in 1979. The prevalence of eating disorders is not increasing but the awareness of these problems by lay people and healthcare professionals has risen exponentially in the past 40 years. The presentation of patients can be slightly different in different cultures and appears to be changing. The emphasis on body image, with adolescent women wanting to be like skinny models and film stars, is declining. Currently the governments and public health professionals in most developed countries are attempting to educate people to try to combat the increasing incidence of obesity in all age groups of people. As a result, more adolescents presenting with eating disorders are aiming to 'eat healthily and exercise more', in contrast to 'lose weight for a perfect body image'.

PREVALENCE

Current information suggests that the figures in Box 47.1 give a reasonable estimate of the prevalence of the eating disorders in women aged 13–30 years. Not all these people have sought treatment for their eating disorder and the majority are not assessed and treated by eating disorder specialists.

The eating disorders occur mostly in post-pubertal women. Approximately 1 in 15 eating-disordered people are male, although an increasing number of young males are being diagnosed with the condition in recent years. Onset is usually during adolescence or early adulthood; the peak incidence of anorexia nervosa is between 14 and 18 years, and the peak incidence for bulimia nervosa is from 18 to 25 years. Later appearance suggests that the onset is secondary to another psychiatric or medical illness.

The estimated prevalence of anorexia-nervosa-like problems is probably 3–4% and bulimia-nervosa-like 6–8%. These women are included in the EDNOS prevalence in Box 47.1. The prevalence of binge-eating disorder is thought to be 1–4%, with one in three being male, but this may not include older men and women, and may include adolescent sufferers of any or all of the other eating disorders.

AETIOLOGY

There is no consensus on why eating disorders occur. There are many explanations and these include genetic, physiological, social and psychological perspectives (Fig 47.1) and involve theories relating to childhood and adolescent development. Weight loss precedes the onset of the eating disorder. The initial weight loss may be intentional and in response to post-pubertal weight gain in women, or it may occur for other reasons such as illness or change in exercise routine.

BOX 47.1 Prevalence of eating disorders by age 30

Anorexia nervosa: 1% (range 0.5–2%)
Bulimia nervosa: 2% (range 1–3%)
EDNOS: 12% (range 8–23%)

(EDNOS: eating disorder not otherwise specified; includes binge-eating disorder.)

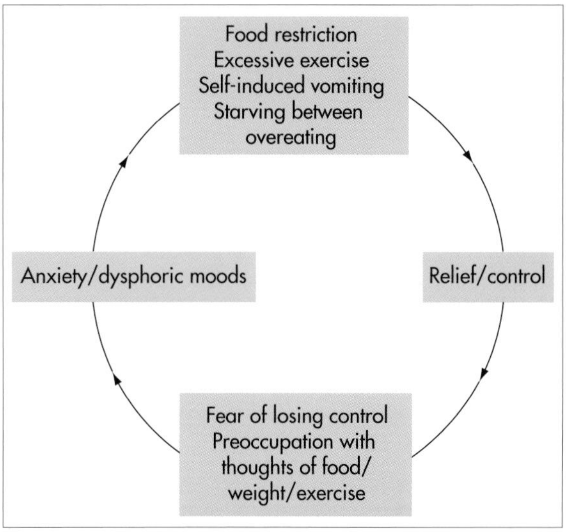

FIGURE 47.1 Psychological factors associated with being in a negative energy balance

After a woman loses weight, particularly if there is a genetic sensitivity or the woman feels 'good' when she experiences the energy-deprived state, she can become preoccupied with thoughts of body weight, eating, food and exercise. She may feel unable to accept the feelings experienced while gaining body weight back to a 'normal' healthy range and continue to lose weight, or she may experience an overwhelming urge to eat—no matter how hard she tries to resist eating, she cannot, and binge eating occurs, only to be replaced by further attempts to lose weight. Being in a negative energy state (too little in or too much expended) helps to control negative moods and feelings.

RISK FACTORS

Risk factors include genetic factors. A genetic contribution of 50–80% is found among sufferers of eating disorders. This appears to be a genetic propensity to develop an eating disorder if other factors are present; this is most likely to be weight loss. Other risk factors are likely to be the simple failure to learn 'normal' regular and sensible eating and exercise patterns as a child, or a more complicated upbringing associated with neglect or abuse. These factors do not cause an eating disorder to occur but do make the person more susceptible to developing disordered eating. Sexually and physically abused women need more intensive treatment and take longer to recover from their eating disorder.

TRIGGER FACTORS

Factors that appear to trigger the onset of the eating disorder may be stressful events such as major school examinations, or losses such as the death of a parent or psychological changes in anxiety and depression. One of the biggest is the body weight increase following puberty in young women (not men). This body image challenge in women and not men may help to explain why eating disorders are more likely to occur in women and during adolescence. Following a woman's first menstrual period she also experiences decreasing self-esteem and increased anxiety and depressive feelings.

PERPETUATING FACTORS

Factors associated with the beginnings of the eating disorder may not be those that cause it to continue for more than a brief period and possibly to become chronic (Fig 47.2) . Simple examples are receiving attention from people, achieving what others cannot, being able to eat anything and not put on weight, or being a scapegoat for family problems.

Some behaviours appear to be self-perpetuating. Being at low weight, self-induced vomiting and excessive exercise are behaviours that become entrenched and may require considerable treatment and even hospitalisation to change. There may be a physiological basis. This is seen for starvation when a certain breed of rat is put into a running cage—as long as it has been well fed, the rat will run and eventually stop when it is tired and the novelty of the activity has decreased; if the rat is starved before being put in the running cage it will keep running until it collapses and dies. It is understood that the changes in brain chemistry associated with starvation result in the animal continuing activity in order to find food at the expense of further energy consumption. Excessive exercise may also be understood in a similar way. Self-induced vomiting is perhaps the most addictive of all and is associated with a poor outcome of treatment; it is thought that the ease of inducing vomiting has a genetic component. In all these cases it is likely that we will understand these behaviours much better when we know more about the neuropeptide neurotransmitter substances of the brain, and the appetite and feeding hormones involved in the energy balance of the body, when these behaviours are present.

All the behaviours are associated with temporary decreases in anxiety and dysphoric moods.

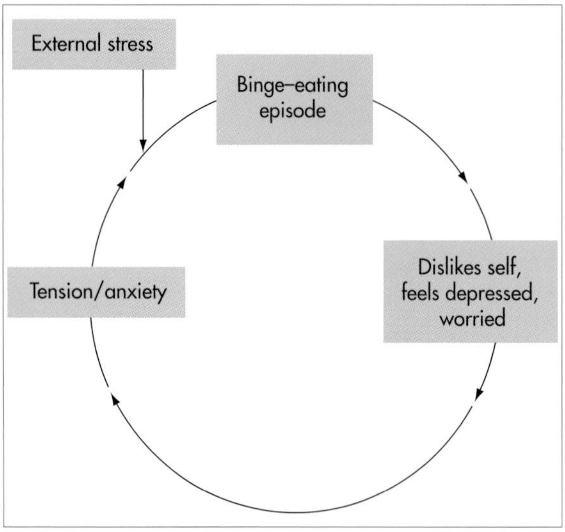

FIGURE 47.2 The psychological circle of binge eating

EATING DISORDERS IN MALES AND AMONG CHILDREN

Anorexia nervosa occurs in males and begins in the same way, and its clinical characteristics and its course are identical to that in females. Why males should pursue thinness so relentlessly is obscure, as adolescent men seek to be muscular rather than thin. Unlike women, men do not experience a rapid unwanted increase in body weight in early adolescence (they lose body fat and gain more muscle) or the accompanying loss of self-esteem. This may explain why males are older at onset of their eating disorder. Compared with female eating disorder, men who are at low weight are more likely to induce vomiting and binge-eat, and men who are at any weight are more likely to exercise excessively than women with eating disorders. Males suffering from eating disorders are likely to have additional problems including obsessive-compulsive disorder, alcohol and substance abuse and personality disorder.

A few male and female children develop eating disorders well before puberty, and again this appears to follow weight loss.

ASSESSMENT

Assessment consists of a thorough physical examination and clinical history. The typical clinical history includes:

- a history of eating, body weight and exercise since first menstruation
- reasons for presenting for help at the time
- past help for problems including anxiety, depression and low self-esteem.

It is helpful to see the family or partner.

The risk factors, trigger factor and perpetuating factors involved in the development and maintenance of the eating disorders (Fig 47.3) give a guide to the history. Family medical and psychiatric histories are necessary.

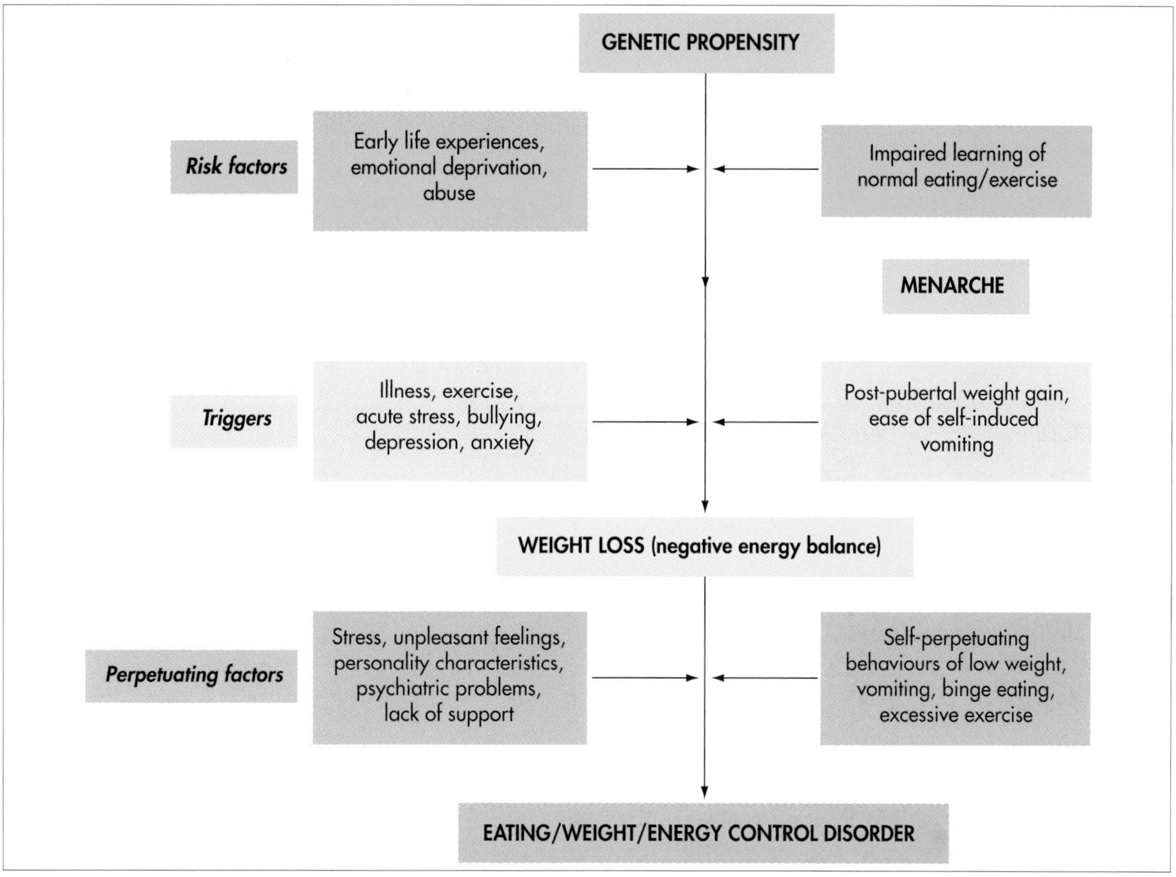

FIGURE 47.3 Risk factors, trigger factors and perpetuating factors involved in the development and maintenance of the eating disorders

COMORBIDITY

Patients with eating disorders can also have other problems. These may need to be treated separately or concurrently with their eating disorder. At times it can be difficult to know whether or not the problem is part of the eating disorder. Most people who are caught up in the preoccupying thoughts of an eating disorder show depressive symptoms but these usually disappear with recovery from the eating disorder. A few will have both a depressive illness and an eating disorder. People prone to develop eating disorders can be more anxious, perfectionistic and obsessional. Obsessional behaviour usually decreases with weight gain but a few have an obsessive-compulsive disorder (OCD) that persists after recovery. Personality disorders with obsessional, avoidant and borderline features are common. Asperger's syndrome and autistic spectrum disorders may be more common than expected in the community, but autistic features for most patients may only be present at low body weight. Any illness that increases awareness and choice of what to eat also appears to make a person more 'at risk' of developing an eating disorder (e.g. diabetes, coeliac disease).

PSYCHOLOGICAL AND PHYSICAL SYMPTOMS

The psychological changes that may accompany low weight are seen in people during starvation (Box 47.2).

BOX 47.2 Psychological symptoms associated with eating disorders

- Irritability
- Indecisiveness
- Poor concentration
- Confusion
- Depressed or dysphoric mood
- Hyperactivity
- Insomnia
- Perfectionism
- Obsessive behaviour, particularly around food
- Withdrawal from people

These same symptoms are seen in women who are not underweight, because they are having episodes of overeating or binge-eating between their periods of severe weight-losing behaviour. Insomnia is thought to be secondary to the hyperactivity, which in turn can be viewed as 'food-seeking behaviour'. The depressed mood is usually described as feelings of hopelessness, guilt and worthlessness. Some cite anger if their binge eating is disturbed. All are anxious around food.

The physical symptoms (Boxes 47.3 and 47.4) associated with eating disorders result from starvation, the extreme methods of weight control employed and excessive binge eating, and hence include the symptoms of low body weight, high body weight, dehydration and electrolyte disturbance.

MENSTRUAL DISTURBANCE

Menstrual disturbances indicate lack of available energy for normal body function. The best predictors of oligomenorrhoea or amenorrhoea are:

- low body weight/fat
- large amount of weight lost (not at low weight)
- excessive exercise
- extreme weight-losing behaviour (e.g. vomiting).

If a patient has restored her body weight to a BMI of 19 or above and her periods have not returned, she is likely to be exercising a great deal, starving in between eating well, continuing to induce vomiting or one of the other eating-disordered behaviours.

Many young women inaccurately believe that when they are taking oral contraception they have 'a normal menstrual cycle', not realising that the bleeding is a 'withdrawal bleed' and that if they cease taking the pill they may have amenorrhoea or irregular cycles.

OSTEOPOROSIS

Oestrogen deficiency results in less new bone being formed, and the high levels of cortisol from starvation mean that existing bone is reabsorbed more quickly. The net effect in anorexia nervosa patients is osteopenia or osteoporosis. The benefits of oral contraception are small, even when calcium supplements are also taken. Improvement and recovery of bone density is associated with weight gain and maintenance of a normal body weight, BMI > 20. This may take several years and depend on the woman's age. A woman who has anorexia nervosa and whose periods have ceased for 6 months should have her bone mineral density and vitamin D levels measured and then be monitored every 12 months.

GASTROINTESTINAL DISTURBANCE

At low weight there is a reduction in time for gastric emptying and transit in general. Constipation and irritable bowel type symptoms are common. Pain, discomfort and bloating occur when eating is attempted. There may be some sensitivity to fructose and sorbitol at low weight. Bloating is a common symptom following eating if the person is eating infrequently. Most functional gastrointestinal diseases associated with the eating disorders—including functional heartburn and

BOX 47.3 Physical examination

External signs

- body weight (under- or overweight)
- clothing loose or tight (reflecting weight change or to disguise)
- dry skin (dehydration), carotenaemia
- overdeveloped muscles (excessive exercise)
- lanugo hair, especially on face, forearms (underweight)
- hands and feet cold and blue (underweight)
- calluses on the back of hands and fingers (from inducing vomiting)
- fingers and face puffy (binge eating)
- enlarged parotid glands (vomiting)
- peripheral oedema (multiple reasons)
- teeth discoloured and damaged (vomiting and poor nutrition)

Examination

- heart rate slow (low weight, excessive exercise)
- blood pressure low (low weight), high (high weight)
- gastrointestinal disturbances (low weight, vomiting, laxatives, binge eating)
- amenorrhoea or irregular menstruation (see menstrual disturbance)
- exercise injuries (excessive exercise)
- osteopenia or osteoporosis (see osteoporosis)
- gastritis, oesophagitis, gastro-oesophageal reflux, blood in vomit (self-induced vomiting)

BOX 47.4 Minimal physical examination and investigations

- Body height and weight
- Heart rate
- Blood pressure
- Full blood count
- Blood glucose
- Serum electrolytes
- Serum creatinine
- Iron and serum ferritin
- Vitamin B_{12} and folate
- Vitamin D
- Calcium
- Magnesium
- Zinc
- Phosphate
- Liver function tests
- Thyroid function
- Electrocardiogram

gastro-oesophageal reflux, which are more likely if the patient is binge eating and vomiting, and IBS—improve as recovery progresses.

TREATMENT

The main focus of treatment is on nutritional rehabilitation, restoration of a 'normal' body weight, education about behaviours involving body weight and exercise, and psychological management.

NUTRITIONAL REHABILITATION

Nutritional rehabilitation consists of learning 'normal structured eating'. A dietician can provide a menu plan (guide) that fulfils the criteria for 'normal eating' (see Box 47.5). This is not a 'diet' and there are no such things as 'bad' foods or 'healthy' foods in a normal eating plan.

The aims of 'normal eating' are to:

- allow the person to eat enough to prevent the drive to eat (thinking of food)
- get used to feeling full and empty
- avoid getting used to eating large amounts of food, and train the body to expect food at regular intervals (no need to eat in order to store energy for the next famine)
- stop depriving the body of nutrients (some fat to absorb vitamins, for normal immunity)
- stop feeling deprived of certain foods (prevent binge eating)
- allow psychological changes in thinking to occur
- allow anxiety around food to decrease
- allow normal behaviour around food and with family and friends.

BOX 47.5 'Normal structured eating'

- Eating three meals and two or three snacks each day
- Usually eating at approximately the same time each day
- Eating a variety of foods
- Learning to eat normal food—i.e. normal fat, normal energy content
- Learning to eat normal amounts of food (not large amounts of low-energy food)
- Eating foods containing protein, carbohydrate and fruit/vegetables at most eating episodes
- Having no 'banned' foods—can have a couple of dislikes that are not associated with weight control
- Being able to eat anywhere—e.g. in any country around the world, home, food courts, fast food outlets, restaurants
- Not having specific rules about eating associated with restricting food—e.g. always eating with a teaspoon, never eating fast food
- Allowing flexibility in eating—e.g. eating at different times with friends, eating what people normally eat at celebrations

It is helpful if there is structured eating in the family and young people learn the patterns associated with 'normal eating' and to be able to be flexible with this structure so it can allow travel, social life and hobbies to be undertaken.

BODY WEIGHT

If a person is underweight, the menu plan must be designed to increase body weight to a BMI > 19 (Asian 18). Some variation may be made if the person is very tall, very short, very muscular or within 12 months of her first menstrual period. A reasonable amount to aim for is an increase of 0.5 kg/week as an outpatient and 1.0 kg/week as an inpatient.

If the patient is at a normal weight, overweight or obese, the menu plan will be the same irrespective of body weight and appropriate for weight maintenance in the normal range. The aim is to prevent weight gain. Any attempts to lose weight are likely to lead to binge eating, which will result in further weight gain or more vomiting or starvation. An overweight or obese patient may need a lot of reassurance but when they find that they stop gaining weight, and even lose weight very slowly by following a normal flexible menu plan, they can learn to change their thinking and their behaviour.

SUPPLEMENTATION

Despite erratic and dysfunctional eating and drinking patterns, most eating-disordered patients do not have vitamin and mineral deficiencies. Patients vary in their compliance with supplements, and may fear the 'real' or 'imagined' energy content of supplementation. The absorption of supplements also varies according to their behaviour, body weight and duration of illness. Weight gain and 'normal eating' are essential for recovery of the bones and reproductive and immune systems, and for improvement in mood and psychological functioning; supplementation alone is not sufficient.

A suggested regimen might include:

- a high-potency combination multivitamin and mineral that includes vitamins A, C and E, B vitamins, iron, zinc, selenium and magnesium
- calcium 600–1200 mg daily and vitamin D 1000 IU daily for bone protection
- omega-3 fatty acids such as fish oil, 1–2 g per day
- vitamin C 1000 mg daily
- coenzyme Q10, 100 mg at night
- amino acid supplementation—can be supportive where there is significant muscle wasting
- additional supplementation of any deficiencies detected—zinc and folate deficiencies may continue after short-term weight recovery and warrant further consideration.

Adjunctive nutritional rehabilitation may include reducing caffeine, tobacco and alcohol intake, as well as addressing deficiencies with supplementation.

EXERCISE

Some patients have an exercise disorder. They feel compelled to exercise excessively and are preoccupied with thoughts about exercise rather than weight or food. Many eating-disordered patients experience this for a few months but some continue for years. At any one time about 14% of eating-disordered patients have problems with disordered and excessive exercise. For some people, their exercise problem can appear to be a primary problem, arising from activities such as sport, dancing or gymnastics rather than an eating or weight disorder, at least in the early years after onset.

Reducing the level of exercise will lead to agitation and anxiety. In normal-weight patients it is helpful to suggest team and social sports rather than solitary sports (running, gym workouts) and having two exercise-free days each week, but these days can include activities with friends and gentle yoga or tai chi.

Decreasing exercise levels in low-weight patients being re-fed can be difficult to achieve. It may require inpatient treatment to achieve 'exercise withdrawal' as the activity and agitation can be overwhelming for the patient without support and supervision. A graded exercise program from gentle yoga or stretching to walking and team activity should be implemented.

PSYCHOLOGICAL AND LIFE SKILLS MANAGEMENT

Supportive psychotherapy needs to be provided throughout treatment and may need to continue for many years. This can provide brief intervention at times of stress and crisis, and general support with daily living and management of relationships and lifestyle. In addition to this is the need to help people as individuals or in groups to:

- change their unhelpful thinking
- correct inaccurate beliefs
- tolerate uncomfortable feelings
- learn a range of relaxation and anxiety management techniques (active and passive)
- learn the limits of acceptable behaviour
- learn how to cope with uncomfortable feelings without resorting to eating-disordered behaviour or weight loss
- learn how to cope with uncomfortable feelings without substituting another inappropriate disorder such as exercise disorder or drug or alcohol abuse
- set goals and learn to work towards these in the short and long term
- explore needs and values and improve self-esteem
- learn to accept and move on without their eating disorder
- practise and develop skills in communicating with friends and family without the eating disorder
- learning problem solving, 'learning resilience'.

The psychological therapies or techniques employed to achieve these aims are mostly based on or modified from cognitive behaviour therapy (CBT) and are:

- schema therapy
- interpersonal therapy (IPT)
- motivational therapy
- family therapy—this may involve assessment, short term intervention for specific problems or total involvement, with a therapist assisting the family to treat the eating disorder. This whole-family approach is very successful for very young patients, especially following hospitalisation for re-feeding, and with highly motivated and well-functioning families.

Mindfulness-based approaches for eating disorders—'mindful eating'—have attracted increasing interest in recent times and have been found to be helpful for a range of eating disorders, particularly binge eating. The more widely used mindfulness approaches include:

- mindfulness-based stress reduction (MBSR)
- mindfulness-based cognitive therapy (MBCT)
- mindfulness, acceptance and commitment therapy (ACT)
- dialectical behaviour therapy (DBT).

Patients also have individual problems that may require additional expertise, such as infertility and sexual or physical abuse.

MEDICATIONS

Antidepressants

Nutritional rehabilitation and establishing normal eating patterns are recommended before medication is considered. Medications play an insignificant part in the management of anorexia nervosa and bulimia nervosa. If an antidepressive drug is needed, one of the selective serotonin reuptake inhibitors (SSRIs) such as fluoxetine or paroxetine is preferred. These drugs are effective for women who are depressed and who suffer from OCD but the results from studies of their use in the treatment of women suffering from anorexia nervosa, both during and after weight gain, are disappointing. Trials with bulimia sufferers suggest that antidepressants are of limited benefit in the treatment of bulimia nervosa. The SSRIs help a small number of women with bulimia nervosa to reduce binge eating in the short term. Interestingly, women who do respond are no more likely to be suffering from symptoms of depression than women who do not respond favourably.

A possible explanation for the ineffectiveness of SSRIs in underweight anorexia nervosa patients is that they may have reduced synaptic 5-HT. 5-HT is derived from tryptophan, and plasma levels are significantly reduced with weight loss and malnourishment in anorexia nervosa.[1] This in turn reduces brain 5-HT synthesis and therefore impairs serotonin activity. A previous study showed that depletion of tryptophan will reverse the effects of antidepressants in depressed patients.[2]

Antipsychotics

When very low weight anorexia nervosa patients find it impossible to accept help to eat sufficient to achieve weight gain, very low doses of a novel antipsychotic drug, such as olanzapine, can help. Patients report that their eating-disordered thoughts are less intense and 'slowed down' so they can make decisions about their treatment. They are also less agitated and restless. Once body weight is increasing and adequate nutrition restored, the medication can be ceased. Because these drugs are known to stimulate appetite in some patients with psychotic illnesses, eating-disordered patients need reassurance that the dose being prescribed is very small and that at these doses the appetite is not stimulated.

HORMONES

There are multiple neuroendocrine–metabolic dysfunctions in anorexia nervosa and bulimia nervosa. All recover with weight gain and maintenance of body weight in the normal range. There is no current evidence to support hormone replacement in the form of oral contraception, and some recent information suggests that it may inhibit recovery of bone.

If amenorrhoea is persistent or if polycystic ovarian syndrome, premature menopause or a pituitary tumour is suspected, appropriate hormones should be measured and further investigations conducted.

TREATMENT BY WHOM AND WHERE?

The general practitioner is usually the first contact and makes the initial assessment and investigations, provides education, discusses misconceptions, helps and encourages the patient to make changes in their behaviour and thinking, and makes a referral to a dietician. This support and information may be sufficient for some young people to initiate changes that lead to recovery. If there is any deterioration, referral to a specialist team as soon as possible is advised. This team usually consists of a dietician, psychiatrist, psychologist, family therapist or social worker and, as required, a physician or paediatrician.

The general practitioner should be part of the multidisciplinary team and coordinate treatment, provide counselling about short- and long-term complications and be the contact and support person when the patient is between treatments. If the general practitioner wants and has some training they may be the main therapist. Different treatments may be beneficial at different stages of the illness—at very low weight, psychological approaches are of limited usefulness (i.e. recovery cannot occur without weight gain). If there is the possibility that a psychiatric illness is present or a strong family psychiatric history, assessment by a psychiatrist is advisable. For example, a very low weight may cover a psychotic illness.

SELF-HELP, SELF-HELP GROUP, INTERNET

For highly motivated people there are good self-help books available, particularly for binge-eating and weight-losing behaviours. 'Guided self-help' is more successful as the general practitioner or other therapist can be contacted when motivation lapses and the person's moods feel out of control. There are also excellent self-help groups run by 'recovering' eating-disordered people. These allow a person to obtain support from other sufferers and to allow them to feel in control of their recovery. Women and men should be assessed by their general practitioner before embarking on any treatment. Treatment should not involve weight-reducing diets.

For people living a long way from help, support with self-help can be done by email. The internet can also provide support in approved programs, but becoming obsessed with anorexic and bulimic sites is not helpful.

OUTPATIENT, DAY PATIENT AND INPATIENT TREATMENT

Outpatient, day patient and inpatient treatment is available in most large cities. Outpatient treatment usually consists of individual visits to healthcare professionals. Day programs include attendance for group nutritional education and psychological therapies one to five days each week for set periods of time.

Hospital admission for emergency and/or specialised treatment may be necessary if:

- the patient does not respond to outpatient or day patient treatment
- the patient is at very low body weight, with serious physiological changes
- the patient has cardiac and electrolyte disturbances
- the patient is at risk of suicide or self-harm
- the patient has other problems, such as diabetes
- the patient lives too far away from a treatment centre, does not have adequate carer support, or prefers hospital
- the patient's family needs 'time out' to recuperate, as living with an eating-disordered patient can be extremely stressful for everyone in the home.

PREVENTION

- Continuing education of young people:
  - general information, e.g. photos of models are airbrushed, most women want to weigh less than they do
  - sensible eating includes snacks and social eating
  - taking care when defining what is 'healthy' eating for an adolescent
  - sensible exercise includes rest days
  - targeting specific health messages to the appropriate people and not those who are already health conscious. 'Eat less fat and exercise more' to a normal-weight, active teenage woman sends the wrong message.
- Easy access to individual discussion and possible referral:
  - easy access to individual discussion and education about eating, binge eating, dieting, and weight and exercise during adolescence
  - if, after discussion, eating or exercise is affecting their quality of life, treatment should be offered.
- Education of adults:
  - Parents need education and help to assess the information available about 'normal structured eating and exercise' for adolescents.
  - Parents and partners need to be firm, supportive and seek help if they are worried about their partner's or children's eating or exercise.
  - Relapse prevention—information about relapse prevention should be available.

OUTCOME

In the first year after treatment, 20–30% of anorexia nervosa patients lose weight and relapse. Later relapses can occur, usually at times of stress when the woman feels helpless to change what is happening in her life, or it may follow a body weight challenge such as pregnancy. Approximately 40–50% of anorexia nervosa sufferers recover completely, and 30–40% recover sufficiently to lead a normal life, although they may continue to have some intermittent or low-level eating-disordered thoughts or behaviours. Treatment at a younger age, no vomiting, no binge eating and a supportive and relatively problem-free family appear to be associated with a good outcome.

The long-term outcome for bulimia nervosa patients is similar: approximately 50% are 'cured', 30% improve and 20% still suffer, although the frequency of binge eating is likely to be decreased. Relapses following treatment are common and the precipitants similar to those for anorexia nervosa. The factors associated with a good outcome are treatment at a younger age, no episodes of anorexia nervosa and no other psychiatric illnesses in the family.

SUMMARY

Eating disorders, weight disorders and energy control disorders are the same. They are psychosomatic illnesses requiring a multidisciplinary approach to assessment and treatment. Most commonly they first occur in post-pubertal women during adolescence. Patients may seek and want help or they may try to avoid treatment, particularly if they associate feelings of loss of control with weight gain, ceasing vomiting or stopping excessive exercise. The behaviours and thinking can respond readily to treatment if this is sought early and there are no major factors perpetuating the behaviour. Or the behaviours and thoughts can be resistant to change and take a chronic or relapsing course. Early commonsense information and intervention shortly after onset appears to offer the best results.

RESOURCES

Janet Treasure, A guide to the medical risk assessment for eating disorders, Section of Eating Disorders, Institute of Psychiatry, South London and Maudsley NHS trust, http://www.iop.kcl.ac.uk/sites/edu/downloads/HP/STUDENT_COUNSELLOR_GUIDE_TO_EATING_DISORDERS.pdf

Suzanne Abraham, Eating disorders: the facts. Oxford: OUP. 6th edn; 2008.

REFERENCES

1 Anderson GH, Kennedy SH, eds. The biology of feast and famine: relevance to eating disorders. San Diego: Academic Press; 1992.

2 Ferguson CP, La Via MC, Crossan PJ. Are serotonin selective reuptake inhibitors effective in underweight anorexia nervosa? Int J Eat Disord 1999; 25:11–16.

part FOUR

Men's health

chapter 48

Men's health

INTRODUCTION AND OVERVIEW

When discussing men's health, it is important to appreciate that there are two aspects to the subject:

- diseases that are common to both men and women, where our responsibility as GPs is to prevent the poorer outcomes that men suffer as a consequence of these diseases
- diseases that affect the male reproductive organs, such as prostate disease, testicular cancer and erectile dysfunction.

Despite the significant advances in healthcare of this century and the previous, men still have poorer health outcomes than women—an example is the current average male life expectancy of 78 years, compared to 83 for females.[1] GPs regularly see male patients ignoring warning symptoms, denying health problems and dying prematurely from heart disease and cancer. Statistics show that, compared with females, males in the 25–64 year age group have four times the risk of dying from heart disease, twice the risk of dying from cancer and three times the risk of dying from alcoholic liver disease.

Males in developed countries have higher rates of the following conditions, which goes a large way to explaining their lower life expectancy:

- malignancy
- ischaemic heart disease (until after women pass through menopause)
- cerebrovascular diseases
- chronic lower respiratory disease
- accidents and violence
- suicide
- diabetes mellitus
- motor vehicle traffic accidents
- alcohol and substance abuse
- work-related injuries.

As to whether these differences are simply due to the presence of a Y chromosome (*nature*) or the result of broader issues such as lifestyle, attitudes, social expectations and upbringing (*nurture*) is a matter of speculation—but the typical male in most cultures is brought up to:

- deal with problems without asking for help—so he doesn't readily seek medical advice
- not let pain or discomfort show—so he ignores signs of 'Dis-ease'.

REGULAR SERVICE PREVENTS BREAKDOWNS

As GPs we face not only the problem of getting men in the community to come and see us when they have symptoms, but also the difficulty of getting male patients to present for a regular check-up.

Men confront a number of challenges and barriers in being more proactive about their health. First, self-awareness and self-care are often not cultivated by men as much as women, and are not part of the traditional male culture. Images of male resilience and strength are more commonly inflexible and independent. Men also tend to be very career focused, in such a way that taking time off for 'non-essential' or 'non-urgent' things like GP consultations does not rate highly on the priority list unless the health matter cannot be ignored. Even then, denial is more common among men. Or men can avoid going to the doctor because they find talking about personal issues or vulnerability a lot more difficult than women do, particularly when those issues are of an emotional nature, regarding relationships, for example, or depression or anxiety. Self-medicating for such problems is an important part of the reason that substance abuse is more common among men. Many men may have a preference for consulting a GP of a particular gender. For example, some men may prefer to discuss emotional issues with women, or relationship or sexual issues with an experienced male practitioner. Often when a man presents with psychological and emotional concerns, he may want to approach the problem in a different way than a woman would—for example, a woman (and female practitioner) may wish to discuss the emotions and issues at greater length, whereas the man may want to discuss more direct and pragmatic solutions to dealing with the 'problem', whatever that may be. Being flexible in consulting style, or knowing how to open up discussion about emotional issues in a non-confronting way, may be an important skill for the healthcare practitioner to have in dealing with health matters for men. Furthermore, women tend to more often take the children and other family members to the doctor for appointments and so will more commonly establish a stronger link with healthcare practitioners and clinics, or are reminded about personal health issues while there. Women's greater role than men in nurturing and caring is partly due to nature (biological and hormonal) and partly due to nurture (culture and upbringing). Therefore, confronting the barriers to men being more active participants in their own healthcare requires not only a healthcare practitioner who is sensitive to the consulting issues and psychology of men, but also a change of societal images of manhood.[2]

Ideally, health checks should be performed regularly through childhood, adolescence and adulthood (see Ch 17, The general check-up)—once men become familiar with the concept of being proactive rather than reactive, the GP can schedule a long consultation and perform the same comprehensive check-up, directed to conditions relevant to the age of the man, for older and younger patients.

In fact, if we as GPs can inculcate in the community—particularly the males in our community—the idea of presenting for an annual check-up in a similar manner to taking their cars for a regular service, then it stands to reason that the incidence of 'breakdowns' will be far less than it is now!

Because most people remember their own birthdays, a useful method is to encourage patients to come for

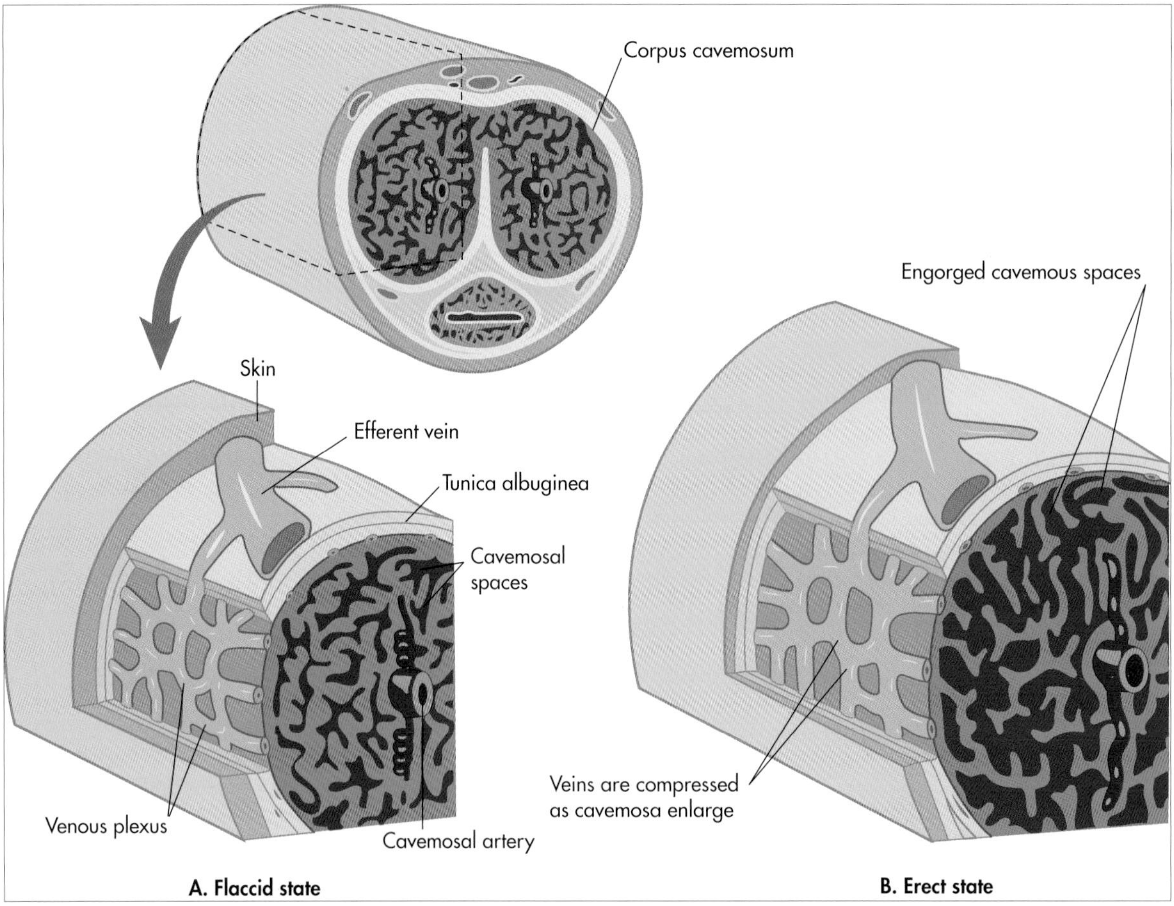

FIGURE 48.1 The corpus cavernosa of the penis, showing how increasing blood flow increases turgor

their check-up during the month of their birthday. As a minimum, in addition to a basic clinical examination (with or without a prostate check), they should have their weight, girth and blood pressure measured, plus blood tests for glucose, lipids and liver function. Based on the results, further examinations and investigations may be indicated. More likely is the situation where the results of the tests provide an opportunity for health education and counselling about appropriate lifestyle interventions—for example, practical steps that could be taken if their cholesterol or blood pressure is outside the expected range.

ERECTILE DYSFUNCTION

Erectile dysfunction is discussed in detail in Ch 49, Erectile dysfunction.

With the advent of medications for erectile dysfunction and media attention focusing on prostate cancer, GPs are now seeing more men presenting for advice about these conditions, which in the past were either suffered in silence or accepted as the price one paid for growing old. Impotence, now known as erectile dysfunction (ED), is defined as the persistent inability to attain and/or maintain an erection adequate to permit satisfactory sexual intercourse.

It is important to be aware that ED is common, and in most men is not caused by a deficiency of male hormones or a lack of masculinity. Despite its common incidence, only about a third of men affected have consulted a doctor about it. Erection is essentially a vascular phenomenon, brought about by increasing blood flow to the penis, so anything that inhibits the augmentation of blood flowing into the corpora cavernosa can stop the erection.

The strong association of ED with a diseased cardiovascular system is easy to understand if one appreciates that the inadequacy of blood flow in the penile arteries is simply a manifestation of what is happening in other similar-sized blood vessels. This explains why ED is more common in patients with conditions such as hypertension, high cholesterol, diabetes and ischaemic heart disease. Although ED is a common cause of emotional stress and relationship issues, one should also remember that stress and relationship issues are also common causes or exacerbating factors for ED. A significant finding by Thompson and colleagues was that men diagnosed with ED at the start of their study who were followed over 9 years had a higher incidence of heart attacks and strokes than a control population.[3]

ED can present to GPs in one of two ways:

- A patient presents with a complaint of erectile inadequacy—our task is not only to treat the problem but also to identify any associated diseases.
- A patient has chronic disease that puts them at risk of ED—our task is to ascertain whether they have ED and, if so, to help them achieve satisfactory erectile function if they so desire.

In the case of the former, it is important to confirm that the symptoms are actually caused by ED rather than low libido, premature ejaculation or relationship difficulties, and to ensure that the dysfunction is not caused by undue anxiety to perform. Using the IIEF-5 questionnaire[4] (described in Ch 49) can be useful in helping to ascertain whether the patient's problem really is ED.

With patients who suffer from the chronic diseases that damage blood vessels, it may be difficult to tactfully broach the topic of ED during a routine consultation. One technique is to provide a brief preliminary explanation about how diabetes (or high cholesterol or high blood pressure) damages the small blood vessels and affects the circulation to the eyes, kidneys, penis, heart and limbs—and then say, 'Many men with diabetes experience problems with getting an erection—have you ever had this problem yourself?'. This allows the patient to identify with the 'majority' rather than labouring under the misconception that he has a unique and embarrassing ailment.

The management of ED is discussed at length in Ch 49. The important message here is that ED is common, can be effectively and easily treated in the majority of men, and *may* be the first symptom indicating more generalised serious disease.

TESTICULAR CANCER

Responsible for 10% of all cancer deaths in the 15–35 year age group, testicular cancer is the most common cancer affecting young men. Ninety per cent of these tumours originate from germ cells, and are divided into seminomas (40%), non-seminoma germ cell tumours (NSGCT, 35%) and mixed tumours (seminoma plus NSGCT, 15%). The remaining 10% of testicular tumours are non-germ cell tumours.

Over the past 30 years, the annual incidence has risen. Mortality rates, however, have declined dramatically (5-year relative survival today is about 95%) as a consequence of earlier diagnosis and new treatment techniques, such as platinum-based chemotherapy.

Identified risk factors include:

- first-degree family members with testicular cancer
- previous history of undescended testes
- low birth weight
- low semen quality
- cancer in the opposite testis.

A testicular cancer typically presents as a painless, hard, enlarged testis. Pain, if at all, occurs due to a bleed into the lesion—and this may delay diagnosis by mimicking epididymo-orchitis.

If a man is suspected to have a cancer in his testis, it is mandatory to perform an ultrasound scan, which can usually differentiate a solid (cancer) from a cystic (benign) swelling. Such a patient should undergo thorough clinical examination as well as CT scans for features of metastatic cancer in the retroperitoneal nodes and lungs. The basic management of the primary tumour is orchidectomy through an inguinal incision.

Seminomas are exquisitely radio-sensitive, so early-stage disease is currently treated with postoperative radiotherapy to the draining nodes—although some centres use a single dose of carboplatin chemotherapy followed by active surveillance. Opinions differ as to the best method of dealing with NSGCT. Some centres advocate radical removal of the para-aortic lymph nodes at the time of orchidectomy; others adopt a surveillance approach, monitoring the patient with regular measurement of tumour markers and CT scans.

Our task as GPs is to get the simple message out into the community that any man who detects a lump in the testis should have it examined by his doctor—who will, after examination, arrange an ultrasound scan (with or without other investigations) to distinguish a testicular cancer from the more common benign causes of testicular lumps.

PROSTATE DISEASE

General practitioners now see more older men presenting with urinary symptoms. This is most likely due to the increasing lifespan of our patients. Previously termed *prostatism*, lower urinary tract symptoms (LUTS) include obstructive symptoms (straining to pass urine, difficulty in initiating micturition and poor urinary stream) and irritative symptoms (frequency, urgency and nocturia). The last can often be due to other factors that cause over-activity of the bladder (OAB)—and in this situation, bladder ultrasound and urine cytology are important investigations that help exclude bladder calculi and early bladder cancer. If a post-micturition scan shows that that the bladder empties well, treatment with anticholinergic drugs can be considered.

The term *benign prostatic hypertrophy* (BPH) is used to denote the pathological condition, while *bladder outlet obstruction* (BOO) describes the clinical syndrome, which may also be caused by other conditions such as bladder neck hypertrophy or urethral stricture. BPH was originally and impractically defined histopathologically as 'a prostate larger than 20 g plus either elevated symptom score or reduced peak flow', although no single definition has gained universal acceptance.[5]

Fifty per cent of men aged over 60 years suffer from BPH.[6] We now know that BPH is not necessarily progressive; symptoms stay the same or regress spontaneously in at least half these men. Moreover, the impact of the symptoms is variable, and although there is a small risk of acute retention, in many cases all the GP need provide is reassurance, together with periodic monitoring of symptoms.

TREATMENT

Should symptoms deteriorate, medication in the form of 5-alpha-reductase inhibitors (finasteride, dutasteride) or alpha-blockers (prazosin, tamsulosin) can be helpful. Herbal remedies such as saw palmetto, stinging nettle and red clover (isoflavones) have also been used with benefit in some studies. Where medical therapy is ineffective, surgery (transurethral resection of the prostate, TURP) usually proves effective.

PROSTATE CANCER

Prostate cancer is discussed in detail in Ch 50, An integrative approach to prostate cancer.

Contrary to popular misconception, prostate cancer does not present with urinary symptoms. By the time the characteristic symptoms of bone pain and haematuria appear, the disease is too advanced for cure. Early detection is essential but thus far no foolproof test is available. Until we have more definitive studies, population screening for prostate cancer is not recommended—but a form of screening, termed 'case finding', is used whereby asymptomatic men in the susceptible age group are offered the best test currently available to detect the condition.

At present, measurement of serum PSA (prostate-specific antigen) is combined with a rectal examination—PR (per rectum) or DRE (digital rectal examination)—to feel for nodules in the prostate gland. PSA is a glycoprotein produced by the normal prostate gland, and is normally present at very low levels in the blood. Prostate cancer cells produce increased amounts of PSA, so an increase in the level of PSA in the blood is suggestive (although not diagnostic) of prostate cancer. Twenty per cent of prostate cancers do not produce an elevated PSA, so both components (blood test for PSA as well as DRE) are essential. It is also important to note the age-specific ranges for normal PSA, as the previously accepted 'cut-off point' of 4.0 ng/L is no longer accurate. (See Ch 50 for discussion of PSA levels.)

SUMMARY

It is only recently that we as doctors have come to realise that men suffer a considerable degree of morbidity as well as mortality from andrological causes. Awareness of the unique health needs of men and cognisance of the latest information about the management of these conditions, as well as community education to encourage men to consult their doctors for preventive healthcare as well as when they develop symptoms, will go a long way towards improving male health in the twenty-first century.

Take-home messages:

- Men should be encouraged to get an annual check-up, just as regularly as they get their cars serviced!
- Erectile dysfunction is treatable in most patients, and may be an indicator of hitherto asymptomatic cardiovascular disease (see Ch 49).
- Lower urinary tract symptoms are not always due to benign prostate hypertrophy, and may remain stable (or even improve) over time.
- Early detection of prostate cancer relies on a PAP test (**P**SA **A**nd **P**R examination) (see Ch 50).

RESOURCES

Andrology Australia, http://www.andrologyaustralia.org
Mensline, http://www.menslineaus.org.au

REFERENCES

1 Australian Bureau of Statistics. Deaths Australia, 2004. ABS (2005) Cat. No. 3302.0. Canberra.
2 Malcher G. Engaging men in health care. Aust Fam Physician 2009; 38(3):92–95.
3 Thompson IM, Tangen CM, Goodman PJ et al. Erectile dysfunction and subsequent cardiovascular disease. JAMA 2005; 294:2996–3002.
4 Rosen RC, Cappelleri JC, Smith MD et al. Development and evaluation of an abridged, 5-item version of the International Index of Erectile Function (IIEF-5) as a diagnostic tool for erectile dysfunction. Int J Impot Res 1999; 11:319–326.
5 Walsh PC. Editorial: treatment of benign prostatic hyperplasia. N Engl J Med 1996; 335:587.
6 Kooner R, Stricker P. Benign prostatic hyperplasia. Med Today 2000; 1:317–324.

chapter 49

Erectile dysfunction

INTRODUCTION AND OVERVIEW

Erectile dysfunction (ED) was defined by the 1992 National Institutes of Health Consensus Development Panel on Impotence as the persistent inability to achieve and/or maintain an erection sufficient for satisfactory sexual intercourse. It is a symptom that causes significant psychological and relationship stress and is often not investigated or treated, as a significant majority of men do not report it to their doctor.

Until the late 1980s, ED was regarded as mainly psychological in origin. We now understand that ED is a complex process requiring a combination of urological, endocrinological, psychological, vascular and biochemical factors for satisfactory function.

EPIDEMIOLOGY

In recent times there have been many epidemiological studies of erectile dysfunction, the hallmark study being the 1987 Massachusetts Male Aging Study.[1] This study found that ED occurred in 52% of men aged between 40 and 70 years. It confirmed that ED increases in frequency as men grow older, and that age is not a cause but an association of this condition. The study found that the most common pathological factor in ED is vascular disease, found in diabetes, hypertension, obesity and hyperlipidaemia (metabolic syndrome).

Thus the incidence of ED is highly correlated with health conditions such as metabolic syndrome, and with lifestyle factors such as smoking and lack of exercise.

The first Australian-based community study of ED was carried out by Chew and colleagues from the Keogh Institute for Medical Research, Perth, in 1997.[2] This study found that some degree of ED was present in almost 40% of men aged 18 years or older. Complete ED occurred in 18.6% of men. The prevalence of complete ED increased with age. Despite the frequency of ED, this study found that only 11.6% of men with ED had received treatment.

ANATOMY

The basic anatomy of the penis (Fig 49.1) consists of vascular cavernosal tissue that responds to neurological impulses, resulting in penile rigidity.

Each corpus cavernosum contains blood-filled compartments called sinusoids or lacunar spaces and is surrounded by a fibrous sheath called the tunica albuginea. The endothelium and integrity of the smooth muscle cells play an important role in the vascular events of erection.

The corpus spongiosum surrounds the urethra and distally forms the glans penis. The arterial inflow arises from the internal pudendal artery, which provides a cavernosal artery for each corpus.

Venous drainage occurs through emissary veins passing through the tunica albuginea. The rigidity during tumescence compresses these veins, causing veno-occlusion. When this mechanism functions poorly, it is often described as venous leakage.

Parasympathetic nerves from the S2 to S4 nerve root control erectile function, and sympathetic nerves from T11 to L2 control detumescence and ejaculation. Penile erection is thus a neurovascular event. Sexual stimulation results in increased parasympathetic activity, leading to release of neurotransmitters from the cavernous nerve terminals and relaxing factors from the endothelial cells in the penis. The neurotransmitters are acetylcholine, vasointestinal peptide and nitric oxide.

PATHOPHYSIOLOGY

Cyclic guanosine monophosphate (cGMP), which arises from the precursor L-arginine by the action of nitric oxide synthase, controls nitric oxide function. Calcium efflux mediated by cGMP leads to smooth

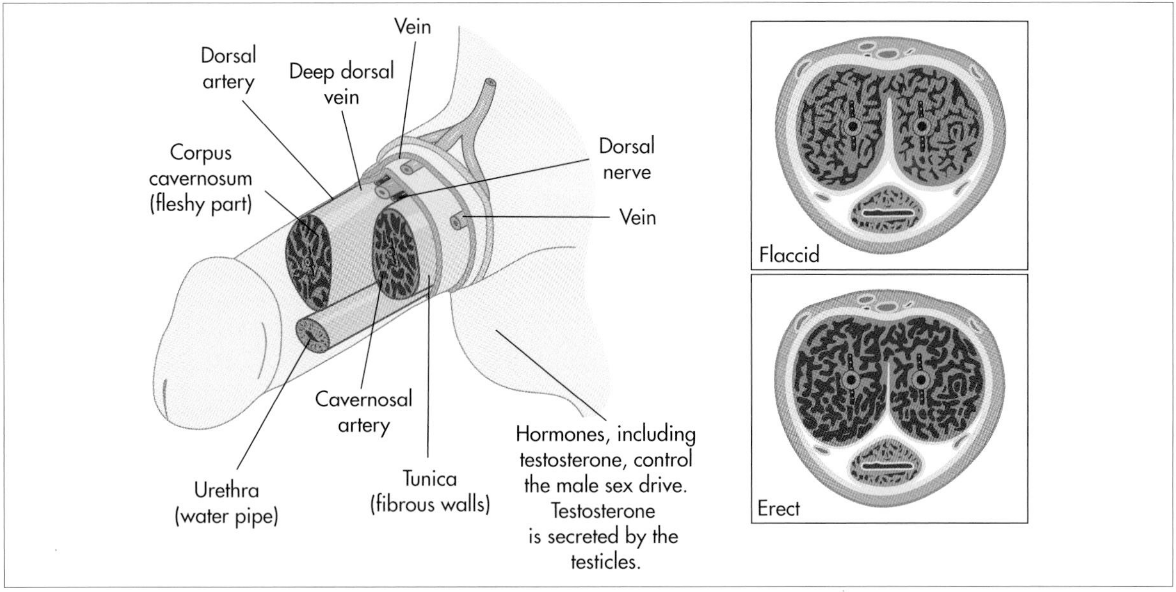

FIGURE 49.1 Basic anatomy of the penis

muscle cell relaxation in the arteries and arterioles supplying the erectile tissue, increasing blood flow and causing the erection (Fig 49.2). This action is ended by phosphodiesterase type 5 (PDE-5), which leads to detumescence. Additional smooth muscle relaxation via the cyclic adenosine monophosphate (cAMP) pathway is mediated by prostaglandin E_1 and vasointestinal peptide. Availability of nitric oxide in the endothelium decreases with age. Endothelial dysfunction occurs in both coronary artery disease and ED when the action of nitric oxide is affected. Impaired nitric oxide synthesis reduces the capacity of vasodilation and increases the risk of platelet aggregation. Atherosclerosis has a greater effect in ED than the ageing process. Diabetes is associated with both vascular and neurological effects that interfere with the interaction between the endothelium and the smooth muscle cells.

AETIOLOGICAL FACTORS

As mentioned, the prevalence of ED increases with age; generally 70% of men at the age of 70 years describe a form of erectile dysfunction. Men with sexual dysfunction may have physical and psychological health problems (Box 49.1).

Psychological factors may be the primary cause of the ED or can arise secondary to the distress caused by its presence. Psychological factors include anxiety, stress, depression, relationship issues and other presentations of mental illness.

Erectile dysfunction may be associated with many medical conditions; it is strongly associated with atherosclerosis, making ED a marker of potential coronary artery disease. Because of the smaller size of the penile arteries compared to the coronary arteries, erectile dysfunction may precede coronary artery disease by 3–5 years. Thus a high level of total cholesterol with a low HDL is an important risk factor for ED causing both arterial and venous dysfunction due to endothelial injury and smooth muscle cell changes.

Smoking has been shown to be an important risk factor for ED. Smoking may result in the arterial inflow problems or faulty veno-occlusive mechanism. Obstructive sleep apnoea has been associated with reduced nocturnal erections.

Diabetes may involve vascular and neurological problems involving vascular insufficiency and sensory and autonomic neuropathy. Men with diabetes experience the onset of ED 10–15 years earlier than those without diabetes. More than 50% of these will have ED at some time, and 39% suffer from the condition all the time. The Massachusetts Male Aging Study showed a 28% probability of complete ED among men with diabetes, compared with a 9% probability in those without diabetes.[1] The risk may depend on the duration of diabetes and the presence of poor glycaemic control.

The neurological causes of ED include multiple sclerosis, temporal lobe epilepsy, Parkinson's disease, stroke, Alzheimer's disease and spinal cord injury. Hypoxia associated with respiratory disease may result in the aggravating vascular causes of ED. Renal insufficiency may result in ED in up to 50% of patients due to multiple causes, including vascular, neurological, endocrine and electrolyte and mineral issues.

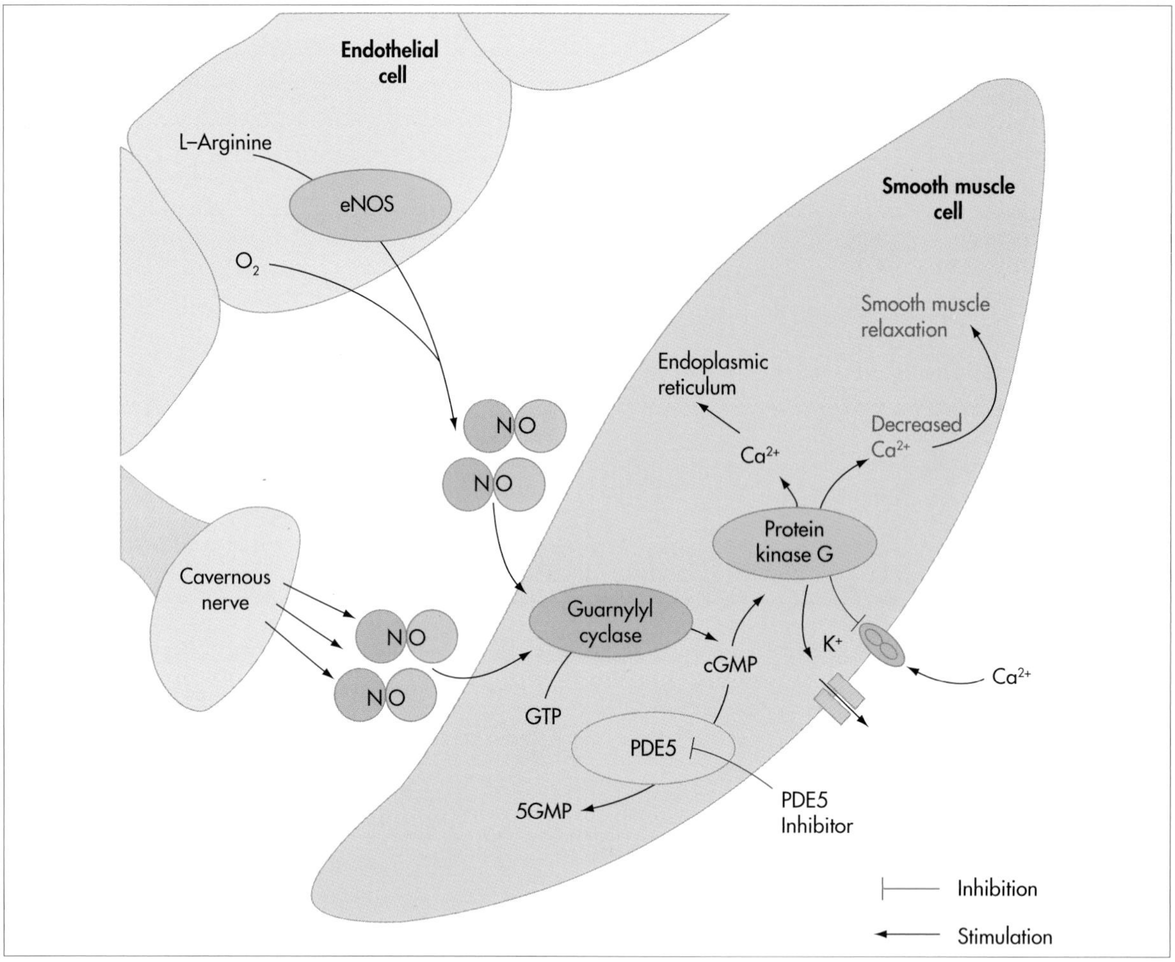

FIGURE 49.2 Biochemical pathway of erection

The medications implicated in ED include blood pressure tablets containing thiazide diuretics and beta-blockers. Antidepressant medication may affect libido and ejaculation more so than erection. Cardiac medication includes digoxin and amiodarone. Many psychotropic medications affect the erection, including the older major tranquillisers and the more modern atypical antipsychotics. An important part of the patient history is to check all prescribed and over-the-counter medications to check for ED as a side effect.

Most of the illicit recreational drugs are associated with erectile dysfunction. Because of its disinhibiting effect, alcohol may occasionally result in enhanced sexual function and is often used by men with premature ejaculation to delay ejaculation.

METABOLIC SYNDROME

The combination of obesity, diabetes, raised lipids and hypertension is known as the metabolic syndrome. This condition is often associated with ED and a low level of testosterone. ED in this situation arises from endothelial dysfunction, which is deterioration of the lining of small blood vessels known as the endothelium. Specific treatment of these four components plus lifestyle modification is an important aspect of the treatment of metabolic syndrome to improve endothelial function. The improvement of weight, blood pressure, lipid levels and glucose control may improve testosterone levels and the symptoms of ED.

Low testosterone, or hypogonadism, remains a controversial topic. Testosterone production falls by 1% per year from the age of 40 years. As men age, high levels of sex hormone binding globulin reduce the amount of a bioavailable testosterone. However, many older men with low-ish testosterone levels remain sexually functional. The role of testosterone in male sexual function was regarded in the past as only essential for libido and general sense of wellbeing, although recently there is

BOX 49.1 Aetiological factors in erectile dysfunction

Social
- age
- education
- occupation
- socioeconomic
- family of origin
- relationship
- psychological health

Lifestyle
- alcohol
- smoking
- obesity
- substance abuse
- sedentary lifestyle
- lack of exercise

Medical
- medication
- acute surgery & trauma
- chronic medical conditions
  - metabolic syndrome, diabetes
  - hypogonadism
  - kidney disease
- cardiac disease, hypertension, raised lipids
- cerebrovascular disease
- neurological disorders
- prostate disease/Peyronie's disease
- psychiatric issues—anxiety, stress, depression

evidence that some level of testosterone is required for normal erectile function. Testosterone also plays an important role in the maintenance of bone density, muscle mass, maintenance of male characteristics and a general sense of wellbeing.

LOWER URINARY TRACT SYMPTOMS

Lower urinary tract symptoms are associated with increasing severity of ED, possibly through altered nitric oxide levels in the smooth muscle of the prostate and penis. Radical prostatectomy surgery for prostate cancer (open or robotic) usually results in ED. Even when the neurovascular bundles are saved, and these are the requirement for erectile function, the nerves may take 6–36 months to recover, if ever. Any other form of pelvic injury or surgery has the potential to damage the pelvic nerves and result in ED.

PEYRONIE'S DISEASE

Peyronie's disease is a fibrotic condition of the corpora cavernosa that results in penile shortening, the presence of a plaque, curvature of erection and occasionally ED. The disease may be self-limiting, taking up to 18 months to resolve. However, sometimes the condition is progressive, resulting in increasing curvature of the erection and requiring surgical straightening. Peyronie's disease can arise from penile trauma during sexual activity. It can be associated with Dupuytren's contracture and the HLA-B27 antigen.

DIAGNOSIS

The diagnosis of ED arises from a medical and sexual history and the use of various questionnaires and instruments. An abbreviated version of the international index of erectile function (IIEF) is the five questions of sexual health inventory for men (SHIM). These questions are:

- Do you have the regular confidence that you can get and keep an erection?
- When you have erections with sexual stimulation, are the erections enough for penetration?
- During sexual intercourse, how often are you able to maintain an erection after you have penetrated your partner?
- During sexual intercourse, how difficult is it to maintain your erection to completion of intercourse?
- When you attempt sexual intercourse, how often is it satisfactory for you?

It is important to take a general history and a sexual history. Taking a general history may provide clues to the presence of risk factors that can be revealed by the patient's medical history. Other important factors are the use of medications, tobacco, alcohol and other recreational drugs, and psychological and relationship issues.

The sexual history should establish the exact nature of the problem, whether it is one of erectile dysfunction, libido or ejaculation. It is important to ask:

- how long the problem has been present
- whether the change was sudden or gradual
- whether the problem occurs in all situations or varies
- whether nocturnal and morning erections occur
- whether the problem is the same with masturbation
- whether penile curvature has developed
- whether the problem has ever been present before
- about details of the current relationship.

NORMAL CHANGES OF AGEING

It is important to differentiate the normal changes of ageing that occur with men and provide reassurance that these do not necessarily require treatment. Ageing men require reassurance that change in erectile function is a natural process. Older men require more stimulation to achieve an erection, they experience a less intense orgasm, reduced ejaculatory volume and a longer refractory period (the time it takes to repeat sexual activity). Older men may therefore have difficulty using condoms, as their erections are not as robust.

EXAMINATION

The examination of men with ED should be general as well as paying specific attention to the genitals, secondary sexual characteristics, peripheral pulses and prostate.

Examination of the penis may reveal Peyronie's disease. Examination of the testis may indicate hypogonadism or the presence of Klinefelter's syndrome. The character of limb pulses indicates peripheral vascular status. Digital rectal examination reveals the presence of anal tone, the bulbocavernosus reflex and the state of the prostate.

Ideally, the partner of the man with ED should be present, as the partner often reveals information that is relevant to the potential cause, such as the state of the relationship, and the man's and the partner's expectations.

INVESTIGATIONS

Investigations include routine blood testing for fasting lipids and glucose, liver function, creatinine, morning total testosterone and a PSA prostate blood test if indicated. Some centres perform more sophisticated testing, which includes an office prostaglandin E_1 (PGE_1) injection test, a duplex Doppler ultrasound scan of the penile blood flow and, when indicated, overnight erection testing with a Rigiscan monitor. For men who may be considered for vascular surgery, investigations such as cavernosometry and selective pudendal arteriography may reveal vascular lesions, especially in the case of trauma.

TREATMENT

FIRST-LINE THERAPY

Psychological and relationship factors should always be included in the initial assessment, as well as lifestyle issues, with particular emphasis on diet, weight loss and exercise. Men are often reluctant to undergo psychological and lifestyle counselling, as they generally seek a quick fix. However, when psychological issues predominate as the cause of ED, a medical treatment may not be overly effective.

Yoga and meditation can reduce the effects of stress and relieve anxiety about the condition. Exercising the pelvic floor muscles may result in improved quality of erection and ejaculation.

Oral PDE5 inhibitors (sildenafil, tadalafil, vardenafil) are effective in up to 70–80% of men with ED. Side effects may include flushing of the face, headache, blocked nose, gastric reflux and some muscle and lower back pain. These medications enhance penile blood flow via the cGMP cycle, prolonging smooth muscle cell relaxation by inhibiting the PDE5 action.

PDE5 inhibitors may not be effective in the presence of low testosterone, and so replacement of testosterone may result in an improved response. PDE5 inhibitors are generally taken orally one hour before planned sexual activity on an as-required basis. These medications are effective with the treatment of vascular causes of ED, and are being assessed for their effectiveness in recovery of erectile function following treatment for prostate cancer with daily dosing of the lowest dose of a PDE5 inhibitor.

Non-arteritic anterior ischaemic optic nerve neuropathy (NAION) is a condition resulting in visual loss often seen in older men in the age group of those who take PDE5 inhibitors. No direct cause or link has been found. These men have the vascular risk factors for NAION in that they are older men, with a history of hypertension, diabetes and smoking.

SECOND-LINE THERAPY

Before the discovery of PDE5 inhibitors, intracavernosal self-injection was the main medical treatment for ED. In the 1980s, papaverine was used until the discovery of prostaglandin E_1 (PGE_1, or alprostadil). Penile injection therapy works through the cAMP cycle and is effective in more serious cases of ED and in men with neurogenic ED. PGE_1 can be mixed with papaverine and phentolamine to form a preparation known as TriMix when PGE_1 on its own is ineffective in severe cases of ED. PGE_1 can produce some delayed pain in some men, but generally it is well tolerated. Overdosing with PGE_1 may result in a prolonged erection known as priapism. This requires emergency treatment, for detumescence of the penis. Regular use of penile injection therapy may result in penile fibrosis, which may result in similar symptoms to those of Peyronie's disease, such as curvature of the erection.

An intraurethral therapy with PGE_1 was briefly available in Australia, with a product called medicated urethral system for erection (MUSE). This has not been found to be an overly effective medication. Another second-line treatment is the use of a vacuum erection device, a non-invasive treatment that is a useful alternative for those who do not wish to or are unable to take oral or injectable medication. The vacuum device applies a negative pressure to the penis, drawing venous blood into the penis, which is then retained by the application of an elastic constriction band to the base of the penis.

THIRD-LINE THERAPY

Surgical implantation of a penile prosthesis or implant is considered when other treatments have failed. The three-piece penile prosthesis is a highly engineered product, is well concealed and has a low rate of mechanical failure.

Vascular surgery consists of venous ligation or dorsal vein arterialisation. Because of its poor long-term prognosis, this type of surgery is now mainly relegated to younger men with traumatic arterial lesions with no evidence of atherosclerosis.

TESTOSTERONE

Should the man with ED be shown to be deficient in testosterone, consideration is given to testosterone supplementation. Testosterone may improve libido and play some role in improving erectile function. Caution should be exercised with testosterone therapy in the presence of an enlarged prostate and when there is a risk of prostate cancer. Testosterone replacement therapy is available as oral capsules, skin patches, skin gel, injection therapy and skin implants. There is much controversy over the level of testosterone that is regarded as being low for both sexual and general health matters. A level of total testosterone ≤ 8 nmol/L has always been regarded as the point where testosterone treatment is commenced. A 'grey area' of testosterone level between 8 and 12 nmol/L is now under research for consideration of treatment of sexual and general health problems.

NON-PRESCRIPTION TREATMENTS

The most effective treatments remain the prescription oral and injectable medications. Their use has been undermined by massive internet promotions to obtain similar products without prescription or assessment. Often these products are counterfeit.

Some men prefer treatment for ED to be complementary based, but no studies have yet shown any to be as effective as the prescription medications. However, a practitioner prescribing safe complementary medications for ED may be of much benefit through counselling skills and a genuine interest in helping the patient.

Herbal

Herbal medicines have much to offer in improving stress management, and increasing energy, libido and testosterone levels. Improving peripheral circulation may also be of benefit. All these have a role to play in improving erectile dysfunction, although the evidence is inconsistent.

Common herbs used are:[3]

- puncture vine fruit (*Tribulus terrestris*[4])—increases libido, aphrodisiac
- saw palmetto seed (*Serenoa repens*)—male tonic
- Korean ginseng root (*Panax ginseng*)—adaptogen, regulates HPA axis, may increase testosterone levels[5,6]
- damiana leaf (*Turnera diffusa*[7])—male tonic, aphrodisiac, anti-inflammatory
- *Ginkgo biloba* leaf[8]—peripheral circulation stimulant.

Traditional Chinese medicine

Erectile dysfunction belongs to 'Yang Wei' in traditional Chinese medicine (TCM). In TCM normal sexual functioning depends on the health of the kidney and the liver. Kidney yang controls the functional aspect of an erection and kidney jing the ability to reproduce, while the liver channel passes through the external genitals. Weakness of the kidney reduces the physiological 'Fire of desire', while stagnation of liver qi reduces the physical ability.

In general, TCM treatment for this condition is to strengthen the kidney and liver, and the treatment should be combined with psychological treatment.

SUMMARY

Erectile dysfunction may be a presenting sign of undiagnosed vascular disease elsewhere in the body. Even when vascular causes of ED predominate, the psychological issues that are inevitably present should also be addressed. Low testosterone level may be a cause of ED, although it is usually associated with low libido. Low libido can be also a presenting sign of depression and relationship issues.

The increasing incidence of ED together with the ageing population will result in increasing requests for treatment because of people's expectations of maintaining good quality of life in their senior years. The man must be fit enough to engage in sexual intercourse to be considered suitable for any ED treatment. Patients often have misguided fears of the risks of oral ED medication. Counselling can be an effective treatment on its own and can improve the effectiveness of medical treatment. Involvement of the partner improves the outcome of the combined counselling and medical treatment.

Men should be encouraged to have an annual health check, particularly in the middle years when there is a family history of diabetes, hypertension, hyperlipidaemia and bowel and prostate cancer. These check-ups allow men to be assessed for metabolic syndrome, physical fitness, mental health and sexual function. They may also encourage men to be more aware of their general health and the benefits of a healthy lifestyle, and prevent ill health at an earlier stage. Regular checks may allow interventions to be more effective for smoking, excessive alcohol intake, illicit drug use and weight and exercise issues.

RESOURCES

Andrology Australia, http://www.andrologyaustralia.org.au

Braun L, Cohen M. Herbs and natural supplements. An evidence-based guide. 2nd edn. Sydney: Elsevier; 2007.

Ernst E, Pittler M, Wider B, eds. The desktop guide to complementary and alternative medicine. An evidence-based approach. 2nd edn. Sydney: Elsevier; 2006.

Hackett G et al., for the British Society for Sexual Medicine. British Society for Sexual Medicine Guidelines on the Management of Erectile Dysfunction. J Sex Med 2008; 5:1841–1865.

Impotence Australia, http://www.impotenceaustralia.com.au

Porst H, Buvat J, eds. Standard practice in sexual medicine. International Society for Sexual Medicine. Oxford: Blackwell; 2006.

REFERENCES

1 Feldman HA, Goldstein I, Hatzichristou DG et al. Impotence and its medical and psychological correlates: Results of the Massachusetts Male Aging Study. J Urol 1994; 151:54–61.

2 Chew KK, Earle CM, Stuckey BGA et al. Erectile dysfunction in general medicine practice: prevalence and clinical correlates. Int J Impotence Res 2000; 12:41–45.

3 McKay D. Nutrients and botanicals for erectile dysfunction: examining the evidence. Alt Med Rev 2004; 9(1):4–16.

4 Ademoelja A. Phytochemicals and the breakthrough of traditional herbs in the management of sexual dysfunctions. Int J Androl 2000; 23(Suppl 2):82–84.

5 Price A, Gazewood J. Korean red ginseng effective for treatment of erectile dysfunction. J Fam Pract 2003; 52(1):20–21.

6 Jang DJ, Lee MS, Shin BC et al. Red ginseng for treating erectile dysfunction: a systematic review. Br J Clin Pharmacol 2008; 66(4):444–450.

7 Estrada-Reyes R, Ortiz-López P, Gutiérrez-Ortiz J et al. *Turnera diffusa* Wild (Turmeraceae) recovers sexual behaviour in sexually exhausted males. J Ethnopharmacol 2009; 123(3):423–429.

8 Cohen AJ, Bartlik B. *Ginkgo biloba* for antidepressant-induced sexual dysfunction. J Sex Marital Ther 1998; 24(2):139–143.

chapter 50

An integrative approach to prostate cancer

INTRODUCTION AND OVERVIEW

Prostate cancer is a major health issue for men around the world, particularly in developed countries. In Australia, for example, over 18,000 men are diagnosed with it per year and it kills over 3000 patients each year.[1] There were 679,000 new cases of prostate cancer worldwide in 2002, making it the fifth most common cancer in the world and the second most common in men (11.7% of new cancer cases overall; 19% in developed countries and 5.3% in developing countries).[2] It is the most common cause of cancer-related death in men.[3] It is the most common non-cutaneous malignancy and there are around 250,000 prostate cancer deaths each year worldwide.[4]

AETIOLOGY

The causes of prostate cancer are essentially unknown, although it is estimated that up to 40% of prostate cancers may have an inherited component, according to twin studies.[5] Furthermore, there is approximately a 40-fold difference in the reported incidence and a 12-fold difference in mortality rate of prostate cancer between various geographic and ethnic populations.[6] The highest reported incidence of prostate cancer is in Afro-American men.[7] Men with a family history of prostate cancer also have an increased risk of developing prostate cancer.[8] There is a two-fold risk with one first-degree relative and a five-fold risk with two first-degree relatives.[8] Results from migrant studies provide strong

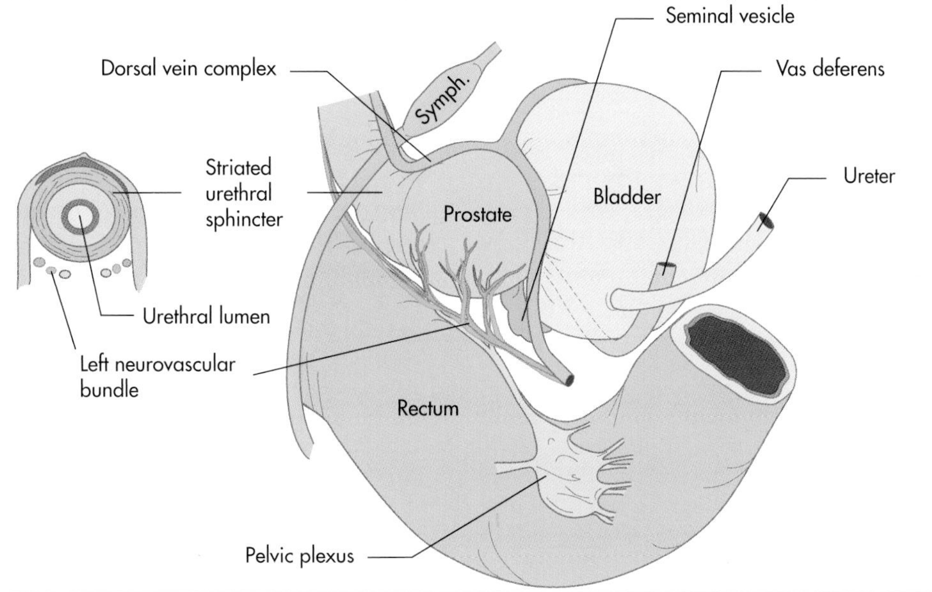

FIGURE 50.1 Anatomy of normal prostate

evidence of the importance of environmental and lifestyle factors in the development of prostate cancer.[9] Recently, there has been considerable interest in the role of diet and other lifestyle factors in the initiation, promotion and progression of prostate cancer.[10]

PREVENTION

A few studies have been undertaken to determine whether prostate cancer can be prevented by taking 5-alpha-reductase inhibitors (finasteride and dutasteride).[11–13] The finasteride (Proscar®) trial showed a 25% reduction in the prevalence of prostate cancer over a 7-year period; however, there has been some concern that there may be a slight increase in the incidence of more aggressive tumours, but subsequent, more careful analyses have not supported this.[12,14] Currently, chemo prevention with finasteride is therefore not recommended by most urologists.

Further major studies that have recently been reported include a prevention study using dutasteride (Avodart®) and another study, the SELECT trial, using selenium and vitamin E, and studying 30,000 men. The dutasteride study (REDUCE trial) reported a 20% decrease in the detection of prostate cancer after only 4 years of follow-up in a slightly higher-risk group of men without any increase in detection of high-grade disease. There was a 4% increased incidence of reduced libido, similarly to the finasteride study. The SELECT trial reported no benefit in taking selenium and vitamin E in the prevention of prostate cancer. It was, however, performed in a country not deficient in selenium.[15–18]

Other medications that have been implicated in possible prevention are the statins, for which there is currently low-level evidence of a possible risk reduction[19–21] and toremifene, a selective oestrogen receptor modulator that has shown some experimental evidence in animals for a reduction in incidence.[22]

There is now some evidence-based dietary advice that GPs can give their patients on how to reduce their risk of prostate cancer (Box 50.1). Obesity, high saturated fat intake and high calorie intake may increase the risk of developing prostate cancer.[23,24]

In countries where the soil is deficient in selenium (e.g. Australia), 100–200 μg of selenium daily is considered safe and appears to reduce the incidence of prostate cancer.[25,26] Lycopene, found in the red part of tomatoes, and, in the new world, red wines, also seem to be a possible factor.[27,28] Adequate vitamin D intake is to be encouraged, usually by natural means, but possibly by supplementation.[29] Vitamin E supplementation may help some patients if the dose is limited to < 400 IU per day, although the SELECT trial has raised doubt about this.[30] A dosage higher than this may increase the risk of heart attack or stroke.

BOX 50.1 Evidence-based dietary advice on how to reduce prostate cancer risk

- Healthy heart diet (Mediterranean)
- Low saturated fats
- Low calorie intake
- No obesity
- Selenium (100 μg/day) if the country is deficient
- High lycopenes
- Vitamin D_3 (adequate dosage to correct deficiency)
- Fish oil/ omega-3 fatty acids—considered to provide a protective role; can be taken as 4000 mg/ day or > 3 serves of fish a week
- Soy isoflavones
- Pomegranate
- Antioxidants (e.g. green tea, moderate intake of red wine, soy protein, red clover; all have low-level evidence)

Avoid:

- Saturated fats
- Excessive zinc, calcium and dairy products
- Excessive multivitamins
- Excessive red meat (more than 500 g per week)

Vasectomy and sexual activity do not appear to be major factors in the aetiology of prostate cancer.[31,32]

Herb and plant extracts have also been implicated in some studies, but there is currently no evidence for the use of saw palmetto, pygeum, pumpkin or stinging nettle, all of which have traditionally been used for benign prostatic hyperplasia. There is, however, some experimental evidence that isoflavones, such as red clover, which has a phyto-oestrogenic effect, as well as milk thistle, may have some benefit, but this has only been shown in experimental models and has been extrapolated from low-risk Asian populations.[33,34]

DIET SUPPLEMENTS AND PROSTATE CANCER

There is now considerable evidence that environmental factors, particularly dietary factors, may have a profound influence on the incidence of, and effect on, the natural history of prostate cancer.[35–37] Current research into prostate cancer suggests that changes in so-called modifiable risk factors, such as diet and supplements, may translate into very meaningful benefits.[38–43] The level of evidence for each component of the diet and supplement varies, and is still evolving. Having said that, many of the dietary modifications also have a general benefit.

DIET

The information on diet currently suggests that a healthy heart diet, or Mediterranean diet, appears to be beneficial to prostate cancer patients.[44–46] Limited caloric intake, as well as reduction in saturated fats and a high intake of fish, appear to be beneficial.[39] A diet high in cruciferous vegetables and plant-based foods appears to be beneficial not only to the heart, but also to the prostate.[43,47]

SUPPLEMENTS

The recently published large randomised control trial (SELECT) looking at the effects of selenium and vitamin E in prostate cancer concluded that there was no statistically significant benefit in the use of either selenium or vitamin E (alone or in combination) in the prevention of prostate cancer in relatively healthy men.[18] Excessive use of multivitamins has recently been shown to increase the rate of advanced and fatal disease.[48] Fish oil appears to be a good source of omega-3, particularly if fish is not a common part of one's diet. Pomegranate has recently also shown some potential benefit.[49–52]

PHYTOMEDICINE

Herbs and spices, such as garlic, turmeric, rosemary and lemongrass, have been variously recommended, but most evidence for any general benefit appears to come from studies of garlic.[53] For most of these, however, there is no reliable evidence in humans in vivo at normal intake levels.

There has also been evidence for polyphenols, such as green tea and red wine. Again, results have been mixed. A Chinese control study showed a protective effect of green tea with synergy for lycopene, but no benefit for green tea in a Japanese study.[54,55] There appeared to be a combined inhibitory effect of green tea and COX-2 inhibitors.[56,57] The benefit of red wine appears to come from the polyphenol resveratrol, and a moderate intake (< 4 glasses of red wine per week) appeared to have some benefit in the healthcare professional follow-up studies.[58,59] Other plant extracts, such as soy and red clover, appeared to induce their effect through their oestrogenic content. These have been shown, in some population and experimental studies, to have a benefit, but not in vivo.[60]

LIFESTYLE FACTORS

Other aspects of supportive care include stress management and regular exercise and, certainly, there is now a lot of evidence to suggest that regular moderate exercise has benefits in many of the stages of prostate cancer and, in particular, in the more advanced stages, when patients are on hormone therapy.[61,62] For example, elderly men with prostate cancer are about a third as likely to progress to more aggressive prostate cancer if they exercise regularly.[63] It is, however, important to avoid certain dietary and supplementary treatments and, in particular, an excessive intake of calcium and zinc; and dietary fat, particularly saturated dietary fat, is to be avoided.[46,64]

The data on diet, as they relate to prostate cancer, are incomplete. As a general principle it is currently recommended that a healthy-heart diet, low in saturated fat and rich in omega-3 fatty acids, as well as judicious use of supplements, such as lycopene, selenium, vitamin D_3, soy isoflavones, limited vitamin E and, possibly, pomegranate, are potentially useful.[30,41,46,52,65] This should always be combined with appropriate stress management as well as regular exercise. The further benefit of this is that it empowers the patient to do something for himself.

The Ornish program was mentioned in some detail in Chapter 24. It was trialled on men with early prostate cancer who chose to watch and wait, and over 2 years showed that men who adopted the Ornish program had only a fifth the rate of progression to more aggressive cancer of those who had maintained their usual lifestyle. The Ornish program included all the elements of the ESSENCE model (see Ch 6):

- vegan diet
  - fruits, vegetables, whole grains, legumes and soy
  - low fat (10% calories from fat), particularly saturated/animal product fats
  - supplemented by soy (tofu), fish oil (3 g daily), vitamin E (400 IU daily), selenium (200 μg daily), vitamin C (2 g daily)
- exercise
  - walking (30 min, 6 times weekly)
- stress management
  - gentle yoga, meditation, breathing and progressive muscle relaxation
- support group 1 hour weekly.

Since the data from the outcome studies have been reported there has also been interesting data on the possible mechanisms underlying the positive outcomes. Healthy lifestyle change along the lines of the Ornish program have been found to improve telomerase activity[66]—an indicator of improved genetic repair—and also down-regulation of prostate cancer gene expression.[67] These studies indicate a number of things:

- Watching and waiting is not an unreasonable option for men with less aggressive forms of prostate cancer if it is undertaken along with substantial and healthy lifestyle change.
- Healthy lifestyle change is important regardless of whether a man chooses to watch and wait or have interventional treatment, to both improve outcomes and enhance quality of life.
- Although the data are yet to come, healthy lifestyle change is likely to improve outcomes for men with more advanced prostate cancer.

The extensive discussion on lifestyle change and cancer using the ESSENCE model should also be reviewed in Chapter 24, Cancer.

SCREENING

WHY?

There is increasing evidence that prostate cancer testing and early aggressive treatment of appropriately selected cases is likely to save lives.[68–70] This evidence includes the European randomised trial (described below), which reported in 2009.[69] Prostate-specific antigen (PSA) testing has been responsible for the earlier detection of prostate cancer, which has led to the increased success of curative treatment. There is increasing evidence that use of PSA testing leads to the detection of cancers at an earlier and more curable stage, and that the falling death rate from prostate cancer can, at least in part, be attributed to the efforts of testing and early treatment. Also, in countries with a high uptake of PSA testing, there has been a consistently lower death rate from prostate cancer.

Recently, the European Randomised Study of Screening for Prostate Cancer published its results in the *New England Journal of Medicine*.[69] This landmark study demonstrated unequivocally that PSA screening saves lives. This enormous undertaking was carried out in seven European countries and involved about 162,000 men aged between 55 and 69 years, who were screened with PSA testing every 4 years (with a cut-off value of 3 ng/mL, indicating the need for biopsy) versus no screening. It was scheduled to report in 2 years' time, but was published early because a statistically significant reduction in the death rate from prostate cancer was found in the screened group. The median follow-up in this group was 9 years, with up to 14 years of follow-up.

Patients who underwent screening experienced a 71% increase in the incidence of prostate cancer detected compared with patients who did not undergo screening, and a 41% reduction in advanced disease; and a 20% reduction in deaths from prostate cancer was seen in all men at study entry. If only men who actually underwent screening were included in the results, the reduction in deaths from prostate cancer was 27%. It is highly likely that, as this study matures, the mortality benefit will increase further. This result is very similar to the 30% reduction in mortality in patients with breast cancer following screening with mammography[71] and the 33% reduction in prostate-cancer-specific mortality that occurred in the United States from 1994 to 2003, following the introduction of PSA screening.[72]

The authors of the European study point out that, to prevent one prostate cancer death at 10 years of follow-up, 1410 men would need to be screened and 48 additional men would need to be treated. These numbers are very similar to those that need to be screened with mammography for breast cancer, and faecal occult blood testing for colorectal cancer, to prevent one death. The European study has come under criticism because of the side effects associated with the treatment of prostate cancer which, in many men, might have been unnecessary. It is for this reason that controversy over prostate cancer screening continues.

The controversy about PSA testing is further compounded by another trial, published in the same edition of the *New England Journal of Medicine*.[73] The conclusion of this US study, after 7–10 years of follow-up, was that the rate of death from prostate cancer was very low in both groups of screened and unscreened patients and did not differ significantly between the two study groups. This study has been criticised because not only did it have a poor method of testing, but 52% of the controls were screened, follow-up was too short, it was compared with a background of a heavily screened population and very few people underwent biopsies.[73]

PSA testing, therefore, is not a perfect science, for the following reasons:

- A PSA test can be abnormal when cancer is not present.
- A PSA test can be normal, even when cancer is present.

If prostate cancer is found to be present after an abnormal PSA test, the following issues may arise:

- Some cancers are latent and slow growing, and do not require treatment (over-diagnosis and possibly over-treatment).
- Some cancers are incurable, even with early detection (under-diagnosis).
- All treatments have potential side effects.

Furthermore, there is evidence to suggest that use of the PSA test leads to detection of cancers at an earlier, and more curable, stage.[74] This is supported by a falling death rate from prostate cancer which can, at least in part, be attributed to the efforts of testing and early treatment, particularly in areas that have been testing for more than 15 years in a high proportion of the community (e.g. in Tyrol, Austria).[75,76] A 10-year study comparing surgery for early prostate cancer versus watchful waiting showed a clear benefit in terms of prostate cancer survival and the incidence of metastatic disease.[77]

Even less-aggressive tumours have been shown, after 15–20 years, to metastasise and lead to prostate cancer death.[78]

There is now increased effort to avoid treating latent tumours by putting the patient on active surveillance to avoid over-treatment, particularly in older patients.[79–82] With improved clinical judgment, these less-threatening cancers are more likely to be identified at the time of diagnosis and less likely to be treated.

The side-effect profiles of treatments have decreased markedly in recent times.[83,84]

The official position of the Urological Society of Australia and New Zealand is that PSA-based testing together with digital rectal examination should be offered to men between the ages of 55 and 69 years, after providing information about the risks and benefits of such testing. Men under 55 years of age are less likely to be diagnosed with prostate cancer, but if they are diagnosed they are more likely to die from prostate cancer than men over 55 years of age, due to a reduced likelihood of dying from comorbid illnesses.

Men in the younger age group who are interested in their prostate health could have a single PSA test and digital rectal examination performed at or beyond the age of 40 years, to provide an estimate of their prostate cancer risk over the next 20 years. At this stage, population screening in asymptomatic men is not recommended as a public health policy. A complete executive summary of the position of the Urological Society of Australia and New Zealand is available on its website (see the Resources list). In the interim, informed consent prior to testing will remain necessary.

HOW?

PSA testing and digital rectal examination currently form the cornerstone of prostate cancer testing. A raised PSA level can detect a non-palpable tumour, and an abnormal digital rectal examination can detect a non-PSA-producing tumour. Any older patient with haemospermia should also be tested for prostate cancer. Increasingly, PSA velocity is being used to detect cancer at an earlier stage by monitoring the PSA and recommending biopsy when the velocity increases (when the PSA goes up by > 0.75 ng/mL per year for two consecutive years).[85,86] This is particularly useful in younger patients with a family history.

A biopsy should be performed if the digital rectal examination is abnormal or if the PSA reading is greater than the reference range for age on two consecutive occasions and there is no other explanation for the elevated PSA, such as severe prostatic enlargement,

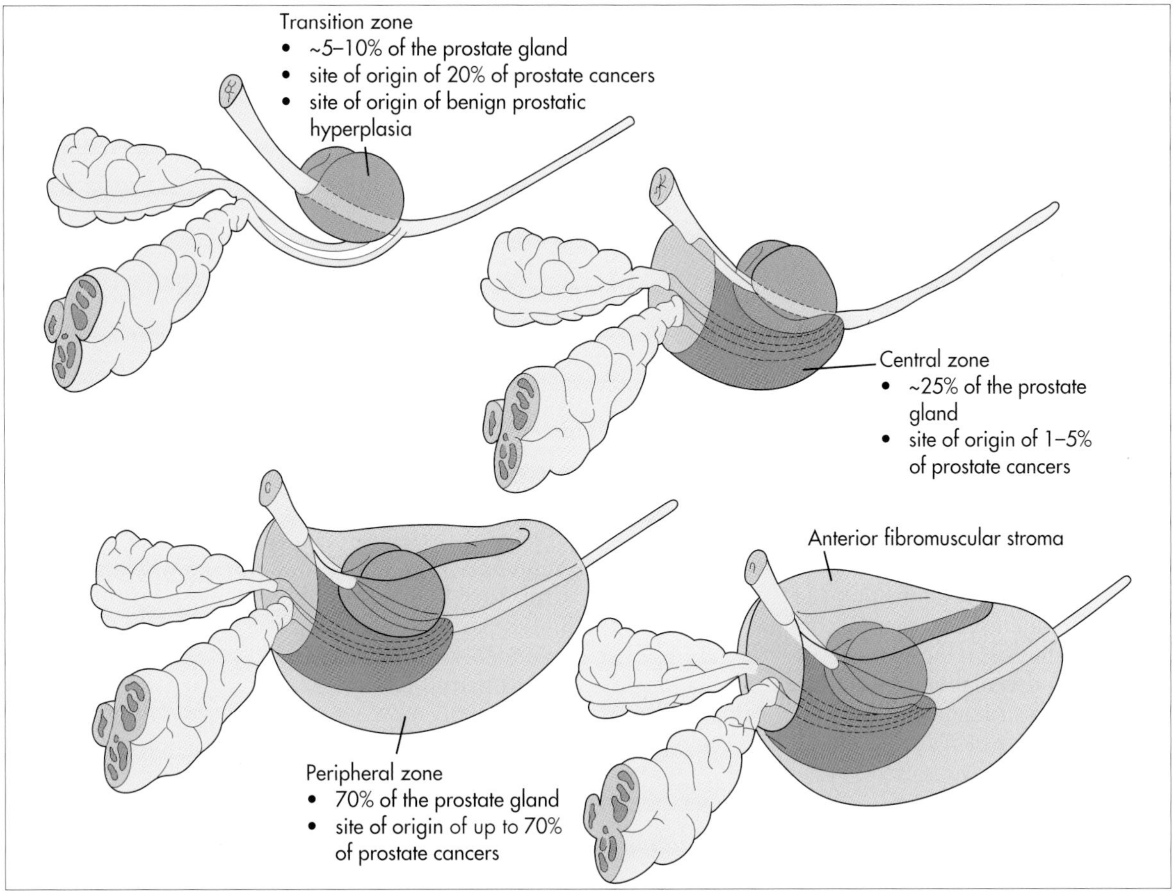

FIGURE 50.2 Zones affected by prostate cancer

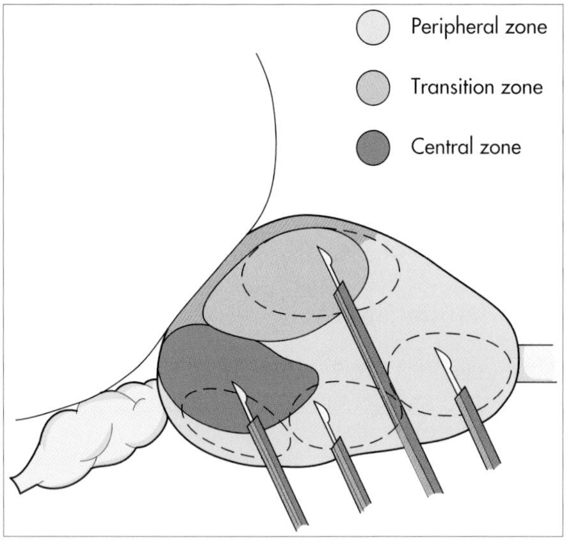

FIGURE 50.3 Prostate biopsy

prostatitis, recent ejaculation or recent instrumentation. Biopsies should also be recommended if the PSA velocity starts to increase after a baseline of minimal PSA velocity.

WHO?

Assessing a patient's preferences and determining the likelihood that he will benefit from screening is part of the physician's responsibility. Generally, a patient should have a life expectancy of > 15 years.

Screening should include:

- patients at high risk (family history)
- patients who are particularly anxious about prostate cancer
- symptomatic and asymptomatic patients aged between 40 and 70, after informed consent.

WHEN?

Although advice varies in different countries and at different times,[87] the current position of the Urological Society of Australasia is that individual men, aged between 50 and 70, with at least 10 years' life expectancy, should be able to be screened by annual digital rectal examination and PSA testing, after appropriate counselling regarding the potential benefits of investigations and the controversy of treatment. The age at which screening commences should be reduced to 40 if there is a strong family history.[69] The effectiveness of this screening in reducing mortality from prostate cancer is not entirely resolved.[69]

Guidelines on PSA and DRE testing vary from country to country and are likely to keep changing as evidence continues to come in. For example, the current recommendations from the United States and the United Kingdom are given below.

- 'The US Food and Drug Administration (FDA) has approved the use of the PSA test along with a digital rectal exam to help detect prostate cancer in men age 50 and older.' That age recommendation drops to 45 in the case of men at high risk of prostate cancer.[88]
- 'PSA alone is not recommended for screening in the UK, as the evidence of its reliability is still very unclear. At the moment the NHS policy is that if a man asks for a PSA test, he should be given information about the advantages and disadvantages of having the test and a chance to discuss this with his doctor.'[89]

GPs will therefore need to make their own informed decisions on the recommendation or otherwise of PSA and DRE screening, bearing in mind that clinical decisions are often made on the basis of a combination of evidence, personal experience and the individual patient's concerns and clinical background.

There is some evidence that an isolated PSA test at the age of 40 can predict the likelihood of a man developing prostate cancer in his lifetime.[90] For example, a PSA level of > 0.6 ng/mL at 40 years of age suggests that the man is seven times more likely to develop prostate cancer than a man with a PSA level of < 0.3 ng/mL. This has useful implications for how frequently a PSA should be performed.

Generally, PSA tests should be done annually between the ages of 50 and 70, but can be reduced to every 4 years if the PSA is < 1 ng/mL.

ACCURACY OF PSA SCREENING

Approximately 30% of patients with a PSA level of 4–10 ng/mL have cancer. When PSA is above 10, approximately 50% of prostate cancers have broken through the capsule.

Detection of prostate cancer in its curable stages therefore requires the use of relatively low PSA cut-off levels, which leads to unnecessary biopsies in approximately 70% of patients. This can be minimised by the use of age-specific reference ranges, free/total PSA ratio and PSA velocity and density.[91] For example, if patients with a free/total PSA ratio of > 25% (for PSA range 4–10) are not biopsied, 8% of cancers will be missed but up to 30% of unnecessary biopsies will be avoided.

Furthermore, if the PSA goes up by > 0.75 ng/year for two consecutive years, this is highly suggestive, even at low PSA levels, of an underlying cancer.

ISSUES WITH PSA TESTING AND REFERRAL

PSA testing

- *Elevated PSA*—treat prostatitis (if suspected, give 4 weeks of a quinolone antibiotic). Exclude recent ejaculation, repeat test with free/total PSA ratio; if still elevated and above age-specific reference range, refer.

- *PSA and urinary tract infection*—PSA takes up to 3–6 months to return to normal after a significant infection in the prostate or bladder.
- *PSA and extent of cancer*—once the PSA is > 10 ng/mL there is a 50% chance that the cancer is outside the capsule.
- *PSA and treatments*—after prostatectomy, the PSA should be < 0.1 ng/mL and after radiotherapy it should slowly fall, over 2–3 years, to below 0.5 ng/mL and certainly should not rise to > 2 ng/mL after that.

Referral

All patients with an abnormal digital rectal examination should be referred to a urologist for biopsy, irrespective of their PSA level. In the presence of a normal digital rectal examination, patients with a PSA above the age-specific reference range and free/total PSA ratio of < 25% should be referred if a repeat test confirms an elevated PSA level. Patients being monitored, with a PSA rise of > 0.75 ng/mL per year for two consecutive years, should also be referred.

DIAGNOSIS AND STAGING

To diagnose prostate cancer, a transrectal ultrasound-guided or transperineal biopsy of the prostate is performed, under a light anaesthetic or local anaesthesia. The transperineal approach may reduce the risk of septicaemia (approximately 1–2% with the transrectal technique). Modern biopsy techniques have a minimum of 12, and preferably 18–24, biopsies of the prostate. This minimises the chance of a false negative result.

If prostate cancer is diagnosed, it can generally be grouped into localised or metastatic disease, and localised cancer can be grouped into low-, intermediate- and high-risk disease.

From the biopsy, the pathologist can assess the Gleason Score of the tumour. Generally, if the Gleason Score is 6 or below, it is a slow-growing tumour; if it is 7, it is intermediate grade; and if it is 8–10, it is high-grade. Within the 7 category, a Gleason 3+4 behaves far less aggressively than a Gleason 4+3.[92]

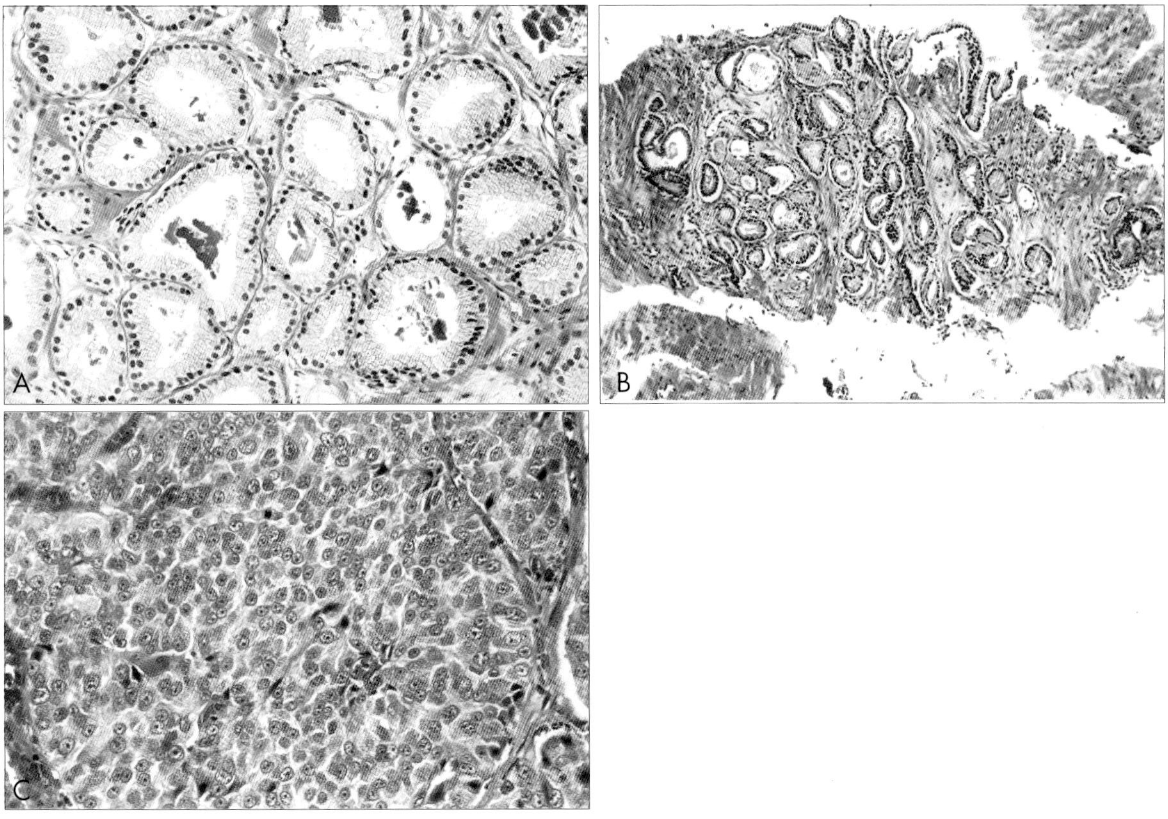

FIGURE 50.4 Prostate cancers. **A** Low grade (Gleeson score 1 + 1 = 2), consisting of back-to-back, uniformly sized malignant glands. **B** Needle biopsy of moderately differentiated adenocarcinoma (Gleeson 3 + 3 = 6), glands variably sized and widely dispersed. **C** Poorly differentiated adenocarcinoma (Gleeson 5 + 5 = 10), composed of sheets of malignant cells.

It is now known that Gleason 6, or lower, tumours generally grow very slowly and only carry a 20% chance of spreading and causing death, even after 20 years with no treatment. This is why patients with small tumours that are Gleason 6 or below, especially elderly men, are often suitable for active surveillance, to see if they have an active tumour.[80,82,93]

Investigations to assess the extent of a tumour include a bone scan (when the PSA is > 10), an abdomino pelvic CT scan (when the PSA is > 20 or there is a high Gleason Score) and, increasingly, MRI, preferably with an endorectal coil and a 3-Teslar machine and/or spectroscopy.

TREATMENT OF LOCALISED PROSTATE CANCER

There are now many treatment options for localised prostate cancer, making it difficult to choose the best option. Furthermore, there have been major improvements in all forms of therapy, and results vary from centre to centre.

Options include: radical prostatectomy in all its various forms, radiation therapy, active surveillance, brachytherapy, and newer therapies such as cryotherapy and high-intensity focused ultrasound (HIFU).

As men vary greatly in the value they ascribe to potential outcomes (i.e. survival, potency, continence), treatment should be carefully tailored to fit the individual's values and situation. It is essential to spend adequate time to ensure the correct selection of treatment for the individual. If a patient is uncomfortable with the decision, he should defer his decision.

It is essential that the patient, preferably including his family, is actively involved in the decision-making process and that adequate resources and information are provided on the cure and side effects of each therapy, often with multiple meetings, so that the patient can study the published literature and hand-outs and discuss the information at home.

The prognosis of the cancer should be discussed carefully and not overstated, as the patient's decisions will be governed by this information.

Finally, as the pathology is so integral to the recommendation, the pathology should always be reviewed by an experienced prostate pathologist.

The final decision regarding treatment will depend on the tumour, local factors, patient factors including comorbidities, the type of person and his particular priorities, and the expertise of the institution.

LIFESTYLE THERAPY

Lifestyle issues have been previously discussed, and any men diagnosed with prostate cancer should be advised to make lifestyle modification along the guidelines previously given. The aim is not just to improve survival but also to enhance quality of life and reduce the impact of treatment side effects.

RADICAL PROSTATECTOMY

Technical improvements and experience have markedly improved outcomes. There have now been several publications suggesting that surgical experience has a significant impact on outcomes.[94–96] The aim of surgery is to achieve the 'trifecta' (negative margins, continence and potency). Radical prostatectomy can be performed via the retropubic open route, laparoscopic, perineal and robot-assisted laparoscopic route. The robot-assisted laparoscopic technique is gaining popularity in the United States, where 84% of cases were performed using this technique in 2009.[97,98]

The prognosis is determined by the preoperative Gleason Score, clinical stage, PSA level and PSA velocity. PSA rises of > 2 ng/mL in a calendar year impart a worse prognosis for all therapeutic options.

Cure rates of > 90% for low-risk prostate cancer and > 70% for intermediate-risk prostate cancer are to be expected, and incontinence rates are consistently < 5%.[99–103] Impotence rates are dropping with improved modifications of the nerve-sparing techniques, as well as better patient selection. In younger men who were potent before surgery, 80–90% are capable of intercourse by 2–4 years with or without PDE5 inhibitors.[104–109] Results from large robotic centres are claiming a more rapid recovery of erectile functioning compared with open series, although this needs to be reproduced in other centres.[110]

Robot-assisted radical prostatectomy aims to perform the same operation as a radical prostatectomy through smaller holes and improved magnification. The learning curve for this technique is considerably shorter than the laparoscopic learning curve, and results from mature series consistently show a more rapid return to normal activities with an equal likelihood of the trifecta.[111,112] No direct comparisons, however, have been made between these two procedures. The potential advantages of robot-assisted radical prostatectomy include improved magnification, less bleeding, a shorter hospital stay and a more rapid return to normal activities.[113] The disadvantages are the learning curve for the surgeon, the loss of tactile sensation and the cost.

In deciding between robot-assisted radical prostatectomy, laparoscopic and open prostatectomy performed by an experienced surgeon, patients should focus on the surgeon's results and experience, rather than the technology. Questions should centre on the likelihood of the trifecta (the chance of achieving a negative margin and the long-term chance of preserving urinary control and sexual function).

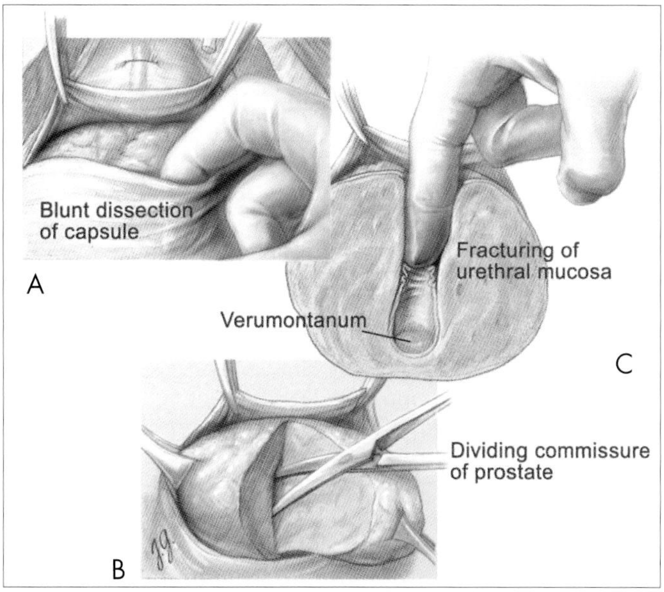

FIGURE 50.5 Retropubic prostatectomy

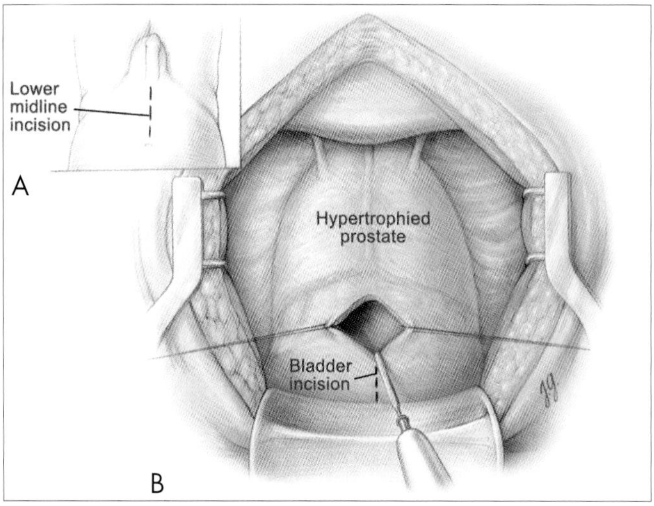

FIGURE 50.6 Suprapubic prostatectomy

RADIATION THERAPY

It has now become clear that external beam radiotherapy was previously not accurate or intense enough to kill many forms of prostate cancer and minimise side effects. Many forms of radiation therapy have therefore evolved, including conformal radiotherapy, IMCRT, low-dose rate brachytherapy (iodine-125 seed therapy) and high dose rate brachytherapy.

Conformal radiotherapy and IMCRT

With the use of careful planning and better machinery, it is now possible to deliver a higher, more accurate, dose of radiotherapy to the prostate, thereby maximising the likelihood of cure and minimising the chance of damaging adjacent organs. Generally, doses of at least 72 gray are needed, and this requires a skilful unit where accurate planning and appropriate machinery are available to deliver the therapy. There still remains a 2–3% chance of ongoing, severe rectal toxicity.

Iodine-125 brachytherapy

This less-invasive therapy involves implanting radioactive seeds into the prostate as a day procedure, but is only suitable for low-risk prostate cancers with minimal urinary symptoms. Cure rates for the select group appear to be comparable to surgical results.[114–117]

Long-term side effects include lower urinary tract irritability and impotence (30–50%).

It is ideal for middle-aged, older men with a fear of surgery who are sexually potent and anxious to retain potency, and have a low-volume, low-staged tumour in a small prostate with no urinary obstruction, particularly if they are also obese.

High dose rate brachytherapy

High dose rate brachytherapy is a more invasive treatment in which a very high dose of radiotherapy can be placed accurately into the prostate by wires, supplementing ordinary radiotherapy, which is also given at a lower radiation dose.

Complications include a 2–3% chance of urethral stricture and a 50% impotence rate. Ten-year results are excellent for patients with more advanced disease, particularly when surgery is unlikely to cure them.[115,118] This is often combined with hormone therapy.

ACTIVE SURVEILLANCE

With increased numbers of biopsies, it may now be possible to predict more accurately whether one has a non-aggressive, low-volume prostate cancer.[93] Increasingly, patients with low-volume, low-grade tumours (less than, or equal to, Gleason 6) are initially being monitored carefully on an active surveillance program and offered treatment only if the cancer shows signs of progressing.[79,80,119] This is particularly so in older patients (aged over 70). Active surveillance involves regular PSA and digital rectal examination monitoring, and periodic biopsies.

OTHER TREATMENTS

Cryotherapy and HIFU

These newer, less-tested technologies are used to either freeze or heat the prostate. Long-term results in both these technologies are not yet known.[120,121] They both appear to have a significant recurrence rate. They are both particularly attractive options for older men who refuse, or are unsuitable for, surgery or radiotherapy. They can also be used, albeit with a high side-effect profile, if radiotherapy fails to cure the cancer locally.[120,122,123]

COMPLICATIONS OF TREATMENTS

Urinary problems, particularly urinary incontinence, are far less common after surgery than in previous decades. It is important to engage a pelvic floor physiotherapist early after surgery, to encourage pelvic floor strength.[124,125] If incontinence continues after 6–12 months, options include injections with collagen and Macroplastique®, urethral slings or, for the more severe types of incontinence, an artificial urinary sphincter.

Sexual problems are still the most common problem after all forms of therapy.[126] The early use of PDE5 inhibitors or prostaglandin E_1 injections after surgery appears to minimise the chance of permanent erection problems.[127] Ideally, a sexual health physician should be involved in the rehabilitation phase. If erection problems do not recover, the use of a PDE5 inhibitor, prostaglandin E_1 injection, a vacuum constriction device or even a penile implant, are options. However, many patients, especially older men, opt for no therapy and engage in other forms of sexual pleasuring.

PSA recurrence can occur after any form of therapy and, if it occurs after surgery, radiotherapy remains a potentially curative treatment if indications suggest that the cancer has recurred locally.[128–131] The PSA doubling time seems to be an accurate predictor of whether this is likely to go on to more advanced disease.[132–135] Many patients who develop a PSA recurrence after any form of therapy should be encouraged to undertake their own personal supportive care with regards to diet, supplements and exercise.

CHOOSING BETWEEN TREATMENTS

The final choice of treatment for localised prostate cancer requires careful tailoring of the treatment to the patient, with appropriate importance placed upon the tumour factors, the patient's local factors, the patient's general wellbeing including comorbidities, the patient's particular priorities, other factors such as geographical and financial considerations, and institutional expertise. During this decision-making process it may be necessary to incorporate a clinical psychologist and even a sexual health physician, to aid in this regard.

TREATMENT OF ADVANCED CANCER

Hormone therapy, either continuous or intermittent, remains the mainstay for this stage of the disease. Generally, if the PSA is > 50 or there is evidence of metastatic disease, it is regarded as incurable or advanced.

Hormone therapy is generally administered by luteinising hormone releasing hormone (LHRH) agonists, such as goserelin, leuprorelin or Eligard®. These may be combined with anti-androgens, including bicalutamide, flutamide, nilutamide or cyproterone.

There is evidence that regular resistance exercise, as well as a carefully planned diet, can prevent many of the side effects, including weight gain, decreased muscle mass, depression and mood swings.[62] Hot flushes can be treated with cyproterone or oestrogen patches and there is some evidence that isoflavones of 100 mg may have a role in this treatment. Depression and mood swings, if mild, may be treated with St John's wort.[136]

Long-term hormone therapy can lead to osteoporosis. This can be prevented by regular resistance exercise, adequate vitamin D and calcium supplements.[137–140] People on long-term hormone therapy need to be monitored with bone mineral density (BMD) tests and, if BMD significantly deteriorates to the osteoporotic range, bisphosphonate therapy will need to be commenced. Patients need to be aware that this therapy is associated with a small risk of osteonecrosis of the jaw and, prior to commencement of this, appropriate dental hygiene must occur.[141,142] Osteoporosis can also be prevented by reducing alcohol intake and increasing isoflavone intake.[143,144]

The prognosis of a patient with metastatic disease is dependent on the PSA nadir and the PSA doubling time prior to the commencement of hormone treatment.[145,146] A patient with a PSA doubling time of < 3 months prior to the commencement of hormone therapy has only a 1% chance of surviving 10 years.[147,148] Despite having advanced disease, many patients can be maintained on hormone therapy for more than five, and often more than ten, years, particularly if the PSA doubling time is slow.

Many patients with less aggressive cancers use intermittent hormone therapy, which appears to be as effective as continuous therapy, but with some benefits in terms of quality of life.[149]

Docetaxel is the first chemotherapy drug proved to prolong life in patients with metastatic prostate cancer who have failed hormone therapy.[150–152] New potential developments in this area will occur in the angiogenesis and growth factor fields.[153]

RESOURCES

Andrology Australia, http://www.andrologyaustralia.org
Cancer Council Australia, http://www.cancer.org.au
Cancer Council New South Wales, http://www.cancercouncil.com.au
Lions Australia Prostate Health, http://www.prostatehealth.org.au
National Cancer Institute, http://www.cancer.gov/cancertopics/factsheet
National Comprehensive Cancer Network, http://www.nccn.org
Prostate Cancer Foundation of Australia and New Zealand, http://www.prostate.org.au
Urological Society of Australia and New Zealand, http://www.usanz.org.au
Vincent's Prostate Cancer Centre, http://www.prostate.com.au

Books/booklets

Localised prostate cancer, a guide for men and their families, http://cancer.org.au.
Prostate cancer, a guide for people with cancer, their families and friends, http://cancercouncil.com.au.
Rashid P. Prostate cancer: your guide to the disease, treatment options and outcomes, 3rd edn. http://prostate.org.au
Stricker P, Phelps K. Prostate cancer for the general practitioner, 2nd edn. http://prostate.com.au

REFERENCES

1 Council NC. Cancer in New South Wales. Incidence and mortality 2004. Online. Available: http://www.cancercouncil.com.au/editorial.asp?pageid=9, 2007.
2 Parkin DM, Bray F, Ferlay J et al. Global cancer statistics, 2002. Cancer J Clin 2005; 55:74–108.
3 Parkin DM, Bray FI, Devesa SS. Cancer burden in the year 2000. The global picture. Eur J Cancer 2001; 37(Suppl 8):S4–S66.
4 Garcia M, Jemal A, Ward EM et al. Global cancer facts and figures 2007. Atlanta, GA: American Cancer Society; 2007. Online. Available: http://www.cancer.org/downloads/STT/Global_Cancer_Facts_and_Figures_2007_rev.pdf
5 Page WF, Braun MM, Partin AW et al. Heredity and prostate cancer: a study of World War II veteran twins. Prostate 1997; 33(4):240–245.
6 Jemal A, Siegel R, Ward E et al. Cancer statistics 2007. CA Cancer J Clin 2007; 57(1):43–66.
7 Ghafoor A, Jemal A, Cokkinides V et al. Cancer statistics for African Americans. CA Cancer J Clin 2002; 52(6):326–341.
8 Bratt O. Hereditary prostate cancer: clinical aspects. J Urol 2002; 168(3):906–913.
9 Kenfield SA, Chang ST, Chan JM. Diet and lifestyle interventions in active surveillance patients with favorable-risk prostate cancer. Curr Treat Options Oncol 2007; 8(3):173–196.
10 Morton MS, Turkes A, Denis L et al. Can dietary factors influence prostatic disease? BJU Int 1999; 84(5):549–554.
11 Lotan Y, Cadeddu JA, Lee JJ et al. Implications of the prostate cancer prevention trial: a decision analysis model of survival outcomes. J Clin Oncol 2005; 23(9):1911–1920.
12 Lucia MS, Epstein JI, Goodman PJ et al. Finasteride and high-grade prostate cancer in the Prostate Cancer Prevention Trial. J Natl Cancer Inst 2007; 99(18):1375–1383.
13 Thompson IM, Goodman PJ, Tangen CM et al. The influence of finasteride on the development of prostate cancer. N Engl J Med 2003; 349(3):215–224.
14 Rubin MA, Kantoff PW. Effect of finasteride on risk of prostate cancer: how little we really know. J Cell Biochem 2004; 91(3):478–482.

15 Andriole GL, Roehrborn C, Schulman C et al. Effect of dutasteride on the detection of prostate cancer in men with benign prostatic hyperplasia. Urology 2004; 64(3): 537–541; discussion 42–43.

16 Klein EA, Thompson IM, Lippman SM et al. SELECT: the next prostate cancer prevention trial. Selenium and Vitamin E Cancer Prevention Trial. J Urol 2001; 166(4):1311–1315.

17 Kerr M. AUA 2009: Dutasteride lowers risk for prostate cancer. American Urological Association, 104th Annual Scientific Meeting: Late Breaking Abstract 1. Partial results presented 27 April 2009; full results presented 28 April 2009.

18 Lippman SM, Klein EA, Goodman PJ et al. Effect of selenium and vitamin E on risk of prostate cancer and other cancers. The Selenium and Vitamin E Cancer Prevention Trial (SELECT). JAMA 2009; 301(1):39–51.

19 Hoque A, Chen H, Xu XC. Statin induces apoptosis and cell growth arrest in prostate cancer cells. Cancer Epidemiol Biomarkers Prev 2008; 17(1):88–94.

20 Moyad MA. Why a statin and/or another proven heart healthy agent should be utilized in the next major cancer chemoprevention trial: part II. Urol Oncol 2004; 22(6):472–477.

21 Moyad MA, Merrick GS, Butler WM et al. Statins, especially atorvastatin, may favorably influence clinical presentation and biochemical progression-free survival after brachytherapy for clinically localized prostate cancer. Urology 2005; 66(6):1150–1154.

22 Price D, Stein B, Sieber P et al. Toremifene for the prevention of prostate cancer in men with high grade prostatic intraepithelial neoplasia: results of a double-blind, placebo controlled, phase IIB clinical trial. J Urol 2006; 176(3):965–970.

23 Efstathiou JA, Bae K, Shipley WU et al. Obesity and mortality in men with locally advanced prostate cancer: analysis of RTOG 85-31. Cancer 2007; 110(12):2691–2699.

24 Gong Z, Agalliu I, Lin DW et al. Obesity is associated with increased risks of prostate cancer metastasis and death after initial cancer diagnosis in middle-aged men. Cancer 2007; 109(6):1192–1202.

25 Etminan M, FitzGerald JM, Gleave M et al. Intake of selenium in the prevention of prostate cancer: a systematic review and meta-analysis. Cancer Causes Control 2005; 16(9):1125–1131.

26 Pourmand G, Salem S, Moradi K et al. Serum selenium level and prostate cancer: a case-control study. Nutr Cancer 2008; 60(2):171–176.

27 Ivanov NI, Cowell SP, Brown P et al. Lycopene differentially induces quiescence and apoptosis in androgen-responsive and -independent prostate cancer cell lines. Clin Nutr 2007; 26(2):252–263.

28 Vaishampayan U, Hussain M, Banerjee M et al. Lycopene and soy isoflavones in the treatment of prostate cancer. Nutr Cancer 2007; 59(1):1–7.

29 Autier P, Gandini S. Vitamin D supplementation and total mortality: a meta-analysis of randomized controlled trials. Arch Intern Med 2007; 167(16):1730–1737.

30 Peters U, Littman AJ, Kristal AR et al. Vitamin E and selenium supplementation and risk of prostate cancer in the Vitamins and Lifestyle (VITAL) study cohort. Cancer Causes Control 2008; 19(1):75–87.

31 Cox B, Sneyd MJ, Paul C et al. Vasectomy and risk of prostate cancer. JAMA 2002; 287(23):3110–3115.

32 Lynge E. Prostate cancer is not increased in men with vasectomy in Denmark. J Urol 2002; 168(2):488–490.

33 Bemis DL, Capodice JL, Desai M et al. A concentrated aglycone isoflavone preparation (GCP) that demonstrates potent anti-prostate cancer activity in vitro and in vivo. Clin Cancer Res 2004; 10:5282–5292.

34 Ganry O. Phytoestrogens and prostate cancer risk. Prev Med 2005; 41(1):1–6.

35 Hayes RB, Ziegler RG, Gridley G et al. Dietary factors and risks for prostate cancer among blacks and whites in the United States. Cancer Epidemiol Biomarkers Prev 1999; 8(1):25–34.

36 Kavanaugh CJ, Trumbo PR, Ellwood KC. The US Food and Drug Administration's evidence-based review for qualified health claims: tomatoes, lycopene, and cancer. J Natl Cancer Inst 2007; 99(14):1074–1085.

37 Kirsh VA, Peters U, Mayne ST et al. Prospective study of fruit and vegetable intake and risk of prostate cancer. J Natl Cancer Inst 2007; 99(15):1200–1209.

38 Moyad MA. Emphasizing and promoting overall health and nontraditional treatments after a prostate cancer diagnosis. Semin Urol Oncol 1999; 17(2):119–124.

39 Moyad MA. Dietary fat reduction to reduce prostate cancer risk: controlled enthusiasm, learning a lesson from breast or other cancers, and the big picture. Urology 2002; 59(4 Suppl 1):51–62.

40 Moyad MA. Is obesity a risk factor for prostate cancer, and does it even matter? A hypothesis and different perspective. Urology 2002; 59(4 Suppl 1):41–52.

41 Moyad MA. Heart healthy equals prostate healthy equals statins: the next cancer chemoprevention trial. Part I. Curr Opin Urol 2005; 15(1):1–6.

42 Moyad MA, Carroll PR. Lifestyle recommendations to prevent prostate cancer, part II: time to redirect our attention? Urol Clin North Am 2004; 31(2):301–311.

43 Moyad MA, Carroll PR. Lifestyle recommendations to prevent prostate cancer, part I: time to redirect our attention? Urol Clin North Am 2004; 31(2):289–300.

44 Escrich E, Moral R, Grau L et al. Molecular mechanisms of the effects of olive oil and other dietary lipids on cancer. Mol Nutr Food Res 2007; 51(10):1279–1292.

45 Escrich E, Solanas M, Moral R et al. Are the olive oil and other dietary lipids related to cancer? Experimental evidence. Clin Transl Oncol 2006; 8(12):868–883.
46 Stamatiou K, Delakas D, Sofras F. Mediterranean diet, monounsaturated: saturated fat ratio and low prostate cancer risk. A myth or a reality? Minerva Urol Nefrol 2007; 59(1):59–60.
47 Moyad MA. Step-by-step lifestyle changes that can improve urologic health in men, part I: What do I tell my patients? Prim Care 2006; 33(1):139–163.
48 Lawson KA, Wright ME, Subar A et al. Multivitamin use and risk of prostate cancer in the National Institutes of Health—AARP Diet and Health Study. J Natl Cancer Inst 2007; 99(10):754–764.
49 Hong MY, Seeram NP, Heber D. Pomegranate polyphenols down-regulate expression of androgen-synthesizing genes in human prostate cancer cells overexpressing the androgen receptor. J Nutr Biochem 2008; 19(12):848–855.
50 Malik A, Mukhtar H. Prostate cancer prevention through pomegranate fruit. Cell Cycle 2006; 5(4): 371–373.
51 Pantuck AJ, Leppert JT, Zomorodian N et al. Phase II study of pomegranate juice for men with rising prostate-specific antigen following surgery or radiation for prostate cancer. Clin Cancer Res 2006; 12(13): 4018–4026.
52 Seeram NP, Aronson WJ, Zhang Y et al. Pomegranate ellagitannin-derived metabolites inhibit prostate cancer growth and localize to the mouse prostate gland. J Agric Food Chem 2007; 55(19):7732–7737.
53 Tapsell LC, Hemphill I, Cobiac L et al. Health benefits of herbs and spices: the past, the present, the future. Med J Aust 2006; 185(4 Suppl):S4–S24.
54 Jian L, Xie LP, Lee AH et al. Protective effect of green tea against prostate cancer: a case-control study in southeast China. Int J Cancer 2004; 108(1):130–135.
55 Kikuchi N, Ohmori K, Shimazu T et al. No association between green tea and prostate cancer risk in Japanese men: the Ohsaki Cohort Study. Br J Cancer 2006; 95(3):371–373.
56 Gupta S, Mukhtar H. Green tea and prostate cancer. Urol Clin North Am 2002; 29(1):49–57.
57 Srinath P, Rao PN, Knaus EE et al. Effect of cyclooxygenase-2 (COX-2) inhibitors on prostate cancer cell proliferation. Anticancer Res 2003; 23(5A):3923–3928.
58 Anon. Red wine may lower prostate cancer risk. Health News (Waltham, Mass.) 2005; 11(3):15.
59 Sutcliffe S, Giovannucci E, Leitzmann MF et al. A prospective cohort study of red wine consumption and risk of prostate cancer. Int J Cancer 2007; 120(7):1529–1535.
60 Hamilton-Reeves JM, Rebello SA, Thomas W et al. Effects of soy protein isolate consumption on prostate cancer biomarkers in men with HGPIN, ASAP, and low-grade prostate cancer. Nutr Cancer 2008; 60(1):7–13.
61 Barnard RJ, Leung PS, Aronson WJ et al. A mechanism to explain how regular exercise might reduce the risk for clinical prostate cancer. Eur J Cancer Prev 2007; 16(5):415–421.
62 Galvao DA, Taaffe DR, Spry N et al. Exercise can prevent and even reverse adverse effects of androgen suppression treatment in men with prostate cancer. Prostate Cancer Prostatic Dis 2007; 10(4):340–346.
63 Giovannuci EL, Liu Y, Leitzmann MF et al. A prospective study of physical activity and incident and fatal prostate cancer. Arch Intern Med 2005; 165(9):1005–1010.
64 Gallus S, Foschi R, Negri E et al. Dietary zinc and prostate cancer risk: a case-control study from Italy. Eur Urol 2007; 52(4):1052–1057.
65 Badger TM, Ronis MJ, Simmen RC et al. Soy protein isolate and protection against cancer. J Am Coll Nutr 2005; 24(2):146S–149S.
66 Ornish D, Lin J, Daubenmier J et al. Increased telomerase activity and comprehensive lifestyle changes: a pilot study. Lancet Oncol 2008; 9(11):1048–1057.
67 Ornish D, Magbanua MJ, Weidner G et al. Changes in prostate gene expression in men undergoing an intensive nutrition and lifestyle intervention. Proc Natl Acad Sci USA 2008; 105(24):8369–8374.
68 Roobol MJ, Kerkhof M, Schroder FH et al. Prostate cancer mortality reduction by prostate-specific antigen-based screening adjusted for nonattendance and contamination in the European Randomised Study of Screening for Prostate Cancer (ERSPC). Eur Urol 2009; 56(4):584–591.
69 Schroder FH, Hugosson J, Roobol MJ et al. Screening and prostate-cancer mortality in a randomized European study. N Engl J Med 2009; 360(13): 1320–1328.
70 van Leeuwen PJ, Connolly D, Gavin A et al. Prostate cancer mortality in screen and clinically detected prostate cancer: estimating the screening benefit. Eur J Cancer 2010; 46(2):377–383.
71 Shapiro S, Venet W, Strax P et al. Selection, follow-up, and analysis in the Health Insurance Plan Study: a randomized trial with breast cancer screening. Natl Cancer Inst Monogr 1985; 67:65–74.
72 Ries LAG, Melbert D, Krapcho M et al, eds. SEER Cancer Statistics Review, 1975–2005. Bethesda, MD; National Cancer Institute; 2008. Online. Available: http://seer.cancer.gov/csr/1975_2005 October 2009.
73 Andriole GL, Crawford ED, Grubb RL III et al. Mortality results from a randomized prostate-cancer screening trial. N Engl J Med 2009; 360(13):1310–1319.

74 Jang TL, Han M, Roehl KA et al. More favorable tumor features and progression-free survival rates in a longitudinal prostate cancer screening study: PSA era and threshold-specific effects. Urology 2006; 67(2):343–348.
75 Bartsch G, Horninger W, Klocker H et al. Tyrol Prostate Cancer Demonstration Project: early detection, treatment, outcome, incidence and mortality. BJU Int 2008; 101(7):809–816.
76 Horninger W, Berger A, Pelzer A et al. Screening for prostate cancer: updated experience from the Tyrol study. Can J Urol 2005; 12(Suppl 1):7–13.
77 Bill-Axelson A, Holmberg L, Filen F et al. Radical prostatectomy versus watchful waiting in localized prostate cancer: the Scandinavian prostate cancer group-4 randomized trial. J Natl Cancer Inst 2008; 100(16):1144–1154.
78 Sandblom G, Dufmats M, Varenhorst E. Long-term survival in a Swedish population-based cohort of men with prostate cancer. Urology 2000; 56(3): 442–447.
79 Klotz L. Active surveillance versus radical treatment for favorable-risk localized prostate cancer. Curr Treat Options Oncol 2006; 7(5):355–362.
80 Klotz L. Active surveillance for favorable-risk prostate cancer: what are the results and how safe is it? Curr Urol Rep 2007; 8(5):341–344.
81 Klotz L. Active surveillance for favorable risk prostate cancer: what are the results, and how safe is it? Semin Radiat Oncol 2008; 18(1):2–6.
82 Klotz L. Low-risk prostate cancer can and should often be managed with active surveillance and selective delayed intervention. Nat Clin Pract Urol 2008; 5(1):2–3.
83 Edgren M, Lennernas B, Haggman M et al. Postoperative radiotherapy after prostatectomy can be associated with severe side effects. Anticancer Res 2001; 21(3C):2231–2235.
84 von Knobloch R, Wille S, Hofmann R. Clinical side effects after radical prostatectomy. Front Radiat Ther Oncol 2002; 37:191–195.
85 Perrin P. PSA velocity and prostate cancer detection: the absence of evidence is not the evidence of absence. Eur Urol 2006; 49(3):418–419.
86 Sun L, Moul JW, Hotaling JM et al. Prostate-specific antigen (PSA) and PSA velocity for prostate cancer detection in men aged <50 years. BJU Int 2007; 99(4):753–757.
87 National Conference of State Legislatures. Prostate cancer screening mandates; 2009. Online. Available: http://www.ncsl.org/programs/health/prostate.htm
88 US National Institutes of Health, National Cancer Institute. Prostate-specific antigen (PSA) test. Online. Available: http://www.cancer.gov/cancertopics/factsheet/Detection/PSA
89 CancerHelp UK, Why isn't there UK PSA screening? Online. Available: http://www.cancerhelp.org.uk/about-cancer/cancer-questions/why-isnt-there-uk-psa-screening
90 Gerber GS. Biopsies for 'normal' PSA? Certain relatively young, healthy men with PSA levels below 4 should consider having a biopsy. Health News (Waltham, Mass.) 2004; 10(7):4.
91 Schroder FH. Diagnosis, characterization and potential clinical relevance of prostate cancer detected at low PSA ranges. Eur Urol 2001; 39(Suppl 4):49–53.
92 Mitchell RE, Shah JB, Desai M et al. Changes in prognostic significance and predictive accuracy of Gleason grading system throughout PSA era: impact of grade migration in prostate cancer. Urology 2007; 70(4):706–710.
93 Abouassaly R, Lane BR, Jones JS. Staging saturation biopsy in patients with prostate cancer on active surveillance protocol. Urology 2008; 71(4):573–577.
94 Bianco FJ Jr, Riedel ER, Begg CB et al. Variations among high volume surgeons in the rate of complications after radical prostatectomy: further evidence that technique matters. J Urol 2005; 173(6):2099–2103.
95 Brausi M. High surgical volume, high quality, and low costs: a perfect combination. Is it always possible in patients who need radical prostatectomy? Eur Urol 2006; 50(1):17–19.
96 Ramirez A, Benayoun S, Briganti A et al. High radical prostatectomy surgical volume is related to lower radical prostatectomy total hospital charges. Eur Urol 2006; 50(1):58–62; discussion 63.
97 Menon M, Muhletaler F, Campos M et al. Assessment of early continence after reconstruction of the periprostatic tissues in patients undergoing computer assisted (robotic) prostatectomy: results of a 2 group parallel randomized controlled trial. J Urol 2008; 180(3):1018–1023.
98 Patel HR, Arya M, Joseph JV. Robotic versus nonrobotic surgery: experts, toys and prostatectomy. Expert Rev Anticancer Ther 2008; 8(6):843–847.
99 Khan MA, Han M, Partin AW et al. Long-term cancer control of radical prostatectomy in men younger than 50 years of age: update 2003. Urology 2003; 62(1):86–92.
100 Walsh PC. Patient-reported urinary continence and sexual function after anatomic radical prostatectomy. J Urol 2000; 164(1):242.
101 Walsh PC. Sexual function and bother after radical prostatectomy or radiation for prostate cancer: multivariate quality-of-life analysis from CaPSURE. J Urol 2000; 163(1):370.
102 Walsh PC. Prospective comparison of radical retropubic prostatectomy and robot-assisted anatomic prostatectomy: the Vattikuti Urology Institute experience. J Urol 2003; 170(1):318–319.

103 Walsh PC. A randomized trial comparing radical prostatectomy with watchful waiting in early prostate cancer. J Urol 2003; 169(4):1588–1589.
104 Dubbelman YD, Dohle GR, Schroder FH. Sexual function before and after radical retropubic prostatectomy: a systematic review of prognostic indicators for a successful outcome. Eur Urol 2006; 50(4):711–718; discussion 718–720.
105 Katz R, Salomon L, Hoznek A et al. Patient reported sexual function following laparoscopic radical prostatectomy. J Urol 2002; 168(5):2078–2082.
106 Michl UH, Friedrich MG, Graefen M et al. Prediction of postoperative sexual function after nerve-sparing radical retropubic prostatectomy. J Urol 2006; 176(1):227–231.
107 Noldus J, Michl U, Graefen M et al. Patient-reported sexual function after nerve-sparing radical retropubic prostatectomy. Eur Urol 2002; 42(2):118–124.
108 Smith JA Jr. Editorial: sexual function after radical prostatectomy. J Urol 2003; 169(4):1465.
109 Zucchi A, Arienti G, Mearini L et al. Recovery of sexual function after nerve-sparing radical retropubic prostatectomy: is cavernous nitric oxide level a prognostic index? Int J Impot Res 2006; 18(2):198–200.
110 Menon M, Kaul S, Bhandari A et al. Potency following robotic radical prostatectomy: a questionnaire based analysis of outcomes after conventional nerve sparing and prostatic fascia sparing techniques. J Urol 2005; 174(6):2291–2296.
111 Ahlering TE, Eichel L, Edwards RA et al. Robotic radical prostatectomy: a technique to reduce pT2 positive margins. Urology 2004; 64(6):1224–1228.
112 Ahlering TE, Skarecky D, Lee D et al. Successful transfer of open surgical skills to a laparoscopic environment using a robotic interface: initial experience with laparoscopic radical prostatectomy. J Urol 2003; 170(5):1738–1741.
113 Patel VR, Thaly R, Shah K. Robotic radical prostatectomy: outcomes of 500 cases. BJU Int 2007; 99(5):1109–1112.
114 Ferrer M, Suarez JF, Guedea F et al. Health-related quality of life 2 years after treatment with radical prostatectomy, prostate brachytherapy, or external beam radiotherapy in patients with clinically localized prostate cancer. Int J Radiat Oncol Biol Phys 2008; 72:421–432.
115 Jo Y, Junichi H, Tomohiro F et al. Radical prostatectomy versus high-dose rate brachytherapy for prostate cancer: effects on health-related quality of life. BJU Int 2005; 96(1):43–47.
116 Namiki S, Satoh T, Baba S et al. Quality of life after brachytherapy or radical prostatectomy for localized prostate cancer: a prospective longitudinal study. Urology 2006; 68(6):1230–1236.
117 Tward JD, Lee CM, Pappas LM et al. Survival of men with clinically localized prostate cancer treated with prostatectomy, brachytherapy, or no definitive treatment: impact of age at diagnosis. Cancer 2006; 107(10):2392–2400.
118 Martinez A, Gonzalez J, Spencer W et al. Conformal high dose rate brachytherapy improves biochemical control and cause specific survival in patients with prostate cancer and poor prognostic factors. J Urol 2003; 169(3):974–980.
119 Klotz LH, Nam RK. Active surveillance with selective delayed intervention for favorable risk prostate cancer: clinical experience and a 'number needed to treat' analysis. Can J Urol 2006; 13(Suppl 1):48–55.
120 Aus G. Current status of HIFU and cryotherapy in prostate cancer—a review. Eur Urol 2006; 50(5):927–934; discussion 934.
121 Wondergem N, De La Rosette JJ. HIFU and cryoablation—non or minimal touch techniques for the treatment of prostate cancer. Is there a role for contrast enhanced ultrasound? Minim Invasive Ther Allied Technol 2007; 16(1):22–30.
122 Chaussy C, Thuroff S, Bergsdorf T. Local recurrence of prostate cancer after curative therapy. HIFU (Ablatherm) as a treatment option. Urologe A 2006; 45(10):1271–1275.
123 Shelley M, Wilt TJ, Coles B et al. Cryotherapy for localised prostate cancer. Cochrane Database Syst Rev 2007; 3:CD005010.
124 Cornel EB, de Wit R, Witjes JA. Evaluation of early pelvic floor physiotherapy on the duration and degree of urinary incontinence after radical retropubic prostatectomy in a non-teaching hospital. World J Urol 2005; 23(5):353–355.
125 Tarcia Kahihara C, Ferreira U, Nardi Pedro R et al. Early versus delayed physiotherapy in the treatment of post-prostatectomy male urinary incontinence. Arch Esp Urol 2006; 59(8):773–778.
126 Dalkin BL, Christopher BA. Potent men undergoing radical prostatectomy: a prospective study measuring sexual health outcomes and the impact of erectile dysfunction treatments. Urol Oncol 2008; 26(3):281–285.
127 McCullough AR. Sexual dysfunction after radical prostatectomy. Rev Urol 2005; 7(Suppl 2):S3–S10.
128 Boehmer D, Maingon P, Poortmans P et al. Guidelines for primary radiotherapy of patients with prostate cancer. Radiother Oncol 2006; 79(3):259–269.
129 Bolla M, Van Poppel H, Collette L. Preliminary results for EORTC trial 22911: radical prostatectomy followed by postoperative radiotherapy in prostate cancers with a high risk of progression. Cancer Radiother 2007; 11(6/7):363–369.
130 Bolla M, van Poppel H, Collette L et al. Postoperative radiotherapy after radical prostatectomy: a randomised

controlled trial (EORTC trial 22911). Lancet 2005; 366(9485):572–578.

131 van der Kwast TH, Collette L, Bolla M. Adjuvant radiotherapy after surgery for pathologically advanced prostate cancer. J Clin Oncol 2007; 25(35):5671–5672.

132 Heidenreich A. Identification of high-risk prostate cancer: role of prostate-specific antigen, PSA doubling time, and PSA velocity. Eur Urol 2008; 54:976–977.

133 Khatami A, Aus G, Damber JE et al. PSA doubling time predicts the outcome after active surveillance in screening-detected prostate cancer: results from the European randomized study of screening for prostate cancer, Sweden section. Int J Cancer 2007; 120(1): 170–174.

134 Klotz L. Active surveillance with selective delayed intervention using PSA doubling time for good risk prostate cancer. Eur Urol 2005; 47(1):16–21.

135 Tewari A, Horninger W, Badani KK et al. Racial differences in serum prostate-specific antigen (PSA) doubling time, histopathological variables and long-term PSA recurrence between African-American and white American men undergoing radical prostatectomy for clinically localized prostate cancer. BJU Int 2005; 96(1):29–33.

136 Vanoni C. Treatment of depression with St. Johns wort in general practice. Praxis (Bern 1994) 2000; 89(51/52):2163–2167.

137 Alibhai SM, Rahman S, Warde PR et al. Prevention and management of osteoporosis in men receiving androgen deprivation therapy: a survey of urologists and radiation oncologists. Urology 2006; 68(1):126–131.

138 McLeod N, Huynh CC, Rashid P. Osteoporosis from androgen deprivation therapy in prostate cancer treatment. Aust Fam Physician 2006; 35(4):243–245.

139 Morote J, Morin JP, Orsola A et al. Prevalence of osteoporosis during long-term androgen deprivation therapy in patients with prostate cancer. Urology 2007; 69(3):500–504.

140 Yee EF, White RE, Murata GH et al. Osteoporosis management in prostate cancer patients treated with androgen deprivation therapy. J Gen Intern Med 2007; 22(9):1305–1310.

141 Diamond TH, Higano CS, Smith MR et al. Osteoporosis in men with prostate carcinoma receiving androgen-deprivation therapy: recommendations for diagnosis and therapies. Cancer 2004; 100(5):892–899.

142 Smith MR. Osteoporosis during androgen deprivation therapy for prostate cancer. Urology 2002; 60(3 Suppl 1):79–85; discussion 86.

143 Kogawa M, Wada S. Osteoporosis and alcohol intake. Clin Calcium 2005; 15(1):102–105.

144 Sampson HW. Alcohol, osteoporosis, and bone regulating hormones. Alcohol Clin Exp Res 1997; 21:400–403.

145 Bates AT, Pickles T, Paltiel C. PSA doubling time kinetics during prostate cancer biochemical relapse after external beam radiation therapy. Int J Radiat Oncol Biol Phys 2005; 62(1):148–153.

146 Hanlon AL, Horwitz EM, Hanks GE et al. Short-term androgen deprivation and PSA doubling time: their association and relationship to disease progression after radiation therapy for prostate cancer. Int J Radiat Oncol Biol Phys 2004; 58(1):43–52.

147 Anscher MS. PSA kinetics and risk of death from prostate cancer: in search of the Holy Grail of surrogate end points. JAMA 2005; 294(4):493–494.

148 Robinson D, Sandblom G, Johansson R et al. PSA kinetics provide improved prediction of survival in metastatic hormone-refractory prostate cancer. Urology 2008; 72:903–907.

149 de Leval J, Boca P, Yousef E et al. Intermittent versus continuous total androgen blockade in the treatment of patients with advanced hormone-naive prostate cancer: results of a prospective randomized multicenter trial. Clin Prostate Cancer 2002; 1(3):163–171.

150 Berthold DR, Pond GR, Roessner M et al. Treatment of hormone-refractory prostate cancer with docetaxel or mitoxantrone: relationships between prostate-specific antigen, pain, and quality of life response and survival in the TAX-327 study. Clin Cancer Res 2008; 14(9):2763–2767.

151 Naito S, Tsukamoto T, Koga H et al. Docetaxel plus prednisolone for the treatment of metastatic hormone-refractory prostate cancer: a multicenter Phase II trial in Japan. Jpn J Clin Oncol 2008; 38(5):365–372.

152 Petrylak DP. Docetaxel (Taxotere) in hormone-refractory prostate cancer. Semin Oncol 2000; 27 (2 Suppl 3):24–29.

153 Liu B, Lee KW, Anzo M et al. Insulin-like growth factor-binding protein-3 inhibition of prostate cancer growth involves suppression of angiogenesis. Oncogene 2007; 26(12):1811–1819.

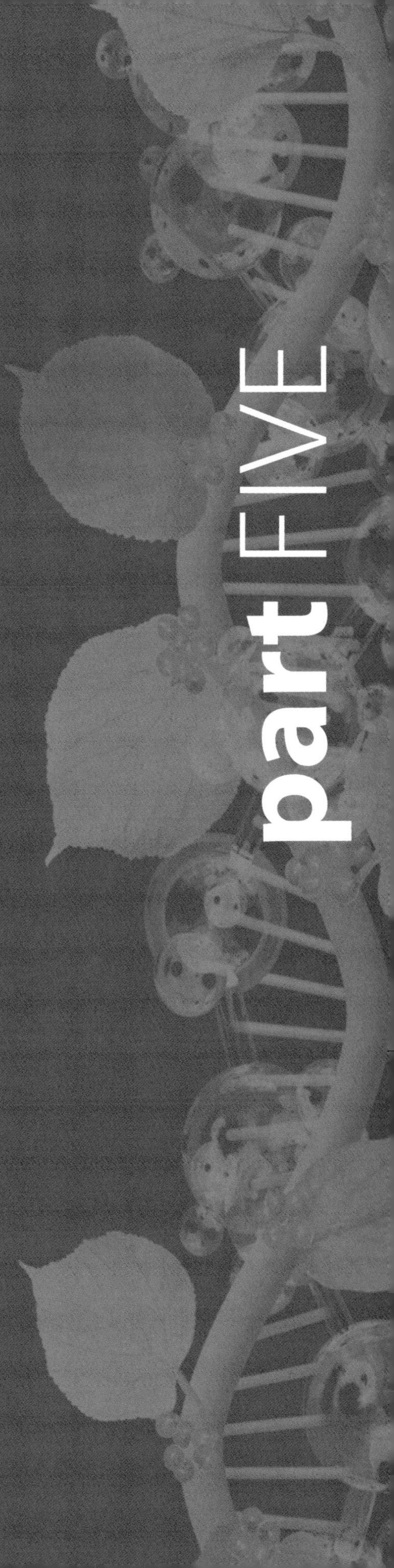

part FIVE

Women's health

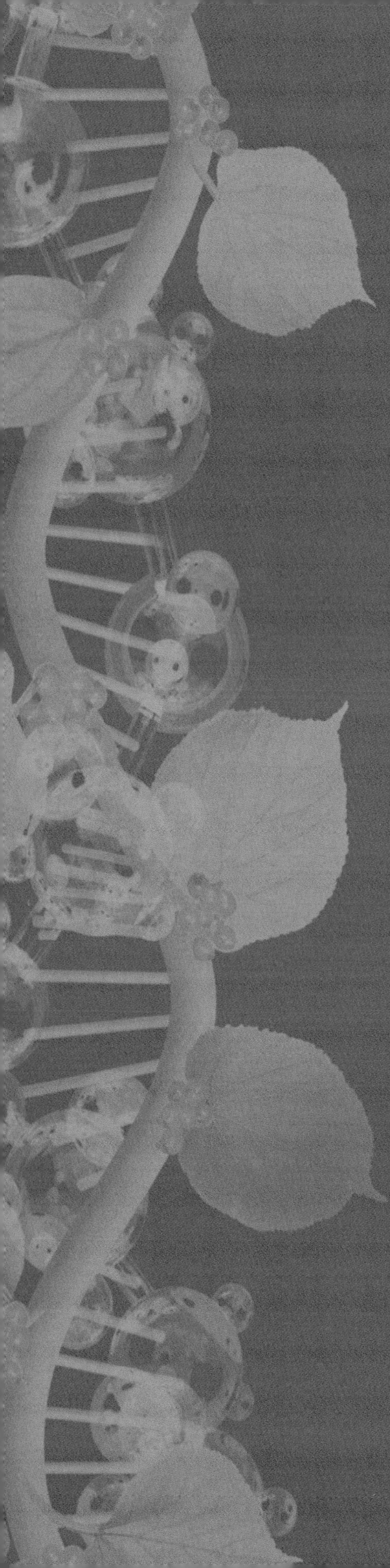

chapter 51

Breast disease

INTRODUCTION AND OVERVIEW

There are approximately 400,000 consultations for breast symptoms each year in general practice in Australia. The vast majority of these will be due to hormonal or benign breast changes. The general practitioner is the first port of call for the effective investigation of these symptoms and, importantly, to exclude or confirm breast cancer. For the thousands of women who are diagnosed with breast cancer each year, whether through mammographic screening or as a result of the investigation of a breast change, the GP provides information, treatment, surveillance and support throughout the patient's journey, as a member of the patient's treatment team.

BREAST HEALTH

Women of all ages should know the normal look and feel of their breasts—this is known as 'breast awareness'. There is no evidence to support any specific technique for breast self-examination. For many women there is also a psychological barrier to conducting a technical systematic examination, often suggesting they are not confident in their technique. For these reasons women should be encouraged to get to know what is normal for them through normal activities such as showering, dressing, putting on body lotion, looking in the mirror. Most importantly, women should be encouraged to present early to their GP if they find a change in their breasts—they are not wasting their doctor's time. This

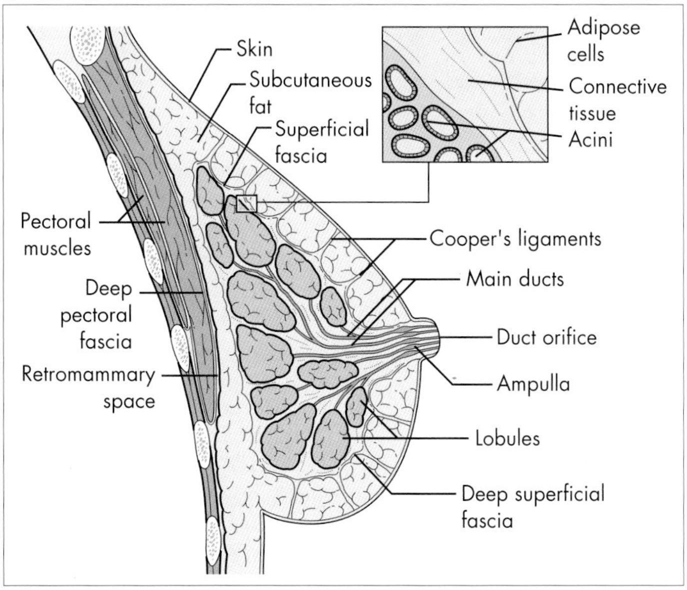

FIGURE 51.1 Gross anatomy of the breast

is important even if they have had a recent 'normal' mammogram.

In Australia, two-yearly mammographic screening is available free to all women aged 40 years and over through BreastScreen Australia. For women aged 50–69 years, there is strong evidence from international randomised trials for the effectiveness of mammographic screening in reducing mortality from breast cancer by about 30%. For women aged 40–49 years, the benefit may be smaller, as the effectiveness of mammography in detecting cancer is affected by the density of the individual woman's breast tissue. BreastScreen does not actively target women aged over 70 years. However, given that risk for breast cancer increases with age, it is important that older women do not presume they are no longer at risk. For women aged 70 years or over, the benefits of mammographic screening will depend on whether there are any significant medical comorbidities.

Women who have a significant family history should be referred to a familial cancer or genetics clinic, where an individual surveillance program and management advice can be provided and, if appropriate, genetic testing can be conducted.[1]

BENIGN BREAST DISEASES

During a woman's life there are three main phases of breast change. Breast development and early reproductive life is followed by mature reproductive life and finally by involution.

There are regular changes in relation to the menstrual cycle. Pregnancy causes a doubling of the breast weight at term, and the breast involutes after pregnancy.

In nulliparous women, breast involution commences at around age 30 years. During involution the breast stroma is replaced by fat and the breast becomes softer and less radio-dense. Changes in the glandular tissue during involution include the development of areas of fibrosis, the formation of small cysts and an increase in the number of glandular elements (adenosis).

Most presentations to healthcare professionals are benign and are the result of aberrations of these normal physiological processes. The most common presenting symptoms are:

- breast nodularity
- pain
- breast lumps
- nipple discharge.

Despite the above statement, the most important consideration for the GP is to exclude cancer as the cause of the presenting symptom.

BREAST PAIN AND FOCAL BREAST NODULARITY

Premenstrual breast pain and nodularity, improving with the onset of menstruation, are so common in women as to be considered physiological, rather than being a disease. Severe pain and nodularity are aberrations of these normal cyclical changes, which occur in the breasts of all women during their reproductive years. Bilateral focal breast nodularity, sometimes referred to as fibroadenosis or fibrocystic disease, is the most common cause of a breast lump. If excised, these areas show either no pathological abnormality, or aberrations of the normal involutional process, such as focal areas of fibrosis or sclerosis.

Breast pain

The causes of breast pain can be cyclical or non-cyclical. The best way to assess whether pain is cyclical is to ask the patient to complete a breast pain record chart.

Cyclical mastalgia is the more common. It shows a definite relationship to the menstrual cycle and is often associated with nodularity of varying degree, maximal in the upper outer quadrant and showing similar cyclicity.

Non-cyclical mastalgia affects older women. The origin of the pain can be from the chest wall, as in costochondritis, the breast itself or outside the breast. The pain may be continuous or random in its time pattern. A careful history and examination is required, to exclude non-breast causes.

The aetiology of mastalgia is unclear. Abnormalities in the control mechanisms of the pulsatile secretion of gonadotrophins and/or prolactin are likely. Women with mastalgia have also been found to have abnormal fatty acid profiles, but the role of dietary factors such as caffeine and fats in the aetiology of breast pain is unclear.

Management

For the management of cyclical breast pain, diuretics, progestogens and vitamin B_6 have not been shown to be any more efficacious than placebo. After excluding cancer, reassurance that the pain is not related to cancer, and an explanation of the hormonal basis of breast pain, may be the only treatment required. A soft support bra worn at night may also assist. Some women find stopping the Pill or changing formulations may assist.

Evening primrose oil (gamma-linolenic acid) has been shown to reduce pain, nodularity and tenderness, at a dose of 3 g daily.[2] It has only minor side effects, including headache, nausea, gastrointestinal upset and possible drug interactions with anticoagulant and antiplatelet agents and phenothiazines. A trial of treatment should last 4 months and be monitored with a pain chart. It does not interact with oral contraceptives.

Several clinical studies in women have suggested that chasteberry (*Vitex agnus castus*) is efficacious in reducing symptoms associated with premenstrual symptoms (PMS) including mastalgia.[2,3] This herb contains steroidal precursors and active moieties including progesterone, testosterone and androstenedione. Chasteberry may interact with oral contraceptives, other hormonal therapy and dopazmine antagonists such as haloperidol and prochlorperazine. Adverse effects reported include nausea, rash, headache and agitation.

If symptoms remain unresponsive to these therapies, consider referral. A range of medications are available to specialist practitioners, including bromocryptine, danazol, tamoxifen and goserelin.

Benign breast lumps

Fibroadenomata

Fibroadenomata result from a focal proliferation of benign breast elements, both epithelial and stromal, and are influenced by hormonal factors. They may fluctuate during the menstrual cycle and pregnancy. They are most common in the 20–30 year age group and are uncommon post menopause.

On clinical examination they are typically smooth, mobile, rubbery masses, which may be tender, especially premenstrually. They may be single or multiple. On breast ultrasound they appear as a well-defined ovoid homogenously hypoechoic mass with smooth margins and increased through transmission.

Diagnosis is confirmed by non-excisional biopsy. Ultrasound-guided core biopsy is used more commonly because of the high proportion of fibrous tissue to epithelial tissue, which increases the risk of not sampling the epithelial cells on fine needle aspiration.

Once the diagnosis is confirmed, fibroadenomata may be managed by either surgical excision or regular clinical and imaging review over 12–18 months until the lesion is proved to be stable. Should the lesion significantly increase in size or develop atypical features on imaging, it should undergo excision biopsy. New palpable fibroadenomas in women aged over 40 years should be referred to a breast surgeon for consideration of excision biopsy, because the likelihood of a new lump being cancer increases with age.[4]

Phyllodes tumour is a rare fibroepithelial tumour that produces a spectrum of diseases ranging from benign (with a significant risk of local recurrence) to malignant (sometimes with rapidly growing metastases). Clinically they may be indistinguishable from fibroadenoma, presenting as a smooth, rounded, painless breast lump that has continued to increase in size. Their appearance on mammogram and ultrasound may also resemble fibroadenomata. Diagnosis is confirmed by histology following excision biopsy.

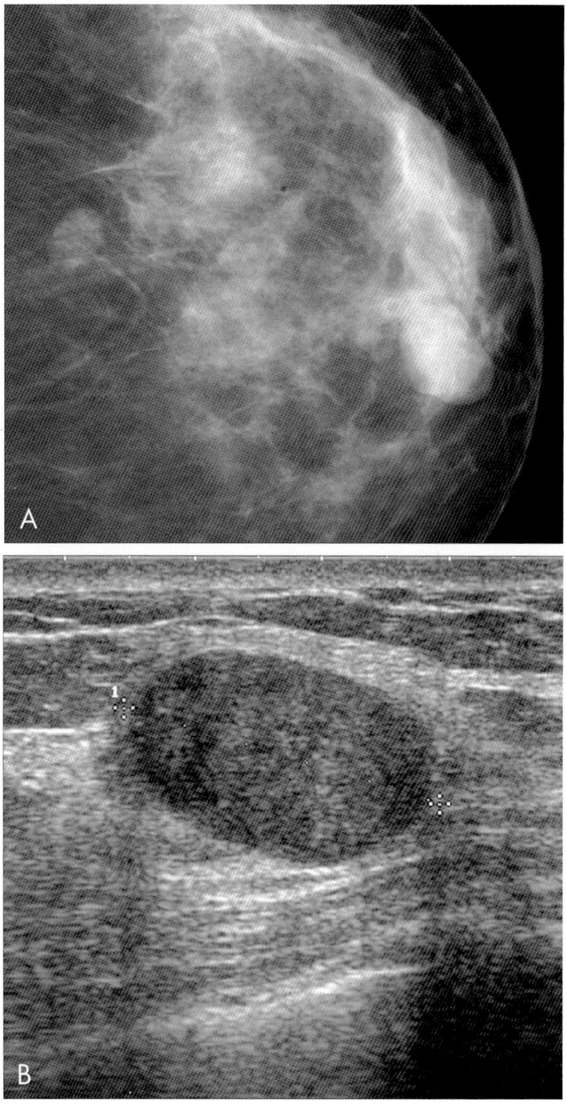

FIGURE 51.2 Fibroadenoma: **A** Mammogram showing two well-defined masses; **B** Ultrasound of the lesion nearer the nipple in **A**

Breast cysts

Breast cysts are distended and involuted lobules. They are hormonally responsive and may fluctuate in size during the menstrual cycle. They occur less commonly in postmenopausal women unless the woman is on hormone therapy.

Most breast cysts are impalpable and asymptomatic and are an incidental finding on breast imaging. They may present as a smooth and sometimes painful discrete

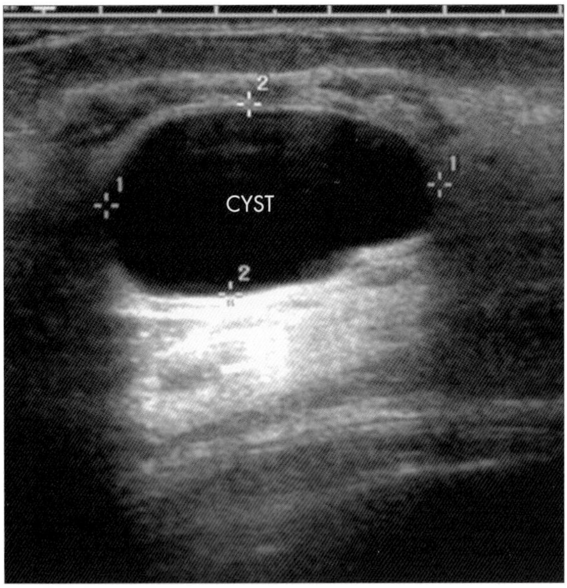

FIGURE 51.3 Breast cyst visible on ultrasound

breast lump. A cluster of cysts may present as a tender area of nodularity.

Cysts have characteristic halos on mammography, and on ultrasound appear as an anechoic lesion with smooth, defined borders and thin capsule with enhancement deep to the lesion, due to the transmission of the ultrasound through the fluid.

Large, painful cysts may be aspirated. The aspirate should be sent to cytology if the lump does not resolve completely with aspiration, if the aspirate is bloodstained or if the cyst has suspicious features on ultrasound, such as internal echoes or an intracystic lesion.

After aspiration, the breast should be re-examined to check that the mass has disappeared. Any residual mass needs full assessment by mammography and non-excisional biopsy to exclude cancer.

BREAST CANCER

BACKGROUND AND PREVALENCE

Breast cancer is the most common invasive cancer diagnosed in women in developed countries and the greatest cause of cancer-related death in women.[1,5] There is very good evidence that survival is related to the size and stage of the disease at diagnosis: the earlier the cancer is diagnosed, the greater the chance of effective treatment.[1,5]

However, even with a fully implemented mammographic screening program, more than 50% of the cancers diagnosed each year will be found as a result of a change in the breast detected by the woman or her doctor. Symptoms of breast cancer include:

- a new or unusual lump/thickening or lumpiness in one breast
- nipple discharge (especially if bloody or serous)
- new nipple inversion or change, such as crusting or ulceration of nipple
- redness, dimpling or puckering of the skin overlying the breast
- unusual and persistent breast pain.

The GP is the first port of call for women with a new breast symptom, the vast majority of which will not be due to breast cancer. The challenge for the GP is to effectively investigate these symptoms and determine those that may be due to breast cancer.

AETIOLOGY

Despite much research into causes and risk factors for breast cancer, we have no means of preventing this disease.[6] There are a number of factors that bear on the probability of a particular symptom being due to a breast cancer.

In general, breast cancer is a disease of ageing, with 75% of breast cancers diagnosed in women aged 50 years or older, and about 6% in women aged under 40 years. However, breast cancer can occur at any age and it is important that younger women who present with symptoms have these adequately investigated. Other factors that may increase risk for a particular woman include whether she has a significant family history of breast or ovarian cancer[1] or a relevant inherited gene mutation, whether she has had a previous invasive or in situ breast cancer or a previous biopsy that shows atypical proliferative disease or other marker for increased risk.

A number of other factors associated with risk for breast cancer are not modifiable, such as the age at menarche or menopause. Additionally some potentially modifiable factors are associated with reduced risk but are complex decisions for the individual woman. These include age at first pregnancy, number of children and breastfeeding. However, a number of lifestyle factors affecting risk for breast cancer are readily modifiable.

Lifestyle factors

Alcohol consumption (two or more standard drinks each day) and weight gain after menopause (BMI > 25) have a negative impact on risk, whereas regular exercise has been shown to reduce risk for breast cancer.

All women should be informed of the benefits of a well-balanced diet with low alcohol intake and regular exercise, not only for breast cancer but for other cancers and chronic diseases, and overall good health.

The World Health Organization estimates that 10% of breast cancer worldwide can be attributed to physical inactivity. It has also estimated that about 5% of breast cancers are attributable to alcohol consumption, and that overweight and obesity in postmenopausal women (BMI > 28) increases risk by about 30%.

The risk for breast cancer associated with taking the oral contraceptive pill is small, as the underlying risk for breast cancer is small at the age at which women are generally taking the Pill. The risk associated with HRT increases with increased duration of use, irrespective of the preparation or mode of administration. The decision about starting or staying on HRT must be made by the woman after being fully informed and weighing up the risks and benefits in her individual case.[7,8]

There are also a number of myths about risks for breast cancer that have no basis in evidence. For example, there is no evidence that wearing underwire bras or using antiperspirant deodorant can increase risk.

PATHOLOGY

The mature female breast contains thousands of potentially milk-producing lobules. Each lobule is drained by a terminal duct attached to the main duct system. Most breast diseases, including cancer, arise from this terminal ductal-lobular unit. About 65% of cancers are invasive ductal, and about 15% are invasive lobular. Tubular, medullary and mucinous breast cancers are less common. About 15% of breast cancers are preinvasive at diagnosis.

The pathological features of the cancer are vital in determining the extent of disease and the potential aggressiveness of the tumour, and in informing treatment decisions.

It is recommended that pathologists provide all relevant information in a synoptic pathology report, such as:

- size
- grade
- margins
- lymphovascular invasion
- hormone receptors
- HER 2
- lymph node status.

DIAGNOSTIC APPROACH

For the GP charged with assessing the presenting symptom, it is important to pursue a systematic approach to investigation that minimises the risk of missing a breast cancer. The 'triple test' is universally accepted as the most effective way to maximise the detection of cancer and to provide an accurate diagnosis for an abnormality. The correct sequencing of tests is important to the overall interpretation of the results.

The triple test refers to:

1. taking a history and performing clinical breast examination
2. diagnostic breast imaging, which may be mammography and/or breast ultrasound
3. non-excisional biopsy, which may be fine needle aspiration cytology or core biopsy.

The sensitivity of the triple test approaches 100%. Triple test negative, where no test results are positive (that is, no suspicious or malignant results), provides very good reassurance that the symptom is not due to cancer. Less than 1% of women will be falsely reassured that they do not have cancer, based on correlation of all three test results that are negative.

If any of the tests is suspicious for cancer or malignant (a triple test positive result), *or* if the results do not correlate with one another, irrespective of whether there are normal or benign test results, further evaluation and referral to a breast surgeon or specialist breast clinic is required.

However, not all women will require investigation with all three tests. Indeed, as the majority of symptoms are due to normal physiological changes, most women will be able to be reassured after providing a history and having a clinical breast examination—for example, where a woman presents with bilateral breast pain that occurs cyclically before her menstrual period and there is no clinical abnormality on examination. Imaging may additionally support this diagnosis.

The sensitivity of each component of the triple test for any individual woman will depend on a number of factors, including the age and history of the patient, the characteristics of the woman's breast tissue and the characteristics of the breast lesion. For example, the evaluation by clinical breast examination of a small lesion within lumpy breast tissue will be limited; and mammography in a young woman is less sensitive because of the increased density of the breast tissue.

History and clinical breast examination

A detailed history and clinical examination provide valuable information and should be accurately documented. Patient history should include details of menstrual history/hormonal status, relevant medications, family history, previous breast problems and results of relevant investigations. History of the presenting symptom includes site, duration, relationship to cycles, associated symptoms and any changes over time. Clinical breast examination includes inspection in good light and palpation of both breasts, with particular attention to the area of patient concern. Details of any clinical findings, including exact position, size, shape, consistency, mobility, fixation or tenderness, should be recorded.

Breast imaging

Patient age is a factor in determining the most appropriate imaging modality. The sensitivity of mammography increases with increasing age. Mammography is recommended as the first imaging modality in women

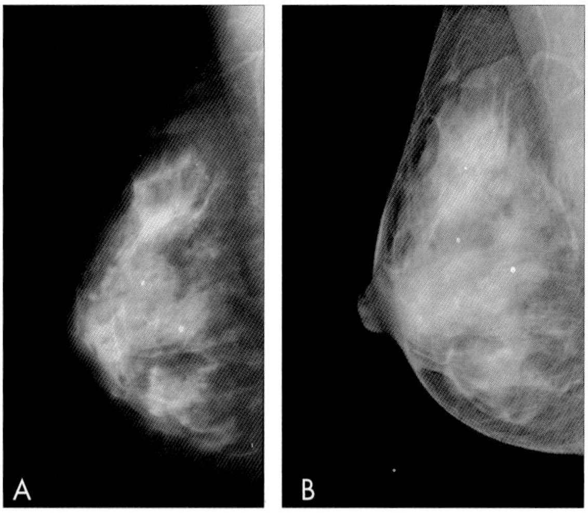

FIGURE 51.4 Screening mammogram: **A** conventional screen/film; **B** digital system

aged over 50 years and should only be used in women under 25 years if the clinical or ultrasound findings are suspicious for malignancy. Ultrasound is more sensitive in detecting cancer in younger women, and is recommended as the first imaging modality in women aged under 35 years. In practice, both mammography and ultrasound are often used to provide complementary information in the evaluation of symptoms.

Non-excisional biopsy

Both fine needle aspiration (FNA) cytology and core biopsy have high specificity and sensitivity for palpable and impalpable lesions. While there are no absolute rules to determine which is the more appropriate investigation, it is important to note that core biopsy can demonstrate invasive cancer, whereas FNA cannot differentiate between in-situ and invasive disease.

These procedures are usually performed under imaging guidance by a radiologist, breast physician or breast surgeon. It may be appropriate, therefore, with prior discussion with the patient, to include the option of performing biopsy if required in the referral for imaging.

TREATMENT

The vast majority of breast cancers are diagnosed 'early'—that is, they are confined to the breast with or without local lymph node involvement, and have not metastasised to other organs. The primary goal of treatment of early breast cancer is to control the disease with the aim of achieving cure. The initial management of breast cancer offers the best hope of cure. There are significant differences in women's views about, and need for, information, choice and support. The patient should be provided with adequate and appropriate information about treatment options in order to make an informed decision about her care.

The way in which a clinician relates to and communicates with a cancer patient can affect her wellbeing.[9] Communication skills training is available to assist health professionals to manage difficult conversations such as breaking bad news and discussing prognosis.[10]

When organising referral for patients with breast cancer, GPs should consider both the preferences of the patient and the fact that patient outcomes are better if treated by clinicians who are part of a multidisciplinary team.[11]

The usual primary treatment of early breast cancer is surgery. Where appropriate, women should be offered the choice of either breast-conserving surgery followed by radiotherapy, or mastectomy, as there is no difference between them in the rate of survival or distant metastasis. Women who undergo mastectomy should be provided with information about, and the option of, breast reconstruction, either immediate or delayed.

Determining the extent of spread of disease is vital to informing treatment choices. Sentinel node biopsy is increasingly becoming the standard of care for the assessment of the axilla, as it has been shown to be as effective as axillary dissection in predicting lymph node involvement and has less morbidity.

The pathological features of the cancer and the involvement of lymph nodes will provide valuable information to guide decisions about the use of systemic adjuvant therapy, which includes all forms of hormonal and cytotoxic chemotherapy. The aim of this treatment is to treat undetectable remaining cancer and reduce the risk of recurrence.

New targeted systemic therapies, such as tamoxifen for oestrogen receptor positive breast cancer, are constantly evolving and have had a significant impact on breast cancer survival rates over the past two decades. The decisions about adjuvant systemic therapy are most appropriately made in a multidisciplinary setting, and will take into consideration both tumour factors and patient factors such as age and overall health, as well as patient preferences, if known. The suggested treatment plan should then be discussed with the patient such that she has an understanding of the side effects and potential benefits in her individual case. Issues that may affect younger patients' decision-making, such as infertility and premature menopause, should be discussed and relevant referrals provided if necessary, prior to treatment commencing.

Note that where a woman has had surgery or radiotherapy involving the axillary lymph nodes, thereafter procedures including measurement of blood pressure or venepuncture should be avoided on that side.

Integrative management

Many patients who have been diagnosed with cancer use complementary and alternative therapies as adjuncts to their medical treatment. Most of these patients find this a way of maintaining a sense of control, particularly in relieving side effects of treatment and improving health-related quality of life, as well as facilitating physical and psychological rehabilitation.

Beyond the stage of active medical and surgical treatment and rehabilitation comes the question of enhancing wellbeing and, ultimately, longevity.

It is important to encourage patients to discuss any adjunctive therapies they may be considering or taking during treatment, as some interfere with conventional therapies and may cause harm. Other complementary therapies can work effectively alongside conventional treatment.

Many patients raise the question of antioxidant use during chemotherapy. Despite the concerns of some oncologists, no trials have reported evidence of significant decreases in efficacy from antioxidant supplementation during chemotherapy.[12]

Many of the studies indicated that antioxidant supplementation resulted in either increased survival times, increased tumour responses, or both, as well as less toxicity than controls; however, lack of adequate statistical power was a consistent limitation.

Patients enquiring about using supplements to control radiation side effects should be informed that they must abstain from smoking tobacco if they take antioxidants during radiotherapy.

It is important that patients discuss their motivation for enquiring about antioxidant and other supplement use, and discuss with their oncologist or radiotherapist. It is equally important for oncologists and radiotherapists to provide well-informed, evidence-based advice for patients, rather than a blanket 'take nothing'.

Hormone therapies for breast cancer can result in a significantly increased risk of cardiovascular disease, obesity, type 2 diabetes, osteoporosis and sarcopenia, so active risk factor management is essential in this group.

General advice includes:

- Encourage a balanced diet with fresh fruit and vegetables and a variety of low-fat protein sources. Include lean organic meat and eggs, fish, tofu, beans. Protein supplements help maintain muscle mass if diet is inadequate.
- Reduce dietary saturated fats.
- Maintain BMI in the healthy range.
- Avoid alcohol.[13]
- Avoid tobacco.
- Exercise, preferably with advice of an exercise physiologist, at least 5 days a week to reduce chronic disease risk factors, overcome side effects of treatment and improve breast cancer survival.[14]
- Reduce or eliminate trans-fatty acids, found in commercial processed foods, and use healthy cooking oils such as olive oil or vegetable oil in food preparation.[15]
- Establish and maintain a regular routine of adequate sleep.[16]
- Avoid HRT for menopause symptoms. Many countries reported significant drops in breast cancer incidence after the sharp reduction in HRT use early this century.[17,18]

Supplements

Supplements may be recommended as adjunctive therapy for nutritional and immune system support, and for reducing the side effects and toxicity of cancer treatment (see Ch 24, Cancer).

Beyond the medical and surgical treatment for cancer, patients usually become very focused on measures to improve their wellbeing and longevity.

The individual requirement for nutritional supplements will be determined by the woman's general state of health, her age, stage of cancer treatment, diet, specific deficiencies and personal preferences.

- A *multivitamin*[19]—daily, containing the antioxidant vitamins A, C, E, the B-complex vitamins, and trace minerals such as magnesium, calcium, zinc and selenium.
- *Probiotic supplement*—containing *Lactobacillus acidophilus*, daily for maintenance of gastrointestinal and immune health. Laboratory and animal studies suggest that probiotics may slow the growth of breast cancer cells. However, human studies are needed before we know what role probiotics have in preventing or treating breast cancer.
- *Omega-3 essential fatty acids (EFA)*—the average Western diet is low in omega-3 EFA. As fish oil, 1–2 g daily.
- *Calcium*—for bone health, particularly in menopausal women and those on aromatase inhibitor adjunctive therapy.[20]
- *Vitamin D*—women who have less exposure to sunlight and have lower levels of vitamin D as a result are more likely to develop breast cancer and other forms of cancer. Vitamin D receptors have been found in up to 80% of breast cancers, and vitamin D receptor polymorphisms have been associated with differences in survival. Although ongoing studies have investigated a possible link between adequate levels of vitamin D and improved cancer prognosis, breast cancer survivors may derive additional, non-cancer-related

benefits from adequate vitamin D levels, including improvements in bone mineral density, quality of life, and mood. Maintaining adequate vitamin D stores is recommended for breast cancer survivors throughout their lifetime.[21]
- *Melatonin*—2–6 mg nocte, for immune support and sleep. Some studies have found that women with lower levels of melatonin, such as those who work night shift or sleep fewer hours, have a higher risk of developing breast cancer. Whether melatonin supplements can help prevent or even treat breast cancer is yet to be determined.[22] More research is needed.
- Black cohosh may help to reduce hot flushes in women on tamoxifen and aromatase inhibitors.

Psychosocial care

Psychosocial care should be considered alongside medical care for all patients with cancer, whose information and supportive care needs may change over time and should be monitored. It has been estimated that, at 3 months after diagnosis, 10–17% of women meet the criteria for major depression. Patients should be monitored for risk or symptoms of anxiety or depression, and referred to a clinical psychologist or psychiatrist for assessment. Psychological therapies have been shown to improve emotional adjustment and social functioning, reduce stress, and improve quality of life for patients with cancer.[11]

A range of therapies is available to improve quality of life for women undergoing treatment for breast cancer. The effectiveness of many of these therapies is influenced by the attitudes, beliefs and psychological make-up of the patient, and will need to be tailored accordingly. It is also important to enquire about the psychosocial needs of the woman's partner and her family.

Psychoeducational programs, which provide both support and information, delivered on an individual or group basis, may reduce anxiety and depression. Patients have also reported feeling less anxious and more optimistic about the future after involvement in peer support programs, but they may not be universally helpful.

Cognitive behavioural techniques such as relaxation therapy, guided imagery, systematic desensitisation and problem solving have been demonstrated to be effective in reducing anxiety. Prayer and laughter are also effective for some individuals.[11] Chemotherapy-induced nausea and vomiting may benefit from psychological interventions, including cognitive behavioural techniques, relaxation and meditation.[11]

Education, nutrition, exercise

Education and nutrition therapies are useful in improving nutritional status and quality of life. Exercise may be effective in reducing fatigue, improving physical functioning and quality of life. Exercise may also be helpful in reducing weight loss when a problem.

Traditional Chinese medicine

Chinese medicinal herbs, when used together with chemotherapy, may improve bone marrow function and quality of life.[23] Other complementary botanicals are commonly used by cancer patients, although most have not been tested in rigorous clinical trials.

Acupuncture

Substantial research supports the value of acupuncture for pain relief and management of nausea. Self-administered acupressure appears to have a protective effect for acute chemotherapy-induced nausea and can be readily taught to patients.[24]

A helpful website providing information on specific complementary botanicals is provided by the Memorial Sloan-Kettering Cancer Center (see Resources list).

Lymphoedema management

Lymphoedema of the upper limb is a possible complication of breast cancer treatment, particularly where there has been surgery or radiotherapy affecting the axillary lymphatics. It involves swelling of the soft tissues of the arm, hand and fingers.

There may be associated numbness, discomfort and an increased risk of infection.

Lymphoedema management is best undertaken with a lymphoedema therapist, who will use specialised massage techniques, exercises and compression bandaging.

Low-level laser therapy may be helpful.[25]

The following medications can exacerbate lymphoedema and should be avoided where possible:
- calcium channel blockers
- non-steroidal anti-inflammatory agents
- hormone replacement therapy
- corticosteroids
- oral hypoglycaemic agents (glitazones).

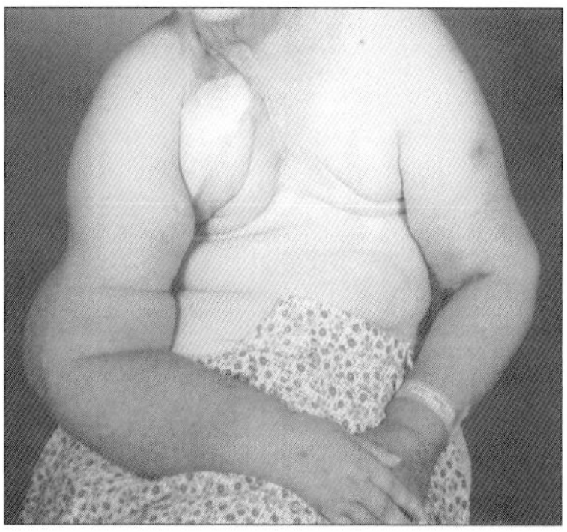

FIGURE 51.5 Lymphoedema

RESOURCES

Memorial Sloan-Kettering Cancer Center, About herbs, botanicals and other products, http://www.mskcc.org/mskcc/html/11570.cfm

Pye JK, Mansel RE, Hughes LE. Clinical experience of drug treatment for mastalgia. Lancet 1985; 2:373–377.

REFERENCES

1 National Breast Cancer Centre. Advice about familial aspects of breast cancer and epithelial ovarian cancer: a guide for health professionals. Sydney: NBCC; 2006.

2 Newall C. Herbal medicines: a guide for health care professionals. London: Pharmaceutical Press; 1997.

3 Schellenberg R. Treatment for premenstrual syndrome with agnus fruit extract: prospective, randomised, placebo-controlled study. BMJ 2001; 322:134–137.

4 Houssami N, Cheung MN, Dixon JM. Fibroadenoma of the breast. Med J Aust 2001; 174:185–188.

5 Australian Institute of Health and Welfare & National Breast Cancer Centre. Breast cancer in Australia: an overview 2006. Cancer Series No. 34. Cat. no. CAN 29. Canberra: AIHW; 2006.

6 National Breast Cancer Centre. Risk factors report. Sydney: NBCC; 2007.

7 National Health and Medical Research Council. Making decisions: should I use hormone replacement therapy? Canberra: NHMRC; 2005.

8 National Breast and Ovarian Cancer Centre. Hormone replacement therapy (HRT) and risk of breast cancer. NBOCC Position Statement.

9 National Breast Cancer Centre. A guide for women with early breast cancer. Sydney: NBCC; 2003.

10 National Breast Cancer Centre. Communication Skills Training Initiative; 2007. Online. Available: http://www.nbcc.org.au/bestpractice/commskills/ 10 October 2007.

11 National Breast Cancer Centre and National Cancer Control Initiative. Clinical practice guidelines for the psychosocial care of adults with cancer. Sydney: NBCC/NCCI; 2003.

12 Block KI, Koch AC, Mead MN et al. Impact of antioxidant supplementation on chemotherapeutic efficacy: a systematic review of the evidence from randomized controlled trials. Cancer Treat Rev 2007; 33(5):407–418.

13 Berstad P, Ma H, Bernstein L et al. Alcohol intake and breast cancer risk among young women. Breast Cancer Res Treat 2008; 108(1):113–120.

14 Ibrahim EM, Al-Homaidh A. Physical activity and survival after breast cancer diagnosis: meta-analysis of published studies. Med Oncol 2010; Apr 22 [Epub ahead of print].

15 Chajès V, Thiébaut AC, Rotival M. Association between serum trans-monounsaturated fatty acids and breast cancer risk in the E3N-EPIC Study. Am J Epidemiol 2008; 167(11):1312–1320.

16 Blask DE. Melatonin, sleep disturbance and cancer risk. Sleep Med Rev 2009; 13(4):257–264.

17 Lambe M, Wigertz A, Holmqvist M. Reductions in use of hormone replacement therapy: effects on Swedish breast cancer incidence trends only seen after several years. Breast Cancer Res Treat 2010; 121(3):679–683.

18 Katalinic A, Rawal R. Decline in breast cancer incidence after decrease in utilisation of hormone replacement therapy. Breast Cancer Res Treat 2008; 107(3):427–430.

19 Harvard School of Public Health. The nutrition source. Vitamins: the bottom line. HSPH; 2010. Online. Available: http://www.hsph.harvard.edu/nutritionsource/what-should-you-eat/vitamins/index.html

20 Nogues X, Servitja S, Peña MJ. Vitamin D deficiency and bone mineral density in postmenopausal women receiving aromatase inhibitors for early breast cancer. Maturitas 2010; 14 Apr [Epub ahead of print].

21 Hines SL, Jorn HK, Thompson KM et al. Breast cancer survivors and vitamin D: a review. Nutrition 2010; 26(3):255–262.

22 Stevens RG. Circadian disruption and breast cancer: from melatonin to clock genes. Epidemiology 2005; 16(2):254–258.

23 Zhang M, Liu X, Li J et al. Chinese medicinal herbs to treat the side effects of chemotherapy in breast cancer patients. Cochrane Database Syst Rev 2007; 2:CD004921.

24 Ezzo J, Richardson M, Vickers A et al. Acupuncture-point stimulation for chemotherapy-induced nausea or vomiting. Cochrane Database Syst Rev 2006; 2:CD002285.

25 Carati CJ, Anderson SN, Gannon BJ et al. Treatment of postmastectomy lymphoedema with low-level laser therapy: a double blind, placebo-controlled trial. Cancer 2003; 98(6):1114–1122.

chapter 52

Gynaecology

INTRODUCTION AND OVERVIEW

Gynaecology is a large part of any general practice, and the conditions described below are part of a general practitioner's everyday experience. While we owe our female patients effective care in their own right, society also benefits when women are healthy and happy in their daily lives. Women are central to the mental, physical, nutritional, educational and, frequently, economic health of their families and communities. By managing the woman's care effectively, we also benefit the health of her children, her partner and, often, her parents.

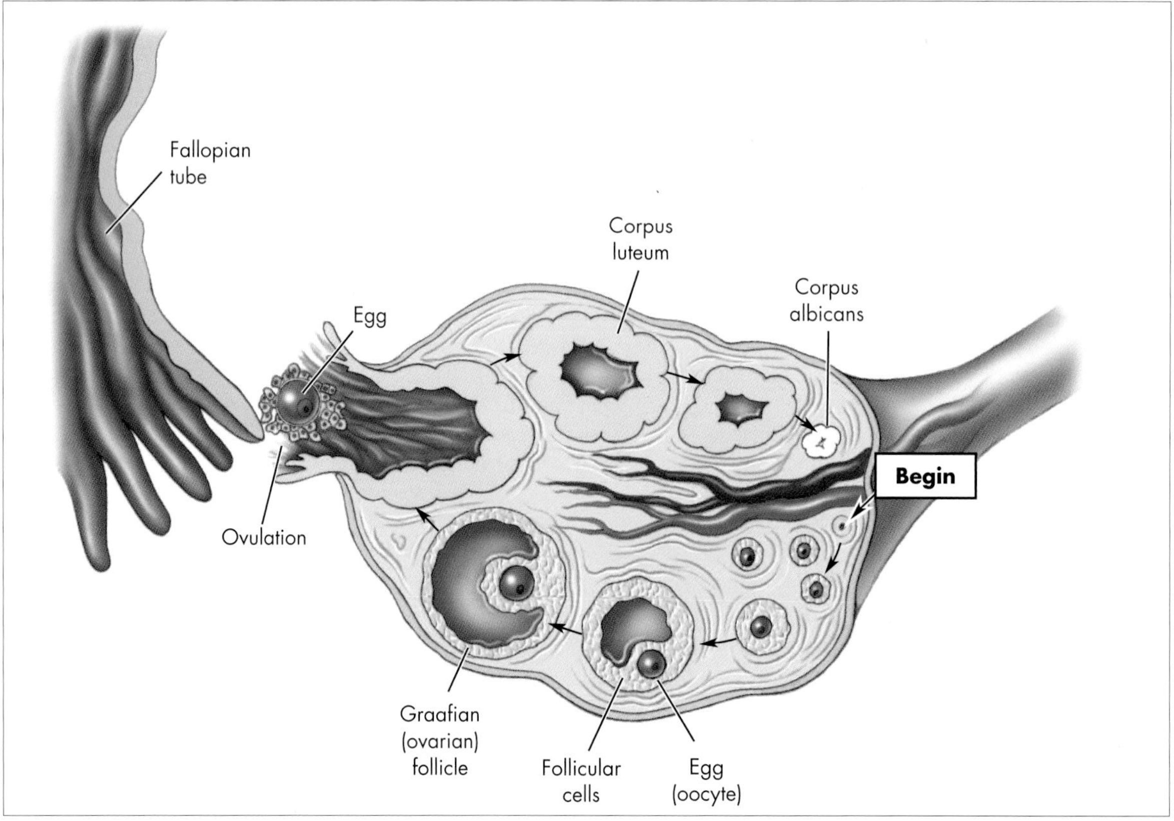

FIGURE 52.1 The female reproductive system

ANATOMY AND DEVELOPMENT OF THE UTERINE CERVIX

The ectocervix is covered by pink squamous epithelium, which changes suddenly to the red columnar (glandular) epithelium of the endocervix at the *squamocolumnar junction* (SCJ) (Fig 52.2). The columnar epithelium is shorter in height than squamous epithelium and appears red because the thin cell layer allows the underlying blood vessels to be easily seen. Columnar epithelium invaginations into the cervical stroma form *endocervical glands*.

Before puberty, the squamocolumnar junction lies close to the external cervical os. As oestrogen levels rise after menarche and during pregnancy, the columnar epithelium everts further out onto the ectocervix to form an '*ectropion*'. Older terms including 'erosion' or 'ulcer' should not be used. Over time, the columnar epithelium exposed to the acid environment of the vagina is replaced by squamous epithelium (*squamous metaplasia*) and a new SCJ closer to the external os is formed. The area between the old and new SCJs where squamous metaplasia occurs is called the *transformation zone*. This is where most carcinogenesis occurs.

Newly formed immature metaplastic epithelium may develop into either:

- normal mature squamous metaplastic epithelium or, occasionally,
- atypical, *dysplastic* epithelium if persistent human papillomavirus (HPV) infection is present—this dysplastic epithelium may regress to normal, persist as dysplasia or progress into invasive cancer.

As oestrogen levels fall at menopause, the cervix shrinks and the new SCJ moves back towards the external os and into the endocervical canal. The epithelium becomes thin, pale and atrophic, with subepithelial petechial haemorrhagic spots.

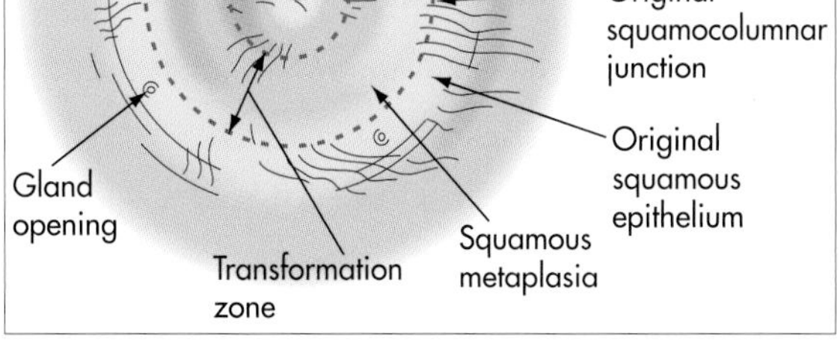

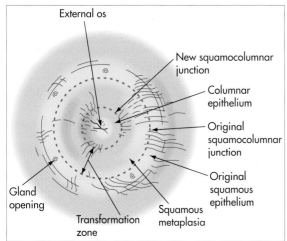

FIGURE 52.2 The uterine cervix

The external os is small and circular in nullipara or in women who have delivered only by caesarean section, and gaping and transverse in parous women. *Nabothian cysts* are retention cysts that develop when endocervical crypt openings are occluded by the overlying metaplastic squamous epithelium.

Endocervical polyps can form at any age after menarche, and arise from the endocervix. They may cause intermittent vaginal or postcoital bleeding, a discharge or, in older women, postmenopausal bleeding.

CERVICAL CANCER SCREENING

Routine screening:

- begins at 1–2 years after first sexual contact with a male or female partner
- is not necessary for women who have never been sexually active
- continues 2-yearly for asymptomatic women with normal smear histories
- may cease at age 70 with two normal smears within the past 5 years
- should continue after hysterectomy if the smear history or histology of the cervix was abnormal, or the cervix was retained.

Technique:

- Examine the vulva, vagina and cervix for visible abnormalities. Suspicious lesions should be referred for colposcopy regardless of the cervical cytology result.
- Sample from the SCJ using the tools most applicable to the site of the transformation zone, e.g. broom for most women, brush where the SCJ is inside the canal, or spatula where the SCJ is on the outer ectocervix.
- Correct sampling requires both endocervical and ectocervical cells to be present on the smear.
- Liquid-based cytology screening may reduce false negatives and avoid unsatisfactory collection where blood is present.

Cytological signs of dysplasia (*cervical intraepithelial neoplasia, CIN*) include nuclear enlargement, increased nuclear–cytoplasmic ratio, hyperchromasia, irregular chromatin distribution and increased mitotic figures.

Koilocytes are atypical cells with perinuclear cytoplasmic cavitation (halo) typical of HPV infection.

Histological signs of dysplasia (CIN) are categorised according to the proportion of the epithelium showing undifferentiated (dysplastic) cells:

- CIN 1—undifferentiated cells confined to the lower third of the epithelium
- CIN 2—undifferentiated cells in the lower two-thirds of the epithelium
- CIN 3—differentiation may be absent or present only in the superficial quarter of the epithelium.

Since 1990, a simplified two-grade histological system using the term 'squamous intraepithelial lesion' (SIL), known as *The Bethesda System*, has been used.

- Low-grade squamous lesion (LSIL)—includes koilocytic atypia (HPV infection) and CIN 1 lesions.
- High-grade squamous lesion (HSIL)—includes CIN 2 and 3; considered a true precursor of invasive cancer.

MANAGEMENT OF ABNORMAL SMEARS

The NHMRC booklet, 'Screening to prevent cervical cancer: guidelines for the management of asymptomatic women with screen detected abnormalities' (see Resources list) contains information on:

- management of women with abnormal cytology
- the Australian Modified Bethesda system (AMBS 2004)
- less common cytological descriptions and their interpretation.

In general:

- Low-grade lesions may be transient. Their management varies and is discussed in the NHMRC booklet. However, women with low-grade lesions on cytology may have high-grade lesions found at colposcopy. CIN or any repeat low-grade lesions should be referred for colposcopy.
- High-grade lesions, including 'possible high grade lesion', may indicate an underlying invasive carcinoma and should be referred immediately for colposcopy.
- Invasive squamous cell carcinoma or adenocarcinoma should be referred immediately to a gynaecological oncologist.

Abnormal cytology results frequently cause significant fear and anxiety for the woman, including:

- embarrassment—at her condition, at having a 'sexually transmitted disease', at the diagnostic procedures involved or lack of privacy
- fear—of infertility, pain, putting her partner at risk or the outcome of investigations.

An explanation of the procedure, reassurance and information to read will help allay her fears and allow her to relax during the procedure. There are no specific symptoms that indicate dysplasia.

Colposcopy

A colposcope is a stereoscopic, binocular microscope with a powerful light source used to view the cervix:

- with green light to show the vascular pattern, and
- after 3–5% acetic acid solution, which stains dysplastic cells or squamous metaplasia 'acetowhite' by coagulating their higher nuclear protein content

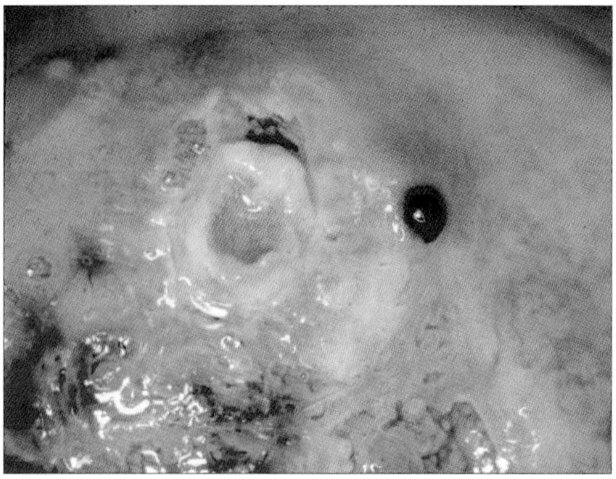

FIGURE 52.3 Colpophotograph after cervical biopsy

- after Lugol's iodine solution, which stains the glycogen in normal oestrogenised squamous epithelium brown/black. Abnormal, oestrogen-deficient or columnar epithelium lacks glycogen and does not stain.

Neoplastic lesions are 'acetowhite' and 'iodine-negative' with abnormal vasculature. Any abnormal areas may be biopsied for histological confirmation.

Colposcopy during pregnancy requires skill and experience, due to progressive oedema, increased eversion, increased vascularity and the risk of significant bleeding with biopsy.

HUMAN PAPILLOMAVIRUS INFECTION

Human papillomavirus (HPV) infection is common. Most infections are transient and resolve over 12–18 months. However, persistent infection with an oncogenic serotype of HPV increases the risk of invasive cancer. Types 16 and 18 cause 70% of cervical cancer cases, and types 31, 33, 35, 39, 45, 51, 52, 56, 58, 59 and 68 are also oncogenic. HPV types 6 and 11 cause 90% of genital warts.

Oncogenic HPV infection is also associated with:

- adenocarcinoma in situ (AIS) of the cervix and invasive adenocarcinoma
- vulval intraepithelial neoplasia (VIN) and invasive cancer
- vaginal intraepithelial neoplasia (VAIN) and invasive cancer
- anal intraepithelial neoplasia (AIN) and invasive cancer.

PREVENTION OF CERVICAL DYSPLASIA

Prevention options include:

- minimising partner numbers
- consistent condom usage, which lowers the risk of HPV infection

- vaccination against HPV prior to infection—there are currently two commercially available recombinant vaccines, both involving a series of three injections over 6 months:
  - Gardasil® (Merck) against HPV 6, 11, 16 and 18. TGA approval covers females aged 9–26 years (subsidised) and males aged 9–15 years (unsubsidised)
  - Cervarix® (GlaxoSmithKline) against HPV 16, 18, 45 and 31
- optimising co-factors such as smoking and chronic inflammation, and correcting micronutrient deficiencies, which may affect disease progression.

TREATMENT OF CONFIRMED CERVICAL DYSPLASIA

Treatment options include:

- colposcopic review only, with treatment if the lesion persists or progresses over 18–24 months
- cryotherapy—healing occurs over 6 weeks, with a watery discharge for 3–4 weeks. No specimen is available for histology and lesions in glandular crypts may be missed. Can be performed without analgesia
- large loop excision of transformation zone (LLETZ, or LEEP)—provides a histological specimen. Severe postoperative bleeding occurs occasionally and must be managed promptly
- cold knife conisation where significant lesions inside the endocervical canal are suspected.

After surgery, women should avoid strenuous exercise, vaginal douche, tampons or intercourse until the vaginal discharge has settled (usually 2–4 weeks). Recurrent lesions occur in 5–10% of women.

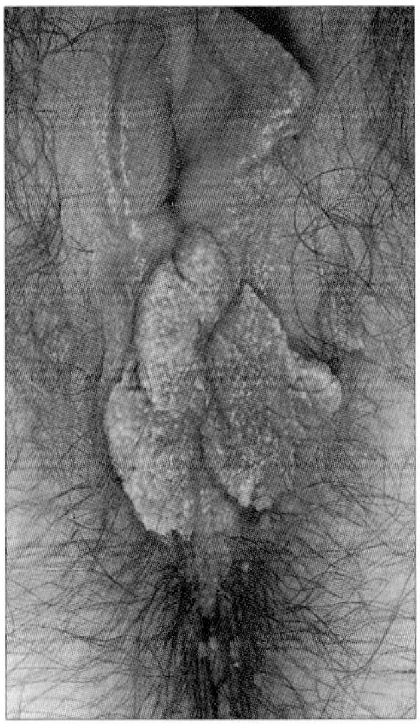

FIGURE 52.4 Vulval warts

Treatment on the day of colposcopy without confirmatory biopsy may be considered in women who may fail to return for follow-up. This risks over-treatment of lesions.

Post-procedure follow-up depends on the severity of the lesion, the completeness of excision and other individual features.

Treatment can remove dysplasia but not cure HPV infection. HPV testing 12 months after treatment of a high-grade lesion may be useful as a 'test of cure'.

Other measures include:

- Avoid tobacco smoke.
- The few studies of HPV persistence showed a possible protective effect of fruits, vegetables, vitamins C and E, beta- and alpha-carotene, lycopene, luterin/zeaxanthin and cryptoxanthin.[1] Evidence for a protective effect of cervical neoplasia was probable for folate, retinol and vitamin E, and possibly for vegetables, vitamins C and B_{12}, alpha-carotene, beta-carotene, lycopene, lutein/zeaxanthin and cryptoxanthin. Evidence for an increased risk of cervical neoplasia associated with high blood homocysteine was probable, although the evidence is still inconclusive. Patients with an abnormal Pap smear should be advised to eat a diet rich in beta-carotene, vitamin C and folate (vitamin B_9) from fruits and vegetables.
- Exercise regularly.
- Reduce avoidable stress. Higher levels of perceived stress have been associated with impaired HPV-specific immune response in women with cervical dysplasia.[2]

ABNORMAL UTERINE BLEEDING

A normal menstrual cycle occurs every 21–35 days, with bleeding for 2–7 days. Normal blood loss is 20–60 mL per period, with > 80 mL described as heavy.

The process of normal regular menstruation requires:

- sufficient oestrogen to induce 'follicular phase' endometrium
- ovulation with formation of a corpus luteum, production of progesterone and induction of 'secretory phase' in the endometrium
- withdrawal of progesterone as the corpus luteum declines. Declining progesterone is the trigger for menstruation
- synchronous breakdown and repair of the endometrium at menses
- breakdown factors including prostaglandins, interleukin-1, matrix metalloproteinase (MMP)-1 and MMP-7
- endometrial repair factors including epidermal growth factor-alpha, endothelins and vascular endothelial growth factor (VEGF).[3]

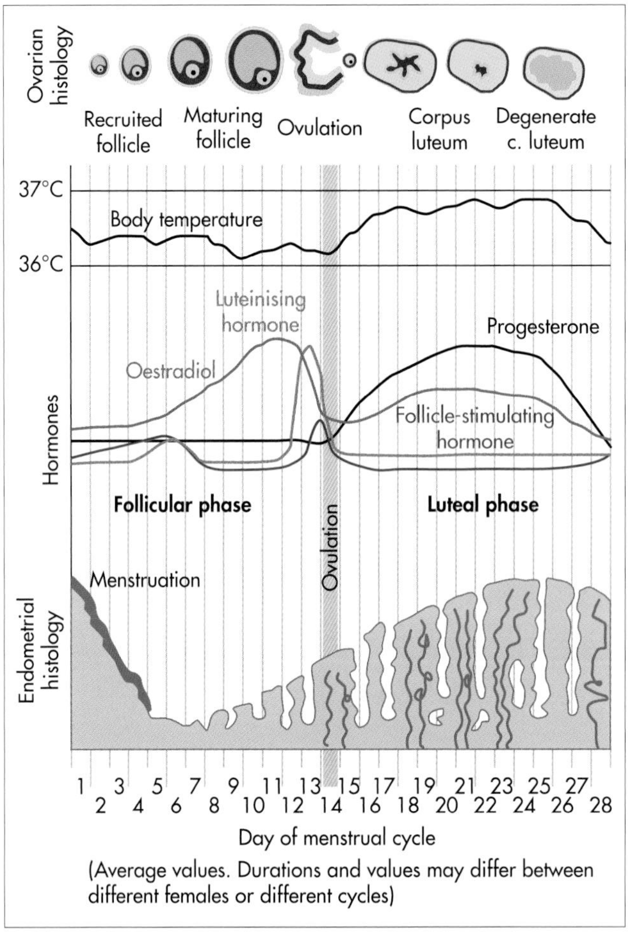

FIGURE 52.5 The menstrual cycle and hormonal levels

TERMINOLOGY

Terms such as menorrhagia, metrorrhagia, polymenorrhoea, oligomenorrhoea and metropathia haemorrhagica should be replaced by descriptions of the frequency, heaviness and length of bleeding.

Abnormal uterine bleeding (AUB) covers all vaginal bleeding apart from regular ovulatory normal menses.

AETIOLOGY

Abnormal uterine bleeding is most common soon after menarche or in the years before menopause. It may be:

- *anovulatory*—without ovulation, a corpus luteum does not form. The resulting lack of progestogen and unopposed oestrogen stimulates the endometrium. Bleeding occurs when oestrogen levels fall or the endometrium becomes unstable:
  - *post-menarche*—oestrogen levels rise but the immature hypothalamic-pituitary axis is unable to trigger ovulation. Menses may be infrequent but very heavy, often resulting in anaemia
  - *perimenopausal*—ovarian follicle quality declines, resulting in variable oestrogen levels and variable menstrual flow. A dyssynchronous endometrium with irregular menstrual shedding results in prolonged menses with eventual amenorrhoea
  - *chronic anovulation*—e.g. polycystic ovarian syndrome or hypothalamic dysfunction associated with low body weight, excessive exercise or stress. Oestrogen levels are variable. The corpus luteum does not form or is inadequate to maintain endometrial stability. Unopposed oestrogen stimulates the endometrium, which ultimately becomes unstable and bleeds irregularly
- *ovulatory*—periods are heavy but regular, due to:
  - uterine pathology, e.g. fibroids
  - abnormal endometrial function[4] or
  - systemic causes, e.g. obesity (endogenous oestrogen), clotting disorders (including von Willebrand's disease), hypothyroidism

- *iatrogenic*—an imbalance between oestrogen and progestogen associated with the oral contraceptive pill (OCP), hormone replacement therapy (HRT) or progestins results in abnormal bleeding:
  - light or absent periods, often with irregular bleeding due to excess progestogen effect
  - premenstrual bleeding with inadequate progestogen
  - intermenstrual bleeding with triphasic contraceptives
  - heavier periods with excess oestrogen effect
  - midcycle bleeding with inadequate oestrogen.

Medications associated with bleeding include anticoagulants, selective serotonin reuptake inhibitors, antipsychotics, corticosteroids, tamoxifen.

Medications that interact with the OCP/HRT, including liver enzyme inducers, antibiotics, anti-tuberculous drugs and antifungals, may also cause bleeding.

Herbal substances associated with bleeding include ginseng, ginkgo and soy supplements.

Causes of abnormal uterine bleeding are listed in Box 52.1.

HISTORY

The history should include:

- menstrual history—last menstrual period (LMP), flow, 'accidents', 'flooding', length of cycle, number of days of bleeding, frequency of pad/tampon changes (more than 2-hourly is heavy), limitations on daily activities, use of double pads, changing at night
- features of polycystic ovarian syndrome
- reproductive history—contraceptive use, pregnancies, fertility plans
- lifestyle factors—change in exercise, stress, weight
- symptoms of anaemia—tiredness, palpitations
- medical history—thyroid function, bleeding disorders
- drug history—anticoagulants, hormone use, aspirin, anticonvulsants, SSRIs, antibiotics, alternative and complementary therapies.

EXAMINATION

Examination may be normal but should include:

- signs of anaemia, thyroid disease, bleeding disorder, hyperprolactinaemia

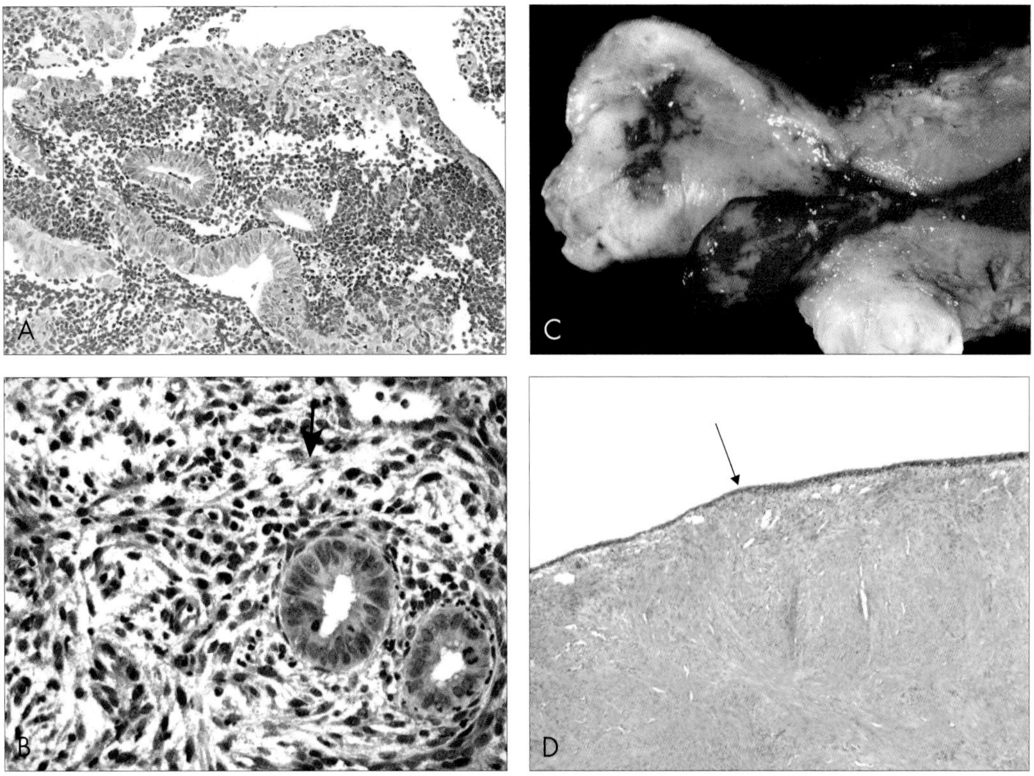

FIGURE 52.6 Main causes of uterine bleeding: **A** Anovulatory endometrium with stromal breakdown; **B** Chronic endometriosis with numerous plasma cells (arrow); **C** Endometrial polyp; **D** Submucosal leiomyoma with attenuation of the endometrial lining (arrow)

BOX 52.1 Causes of abnormal uterine bleeding

Endocrine:
- immature hypothalamic–pituitary axis
- menopause
- obesity
- polycystic ovarian syndrome
- premature ovarian failure
- Cushing's disease
- hyperprolactinaemia
- hypothyroidism
- weight loss

Infections:
- chlamydia
- gonorrhoea
- PID
- cervicitis

Uterine lesions:
- adenomyosis
- endometrial or cervical polyps
- endometrial or cervical malignancy
- leiomyomas

Pregnancy:
- ectopic pregnancy
- incomplete abortion

Medications:
- oral contraceptive pill (especially low dose, missed pills or drug interactions)
- progestogen-only contraceptives
- intrauterine devices
- tamoxifen
- warfarin

Other conditions:
- bleeding disorders (including thrombocytopenia, von Willebrand's disease)
- endometriosis
- trauma
- excessive exercise
- stress

- signs of polycystic ovarian syndrome (i.e. hyper-androgenism, hirsutism, acne, obesity and palpable enlarged ovaries; see Fig 52.7)
- speculum examination to exclude cervical and vaginal causes, especially if bleeding is post-coital
- bimanual examination to exclude fibroids and adnexal masses.

INVESTIGATIONS

Investigations include:
- pregnancy test
- Pap smear, STD screen
- haematology where loss is heavy:
  - complete blood picture
  - iron studies
  - prothrombin time, activated partial thromboplastin time, von Willebrand screen—if bleeding heavy since menarche or suggestive history
  - follicle-stimulating hormone, prolactin, thyroid-stimulating hormone
- transvaginal ultrasound—uterine lesions, polycystic ovarian syndrome (PCOS), retained products of conception, ovarian tumours. An endometrial thickness ≤ 4 mm virtually excludes endometrial cancer[5]
- endometrial biopsy—does not allow visual inspection of cavity and will not allow removal of polyps, resection of fibroids or endometrial ablation
- hysteroscopy and curettage, if required—exclusion of malignancy, removal of endometrial polyp, resection of submucosal fibroid.

MANAGEMENT

Management depends on the cause of bleeding, the woman's plans for fertility and the impact that periods have on her life. In addition to bleeding, periods may involve dysmenorrhoea, sore breasts, mood disorder, migraines or an aggravation of pelvic symptoms.

Some women may request minimal treatment. Others may wish to avoid periods entirely. Different women may choose very different treatment options.

Teenagers presenting acutely with prolonged heavy bleeding (anovulatory cycles):
- Exclude anaemia, iron deficiency, pregnancy, bleeding disorders (including von Willebrand's disease).
- Consider options including:
  - *Vitex agnus castus* (chaste tree) 1000 mg daily.[6] Although few randomised controlled trials (RCTs) exist, *Vitex* is commonly prescribed for menstrual irregularities, based on data collected by the German Commission E.[7] Menstrual cycle irregularities due to hyperprolactinaemia, corpus luteum insufficiency, oligomenorrhoea and secondary amenorrhoea have been effectively treated with *Vitex* extract in open-label, uncontrolled studies
  - combined 30–35 μg OCP q.d. with antiemetic until bleeding stops (within 72 hours). Follow with 1 tablet daily without placebo for 3–6 weeks, then withdrawal bleed for 5 days, then OCP[8]
  - norethisterone 5–15 mg daily until bleeding stops, then 5–10 mg daily for 3–6 weeks
  - IV conjugated oestrogen (Premarin®) 25 mg. Repeat 4-hourly until bleeding stops, usually

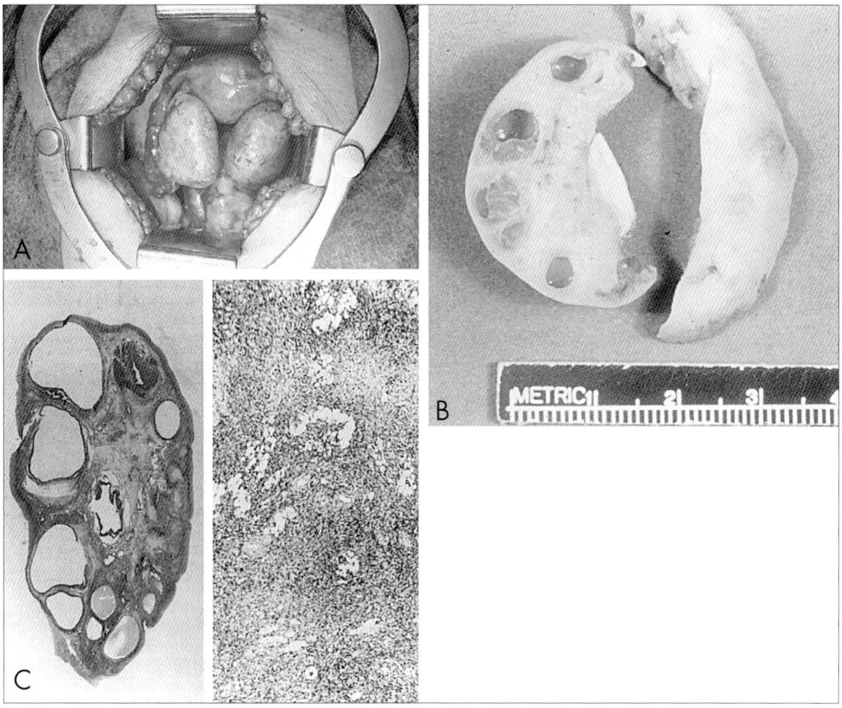

FIGURE 52.7 Polycystic ovaries: **A** Operative findings of classical enlarged polycystic ovaries. The uterus is located adjacent to the two enlarged ovaries. **B** Sectioned polycystic ovary with numerous follicles. **C** Histological section of a polycystic ovary with multiple subcapsular follicular cysts and stromal hypertrophy (low power, left). At higher power (×100, right), islands of luteinized theca cells are visible in the stroma.

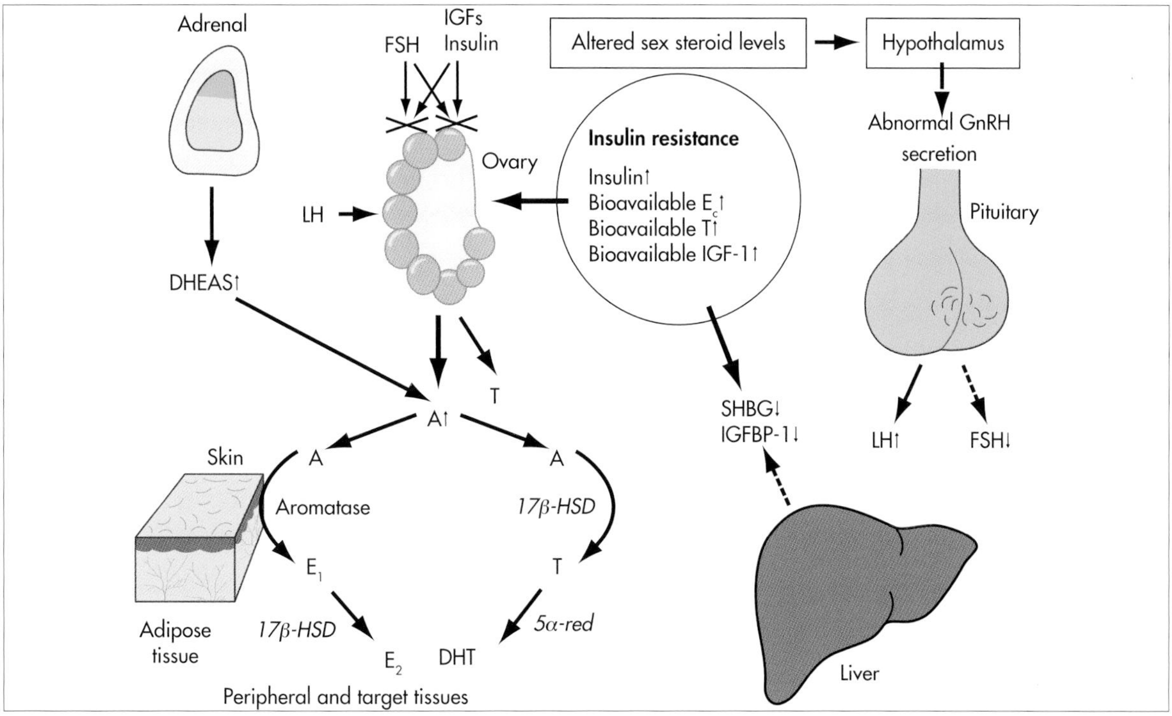

FIGURE 52.8 Pathology of polycystic ovarian syndrome

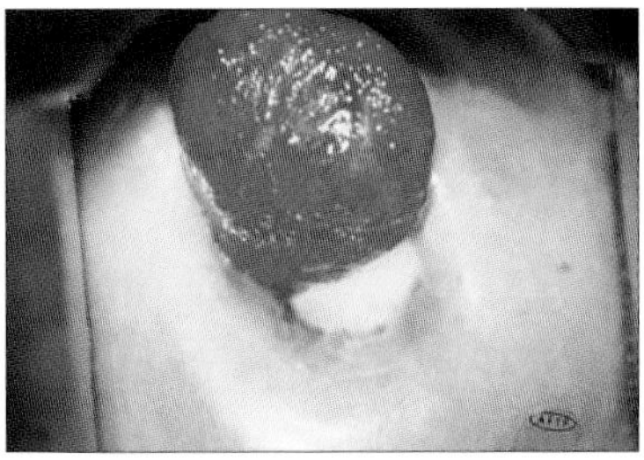

FIGURE 52.9 Cervical polyp

within three doses. Follow with a combined OCP or progestin for 3–6 weeks[9]
  - intracavity tamponade with 30–50 mL Foley catheter for 2–48 hours[10]
- Iron therapy until ferritin level is in normal range and for 3 months after bleeding becomes normal.

Ovulatory, regular, heavy periods:
- Exclude anaemia, hypothyroidism, iatrogenic causes, uterine disease (ultrasound).
- Where dysmenorrhoea is present, consider endometriosis or adenomyosis.
- Consider options including:
  - *Vitex agnus castus* 1000 mg daily
  - progestogen-dominant OCP
  - NSAIDs (e.g. naproxen 500 mg b.i.d. or mefenemic acid 2 capsules t.d.s. during menses)
  - tranexamic acid (i.e. 1–2 capsules q.i.d. during menses. Reduce dose if nauseated)
  - levonorgestrel IUD—will also treat dysmenorrhoea
  - danazol (i.e. 200 mg daily continuously). Treatment beyond 6 months is controversial. Treats mastalgia effectively
  - endometrial ablation—less effective for pain. Contraception is required
  - hysterectomy.

Perimenopausal women with frequent irregular periods and variable flow:
- Exclude anaemia, hypothyroidism, hyperprolactinaemia, iatrogenic causes.
- Exclude uterine and cervical disease—ultrasound and cervical smear.
- Consider the woman's general wellbeing—oestrogen/testosterone deficiency symptoms, increased exercise, dietary review, weight loss assistance, psychological support.
- Consider options:
  - *Vitex agnus castus* 1000 mg daily
  - low-dose OCP—if low risk, non-smoker < 50 years
  - cyclical progestins, e.g. norethisterone 5 mg day 1–12 each calendar month until menses cease
  - sequential HRT—especially with menopausal symptoms
  - levonorgestrel IUD—will reduce volume but not change timing of periods
  - hysterectomy.

DYSMENORRHOEA

Dysmenorrhoea can be considered 'normal' if:
- it is only present on day 1–2 of the cycle
- it resolves with the OCP, or anti-inflammatory medications, *and*
- the woman is nulliparous.

MANAGEMENT

Management options for 'normal period pain' include:
- acupuncture and acupressure
- vitamin B_1, 100 mg daily[11]
- magnesium supplement
- strenuous physical exercise.

Herbal

- Common herbal treatments include:
- Chinese herbal therapies[12]
- chaste tree (*Vitex agnus castus*) 1000 mg daily before breakfast.

Diet

- Reduce red meat, to reduce levels of arachidonic acid.
- Increase consumption of omega-3 fatty acids, including fish and fish oil supplements.

Pharmacological

- Monophasic progestogen-dominant OCP (e.g. 30–35 μg ethinyl oestradiol with 500–1000 mg norethisterone or 150 mg levonorgestrel)—continuous-use OCP with menses every 2–3 months (skipping periods) may be beneficial.
- NSAID medications taken early in the pain, then regularly with food—consider suppositories for longer duration of action. The most effective NSAID varies between individuals. Can be taken with an H_2-antagonist where there is a risk of gastritis.
- A levonorgestrel-releasing IUCD (Mirena®)—frequently most effective. Suitable for nulliparae, virgins and teens, after consideration of risks/benefits. Consider insertion under general anaesthesia. Three months of irregular bleeding ± crampy pain is common while it settles.
- Etonorgestrel implant (Implanon®)—less effective than levonorgestrel IUCD.

Dysmenorrhoea that does not resolve with the OCP or anti-inflammatories requires investigation. Common causes include endometriosis and adenomyosis. Any woman old enough to have periods is old enough to have

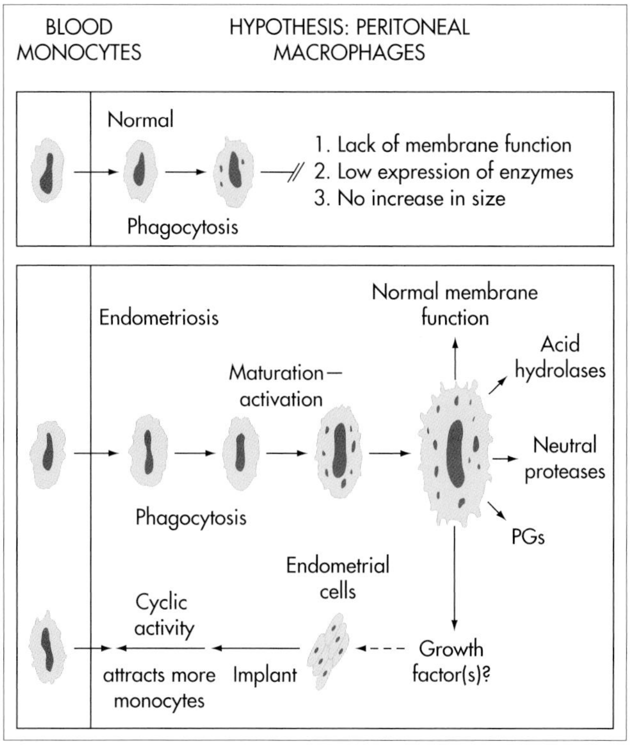

FIGURE 52.10 Pathology of endometriosis

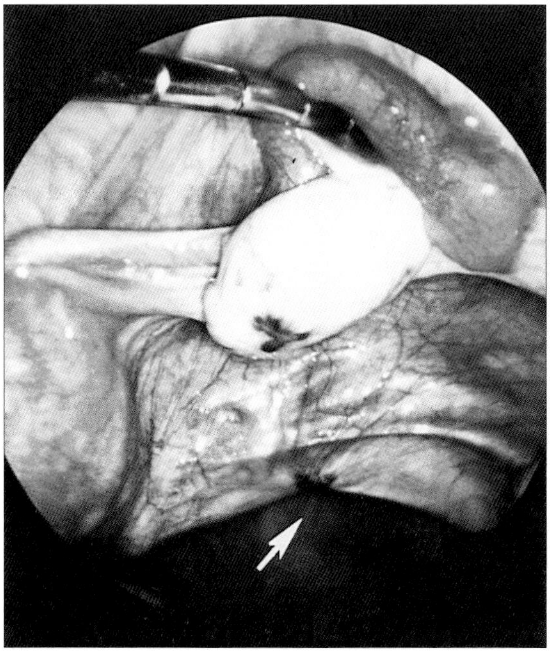

FIGURE 52.11 Intraoperative photo of endometriosis

endometriosis. While pregnancy frequently improves day 1–2 period pain in normal nulliparae, it seldom improves dysmenorrhoea in women with endometriosis and is inappropriate to recommend outside a suitable social setting.

ENDOMETRIOSIS

DEFINITION

Endometriosis is the presence of endometrial glands and stroma outside the uterus.

AETIOLOGY

The aetiology of endometriosis is unknown. It is increasing in prevalence. A tendency to develop endometriosis is inherited as a complex genetic trait influenced by environmental factors.[13] Established lesions include inflammatory cells, fibrosis, neovascularisation and aberrant innervation. It has been associated with environmental toxins including organochlorines (polychlorinated biphenyls and dioxin-like compounds).[14]

Risk is increased with nulliparity and early menarche.[15]

SYMPTOMS

In the past, endometriosis was considered an uncommon condition of women in their thirties and forties. We now know it to be a common condition (5–10%) of women in their teens and twenties.

While some women are asymptomatic, common symptoms include:

- period pain resistant to OCP or anti-inflammatories
- period pain present for more than 1–2 days
- period pain felt on one side or in the lower back
- period-like pain during the month
- ovulation pain always felt on one side
- deep dyspareunia
- progression to chronic pelvic pain
- infertility—this is variable; many women become pregnant easily, so contraception is required
- fatigue.

Dysmenorrhoea is usually a combination of pain from the endometriosis and pain from the uterus. The endometrium of women with endometriosis has nerve fibres (pain receptors) not present in women without endometriosis.[16] Optimal outcome requires management of both endometriotic lesions and the uterine component of pain.

HISTORY

Typical histories include:

- a teenager in whom periods have always been painful. Initial improvement on the OCP is followed by worsening pain resistant to NSAIDs
- a young woman with period pain on more than 1–2 days of a period, pain leading up to a period or pain that feels like period pain at other times of the cycle
- a woman who has had period pain for some time, but now has pain on most days (chronic pain), often with several different pain symptoms
- a woman whose severe period pain as a young woman did not resolve after pregnancy.

DIAGNOSIS

Reliable diagnosis requires laparoscopy. Diagnostic delay averages 6 years in Australia, due to a mixture of:

- Late presentation to a doctor. The woman or her family may believe that severe pain is normal. Her pain may be considered unimportant or exaggerated.
- Lack of investigation by the woman's doctor, who may:
  - fail to recognise a suggestive history
  - believe she is too young for endometriosis
  - underestimate the severity of her pain
  - persist with failed treatments, or
  - believe that a normal ultrasound excludes endometriosis.
- Lack of a non-invasive test for endometriosis.
- Missed diagnosis at laparoscopy. Lesions may be subtle, clear blebs in teenagers. White lesions may be misdiagnosed as scar tissue of unknown cause. The diagnosis of endometriosis requires a skilled laparoscopist.

INVESTIGATIONS

CA 125

- Rarely used. Not useful for screening.
- Mildly elevated in some cases.

Ultrasound

- *Usually normal* unless endometriomas are present.
- Transvaginal ultrasound is preferred, except in virgins or where the vaginal probe would cause pain or distress.
- An endometrioma has a grey, homogeneous, 'ground glass' appearance.
- The differential diagnosis of an endometrioma is a haemorrhagic corpus luteum. Repeat scan in 2–3 months will show persistence of an endometrioma or resolution of a corpus luteum.
- 99% of women with an endometrioma on ultrasound will have additional peritoneal deposits found at laparoscopy.[17]
- An endometrioma may be a marker for severe peritoneal or rectosigmoid disease.

MRI

Rarely required. May be used to investigate rectosigmoid disease or diagnose coexistent adenomyosis.

Laparoscopy

- Required for definitive diagnosis and treatment.
- Lesions may be clear, pink, yellow, brown, white, red or bluish black. May show only as increased vascularity, white scarring or adhesions. Frequently under-diagnosed.
- Histological confirmation of lesions is required.
- Areas of inflammatory tissue are common, but rare in women without pain.

TREATMENT OPTIONS

The treatments chosen will depend on the woman's individual symptoms, preference, desire for fertility and coexistent conditions.

Explanation and support

- Ensure she knows you believe in her pain. Many women have been told that their pain is exaggerated, it is all in their head or their pain is normal.
- Provide education regarding endometriosis, her specific situation and the treatment options.

- Provide a management plan for when pain is severe, to allow her to control her pain. Anticipation of severe uncontrolled pain causes distress and anxiety as the period approaches.
- Involve a psychologist/counsellor where possible. The psychological, educational, financial, employment and relationship sequelae of pain, low self-esteem and self-doubt are common.

Laparoscopy

Once the diagnosis has been made, options include:

- excision of the endometriosis lesions if an experienced laparoscopic surgeon is present. Conservation of the uterus and ovaries is usual unless the woman is older and removal of these organs has been discussed
- documentation of the lesions and referral to a laparoscopic surgeon for repeat laparoscopy with excision
- diathermy to the endometriosis lesions—this is suitable for superficial ovarian lesions and some superficial peritoneal lesions. It is less effective than excision as deep lesions are incompletely removed and lesions close to the bowel or ureter cannot be safely diathermied
- no surgical treatment, with consideration of medical therapies.

Dietary and complementary therapies

These aim to:

- reduce oestrogen dominance
- reduce inflammation
- block aromatase activity in the endometriosis lesion.

Management includes:

- reducing dietary saturated fats
- avoiding trans fats (found in many processed foods)[18]
- maintaining healthy weight range
- reducing caffeine and alcohol intake
- engaging in regular strenuous exercise.

Herbs and supplements:[19]

- *Vitex agnus castus* 1000 mg daily
- anti-inflammatory—*Boswellia*, cat's claw, turmeric, bromelain
- magnesium
- vitamin C 500 mg daily, vitamin E 400 IU daily[20]
- fish oil 1–2 g daily
- traditional Chinese medicine[21]—herbs often prescribed include corydalis, cnidium, bupleurum, dong quai and perilla, sometimes accompanied by acupuncture.

Medical treatments

Medical treatments do not improve fertility, will not divide adhesions or remove scar tissue, will not resolve an endometrioma and will not resolve deep endometriotic lesions. They may improve symptoms in the short term. *Medical treatments are not required where excision of endometriotic lesions is complete.* However, endometriosis surgery is challenging and requires advanced laparoscopic surgical skills and equipment. Medical treatments include:

- gonadotrophin-releasing hormone (GnRH) analogues—by daily nasal spray or monthly depot injection, for 3–6 months. Hypo-oestrogenic side effects include hot flushes, poor sleep, tiredness, dry vagina and loss of bone density. May be used with combined HRT to minimise side effects without decreased efficacy
- progestins (e.g. norethisterone 5–10 mg daily)—can be used in the long term if effective
- danazol or dimetriose—used less now due to androgenic side effects
- aromatase inhibitors.

Consider treatment of coexistent causes of pelvic pain at the laparoscopic procedure. For example:

- insertion of levonorgestrel IUCD to manage uterine aspect of dysmenorrhoea
- cystoscopy with hydrodistension to diagnose interstitial cystitis
- starting a medication for neuropathic pain
- providing photographs to allay fears and increase understanding.

A full discussion of the management of endometriosis is available in textbooks on this topic.[22]

MANAGEMENT OF OVARIAN ENDOMETRIOMAS / SEVERE ENDOMETRIOSIS

Effective treatment of endometriomas requires removal of the cyst wall from inside the ovary, by either 'stripping' cystectomy or diathermy (less effective). Drainage alone is rapidly followed by recurrence. Where endometriosis is severe, the pouch of Douglas may be obliterated, and endometrosis may invade the muscularis of the rectum.

Where laparoscopy does not help her pain

Either the endometriosis was incompletely removed, or the pain is due to another condition (e.g. uterine pain, pelvic muscle pain, interstitial cystitis or neuropathic pain). Even when present, the endometriosis may not be the main cause of pain.

Recurrent pain after previously successful surgery

Where the current pain is the same as the pain that resolved with surgery, review laparoscopy is reasonable. Where the pain is different, consider other causes of pain (e.g. uterine pain, interstitial cystitis, neuropathic pain).

ADENOMYOSIS

Adenomyosis is the presence of endometrial glands and stroma in the myometrium with adjacent smooth muscle hyperplasia. It is generally diffuse but may form an adenomyoma locally. The aetiology is unknown, but it is more common in women with endometriosis.

SYMPTOMS

Symptoms where present include:

- dysmenorrhoea, often with back pain
- heavy periods
- dyspareunia.

Suggestive histories include:

- dysmenorrhoea due to endometriosis as a young woman, few problems during childbearing years, then increasing dysmenorrhoea due to adenomyosis once childbearing complete
- trouble-free periods when young, with worsening dysmenorrhoea after the birth of a child.

DIAGNOSIS

Diagnosis requires histology but is likely with:

- suggestive symptoms and the absence of endometriosis at laparoscopy
- a bulky uterus on vaginal examination
- ultrasound features of:
  - bulky, rounded uterus with asymmetrical thickness of the anterior and posterior myometrium
  - subendometrial myometrial microcysts
  - subendometrial echogenic linear striations
  - poor definition of the endometrial myometrial junction
  - heterogeneous myometrium
- MRI changes consistent with adenomyosis.

TREATMENT

If asymptomatic, no treatment is required. Treatment options include:

- levonorgestrel-releasing IUCD
- NSAIDs with back-up narcotic-based analgesia for dysmenorrhoea
- progestogens, e.g. norethisterone 5 mg daily continuously or progestogenic OCP
- treatment of coexisting menorrhagia, to minimise the contribution from 'clot colic'. Endometrial ablation may worsen adenomyosis
- treatment of coexisting menstrual symptoms, to minimise the number of symptoms the woman must

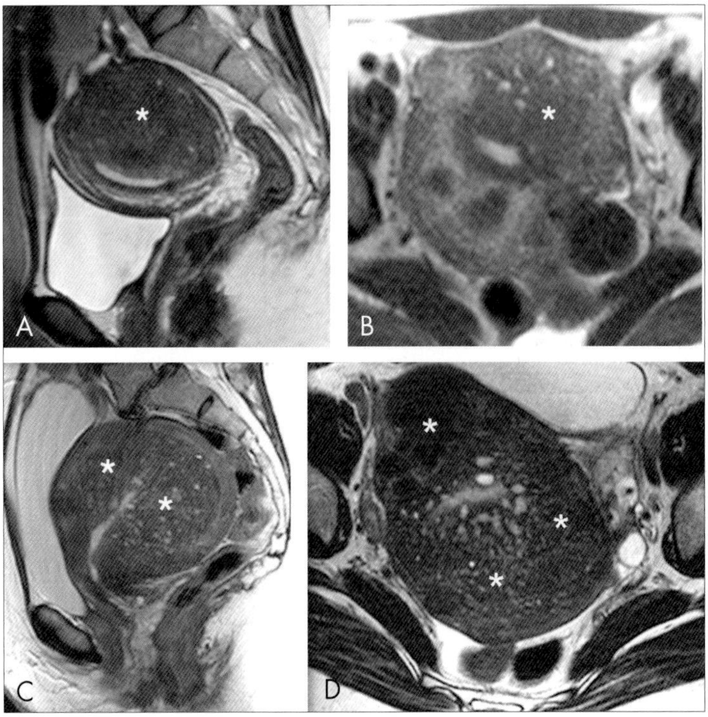

FIGURE 52.12 Pathology of adenomyosis: Sagittal (**A**) and axial (**B**) MR images through the pelvis show focal junctional zone widening and characteristic thickened areas (*); Sagittal (**C**) and axial (**D**) MR images in a different patient show widening of the entire junctional zone (*) which contains endometrial rests

cope with during menses (e.g. premenstrual mood disorder, menstrual migraine, bloating, lethargy)
- hysterectomy.
- A danazol-loaded IUCD has been investigated in Japan.[23]

CHRONIC PELVIC PAIN

While some women with endometriosis improve over time and others persist with dysmenorrhoea over the long term, a proportion progress to chronic pelvic pain. Pain becomes a mixture of pelvic symptoms and central sensitisation with neuropathic pain. Symptoms include some or all of:
- dysmenorrhoea present before the chronic pain began, that now affects more days per month
- urinary symptoms of frequency, urgency, nocturia and bladder pain
- variable bowel symptoms, often with food intolerance and bloating
- sharp, stabbing, burning or aching pains that occur spontaneously, often at night
- painful pelvic muscles with dyspareunia
- other pain conditions, including migraine, muscle trigger points, generalised muscle aches or vulvodynia
- hypersensitivity of the abdomen or pelvis
- poor sleep, fatigue, anxiety and diminished quality of life.

These symptoms may develop even when all her endometriosis has been removed and after hysterectomy. In women with pain on most days, a central chronic pain process is likely, and management usually includes neuropathic pain medications, cognitive behavioural lifestyle changes, and management of the local pelvic symptoms.[24]

MANAGEMENT

Pain is now complex. No single treatment and no surgery will resolve all the woman's pain. While complete cure is unlikely, substantial improvement can be achieved by managing local pain symptoms, treating central sensitisation and rehabilitation of the sequelae of her chronic pain condition.
- Make a list of each pain she has, what it feels like, where it is and when it happens. Ask specifically about sharp pains, bladder function, bowel function, dyspareunia and pain in other areas of the body.
- Diagnose pain from pelvic muscles with a one-finger examination of the muscles just inside the vagina posteriorly and laterally. Diagnose a painful bladder by pressure with one finger anteriorly with suggestive symptoms.
- Plan treatment for each pain.
- At each follow-up visit, return to the initial list of pains and ask about each one, to assess the benefit of the treatments used. Many women forget a particular pain once it resolves and may feel that they have made little progress because another pain remains.
- Treat coexisting health problems, to allow her more energy to cope with any remaining problems.

SPECIFIC PAIN SYMPTOMS AND THEIR MANAGEMENT

Urgency, frequency and nocturia

These are commonly due to interstitial cystitis (IC) or painful bladder syndrome (PBS). IC commonly coexists with endometriosis.[25] There is often a history of 'frequent UTI' managed with antibiotics, but with negative urine culture. Urine may show WBC or RBC. Pelvic floor dysfunction secondary to IC, with painful intercourse, cervical smear tests and tampon use is common.

General measures:
- Explain that the bladder is inflamed rather than infected.
- Explain that the woman should drink enough that urine is not concentrated—approximately 2 litres daily.
- Consider dietary triggers. May require exclusion diet with dietician. Where triggers can be identified and avoided, medication may not be necessary. Common triggers include:
  - foods high in acid, such as citrus fruit, cranberry juice, vitamins B and C, teas including green teas and some herbal teas, coffee including decaffeinated coffee, tomatoes
  - foods that stimulate nerves, such as caffeine, cola drinks
  - foods high in histamine, such as chocolate
  - artificial sweeteners, carbonated drinks, spicy foods, alcohol and cigarettes
- Urine culture to exclude UTI.

Herbal:
- A TCM combination of *Rosa laevigata* (Cherokee rose), *Smilax china* (China root) and *Lygodium japonicum* (Japanse climbing fern) can have a urinary analgesic and anti-inflammatory effect.

Medications:[26]
- amitriptyline 5–50 mg taken early evening. Also helps sharp pains, sleep and some migraines
- hydrozine 10–50 mg at night, especially if the woman has allergies
- oxybutinin 5 mg 1–3 times daily, solifenacin 5 mg (or half a 10 mg tablet) daily, or tolterodine 1–2 mg daily, which cause less sedation. Consider long-acting formulations.

BOX 52.2 Self-management plan for acute bladder symptoms

- Drink 500 mL water mixed with 1 tsp of bicarbonate soda or 2 sachets urinary alkaliniser with paracetamol 500 mg and an anti-inflammatory.
- Follow with 250 mL water every 20 minutes, up to 500 mL.
- If no better, then urine culture (provide her with urine culture request form in case of symptoms).
- Antibiotics only if culture confirms infection.

Other treatments:

- cystoscopy with hydrodistension under anaesthesia. Plain cystoscopy is normal in most cases. View after hydrodistension shows typical bleeding glomerulations. Excludes other pathology
- pelvic floor physiotherapy for pelvic floor dysfunction. Bladder retraining is only useful where pain has already been managed
- sodium pentosan polysulfate 100 mg t.d.s.
- self-management plan for exacerbations (Box 52.2)
- intravesical heparin and lignocaine for acute exacerbations
- intravesical dimethyl sulfoxide (DMSO).

Sharp, stabbing, burning or aching pain (neuropathic pain)

This pain is commonly neuropathic in origin. Frequently there is a history of endometriosis, although current laparoscopy may be normal. Surgery is rarely effective and may induce de novo symptoms.

Typical symptoms include:

- hyperalgesia—sensations that would normally be painful become more painful
- allodynia—sensations that would not normally be painful become painful
- wind-up pain—pain felt over a larger area when severe
- unusual sensations—sharp, stabbing, burning pains
- worse pain when tired, stressed, exercise decreases or over-exercised.

On examination, there may be reduced cold sensation or other sensory changes in the area of maximal pain.

Management options include:

- explaining that pain is due to a change in pain processing by nerves, rather than weakness on her part. Nerves may generate pain impulses spontaneously. Pain is not curable and cannot be treated with surgery, but can be managed effectively
- acupuncture[27]
- amitriptyline 5–25 mg taken early evening; 10 mg is often effective. Start with 5 mg nocte (half a 10 mg tablet) and increase slowly, to avoid sedation
- pregabalin 75–600 mg daily. Initially 37.5 mg dose, dissolve contents of 75 mg capsule in water and drink half (100% soluble)
- regular sleep—tired nerves are irritable
- regular gentle exercise—start slowly
- stress management—stress exacerbates but does not cause the pain
- pain clinic referral if symptoms persist.

Where effective medication has ceased, pain may not recur immediately. When pain recurs, re-commence medication. Increase or reduce doses slowly. The woman may decide to use the medication for episodes of weeks/months, then cease it until pain recurs. An exacerbation of pain may be due to increased stress, overwork, tiredness or a decrease in regular exercise.

SSRI medications and narcotics are usually ineffective. Stabbing pains may also be due to pelvic muscle spasm.

Dysmenorrhoea and 'period-like' pain

Day 1–2 dysmenorrhoea is usually uterine pain.

- Excision of endometriosis is often ineffective for day 1–2 pain (uterine pain).
- Consider dysmenorrhoea treatment options.
- Allow the woman to control her pain with:
  - the option of NSAIDs suppositories for longer action and where there is nausea/vomiting
  - back-up narcotic-based analgesia for the worst days, rather than chronic use. Consider an oral narcotic with doxylamine for nighttime use
  - H_2 antagonist medications with NSAIDs where gastritis is a concern
  - hysterectomy—reasonable in older women with completed families.

Dysmenorrhoea symptoms during the month or premenstrually are frequently due to endometriosis lesions. Complete surgical excision is the most effective treatment.

Bowel dysfunction

(See Ch 30, Gastroenterology.)

Women with chronic pelvic pain have more to gain from a good diet, and more to lose from a bad diet, than other women. Sensitisation of the bowel means that any dietary indiscretion may result in pain. Food intolerance of certain carbohydrates is common.

General measures:

- Consider lifestyle factors such as alcohol, stress, hurried meals, irregular sleep and cigarettes.
- Review her medications and herbal supplements.
  - Antibiotics, antacids, laxatives, thyroid medicines, magnesium, some blood pressure tablets and several herbal therapies can worsen diarrhoea.

- Amitriptyline, iron tablets, pain killers, sedatives and other blood pressure tablets can worsen constipation.
- Consider bloods for ESR, CRP (inflammatory bowel disease), iron studies, coeliac screen.
- Consider comprehensive stool pathogen analysis by a specialised laboratory (organisms such as *Blastocystis hominis*, *Giardia lamblia* and *Dientamoeba fragilis* can cause persistent bowel dysfunction).
- Breath test for lactose intolerance or other food intolerances.
- Gastroenterology review for colonoscopy/ endoscopy where constipation is unmanageable, there is bleeding from the bowel, inflammatory bowel disease is possible or the presence or absence of coeliac disease is uncertain.

Treat constipation:

- Increase exercise and water intake.
- Dietary fibre—consider sterculia (a low-flatus fibre supplement).
- Magnesia S. Pellegrino daily.[28]

Treat bowel spasms and indigestion:

- peppermint oil capsules t.d.s./q.i.d. half an hour before meals for bloating and pain (may aggravate indigestion)
- anti-spasm medications such as mebeverine
- anti-diarrhoeal medications such as loperamide.

Bloating

Dietary bloating is frequently due to slow absorption of certain carbohydrates in the small intestine. If these substances reach the large intestine, they are fermented by large intestine bacteria and result in flatus, bloating, distension of the bowel and sometimes pain. Common foods of this type include:

- *fructose* (fructose malabsorption)—fruits with more fructose than glucose (such as apples, pears, dried fruit, fruit juice, coconut, honey) cause problems for people who absorb fructose slowly. Fruits with more glucose than fructose (such as citrus fruit, berry fruit, pineapples, kiwifruit, bananas and stone fruit) do not cause problems because the glucose facilitates fructose absorption across the bowel wall
- *fructans*—these are foods that release fructose when digested in the bowel. They include onions, artichokes, corn syrup, inulin (in 'fibre-enriched' foods) and all wheat products such as bread, biscuits, pastas, breakfast cereals and pizzas. This is another form of 'fructose malabsorption' and explains why some people without coeliac disease feel well on a low-gluten (i.e. low-fructan) diet
- *lactose* (lactose intolerance)—cottage cheese or yoghurt causes fewer problems. Alternatively, use lactose-free products or oral lactase when milk products are consumed
- *raffinose and galactans*—these sugars are found in brussel sprouts, cabbage, beans, cauliflower, broccoli, beans and some whole grains. Most people absorb these foods slowly, so flatus with these foods is normal
- *polyols*—these are artificial sweeteners such as sorbitol in chewing gum or diabetic food

Exclude coeliac disease.

Premenstrual bloating is common before a period and should resolve post menses.

A bloated feeling, associated with hypersensitivity, and sharp pains may be a feature of neuropathic pain.

For all bloating, exclude an ovarian tumour with vaginal examination or ultrasonography.

Dyspareunia

Possible causes include:

- *vulvovaginal infections*—vaginal swab, STD screen
- dermatological causes—lichen sclerosis, lichen planus, dermatitis, allergy, vulvar vestibulitis (tender to touch with cotton swab at posterior fourchette); consider biopsy, vulval dermatologist
- *interstitial cystitis*—urinary symptoms, tender anterior vagina
- *pelvic floor dysfunction /vaginismus*—tender, tight pelvic floor muscles. Examine with one finger pushing posteriorly on pelvic floor *before* speculum examination. Often secondary to another cause of pain or bladder dysfunction. Treat primary cause of pain, continence physio review to teach pelvic floor muscle relaxation, vaginal dilators, sexual counsellor, botox injection
- *neuropathic pain* with sensitisation of the vagina
- *endometriosis in pouch of Douglas*—deep dyspareunia; requires laparoscopic excision by experienced laparoscopic surgeon
- *psychological causes* and relationship difficulties
- *other pelvic pathology*.

Pelvic muscle pain

Painful pelvic muscles may mimic pelvic pathology. It is common but often misdiagnosed. Typical symptoms include:

- a chronic pain deep in the pelvis, with stabbing exacerbations, often after movement, intercourse, use of tampons or cervical smear tests. May wake her at night
- painful intercourse and a feeling that the vagina is 'too tight'. Pain often persists next day
- pain on moving, lying flat in bed, prolonged sitting, or sometimes getting up out of a chair

- inability to pass urine at times, despite a strong urge, due to tight periurethral muscles
- pain as a bowel action is passed through the anus, due to tight perianal muscles
- possible urinary incontinence, due to urge and pelvic floor dysfunction.

On examination:

- narrowed vaginal introitus due to muscle tightness
- pain reproduced with pressure backwards on pelvic floor muscle at vaginal introitus, or laterally along pubococcygeus
- limited range of muscle movement on voluntary contraction or relaxation (short, tight muscles)
- pain on palpation laterally out to pelvic side wall (obturator internus).

Treatment options include:

- treating the precipitating causes (e.g. bladder or neuropathic)
- hot pack or hot bath for acute pain
- encouraging regular gentle exercise, starting slowly
- improving general health and posture
- pelvic floor physiotherapist for pelvic muscle relaxation training, possibly with the use of vaginal dilators
- relaxation techniques
- amitriptyline 5–25 mg in the early evening (mildly effective)
- botox injection to affected muscles.

Other musculoskeletal conditions may also cause pelvic pain. These may include trochanteric bursitis, gluteus tendinopathy, labral hip tears, iliopsoas tendinopathy. Consider physiotherapy review and MRI of hip.

WHEN TO REFER FOR LAPAROSCOPY

Many women with pelvic pain undergo multiple laparoscopies, frequently without long-term benefit. Laparoscopy is useful to:

- diagnose the presence of endometriosis
- excise endometriosis where present. This is usually beneficial for:
  - dysmenorrhoea lasting longer than 2–3 days per month
  - dysmenorrhoea-like pain during the month
  - pain on opening bowels with periods
  - deep dyspareunia where other causes of dyspareunia have been excluded
  - back pain with periods (uterosacral ligament endometriosis or adenomyosis)
- provide a review of the pelvis at a later date, to manage recurrence if pain consistent with endometriosis persists and other causes of pain have been excluded.

Repeated laparoscopy with diathermy only or incomplete excision should be avoided. Endometriosis excision, particularly in the pouch of Douglas, requires advanced laparoscopic skills and equipment. Laparoscopy rarely improves:

- day 1 period pain (uterine pain)
- pelvic muscle pain
- urinary symptoms of frequency, urgency, nocturia (IC)
- superficial dyspareunia (vulvar vestibulitis, dermatological conditions, vaginal infections or neuropathic pain)
- bowel symptoms such as irritable bowel syndrome, constipation or food intolerance
- sharp, stabbing, burning pain (neuropathic pain).

PSYCHOLOGICAL SUPPORT / PSYCHOLOGIST

- Encourage the woman to become involved in her own care and take ownership of her pain. This avoids dependency and a feeling of helplessness.
- Discuss her fears, and how they apply to her situation, including:
  - fear of infertility and letting her partner down
  - fear of cancer; photographs taken at laparoscopy may be reassuring
  - fear that she will have uncontrollable pain with no assistance
  - fear that her condition will worsen and she will become dependent.
- Treat depression where present.
- Encourage her to remain involved or re-start activities she enjoys and can do, rather than concentrate on what she cannot do.
- Ensure that her family understand her condition and will support her.
- Encourage regular exercise, but start modestly to avoid pain exacerbation.
- Anticipate that even where pain is completely resolved, full recovery of confidence, optimism and independence will take some time. Regular 'health review' is beneficial.

MENSTRUAL MIGRAINE

Migraines are more common in women, in families and in women with endometriosis.[29] Menstrual migraines are migraines occurring with periods. Commonly there is a chronic low-grade headache at other times of the month too (chronic migraine), which may not be recognised as a migraine process. Headaches at the back of the head, associated with nausea, one-sided pain when severe, tender areas near the temples, pain behind the eyes, headaches on waking or pain worse with movement are all suggestive of a migraine-like process. Migraines in young children are common, and in girls they become even more common after menarche.

AETIOLOGY

There are two known causes of menstrual migraine:

- the fall in oestrogen levels at the beginning of a menses—a smaller fall in oestrogen at ovulation may trigger similar headaches in women not using the OCP. These headaches do not usually respond to NSAIDs
- high levels of prostaglandins at menses—these headaches respond to NSAID medications.

INVESTIGATIONS

A typical history of migraine at menses does not require further investigation, unless:

- the headaches have changed or started recently
- there are new sensory changes (e.g. double vision, loss of hearing, loss of feeling, weakness or abnormal movements in part of the body)
- the headache starts suddenly, is unusually painful or lasts more than 72 hours
- the headaches start after a head injury
- the woman has a stiff neck or a fever
- no one in the woman's family has migraine headaches.

TREATMENT

Treatment involves:

- avoiding migraine triggers
- specific treatments for menstrual migraine
- preventive medications for women with chronic headache
- management of an acute migraine if it occurs.

Avoiding migraine triggers

Common triggers include:

- becoming overtired or oversleeping
- dehydration
- low blood sugar (suggest small frequent meals)
- alcohol
- hormone changes—migraines may become more frequent or severe at perimenopause, with improvement post-menopausally
- stress, or relaxation after stress (weekend migraines)
- a 'head forward' position of the neck
- foods containing vasoactive substances—these include:
  - monosodium glutamate (MSG) (in processed and take-away food)
  - nitrites (preservatives in salami/bacon/ham and some aged cheese)
  - amines (many fruits and vegetables including avocados, bananas, chocolate.
  - alcohol
  - caffeine (may be used to treat a migraine in some cases).

An elimination–rechallenge diet may help identify triggers.

A migraine diary that records the time of the menstrual cycle, foods and drinks consumed, activities when the headache started, unusual stress and treatments used will help identify triggers.

Specific treatments for menstrual migraine

For women whose menstrual migraines are due to high prostaglandin levels (i.e. they respond to NSAIDs):

- an anti-inflammatory medication started 2–3 days before the period is due, and continued regularly for the first 2–3 days of the period, or a diclofenac 100 mg suppository early in the headache process
- a levonorgestrel-releasing IUCD (Mirena®)—will also treat painful or heavy periods and provide contraception, but will not help women with migraines triggered by a fall in oestrogen
- norethisterone 5 mg or desogestrel 75 μg *every day*, aiming at amenorrhoea.

For women whose menstrual migraines are due to a fall in oestrogen levels at menses:

- a 100 μg oestrogen patch at period time to stop oestrogen levels from falling at period time. Suitable for women with regular periods or who use the OCP. Use a 100 μg oestrogen patch from 5 days before menses until day 5 of the period. For the last 3 days of treatment, cut the patch in half (50 μg equivalent) so the dose decreases slowly. Where a migraine occurs at the end of the cycle, continue the patch until day 7 of the period[30]
- oral contraceptive pill taken continuously to avoid periods
- continuous hormone replacement therapy for women close to menopause
- a GNRHa medication with 'add-back therapy'—usually 6 months therapy only.

The oral contraceptive pill (OCP) is relatively contraindicated in:

- women with migraine and aura
- women with migraine without aura but with one additional risk factor: age 35 years or over, diabetes, a close family member who has had a stroke, heart attack or similar 'vascular' disease before they were 45 years old, a high lipid (cholesterol) level, hypertension, obesity, smoking.

Management of chronic migraine

Women with migraine headaches frequently describe milder headaches at other times, and may have a headache for much of the time. This is described as *chronic migraine*, and results in a significantly lower quality of life.

Diet

Magnesium

Intracellular magnesium levels are lower in people with migraine headaches, and magnesium deficiency is common. Two RCTs found that high-dose magnesium reduced the frequency and duration of migraine headaches.[31,32]

Magnesium can help prevent migraine in women with cyclic headaches related to periods, and is also used in treatment of conditions involving muscle spasm or tension, fibromyalgia, anxiety states and tension headaches.

Riboflavin (vitamin B_2)

Regular riboflavin may help reduce the frequency and shorten the duration of migraine headaches through anti-nociceptive and anti-inflammatory effects.

Dose: 400 mg/day for at least 3 months, to assess the effect in combination with feverfew and magnesium.

Herbal

Vitex agnus castus (chaste tree)

Vitex agnus castus is an effective treatment for common PMS symptoms, including headache.[33]

Feverfew (*Tanacetum parthenium*)

A systematic review of six RCTs concluded that evidence favours feverfew as an effective preventative treatment against migraine, and that it is well tolerated.[34]

Dose:

- dried leaf: 50–200 mg daily
- fresh plant tincture (1:1): 0.7–2.0 mL daily
- dried plant tincture (1:5): 1–3 mL/day

Note: There is significant variation in the amount of active ingredient in commercially available feverfew preparations.

Contraindicated in pregnancy.

Pharmacological

There are several medications used for headache prophylaxis. As none help all women, it may be necessary to try a few different medications to find one that is effective. These medications work best for chronic migraine, rather than menstrual migraine.

Common medications useful in young women include:

- *amitriptyline* (5–25 mg daily)—taken early in the evening to avoid morning sedation. Start with 5 mg and increase slowly. Especially suitable for women with chronic pelvic pain, bladder overactivity or poor sleep
- *cyproheptadine*—start with 2 mg nocte, then increase to 4 mg nocte, then 4 mg b.i.d. if needed. Useful if the woman also has allergies. Sleepiness wears off within a few days
- *topiramate*—start with 25 mg at night, then b.i.d. and increase if necessary. Reduces appetite, so may cause weight loss
- *venlafaxine*—start with 37.5 mg nocte, which may be sufficient. May cause sexual dysfunction
- *pizotifen* (0.5 mg daily)—weight gain and sleepiness are common
- *beta-blockers*—help hypertension or tachycardia, but cause reduced exercise tolerance and fatigue, and may cause sexual dysfunction.

Management of acute migraine

General measures:

- Relax in a dark, quiet room. Sleep if possible.
- Use a hot or cold pack on the head/neck or a warm shower/bath to relax tense muscles.
- Massage painful areas in the scalp, temples or shoulders.
- Relax jaw and facial muscles.
- Eat starchy food such as biscuits, rice or bread.
- Drink some water if dehydrated.

Simple medications to try:

- a single caffeinated drink—this is often helpful. Excess caffeine may cause rebound headache later, or trigger headaches in some people
- three soluble aspirin, 400 mg ibuprofen, 500 mg naproxen or diclofenac 100 mg rectal suppository (often most effective)—many women find three soluble aspirin and a cola drink taken *early* in a migraine very effective
- paracetamol 1 g
- metoclopramide 10 mg or prochlorperazine 5 mg for nausea.

Stronger medications:

- triptans—these are the *most* effective treatments available and can stop a migraine within 30 minutes if taken early. They affect the serotonin molecule in the brain and can be taken as a nasal spray, tablet or injection. The nasal spray is convenient, especially if there is nausea
- narcotic medications, often with paracetamol, an NSAID or a sedative such as doxylamine to promote sleep
- cafergot (an ergotamine compound).

While triptan medications may manage the severe headache, background 'unwell feelings' or milder headache may remain. Combining a triptan with one of the simpler medications or non-medication options may give the best effect.

Advise the woman to keep a dose of her medication, some food and a drink with her in case of migraine, to allow prompt treatment of a migraine if it occurs.

LEIOMYOMAS (FIBROIDS)

Leiomyomas are benign tumours of smooth muscle, commonly found in the uterus.

INCIDENCE AND NATURAL HISTORY

Myomas:

- are rare before puberty and diminish after menopause
- occur in 40% of Caucasian women by age 35[35] and higher in Negro women
- increased by obesity, early menarche, family history (2.5 times in first-degree relatives)[36]
- decreased with increasing parity, increased exercise and possibly smoking[37]
- will grow at variable rate until hormone levels fall.

There is no relationship with sexually transmitted infections including chlamydia, IUD use, talc exposure or number of sexual partners.

During pregnancy, myomas usually grow little and do not affect the pregnancy.

AETIOLOGY

The aetiology is unknown. Myomas are monoclonal. Chromosomal abnormalities are common (e.g. 12, 14 translocations, 7 deletions and trisomy 12), especially in cellular, atypical or large myomas.[38]

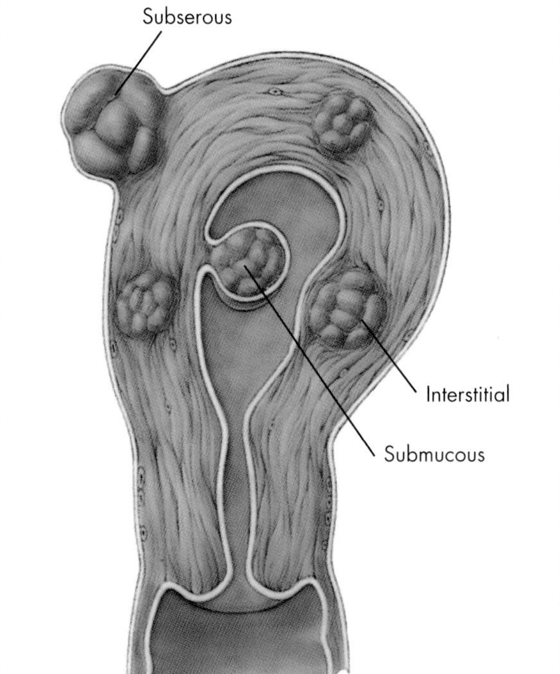

FIGURE 52.13 Pathology of fibroids; locations of leiomyomas

Myoma *initiation* may involve intrinsic abnormalities of the myometrium, congenitally elevated myometrial oestrogen receptors, hormonal changes or a response to ischaemic injury at the time of menstruation.[39]

Myoma *growth* is promoted by smooth muscle proliferation growth factors, oestrogen and progesterone. Intracellular aromatase converts androgens to oestrogens to increase intracellular oestrogen further.

Myoma size decreases with GnRH analogues or mifepristone (progesterone receptor modulator), but the myoma returns to its original size after treatment ceases.

There is no definite relationship between myoma initiation/growth and the OCP. Growth with HRT is uncommon, and where present may be due to progestin.

MYOMA CLASSIFICATION

- *Submucosal*—lie beneath the endometrium and bulge into the endometrial cavity. Can be seen hysteroscopically.
- *Intramural*—lie within the uterine wall.
- *Subserous*—lie on the outer (serosal) surface of the uterus. Easily seen laparoscopically.
- *Pedunculated*—a serosal myoma attached to the uterus by a thin pedicle. Submucosal myomas may also become pedunculated.
- Myomas of the ovaries, round ligament and cervix are less common.

SYMPTOMS

Most uterine myomas are asymptomatic.

Symptoms include:

- menorrhagia—the relationship to menorrhagia is variable; many women with fibroids have normal periods. Where menorrhagia is present, it may be due to vasoactive growth factors or to mechanical compression of veins
- pelvic pressure symptoms—e.g. heaviness in lower abdomen, urinary frequency and urgency, constipation
- dyspareunia—especially where myomas are low and posterior
- pelvic pain—uncommon; it is more common where the myoma extends laterally towards the pelvic side wall
- bleeding between periods—uncommon
- low back pain—especially after prolonged standing.

EXAMINATION

A firm, irregular, non-tender mass arising from the pelvis. May be palpable abdominally where uterine size exceeds approximately 12 weeks pregnancy size and myomas are anterior.

INVESTIGATIONS

Investigations include:

- vaginal ultrasound scan—combined abdominovaginal ultrasound for large myomas. Myomas are rounded, hyp*o*echoic, heterogeneous, well-defined masses on ultrasound. Hyp*er*echoic where calcification or haemorrhage is present. Anechoic in cystic areas
- saline infusion sonogram or hysteroscopy to delineate submucous myomas and assess uterine cavity
- MRI—accurate assessment of submucous myomas. Differentiates adenomyomas and presence of adenomyosis.[40]

TREATMENT

Treatment options include:

- No treatment. Asymptomatic myomas where malignancy has been excluded do not require treatment.
- Exclude other causes of symptoms, e.g. other causes of menorrhagia, endometriosis, adenomyosis, ovarian mass.
- Surgical options:
  - hysteroscopic resection of submucous myoma—requires > 50% myoma into endometrial cavity
  - myomectomy—laparoscopic or abdominal. Allows subsequent pregnancy, but with small risk of uterine rupture and increased likelihood of caesarean section[41]
  - myolysis—uncommon. Cautery, laser or cryotherapy laparoscopically to decrease myoma size
  - hysterectomy.
- Medical options do not improve fertility. They include:
  - levonorgestrel-releasing IUCD. Decreased menorrhagia. No decrease in myoma size
  - GnRH analogues. Decreased myoma size while on treatment
  - progesterone receptor modulators, e.g. mifepristone (RU 486) and asoprisnil
  - androgenic steroid hormones, e.g. danazol for menorrhagia
  - raloxifene—postmenopausal women only.
- Uterine artery embolisation (experimental radiological procedure):
  - Beads of polyvinyl alcohol are injected via radiological catheter to block both uterine arteries. Risks include infected necrotic myomas, premature ovarian failure from ovarian artery obstruction and uterine rupture with subsequent pregnancy.

MYOMAS, FERTILITY AND PREGNANCY

Growth during pregnancy or obstetric complications are uncommon. However:

- Submucous or intramural myomas with an intracavity component are associated with reduced fertility and increased miscarriage. Hysteroscopic removal of the submucous myoma returns fertility to normal.
- The relationship between intramural or subserous myomas and fertility is controversial.[42]
- Incidence of caesarean section, malpresentation, preterm delivery, placenta praevia and postpartum haemorrhage are all slightly elevated.[43]
- Myoma degeneration occurs in 5% of myomas during pregnancy, often with severe abdominal pain.

LEIOMYOSARCOMA

Leiomyosarcoma are a distinct entity, genetically different from benign myomas. Sarcomatous change in a benign myoma is very rare.

Features suggestive of leiomyosarcoma include:

- age 40–60 years
- previous pelvic radiotherapy
- *post*menopausal growth of a myoma
- lack of shrinkage of myoma with GnRH analogues
- recent onset of symptoms
- raised lactate dehydrogenase, specifically LDH isozyme 3[44]
- indistinct tumour margins and rich vasculature on contrast MRI.

Rapid myoma growth in a *pre*menopausal woman rarely means sarcoma.

OVARIAN CYSTS (EXCLUDING POLYCYSTIC OVARIAN SYNDROME)

The ovary may contain a wide variety of cysts or tumours. Commonly, they include:

- functional cysts
- benign tumours—including cystadenomas derived from epithelial cell lines, germ cell tumours such as teratomas (dermoids) derived from germ cells and stromal tumours derived from ovarian stromal cells
- endometriomas
- para-ovarian (e.g. fimbrial) cysts
- malignant tumours
- tumours of low malignant potential.

PRIMARY PREVENTION

Functional cysts are common in premenopausal women. Pregnancy, breastfeeding and the OCP suppress ovulation and reduce their incidence.

SYMPTOMS

Many functional cysts are asymptomatic. Hormonal effects including menstrual irregularity, nausea, vomiting or breast tenderness are common and mimic early pregnancy. Ovarian cyst rupture may occur, with sudden acute pain spontaneously or after intercourse. The pain improves over a few hours but may be followed by an ache for a few days.

Ovarian cysts of any kind may cause:

- pressure symptoms, e.g. urinary frequency, constipation, fullness in abdomen, tighter clothing
- menstrual irregularities
- dyspareunia
- pelvic pain
- ovarian torsion—sudden acute pain with vomiting, raised pulse rate and sometimes fever. Commonly involves a benign cyst of moderate size on a long ovarian pedicle. *Torsion is an acute medical emergency similar to torsion of the testis. It requires urgent laparoscopy to untwist the ovarian pedicle and avoid loss of the ovary.*

Women with endometriomas may describe typical symptoms of endometriosis or be asymptomatic.

Women with ovarian cancer present with non-specific symptoms that include abdominal pain, bloating, difficulty eating/feeling full, urinary frequency or abdominal distension. There may be changes in bowel habit frequently misdiagnosed as irritable bowel syndrome. *Ovarian cancer should always be considered in women with recent-onset non-specific abdominal symptoms.*

Hormone-producing tumours are uncommon. Symptoms depend on the hormone produced, e.g. oestrogen from granulose cell tumours, testosterone from an androblastoma.

EXAMINATION

A mass separate from the uterus arising from one or both adnexae may be palpable. Large ovarian cysts may be palpable abdominally, especially in thin women. Any postmenopausal woman with a palpable ovary vaginally requires ultrasound assessment.

INVESTIGATIONS

Radiological

Ultrasound examination:

- Functional cysts should be < 5 cm in diameter, thin walled, fluid filled, perfectly round, with no intracellular debris or septae and resolve within 3 months.
- Haemorrhage in a functional cyst may result in a larger cyst with bizarre intracystic echoes that may mimic an endometrioma but resolve within 3 months.
- Endometriomas have a grey, homogenous 'ground glass' appearance.
- Teratomas (dermoids) contain highly echogenic sebaceous or calcium-containing tissue.
- Serous cystadenomas are typically unilocular.
- Mucinous cystadenomas are typically multilocular.
- Complex cysts (unilateral or bilateral) or the presence of increased abdominal fluid/ascites must have malignancy excluded.
- The ovarian crescent sign (OCS) has been proposed, to differentiate benign and malignant disease. The OCS is defined as a rim of visible healthy ovarian tissue in the ipsilateral ovary. Where absent, invasive cancer is more likely.[45]

Vaginal ultrasound provides a clearer view of the ovaries than abdominal ultrasound in most women. Abdominal ultrasound scans are appropriate for children, virgins, very large ovarian cysts or where vaginal ultrasound would cause pain or distress.

It is normal to see a 2–3 cm fluid-filled ovulation cyst/corpus luteum from ovulation until menses. To minimise false positive results, request ultrasound scans in the early follicular phase.

CT scans assess the extent of metastatic disease.

MRI may be used to assess bowel or bladder infiltration in the presence of endometriomata.

Abdominal X-ray is rarely indicated but will show the teeth or bone frequently present in a teratoma (dermoid). Radiation to the ovaries of young women should be minimised.

TABLE 52.1 Risk of malignancy index

	RMI 1 score	RMI 2 score
Ultrasound features: • multilocular • solid areas • bilateral lesions • ascites • intra-abdominal metastases	0 = no abnormalities 1 = 1 abnormality 3 = 2 or more abnormalities	0 = no abnormalities 1 = 1 abnormality 4 = 2 or more abnormalities
Premenopausal	1	1
Postmenopausal	3	4
CA 125 level	U/mL	U/mL

Biochemical

Pregnancy test

Where positive, consider haemorrhage in the corpus luteum of pregnancy or ectopic pregnancy.

Cancer antigen 125

Normal level is < 35 U/mL.

Cancer antigen 125 (CA 125) levels are frequently raised in:

- serous, clear cell and endometrioid cystadenocarcinoma, but not mucinous cystadenocarcinoma
- endometriosis—mild elevation
- other benign conditions including fibroids, adenomyosis, diverticulitis, pelvic inflammatory disease, normal menstruation and liver disease
- other malignant conditions including cancer of the pancreas, breast, lung and colon.

As CA 125 is raised in a wide variety of benign conditions, it should not be used for screening, or for cysts with benign features. It is of most use in:

- postmenopausal women with an ovarian cyst, where malignancy is possible. CA 125 levels are raised in 80% of advanced ovarian cancers, but only 50% of stage 1 disease[46]
- follow-up of known ovarian malignancy to assess treatment response.

Other tumour markers used to distinguish benign from malignant disease are discussed below.

Risk of malignancy index

The risk of malignancy index (RMI, Table 52.1) combines menopausal status, CA 125 level and ultrasound features to predict the risk of ovarian malignancy in a known cyst. Two scores have been used: RMI 1 and RMI 2.

An RMI 1 score > 200 has a sensitivity of 80%, specificity of 92% and positive predictive value of 83%[47] for ovarian malignancy.

For example:

- RMI 1 for a postmenopausal woman with a multilocular cyst and Ca 125 level of 100 is $1 \times 3 \times 100 = 300$
- RMI 1 for a premenopausal woman with a multilocular cyst and a Ca 125 level of 100 is $1 \times 1 \times 100 = 100$.

TREATMENT

Before treatment, it is important to explain the nature of the cyst (as far as is known) and specifically discuss common concerns the woman may have. These include:

- fear that the cyst may be cancer
- fear that her fertility may be affected, or that she will lose an ovary
- fear of surgery
- embarrassment at having a 'gynaecological condition'.

Where pain is present, this will add to her distress.

Medical treatment options

Repeat ultrasound

Repeat ultrasound in the early follicular phase after 2–3 months allows a functional cyst, if present, to resolve, and is appropriate in:

- a premenopausal woman with a single fluid-filled cyst < 5 cm diameter
- a single cyst with the grey homogeneous 'ground glass' appearance of an endometrioma and few symptoms. Haemorrhage in a corpus luteum will resolve over this time. Endometriomas will persist and require surgery
- a postmenopausal woman with a single, round, thin-walled, fluid-filled cyst < 2 cm in diameter. Such cysts are frequently fimbrial (para-ovarian) rather than ovarian.

Laparoscopy

Laparoscopy is used to diagnose and remove the cyst. Conservation of the ovary by laparoscopic cystectomy is frequently possible, although oophorectomy may be required. Laparoscopic surgery allows good visualisation of the cyst, excision of other coexisting abnormalities such as endometriosis, faster postoperative recovery and minimisation of post-surgical adhesions. Laparoscopy is appropriate where:

- the cyst has persisted at repeat ultrasound or is enlarging
- ultrasound suggests that it is unlikely to be a functional cyst, or symptoms are troublesome
- pregnancy has been excluded
- malignancy is unlikely.

Laparotomy

Laparotomy is appropriate where:

- the chance of malignancy is high. Ovarian cancer requires staging surgery and cytoreduction
- a large teratoma is present. This avoids spillage of irritant contents through the pelvic cavity. Smaller teratomas remain suitable for laparoscopic removal.

Oral contraceptive pill

Although widely used, the OCP *will not* hasten resolution of an existing cyst.[48] It *will* reduce the incidence of subsequent functional cysts.

OVARIAN CYSTS AFTER MENOPAUSE

The incidence of ovarian cancer increases with increasing age, and functional cysts are less likely, so referral to a gynaecologist without repeat scan is appropriate, especially where ultrasound features are complex.

OVARIAN CYSTS DURING PREGNANCY

Expect a corpus luteum ± intracystic haemorrhage in the first trimester. This provides hormonal support for the pregnancy

Persisting cysts are abnormal and require obstetric review. Where surgery is required, this is performed in the second trimester.

OVARIAN CYSTS IN PREPUBERTAL GIRLS

Frequently, diagnosis is made only when a mass is palpable abdominally. Ovarian cysts in a prepubertal girl are always abnormal and may be malignant.

GYNAECOLOGICAL MALIGNANCIES

(See also Ch 24, Cancer.)

Gynaecological malignancies occur in 9.2% of women. The risk is 1:34 by age 75 years and 1:24 by age 85 years (Table 52.2).[49]

UTERINE CANCER

The histology of uterine cancer includes:

- endometrial cancer—95% (adenocarcinoma, adenosquamous, clear cell and papillary serous)
- sarcomas (carcinosarcomas, mixed müllerian tumours, leiomyosarcomas and endometrial stromal sarcomas)
- gestational trophoblastic tumours (childbearing years).

Risk and protective factors

Most risk factors involve unopposed oestrogen stimulation. They include:

- personal or family history of breast, bowel or endometrial cancer
- age > 40 years; peak incidence in late sixties
- unopposed oestrogen hormone therapy
- hereditary non-polyposis colorectal cancer (HNPCC)
- endometrial hyperplasia, especially where atypia is present
- tamoxifen use
- nulliparity
- high BMI
- diabetes mellitus
- hypertension
- early menarche
- late menopause
- poor diet.

Protective factors include:

- not being overweight
- OCP use
- progestogen medications.

TABLE 52.2 Rate of gynaecological malignancies at ages 75 and 85 years

Type of malignancy	Incidence	
	Age 75 years	Age 85 years
Ovary	1:123	1:81
Fallopian tube	rare	rare
Uterus	1:74	1:54
Cervix	1:191	1:149
Vagina	1:2715	1:1343
Vulva	1:856	1:406

Hereditary cancer syndromes

The lifetime risk of endometrial cancer is:

- 40% for HNPCC[50]
- possibly slightly increased with BRCA1.

HNPCC (Lynch syndrome) is an autosomal-dominant genetic disorder involving DNA mismatch repair genes MLH1, MSH2, MSH6 and PMS2. Women with HNPCC are at increased risk of colon, endometrial and ovarian cancer. Endometrial cancer may present before colon cancer and 30% are diagnosed before the age of 40 years.

Screening

There are no screening tests currently recommended for endometrial cancer.

Symptoms

Symptoms include:

- postmenopausal bleeding (PMB)
- intermenstrual bleeding, especially where periods are irregular
- lower abdominal pain (uncommon)
- back pain or leg oedema secondary to metastasis (rare).

Growth commonly follows the pattern:

- exophytic, spreading growth within the uterine cavity with early bleeding
- myometrial invasion and extension towards the cervix
- local spread to nearby organs
- lymphatic spread to pelvic, para-aortic and, rarely, inguinal lymph nodes
- haematological spread to lungs, liver, bone and, rarely, brain.

Examination

Commonly the uterus, vagina and cervix are normal to examination. In advanced disease there may be an enlarged uterus or pelvic mass. Exclude other causes of bleeding (e.g. vulval, vaginal and cervical lesions). Take a cervical smear.

Investigations

Transvaginal ultrasound:

- Endometrial thickness ≤ 4 mm in women with PMB on *no* HRT virtually excludes malignancy.[52]
- Endometrial thickness in women on HRT is increased but an agreed cut-off level has not been conclusively determined.
- Pyometra or haematometra suggests cervical obstruction.

Endometrial biopsy:

- is less reliable than curettage
- will not treat endometrial polyps or submucosal fibroids
- will not diagnose atrophic endometritis.

Hysteroscopy and curettage:

- are required where endometrial thickness is > 4 mm, ultrasonography is inconclusive, endometrial biopsy is inadequate or unsuitable, bleeding persists or recurs, or suspicious symptoms are present.

Chest X-ray and CT abdomen:

- to assist staging of confirmed disease.

Treatment

Treatment of confirmed malignancy is optimised by involvement of a gynaecological oncologist. It includes:

- surgical staging and removal of disease—hysterectomy, bilateral salpingo-oophorectomy, lymphatic node sampling with additional procedures as required using an abdominal or laparoscopic approach
- adjuvant treatments, if required, depending on the stage, grade and histology of the malignancy. Adjuvant treatments include radiotherapy, medical treatments including progestogens and, less commonly, chemotherapy (see Ch 24, Cancer).

HRT and endometrial cancer risk

Unopposed oestrogen replacement significantly increases the risk of endometrial cancer.

HRT after endometrial cancer

Current knowledge suggests that there is no increased risk of recurrence with oestrogen replacement after treatment for endometrial cancer, although this should be discussed with the treating gynaecological oncologist.[52]

GESTATIONAL TROPHOBLASTIC DISEASE

Gestational trophoblastic disease includes a spectrum, from benign hydatidiform mole, through invasive mole, to choriocarcinoma. Clinical features include:

- reproductive age group
- positive hCG
- uterine size 'large for dates'
- increased hyperemesis
- first-trimester bleeding
- passage of grapelike vesicles from the vagina
- potential for severe eclampsia
- small hypoechoic cysts filling the uterine cavity on ultrasound, often with bilateral theca lutein ovarian cysts induced by the high hCG.

OVARIAN TUMOURS

A wide variety of tumours develop in the ovary. Each histological type may be benign or malignant. Tumours derived from epithelial cells may also be of borderline malignancy (low malignant potential).

Ovarian tumours include:

- Epithelial tumours derived from surface epithelium of the ovary—serous, mucinous, endometrioid, clear cell, Brenner. Seventy-five per cent of ovarian tumours and 95% of ovarian cancer are epithelial. Approximately 15% of all epithelial ovarian tumours are of 'borderline' malignancy.
- Germ cell tumours derived from primitive germ cells—teratomas (dermoids), dysgerminoma, endodermal sinus tumour, choriocarcinoma. Most are benign. Fifteen to twenty per cent of ovarian tumours and < 5% of ovarian cancers are germ cell. More common in younger women.
- Sex cord stromal tumours derived from ovarian stroma—granulosa cell, theca cell, thecoma, fibroma, Sertoli-Leydig cell, lipid cell, gynandroblastoma. Most are benign. Risk is increased with Peutz-Jeghers, Gorlin's, Cushing's and Meigs' syndromes.
- Metastatic cancer from other organs, commonly breast, gastrointestinal tract (stomach, colon, pancreas, appendix) or haemopoietic system. Five per cent of ovarian cancers are secondary.

RISK AND PROTECTIVE FACTORS FOR OVARIAN CANCER

Ninety-five per cent of ovarian cancer is epithelial in histology. Risk factors include the hereditary cancer syndromes, repeated ovulatory cycles, environmental and dietary factors. Specific risk factors:

- family history of ovarian cancer and the hereditary cancer syndromes—this is the major risk factor
- age > 50 years
- increased number of ovulatory cycles
- nulliparity
- environmental factors, including use of talc on the vulva, asbestos and possibly mumps
- dietary factors, including high-fat diet, obesity and possibly lactose consumption

- past history or family history of breast cancer
- endometriosis, especially if severe,[53] especially endometrioid or clear cell malignancies
- Jewish descent (higher carriage of BRCA1 and 2 genes)
- HRT use after menopause—possible small increased risk
- Sedentary lifestyle.

Initial concern regarding the use of clomiphene for ovulation induction and risk of ovarian cancer has not been substantiated[54] but remains under review.

Protective factors include:

- factors that reduce the number of ovulatory cycles, including:
  - parity—risk decreases with each childbirth[55]
  - breastfeeding
  - OCP use
- tubal ligation
- hysterectomy
- oophorectomy—does not protect against primary peritoneal cancer.

HEREDITARY CANCER SYNDROMES

The lifetime risk of ovarian cancer is:

- 40–50% for BRCA 1
- 20–30% for BRCA 2
- 10% for HNPCC.

By the age of 60, a woman with BRCA1 or 2 genes has a higher chance of developing cancer of the ovary in the next year than cancer of the breast.[50]

SCREENING

The value of screening in women in the general population is not established.[56] Screening in women at high risk may be beneficial. Screening options include:

- annual cancer cell surface antigen 125 (CA 125) estimation—CA 125 is formed by:
  - most epithelial ovarian cancers, including most serous, endometrioid and clear cell types. Less common with mucinous tumours. Approximately 90% of ovarian cancer is 'epithelial' and produces CA 125
  - some endometrial, fallopian tube, pancreatic, breast, colon or lung cancers
  - benign gynaecological conditions including endometriosis, leiomyomas, benign ovarian tumours and fallopian tube disease
  - other benign conditions, including liver cirrhosis
- annual transvaginal ultrasound with colour Doppler
- annual bimanual pelvic examination.

A combination of all three methods may be the most effective.

OVARIAN TUMOUR MARKERS

Although only CA 125 is widely used, tumour markers in current clinical use for diagnosis or to monitor treatment progress include:

- markers for epithelial tumours:
  - CA 125—epithelial
  - carbohydrate antigen 19-9 (CA 19-9)—mucinous. It is also increased with diseases of the liver and pancreas, and occasionally dermoid tumours
  - carcinoembryonic antigen (CEA)—Brenner, endometrioid, clear cell and serous. It is also increased with diseases of the liver, colon, pancreas, stomach, lung and breast
- markers for germ cell tumours:
  - alpha-fetoprotein (AFP)—endodermal sinus/yolk sac tumours
  - hCG—dysgerminoma, choriocarcinoma
  - lactate dehydrogenase (LDH)—dysgerminoma
- markers for sex cord stromal tumours:
  - inhibin—granulosa cell
  - oestrogen—granulosa cell
  - androgens—virilising tumours.

SYMPTOMS

Many ovarian tumours are initially asymptomatic. Symptoms include:

- non-specific symptoms such as bloating, abdominal swelling, urinary symptoms, dyspepsia, early satiety, lack of appetite, malaise, weight gain, palpable mass or loss or changes in bowel function. *Women presenting with these symptoms, especially with recent onset, require exclusion of ovarian tumours.*
- less common presentations, including:
  - postmenopausal bleeding, menorrhagia, amenorrhoea, endometrial hyperplasia or cancer or fibrocystic breast disease—oestrogen-producing sex cord stromal tumours
  - precocious puberty—granulosa cell tumour in girls
  - virilisation—androgen-producing sex cord stromal tumours
  - abnormal thyroid function where a dermoid includes significant functioning thyroid tissue.

EXAMINATION

A firm, fixed, nodular, non-tender pelvic mass, possibly with ascites, suggests malignancy. Both borderline and malignant tumours of the ovary are often bilateral.

INVESTIGATIONS

The risk of malignancy index can be estimated by combining the ultrasound features, CA 125 level and menopausal status.

A CT abdomen and chest X-ray will aid staging of malignant disease.

MANAGEMENT

For benign tumours, surgical removal alone is usually sufficient.

Where malignancy is likely, the outcome is improved when managed by a gynaecological oncologist. Management depends on the stage and histological type of tumour, and the woman's age and fertility requirements.

- *Epithelial tumours*—debulking surgery (hysterectomy, bilateral salpingo-oophorectomy, omentectomy, lymph node sampling and peritoneal resection of visible lesions) followed by chemotherapy with a platinum compound is usual. Fertility-sparing surgery can be considered where:
  - early-stage cancer is confined to the ovary
  - histology is borderline.
- *Germ cell tumours*—highly chemo- or radiosensitive. Fertility-sparing surgery is frequently possible and cure rates are high.
- *Sex cord stromal tumours*—surgery alone may be sufficient. Chemotherapy or radiotherapy may be used.
- *Metastatic cancer*—management depends on the nature of the primary malignancy.

Where fertility is possible, contraception should be used throughout treatment, even with amenorrhoea, to avoid damage to a developing fetus.

Where tumour markers have been elevated, these can be used to assess response to treatment, relapse and survival. A rapid decrease in CA 125 levels during initial treatment correlates with longer progression-free intervals and survival.

For further information on integrative and lifestyle management, see Ch 24, Cancer.

HRT AND OVARIAN CANCER RISK

A low increased risk of one extra ovarian cancer per 2500 HRT users has been suggested. This risk is lower than that attributable to nulliparity, obesity or inactivity.[57,58]

HRT AFTER OVARIAN CANCER

There are currently no data to suggest that HRT should be avoided after ovarian cancer.

PRIMARY PERITONEAL CANCER

Primary peritoneal cancer is rare. It develops from the epithelial cells of the peritoneum. Management is as for cancer of the ovary.

CANCER OF THE FALLOPIAN TUBE

Cancer of the fallopian tube is rare. An adenocarcinoma, it is more common in women with BRCA 1 and 2 genes.

It may present as vaginal discharge or bleeding in a woman with a positive cervical smear but no abnormality of the endometrium or cervix found. CA 125 is frequently high.

CERVICAL CANCER

HISTOLOGICAL TYPES

Histological types include:

- squamous cell carcinoma (~95%)
- adenocarcinoma (~5%).

RISK AND PROTECTIVE FACTORS

Risk factors include:

- HPV infection, especially serotypes 16, 18, 31—this is the major risk factor
- coexistent sexually transmitted diseases, including herpes and chlamydia
- smoking—benzpyrene has been isolated in the cervical mucus of smokers
- lowered immunity
- poor diet
- possibly the OCP—the relationship with the Pill may reflect increased sexual activity rather than a pill effect
- high number of sexual partners—this increases the likelihood of HPV infection.

Protective factors include:

- factors that reduce HPV infection—i.e. condoms, fewer sexual partners
- vaccination against HPV serotypes.

It is beneficial to teach young women:

- how to use a condom
- to avoid intercourse when young
- how to negotiate safe sex with a new sexual partner.

Hereditary cancer syndromes

The risk of cervical cancer is *not* increased in women with a family history of cervical, vaginal or vulval cancer, or in women who carry the BRCA 1, 2 or NHPCC gene.

SYMPTOMS

Most women with cervical cancer are asymptomatic. Symptoms where present include:

- intermenstrual bleeding
- post-coital bleeding
- foul-smelling or seropurulent discharge
- heavier periods
- urinary symptoms of frequency, urgency and recurrent cystitis.

Advanced cases may present with breathlessness due to severe anaemia, obstructive uropathy, oedema of the lower limbs, haematuria, bowel obstruction and cachexia.

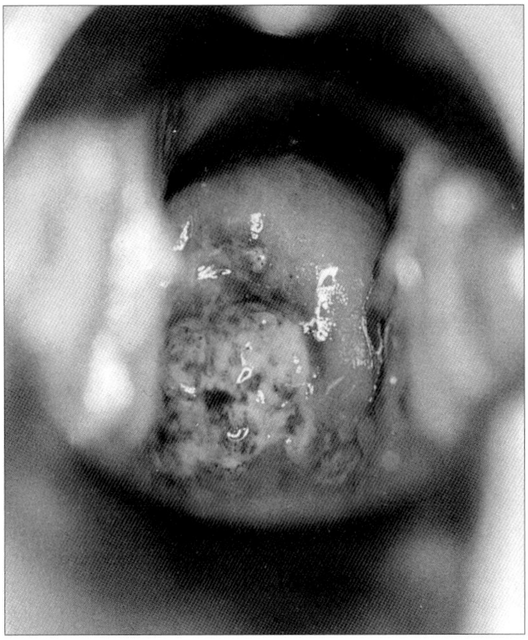

FIGURE 52.14 Cervical herpes

EXAMINATION

Very early lesions appear as a rough, reddish, area that bleeds on touch.

- Cervical growth may be exophytic with an obvious lesion, or endophytic with an enlarged, barrel-shaped cervix. The lesion is often ulcerated.
- Further invasion is to:
  - parametrium, surrounding vagina, bladder or rectum. Ureteric compression may cause hydronephrosis with renal failure
  - pelvic lymph nodes
  - para-aortic nodes, lungs, liver, late in disease.

MANAGEMENT

Management depends on surgical staging, which frequently requires examination under anaesthesia.

- Microinvasive cancer (Stage IA), where the cancer has invaded no more than 5 mm deep and 7 mm wide into the underlying stroma, may be treated with conisation (preserves fertility) or hysterectomy.
- Cancer confined to the cervix is treated with either a radical (Wertheim) hysterectomy and pelvic lymphadenectomy, or with radiotherapy. In selected early cases, radical trachelectomy (removal of the cervix alone) combined with lymphadenectomy has been used to preserve fertility.
- More extensive cancer is treated with radiotherapy.
- Chemotherapy has been used for late-stage disease.

HRT AND CERVICAL CANCER

HRT does not increase the risk of cervical cancer.

There is no contraindication to HRT use in women with cervical cancer (see Ch 53, Menopause).

VAGINAL CANCER

Histological types:

- squamous cell carcinoma (85%)—spreads superficially within the vaginal wall and later invades the paravaginal tissues and the parametria. Distant metastases occur most commonly in the lungs and liver
- adenocarcinoma (15%)—peak incidence is between 17 and 21 years of age. It differs from squamous cell carcinoma by an increase in pulmonary metastases and supraclavicular and pelvic node involvement
- other tumours, including sarcoma, melanoma, lymphoma and carcinoid tumours
- clear cell carcinoma (rare)—most common in women under 30 years of age with a history of DES exposure.

RISK FACTORS

Risk factors include:

- presence of HPV infection
- previous CIN or cancer
- presence of VAIN
- diethylstilboestrol (DES) exposure
- cigarette smoking.

MANAGEMENT

Early-stage cancer of the vagina is managed by surgery or radiotherapy. Radiotherapy is preferred in later-stage disease.

HRT AND VAGINAL CANCER

HRT does not increase the risk of vaginal cancer.

There is no contraindication to HRT use in women with vaginal cancer.

CANCER OF THE VULVA

HISTOLOGY

Histological types include:

- squamous cell carcinoma (95%)
- melanoma or adenocarcinoma.

RISK FACTORS

Risk factors include:

- HPV infection, especially serotypes 16, 18 and 31

- lichen sclerosis—2–3% of women with lichen sclerosis develop vulval cancer
- lichen planus
- presence of VIN—linked to HPV infection
- age > 50 years
- cigarette smoking.

SYMPTOMS
Symptoms include:
- a lump in the vulva
- an itchy or tender area
- a lesion that bleeds.

EXAMINATION
- Women with lichen sclerosis or lichen planus require regular review.
- Intraepithelial neoplasia may affect the cervix, vagina, vulva or anus, so all areas should be examined.
- Vulval cancer may appear as a white, pink or red lesion (pigmented if melanoma).
- Any lesions found require colposcopy and biopsy or excision.
- Lymphatic spread involves the inguinal or femoral nodes.

MANAGEMENT
Management depends on the stage of the disease. Early-stage disease may be cured by wide surgical excision. Vulvectomy with inguinal/femoral lymphadenectomy may be required.

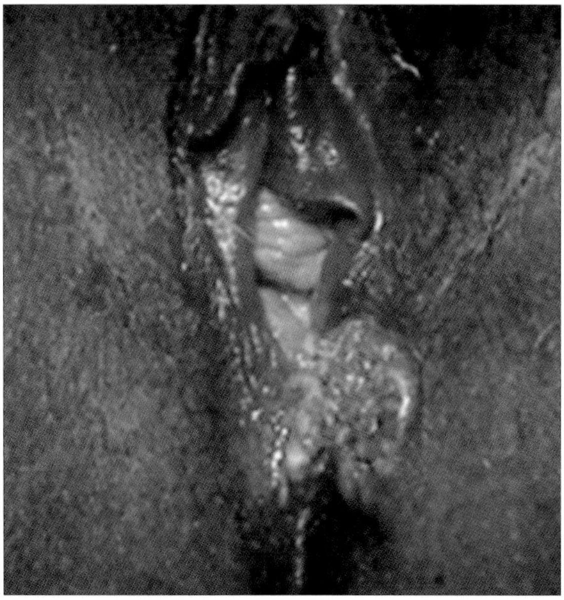

FIGURE 52.15 Cancer of the vulva

HRT AND VULVAL CANCER
HRT does not increase the risk of vulval cancer.

There is no contraindication to HRT use in women with vulval cancer.

DIETHYLSTILBOESTROL EXPOSURE
Diethylstilboestrol (DES) was prescribed in the 1950s and 1960s to women at increased risk of miscarriage. Its use ceased in 1971. Women exposed to DES in utero before 18 weeks gestation have an increased risk of:
- clear cell adenocarcinoma of the vagina. This is a rare cancer that occurs in women aged < 30 years. As it is now > 30 years since DES use was ceased, further cases are unlikely
- vaginal adenosis—an area of glandular epithelium in the vagina. Progression to adenocarcinoma is possible
- T-shaped uterine cavity
- CIN
- breast cancer
- infertility
- premature labour.

Women exposed in utero to DES require regular gynaecological review.

CARE OF WOMEN WITH GYNAECOLOGICAL CANCER
PSYCHOLOGIST
In addition to the concerns that all cancer patients share, specific gynaecological issues include:
- infertility
- premature menopause
- sexual concerns
- altered genital appearance and body image.

These issues have a continuing influence well after medical treatment is completed. Fear and insecurity may worsen after treatment, as medical visits become less regular and the woman feels less supported.

SEXUAL CONCERNS
Sexual concerns are frequent and include:
- tiredness and low libido with mismatched desire
- altered or diminished orgasm due to:
  - division of nerves during extensive surgery; minimised by 'nerve-sparing surgery'
  - removal of the clitoris, if required, for vulval cancer
- dyspareunia:
  - narrowed, tender and less flexible vagina after radiotherapy. Initial tenderness followed by scar tissue. Minimise with prophylactic oestrogen vaginal cream and either regular intercourse or vaginal dilators

- shortening of the vagina where a vaginal cuff is removed for cervical malignancy. Positions with the woman superior will allow her more control over depth of penetration
- distortion, delayed healing and pain after vulvectomy
- vaginal candida infections where steroids and antibiotics are used to avoid infection during chemotherapy
- vaginal ulcers with radiotherapy
- contraception:
  - treatment alone may not prevent conception.

FERTILITY SPECIALIST

All women of childbearing age, and girls, should be counselled regarding available fertility-preservation techniques. These will depend on which organs are involved, the stage of disease, the woman's age, availability of a partner and availability of expertise. Techniques may include:

- conservative surgery with chemotherapy for germ cell tumours, sex cord stromal tumours or early-stage epithelial ovarian tumours
- cryopreservation of embryos (requires a partner or donor sperm), oocytes (requires ovarian stimulation) and possibly ovarian tissue (currently experimental)
- ovarian transposition to move the ovaries out of the radiation field
- radical vaginal trachelectomy (removal of the cervix) with conservation of the uterus for early-stage cervical cancer
- gonadal shielding during radiotherapy
- ovarian suppression during chemotherapy or radiotherapy.[59–61]

CONTRACEPTION, PREGNANCY AND CANCER

Radiotherapy and chemotherapy do not reliably prevent conception, and can damage an unborn child, so effective contraception should be used throughout treatment in women who may become pregnant.

In women who are pregnant when the cancer is diagnosed, the decision when to start treatment should be discussed with the gynaecological oncologist.

RESOURCES

Australian Government, National Health and Medical Research Council (NHMRC), Screening to prevent cervical cancer: guidelines for the management of asymptomatic women with screen-detected abnormalities, http://www.nhmrc.gov.au/publications/synopses/wh39syn.htm

Endometriosis Association (Qld) Inc. (QENDO), support line, website and information, http://www.qendo.org.au/

Endometriosis.org website, http://www.endometriosis.org

Evans S, Bush D. Endometriosis and other pelvic pain. Adelaide, Australia: authors; 2009. For information: http://www.drsusanevans.com

Interstitial Cystitis Association, http://www.ichelp.com

Interstitial Cystitis Network, http://www.ic-network.org

REFERENCES

1 García-Closas R, Castellsagué X, Bosch X et al. The role of diet and nutrition in cervical carcinogenesis: a review of recent evidence. Int J Cancer 2005; 117(4):629–637.

2 Fang CY, Miller SM, Bovbjerg DH et al. Perceived stress is associated with impaired T-cell response to HPV16 in women with cervical dysplasia. Ann Behav Med 2008; 35(1):87–96.

3 Salamonsen LA. Tissue injury and repair in the female human reproductive tract. Reprod 2003; 125(3):301–311.

4 Hickey M, Crewe J, Mahoney LA et al. Mechanisms of irregular bleeding with hormone therapy: the role of matrix metalloproteinases and their tissue inhibitors. J Clin Endocrinol Metab 2006; 91(8):3189–3198.

5 Bakour SH, Dwarakanath LS, Khan KS et al. The diagnostic accuracy of ultrasound scan in predicting endometrial hyperplasia and cancer in postmenopausal bleeding. Acta Obstet Gynecol Scand 1999; 78(5):447–451.

6 Roemheld-Hamm B. Chasteberry. Am Fam Physician 2005; 72:821–824.

7 Blumenthal M. German Federal Institute for Drugs and Medical Devices. Commission E. The complete German Commission E monographs: therapeutic guide to herbal medicines. Austin, TX: American Botanical Council; 1998.

8 Munro MG, Mainor N, Basu R et al. Oral medroxyprogesterone acetate and combination oral contraceptives for acute uterine bleeding: a randomized controlled trial. Obstet Gynecol 2006; 108(4):924–929.

9 deVore GR, Owens O, Kase N. Use of intravenous Premarin in the treatment of dysfunctional uterine bleeding—a double-blind randomized control study. Obstet Gynecol 1982; 59(3):285–291.

10 Goldrath MH. Uterine tamponade for the control of acute uterine bleeding. Am J Obstet Gynecol 1983; 147(8):869–872.

11 Proctor ML, Murphy PA. Herbal and dietary therapies for primary and secondary dysmenorrhoea. Cochrane Database Syst Rev 2001; 3:CD002124.

12 Zhu X, Proctor M, Bensoussan A et al. Chinese herbal medicine for primary dysmenorrhoea. Cochrane Database Syst Rev 2007; 4:CD005288.

13 Treloar SA, O'Connor DT, O'Connor VM et al. Genetic influences on endometriosis in an Australian twin sample. Fertil Steril 1999; 71:701–710.

14 Heilier JF, Donnez J, Lison D. Organochlorines and endometriosis: a mini-review. Chemosphere 2008; 1(2):203–210.

15 Missmer SA, Hankinson SE, Spiegelman D et al. Reproductive history and endometriosis among premenopausal women. Obstet Gynecol 2004; 104(5 Pt 1):965–974.

16 Tokushige N, Markham R, Russell P et al. Different types of small nerve fibers in eutopic endometrium and myometrium in women with endometriosis. Fertil Steril 2007; 88(4):795–803.

17 Redwine DB. Ovarian endometriosis: a marker for more extensive pelvic and intestinal disease. Fertil Steril 1999; 72(2):310–315.

18 Missmer SA, Chavarro JE, Malspeis S. A prospective study of dietary fat consumption and endometriosis risk. Hum Reprod 2010; 23 Mar [Epub ahead of print].

19 Wieser F, Cohen M, Gaeddert A. Evolution of medical treatment for endometriosis: back to the roots? Hum Reprod Update 2007; 13(5):487–499.

20 Mier-Cabrera J, Aburto-Soto T, Burrola-Méndez S. Women with endometriosis improved their peripheral antioxidant markers after the application of a high antioxidant diet. Reprod Biol Endocrinol 2009; 7:54.

21 Flower A, Liu JP, Chen S et al. Chinese herbal medicine for endometriosis. Cochrane Database Syst Rev 2009; 3:CD006568.

22 Evans S, Bush D. Endometriosis and pelvic pain. Adelaide, Australia: authors; 2009.

23 Cobellis L, Razzi S, Fava A et al. A danazol-loaded intrauterine device decreases dysmenorrhea, pelvic pain, and dyspareunia associated with endometriosis. Fertil Steril 2004; 82(1):239–240.

24 Gillett W, Jones D. Chronic pelvic pain in women: role of the nervous system. Expert Rev Obstet Gynecol 2009; 4(2):149–163.

25 Paulson JD, Delgado M. The relationship between interstitial cystitis and endometriosis in patients with chronic pelvic pain. J S Lab Surg 2007; 11(2): 175–181.

26 Forrest JB, Mishell DR Jr. Breaking the cycle of pain in interstitial cystitis/painful bladder syndrome: toward standardization of early diagnosis and treatment: consensus panel recommendations. J Reprod Med 2009; 54(1):3–14.

27 White AR. A review of controlled trials of acupuncture for women's reproductive health care. J Fam Plann Reproduct Health Care 2003; 29:233–236.

28 Levitt M. The other women's movement. Osborne Park, Western Australia: Michael Levitt Balance Publications; 2008.

29 Nyholt DR, Gillespie NG, Merikangas KR et al. Common genetic influences underlie comorbidity of migraine and endometriosis. Genet Epidemiol 2008; 33(2):105–113.

30 MacGregor A. Menstrual migraine. Fact sheet. City of London Migraine Clinic. Online. Available: http://ww2.migraineclinic.org.uk/wp-content/uploads/2009/07/menstrual-migraine.pdf

31 Taubert K. Magnesium in migraine. Results of a multicentre pilot study. Fortschr Med 1994; 112(24):328–330.

32 PeikertA, Wilimzig C, Kohne-Volland R et al. Prophylaxis of migraine with oral magnesium: results from a prospective multi-center, placebo-controlled and double-blind randomized study. Cephalalgia 1996; 16(4):257–263.

33 Schellenberg R. Treatment for the premenstrual syndrome with agnus castus fruit extract: prospective, randomised, placebo controlled study. BMJ 2001; 322(7279):134–137.

34 Ernst E, Pittler MH. The efficacy and safety of feverfew (*Tanacetum parthenium*): an update of a systematic review. Public Health Nutr 2000; 3(4A):509–514.

35 Day Baird D, Dunson DB, Hill MC et al. High cumulative incidence of uterine leiomyomas in black and white women: ultrasound evidence. Am J Obstet Gynecol 2003; 188(1):100–107.

36 Schwartz SM, Marshall LM, Baird DD. Epidemiologic contributions to understanding the etiology of uterine leiomyomata. Review. Environ Health Perspect 2000; 108(Suppl 5):821–827.

37 Baird DD, Dunson DB. Why is parity protective for uterine fibroids? Epidem 2003; 14(2):247–250.

38 Walker CL, Stewart EA. Uterine fibroids: the elephant in the room. Review. Science. 2005; 308(5728):1589–1592.

39 Parker WH. Etiology, symptomatology, and diagnosis of uterine myomas. Review. Fertil Steril 2007; 87(4):725–736.

40 Dueholm M, Lundorf E, Hansen ES et al. Magnetic resonance imaging and transvaginal ultrasonography for the diagnosis of adenomyosis. Fertil Steril 2001; 76(3):588–594.

41 Sizzi O, Rossetti A, Malzoni M. Italian multicenter study on complications of laparoscopic myomectomy. J Minim Invasive Gynecol 2007;14(4):453–462.

42 Pritts EA. Fibroids and infertility: a systematic review of the evidence. Review. Obstet Gynecol Surv 2001; 56(8):483–491.

43 Qidwai GI, Caughey AB, Jacoby AF. Obstetric outcomes in women with sonographically identified uterine leiomyomata. Obstet Gynecol 2006; 107(2 Pt 1):376–382.

44 Goto A, Takeuchi S, Sugimura K. Usefulness of Gd-DTPA contrast-enhanced dynamic MRI and

serum determination of LDH and its isozymes in the differential diagnosis of leiomyosarcoma from degenerated leiomyoma of the uterus. Int J Gynecol Cancer 2002; 12(4):354–361.
45 Yazbek J, Aslam N, Tailor A et al. A comparative study of the risk of malignancy index and the ovarian crescent sign for the diagnosis of invasive ovarian cancer. Ultrasound Obstet Gynecol 2006; 28(3):320–324.
46 Jacobs I, Bast RC Jr. The CA 125 tumour-associated antigen: a review of the literature. Hum Reprod 1989; 4(1):1–12.
47 Tingulstad S, Hagen B, Skjeldestad FE et al. Evaluation of a risk of malignancy index based on serum CA 125, ultrasound findings and menopausal status in the pre-operative diagnosis of pelvic masses. Br J Obstet Gynaecol 1996; 103(8):826–831.
48 Grimes DA, Jones LB, Lopez LM et al. Oral contraceptives for functional ovarian cysts. Cochrane Database Syst Rev 2006; 4:CD006134.
49 Australian Institute of Health and Welfare. Cancer in Australia: an overview. AIHW; 2006.
50 South Australian Familial Cancer Unit Publication. Adelaide, Australia: Royal Adelaide Hospital; 2006.
51 Bakour SH, Dwarakanath LS, Khan KS et al. The diagnostic accuracy of ultrasound scan in predicting endometrial hyperplasia and cancer in postmenopausal bleeding. Acta Obstet Gynecol Scand 1999; 78(5): 447–451.
52 Creasman WT. Hormone replacement therapy after cancers. Curr Opin Oncol 2005; 17(5):493–499.
53 Melin A, Sparén P, Bergqvist A. The risk of cancer and the role of parity among women with endometriosis. Hum Reprod 2007; 22(11):3021–3026.
54 Brinton LA, Lamb EJ, Moghissi KS et al. Ovarian cancer risk after the use of ovulation-stimulating drugs. Obstet Gynecol 2004; 103(6):1194–1203.
55 Riman T, Nilsson S, Persson IR. Review of epidemiological evidence for reproductive and hormonal factors in relation to the risk of epithelial ovarian malignancies. Acta Obstet Gynecol Scand 2004; 83(9):783–795.
56 van Nagell JR Jr, dePriest PD, Ueland FR et al. Ovarian cancer screening with annual transvaginal sonography: findings of 25,000 women screened. Cancer 2007; 109(9):1887–1896.
57 Beral V, Million Women Study Collaborators, Bull D, Green J, Reeves G. Ovarian cancer and hormone replacement therapy in the Million Women Study. Lancet 2007; 369(9574):1703–1710.
58 Neves E, Castro M. An analysis of ovarian cancer in the Million Women Study. Gynecol Endocrinol 2007; 23(7):410–413.
59 Donnez J, Martinez-Madrid B, Jadoul P et al. Ovarian tissue cryopreservation and transplantation: a review. Hum Reprod Update 2006; 12(5):519–535.
60 Seli E, Tangir J. Fertility preservation options for female patients with malignancies. Curr Opin Obstet Gynecol 2005; 17(3):299–308.
61 Oktay K, Sönmezer M. Fertility preservation in gynecologic cancers. Curr Opin Oncol 2007; 19(5):506–511.

chapter 53

Menopause

INTRODUCTION AND OVERVIEW

The menopause transition can be a time of great change and disturbance for some women. Symptoms such as hot flushes, night sweats, mood swings and vaginal dryness can greatly affect quality of life and, in most Western countries, around a quarter to a third of such affected women will seek medical attention. More controversially, the postmenopausal phase of life may be associated with adverse long-term sequelae such as increased bone loss, and perhaps an increased risk of cardiovascular disease and even dementia.

One of the basic sex differences is that women obtain all their eggs in fetal life and then start to lose them, in contrast to males, who do not produce sperm until puberty and then continue to make them, even into advanced old age. Oocyte number peaks at around 6–7 million at 20 weeks of gestational age, and even by birth a baby girl has lost about half her eggs. The production of sex hormones is linked to the presence of oocytes and so menopause, or 'last period', signifies the permanent cessation of menstrual periods and the loss of the final egg.

DEFINING THE MENOPAUSE TRANSITION

Over the past two decades there has been much discussion about defining the terminology surrounding the last period. Sherry Sherman has aptly summarised some of the terminology, drawing together the WHO and International Menopause Society (IMS) recommendations (Box 53.1).[1]

BOX 53. 1 Menopause terminology

1. *Natural menopause* is defined as the permanent cessation of menstruation resulting from the loss of ovarian follicular activity. The final menstrual period (FMP) is recognised to have occurred after 12 consecutive months of amenorrhoea, for which there is no other obvious pathological or physiological cause.
2. *Perimenopause* should include the period immediately before the menopause (when the endocrinological, biological and clinical features of approaching menopause commence) and the first year after menopause. The term 'climacteric' should be abandoned, to avoid confusion.
3. *Menopausal transition* should be reserved for that period before the FMP when variability in the menstrual cycle is usually increased.
4. *Premenopause* is often used ambiguously either to refer to the 1 or 2 years immediately before the menopause or to refer to the whole of the reproductive period before the menopause.
5. *Induced menopause* is defined as the cessation of menstruation that follows either surgical removal of both ovaries (with or without hysterectomy) or iatrogenic ablation of ovarian function (e.g. by chemotherapy or radiation).
6. *Postmenopause* is defined as the period dating from the FMP, regardless of whether the menopause was induced or spontaneous.
7. *Premature menopause* ideally should be defined as menopause that occurs at an age two standard deviations below the mean estimated for the reference population. In practice, the age of 40 years is frequently used as an arbitrary cut-off point, below which menopause is said to be premature.

Source: adapted from Sherman 2005[1]

EPIDEMIOLOGY

In Western countries, the average age at FMP is 51 years, with a normal range of 40–60 years.[2] The four or five years leading up to the FMP are characterised by menstrual irregularity, often initially cycle shortening, followed by cycle lengthening, although there is much normal variability. There are some minor variations

BOX 53.2 Symptoms that might be due to the menopause transition

Hot flushes
Night sweats
Insomnia
Mood swings
Aches and pains
Formication (a sensation of 'ants' crawling on the skin)
Vaginal dryness
Light-headedness
Headache

in cycle patterns across different cultures but, as will be discussed later, quite marked differences in the symptoms are experienced across the menopause transition.

SYMPTOMS

Some of the symptoms experienced by women in the menopause transition are listed in Box 53.2.

The Melbourne Women's Midlife Health Project is a prospective, longitudinal study of healthy women passing through the menopause transition.[3] The study began in 1991 and used random telephone dialling to recruit Australian-born women aged 45 to 55 years. One hundred and seventy-two women were premenopausal at the time at baseline, and by the end of the seventh year of annual follow-up had advanced to the peri- or postmenopausal interval.

By the postmenopausal period, almost all had recorded at least one symptom—the most common being hot flushes. As women transited from the premenopausal to the postmenopausal phase, they noted significantly less breast pain, but significantly more hot flushes, night sweats and vaginal dryness.

CULTURAL DIFFERENCES

There appear to be marked cultural differences in attitudes to menopause. In a study of Sydney women, Asian women generally appeared to view menopause in a more favourable light than Western women, who linked menopause with 'getting older'. Asian women were also less likely to admit to a healthcare professional that they were suffering from vaginal dryness, but if a doctor raised the issue, they were very grateful.[4,5]

Among Indian women, only 34% complained of hot flushes; more were concerned about depression and memory loss.[6] Unemployment was associated with more flushing and depression. Lebanese Muslim women reported high rates of feeling tired and worn out, as well as aches and pains, as they went through the menopause transition.[7] Sixty-three per cent reported hot flushes and more than half had noticed vaginal dryness during intercourse.

Chinese women largely see menopause as a natural process.[8] A group of Sydney-based Chinese women had more vasomotor symptoms (34%) than those women who live in mainland China (10.5%) or in Hong Kong (10–20%). The top three symptoms reported by Sydney-based Chinese women were poor memory (76.4%), dry skin (69.1%) and aching in muscles and joints (68.3%). Some told the interviewers that their vaginal dryness problem was so severe that they had given their husbands permission to have sex with someone else.

Among Greek women, most were more concerned about back pain, aches, pains and fatigue than about hot flushes.[9] Seventy-nine per cent of the postmenopausal Greek women had vaginal dryness, and there was a high rate of sexual problems.

THE MENOPAUSE CONSULTATION

HISTORY

The initial menopause consultation is a long session and often takes at least 30 minutes. It might be facilitated by some pre-reading and by using one of the many menopause-scoring charts that are available, such as the MENQOL (Menopause-specific Quality of Life Questionnaire, Table 53.1).[10]

The following should be particularly considered while taking a 'menopause' history:

- *The menstrual cycle.* During the last 5 years of menstrual life, the cycle often shortens from 28 to even 21 days. Skipping months usually occurs during the last few years of menstruation. Variability is the norm. Some periods might be heavy with clotting, and others light. Bleeding lasting longer than seven days or continual bleeding needs to be investigated. Usually this means a transvaginal ultrasound scan and a referral for hysteroscopy and endometrial biopsy. Endometrial hyperplasia and cancer are increasingly common after the age of 40 years.
- *Menopause symptoms* (see Table 53.1)
- *Contraception.* Is the patient worried that she might 'accidentally' become pregnant? Has she used the oral contraceptive pill (OCP) in the past? If so, did she have any side effects? For example, if she became depressed on the Pill, this is a progestin side effect. Women who had 'PMT-type' side effects with levonorgestrel-containing OCP are usually also intolerant of other progestins such as norethisterone, cyproterone and medroxyprogesterone acetate (MPA), but may tolerate dydrogesterone.
- *Sleep patterns.* Sleep lightens with ageing, but at this time of life, sweats and flushes at night will often disturb sleep.

TABLE 53.1 Oestrogen deficiency symptom score, using MENQOL[11]

The following symptoms are rated as follows:
Not bothered at all 0 1 2 3 4 5 6 Extremely bothered

	0	1	2	3	4	5	6
1 Hot flushes or flashes							
2 Night sweats							
3 Sweating							
4 Being dissatisfied with my personal life							
5 Feeling anxious or nervous							
6 Experiencing poor memory							
7 Accomplishing less than I used to							
8 Feeling depressed, down or blue							
9 Being impatient with other people							
10 Feelings of wanting to be alone							
11 Flatulence (wind) or gas pains							
12 Aching in muscles and joints							
13 Feeling tired or worn out							
14 Difficulty sleeping							
15 Aches in the back of neck or head							
16 Decrease in physical strength							
17 Decrease in stamina							
18 Feeling a lack of energy							
19 Drying skin							
20 Weight gain							
21 Increased facial hair							
22 Changes in appearance, texture or tone of my skin							
23 Feeling bloated							

- *Bladder and vaginal symptoms.* Incontinence is common and, after menopause, vaginal dryness increases in prevalence; and apart from making vaginal intercourse uncomfortable and even painful, urinary tract infections increase in frequency.
- *Mood.* Severe depression and anxiety are not more common during the menopause transition, but those women with a pre-existing history of mood disorder commonly find that it worsens.
- *Skin sensations.* About one-third of perimenopausal women notice a peculiar skin sensation (no rash) called 'formication' or 'ants under the skin'. Some describe it as like insects moving over the skin. It can be very unpleasant. The cause is not completely understood, but it does seem to be due to an effect of swinging hormone levels on nerve endings and usually passes after some months.

EXAMINATION

A woman may present to her doctor with a concern about menopause because of symptoms that she feels may be hormonally based. It is essential to have the diagnostic radar well-tuned for other possible explanations for symptoms. It is worth taking the opportunity to do a general physical examination and identify any possible risk factors for middle age and beyond. At the very least, it is prudent to check the woman's blood pressure and weight, ensure that her Pap smears are up to date, and examine the breasts for abnormal lumps.

TESTS

A woman aged in her forties with amenorrhoea or slight periods should be tested for pregnancy. If a woman has 'hot flushes' and her blood pressure is elevated, a 24-hour ambulatory blood pressure monitor will reveal whether the flushes are symptomatic of hypertension.

All that flushes is not menopause. Consider the differential diagnosis of 'night sweats' (see below) including viral infection, tuberculosis, neoplasm, hyperthyroidism, sleep apnoea, gastro-oesophageal reflux disease, alcohol excess and hypoglycaemia.[12]

There is no place for the routine measurement of hormone levels (e.g. FSH and oestradiol (E2)). During the normal menstrual cycle, E2 levels fluctuate from very low (below 100 pmol/L) to 500–1000 pmol/L at ovulation. FSH levels more than 20 U/L suggest that the patient is perimenopausal. The problem is that perimenopausal women can have even more variation than usual. It is not unusual for E2 levels to be greater than 2000 pmol/L and FSH levels can vary from less than 10 U/L to more than 40 U/L. The typical patient who is over 40 years of age with irregular periods and typical symptoms does not need her FSH and E2 measured.

If early menopause is suspected in a woman under 30 years of age, it might be prudent to measure her FSH levels three times over 2–3 months. In this way, the diagnosis is usually readily confirmed. Antimüllerian hormone (AMH) is a relatively new blood test that may give some information on ovarian reserve.

Use this opportunity to check the results of her last Pap smear, mammogram, bone density, lipids and blood glucose measurement, and ensure that a regular testing protocol is established for the perimenopause and postmenopausal phase.

MANAGING MENOPAUSE

There are a number of important issues for a woman and her doctor to be mindful of in managing the menopause but there are also a wide range of options available to a woman in managing those issues. The management objectives include ameliorating symptoms associated with menopause as well as making efforts to minimise the risk of other illnesses that become more common after menopause, such as heart disease, cancer and osteoporosis. The management approaches outlined below focus on lifestyle issues and specific medical and complementary therapies.

LIFESTYLE ISSUES: THE ESSENCE MODEL

Education

Being educated about the changes associated with menopause will be very useful in helping a woman to appreciate that many of the symptoms she might be experiencing are natural and that she is not alone. It will help to allay many concerns, may motivate her to consider the need for other lifestyle changes, and also help to improve her understanding of and compliance with any management strategies undertaken.

Stress management

Mental and emotional support is vital at such an important life transition as menopause. Such times are associated with an increased risk of mental and emotional problems. Emotional state will not only affect coping but can affect hormonal balance and exacerbate the effect of symptoms enormously. Poor mental health can also accelerate the progression of chronic illnesses including heart disease, metabolic syndrome, dementia and osteoporosis, due to the effects of allostatic load and its sequelae, such as elevated cortisol levels.

Spirituality

What meaning a woman makes of a life-changing event like menopause can affect how easy or difficult that transition is. It can be seen in a very positive light, as it has been for millennia in many traditional cultures, or it can be seen in a very negative light, particularly in our youth-obsessed contemporary society. Questions of spirituality or meaning can arise when one's life role is being redefined, along with changes in relationships and life priorities. Also, for some, it is a time when ageing and mortality come into view.

Exercise

Regular exercise is particularly important during and after menopause, not only to help manage symptoms but also to help prevent a range of chronic conditions such as heart disease, cancer, dementia and osteoporosis. Regular moderate activity will help weight management and can help to improve sleep and maintain mental and physical vitality and performance in menopausal women.[13,14] Vigorous aerobic exercise can precipitate hot flushes, in some women.

Nutrition

Apart from maintaining a healthy diet generally, a range of foods can be helpful for menopause. To reduce the incidence of hot flushes, advise women to try to avoid caffeine, spicy foods and smoking. Encourage soy foods such as tofu, miso and tempeh. Ensure adequate calcium and vitamin D either naturally or through supplementation. Advise on achieving a healthy weight range with a balanced, high-fibre, low-fat diet as well as calorie restriction (i.e. avoiding excess empty calories while maintaining a varied and nutritious diet).

Connectedness

As with any time of life, relationships matter enormously during menopause. Not feeling isolated and having the support of partner, friends, family, work colleagues and health practitioners can all make an enormous difference. Menopause corresponds with a time when many women find themselves with an 'empty nest', which can be a time of rejoicing for some, but grief for others. Staying connected to and engaging with one's community as well as personal relationships can also help to provide new meaning and purpose at this important time.

Environment

Much has been said about environment in previous chapters. Particular things to note are the need for regular moderate doses of sunlight for mood and vitamin D, as well as helping to facilitate exercise. An unhealthy environment, physically or emotionally, can affect health in a variety of ways.

MANAGING HOT FLUSHES

In Western culture, the most common menopause symptom is the hot flush (referred to as 'hot flash' in American literature). This typically begins as a feeling of intense heat in the chest and neck which soon rushes up over the head and then over the rest of the body. It lasts a few minutes and might be associated with feelings of nausea, palpitations, dizziness and formication. The sufferer usually goes bright red and ends up with a drenching sweat, often followed by chills and shivering. The menopausal hot flush can be extremely unpleasant. The frequency varies considerably, from 1–2 a day to 10–20 an hour, day and night. During the flush, central temperature does not rise, but skin temperature goes up by 5–7°C.

Most women will have mild flushes for a couple of years, and then the temperature centre adapts and the flushes settle. In a significant minority (10–20%), flushes continue forever.

DIFFERENTIAL DIAGNOSIS

Not all flushing is due to menopause, and so it is important to ask the patient to describe her hot sensation. The differential diagnosis includes:

- *fever*—if the patient takes her central (mouth) temperature during a flush, it will be less than 37°C. If her temperature is more than 37.5°C, she has a fever and that will need to be investigated
- *hyperhydrosis*—these patients sweat all the time. It often especially affects the upper body and can be confused with hot flushes
- *hypertension*
- *anxiety*
- *acne rosacea*—causes facial flushing and can coexist with menopausal flushing
- *hyperthyroidism*—causes an increase in sweating, not flushes as such
- *phaeochromocytoma*—most of these secrete noradrenaline and so the sufferer will go pale and white because of vasoconstriction. During an attack they will be hypertensive and feel dreadful ('like they are going to die')
- *carcinoid tumours*—these secrete serotonin and the usual primary site is the bowel. During an attack, the patient may turn red, but they often have diarrhoea too and the attack usually lasts longer than a few minutes. If the patient had a colonic carcinoid tumour and has serotonin-symptoms, this usually indicates the presence of liver metastases
- *some drugs*—high doses of SSRIs, SNRIs and vasodilators can cause sweating and flushing
- *very rare causes*—mast-cell tumours secrete histamine (producing urticaria) and some rare parathyroid tumours secreting calcitonin can also elicit flushes.

The menopause flush is caused by disruption of the thermoregulatory system in the anterior hypohalamus.[15] Basically, there are two 'thermostats': if core temperature goes above the high one, flushes occur; and if core temperature goes below the lower thermostat, shivering happens. For those with severe vasomotor symptoms, the two thermostats are close together, and thus sweating and shivering are more easily triggered in these women. Neurotransmitters such as serotonin and noradrenaline are involved, which, as we shall see shortly, has implications for therapy.

LIFESTYLE MODIFICATIONS

Avoidance of triggers can be helpful for some. Such triggers include stress, hot drinks, spicy foods, alcohol, over-heating and hot weather. There is some evidence that a diet high in soy and cereal can help those with mild flushes.[16] Vigorous exercise can make flushes worse by overheating the body.

HERBAL

Most of the over-the-counter herbal therapies either have been shown not to be more effective than placebo or have not been formally tested.[17] Sage (*Salvia officinalis*), dong quai (*Angelica sinensis*), red clover (*Trifolium pratense*), Asian ginseng (*Panax ginseng*) and kudzu (*Pueraria lobata*) are commonly recommended, but evidence for their effectiveness is lacking.

Nelson and colleagues performed a meta-analysis of non-hormonal therapies for menopausal hot flushes.[18] They found that red clover extracts were no more effective than placebo but that there was some evidence that some soy extracts are effective (e.g. Phyto Soya®).

By far the most effective and tested herbal is a standardised extract of black cohosh. It has been submitted to several randomised controlled trials (RCTs). Osmers and colleagues performed a RCT of 304 women randomised to two tablets a day versus placebo.[19] The active treatment was statistically significant for a global menopause score and specifically for vasomotor, mood and vaginal symptoms, despite the fact that the extract is not oestrogenic.

Uebelhack and colleagues performed a RCT of black cohosh and St John's wort extract among 301 women.[20] Again the active compound was found to be superior to placebo for vasomotor and mood symptoms. St John's wort can be combined with black cohosh. Palacio and colleagues reviewed trials of black cohosh.[21] Most placebo-controlled trials showed that black cohosh was superior to placebo and equivalent to low-dose HRT and even tibolone. One trial even compared black cohosh with fluoxetine 40 mg and found that black cohosh was better for flushes and fluoxetine superior for moods.

Trials with black cohosh extracts have largely found no greater risk of side effects than placebo. However, there have been case reports of hepatic failure, probably autoimmune and idiosyncratic, associated with black cohosh. The incidence appears to be less than 1 in 100,000 cases.

Vitex agnus castus (chasteberry) 20 mg daily may help perimenopausal symptoms such as irregular menses and mastalgia.

OTHER COMPLEMENTARY AND ALTERNATIVE THERAPIES

Nedrow and colleagues have systematically reviewed complementary and alternative medicines (CAMs) used for menopausal symptoms.[22] It can be challenging to design placebo for physical CAMs such as reflexology and acupuncture, but some researchers have managed to do so. One trial compared reflexology and 'routine' foot massage; and four trials used sham acupuncture needles. None of these treatments was found to be superior to sham treatment for the relief of menopausal symptoms. Nedrow and colleagues also reviewed six RCTs of Chinese herbal mixtures—all the RCTs were negative.

Slow, deep breathing—'paced respiration'—can reduce the severity of a hot flush.[15]

NON-HORMONAL DRUGS FOR FLUSHES

An increasing number of 'brain drugs' are being used to treat menopausal symptoms. Intuitively this makes sense, because the vasomotor and mood symptoms are brain in origin. Currently, the most popular non-hormonal drugs (or, more correctly, 'non-sex-hormonal', as these drugs act primarily on brain 'hormones') for managing menopausal brain symptoms are listed below.

- *SSRIs and SNRIs*—Nelson and colleagues' review examined seven RCTs and clearly showed evidence of efficacy.[18] Typically the lowest tablet size was the most effective for treating hot flushes. High doses of these agents can actually cause hot flushes and sweats as a side effect. This is not unusual for hormonal agents. Many hormones in low pulsatile doses stimulate the target receptor, in contrast to high continuous doses, which often down-regulate the receptor. Typical doses used to treat flushes and mood swings of menopause include venlafaxine 75XR and citalopram 20 mg daily. The side effects of these agents are discussed elsewhere in this book.
- *clonidine*—most of the clonidine RCTs used doses of 0.05–0.15 mg daily.[18] These doses were more effective than placebo. Side effects include hypotension, dry mouth, sedation and, in high doses, depression. Clonidine might be useful to manage both hypertension and flushes. It can also be used as a prophylactic migraine drug. It is not unusual for migraine frequency to increase at around the time of perimenopause, and to then settle after the last period.
- *gabapentin*—Toulis and colleagues[5] published a meta-analysis of studies trialling gabapentin (dose range 900–2400 mg) for treating hot flushes. This systematic review included seven trials. Gabapentin was found to be superior to placebo for reducing hot flushes. The main side effects can be headache, drowsiness, dizziness, nausea, disturbed sleep, fluid retention and weight gain. When the patient is coming off gabapentin, the dose should be reduced by 300 mg at a time every 3 days.

It is certainly helpful to have these agents available to the clinician and the patient. For example, consider a woman who has just completed chemotherapy for breast cancer and is now rendered menopausal. Her oncologist starts her on tamoxifen or an aromatase inhibitor and, not surprisingly, her flushes increase dramatically. Black cohosh, perhaps even combined with an SNRI, will help around 70–80%. These women are often grateful for a reduction in symptom severity, rather than complete resolution of their symptoms. It can be clinically useful to temporarily cease the endocrine therapy for 2–4 weeks to examine the impact of the drug on flushing severity.

A migrainous, hypertensive perimenopausal woman might choose to try clonidine. A patient suffering from trigeminal neuralgia and significant flushing might wish to try gabapentin, for both problems.

HORMONE THERAPY

Hormone therapy (HT), also known as hormone replacement therapy (HRT), remains controversial and should be reserved for women who are unable to tolerate symptoms of menopause and have not responded to other measures. The woman should be informed of the potential risks and side effects. If the decision is made to proceed with HT, the lowest effective dose should be prescribed, and reviewed regularly.

For the interested reader, Blake[2] and Grady[15] have recently reviewed the evidence base for managing menopause. HT has been around for a very long time—oestradiol implants since the mid-1930s and Premarin® (conjugated oestrogens) since 1942.

In Grady's review, she demonstrates that 0.625 mg Premarin® and 1–2 mg E2 orally reduce hot flushes by around 90–95%, with a placebo effect of 45%.[15] Relief is usually substantial within 4 weeks. Lower doses (e.g. 1 mg E2 daily) take longer to work but have a lower rate of side effects. Progestins are added to prevent endometrial hyperplasia. These are given either cyclically for 10–14 days or continuously, on a daily basis.

Using hormone therapy

The healthy perimenopausal woman seeking HT usually begins with a cyclical HT. Continuous HT does not suppress the cycle, and so breakthrough bleeding is

TABLE 53.2 Risks and benefits of combined hormone therapy in older women*

Adverse effects	Benefits
8 extra breast cancers 7 extra episodes of cardiovascular disease** 8 extra cases of pulmonary embolism 8 extra strokes	6 fewer bowel cancers 2 fewer uterine cancers 10 fewer hip & spine fractures

*Risk and benefits after 5 years of combined HT (compared with placebo). All rates are per 10,000 women per year.
**Not statistically significant.

common and can be troublesome. A short course of a low-dose OCP might be considered for a healthy, non-smoking, non-migrainous, normotensive woman under 50 years of age.

No matter what the regimen is, initial breast soreness and irregular vaginal bleeding are common, and usually settle with time. Around 10–15% will have progestin side effects—bloatedness, mood swings, even depression. Dydrogesterone is the best-tolerated oral progestin and, for some, the Mirena® intrauterine device might suit. If heavy menstrual periods need treatment, a Mirena® intrauterine device could be used to both control the menstrual problem and give endometrial protection, while giving a tablet or patch of oestrogen to control flushes and sweats.

Postmenopausal women are usually offered continuous HT to help minimise bleeding. Even with low-dose regimens, around one-third to half will have spotting and bleeding, at least for a month or two.

There are surprisingly few trials on stopping HT. Most clinicians would treat initially for 2 years and then wean the woman slowly off the HT over 3–6 months, although there is no evidence to support this practice. If flushes return, some will go back on HT—often on a lower dose than initially. A significant minority have great trouble coming off HT, and these are probably the same women who 'flush forever'.

Risks and benefits of long-term hormone therapy

In the 1990s there was a hope that HT might be a useful long-term preventive agent for women over 50 years of age—reducing heart and fracture risks. However, since 2002, the Women's Health Initiative (WHI) study has had high media profile, and has caused enormous fear in the community because of a link between HT and breast cancer.

The WHI was an NIH-funded study into strategies to help older women. It had two HT arms, both tested in women whose average age was late sixties. The combined HT arm (Premarin®–Provera®) has been summarised by MacLennan (Table 53.2 and Figure 53.1).[23]

When the WHI data were re-analysed in 2007, to examine risks in the usual age group who take HT—those aged under 60 years—no increased risks were found.[23] It was disappointing that the authors took 5 years to release these data, and unfortunately this important message has not reached the general community. MacLennan also points out that there are emerging data that side effects are reduced by using lower HT doses, minimising systemic progestin exposure by using a Mirena® device, using non-oral HT in some women and initiating HT near menopause.

Several studies have examined the population rates of breast cancer since the decline in HRT use following the release of the WHI data. Breast cancer incidence decline and decreased HRT use showed a high correlation. The decline of breast cancer incidence started about 2 years after the HRT decline.[24]

The woman who has had a hysterectomy

The woman who has had a hysterectomy and who makes an informed decision to take HT should be treated with oestrogen only. The oestrogen-only arm of the WHI (Premarin® 0.625 mg daily versus placebo) enrolled 10,739 women aged 50–79 years and continued the trial for 7 years. The risk of breast cancer was decreased in the Premarin® arm and a non-significant increased risk of stroke was demonstrated.[25,26] There is some evidence of decreased risk of thrombosis with transdermal oestrogen.[2,15]

Tibolone

Tibolone is not a traditional HT, but a steroid with oestrogenic, progestational and androgenic actions. Its effect on a target tissue depends on its final metabolism. For example, the endometrium converts tibolone to a progestational metabolite. When given to postmenopausal women, it has a lower rate of breakthrough bleeding and breast pain than standard HT and appears to have no impact on mammographic density, unlike HT, which usually increases breast density.[2,15,23] However, weight gain is a common side effect and this tends to limit its appeal.

A randomised placebo-controlled trial of tibolone 1.25 mg (4538 women aged 60–85 years) was published in 2008.[27] Women receiving the active treatment had significantly fewer vertebral and non-vertebral fractures

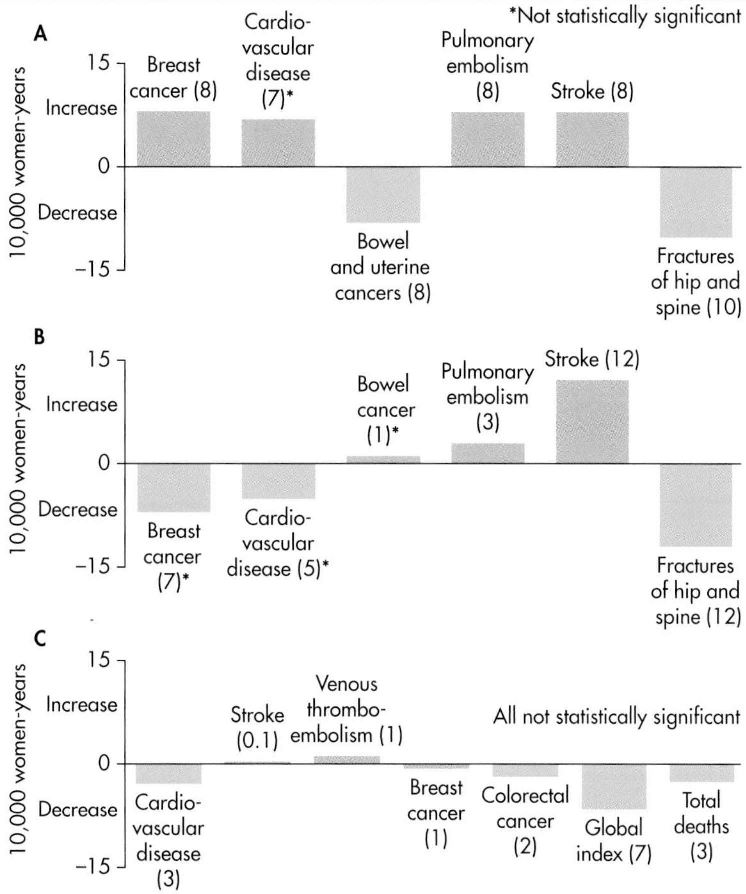

FIGURE 53.1 Risks and benefits of long-term HRT: **A** After 5 years of combined HRT; **B** after 7 years of oestrogen-only HRT; **C** oestrogen-only HRT initiated at age 50–59 years. Complete data for women under age 60 years in the WHI have only been published for the oestrogen-only arm. The WHI was not powered for such subanalyses, as major morbidities are uncommon in this age group. Global index: a global index of risks and benefits. (from MacLennan 2007[23])

and less breast and bowel cancer than the placebo group. However, the tibolone group had a doubled risk of stroke.

The LIBERATE trial[28] randomised 3148 women with breast cancer to tibolone 2.5 mg or placebo. Fifty-eight per cent were node positive, 71% were oestrogen receptor (ER) positive, 67% used tamoxifen and 7% used aromatase inhibitors. Tibolone improved vasomotor symptoms and bone density in this cohort but, unfortunately, it was also associated with an increased risk of metastases. Therefore, tibolone cannot be recommended for women who have had breast cancer.

MANAGING THE WOMAN WHO FLUSHES FOREVER

If a patient is still having significant flushes after 5–6 years, she is probably in the small group who flush forever.[2] Properly counselled, some of these women will persist with non-pharmacological methods of coping with the symptoms and some will choose to stay on low-dose HT—at least until a better choice is available—and accept the small risks. Theoretically, it may be appropriate to treat these women with transdermal oestrogen (e.g. a dot-patch) to minimise the risk of thrombosis, and consideration should be given to fitting her with a Mirena® device to minimise systemic progestin exposure. However, it should be pointed out that, at the moment, there is no evidence to support such an approach—and there will probably never be such data available.

DEPRESSION AND MENOPAUSE

Feeling sad or blue is a common symptom of menopause, affecting 19–29%, but studies have shown that clinical depression per se is not more common at menopause,[2] except perhaps for those who have longstanding depression/anxiety. CBT and St John's wort may assist with mood stabilising. HT might help stabilise the mood of some symptomatic perimenopausal women, but not those who are postmenopausal and flush-free.[2]

MANAGING GENITOURINARY SYMPTOMS

After menopause, most women will have unpleasant genitourinary symptoms. These include bladder irritability, vaginal dryness, pain during intercourse and recurrent urinary tract infections. Physiologically, after menopause the vaginal epithelium thins dramatically, *Lactobacillus* disappears, vaginal pH rises from around 4.0 to neutral and the vagina becomes colonised by enteric bacteria.

These symptoms can be managed by the use of non-hormonal moisturisers such as Replens®, avoiding soap (and instead washing with soap-free washes or sorbolene) and the use of lubricants. However, for some the symptoms are so severe that the only real option is oestrogen therapy. Rather than giving HT, topical oestrogens can be tried.[15] There is scant long-term safety data on these products, but there is probably some minimal absorption in the first few weeks of usage while the vaginal epithelium is thin, but little absorption after that.

Vaginal insertion of a *Lactobacillus* capsule once or twice a week replenishes the vaginal *Lactobacillus* population and reduces the incidence of vaginal candidiasis.

Continence training with an experienced continence therapist can assist bladder control.

Unfortunately, no CAM has been shown to help genitourinary symptoms.

THE ROLE OF ANDROGENS FOR WOMEN

Testosterone is more abundant in female serum than oestrogen, and serum testosterone levels appear to fall with age, not menopause, unless the ovaries are removed. In blood, testosterone is avidly bound to sex-hormone-binding globulin (SHBG) and only the small 'free' fraction is biologically active. Normally, the postmenopausal ovary continues to produce some androgens.[2] Population studies have failed to link a decline in sexual activity with serum androgen levels. There are also technical problems with the measurement of testosterone. The commercially available assays are designed for the male normal range and not accurate for women or children. In some laboratories, a 'sensitive testosterone' assay is available, but even these have poor correlation with sexual desire and responsiveness. Clinical trials have been more helpful than laboratory-based studies.

Oestrogen therapy has been shown to improve vaginal lubrication; even oral HT, despite its adverse effects on SHBG (oral oestrogens increase SHBG levels and so lower free, bioactive testosterone levels), has been shown to improve sexual desire and arousal.[2] There have been several RCTs of transdermal testosterone for women, usually as patches. In most of the trials, women received adequate oestrogenisation first. These studies have shown a significant improvement in sexual desire and more satisfying sex than placebo. Although serum testosterone levels are of no value in diagnosing hypoactive sexual disorders, they are useful in ensuring that patients are not over-treated, so that androgenic side effects can be minimised. Panay and colleagues published a trial using testosterone patches designed for women without oestrogen replacement, and showed a statistically beneficial effect on sexual desire with minimal side effects.[29] It is important to explore possible reasons for low libido before reaching for the prescription pad. These might include relationship problems, emotional issues, over-commitment to responsibilities, and more.

BIO-IDENTICAL HT

Some doctors, working with compounding chemists, 'hand-make' hormonal mixtures and call them 'bio-identical HT'. Typically these treatments are presented as 'troches' or lozenges that are sucked, or sometimes prescribed as creams to be rubbed into the skin. They usually contain three oestrogens, progesterone, DHEA, testosterone and sometimes other steroids such as pregnenolone.

Cirigliano has reviewed the scant medical literature on these products.[30] These treatments do not undergo stringent quality control, their pharmacokinetics are largely unknown and there are no medium- or long-term safety studies. Often these expensive treatments are monitored using salivary and blood hormone levels that have not been validated.[30] It is well known in clinical practice that, unlike monitoring thyroid function, where blood tests are exquisitely sensitive and useful, as already discussed, many of the main symptoms of menopause relate to the brain, rather than blood levels of any particular hormone.

Three cases of uterine cancer were described in Australian women using troches.[31] The Australasian Menopause Society[32] and the North American Menopause Society[33] oppose the use of bio-identical HT, and the medical defence organisations are unlikely to cover the prescribing medical practitioner if there is an adverse patient outcome. However, if a patient has been using this treatment for more than a few months, it may be prudent to perform endometrial surveillance (e.g. transvaginal ultrasound and perhaps an endometrial biopsy[31]).

PREMATURE MENOPAUSE

Around 1–2% of women will be spontaneously menopausal before the age of 40 years.[34] Some of the causes of premature ovarian failure (POF) are summarised in Box 53.3.

Patients with POF may present with primary or secondary amenorrhoea. Not all will have hot flushes. Many will have oligomenorrhoea before amenorrhoea. A high index of suspicion is required and the diagnosis is confirmed by finding elevated levels of FSH (> 20 U/L, usually > 40 U/L). It is prudent to repeat the FSH measurement to confirm the diagnosis. In a patient under the age of 30 years, chromosomal analysis, bone mineral density and an autoantibody screen (e.g. thyroid, adrenal, ovarian, parietal cell autoantibodies, antinuclear antibodies) are useful tests, and referral to a reproductive endocrinologist is prudent as these women need specialist care. For example, if the woman has not had any breast development yet, very low doses of oestrogen need to be given initially, and then the dose slowly increased. If the woman is commenced on an OCP, for example, the breasts usually remain small and misshapen. From a fertility perspective, sporadic cases of spontaneous pregnancy have been reported, but most will need egg donation to achieve pregnancy.

BOX 53.3 Causes of premature ovarian failure

Apparently healthy women with POF

Genetic causes:
- fragile X syndrome
- partial deletions of the X chromosome
- mosaicism (e.g. 45X0 and 47XXX cell lines in the same patient)

Autoimmune:
- ovarian autoantibodies

Mutations in FSH or LH (very rare)

Mumps oophoritis (may or may not remember pelvic pain)

Women with a significant medical history and POF

Genetic causes:
- above, and Turner's syndrome
- rare genetic syndromes (e.g. Swyer's syndrome, Perrault's syndrome, blepharophimosis)

Ovarian antibodies associated with other autoimmune conditions:
- Addison's disease
- diabetes mellitus
- thyroid disease
- myasthenia gravis
- systemic lupus erythematosus
- rheumatoid arthritis

Infiltrative disease:
- iron overload (e.g. thalassaemia major)
- sarcoid

Chemotherapy

Radiotherapy to the pelvis

Galactosaemia

Severe enzyme deficiencies (e.g. cholesterol demolase deficiency)

LONG-TERM ISSUES

Hormone therapy remains a valid treatment option for some women with osteopenia or osteoporosis, although evidence suggests that HT would need to be taken for over 10 years, by which time the risks may outweigh the benefits. The RCTs to date suggest that HT has no role in the prevention of heart disease or dementia.[2,12,22]

CONCLUSION

For many women, menopause will not present any great difficulties. Most women with mild to moderate symptoms will be content in the knowledge that menopause is another natural stage in their life, perhaps combined with some lifestyle changes and a herbal therapy such as black cohosh. For some, however, severe flushes and sweats severely disrupt their lives, and these women should be offered medical treatment, based on each woman's individual situation. For a small number, menopause symptoms will continue forever. The long-term management of these patient remains a challenge, but the key is quality medical information and presenting the women with well-informed choices.

RESOURCES

Australasian Menopause Society, http://www.menopause.org.au

International Menopause Society, http://www.imsociety.org

Jean Hailes Foundation for Women's Health, http://www.jeanhailes.org.au

North American Menopause Society, http://www.menopause.org

Women's Health and Research Institute of Australia, http://www.whria.com.au

REFERENCES

1 Sherman S. Defining the menopause transition. Am J Med 2005; 118(12B):35–75.

2 Blake J. Menopause: evidence-based practice. Best Pract Res Clin Obstet Gynaecol 2006; 20(6):799–839.

3 Dennerstein L, Dudley EC, Hopper JL et al. A prospective population-based study of menopausal symptoms. Obstet Gynecol 2000; 96:351–358.

4 Peeyananjarassri K, Cheewadhanaraks S, Hubbard M et al. Menopause symptoms in a hospital-based sample

of women in southern Thailand. Climacteric 2006; 9:23–29.

5 Toulis KA, Tzellos T, Kouvelas D et al. Gabapentin for the treatment of hot flashes in women with natural or tamoxifen-induced menopause: a systematic review and meta-analysis. Clin Therapeutics 2009; 31(2):221–235.

6 Hafiz I, Lui J, Eden J. A quantitative analysis of the menopause experience of Indian women living in Sydney. Aust NZ J Obstet Gynaecol 2007; 47:329–334.

7 Lu J, Lui J, Eden J. The experience of menopausal symptoms by Arabic women in Sydney. Climacteric 2007; 10:72–79.

8 Liu J, Eden J. Experience and attitudes toward menopause in Chinese women living in Sydney—a cross-sectional survey. Maturitas 2007; 58(4): 359–365.

9 Liu J, Eden J. The menopausal experience of Greek women living in Sydney. J North Am Menopause Soc 2008; 15(3):476–481.

10 Hilditch JR, Lewis J, Peter A et al. A menopause-specific quality of life questionnaire: development and psychometric properties. Maturitas 1996; 24:161–175.

11 Australian Menopause Society. Oestrogen deficiency symptom score, using MENQOL. Online. Available: http://www.menopause.org.au /education/Edu_html.asp?ID=89

12 Viera A, Bond M, Yates S. Diagnosing night sweats. Am Family Physician. March 2003. Online. Available: http://www.aafp.org/afp/2003/0301/p1019.html.

13 Daley AJ, Stokes-Lampard HJ, Macarthur C. Exercise to reduce vasomotor and other menopausal symptoms: a review. Maturitas 2009; 63(3):176–180.

14 Villaverde-Gutierrez et al. Quality of life of rural menopausal women in response to a customized exercise programme. J Adv Nurs 2006; 54(1):11–19.

15 Grady DG. Management of menopausal symptoms. N Engl J Med 2007; 356:1176–1178.

16 Brzezinski A, Adlercreutz H, Shaoul R et al. Short-term effects of phytoestrogen-rich diet on postmenopausal women. Menopause: J North Am Menopause Soc 1997; 4:89–94.

17 Eden JA. Herbal medicines for menopause: do they work and are they safe? Med J Aust 2001; 174(2): 63–64.

18 Nelson HD, Vesco KK, Haney E et al. Non-hormonal therapies for hot flushes. Systematic review and meta-analysis. J Am Med Assoc 2007; 295(17):2057–2071.

19 Osmers R, Friede M, Liske E et al. Efficacy and safety of isopropanolic black cohosh extract for climacteric symptoms. Obstet Gynecol 2005; 105:1074–1083.

20 Uebelhack R, Blohmer JU, Graubaum HJ et al. Black cohosh and St John's wort for climacteric complaints. Obstet Gynecol 2006; 107:247–255.

21 Palacio C, Masri G, Arshag D. Black cohosh for the management of menopausal symptoms. A systematic review of the clinical trials. Drugs Aging 2009; 26(1):23–36.

22 Nedrow A, Miller J, Walker M et al. Complementary and alternative therapies for the management of menopause-related symptoms. Arch Intern Med 2006; 166:1453–1465.

23 MacLennan AH. HRT: a reappraisal of the risks and benefits. Med J Aust 2007; 186(12):643–646.

24 Katalinic A, Rawal R. Decline in breast cancer incidence after decrease in utilisation of hormone replacement therapy. Breast Cancer Res Treat 2008; 107(3):427–430.

25 Rossouw JE, Prentice RL, Manson JE et al. Postmenopausal hormone therapy and risk of cardiovascular disease by age and years since menopause. J Am Med Assoc 2007; 297(13):1465–1477.

26 The WHI steering committee. Effects of conjugated equine estrogen in postmenopausal women with hysterectomy. J Am Med Assoc 2004; 291:1701–1712.

27 Cummings SR, Ettinger B, Delmas PD et al. The effects of tibolone in older postmenopausal women. N Engl J Med 2008; 359:697–708.

28 Kenemans P, Bundred NJ, Foidart JM et al. Safety and efficacy of tibolone in breast-cancer patients with vasomotor symptoms: a double-blind, randomised, non-inferiority trial. Lancet Oncol 2009; 10(2): 135–146.

29 Panay N, Al-Azzawi F, Bouchard C et al. Testosterone treatment of HSDD in naturally menopausal women: the ADORE study. Climacteric 2010; 13(2):121–131.

30 Cirigliano M. Bioidentical hormone therapy: a review of the evidence. J Women's Health 2007; 16(5):600–631.

31 Eden JA, Hacker NF, Fortune M. Three cases of endometrial cancer associated with 'bioidentical' hormone replacement therapy. Med J Aust 2007; 187(4):244–245.

32 Australasian Menopause Society. Bioidentical hormones (troches) advice to consumers. 29 November 2003. Online. Available: http://www.menopause.org.au/content/view/211/102/

33 North American Menopause Society. Bioidentical hormone therapy. Online. Available: http://www.menopause.org/bioidentical.aspx

34 Meskhi A, Seif MW. Premature ovarian failure. Curr Opin Obstet Gynecol 2006; 18:418–426.

part SIX

Lifecycle health

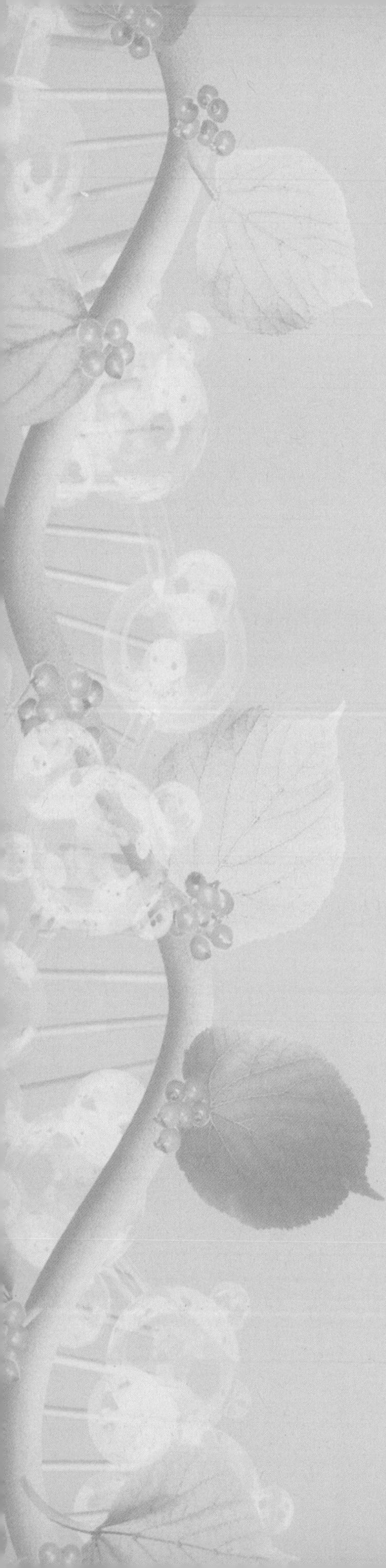

chapter 54

Pregnancy and antenatal care

INTRODUCTION AND OVERVIEW

General practitioners see patients throughout their life cycle, and integrative healthcare begins before conception and continues throughout pregnancy. Depending on your practice environment, you may be the sole practitioner responsible for the patient's antenatal care as a GP/obstetrician, part of the antenatal shared care team including hospital-based midwives and an obstetrician, or see the patient for preconception advice, and then less frequently during the pregnancy if the patient is seeing an obstetrician for their antenatal care through personal preference or medical best practice.

PRECONCEPTION COUNSELLING

Comprehensive pregnancy care begins with the first discussion of conception, particularly for nulligravida. Ideally this consultation should occur 6–12 months before starting to attempt to conceive.

It may take the form of a formal preconception consultation, or begin with opportunistic questioning by the GP at the routine check-up of a woman of childbearing age (approximately 15–49 years), such as:

- Are you planning a pregnancy at some time in the future?
- Are you currently using contraception?
- How many babies do you think you will have?
- What spacing do you anticipate?
- What is your expected timing?

Enquire about previous pregnancies and the outcomes, including infant death, fetal loss, birth defects, low birth weight, preterm birth, or gestational diabetes or other maternal complications.

Chronic medical conditions such as diabetes need to be fully assessed and management optimised.

Immunisation status needs to be checked, particularly for preventable infectious diseases likely to affect a pregnancy, such as rubella, varicella, hepatitis B and measles. If non-immune, rubella and varicella immunisation need to be given at least 28 days before planned conception.

Influenza vaccination can be given at any time in pregnancy, particularly if the second or third trimester falls in influenza season.

Diphtheria/tetanus/pertussis combined vaccine should be given if a booster dose is due. This helps to protect the newborn from pertussis before they are old enough to have their immunisations.

Investigations might include:

- full blood examination and blood group
- iron studies
- serology for rubella, varicella, hepatitis B and measles immunity
- HIV status
- folate
- urine protein
- urinary iodine
- blood glucose
- vitamin D.

The genetic history should explore any congenital abnormalities in the extended biological family and, if necessary, genetic counselling arranged.

An important principle to remember is that any investment in the mother's wellbeing—and the wider family, for that matter—is an investment in the wellbeing of the pregnancy and the future of the child. Preparation for pregnancy needs to address the woman's physical, emotional and spiritual situation, including her beliefs about her relationship, parenting and lifestyle. It is helpful to consider the elements using the ESSENCE model, as discussed below (also see Ch 6).

EDUCATION

Planning a pregnancy is the time when women are arguably the most interested they have ever been in optimising their health, in the interests of having a healthy baby. It is also an opportunity to discuss the potential father's lifestyle and general health. The advice provided at the preconception consultation may be the last chance to see the patient before she becomes pregnant, so this consultation needs to address issues that will be important in the early stages of pregnancy, even before she knows she is pregnant.

Women can be informed that the optimum biological age for pregnancy is between 20 and 35 years. Beyond that age, the risk of infertility, miscarriage, multiple pregnancy, pregnancy complications and fetal abnormalities increases statistically. However, many women are delaying conception until their late thirties and early forties, and deliver healthy babies.

Advice should include avoiding any prescribed or over-the-counter medications likely to affect early pregnancy, exercising regularly and avoiding alcohol, tobacco and illicit drugs. Any household members should be encouraged to stop smoking.

Preconception education will involve answering the questions posed, but also providing information to assist in optimising the health of the parents and opening a discussion about parenting ideas and philosophies.

STRESS MANAGEMENT

Because the mother's stress hormones (including cortisol and catechols) cross the placenta, maternal stress also affects fetal neurological, physiological and metabolic development. For example, significant and prolonged maternal stress,[1,2] particularly in the first trimester, is associated with poorer fetal growth, developmental problems, an increased risk of mental illness and a higher risk of cardiovascular disease in the offspring.

The work and home environment will have a significant impact on the potential mother's stress levels.

Planning a pregnancy brings with it many anxieties about whether the woman will be able to become pregnant, inevitable life change, financial pressure, changes to career path and more. Information and an opportunity to talk through these concerns is helpful. Therefore, putting in place effective strategies for managing stress is an important part of preparing for pregnancy. Stress management activities such as regular sleep patterns, reducing reliance on substances and practising yoga, T'ai chi, meditation and relaxation exercises, as well as planning staged modifications to the mother's work schedule, can provide benefits to emotional health. Counselling, cognitive behaviour therapy and mindfulness-based stress management may be helpful for some women where needed.

SPIRITUALITY

Starting a family affects a woman, her family and her work in profound ways. Asking about what all this means for her and how she will adjust may be an important conversation. A preliminary discussion of a patient's religious or spiritual beliefs may be appropriate, particularly if there is a problem with fertility, if the pregnancy fails to proceed or if antenatal testing reveals a fetal abnormality.[3] A discussion of the parents' religious views about circumcision, should they have a male child, may be appropriate in the planning stages.

EXERCISE

Optimum fitness is a desirable goal prior to conception. Pregnancy adds a significant physical and physiological load, so aerobic and resistance training to help build fitness and muscle strength, and a back care program, will help her to cope with the pregnancy and childbirth far more effectively. She will also be able to reduce the risk of hypertension and diabetes during pregnancy, improve immunity and mental health and minimise complications. It should also be remembered that exercising to excess during pregnancy can be as much of a problem as being inactive.

Stretching and yoga improve flexibility. Patients with low back problems can be referred for back rehabilitation programs such as those supervised by physiotherapists or exercise physiologists.

Once the patient is pregnant, she can continue or adjust her current exercise program (Box 54.1).

NUTRITION

Assess the patient for possible nutritional risk, especially if the patient is vegan, lactose-intolerant, has coeliac disease or other gut problems or an eating disorder likely to affect nutritional status. If the woman's body weight is in the normal range, then dietary advice will focus on the quality and balance of foods she is eating.

However, women who are either significantly overweight or underweight need to address this risk factor. Obese women are 2.7 times more likely to be infertile than women in the healthy weight range. Obesity in women can also increase the risk of miscarriage and impair the outcomes of assisted reproductive technologies and pregnancy.[4] It is also associated with an increased rate of caesarean section.[5]

Being underweight is associated with reduced conception rates among nulliparous women and increased likelihood of conception among parous women.[6]

Some foods are to be avoided because of the risk of listeriosis, which causes a risk of miscarriage. These foods include raw seafood, pre-prepared (salad bar) salads, delicatessen meats, leftovers, soft cheeses and

BOX 54.1 Exercise advice for women with a normal pregnancy

- Swimming, walking and jogging are considered safe throughout pregnancy. Minimal contact sports such as tennis and netball are considered safe for at least the first 12 weeks and beyond, depending on the level of competition, the state of the pregnancy and the mother's fitness level.
- Collision sports such as basketball and soccer are considered safe only up to 12 weeks, although there is no evidence that the type of impact that would occur from a sport-related collision or fall has ever injured an unborn baby.
- If a woman was not active before she became pregnant, she should start with gentle exercise such as walking or swimming.
- Assess whether there is any particular risk related to specific patients or their choice of sport(s). Refer to an exercise physiologist for specific advice.
- Review the training program regularly.
- Always work at less than 75% of the maximum heart rate (140 beats per minute or less, depending on the patient's age).
- Patients need to know not to expect the same level of athletic performance when they are pregnant. They should stop exercising when tired and should avoid getting exhausted.
- Ensure a gentle cool-down period after strenuous exercise.
- Drink plenty of fluids and avoid getting over-heated.
- Advise patients to call you or their obstetrician urgently if they notice bleeding, abdominal pain or cramps, chest pain, oedema, dizziness, dyspnoea, insufficient weight gain or reduced fetal movements.

Activities to be avoided in pregnancy:

- gymnastics
- heavy weight-lifting
- horse riding
- martial arts
- mountain climbing
- parachuting
- saunas
- scuba diving
- trampolining
- water skiing

pâté. All fruit and vegetables should be washed in filtered water before eating.

Eating a fresh, varied and healthy diet is important during pregnancy, as it is at any other time. Supplementation, particularly for those with poor vegetable intake, with a multivitamin containing 500 μg folate should commence prior to conception. Iron, zinc, vitamin D, calcium and iodine are all essential nutrients that may be lacking, and should be included in the choice of a high-quality antenatal supplement. A good intake of omega-3 fatty acids is also important for fetal development, and supplements of 3 g daily should be considered for those with a poor intake.

Some women think that 'if one supplement is good, then more is better'. Check the contents of any supplements or over-the-counter preparations that are being taken, and be sure to avoid excess. This may particularly be the case for substances such as vitamin A.

CONNECTEDNESS

Relationships and social support are important not only for practical reasons but also because they have such a profound effect upon maternal emotional wellbeing and coping. Discuss the social connections the patient has with family and friends. Encourage development of a network of parents with babies, particularly if there are no family members likely to be around once the baby arrives.

ENVIRONMENT

The patient should be advised to avoid contact with household or occupational chemicals. Clear any toxic chemicals out of the house and replace with non-toxic alternative cleaning products.

If the family has a cat, advise that someone other than the pregnant (or intending to be pregnant) woman should empty the litter tray, to minimise the risk of toxoplasmosis. She should avoid contact with garden soil, wash all fruit and vegetables before consumption and avoid undercooked or raw meat or unpasteurised milk products. She should also limit the consumption of large fish likely to contain higher levels of mercury.

Discuss the potential for transmission of parvovirus B19 and cytomegalovirus. Childcare workers should wear gloves when changing children's nappies and wash their hands frequently. Regular, moderate sun exposure will also be helpful for adequate vitamin D levels.

ANTENATAL CARE

Women suitable for shared antenatal care with their general practitioner (GP) include those defined as healthy women having a normal pregnancy. Complications usually requiring additional care by an obstetrician or other specialist are summarised in Box 54.2. Some of these women may still be suitable for shared care, with some modification of the usual schedule of visits.

SCHEDULE OF VISITS

The traditional schedule of antenatal visits was developed in the United Kingdom in the 1920s and consists of 14 visits based on first presentation early in pregnancy, monthly visits until 28 weeks' gestation, fortnightly visits until 36 weeks' gestation and weekly visits thereafter until delivery. Observational studies

BOX 54.2 Complications of pregnancy requiring specialist advice

- Cardiac (heart) disease, including hypertension (high blood pressure)
- Renal (kidney) disease
- Endocrine disorders or diabetes requiring insulin
- Psychiatric disorders (on medication)
- Haematological (blood) disorders, including thromboembolic disease
- Epilepsy requiring anticonvulsant drugs
- Malignant disease (such as cancer)
- Severe asthma
- Chemical dependency
- HIV positive
- HBV positive
- Autoimmune disorders
- Significantly overweight or underweight
- Significant environmental factors and lack of social support
- Recurrent miscarriage or mid-trimester loss
- Previous preterm delivery < 30 weeks of gestation
- More than five previous pregnancies (grand multiparity)
- Severe preeclampsia
- Rhesus isoimmunisation or other significant blood group antibodies
- Uterine surgery including caesarean section or cone biopsy
- Antenatal or postpartum haemorrhage on two or more occasions
- Retained placenta on two or more occasions
- Intrauterine growth restriction (IUGR)
- Stillbirth or infant (neonatal) death
- Birth weight < 2500 g, or > 4500 g
- Congenital abnormality, e.g. Down syndrome
- Postnatal depression or puerperal psychosis

Source: 3 Centres Collaboration[7]

have demonstrated a beneficial effect of regular antenatal care on perinatal outcomes. Despite varying schedules, the overall aims of antenatal care can be summarised as described below.

- *First trimester*—from a carer's perspective, the main aim of the first trimester antenatal visits is to identify potential risks to maternal and fetal wellbeing. The risk assessment includes careful history-taking, establishment of expected date of confinement, discussing illicit drug-taking, alcohol intake and smoking behaviour and establishing care options. Visits are usually timed to coincide with recommended screening tests where these occur at specific times, such as Down syndrome screening.
- *Second trimester*—the aim of second trimester visits is primarily to monitor fetal growth and maternal wellbeing, and monitor for early-onset preeclampsia. Routine tests in this trimester include an ultrasound for morphology at 18–22 weeks' gestation and glucose screening at 24–28 weeks' gestation.
- *Third trimester*—third trimester visits are primarily for the assessment of fetal growth and presentation, and of maternal wellbeing, detection of preeclampsia, and preparation of the woman for admission to the birthing facility and labour. Bacteriological screening for group B streptococcus takes place at around 35–37 weeks' gestation.

Two reviews of the literature[8,9] have suggested that reducing this schedule of visits to 10 is equally effective in achieving positive perinatal outcomes in low-risk gravidas, although it may be associated with a decrease in satisfaction with care. In particular, there was no difference in perinatal outcomes between primigravidas and multigravidas.

Early in her pregnancy, the woman should be given information regarding the schedule of visits and testing that she can expect. The number and timing of visits should be flexible, to suit her needs. Additional visits should be provided if complications arise.

MODELS OF CARE

Routine involvement of specialist obstetricians in low-risk maternity care is not associated with any improvement in perinatal outcomes compared to involving obstetricians when complications arise.[9] Midwifery and GP-led models of care are safe for low-risk women. Women are more likely to be satisfied with their care where there is continuity of care, or carer. At each antenatal visit, midwives and doctors should offer information, consistent advice and clear explanations and provide the opportunity to ask questions.

INITIAL RECOMMENDED TESTS

- *FBE including mean cell haemoglobin concentration (MCHC)/mean cell volume (MCV)*—ferritin and thalassaemia screening by Hb electrophoresis is indicated on the basis of low MCV. Thalassaemia screening may also be indicated by family history or ethnicity. Women at risk of a severely affected fetus should be offered partner screening.
- *Blood group/antibody screen*—although Rhesus status may be known, a screen for antibodies should be performed in every pregnancy. Anti-Kell antibodies, for example, although rare (incidence approximately 0.5 per 1000), are associated with poor perinatal outcomes.[10]
- *HIV antibodies* (level 1 evidence)—the prevalence of HIV among pregnant women in Australia is unknown but has been estimated at 0.23 per

1000. It has been reported that 48% of Australian mothers whose children were exposed perinatally to HIV infection reported no other risk factors apart from heterosexual contact. Four interventions have been shown to significantly reduce vertical transmission rates: antiretroviral therapy to the pregnant woman and the child in the first 6 weeks of life; elective Caesarean section; avoidance of invasive obstetric procedures; and alternatives to breastfeeding. Evidence supports universal offering of HIV screening to pregnant women with appropriate pre- and post-test counselling.[11]

- *Hepatitis B serology*—vertical transmission of HBV can be prevented by prompt immunoprophylaxis at birth. Existing evidence supports screening at the first antenatal visit for hepatitis B surface antigen.
- *Syphilis serology*—congenital syphilis results in serious sequelae in liveborn infected children, and is also associated with long-term morbidity for women and increased pregnancy complications including non-immune hydrops. Although the prevalence of syphilis in the general population is low, universal screening programs have been shown to significantly increase the detection of syphilis in pregnant women compared with selective screening of those thought to be at high risk. In populations of high prevalence it may be repeated in the third trimester.
- *Rubella immunity*—pregnant women found not to be immune to rubella should be advised to avoid any potential risks, such as children with an unknown febrile illness. Vaccination should be given post partum.
- *Asymptomatic bacteriuria (ASB)*—routine screening between 12 and 16 weeks is recommended, to prevent urinary tract infections, preterm birth and low birth weight. Mid-stream urine for microscopy and culture is more sensitive than any other method and also more cost-effective in terms of outcomes. A full ward test may be used in addition to screening for chronic renal disease.
- *PAP smear*—if the woman is due and presenting in the first trimester.

OTHER TESTS TO BE CONSIDERED

- *Hepatitis C*—screening for hepatitis C by testing for HCV antibodies should be offered to all women at increased risk (Box 54.3). Unlike hepatitis B, however, universal screening has not been recommended from the point of view of antenatal care as the prevalence in the community is low, vertical transmission rates are low (6%) and there are no techniques to reduce vertical transmission rates. A positive HCV antibody test should be further investigated with HCV viral studies by polymerase chain reaction (PCR). Two negative PCR studies suggest that the patient is not a chronic carrier.

BOX 54.3 High-risk factors for hepatitis C

- History of injecting drugs (~40% of infected mothers)
- Partner who injected drugs
- Tattoo or piercing
- Been in prison (~67% of women in prison)
- Blood transfusion, later positive for hepatits C
- Migration from a country with a high endemic rate

- *Ferritin*—iron deficiency is common in pregnancy, particularly in multigravidas or with a history of recurrent miscarriage. A ferritin of 50 (reference range 9–150) is thought to be adequate at the start of a pregnancy. Ferritin can be elevated in the presence of infection.
- *Vitamin D*—during pregnancy, sufficient vitamin D concentrations are needed not only to supply the growing demand for calcium on the part of the fetus, but also to participate in fetal growth, development of the nervous system, lung maturation and fetal immune system function. Hypovitaminosis D has been related to the development of fetal neurological and skeletal disorders. It is advisable for pregnant and lactating women to maintain adequate levels of vitamin D. If sun exposure is insufficient, which may be seen in darker-skinned women who have migrated to more temperate areas or through excessive covering up, supplements may be required.[12]
- *Thalassaemia screen*
- *Dating ultrasound*—a first-trimester ultrasound has been consistently shown to be more accurate than last menstrual period dates.

Other recommended tests

26 weeks

- Antibody screen
- FBE ± Fe studies
- *Gestational diabetes screening*—strategies for screening for gestational diabetes vary widely. Women are most commonly screened using a glucose challenge test, which does not require them to fast and consists of a single blood glucose 2 hours after the glucose load. If abnormal, this requires a full glucose tolerance test (GTT) for confirmation of the diagnosis. High-risk patients such as those with previous gestational diabetes should have the latter test only. Any suspicion that the woman may have undiagnosed prepregnancy

BOX 54.4 Recommendations for intrapartum antibiotics in prevention of GBS disease

Intrapartum antibiotics recommended if:
- < 37 weeks
- ruptured membranes > 18 weeks before delivery
- maternal temperature ≥ 38°C
- previous GBS colonisation, bacteriuria or infant with GBS

diabetes requires investigation with a GTT in the first trimester; however, this does not replace the 26-week GTT, which should still be performed.

36 weeks

- *Group B Streptococcus (GBS) screening*—about 25% of pregnant women are thought to be carriers of GBS. Transmission to the newborn may occur during labour, resulting in pneumonia, septicaemia and, occasionally, mortality. The incidence of GBS disease is 1–3 per 1000 live births and can be reduced to 0.6 per 1000 live births by universal screening. The death rate for newborn GBS disease is estimated at 4.7–9%.[13] Swabs should be taken between 35 and 37 weeks' gestation. Recommendations for intrapartum prophylaxis are given in Box 54.4.

  GBS is part of the intestinal flora. Treatment with oral antibiotics will not clear it from the bowel, and clearance from the vagina occurs spontaneously, as does the inevitable reinfection. The strategy is to provide chemoprophylaxis to the baby at the time that the baby is likely to come into contact with the organism.
- *Repeat antibody screen* for Rh-negative women unless the woman earlier received antenatal anti-D prophylaxis at 28 and 34 weeks' gestation as the National Health and Medical Research Council recommends.[14] If prophylaxis has been administered, the identification of passive anti-D from immunisation may cause confusion.

PRENATAL SCREENING FOR ANEUPLOIDY

Prenatal screening should be offered to all pregnant women irrespective of maternal age. Counselling should explore the woman's current knowledge of chromosomal disorders. Most people are aware of the most common of the trisomies, trisomy 21 or Down syndrome. It should be emphasised that participation in screening is voluntary. The three commonly available screening tests—the first-trimester combined screen, nuchal translucency alone, and the second-trimester biochemical screening test or 'quadruple test'—all give a 'high risk' or 'low risk' result rather than a definitive answer. Women should be made aware that they would be referred for genetic counselling following a 'high risk' result, with the option of having a subsequent invasive definitive test such as chorionic villus sampling or amniocentesis. Both of these invasive tests carry a risk of miscarriage of 1:100 or 1:200 respectively. The woman may elect not to have definitive testing. Following definitive testing, the woman could expect to receive further counselling about the result. A woman who has a diagnosis of aneuploidy confirmed may, after further counselling, be offered a termination of the pregnancy, depending on local laws and the views of the patient and doctor.

A 'high risk' result in the screening tests results in considerable anxiety for the mother and also her close supports. These women should be offered appropriate counselling and further testing as soon as possible. A quick result may be available after 24 hours through the technique of fluorescence in situ hybridisation (FISH).

The first-trimester combined screen consists of nuchal translucency in combination with maternal age and serum markers, pregnancy-associated plasma protein A (PAPP-A) and the free beta subunit of human chorionic gonadotrophin (fβhCG). Trisomy 21 detection rates are estimated at about 87% for a false-positive rate of 5%.[15,16] This rate depends on the timing of the individual components. The test is most informative when the serum markers are performed during the ninth week of gestation and the nuchal translucency component during the twelfth week. The advantages of the first-trimester test include higher detection rates, more straightforward termination procedures for those choosing to terminate an aneuploid pregnancy, and earlier reassurance.[16]

Nuchal translucency can be used alone. This approach is often taken for multiple gestations.

Second-trimester maternal serum screening using a combination of markers that include alpha-fetoprotein (AFP), human chorionic gonadotrophin (hCG), unconjugated oestriol (uE3) and inhibin A. Detection rates for trisomy 21 are usually quoted as 80% for a false-positive rate of 5%. Screening can be undertaken between 15 and 20 weeks' gestation.

A number of 'soft' markers have been described which increase the risk of aneuploidy when present. These include nasal bone hypoplasia, cystic hygroma, abnormal ductus venosus flow and tricuspid regurgitation at the first-trimester ultrasound. Markers identified at the routine second-trimester morphology scan include nuchal translucency, short femur or humerus, pyelectasis, echogenic bowel, echogenic intracardiac focus, single vessel cord and any major structural malformation. Definitive testing is usually offered to women with two or more of these markers, which in studies were observed in 15.1% of cases and 1.6% of normal controls.[17]

It is worth noting that many people have a somewhat misplaced confidence in the ability of the second-trimester morphology scan to detect chromosomal abnormalities. Detection rates based on this ultrasound alone have been quoted at around 30%. The focus of this scan is really directed at the detection of structural abnormalities. Even these detection rates differ, being highest for spinal anomalies and lowest for cleft lip and digit anomalies.

THE STANDARD ANTENATAL CHECK

Smoking

Evidence indicates serious fetal risks associated with maternal smoking. Meta-analysis has demonstrated twice the normal risk of low birth weight for babies of mothers who smoke (RR 2.04). Preterm birth is a third more likely (RR 1.34) and IUGR risk is more than doubled (RR 2.28). The risk of sudden infant death syndrome is almost three times higher (RR 2.76), and maternal smoking is associated with 10% of stillbirths (RR 1.33) and spontaneous abortions (RR 1.36).[18,19]

Evidence clearly supports the effectiveness of smoking cessation interventions in reducing smoking rates in pregnant women, as well as reducing preterm birth and low birth weight. Women should be asked about their smoking behaviour at every antenatal visit, using multiple-choice or open-ended questions. The response should be documented in the antenatal record. Smoking cessation interventions should be offered to all pregnant women who smoke or who have recently quit. At every visit, women should be advised about the risks to their own and their babies' health, and the benefits of quitting at every stage should be emphasised. The five-step strategy includes *Ask*, *Advise*, *Assess*, *Assist* and *Ask again* at each antenatal visit. The cycle should be repeated throughout pregnancy, due to high relapse rates in quitters, inaccurate reporting by women of their smoking status and the impact of changed circumstances on women's motivation.

The evidence regarding the relative risks and benefits of nicotine replacement therapy or other pharmacotherapies is currently insufficient. A cognitive-behavioural approach remains the approved intervention.

Blood pressure measurement

Blood pressure should be recorded at every antenatal visit. Measurements should be taken after 2–3 minutes of the woman sitting, with her feet supported. A standard-size cuff should be used for women with an arm circumference less than 33 cm and a large cuff for an arm circumference greater than this. Diastolic blood pressure readings should be recorded using the Korotkoff V sound (disappearance). If Korotkoff V is not present, then phase IV should be recorded.

Hypertension is defined as systolic blood pressure of 140 mmHg and/or diastolic blood pressure of 90 mmHg. Previous definitions included an incremental rise of 30 mmHg systolic or 15 mmHg diastolic compared to blood pressure as measured in the first trimester; however, most recent definitions have excluded the incremental rise in favour of the former definition. Automated devices should not be used and the role of ambulatory monitoring is currently uncertain. Elevated blood pressure is one of the early signs of preeclampsia, a major cause of maternal and perinatal morbidity (see Fig 54.1). Early detection is important, as the condition can progress rapidly. Hypertension in pregnancy without preeclampsia is also associated with adverse perinatal outcomes. A diagnosis of hypertension in pregnancy requires early assessment by a specialist obstetrician. A clinical diagnosis of preeclampsia is usually made when hypertension occurs with one or more of proteinuria, renal insufficiency, biochemical liver abnormalities, neurological signs, haematological disturbances or fetal growth restriction, and again it requires early assessment by a specialist obstetrician.

Blood pressure greater than 170/110 mmHg requires immediate admission to hospital.

Measurement of the symphyseal–fundal height

The symphyseal–fundal height is an indirect measure of fetal growth. If the measurement is larger or smaller than expected, an ultrasound assessment may be required. Possible causes include macrosomia, intrauterine growth restriction (IUGR), polyhydramnios, oligohydramnios, malpresentation and uterine anomalies.

Accurate dates are essential for correct diagnosis. Evidence supports either palpation for fetal size or measurement of the symphyseal–fundal height; however, the latter may provide a greater degree of reliability and consistency when the woman has multiple carers. Measurement of the fundus should start at the variable point (the fundus) to the fixed point (the symphysis pubis) using a non-elastic tape measure. The centimetre markers should be face down during the measurement, to discourage bias on the part of the examiner. Measurements should be recorded in a consistent manner. This clinical assessment of fetal growth is not useful in maternal obesity. Women with BMI over 35 should have a third-trimester ultrasound assessment of fetal growth and wellbeing to detect IUGR, which may otherwise remain undiagnosed.

Intrauterine growth follows a standard curve pattern. The maximum rate of growth occurs between 20 and 32 weeks and is generally 1 cm per week. After 32 weeks'

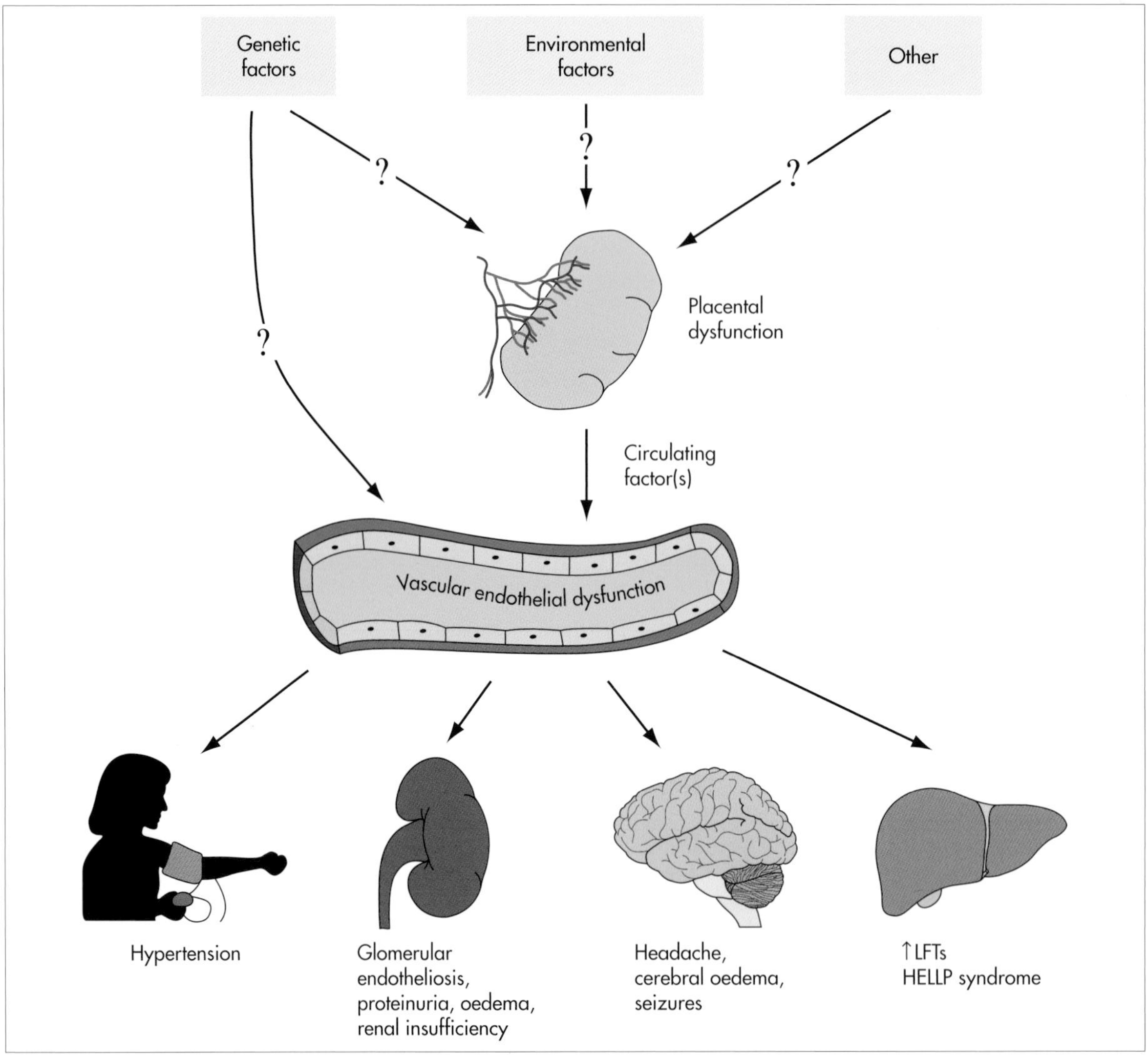

FIGURE 54.1 The clinical effects of preeclampsia

gestation, the rate of growth decreases slightly. Any variation in measurement from the expected may lead to a diagnosis of small for gestational age (SGA) or large for gestational age (LGA). These are somewhat vague terms that relate to the 10th and 90th centiles respectively and may or may not represent pathology. A baby who is SGA may be well and constitutionally small or may have IUGR. The diagnosis of IUGR is very important as these fetuses are at high risk of fetal death in utero, especially in postdates pregnancies. Other risks for these fetuses include perinatal morbidity, neurodevelopmental delay and endocrinological disorders. IUGR is usually further subdivided into symmetrical and asymmetrical, based on measurements of head size compared to body measurements such as abdominal circumference and femur length. Symmetrically small fetuses are more likely to have chromosomal abnormalities or intrauterine infection, as opposed to asymmetric growth restriction, which is more likely to be due to placental insufficiency and reflects the phenomenon of head sparing, by which the fetus attempts to preserve the blood supply to its most important organ, the brain, at the expense of the rest of the body. The diagnosis of IUGR really rests on evidence of slower growth than expected from two scans more than 2 weeks apart, but the diagnosis of placental insufficiency can be inferred at a single examination on the basis of a small baby and the abnormalities of markers of biophysical wellbeing. These include the amniotic fluid index (AFI), Doppler flow studies of the umbilical artery, middle cerebral

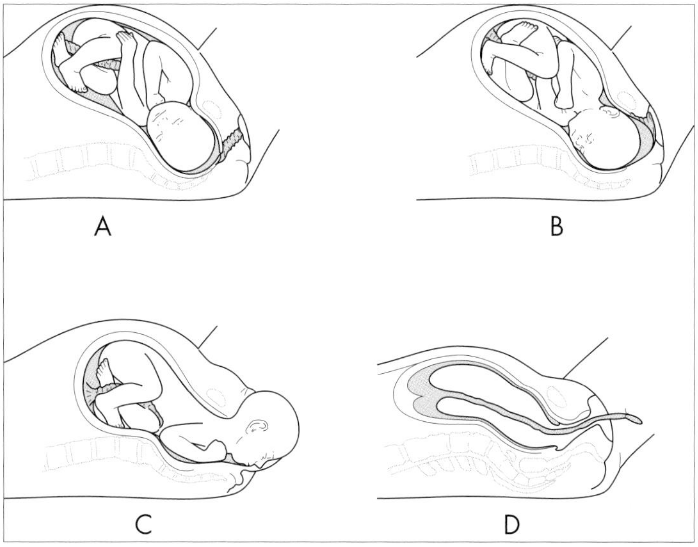

FIGURE 54.2 Normal presentation: **A** Engagement and flexion of the head; **B** Internal rotation; **C** Delivery by extension of the head after dilatation of the cervix; **D** Retraction of the uterus leading to delivery of the placenta

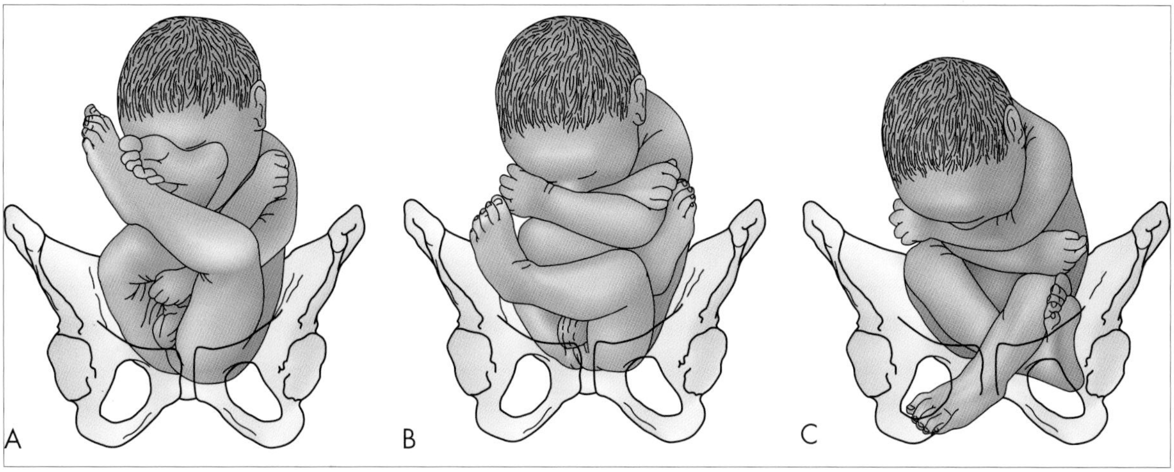

FIGURE 54.3 Breech presentation: **A** frank, **B** complete; **C** incomplete

artery and ductus venosus. Changes in the latter two suggest that the changes in blood flow associated with head sparing are taking place.

Any baby labelled as SGA clinically should receive some kind of ultrasound assessment of growth and wellbeing, depending on the gestation. From 36 weeks' gestation it may be more difficult to obtain an accurate estimation of fetal size due to technical problems such as head engagement, and the full growth assessment may be replaced by a modified biophysical profile consisting of AFI, Doppler studies and cardiotography. If all these tests are within normal range it suggests that the fetus is well and unlikely to be at risk. These tests should be performed weekly for continued reassurance. Most maternity centres offer these services in day assessment format.

The diagnosis of LGA suggests a possible diagnosis of macrosomia. Macrosomia is associated with uncontrolled diabetes and poor outcomes such as increased risk of shoulder dystocia. A diagnosis of macrosomia may alter management decisions during labour—for example, in the setting of vaginal birth after caesarean. Again, ultrasound assessment should be undertaken.

Fetal presentation and descent

A check to determine the presenting part should be performed as part of fetal palpation from about 30 weeks. Malpresentation is more likely with increasing maternal age, probably secondary to increasing incidence of uterine factors such as fibroids, which may alter the shape of the cavity and thus predispose to breech presentation or the uterine laxity associated with multiparity. The Term Breech Trial demonstrated a decrease in perinatal mortality or serious morbidity in developed countries for delivery by planned caesarean section rather than planned vaginal birth with no increase in serious morbidity or mortality for mothers.[20] Following the findings of this trial, practice in general has changed to favour elective caesarean section for all breech presentations at term, both multigravid and primigravid. This has increased the importance of the diagnosis of breech presentation, to allow for appropriate counselling.

The consequence of the Term Breech Trial has been a small but notable increase in the caesarean section rate. The only intervention proved to reduce this increase is external cephalic version (ECV). This has been found to be a safe and well-tolerated procedure which should be offered to women with a breech or transverse presentation in the last few weeks of pregnancy.

A presenting part remaining high at term, and particularly at full term, may be an indicator of cephalopelvic disproportion. If the presenting part is very mobile, there is a small risk of cord prolapse in the event of spontaneous ruptured membranes.

Fetal heart auscultation

Listening to the fetal heart at each visit is of no proven clinical benefit but is widely thought to be of psychological benefit to the mother. It should be offered at least at every visit after 20 weeks' gestation.

Some practices that are *not* useful

Recording the maternal weight at every visit has been standard practice for many years, but there is no conclusive evidence that it is a useful screening tool in the detection of IUGR, macrosomia or preeclampsia. Maternal weight and height should be measured at the first visit and the maternal BMI recorded. BMI < 20 is associated with increased complications including preterm labour and nutritional deficiencies, as well as the possibility of eating disorders. BMI > 35 is associated with increased complications including preeclampsia, hypertension, postdates pregnancy and operative delivery for dystocia.

Routine weighing at each visit should be confined to circumstances where it is relevant.

Routine screening for proteinuria in low-risk women after the first visit is also no longer recommended. Evidence suggests high rates of both false-positive and false-negative samples compared to the gold standard, the 24-hour urine collection. If the woman is noted to be hypertensive, a dipstick urinalysis for proteinuria is still recommended, although most will require 24-hour urine collection for proper assessment of proteinuria. Regular dipstick urinalysis may still be of value in high-risk patients.

RESOURCES

3 centres collaboration, guidelines on antenatal care, http://www.3centres.com.au/guide_frame.htm

Food Standards Australia New Zealand, Advice for women with babies on their minds or in their arms, http://www.foodstandards.gov.au/consumerinformation/adviceforpregnantwomen/

Health Insite, Exercise and pregnancy, http://www.healthinsite.gov.au/topics/Exercise_and_Pregnancy

REFERENCES

1 Bergman K, Sarkar P, O'Connor TG et al. Maternal stress during pregnancy predicts cognitive ability and fearfulness in infancy. J Am Acad Child Adolesc Psychiatry 2007; 46(11):1454–1463.

2 Talge NM, Neal C, Glover V. Antenatal maternal stress and long-term effects on child neurodevelopment: how and why? J Child Psychol Psychiatry 2007; 48(3/4):245–261.

3 Mann Jr, McKeown RE, Bacon J et al. Predicting depressive symptoms and grief after pregnancy loss. J Psychosom Obstet Gynaecol 2008; 29(4):274–279.

4 Pasquali R, Patton L, Gambineri A. Obesity and infertility. Curr Opin Endocrinol Diabetes Obes 2007; 14(6):482–487.

5 Poobalan AS, Aucott LS, Gurung T et al. Obesity as an independent risk factor for elective and emergency caesarean delivery in nulliparous women—systematic review and meta-analysis of cohort studies. Obes Rev 2009; 10(1):28–35.

6 Wise LA, Rothman KJ, Mikkelsen EM et al. An internet-based prospective study of body size and time-to-pregnancy. Hum Reprod 2010; 25(1):253–264.

7 3 Centres Collaboration. Guidelines on antenatal care (last reviewed 2006). Mercy Hospital for Women, Southern Health and Royal Women's Hospital, Melbourne. Online. Available: http://www.3centres.com.au/guide_frame.htm

8 Khan-Neelofur D, Gülmezoglu M, Villar J. Who should provide routine antenatal care for low-risk women, and how often? A systematic review of randomised controlled trials. WHO Antenatal Care Trial Research Group. Paediatr Perinat Epidemiol 1998; 12(Suppl 2):7–26.

9 Villar J, Carroli G, Khan-Neelofur D et al. Patterns of routine antenatal care for low-risk pregnancy. Cochrane Database Syst Rev 2001; 4:CD000934.

10 Moise KJ Jr. Non-anti-D antibodies in red-cell alloimmunization. Eur J Obstet Gynecol Reprod Biol 2000; 92(1):75–81.

11 Giles ML, Mijch AM, Garland SM et al. HIV and pregnancy in Australia. Aust NZ J Obstet Gynaecol 2004; 44(3):197–204.
12 Pérez-López FR. Vitamin D: the secosteroid hormone and human reproduction. Gynecol Endocrinol 2007; 23(1):13–24.
13 Mater Hospital Perinatal Epidemiology Unit and Queensland Council on Obstetric and Paediatric Morbidity and Mortality. Evidence-based clinical practice guidelines for the prevention of neonatal early-onset group B streptococcus disease. MPEU and QCOPMM, Brisbane; 2000 (cited in 3 centres collaboration – see ref 7).
14 Australian Government, National Health and Medical Research Institute. Guidelines on prophylactic use of Rh D immunoglobulin (anti-D) in obstetrics. Online. Available: http://www.health.gov.au/nhmrc/publications/pdf/wh27.pdf
15 Jaques AM, Halliday JL, Francis I et al. Follow-up and evaluation of the Victorian first-trimester combined screening programme for Down syndrome and trisomy 18. BJOG 2007; 114(7):812–818.
16 Breathnach FM, Malone FD. Screening for aneuploidy in first and second trimesters: is there an optimal paradigm? Curr Opin Obstet Gynecol 2007; 19(2):176–182.
17 Bethune M. Literature review and suggested protocol for managing ultrasound soft markers for Down syndrome: thickened nuchal fold, echogenic bowel, shortened femur, shortened humerus, pyelectasis and absent or hypoplastic nasal bone. Australas Radiol 2007; 51(3):218–225.
18 Lumley J, Oliver S, Waters E. Interventions for promoting smoking cessation during pregnancy. Cochrane Database Syst Rev 2000; 2:CD001055.
19 English D, Holman CDJ, Milne Winter MG et al. The quantification of drug-caused morbidity and mortality in Australia 1995: Part 2. Canberra: Commonwealth Department of Human Services and Health; 1995.
20 Hannah ME, Hannah WJ, Hewson SA et al. Planned caesarean section versus planned vaginal birth for breech presentation at term: a randomised multicentre trial. Term Breech Trial Collaborative Group. Lancet 2000; 356(9239):1375–1383.

Acknowledgment

The reference for most of the information provided in this chapter is: 3 Centres Consensus Guidelines on Antenatal Care, Mercy Hospital for Women, Southern Health and Royal Women's Hospital, Melbourne, 2006.

chapter 55

Child health and development

INTRODUCTION AND OVERVIEW

Infancy and childhood are characterised by a range of issues that broadly fall into three categories (Box 55.1):

- acute problems—e.g. infections, trauma
- medium-term problems—e.g. epilepsy, nutritional and feeding problems
- long-term chronic diseases—e.g. diabetes, cerebral palsy, developmental disorders.

Clearly, some cross these boundaries. However, problems in childhood need not extend into adult life even though they may have had major life effects in the short term. A sensitive approach to intervention that includes a holistic or integrative approach may have significant health benefits later. At the same time, a preventative strategy can alter family behaviour to abort important behavioural problems that are likely to lead to a lifetime of social disability.

It is difficult to separate the health of the child from the health of the family and the wider community. The health of the child is based not only upon his or her genetic background but also upon the prenatal environment, which is influenced by the lifestyle and mental and emotional health of the mother. Some of the most important investments in a child's later health can be made by investing in the mental and physical health of the mother during and after pregnancy .

While not an extensive overview of paediatric ill health, this chapter addresses a range of common problems presenting in a primary care setting, to illustrate the role of an integrative approach to children and their families that will support family cohesion and rally mutual physical, psychological and social supports underpinning a healthy approach to living.

BOX 55.1 Examples of chronic lifelong disease issues, and acute and medium-term problems

Acute
- Colic and other feeding problems
- Headaches
- Immunisation
- Infections
- Otitis media
- Pain management

Medium-term
- Asthma
- Allergy
- Cancer
- Constipation
- Enuresis
- Food sensitivity
- Recurrent abdominal pain
- Sleeping problems

Lifelong or chronic
- Behavioural, including autism-spectrum disorders
- Chronic illness
- Diabetes
- Epilepsy
- Obesity

SCREENING

General practitioners are well placed to screen opportunistically for potential health issues when children present for routine immunisations or minor illnesses. Growth monitoring is appropriate at routine visits.

Developmental assessments should include hearing, vision (including strabismus), language acquisition, fine motor skills, social skills and family dynamics. Enquiries need to be made about physical activity, nutrition, time spent watching television, accident prevention and sun protection.[1] Given their high incidence, screen for iron deficiency and vitamin D deficiency in at-risk groups.

Parents should be encouraged to maintain a child's personal health record with entries made by healthcare professionals, and to keep copies of relevant test results.

Children have tended to be the *objects* of healthcare; their opinions have frequently been 'downgraded' by healthcare professionals. Yet children also 'acquire health-related knowledge through informal learning at home … they use their knowledge to promote their own well-being, in the context of and in interaction with social and physical features of their environment'.[2] Children actively participate in the maintenance of healthy lifestyles (their own and others'). A child-to-child approach to health education (albeit with reference to older children) is in operation worldwide, and acknowledges children as active participants in health promotion and maintenance of healthy lifestyles.[3]

GROWTH MONITORING

It is considered good clinical practice to monitor height and weight through childhood, and head circumference for the first 3 years. Most general practice record programs have embedded growth and development charts to assist in identifying deviations from normal that should invoke a second look.

Growth monitoring in children already identified as having a problem is mandatory, but when and how often do you monitor the typically normal child? Importantly, overweight is now considered as important as underweight. In a growth monitoring context it is easier to address developing overweight than to deal with established obesity.

- *Weight* is relatively easy to measure using modern self-zeroing electronic scales on a hard, rather than soft, surface. Babies should be weighed without clothes and nappies, toddlers and children with lightweight vest and pants, and adolescents in very light clothing without shoes.
- *Height* is best measured standing after 2 years using a fixed measuring scale that can be checked regularly with a standard measure (usually 60 cm).

  Between 0 and 18 months, supine length is the best measure and requires two people to accomplish a reliable result. Measuring boards are easy to construct, or more expensive devices are obtainable commercially.
- *Head circumference* is the largest measured length around the head using a disposable plastic or silicon device that does not stretch with repeated use.

Recording the measured growth parameters in the child's personal health record is important, as this is the only record that moves with the child from one healthcare professional to the next.

Most parents are interested in their children's growth and are keen to record progress over time. Maintaining growth records in the child's personal health record beyond infancy can be very informative, particularly if the numbers have been plotted appropriately on the percentile charts. Lack of growth information even after frequent visits to any healthcare professional is a source of considerable frustration for the paediatrician.

Growth monitoring is important as a vehicle for providing health and nutrition advice, together with an opportunity for discussing lifestyle or childcare issues. It may also provide early identification of a range of diseases, including growth hormone deficiency, thyroid insufficiency, emotional or social deprivation and abuse, occult gastrointestinal disease, renal disease and a variety of syndromes including Russell-Silver syndrome, Turner syndrome and atypical mosaicism.

ATOPY

The prevalence of asthma and eczema among children (Fig 55.1) is increasing around the world.[4] The notion of an 'atopic march' from eczema through to rhinitis has been coined,[5] implying that early intervention may reduce the prevalence of disease in later life.

In our striving for cleanliness there is increasing evidence that skin sensitisation to known environmental allergens provokes immune responses that lead to eczema and, later, asthma. Immune provocation in susceptible individuals appears to trigger a cascade of events aggravated by early antibiotic exposure that may lead to medium- and long-term atopy.[6]

ECZEMA

Forty-six per cent of children with eczema have used complementary medicines by the time of presentation to a dermatologist,[7] usually driven by their parents' sense that standard advice has failed. Adverse effects

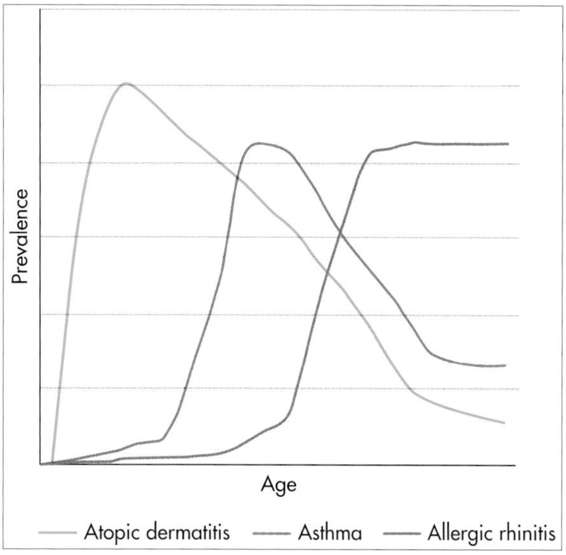

FIGURE 55.1 Incidence of different types of atopy

of eczema include symptoms of itching and soreness, which cause sleeplessness. Sleep deprivation leads to tiredness, mood changes and impaired psychosocial functioning of the child and family, particularly at school and work. At the more severe end of the spectrum, embarrassment, comments, teasing and bullying may cause social isolation and may lead to depression or school avoidance. The child's lifestyle is often limited, particularly with respect to clothing, holidays, staying with friends, owning pets, dietary exclusions, swimming or the ability to play or do sports. Restriction of normal family life, difficulties with complicated treatment regimens and increased work in caring for a child with eczema lead to parental exhaustion and feelings of hopelessness, guilt, anger and depression.[8]

Eczema usually presents by the age of 2 years, initially as an exudative vesicular rash on the face and hands, and later located at the antecubital fossae, neck, wrist and ankles. A generally dry skin is evident, together with signs of scratching and, later, lichenification.

ASSESSMENT

- Ask about:
  - family history
  - comprehensive dietary history
  - irritants or factors that make the rash worse. Assess home and school environment for potential irritants (soaps, shampoos, washing detergents, insecticides, air fresheners, tobacco smoke).
- Also gain a clear understanding of how the eczema is affecting both the child and their family in terms of stress, sleep and intervention.
- Arrange testing for food allergies. This may require a supervised elimination diet, blood tests or skin prick tests.
- Assess for zinc deficiency.

TREATMENT

Intervention is targeted at four levels: resolving any complicating infection, relieving symptoms, reducing triggers and developing a long-term plan. Each of these must be addressed and sustained, for any intervention to be effective. A clear understanding of the triggers by both child and carers, together with a contract of engagement, will ensure likely compliance and a better outcome.

Low-grade infection is common and will retard resolution if not treated. Topical antibiotic cream may be used for localised disease, but for more widespread eczema a systemic, broad-spectrum antibiotic (flucloxacillin, erythromycin) is required.

Medical management includes:

- avoiding irritant clothing (wool etc, which abrades skin and stimulates mast cell degranulation)
- wearing cool and loose cotton garments
- avoiding overheating
- keeping scratching to a minimum (use gloves if necessary and keep fingernails short).

Diet

- Identify likely allergens—using a food and symptom diary.
- Eliminate potential identified food allergens—including, for example, dairy, egg, gluten, colourings, preservatives and food additives. There is limited evidence for these factors but a therapeutic trial can be helpful where eczema is severe or proves resistant to treatment.
- Encourage fresh fruit and vegetables and whole grains.
- Omega-3 fatty acids—for example, fish oil supplementation and introduce fish into the diet.
- Probiotic supplement (containing *Lactobacillus acidophilus*).

Emollients

Use aqueous cream (in a preparation that suits after trying several formulations) as a soap substitute. Greasy preparations are best at night and for particularly dry skin. Creams are best applied during the day and on areas of inflammation. Three to four applications per day are desirable to ensure maximum moisturisation.

Topical steroids

Topical steroids are best used in the short term to suppress inflammation at the beginning of a flare—the intention is to keep the rash under tight control. Parents are often reluctant to use steroids until the condition is more severe; however, parents and carers should be encouraged to use topical steroids at the first sign of redness or itching. Control at this point prevents the inevitable cycle of exacerbation, itch, scratch, infection and worse eczema. Use the minimum concentration to achieve an effect, with an application twice daily.

Chinese herbal medicine

Individualised concoctions of Chinese herbal teas have been shown to be efficacious in a small number of randomised controlled trials from one centre.[9] In general there were about 10 plant extracts in each preparation and few side effects were noted. In other trials there was no clear benefit. However, there have been reports of hepatic and nephro-toxicity, and hypersensitivity reactions.

Other herbal medicines

Calendula, tea tree oil and chamomile have not been shown to be useful in atopic eczema, and may provoke contact dermatitis. Oatmeal baths may reduce pruritis.

Essential fatty acids

Patients with atopic dermatitis are thought to have a reduced rate of conversion from linoleic acid to gamma-linolenic acid (GLA), dihomo-gamma-linolenic acid, or arachidonic acid, compared with healthy subjects. Replacement of GLA, in the form of primrose oil or borage oil, may therefore benefit some patients. There are many randomised controlled studies assessing the effects of GLA, with most studies indicating an improved epidermal barrier on GLA application and others showing no effect, depending on the vehicle used for application.[10,11] Note that, in the latter study, evening primrose oil proved to have a stabilising effect on the stratum corneum barrier, but this was apparent only with the water-in-oil emulsion, not the amphiphilic emulsion for topical use. Oral evening primrose oil capsules do not, however, have a useful effect.

Other therapies

Acupuncture, homeopathy and colon cleansing are recommended by some but have no proven efficacy. Where family stressors appear to exacerbate scratching, these need to be acknowledged and addressed.

PREVENTION AND EDUCATION

Prevention and delay of symptoms are the cornerstones of appropriate management in a family setting, and pregnancy care is particularly relevant in this context.

- Prenatal cessation of smoking reduces allergy risk.
- Maternal omega-3 fatty acid supplementation may reduce the risk of food allergy and IgE-associated eczema during the first year of life in infants with a family history of allergic disease.[12]
- Some studies also suggest that babies whose mothers took probiotics during pregnancy and while breastfeeding were less likely to have eczema at up to 2 years of age[13] and beyond.[14]
- Higher maternal consumption of green and yellow vegetables, citrus fruit and beta-carotene during pregnancy may be protective against the development of eczema in offspring.[15] Prolonged breastfeeding is important but has not been shown to reduce the risk of atopic eczema in the early years.[16,17] Use of low-allergen milk in the first 6 months reduces the severity of eczema up to the age of 2 years in children with significant risk.

Supplementation with the probiotic *Lactobacillus rhamnosus* has been found to substantially reduce the cumulative prevalence of eczema, but not atopy, by 2 years in susceptible individuals with a family history of eczema when given to the mother during pregnancy and for 6 months after birth.[18] Other probiotics are less effective and the choice of *Lactobacillus* in this context seems to be important.[18]

Recent recommendations delay introduction of dairy products, eggs, nuts, fish and shellfish up to 36 months[19,20] in high-risk situations but not for infants with no family history. However, there is a contrary view that suggests that early antigen exposure in small amounts, in an immune tolerance exercise, might prevent disease later.[21]

High-dose steroids and immune modulation

Oral steroids and high-dose topical steroid treatment should be undertaken in consultation with a dermatologist. Topical calcineurin inhibitors (pimecrolimus 1% cream and tacrolimus ointment 0.1% and 0.03%) are potent topical immune modulators for more severe disease. They are non-steroid topical preparations that may reduce the need for potent topical steroids where poor control with standard treatment is evident.

SUMMARY

In summary, eczema is common and increasing. Dietary manipulation has little effect on outcomes except for those with more definitive family histories and where cow's milk proteins are shown to have a causative effect in exacerbating the rash, or where a specific food sensitivity or allergy is identified. Topical treatments, both standard and CAM, are effective in improving skin barrier function and are generally safe. Fastidious attention to skin care, early treatment of emerging patches and appropriate clothing will reduce the stress of eczema in young children and will set the pattern for care later in life if the problem persists beyond childhood.

ALLERGIC RHINITIS

A diagnosis of allergic rhinitis should be considered in children who seem to have a 'perpetual cold', have frequent sore throats, mouth breathing, snoring, headaches, halitosis or poor concentration. Allergic rhinitis commonly occurs intercurrently with asthma, and control of allergic rhinitis may improve asthma control.

There is often a history of allergy in the child (infantile eczema) or the family.

A seasonal pattern of symptoms suggests that pollens or grasses are the allergen. Perennial rhinitis is most likely due to house dust mite or pet dander, mould or cockroaches. Food intolerance may be involved.

DIAGNOSIS

Arrange for radioallergosorbent tests (RAST) to test for specific allergens.

TREATMENT

- Avoid allergens where possible—confirm the allergen before taking action that may be

inconvenient or distressing, such as removal of a household pet.
- Intranasal mometasone furorate spray continued for 3–6 months. Improvement may not be seen for 2 weeks.
- Non-sedating oral antihistamines (loratadine or cetirizine) can be used to relieve itching and sneezing or associated eye symptoms.
- Avoid topical or oral decongestant medication.

ASTHMA

(See also Ch 41, Respiratory medicine.)
Asthma is regarded as an inflammatory disorder of the airways, with oedema, hypertrophy of mucus glands, increased mucus secretion and smooth muscle constriction, resulting in recurrent episodes of cough, wheeze, chest tightness and breathlessness.

Symptoms tend to be worse at night or in the early morning, and may be triggered by exposure to allergens or changes in environmental temperature, emotional stressors or exertion. There is an inherited predisposition.

Between 100 and 150 million people around the globe suffer from asthma, and this number is rising. Worldwide, deaths from this condition have reached over 180,000 annually.[22]
- Around 8% of the Swiss population suffers from asthma, as against only 2% some 25–30 years ago.
- In Germany, there are an estimated 4 million asthmatics.
- In Western Europe as a whole, asthma has doubled in 10 years, according to the UCB Institute of Allergy in Belgium.
- In the United States, the number of asthmatics has leapt by over 60% since the early 1980s, and deaths have doubled to 5000 a year.
- There are about 3 million asthmatics in Japan, of whom 7% have severe and 30% have moderate asthma.
- In Australia, one child in six under the age of 16 years is affected.

Asthma is not just a public health problem for developed countries. In developing countries, however, the incidence of the disease varies greatly.
- India has an estimated 15–20 million asthmatics.
- In the Western Pacific Region of WHO, the incidence varies from over 50% among children in the Caroline Islands to virtually zero in Papua New Guinea.
- In Brazil, Costa Rica, Panama, Peru and Uruguay, prevalence of asthma symptoms in children varies from 20% to 30%.
- In Kenya, it approaches 20%.
- In India, rough estimates indicate a prevalence of 10–15% in children aged 5–11 years.

It is important to distinguish between asthma and other causes of recurrent cough, particularly recurrent infective bronchitis. Misdiagnosis of childhood asthma leads to inappropriate treatment or overtreatment.

DIAGNOSIS

In children aged under 6 years, respiratory function tests are not practical or reliable. Diagnosis depends on careful history taking. A currently asymptomatic child is unlikely to have significant clinical signs.

In a child under the age of 12 months, wheeze is more likely to be due to respiratory syncytial virus (RSV) bronchiolitis or anatomically small airways, and a diagnosis of asthma is best withheld. Bronchodilators tend to be ineffective in this age group.

Once children are over the age of 2 years, persistent or recurrent wheeze or chronic nocturnal cough is more likely to be due to asthma.

Children aged over 6 years can have spirometry testing.

Allergy testing should be organised.

All children diagnosed with asthma will need an asthma management plan carefully developed with the child and their parents or carers, and conveyed to all carers and schools. The asthma action plan (Fig 55.2) chosen should be appropriate for the person's age, educational status, language and culture.

Metered dose inhalers are difficult to administer to a child, so a volume spacer with a face mask is a preferable option (cannot be used in children under the age of 7 years, as coordination is inadequate). Proper use of spacers, preferably large volume, is important, although carrying one of these around is tiresome. A small-volume spacer should be used when out, and a large-volume spacer used when at home.

Management involves a strategy for preventing and relieving attacks, and for recognising deterioration in control and intervening with pre-formulated strategies.

PROPHYLAXIS

- *Pregnancy*—pregnant women should eat a diet rich in omega-3 fatty acids and take a supplement. It is not known definitively whether probiotics taken by pregnant women will have an effect on asthma incidence. Bottle-fed babies should be supplemented with *Lactobacillus*.
- *Diet*—encourage breastfeeding for the first 6 months. If there is a history of allergy or asthma in the family, wait until the baby is 12 months old before introducing cow's milk and other dairy products, soy products, eggs, nut spreads (e.g. peanut butter) and fish. A formal supervised

My Asthma Action Plan

When my asthma is WELL CONTROLLED

- No regular wheeze, or cough or chest tightness at night time, on waking or during the day
- Able to take part in normal physical activity without wheeze, cough or chest tightness
- Need reliever medication less than three times a week (except if it is used before exercise)
- Peak Flow* above ______

What should I do?

Continue my usual treatment as follows:

Preventer

Reliever

Combination Medication

Always carry my reliever puffer

When my asthma is GETTING WORSE

- At the first sign of worsening asthma symptoms associated with a cold
- Waking from sleep due to coughing, wheezing or chest tightness
- Using reliever puffer more than 3 times a week (not including before exercise)
- Peak Flow* between

______ and ______

What should I do?

Increase my treatment as follows:

See my doctor to talk about my asthma getting worse

When my asthma is SEVERE

- Need reliever puffer every 3 hours or more often
- Increasing wheezing, coughing, chest tightness
- Difficulty with normal activity
- Waking each night and most mornings with wheezing, coughing or chest tightness
- Feel that asthma is out of control
- Peak Flow* between

______ and ______

What should I do?

Start oral prednisolone (or other steroid) and increase my treatment as follows:

See my doctor for advice

How to recognise LIFE-THREATENING ASTHMA

Call an ambulance if you have any of the following danger signs:

- extreme difficulty breathing
- little or no improvement from reliever puffer
- lips turn blue

and follow the Asthma First Aid Plan below while waiting for ambulance to arrive.

A serious asthma attack is also indicated by

- symptoms getting worse quickly
- severe shortness of breath or difficulty in speaking
- you are feeling frightened or panicked
- Peak Flow* below ______

Should any of these occur, follow the Asthma First Aid Plan below.

Asthma First Aid Plan

1 Sit upright and stay calm.

2 Take 4 separate puffs of a reliever puffer (one puff at a time) via a spacer device. Just use the puffer on its own if you don't have a spacer. Take 4 breaths from the spacer after each puff.

3 Wait 4 minutes. If there is no Improvement, take another 4 puffs.

4 If little or no improvement **CALL AN AMBULANCE IMMEDIATELY** and state that you are having an asthma attack. Keep taking 4 puffs every 4 minutes until the ambulance arrives.

See your doctor immediately after a serious asthma attack.

FIGURE 55.2 Asthma management plan[23]
*Not recommended for children under 12 years of age
My Asthma Management Plan © Commonwealth of Australia, reproduced with permission.

elimination diet may be indicated where food triggers are suspected.
  - Ensure optimal nutrition. Encourage fresh fruit and vegetables and wholefoods.
  - Eliminate food additives, colourings and preservatives.
- *Medication*—non-steroidal medications will be the preferred first-line preventer. These include sodium chromoglycate and nedocromil sodium (children over 2 years). They are less used in preference to Montelukast, a leukotriene antagonist (LTA), which is particularly useful in intermittent asthma associated with exercise. LTAs orally are an option in children aged over 6 years.
  - If there is no clinical improvement after 4 weeks, consider using the lowest effective dose of inhaled corticosteroids.
  - As in the case of topical steroids for children with eczema, many parents are naturally concerned about giving children with asthma inhaled steroids, and will need accurate information to encourage compliance with preventer medication.
- *Environment*—assess for environmental triggers. Eliminate exposure to tobacco smoke, pet fur and other pollutants. Keep bedrooms and bedding as dust-free as possible, preferably washable hard surfaces on the floor. Contrary to popular belief, feather doonas/duvets and pillows are preferable to synthetic varieties.Wash and thoroughly dry linen regularly. Eliminate cockroaches from the home. Avoid the use of aerosol insecticides.
- *Mind–body*—assess and deal with environmental stressors.
- *Exercise*—ensure regular exercise. Warm up slowly before vigorous activity. Use a bronchodilator before exercise, if exercise is a trigger for acute attacks.

SUPPLEMENTATION

Dietary supplementation with omega-3 fatty acids, zinc and vitamin C has been shown to significantly improve asthma control, pulmonary function tests and pulmonary inflammatory markers in children with moderately persistent bronchial asthma, either singly or in combination.[24] Similarly, adequate intake of vitamin D and sun exposure are important in reducing the risk of asthma.

Magnesium with supportive B-group nutrients assists smooth muscle relaxation, particularly when acutely affected by an asthma attack.

MANAGING ACUTE ASTHMA ATTACKS IN A CHILD

Beta$_2$ agonist inhalers (salbutamol) and a spacer device should be available to the child at all times. Assessment and initial management of a child with acute asthma are summarised in Tables 55.1 and 55.2.

Children who are acutely distressed require immediate oxygen and short-acting beta$_2$ agonist (SABA) before completing a full assessment.

Note that proper use of a spacer is essential: one puff into the spacer, then six breaths, then the next puff and six breaths, and so on. Do not administer six puffs into the chamber at one time.

TABLE 55.1 Assessment of acute asthma in children

Symptoms	Mild	Moderate	Severe and life-threatening*
Altered consciousness	No	No	Agitated Confused/drowsy
Oximetry on presentation (SaO_2)	94%	94–90%	< 90%
Talks in	Sentences	Phrases	Words Unable to speak
Pulse rate	< 100 bpm	100–200 bpm	> 200 bpm
Central cyanosis	Absent	Absent	Likely to be present
Wheeze intensity	Variable	Moderate to loud	Often quiet
PEF**	> 60% predicted or personal best	40–60% predicted or personal best	< 40% predicted or personal best Unable to perform
FEV_1	> 60% predicted	40–60% predicted	< 40% predicted Unable to perform

*Any of these features indicates that the episode is severe. The absence of any feature does not exclude a severe attack.

**Children under 7 years old are unlikely to perform PEF or spirometry reliably during an acute episode. These tests are usually not used in the assessment of acute asthma in children.

Source: National Asthma Council Australia[25]

ANAPHYLAXIS IN CHILDREN

(See also Ch 21, Allergies.)

Anaphylaxis may occur as an acute allergic response to food allergens, medication, envenomation, vaccines, food additives and others.[27] In some cases the causative agent is not identified.

Clinical

Presenting symptoms involve acute onset of:

- skin and/or mucosal changes (flushing, urticaria, angio-oedema, pallor, clamminess) *AND*
- life-threatening **A**irway and/or **B**reathing and/or **C**irculation problems.

Recognition of acute anaphylaxis may involve exposure to a known allergen for the patient and presence of gastrointestinal symptoms (incontinence, abdominal pain).

Common food triggers include nuts, shellfish, eggs, wheat and dairy protein. Prescribed drug reactions are common. There is often a personal history of eczema or atopy.

Investigation

Episodes of anaphylaxis need to be investigated so that identifiable triggers can be assiduously avoided. Skin prick tests for inhaled and food allergens.

TABLE 55.2 Initial management of children with acute asthma

Treatment	Mild episode	Moderate episode	Severe and life-threatening episode
Hospital admission necessary	Probably not	Probably	Yes: consider intensive care
Supplementary oxygen	Probably not required	May be required. Monitor SaO_2	Required. Monitor SaO_2. Arterial blood gases may be required.
Salbutamol*	4–6 puffs (under 6 years) or 8–12 puffs (6 years and over). Review in 20 mins	6 puffs (under 6 years) or 12 puffs (6 years and over). If initial response inadequate, repeat at 20-minute intervals for two further doses. Then give every 1–4 hours.	6 puffs (under 6 years) or 12 puffs (6 years and over) every 20 mins for 3 doses in first hour. If life-threatening episode, use continuous nebulised salbutamol. If no response, bolus IV salbutamol 15 μg/kg over 10 mins then 1 μg/kg/min thereafter.
Ipratropium	Not necessary	Optional	2 puffs (under 6 years) or 4 puffs (6 years and over) every 20 minutes × 3 doses in first hour or nebulised ipratropium
Systemic corticosteroids	Yes (consider)	Oral prednisolone 1 mg/kg daily for up to 3 days	Oral prednisolone 1 mg/kg/dose daily for up to 5 days Methylprednisolone IV 1 mg/kg 6-hourly on day 1, 12-hourly on day 2, then daily
Magnesium	No	No	Magnesium sulfate 50% 0.1 mL/kg (50 mg/kg) IV over 20 mins, then 0.06 mL/kg/h (30 mg/kg/h): target serum Mg 1.5–2.5 mmol/L
Aminophylline	No	No	Only in intensive care: loading dose 10 mg/kg Maintenance 1.1 mg/kg/h if under 9 years, or 0.7 mg/kg/h if 9 years or over
Chest X-ray	Not necessary unless focal signs present	Not necessary unless focal signs present	Necessary if no response to initial therapy or pneumothorax is suspected
Observations	Observe for 20 mins after dose	Observe for 1 hour after last dose	Arrange for admission to hospital

*In children with severe acute asthma that does not respond to initial treatment with inhaled SABA, bolus IV salbutamol 15 μg/kg over 10 mins is effective and can avoid the need for continuous IV salbutamol and ICU admission.

Source: National Asthma Council Australia[26]

Treatment

Whether in or out of hospital, help is called immediately and treatment initiated while awaiting advanced equipment and expertise. As soon as the clinical signs support the diagnosis of anaphylaxis, intramuscular adrenaline should be administered immediately while awaiting advanced equipment and expertise before an ambulance arrives.[28]

In the event of a cardiac arrest following anaphylaxis, cardiopulmonary resuscitation should be commenced, with adrenaline given intravenously or intraosseously according to standard advanced paediatric life support guidelines. Concurrently, high-flow oxygen and intravenous access should be obtained so that rapid fluid resuscitation can be given, to restore intravascular volume.

Bronchospasm should be treated as per the emergency management of severe asthma.

For children at increased risk of anaphylaxis, formal assessment by a paediatric allergy specialist is required before providing an adrenaline auto-injector. All family members, teachers and carers need to be trained in avoidance of triggers, and in the first aid assessment and management of anaphylaxis, as they could be called upon to perform life-saving procedures.

IRON DEFICIENCY

Iron deficiency is the most common nutrient deficiency in preschoolers, despite dietary advice from a wide range of sources. The prevalence varies between 16% and 22%, and it is more common in underprivileged and ethnic minorities. It is also a useful marker for general nutrition, as other nutritional deficiencies often may coexist with iron deficiency.

It is recognised that iron deficiency is associated with a range of developmental and behavioural problems in infancy and childhood that are reversible with iron supplementation and correction of the iron deficiency. Intellectual deficits arising from iron deficiency in infancy do persist into later years, if treatment is delayed. A high degree of suspicion is useful in infancy, as anaemia is a late manifestation of iron deficiency. Risk factors include prolonged breastfeeding without supplementation, more than six breastfeeds per day after 6 months, high cow's milk intake after 12 months and poor solid intake because of high milk intake. Primary prevention of iron deficiency in infants and toddlers can be addressed by a range of measures (Box 55.2), and screening after 12 months is reasonable, particularly in high-risk groups. While prolonged breast feeding is beneficial, without an appropriate solid intake after 6–12 months iron deficiency is much more likely, and so care is required in advising about nutritional supplementation. Some infants become more iron deficient than others, probably because of feeding practices after birth but also because of the degree of intrauterine iron accumulation in the last trimester before birth. Preterm birth and intrauterine growth restriction interrupt normal iron stores and therefore are likely to lead to frank deficiency later if not addressed earlier.

BOX 55.2 Primary prevention for iron-deficiency anaemia

- Iron supplementation for preterm infants until 6 months
- Avoidance of unmodified cow's milk until after 12 months
- Avoidance of tea
- Use of infant formula or follow-on milks that are iron supplemented
- Weaning to mixed-food diet at 6 months
- Ensure a source of vitamin C to aid iron absorption
- Use haem iron (meat) for iron bioavailability
- Iron supplementation as necessary

There are some medical causes of iron deficiency in children that need to be considered in differential diagnosis, particularly where response to iron supplementation is ineffective. These include:

- coeliac disease
- lead poisoning
- gastrointestinal blood loss (Meckel's diverticulum, gastric bleeding).

SCREENING FOR HEARING LOSS

Many states in the United States have passed early hearing detection and intervention legislation. The NHS Newborn Hearing Screening Program (NHSP) offers all new parents the opportunity to have their baby's hearing screened within the first few weeks of life. It is a core service within the NHS in England and part of the family of Antenatal and Newborn Screening Programs.

Universal Neonatal Hearing Screening (UNHS) is now well established in Australia, the United States and Europe. There are slight variations in protocols between states, but overall most use a system of automated auditory brain stem evoked responses (AABAER) using commercial screening apparatus. UNHS detects *congenital sensorineural hearing loss* (SNHL) and ensures that babies are enrolled in a diagnostic pathway leading to early hearing aids or cochlear implantation in a timeframe that ensures language acquisition. Cochlear implantation produces best results when intervention occurs before 6 months. It is essential that babies identified in this way are fast-tracked into hearing services and ENT consultation, and engaged in early signing to ensure meaningful communication. While babies with obvious congenital abnormalities, preterm babies and babies admitted to a neonatal intensive care units can be readily identified as being at high risk of hearing impairment, between 1 and 3 per 1000 live births of otherwise normal babies are congenitally deaf. The results of early intervention programs and cochlear implantation are gratifying[16] and allow these children to move seamlessly into normal schools, achieving normal social and educational skills.

The identification of hearing loss in an otherwise well newborn infant can be catastrophic for parents. There is a period of uncertainty as the diagnosis is confirmed by second-tier testing. Parents require support and accurate information (contact local hearing screening services; see the Resources list).

Acquired conductive hearing loss is more common. At least 50% of preschool children have one or more episodes of otitis media with effusion (OME). About 7% have more frequent episodes leading to significant hearing loss. Risk factors in children include recurrent ear infections, abnormal mucosal immunity and anatomical abnormalities leading to failure of adequate clearance of the eustachian tubes. Children at particular risk are those with Down syndrome, Turner's syndrome, cleft palate and orofacial malformations. The administration of antibiotics for OME is seldom helpful. A combination of antibiotics and steroids is equally unhelpful in the longer term. Most guidelines recommend a period of watchfulness of at least 3 months. In general, OME resolves without significant impact. In children whose hearing is impaired, tympanostomy tubes are indicated. Care should be taken to encourage formal hearing testing. This may indicate the need for hearing aids together with specific educational strategies to assist learning at school.

Acquired sensorineural hearing loss is gaining more interest. Hearing loss due to congenital rubella is seldom seen; however, cytomegalovirus infections are much more common and may lead to progressive SNHL during the first 2 years after birth. Recently, many more children have been diagnosed with unilateral SNHL at birth and later. There is increasing evidence that in these children, hearing in both ears fluctuates over time and may lead to bilateral SNHL later. Moreover, children with unilateral SNHL are being shown to be disadvantaged and frequently have social and developmental problems that reflect unrecognised hearing impairment. Children with known unilateral SNHL must be followed carefully and encouraged to undertake regular hearing testing. Consideration of hearing aids in this group would be prudent and family support in managing these children is important. In particular, families should be encouraged to learn to sign in addition to speaking early in the child's development, to attenuate the impact of fluctuating hearing.

The development of a robust neonatal hearing screening service broadly eliminates the utility of distraction testing during the first year of life.[29] The latter is usually poorly performed in less than ideal settings and has poor sensitivity. Allaying parental concerns about hearing should not be attempted by using this as a screening test.

SCREENING FOR EYE AND VISION PROBLEMS

Amblyopia is a form of cerebral visual impairment caused by abnormal vision, commonly uncorrected refractive error, during a sensitive period of development. Treatment is thought to be effective only during this sensitive period, which varies for different types of amblyopia but most commonly lasts until 7 years of age. The most common forms of amblyopia are monocular, due to squint (strabismic amblyopia), or refractive error, with a prevalence of 2–4%. Such impairment is later a bar to certain occupations, affects binocular vision and stereopsis and causes considerable disability if the normal eye suffers trauma or disease.[30] While definite disabilities caused by vision defects in childhood are largely unknown, more recent attention has focused on the possibility that vision problems contribute to behavioural problems or dyslexia (see below).

Intervention in children with *strabismus* is controversial. Treatment in those with considerably reduced acuity (6/18 and worse) can result in a mean acuity equivalent to 6/9 on the Snellen chart, whereas children with 6/9 or 6/12 show little benefit from treatment.[30] Children whose treatment is deferred from age 4 until age 5 years have the same acuity after treatment, but fewer need patching treatment at all. More than a third of children thought to require treatment after repeat screening do not have acuity loss.[31] Therefore screening is important, and inspection of the eyes in preschool children is useful in detecting squint likely to lead to impairment later. A careful corneal reflection test, cover test and prism test as well as eye movement tests will delineate abnormalities. In children with a family history of squint, children with developmental delays and preterm infants are at particular risk and may need referral to a specialist optometrist or paediatric ophthalmologist.

INFANTILE COLIC

Infantile colic is a condition in which a baby cries constantly at about the same time each day (usually in the evenings) and is very difficult to settle but otherwise healthy. The baby appears to be in pain and may pull their legs up and clench their fists. There may be loud bowel sounds. It usually begins in the first weeks of life, and goes away by 4–5 months of age.[32]

About one in five babies develops colic; it is more common in boys and in firstborn children. Breastfed infants have similar rates of colic as formula-fed infants. The cause is not known.

Medication is ineffective for colic and may have serious side effects, so resist the temptation to prescribe.

Exclude medical causes for symptoms, such as reflux, skin condition or urinary tract infection. Check growth to ensure adequate feeding.

Therapeutic strategies might include having the baby in a sitting position to feed and burp regularly. If the mother is breastfeeding, she can try avoiding caffeine, chocolate, dairy products, citrus fruits, broccoli, cauliflower, cabbage, nicotine and spicy foods in her diet, which may affect the breast milk. Check that formula is being prepared correctly. Elimination of cow's milk protein is effective not only in highly selected subgroups of infants but also in primary care settings.

Acidophilus (especially *bifidus* species) can be given to both the breastfeeding mother and the baby (infant formula).

A warm bath and movement such as slow rocking and gentle abdominal massage may help soothe the baby. Stress management techniques for the parents can be helpful. Parents will need to harness social support from friends or family if the situation becomes difficult for them.

ENURESIS

Nocturnal enuresis can be considered normal up to the age of 5 years. It occurs in up to 20% of 5-year-olds and 10% of 10-year-olds, with a spontaneous remission rate of 14% per year. Weekly daytime wetting occurs in 5% of children, most (80%) of whom also wet the bed.[33]

Primary enuresis refers to the child who has never been dry for more than a few months at a time. Important risk factors for primary nocturnal enuresis include family history, nocturnal polyuria, impaired sleep arousal and bladder dysfunction.

Secondary enuresis refers to a child who has been completely dry for more than 6 months and then starts to wet the bed again. An emotional event, urinary tract infection, diabetes mellitus, social changes or constipation may trigger this kind of bedwetting. Sexual abuse should be considered.

INVESTIGATION

- Urine microscopy and culture to exclude infection.
- A frequency/volume chart (with documentation of the time and volume of all fluid intake and urine output in 24-hour periods) can give objective information about frequency of urination and functional bladder capacity. Overnight urine production (to assess nocturnal polyuria) is measured by adding the volume of the first morning void with the overnight volume, calculated by the before-and-after weight of a nappy worn overnight by the child.

MANAGEMENT

In secondary enuresis management is to treat the underlying cause, and the enuresis tends to cease.

The initial treatment of choice for children with mono-symptomatic nocturnal enuresis is an enuresis alarm. Two types of alarm are available, to be used for a minimum of 14 consecutive dry nights to a maximum of 4 months:

- pad-and-bell alarm—the child lies on a large pad placed in the bed and any liquid triggers the alarm
- personal alarm—the alarm is clipped onto the child's underpants or onto a continence pad placed inside the child's underpants, and any liquid triggers the alarm.

Medication

Desmopressin:

- nasal spray 10–40 μg at night (start with 10 μg nightly and titrate up to 40 μg)
- tablet 200–400 μg at night
- available on authority prescription for children over 6 years who have failed alarm treatment or where alarm therapy is contraindicated.

Referral

Referral for specialist advice is highly recommended for treatment failure after 8–12 weeks for any form of bedwetting or daytime incontinence.

DYSLEXIA

Children whose reading is behind for their expected IQ, and who have symptoms of incoordination, poor sequencing and left-to-right confusion, are termed *dyslexic*. The problem affects 5–10% of children (mainly boys), who may present as depressed or develop compensatory behavioural symptoms that cause them to be labelled as lazy, 'difficult', defiant, 'stupid' or inattentive. Many more children than are diagnosed have dyslexia problems and few receive appropriate interventions in remediation. Inability to recognise the meaning of written words or to interpret unfamiliar words has physiological and anatomical correlates that can readily be identified and mapped to abnormalities in chromosome 6 and others. Recent insights have enabled the development of interventions that will attenuate symptoms and facilitate the child's progress in a mainstream educational environment. The more recent concept of visual stress (Box 55.3) can explain

BOX 55.3 Visual stress symptom questionnaire

Score 0–4 for each item.

Non-critical questions

1 Does reading make your child tired?
2 Does reading become harder the longer he/she reads?
3 Does your child lose his/her place when reading?

Critical questions to ask of the older child

1 Does print move about when you read?
2 Does print become fuzzy or blurry when you read?
3 Does the white page between the lines of print form patterns like rivers?
4 Does the white page glare against the black letters?
5 Do you get sore or tired eyes when reading for a long time?
6 Do you get headaches when reading for a long time?

a number of behaviours that are seen in children with degrees of dyslexia.

Dyslexic children identified as having high visual stress showed significantly higher percentage increases in reading rate with a coloured overlay, and reported significantly higher critical symptoms of visual stress compared to dyslexic children with low visual stress.[34] Thus, while phonological deficits underlie most issues for children with dyslexia, aids to visual interpretation such as coloured overlays or tinted lenses may make a significant difference in about 50%.[35] The other important development is in the arena of fatty acid supplementation. It is increasingly obvious that the diets of today's children are markedly different from those of previous generations. The epidemic of obesity (see below) is serious and coincides with more attention deficit disorders and dyslexia than before. There is mounting evidence that essential fatty acid deficiency may contribute to neurodevelopmental and psychiatric problems including dyslexia, and that supplementation may have significant and long-lasting benefit.[36,37] However, care needs to be taken in delivering essential fatty acids that are likely to be effective. A combination of 80% fish oil and 20% evening primrose oil has been used in most studies.

DEVELOPMENTAL DISORDERS AND DISABILITIES

In considering child development disorders, Hall and Elliman[38] distinguished between low-prevalence high-severity conditions (cerebral palsy, learning disabilities; see Box 55.4) for which a pathological basis can be identified, and high-prevalence low-severity conditions (speech delay, clumsiness; see Box 55.5) for which a pathological basis is rarely found.

BOX 55.4 Low-prevalence, high-severity conditions

- Cerebral palsy (1.5–3 per 1000)
- Duchenne muscular dystrophy (3 per 10,000 males)
- Severe learning disability (3.5–4.5 per 1000)
- Speech and language impairment (2 per 1000)
- Autism (1–2 per 1000)

Less common:

- Osteogenesis imperfecta
- Head injury
- Juvenile arthritis
- Chromosomal abnormalities previously lethal
- Cystic fibrosis

BOX 55.5 High-prevalence, low-severity conditions

- Learning difficulty
- Dyslexia
- Speech delay
- Mild global delay
- Clumsiness
- Mild behaviour difficulties

Low-prevalence, high-severity conditions usually receive attention in current healthcare settings, but high-prevalence, low-severity conditions receive little or cursory attention and yet could lead to more complex problems later. It is essential to respond to parental or carer concerns regarding growth and development. The most useful tests in this environment are the Macarthur communicative developmental inventory (MCDI) up to age 3 years, and the parents' evaluation of developmental status (PEDS) after 4 years.

LANGUAGE DEVELOPMENT

Language development is varied and influenced by both genes and environment. Although delayed language development is common as an isolated problem, many children have other issues including cognitive impairment (low IQ limiting language acquisition), behaviour and conduct disorders acting as comorbid conditions retarding normal language interaction. Parents, under the guidance of speech therapists, can be engaged in interventions that will improve outcome, bearing in mind that most children will eventually communicate reasonably well even after moderate delay. Often therapy involves dealing simultaneously with parenting, behavioural issues and deprivation. Care must be taken in identifying children from socially deprived environments who would benefit from early intervention services, playgroups or preschools.

BEHAVIOUR AND PSYCHOLOGICAL PROBLEMS

The point prevalence for psychological problems in childhood and adolescence is about 20%; it is worse in socially deprived areas. It has been estimated that 68% of preschool children have at least one identifiable problem, and close to one-third have three or more problems. Indeed, such problems characterise 50% of referrals to a paediatrician.[39]

Point prevalences for a range of conditions are shown in Table 55.3.

While some of these might be considered minor or mild, they are the source of considerable misery and reflect a poor quality of existence for many parents and children in our community.[39] These problems interact with physical ill health and produce symptoms that span organic and psychological illness. They are characteristically persistent and polymorphous even though they may have started as discrete single problems.

TABLE 55.3 Point prevalence of a range of childhood conditions

Condition	Prevalence (%)
Preschool children (< 5 years)	
Waking and crying	15
Overactivity	13
Difficulty settling at night	12
Refusal of food	12
Combination behavioural problems	10
Middle childhood (6–12 years)	
Persistent tearful unhappy moods	12
Bedtime behavioural rituals	8
Night terrors and sleep disturbance	6
Bedwetting	5
Inattentive overactivity	5
Faecal soiling	1
Overt psychological disorder	12–25
Overt handicapping psychiatric disorder	7–14
Mild emotional behavioural problems*	5–11
Adolescence (13–18 years)	
Appreciable misery	45
Social sensitivity	30
Evident anxiety	25
Suicidal ideation	7
Complex depressive moods	10
Confirmed psychiatric disorder	2–3

*Including anxious unhappiness, difficult or antisocial behaviour, poor relationships with other children.

Source: adapted from Hall & Elliman 2006[38]

Predisposing factors include:

- poor parenting skills
- inner city
- social deprivation
- boys rather than girls
- children with learning difficulties and delayed speech skills
- other problems of health and development
- adolescence
- in residential or institutional foster care
- marital discord
- mental health problems in other family members
- parental indifference
- poor parental supervision.

Single-issue presentations may reflect a more complex underlying psychopathology and should be addressed with vigour. In many instances this will divert the development of more polymorphous behavioural issues that may be difficult to address later. Established polymorphous presentations will be complex and time consuming. Intervention in single-issue presentations is often successful if other predisposing issues are recognised and addressed at the same time. The role of the general practitioner and the paediatrician in this context is to develop a holistic management strategy that involves structured encounters with locally placed services and supports.

ATTENTION DEFICIT HYPERACTIVITY DISORDER

There is rising concern that the diagnosis of attention deficit hyperactivity disorder (ADHD) in young children is increasing and that intervention using potent stimulant medication is over-used. The causes of ADHD are multifactorial.

- There is certainly a genetic component[40] or a genetic risk factor in most individuals.
- Most children with ADHD have a demonstrable brain-based anatomical/biochemical problem.
- Environment plays a significant part in the expression of ADHD.
- Excessive television watching (screen time) increases the risk.
- Exposure to toxins and dietary deficiencies is increasingly important.

The diagnosis of ADHD is complex and reflects the difficulty of separating comorbidities that may in fact be the primary problem leading to behavioural and educational issues that need addressing. How, then, can the GP intervene and muster allied healthcare services and family support before referring to a paediatrician for consideration of more aggressive pharmacological intervention? There is no doubt that psychostimulant medication is efficacious in the short term in attenuating the symptoms of ADHD in children with uncontrollable or dangerous behaviour. In the long term, children with diagnosed ADHD, whether treated or not, have worse outcomes than those not diagnosed with ADHD. Treatment effect is short term and may allow children to function at home or at school more effectively, reducing stress on affected children and their families and improving social behaviour. However, the long-term results are not positive. The West Australian Raine study[41] found that, by age 14 years, stimulant medication did not significantly improve a child's level of depression, self-perception or social functioning, and that these children were more likely to be performing below their age level at school by a factor of 10.5 times compared with children who had not taken stimulant medication.

Psychological support alone is helpful, and a combination of both modalities provides the best outcome. However, psychosocial support is often lacking or difficult to access, and educational supports are stretched.

INITIAL ASSESSMENT

- Ensure that symptoms cross the school, home and social environments. Confirmatory evidence that behaviours are pervasive is important. Ask parents to obtain letters of concern from teachers and other carers.
- Examine the nutrition of the household. Ask about fast foods and determine the types of meals offered. Discuss breakfast, family meals, TV and computer game culture in the household.
- Assess iron status.
- Assess magnesium status. Magnesium deficiency in children with ADHD occurs more frequently than in healthy children.[44] Supplementation has been shown to reduce hyperactivity.[43]
- Understand the social and family interactions that describe the family. Review behavioural boundaries, expectations of parents for their children and consistency of rules.

ADHD THERAPEUTICS

- Ensure that the child is not iron deficient. Behavioural problems can be attenuated by restoring an adequate iron intake by supplementing and correcting diet.
- Consider a 1-month supervised trial of a diet eliminating gluten, casein, artificial colourings and preservatives.
- Consider fish oil (containing omega-3 and omega-6 fatty acids)[44] and multivitamin supplement.
- Limit time spent watching television and playing computer games.
- Encourage outdoor activities in a natural environment.
- Attention training techniques such as meditation help to ameliorate the symptoms.

There is some evidence that mind–body therapies can assist in modulating activity and oppositional behaviours. This requires the engagement of the family and provides a mechanism to involve them in structural change that provides both containment and restriction of escalation of adverse behaviours. Referral to family therapy, psychologists or educational interventions are beneficial where resources are available.

AUTISM AND AUTISM-SPECTRUM DISORDERS

The spectrum covers a range of neurological disorders characterised by qualitative impairments in social functioning and communication, often accompanied by repetitive and stereotypical behaviours and interests. The condition affects 1 in 150 children in a male–female ratio of 3:1. Autism-spectrum disorders (ASDs) can be diagnosed as early as 18 months, and children identified early benefit from early intervention programs that engage positive behaviours in a therapeutic alliance suppressing more negative ones. Symptoms can range from mild to severe.

- In *autism* the impairments in the social and communication areas are severe and sustained, and clearly present before the age of 3 years. The child is often anxious, has poor attention and motivation, responds unusually to many different stimuli, and is observed as being 'different' from other children. Speech is delayed, or largely absent. A strong reliance on routine is apparent, and the child can have a range of ritualistic behaviours such as toe walking, hand flapping and finger gazing. The child with autism may also be intellectually disabled.
- *High-functioning autism* is a loosely used term (not defined in the diagnostic criteria) to describe a child or adult who meets the criteria for a diagnosis of autism, but is not as severely affected as the more classically autistic person.
- In *Asperger syndrome* there is considerable social impairment, but impairment is not as severe in the language and communication area. Speech usually develops within the normal age range, but the ability to communicate effectively (known as language pragmatics) is impaired. The impairments seem more subtle in the very young child, and become more apparent as the child reaches school

age. Such individuals are usually in the normal intelligence range.

- *Pervasive developmental disorder—not otherwise specified* (PDD-NOS) is a diagnosis given for children who present with some of the characteristics of either autism or Asperger syndrome but not severe enough for a diagnosis of either condition.

Parents often express concern about their child's development and can identify behaviours that are worrying. These should never be dismissed and careful review may inform appropriate referral. The checklist for autism in toddlers (CHAT) (see Table 55.4) can be used to screen for likely ASD traits.

TABLE 55.4 Checklist for autism in toddlers (CHAT)

A screening test designed to be used in children from 18 months to 36 months. Darker-shaded response boxes indicate critical questions most indicative of autistic characteristics.

CHAT Section A: Questions for parents	
	Yes or No
Does your child enjoy being swung, bounced on your knee, etc.?	
Does your child take an interest in other children?	
Does your child like climbing on things, such as chairs?	
Does your child enjoy playing peek-a-boo / hide & seek?	
Does your child ever pretend, for example, to make a cup of tea using a toy cup and teapot, or pretend other things (pouring juice)? [Pretend Play (PP)]	(shaded)
Does your child ever use his or her index finger to point, to ask for something?	
Does your child ever use his or her index finger to point, to indicate interest in something? [Protodeclarative Pointing (PDP)]	(shaded)
Can your child play properly with small toys (e.g. cars or blocks) without just mouthing, fiddling or dropping them?	
Does your child ever bring objects to you (parent), to show you something?	

Shaded boxes indicate critical questions most indicative of autistic characteristics

CHAT Section B: Physician's questions/observations	
	Yes or No
Eye contact: During the appointment, has the child made eye contact with you?	
Gaze monitoring (GM): Get the child's attention, then point across the room at an interesting object and say, 'Oh look! There's a (name of a toy)!' Watch the child's face. Does the child look across to see what you are pointing at? (To record a YES, make sure the child does not just look at your hand, but at the object you are pointing at.)	(shaded)
Pretend play (PP): Get the child's attention, then give the child a miniature toy cup and teapot and say, 'Can you make a cup of tea?' Does the child pretend to pour out tea and drink it? (If you can elicit an example of pretending in some other game, score a YES on this item.)	(shaded)
Protodeclarative pointing (PDP): Say to the child, 'Where's the light?' or 'Show me the light'. Does the child point with their index finger at the light? (Repeat this with, 'Where's the bear?' or some other unreachable object if the child does not understand the word 'light'. To record a YES on this item, the child must have looked up at your face at around the time of pointing.)	(shaded)
Block tower: Can the child build a tower of blocks? (If so, how many?)	

Overall, the more 'NOs' the higher the chance of autism.

In the Baron Cohen studies:

Failing all questions with shaded boxes: risk of autism 80–85%.

Passing all questions with shaded boxes: risk of autism 0%.

Sources: Baron Cohen S et al. 1992[45], 2000[46]; Baird et al. 2000[47]

MANAGEMENT OF AUTISM

Irrespective of the diagnosis or where it fits in the spectrum, each child diagnosed within the autism spectrum is likely to be developmentally delayed and have significant difficulties in participating in day-to-day life. Each child requires sensitive understanding, and specialist support and intervention.

What can the GP do before referral to a paediatrician?

- Refer early for assessment.
- Check chromosomes—high resolution and fragile X.
- Check iron, ferritin and transferrin saturation levels.
- Check thyroid function.
- Arrange carer's allowance and allied health support team.
- Evaluate diet and nutritional status.

There is no medication that can alleviate the symptoms of autism.

The child and family require intensive multidisciplinary support to help with the educational and social development of children with autism. This will require coordination of services such as intensive physiotherapy, occupational therapy, speech therapy and psychological and educational interventions.

There is anecdotal evidence that some (but not all) children respond to dietary change, to varying degrees. It is a low-risk and reasonable strategy to recommend a 1-month trial of:

- a strict gluten-free, casein-free, soy-free diet
- elimination of all artificial colourings, flavourings and preservatives.

Consultation with a dietician is likely to be helpful, to ensure adequate nutrition, particularly if the child is very fussy with their food.

Multivitamin, mineral and omega-3 fatty acid supplementation may be necessary where the diet is deficient.

OBESITY

The epidemic of childhood obesity in the developed world cannot be ignored. Obesity rates for preschool children have doubled internationally, and rates for children aged 6–11 years have tripled since 1996. Overweight adolescents have a 70% chance of becoming obese adults, increasing to 80% where one or more parent is also obese or overweight. Sixty per cent of obese children have one or more additional cardiovascular risk factors (high cholesterol, triglycerides, insulin or blood pressure) identifiable at screening. Serious complications of obesity (type 2 diabetes, metabolic syndrome, fatty liver, slipped epiphyses, hypertension, polycystic ovarian syndrome etc) can be identified in many (Box 55.6).

Body mass index (BMI) is a robust predictor of continuing risk from overweight and obesity into adolescence. Children noted to be overweight at 24, 36 or 54 months are five times more likely to be obese in adolescence than children with normal BMI during infancy.[48] The formula for calculating body mass index (BMI) between 2 and 20 years is shown in Box 55.7. A useful BMI calculator with downloadable BMI curves for children can be found at the Melbourne Royal Children's Hospital website (see Resources list). BMI categories are listed in Table 55.5.

The causes of overweight and obesity are multifactorial (genetic predisposition, overeating, sedentary lifestyle, excessive screen time, fast-food availability, poor overall nutrition, inadequate nutrition knowledge, family role-modelling, school and home environments, food marketing and advertising). The goals of preventing and reversing obesity and overweight appear straightforward—reduce energy intake while maintaining an optimal nutritional intake to support growth and development. Reduce sedentary behaviours, actively engage families, parents, carers and communities in strategies to enhance and apply knowledge and understanding of optimal nutrition during childhood.[49]

BOX 55.6 Physical, social and emotional health consequences of obesity in children and adolescents

Physical health:

- glucose intolerance and insulin resistance
- type 2 diabetes
- hypertension
- dyslipidaemia
- hepatic steatosis
- cholelithiasis
- sleep apnoea
- menstrual abnormalities
- delayed or altered puberty
- impaired balance
- orthopaedic problems

Emotional health:

- low self-esteem
- negative body image
- depression

Social health:

- stigma
- negative stereotyping
- discrimination
- teasing and bullying
- social marginalisation

BOX 55.7 Calculating body mass index (BMI): 2–20 years

$$\text{BMI} = \frac{\text{weight (kg)}}{\text{height (m)} \times \text{height (m)}}$$

Assessment and intervention begins as follows:

- evaluating the child's growth pattern, including plotting BMI for age on an appropriate growth chart
- determining suspected cause(s) of abnormal weight gain
- assessing risk factors and comorbid conditions
- assigning proper diagnosis and excluding known medical syndromes (e.g. Prader-Willi syndrome)
- assessing motivation and readiness to change (see Table 55.6)
- educating parents in nutritional principles and parenting skills.

NUTRITION AND INTEGRATIVE MEDICINE

Integrative medicine is most helpful in obesity management. It is clear that simple interventions for such a complex problem are unlikely to work and that patients identifying as overweight or obese need a nurturing and supportive framework to effect change. It is likely that isolated advice for a single person without involvement of the whole family is thwarted from the outset. If the entire family is ready to engage in change to a better process, there are interventions that can be tailored to each participant based on their own insights and beliefs.

- Diet:
  - Recommend an anti-inflammatory diet[50]
  - Polyunsaturated fatty acid supplement
  - Balanced carbohydrate, protein and fat for age
  - Subsitute energy-dense foods and drinks with wholefoods and water.
- Motivational interviewing:[51,52]
  - Directive counselling
  - Focus on patient's perceptions and motivations
  - Seek to resolve ambivalence
  - Strengthen patient's reasons for positive behaviour change
  - Trigger change aligned with patient's own goals and values.
- Health coaching:
  - Take an active role in patient's progress
  - Keep patient on track
  - Individualised attention
  - Follow-up phone calls, specific appointments.
- Mind–body medicine:
  - Mindfulness
  - Guided relaxation and imagery
  - Clinical hypnosis
  - Yoga
  - Progressive muscle relaxation
  - Biofeedback
  - Cognitive behaviour therapy.
- Acupuncture.

There are adequate data to support the inclusion of these techniques in clinical practice. Their use in paediatrics and paediatric obesity is less researched but intuitively sound and promising.

EXERCISE AND PHYSICAL ACTIVITY

Physical activity is essential in long-term maintenance of weight control in children, and interventions aimed at either increasing physical activity or decreasing physical inactivity or sedentary behaviours) are useful in treating paediatric obesity.[53] There is definitive evidence that obesity is an inflammatory condition characterised by elevated inflammatory markers such as interleukin-6

TABLE 55.5 BMI categories

Category	BMI
Underweight	< 5th percentile for age and gender
Normal weight	≥ 5th percentile to < 85th percentile for age and gender
At risk of overweight	85th percentile to < 95th percentile for age and gender
Overweight	95th percentile for age and gender

TABLE 55.6 Factors associated with readiness for change and engagement

Factor	Family response	Physician response
Pre-contemplation	Not interested	Deliver information about known health risks. Personalise to examination and assessment
Contemplation	Interested in the next 6 months or so	Deliver messages of health risk and identify barriers to change and engagement
Preparation	Willing to try out and plan over the next month	Assist children and family to set reasonable goals—start with one or two easy targets.
Action	Already trying to lose weight	Give positive reinforcement and set new targets
Maintenance	Successful weight management needs help in maintenance	Provide support and monitoring

and C-reactive protein, and that these inflammatory markers diminish with any exercise.[54]

The structure of an exercise program is also important for developing an active lifestyle in treating obesity. Data from several trials incorporating moderate to intense aerobic exercise suggest that school-based exercise interventions may be a promising approach to treating childhood obesity.[55,56] In addition, the family is important to structure and support activity, as parental activity level is a strong predictor of child activity.[57,58] In the healthcare setting, interventions focused on increasing physical activity should be delivered in a nurturing, non-intimidating environment. Obese children respond differently physiologically and emotionally to exercise than do normal-weight children, and experience negative consequences to participation in activities considered appropriate for normal-weight children. In clinical settings, specialised exercise programs that include specific recommendations for obese children have been shown to enhance safety, efficacy and compliance during treatment. Optimal results may be achieved by combining programs to reduce sedentary behaviours with those that increase physical activity,[59] such as walking or cycling to school instead of travelling by car.

A healthcare plan for the treatment of childhood obesity should examine and modify, as necessary, the home environment as it pertains to physical activity. Some children spend more time in front of the television and playing video games than doing any other activity other than sleeping. Watching television often decreases the amount of time spent performing physical activities, and is also associated with increased food consumption either during viewing or as a result of food advertisements.[60] Children who watched 4 or more hours of television per day had significantly greater BMI than those watching less than 2 hours per day.[61] Furthermore, having a television in the bedroom has been reported to be a strong predictor of being overweight, even in preschool-aged children.[62] Note that fatness leads to inactivity, rather than inactivity leading to fatness,[63] but inactivity reduces fitness and increases cardiovascular inflammatory risk, whether fat or thin.

A practical approach to encouraging exercise in children has been outlined by Philpott and colleagues.[64] The easiest way to promote physical activity is to increase movement in daily life. If possible, children should walk or cycle to school, and use stairs instead of lifts. Children allowed to play outdoors usually increase their level of activity spontaneously. Increase participation in household chores from an early age. Involve children in meal preparation and clearing up, thereby reducing potential screen time while increasing responsibility and accountability. Moderate to vigorous activity for 60 minutes each day is the goal that produces the best effect, even if broken down into four 15-minute periods. Plan family activities and use the outdoors. Make practical recommendations for exercise. A written prescription will help to focus goals and stimulate discussion at subsequent visits.

Understand motivational interviewing and use tools for ensuring engagement by children and their families. Individualise the activities to suit the personality of each child—consider their like and dislikes. Consider age-appropriate interventions and recognise particular goals of older children, whether muscle building, endurance or fast exercise. Encourage dance in all its current forms

TABLE 55.7 Immunisation schedule for children up to 4 years old (Australia)

Age	Disease immunised against
Birth	Hepatitis B
2 months	Diphtheria Tetanus Pertussis Polio Hib Hepatitis B Pneumococcal Rotavirus
4 months	Diphtheria Tetanus Pertussis Polio Hib Hepatitis B Pneumococcal Rotavirus
6 months	Diphtheria Tetanus Pertussis Polio Hib Hepatitis B (or at 12 months) Pneumococcal Rotavirus
12 months	Measles Mumps Rubella Hib Hepatitis B (or at 6 months) Meningococcal C
18 months	Varicella
4 years	Diphtheria Tetanus Pertussis Polio Measles Mumps Rubella

Source: Australian Government[65]

and, if necessary, use interactive video games that encourage movement. There is no single 'one-fits-all' solution. Being aware of family dynamics and personal relationships is also important. Engage all the family together, rather than targeting individuals alone.

IMMUNISATION

Specific details of national immunisation programs differ between countries. An indicative schedule for children aged 0–4 years in Australia[54] is given in Table 55.7.

RESOURCES

Infant hearing

Infant hearing program Utah, USA http://www.infanthearing.org/

NHS UK, http://hearing.screening.nhs.uk/

Royal Children's Hospital, Melbourne, http://www.rch.org.au/ccch/research/infanthearing/index.cfm?doc_id=713

Obesity

Royal Children's Hospital, Melbourne, BMI calculator and curves, http://www.rch.org.au/genmed/clinical.cfm?doc_id=2603

The Children's Hospital at Westmead, http://www.chw.edu.au/parents/kidshealth/childhood_obesity/

Autism

Autism Victoria, http://www.autismvictoria.org.au/services/getting_assessed.php

Australian Government, Department of Health and Ageing, http://www.health.gov.au/autism

REFERENCES

1 Royal Australian College of General Practitioners. Red book. Melbourne: RACGP. Online. Available: http://www.racgp.org.au/redbook/download/2009Redbook_7th_ed_chart_children.pdf

2 Mayall B. Children, health and the social order. Buckingham, UK:Open University Press; 1996.

3 Pridmore P, Stephens D. Children as partners for health: a critical review of the child-to-child approach. London: Zed Books; 2000.

4 Innes Asher M, Montefort S, Björkstén B et al., the ISAAC Phase Three Study Group. Worldwide time trends in the prevalence of symptoms of asthma, allergic rhinoconjunctivitis, and eczema in childhood: ISAAC Phases One and Three repeat multicountry cross-sectional surveys. Lancet 2006; 368:733–743.

5 Spergel JM, Paller AS. Atopic dermatitis and the atopic march. J Allergy Clin Immun 2003; 112(6 Suppl 1):S118–S127.

6 Kummeling I, Stelma FF, Dagnelie PC et al. Early life exposure to antibiotics and the subsequent development of eczema, wheeze, and allergic sensitization in the first 2 years of life: the KOALA Birth Cohort Study. Pediatrics 2007; 119(1):e225–e231.

7 Johnston GA, Bilbao RM, Graham-Brown RAC. The use of complementary medicine in children with atopic dermatitis in secondary care in Leicester. Br J Dermatol 2003; 149(3):566–571.

8 Lewis-Jones S. Quality of life and childhood atopic dermatitis: the misery of living with childhood eczema. Int J Clin Pract 2006; 60(8):984–992.

9 Sheehan M, Atherton D. A control trial of traditional Chinese herbal medicinal plants in widespread non-exudative eczema. Br J Dermatol 1992; 126:179–184.

10 Levin C, Maibach H. Exploration of 'alternative' and 'natural' drugs in dermatology. Arch Dermatol 2002; 138(2):207–211.

11 Gehring W, Bopp R, Rippke F et al. Effect of topically applied evening primrose oil on epidermal barrier function in atopic dermatitis as a function of vehicle. Arzneimittelforschung 1999; 49(7):635–642.

12 Furuhjelm C, Warstedt K, Larsson J et al. Fish oil supplementation in pregnancy and lactation may decrease the risk of infant allergy. Acta Paediatr 2009; 98(9):1461–1467.

13 Rautava S, Kalliomäki M, Isolauri E. Probiotics during pregnancy and breast-feeding might confer immunomodulatory protection against atopic disease in the infant. J Allergy Clin Immunol 2002; 109:119–121.

14 Kalliomäki M, Salminen S, Poussa T et al Probiotics and prevention of atopic disease: 4-year follow-up of a randomised placebo-controlled trial. Lancet 2003; 361(9372):1869–1871.

15 Miyake Y, Sasaki S, Tanaka K et al. Consumption of vegetables, fruit, and antioxidants during pregnancy and wheeze and eczema in infants. Allergy 2010; 22 Jan. [Epub ahead of print]

16 Snijders BEP, Thijs C, Kummeling I et al. Breastfeeding and infant eczema in the first year of life in the KOALA birth cohort study: a risk period-specific analysis. Pediatrics 2007; 119(1):e137–e141.

17 Ludvigsson JF, Mostrom M, Ludvigsson J et al. Exclusive breastfeeding and risk of atopic dermatitis in some 8300 infants. Pediatr Allery Immunol 2005; 16(3): 201–208.

18 Probiotic Study Group. Wickens K, Black PN, Stanley TV et al. A differential effect of two probiotics in the prevention of eczema and atopy: a double-blind, randomized, placebo-controlled trial. J Allergy Clin Immunol 2008; 122(4):788–794.

19 Committee on Nutrition. Hypoallergenic infant formulas. Pediatrics 2000; 106(2):346–349.

20 Fiocchi A, Assa'ad A, Bahna S. Food allergy and the introduction of solid foods to infants: a

consensus document. Adverse Reactions to Foods Committee, American College of Allergy, Asthma and Immunology. Ann Allergy Asthma Immunol 2006; 97(1):10–20.
21 Niggemann B, Staden U, Rolinck-Werninghaus C et al. Specific oral tolerance induction in food allergy. Allergy 2006; 61(7):808–811.
22 World Health Organization. Bronchial asthma. Fact Sheet 206; January 2000. Online. Available: https://apps.who.int/inf-fs/en/fact206.html
23 Australian Government, Department of Health and Ageing. My asthma management plan; 2006. Online. Available: http://www.health.gov.au/internet/main/publishing.nsf/Content/957D057CE967D0FECA256F1900136C63/$File/Action%20plan%20form%20page%2020%20Feb%202009.pdf
24 Biltagi MA, Baset AA, Bassiouny M. Omega-3 fatty acids, vitamin C and zinc supplementation in asthmatic children: a randomized self-controlled study. Acta Paediatr 2009; 98(4):737–742.
25 National Asthma Council Australia. Acute asthma. Managing children. Initial assessment. Online. Available: http://www.nationalasthma.org.au/cms/index.php?option=com_content&task=view&id=203&Itemid=151
26 National Asthma Council Australia. Acute asthma. Managing children. Management. Online. Available: http://www.nationalasthma.org.au/cms/index.php?option=com_content&task=view&id=94&Itemid=103 last updated 31 May 2007.
27 Novembre E, Cianferroni A, Bernardini R et al. Anaphylaxis in Children: Clinical and Allergologic Features. Pediatrics. 1998; 101;8-DOI : 10.1542/peds.101.4.e8
28 Tse Y, Rylance G. Emergency management of anaphylaxis in children and young people: new guidance from the Resuscitation Council (UK). Arch Dis Child Educ Pract Ed 2009; 94:97–101.
29 Russ SA, Poulakis Z, Wake M et al. The distraction test: the last word? J Paediatr Child Health 2005; 41(4):197–200.
30 Clarke MP, Wright CM, Hrisos S et al. Randomised controlled trial of treatment of unilateral visual impairment detected at preschool vision screening. BMJ 2003; 327(7426):1251–1254.
31 Williams C, Northstone K, Harrad RA et al. Amblyopia treatment outcomes after screening before or at age 3 years: follow up from randomised trial. BMJ 2002; 324(7353):1549–1551.
32 Lucassen PL. Effectiveness of treatments for infantile colic: systematic review. BMJ 1998; 316(7144):1563–1569.
33 Caldwell PH, Edgar D. Bedwetting and toileting problems in children. Med J Aust 2005; 182(4):190–195.
34 Singleton, Henderson L-M. Computerized screening for visual stress in children with dyslexia. Dyslexia 2007; 13(2):130–151.
35 Whiteley H, Smith C. The use of tinted lenses to alleviate reading difficulties. J Res Reading 2001; 24(1):30–40.
36 Joshi K, Lad S, Kale M et al. Supplementation with flax oil and vitamin C improves the outcome of attention deficit hyperactivity disorder (ADHD). Prostaglandins, Leukot Essent Fatty Acids 2006; 74(1):17–21.
37 Richardson AJ, Montgomery P. The Oxford-Durham Study: a randomised, controlled trial of dietary supplementation with fatty acids in children with developmental coordination disorder. Pediatrics 2005; 115(5):1360–1366.
38 Hall D, Elliman D. Health for all children. Rev. edn. Oxford: OUP; 2006.
39 Hewson PH, Anderson PK, Dinning AH et al. A 12-month profile of community paediatric consultations in the Barwon region. J Paediatr Child Health 1999; 35(1):16–22.
40 Greenhill LL, Pliszka S, Dulcan MK et al. Practice parameter for the use of stimulant medications in the treatment of children, adolescents, and adults. J Am Acad Child Adolesc Psychiatry 2002; 41(2 Suppl):26S–49S.
41 Government of Western Australia, Department of Health. Raine ADHD Study: long-term outcomes associated with stimulant medication in the treatment of ADHD in children. Online. Available: http://www.health.wa.gov.au/publications/documents/MICADHD_Raine_ADHD_Study_report_022010.pdf
42 Kozielec T, Starobrat-Hermelin B. Assessment of magnesium levels in children with attention deficit hyperactivity disorder. Magnes Res 1997; 10(2):143–148.
43 Starobrat-Hermelin B, Kozielec T. The effects of magnesium physiological supplementation on hyperactivity in children with attention deficit hyperactive disorder (ADHD): positive response to magnesium oral loading test. Magnes Res 1997; 10(2):149–156.
44 Johnson M, Ostlund S, Fransson G et al. Omega-3/omega-6 fatty acids for attention deficit hyperactivity disorder: a randomized placebo-controlled trial in children and adolescents. J Atten Disord 2009; 12(5):394–401.
45 Baron-Cohen S, Allen J, Gillberg C. Can autism be detected at 18 months? The needle, the haystack and the CHAT. Br J Psychiatry 1992; 161:839–843.
46 Baron-Cohen S, Wheelwright S, Cox A et al. Early identification of autism by the CHecklist for Autism in Toddlers (CHAT). J R Soc Med 2000; 93:521–525.
47 Baird G, Charman T, Baron-Cohen S et al. A screening instrument for autism at 18 months of age: a 6-year

follow-up study. Am Acad Child Adolesc Psychiatry 2000; 39:694–702.

48 Nader PR, O'Brien M, Houts R et al. Identifying risk for obesity in early childhood. Pediatrics 2006; 118(3):e594–e601.

49 Kirk S, Scott BJ, Daniels SR. Pediatric obesity epidemic: treatment options. J Am Diet Assoc 2005; 105(5 Suppl 1):44–51.

50 Rakel D. Integrative medicine. 2nd edn. Philadelphia: Saunders; 2007.

51 Resnicow K, Davis R, Rollnick S. Motivational interviewing for pediatric obesity: conceptual issues and evidence review. J Amer Diet Assoc 2006; 106(12):2024–2033.

52 Schwartz RP. Motivational interviewing (patient-centred counseling) to address childhood obesity. Pediatr Ann 2007; 39; 3:154–158.

53 Krebs NF, Jacobson MS. American Academy of Pediatrics Committee on Nutrition. Prevention of pediatric overweight and obesity. Pediatrics 2003; 112(2);424–430.

54 Farpour-Lambert NJ, Aggoun Y, Marchand LM et al. Physical activity reduces systemic blood pressure and improves early markers of atherosclerosis in pre-pubertal obese children. J Am Coll Cardiol 2009; 54:2396–2406.

55 Carrel AL, Clark RR, Peterson SE et al. Improvement of fitness, body composition and insulin sensitivity in overweight children in a school-based exercise program. Arch Pediatr Adolesc Med 2005; 159(10):963–968.

56 Evans RK, Franco RL, Stern M et al. Evaluation of a 6-month multi-disciplinary healthy weight management program targeting urban, overweight adolescents: Effects on physical fitness, physical activity, and blood lipid profiles. Int J Pediatr Obesity 2009; 4(3):130–133.

57 Cleland V, Venn A, Fryer J et al. Parental esercise is associated with Australian children's extracurricular sports participation and cardiorespiratory fitness. A cross-sectional study. Int J Behav Nutr Phys Act 2005; 2(1):3.

58 Dowda M,Ainsworth BE, Addy CL et al. Environmental influences, physical activity and weight status in 8–16 year olds. Arch Pediatr Adolesc Med 2001; 155:711–717.

59 Nemet D, Barkan S, Epstein Y et al. Short- and long-term beneficial effects of a combined dietary-behavioural physical activity intenvention for the treatment of childhood obesity. Pediatrics 2005; 115:443–449.

60 Giammattei J, Blix G, Marshak HH et al. Television watching and soft drink consumption. Associations with obesity in 11–13 year old schoolchildren. Arch Pediatr Adol Med 2003; 157:882–886.

61 van Zutphen M, Bell AC, Kremer PJ et al. Association between the family environment and television viewing in Australian children. J Paediatr Child Health 2007; 43:458–463.

62 Dennison BA, Erb TA, Jenkins PL. Television viewing and television in bedroom associated with overweight risk among low income preschool children. Pediatrics 2002; 109:1028–1034.

63 Metcalf BS, Hosking J, Jeffery AN et al. Fatness leads to inactivity, but inactivity does not lead to fatness: a longitudinal study in children (earlybird 45). Arch Dis Child 2010. [epub before print doi.1136/adc2009.175927]

64 Philpott J, Wilson E, Luke A. The importance of exercise: know how to say 'Go'. Pediatr Ann 2010; 39(3):162–171.

65 Australian Government, Medicare Australia. Current immunisation schedule. National Immunisation Program (NIP) Schedule (0–4 years) (from July 2007). Online. Available: http://www.medicareaustralia.gov.au/provider/patients/acir/schedule.jsp

chapter 56

Adolescent health and development

INTRODUCTION AND OVERVIEW

The essence of good adolescent healthcare consists of:

- understanding adolescent development
- recognising the intimate relationship between development, health and behaviour at this time of life
- encouraging self-responsibility and self-care using a resiliency-based approach
- providing a friendly and accessible service.

Adolescent health falls outside biological paradigms, clinical medicine and its usual classifications, and outside the classic distinctions between physical and mental health, between medical and social aspects of health, and between curative and preventive care. Adolescent healthcare is a bio-psychosocial field, one which, by its very nature, requires an integrative approach.

While young people are often considered a relatively healthy population group, current indices are poor for at least 20–30% of young people. Their health problems are mainly psychosocial and, certainly in clinical settings, likely to be overlooked. Young people are notoriously reluctant to seek services to address these social and psychological self-concerns.[1,2] They are also involved in health risk behaviours earlier than in past generations. Many engage in behaviour that threatens their health and wellbeing, and there is increasing evidence that many problem behaviours in young people are interrelated. Young people with conduct disorders, for example, are also likely to engage in tobacco, alcohol and substance use, to engage in high-risk sexual behaviour and to experience academic failure.[3]

A note about terminology: the term *young person* refers to someone aged 12–25 years. The word *adolescent* will be used where it is more appropriate to refer specifically to the developmental processes occurring during these years.

NORMAL ADOLESCENT DEVELOPMENT

Adolescence has been described as:

> a period of personal development during which a young person must establish a sense of individual identity and feelings of self-worth which include an alteration of his or her body image, adaptation to more mature intellectual abilities, adjustments to society's demands for behavioural maturity, internalising a personal value system, and preparing for adult roles.[4]

Adolescence begins with the onset of puberty and ends with the acquisition of adult roles and responsibilities. It is characterised by rapid change in the following domains:[5]

- *physical*—puberty (physical growth, secondary sexual characteristics and reproductive capability)
- *psychological*—development of independence and autonomy
- *cognitive*—moving from concrete to abstract thought, developing more strategic decision-making skills
- *emotional*—shifting from narcissistic to mutually caring relationships
- *social*—peer group influences, formation of intimate relationships, decisions about future vocation
- *cultural*—discovering, negotiating and settling into role/s within cultural context/s.

THE EXPERIENCE OF PUBERTY

Puberty involves the most rapid and dramatic physical changes that occur during the entire lifespan outside the womb. Average duration is about 3 years and there is great variability in time of onset, velocity of change and age of completion. Height velocity and weight velocity increase and peak during the growth spurt.

1 Prepubertal, no pubic hair

2 Sparse growth of minimally pigmented hair, mainly on the labia

3 Considerably darker and coarser hair spreading over the mons pubis

4 Thick adult-type hair that does not yet spread to the medial surface of the thighs

5 Adult-type hair distributed on classical inverse triangle

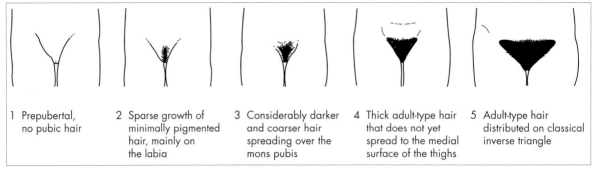

FIGURE 56.1 Tanner stages of pubic hair development in girls

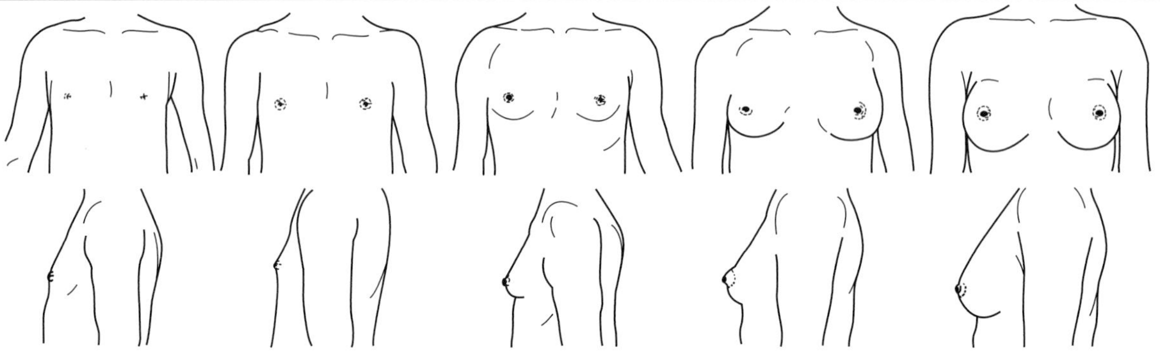

1 Prepubertal, elevation of papilla only

2 Breast buds are noted or palpable, enlargement of the areola

3 Further enlargement of the breast and areola with no separation of the contours

4 Projection of the areola and papilla to form a secondary mound above the level of the breast

5 Adult contour breast with projection of papilla only, areola recesses to breast contour

FIGURE 56.2 Tanner stages of breast development in girls

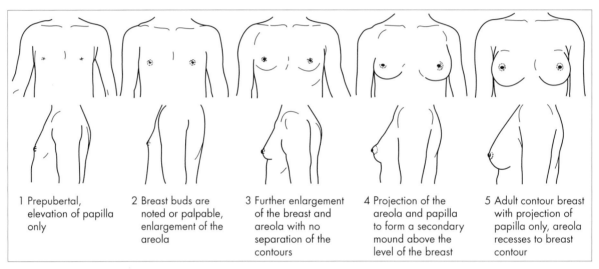

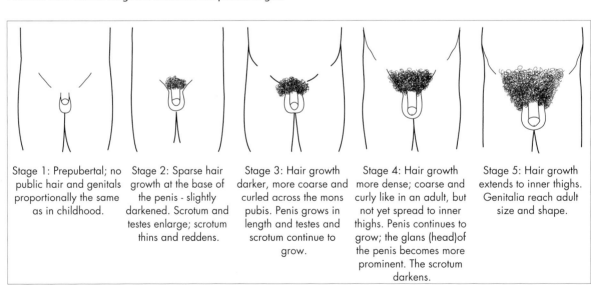

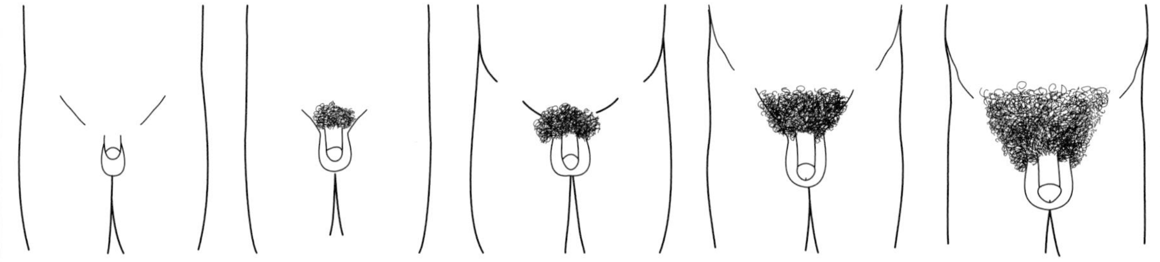

Stage 1: Prepubertal; no public hair and genitals proportionally the same as in childhood.

Stage 2: Sparse hair growth at the base of the penis - slightly darkened. Scrotum and testes enlarge; scrotum thins and reddens.

Stage 3: Hair growth darker, more coarse and curled across the mons pubis. Penis grows in length and testes and scrotum continue to grow.

Stage 4: Hair growth more dense; coarse and curly like in an adult, but not yet spread to inner thighs. Penis continues to grow; the glans (head)of the penis becomes more prominent. The scrotum darkens.

Stage 5: Hair growth extends to inner thighs. Genitalia reach adult size and shape.

FIGURE 56.3 Tanner stages of pubertal development in boys

The classic milestones of puberty are determined by Tanner's sex maturity ratings. Tanner's staging system is based on breast, genital and pubic hair changes, with Stage 1 being prepubertal and Stage 5 adult (Figs 56.1, 56.2 and 56.3).[6] In girls, peak height velocity usually occurs at Stage 2–3 (around 12 years) and menarche (initiation of menstruation) at Stage 4. In boys, peak height velocity occurs at Stage 3–4 (14 years) and semenarche (initial ejaculation) at Stage 3.

The experience of puberty is to have a changing body that feels out of control. Feelings of helplessness or persecution are common and may not abate until about 12 months after the growth spurt has ended. The typical irritability, moodiness and occasional aggressiveness, sexual arousal and unpredictable behaviour of the early adolescent are largely due to hormonal changes. Puberty tends to be conceptualised as a biological event, with emotional and psychological 'side effects'. However, puberty may also be regarded as a cultural phenomenon, with each young person's experience being influenced by the cultural milieu in which it occurs. In many cultures, for example, an event such as menarche remains somewhat taboo, while changing body shape for girls and boys may bring high levels of anxiety in our image-driven society.

The psychosocial impact of the timing of puberty affects girls and boys differently.

For those who mature earlier than average:

- boys seem to benefit—more relaxed, independent, self-confident and physically attractive
- girls seem to be disadvantaged—seen as less popular, appear withdrawn, less positive body image, lack confidence
- both are more likely to engage in more adult behaviours, although they tend to be physically rather than cognitively ready, associating with older peers.

For those who mature later than average:

- boys seem to be disadvantaged—less well liked and viewed as anxious, overly talkative and attention seeking
- girls seem to benefit—regarded by peers and adults as physically attractive, lively, sociable and leaders at school.

STAGES OF ADOLESCENCE

Psychosocial development can also be highly variable in progression from one stage to the next (Table 56.1). Key features are as follows:

- *early*—coming to terms with the physical changes of puberty
- *middle*—establishing oneself among one's peers as a worthwhile individual
- *late*—defining functional roles in terms of work, lifestyle and relationships.

Physical, cognitive and psychological changes may be 'out of sync'. For example, an early-developing, mature-looking girl may be psychologically immature and vulnerable.

NEURODEVELOPMENT

Our understanding of adolescent risk taking has been greatly enhanced by recent findings from neuroscience—research using magnetic resonance imaging (MRI) on the brains of children at 2-year intervals. While some areas of the human brain are mature by the end of childhood, the prefrontal cortex—responsible for such things as impulse control and strategic planning—continues to mature through the teenage years and beyond. This makes sense of adolescence as 'a time of heightened opportunity' (teenagers are more amenable to change), but also 'a time of heightened risk'. An immature brain together with hormones that stir the teenager up and drive them to be a thrill-seeker (especially for boys) is a potentially dangerous mix.

A SNAPSHOT OF HEALTH ISSUES IN ADOLESCENCE[7]

Adolescent health is, ideally, understood via the dual concepts of health and wellbeing. It is estimated that approximately 75% of deaths among young people in developed countries are from preventable causes, mostly non-intentional injury. Drug-related deaths account for almost 25% of all deaths among young people, and youth suicide is another major cause of mortality. Young people are experiencing mental health problems at higher rates than older age groups and retaining their increased risk beyond youth into older age[8]—at any one time, up to 20% of young people will suffer from a mental disorder. Together, mental health and behavioural disorders account for more than half of all afflictions affecting adolescents. Poor nutrition is now also coming to be recognised as a significant risk factor for poor mental health in adolescents.[9]

In most developed countries, over one-third of young people report using marijuana in the previous 12 months, while around 70% of 16–17 year olds report that they consume alcohol. Drug and alcohol use is also of concern because it can seriously exacerbate depression and suicidal behaviour. While teenage smoking rates tend to be on the decline, tobacco use is another prime target for research, with close to 20% of 17-year-olds being established smokers.

Sexual health is another important and challenging issue. The number of notifications for chlamydia among 15–24 year olds has increased by more than 300% between 1999 (when national data have been available) and 2008. Young people, especially young

TABLE 56.1 Adolescent development stages[6]

Early (10–14 years)	Middle (15–17 years)	Late (> 17 years)
	CENTRAL QUESTION	
• 'Am I normal?'	• 'Who am I?' • 'Where do I belong?'	• 'Where am I going?'
MAJOR DEVELOPMENT SERIES		
• Coming to terms with puberty • Struggle for autonomy commences • Same-sex peer relationships all-important • Mood swings	• New intellectual powers • New sexual drives • Experimentation and risk-taking • Relationships have self-centred quality • Need for peer group acceptance • Emergence of sexual identity	• Independence from parents • Realistic body image • Acceptance of sexual identity • Clear educational and vocational goals, own value system • Developing mutually caring and responsible relationships
	MAIN CONCERNS	
• Anxiety about body shape and changes • Comparison with peers	• Influence of peers • Tensions between family and individual • Over-assertion of autonomy • Balancing demands of family and peers • Prone to fad behaviour and risk-taking • Strong need for privacy • Maintaining ethnic identity while striving to fit in with dominant culture	• Self-responsibility • Achieving economic independence • Developing intimate relationships
	COGNITIVE DEVELOPMENT	
• Still fairly concrete thinking • Less able to understand subtlety • Daydreaming common • Difficulty identifying how one's immediate behaviour affects the future	• Able to think more rationally • Concerned about individual freedom and rights • Able to accept more responsibility for consequences of one's own behaviour • Begins to take on greater responsibility within family as part of cultural identity	• Longer attention span • Able to think more abstractly • Better able to synthesise information and apply it to oneself • Able to think about the future and anticipate consequences of their actions
	PRACTICE POINTS	
• Reassure about normality • Ask more direct than open-ended questions • Make explanations short and simple • Base interventions needed on immediate or short-term outcomes • Help identify possible adverse outcomes if they continue the undesirable behaviour	• Address confidentiality concerns • Always assess for health risk behaviour • Focus interventions on short- to medium-term outcomes • Relate behaviours to immediate physical and social concerns, e.g. effects on appearance, relationships	• Ask more open-ended questions • Focus interventions on short- and long-term goals • Address prevention more broadly

women, are more likely to contract STIs and, while rates of teenage childbirth have declined in recent decades, teenage pregnancy remains a major adolescent health concern in developed nations. Restricting our focus to these biological indicators alone, however, ignores the complex, dynamic contexts in which sexuality is being experienced by young people.

In addition, an obesity epidemic is currently affecting 25% of young people, a figure rising every year, and 15–20% of young people have a chronic illness. Chronic illness can have a serious social and emotional impact on young people, who wish to see themselves as 'normal', and can trigger withdrawal from medical care.

THE CLINICAL CONSULTATION

In contrast to most general practice consultations, the aim of the consultation with a young person who you have not seen since they entered adolescence, or who is new to your practice, is to engage them. A relationship of trust must first be established, otherwise many potentially serious health issues can be missed and opportunities for prevention and health promotion forgone.

Adolescent patients have neither the naivety of the child nor the awareness or experience of the adult. However, it probably takes about three seconds for a young person to 'suss out' the kind of encounter it is going to be. Young people have a sixth sense about it and can read the clues: how the doctor greets them, whether or not they are given a chance to talk for themselves, how questions are put and how the physical examination is conducted.

Many healthcare professionals feel ill-equipped to deal with young people in their practices, particularly in relation to sexuality and substance use.[2] Young people want to address health behaviours with their doctor but often feel too embarrassed to initiate discussion in these sensitive areas. And while parents also want clinicians to discuss a broad range of health issues with their adolescent children, many fail to do so.

COMMUNICATION SKILLS WITH YOUNG PEOPLE

Communication skills are essential in general practice. A summary of communication skills that are particularly pertinent to the consultation with a young person is given here.

Negotiating time alone

Within culturally appropriate boundaries, the general practitioner should facilitate the process of a young person taking responsibility for their healthcare by negotiating increasing lengths of time spent alone in a consultation.

Normalise the practice and take charge. For example: 'I start seeing all my teenage patients by themselves for some of the consultation, so I would like to spend a few minutes with X today before seeing both of you together.'

Reassure parents/carers about the importance of their involvement. For example: 'My spending time alone with <your child> helps them develop a relationship with a doctor on their own and is an important part of their growing up. However, your support is essential to <your child's> health and wellbeing, as is your involvement in their healthcare. I will make sure we have time to discuss any concerns you have, at the end of the consultation.'

Confidentiality

Worldwide and within cultures, young people say that confidentiality is the most important aspect of their relationship with a health professional. Maintaining confidentiality reflects respect for the adolescent's privacy and acknowledges their increasing capacity to exercise rational choice and give informed consent. It is important to offer guidance and support and, as appropriate, encourage a young person to seek parental support. While many general practitioners are aware of the importance of confidentiality for young people, they may not routinely discuss it at the beginning of the engagement process.

A suggested form of words is: 'Anything we discuss will be kept confidential. That means that I will not repeat anything you tell me to anyone else, unless I think it would help you and you give me permission to do so. There are, however, a few situations where I will not be able to keep confidentiality, and these are:

- if I am concerned that you could harm yourself or someone else
- if I am concerned that you are being harmed or at risk of being harmed because of somebody else (and you are under 16).

In these situations it would be my duty to ensure that you (or the other person) are safe. I would tell you if I need to notify somebody about something that you've told me, and I would make sure that you have as much support as possible.'

Acknowledge feelings that may hinder communication

Many young people arrive at a consultation feeling anxious, especially if they have come to discuss something sensitive and without their parent's knowledge. Alternatively, if they have been brought to see you by a parent, they may feel resentment or hostility. Acknowledging any obvious affect helps to break down initial barriers. For example:

- 'You seem a bit anxious. Perhaps it's because you're seeing a new doctor on your own or for some other reason. How are you feeling at the moment?'
- 'You look upset or angry. Perhaps it's because your mum made this appointment for you. Can I ask how you're feeling about being here?'

Clarify reasons for attending

This is particularly pertinent when a young person has been brought by a parent or carer and there appear to be confusing or mixed 'agendas'. It can be useful to ask the young person and then their parent why they have come.

Culturally sensitive communication

In exploring cultural issues around diagnosis and treatment:[10]

- ask about the meaning of a young person's symptoms, where relevant, within the context of their culture of origin (e.g. mental health symptoms related to depression, anxiety or eating disorders)
- ask sensitively about experiences that may have adversely affected their development, health and attitude to illness (e.g. refugee experience, exposure to war and trauma, discrimination, racism)
- learn whether cultural difference (e.g. attitudes to sexuality) might affect treatment
- be sensitive to gender issues, particularly the needs of young women, when conducting physical examinations or investigating sexual problems
- develop a management plan that considers the influence of cultural issues and is culturally acceptable.

THE PSYCHOSOCIAL HISTORY AND RISK ASSESSMENT: HEEADSSS

The psychosocial history/risk assessment is the cornerstone of a comprehensive adolescent health assessment and is at the heart of integrative adolescent healthcare.[11] It recognises that adolescent health and wellbeing are mostly influenced by psychosocial and behavioural factors, provides a profile of risk and protective factors that can guide intervention, and also facilitates the development of rapport and trust.

A 'HEEADSSS screen' is one of the recommendations of the RACGP for preventive care among adolescents:[12]

H Home environment
E Education and employment
E Eating and exercise
A Peer Activities
D Drugs
S Sexuality
S Suicide/depression
S Safety from injury and violence.

Simple examples of questions in each domain are given in Table 56.3. For a more comprehensive guide to using HEEADSSS, refer to Goldenring and Rosen.[11]

PHYSICAL EXAMINATION

In contrast to the physical examination of an older or younger patient, young people are more likely to be extremely self-conscious about their changing bodies. All young people should have their weight, height and BMI recorded and skin checked for acne and moles. Blood pressure measurement is recommended for those aged 18 years or over. Other elements of the physical examination will be dictated by the presenting symptoms or concerns.

- Explain what is involved and why you need to conduct a physical examination, and ask permission.
- If undressing is necessary, leave the room while the young person does so.
- Conduct a friendly and reassuring dialogue during the examination.
- Summarise findings after the young person has dressed and is sitting up again.

WRAPPING UP THE CONSULTATION

Closure of a consultation can be a critical part of the engagement process. The goal is to have the young person leave your practice feeling confident about returning if the need arises. Given the likely mismatch between standard consultation times and the time required to develop a relationship of trust, a thorough history may not have been taken, all 'agendas' may not have been explored and all health issues may not yet have been identified. Furthermore, if the presentation was relatively simple (e.g. acute viral illness), wrapping up can include extending the invitation for a further consultation to conduct a more comprehensive assessment and discuss preventive healthcare.

- Summarise your assessment and define the main concerns, leaving the way open for a subsequent consultation.
- Review options/outline management plan, including inviting the young person to return for further assessment, and making the appointment before they leave.
- Invite questions or comments.
- Discuss 'what to tell Mum and/or Dad' before inviting the parent/carer back in.

ENGAGING THE FAMILY

Engaging the family and gaining the trust of parents is critical in treating young people. In many cultures, participation in healthcare is a family responsibility rather than an individual responsibility.[13]

- Respect parents' authority with regard to decision-making, while helping them to understand their child's growing need for developmentally appropriate independence.
- Where the young person is accompanied by a parent, try to spend some time alone with the adolescent. Explain to the parent/s the reasons for doing this and seek their permission.
- Where appropriate, engage the support and involvement of parents and family in treatment, but never use a family member as interpreter.
- Where language is an issue, avoid speaking too loudly or too quickly and keep questions simple; involve the interpreter service.

TABLE 56.3 Questions for HEEADSSS exam

Domain	Questions	Risk/ Protective
Home	• Where do you live? • Who do you live with? • How do you get on with mum/dad/ stepmum/ stepdad/siblings/extended family? • Tell me a bit about your family and cultural background.	*(Protective)* Does the family eat meals together? *(Protective)* Who in the family would you turn to if you had a problem?
Education/ employment	• What school do you go to? • How do you like school? • What is your favourite/least favourite subject? • Who do you sit with at lunchtime?	*(Risk)* Have your grades at school changed recently? *(Protective)* Is there a teacher or adult at school you could turn to if you had a problem?
Eating/exercise	• Do you eat regular meals? • Can you give me an example of what you eat at each meal? • Are there any foods you avoid? • Have you ever worried about your weight? • What exercise do you do in a given week?	
Activities	• What do you like to do outside school—hobbies, sports, on weekends?	*(Protective)* Tell me more about <activity mentioned>. Is it an important part of your life? Who are some of the people involved?
Prior to proceeding to the 'Drugs' and subsequent domains, it is useful to reiterate the confidentiality statement, and to ask permission to ask sensitive questions: 'I am about to ask you some personal questions about drugs, sex and how you feel in general. You don't have to answer them if you don't wish to. I ask these as part of a health assessment with all young people. Is it OK if I proceed?'		
Drugs and alcohol	• A third-person approach can be useful: 'Some young people of your age might have tried cigarettes, alcohol or other drugs. Are there any kids in your year at school who use any of these? What about among your group of friends? What about you?'	Explore motivation to change behaviour if risky
Sexuality	Avoid heterosexist language or assumptions: • 'Have you had any romantic or sexual relationships?' • 'Are you attracted to girls, guys or both?' • 'Have your sexual partners been girls, guys or both?'	Explore feelings around becoming sexual if appropriate
Suicide/depression	• 'On a scale of 1 to 10, how would you rate your mood most of the time, where 1 is feeling really lousy and 10 is as good as you could feel?' • 'Have you ever felt so bad that you thought life wasn't worth living anymore?'	Identify protective factors such as those suggested previously
Safety from injury and violence	• 'Do you feel safe at home, school or any other place where you might hang out?' • 'Is feeling unsafe ever an issue for you?'	

LEGAL ISSUES

The ambiguous legal status of young people aged under 18 years creates unique challenges in the health consultation. Each country, state and territory has its own statutory laws regarding the age at which an individual under 18 years of age can consent to medical treatment, and in relation to child protection and mandatory reporting requirements, both of which have an impact on clinical care.

Even within countries, different state jurisdictions may allow for different legal rights and obligations in relation to medical consultations and mandatory notification by healthcare professionals about issues such as 'children at risk of harm' or the reporting of notifiable diseases. Confidentiality is also a legal requirement in many countries.

Common law allows for the recognition of the 'mature minor' in many countries, a legal concept that arose in the United Kingdom in the 1980s in Gillick *vs* West Norfolk A.H.A. [1984] 1 QB581. This process requires a clinical judgment about the young person's 'intelligence and understanding, to enable full understanding of what is proposed'; this is sometimes referred to the 'Gillick test'.[14]

Full understanding must include understanding of:
- what the treatment is for and why the treatment is necessary
- any treatment options
- what the treatment involves
- likely effects and possible side effects/risks
- the gravity/seriousness of the treatment
- consequences of not treating
- consequences of discovery of treatment by parents/guardians.

Making a competency assessment will include consideration of the young person's age, level of independence, level of schooling, maturity and ability to express their own wishes.

Note that the doctor's assessment of these factors could be influenced by cultural differences between the doctor and the young person. A cognitively mature adolescent may come across as socially or emotionally immature, because of different cultural expectations about their role in the family/society (for example, they may seem less independent), or differences in the way they communicate their thoughts or wishes. If in doubt, seek advice from a colleague or an appropriate agency.

If you are unsure whether a minor is competent, seek the opinion of a colleague, or obtain the consent of the minor's parents/guardians.

CONCLUSION

The entire range of adolescent health problems likely to be seen in general practice is beyond the scope of this chapter. Certain conditions and presentations can be expected: acne and other typical adolescent skin disorders; common menstrual disorders (such as dysmenorrhoea) and sexual health problems including sexually transmitted infections; obesity and eating disorders (anorexia nervosa and bulimia); anxiety, depression and other mental health problems; substance abuse and other health risk behaviours; chronic conditions such as asthma and diabetes, together with challenges related to compliance and transition care. Aspects of these diverse issues and problems are to be found elsewhere in this book as well as in chapters and books dealing specifically with adolescent health and medical care.

Each young person presenting within a general practice setting is hopeful of engaging in a relationship of trust with a caring and insightful adult healthcare professional. By taking a developmental perspective, being sensitive to family and cultural context, and having the skills to elicit a 'psychosocial snapshot' (using the HEEADSSS screen), little of importance will be missed. And, while not all relevant health-related information for that young person can be addressed in a single encounter, the offer of follow-up sends a positive and protective message.

RESOURCES

Alcohol and other drugs

Alcohol and Other Drugs Council of Australia, http://www.adca.org.au

Australian Drug Foundation, http://www.adf.org.au

Depression

beyondblue, National Depression Initiative (advice for parents), http://www.beyondblue.org.au

Getontop, guide to mental health for teenagers, http://www.getontop.org

Headroom, information on mental health for teenagers, parents and friends, http://www.headroom.net.au

Kids' helpline, http://www.kidshelp.com.au

Lifeline, http://www.lifeline.org.au

ReachOut (advice for teenagers), http://www.reachout.com.au

Sexuality

Not So Straight, http://www.notsostraight.com.au

http://www.yoursexhealth.org (young people's sexuality and sexual health)

Smoking

Australian Government, National Tobacco Campaign, http://www.quitnow.info.au

Oxygen (information for young people on smoking), http://www.oxygen.org.au

Teenage pregnancy and sexual health

Sexual Health and Family Planning Australia, http://www.shfpa.org.au/

REFERENCES

1 Kang M, Sanci LA. Primary healthcare for young people in Australia. Int J Adolesc Med Health 2007; 9(3):229–234.

2 Booth M, Bernard D, Quine S et al. Access to healthcare among Australian adolescents: young people's perspectives and their socioeconomic distribution. J Adolesc Health 2004; 34:97–103.

3 Ary D. Development of adolescent problem behaviour. J Abnorm Child Psychol 1999; 27(2):141–150.

4 Ingersoll GM. Adolescents. 2nd edn. Englewood Cliffs, NJ: Prentice-Hall; 1989.

5 Bennett DL, Kang M. Adolescence. In: Oates K, Currow K, Hu W, eds. Child health: a practical manual for general practice. Sydney: MacLennan & Petty; 2001: Ch 12.

6 Bennett DL, Kang M, Leu-Marshall E. Adolescent health. Check program of self-assessment. Melbourne: Royal Australian College of General Practitioners; 2006.

7 Australian Institute of Health and Welfare. Young Australians: their health and wellbeing. AIHW Cat. No. PHE 87. Canberra: AIHW; 2007.

8 Eckersley RM. The health and well-being of young Australians: present patterns, future challenges. Int J Adolesc Med Health 2007; 9(3):217–227.

9 Jacka FN, Kremer PJ, Leslie ER et al. Associations between diet quality and depressed mood in adolescents: results from the Australian Healthy Neighbourhoods Study. Aust NZ J Psychiatry 2010; 44(5):435–442.

10 Bennett DL, Chown P, Kang M. Cultural diversity in adolescent healthcare. Med J Aust 2005; 183(8): 436–438.

11 Goldenring JM, Rosen DS. Getting into adolescent heads: an essential update. Contemp Pediatr 2004; 21:64.

12 Royal Australian College of General Practitioners. Guidelines for preventive activities in general practice. 7th edn. Melbourne, Australia: RACGP; 2009.

13 Reidpath D, Allotey P. Multicultural issues in general practice. Curr Ther 1999/2000; 40(12):35–37.

14 Bird S. Children and adolescents: who can give consent? Aust Fam Physician 2007; 36(3):165–166.

chapter 57

Geriatric medicine

INTRODUCTION AND OVERVIEW

The world's population is ageing rapidly, particularly in developed countries, where life expectancy is over 80 years for women and just under 80 years for men in many countries. Rapid ageing is occurring in less developed countries too, with the number of people aged over 65 years increasing dramatically in many countries. Consequently, much of general practice now involves care of older people in a range of settings—community, residential and acute-care facilities. It is easy to form the impression that ageing normally involves disease, disability and dependency, but while these are more common with increasing age, they are far from inevitable. Most 90-year-olds are not demented, maintain excellent mobility, are independent in personal, domestic and most community activities of daily living and live in their own home.

AGEING

Some changes with normal ageing are generally towards impaired function—for example, maximum heart rate and exercise capacity are reduced, glomerular filtration rate is lower, there is decline in some aspects of cognition and muscle mass is reduced. An emerging concept in geriatric medicine is that of 'frailty', which essentially is a condition in which these normal changes of ageing accumulate and lead to disease, predisposing the person to functional decline. Frailty is not, however, an inevitable part of ageing.

Essentially, most ageing is healthy and most of us age in a mostly healthy way. (Healthy ageing is covered in Ch 58.) However, with time the number of organ systems within an individual that begin to age in an unhealthy way increases, so that by age 90 years it is uncommon to exhibit only healthy ageing. Frailty can be seen as a transition stage between healthy and unhealthy ageing. Factors that increase the chance of healthy ageing include genes, physical activity, cognitive stimulation, social engagement, diet and aggressive detection and management of disease risk factors.

EVALUATION OF THE OLDER PERSON

Comprehensive geriatric evaluation requires a detailed assessment of both physical and cognitive status, but also involves assessment of function (basic and more complex tasks), social environment, psychological/psychiatric status, behavioural issues and support systems.

Particular attention needs to be paid to the features of geriatric medical syndromes, including dementia, impaired mobility and falls, incontinence and medication-related issues. There have been several checklists/proformas developed by GP divisions and individual practices to assist this assessment process. These are particularly useful when carrying out routine comprehensive assessments. A suggested checklist is shown in the appendix. Ideally, this information will then be transformed into a problem list with a management plan—an example is shown in Table 57.1. It will be seen that this is best developed as a dynamic process with additional management of the identified problems added as they occur—so a word processed document on computer would be more appropriate than a single hard copy.

PHARMACOLOGICAL ISSUES, INCLUDING POLYPHARMACY

BACKGROUND AND PREVALENCE

Medication issues in older people include polypharmacy (taking a large number of medications), reduced compliance ('concordance'), drug–drug interactions and adverse drug reactions. Older people consume a disproportionately large number of prescribed drugs, partly

TABLE 57.1 Example of a geriatric medical problem list and management plan

	Problem & date begun		Plan		Date plan begun		Resolved?
Medical/syndromes							
1	Falls with hip fracture 5/2010	A	Improve home safety	A	8/2010: OT visit	A	Completed
		B	Begin bisphosphonate and Vitamin D	B	8/2010: medication begun	B	Ongoing
2	Cognitive impairment since 2009		Refer to geriatrician		9/2010		Yes—diagnosis Mild cognitive impairment, review 6-monthly
3	Urinary incontinence since 2007	A	Investigate—MSU, bladder residual, PR	A	9/2010	A	Completed—no reversible cause
		B	Refer to continence clinic	B	10/2010	B	Completed—diagnosis detrusor instability
		C	Pads, bladder retraining	C	12/2010	C	Ongoing
4	Polypharmacy—on 12 medications as of 7/2010		Cease unnecessary/high risk medications		9/2010		Ongoing—so far indomethacin and diazepam ceased
Functional							
1	Impaired mobility	A	Use a frame	A	10/2010	A	Completed
		B	Physio at CRC	B	10/2010	B	Ongoing
2	Unable to handle finances		Suggest award an EPOA		9/2010		10/2010
3	Unreliable with meals at home		Suggest delivered meals		10/2010		Completed—5 meals delivered weekly
Social/environment							
1	Isolated—family rarely visit	A	Speak to family	A	10/2010	A	Completed—son will visit weekly
		B	Arrange non-family social contact	B	12/2010	B	Completed—'Do Care' visitor coming
Psychological/psychiatric							
1	Depression—positive screen on GDS & diagnosed on further assessment 8/2010		Commence CBT		9/2010		Ongoing—refer to psychiatrist if not improving

because they are more likely to be ill and partly because it can be more difficult to reach a precise diagnosis. On average, an older person in the community takes three prescribed drugs, and this rises to 7–10 in care settings. CAMs and other over-the-counter (OTC) medications are also used extensively by older people. Unfortunately, it is rare for a GP to have a completely accurate list of all the medications their patient consumes—this is partly because the patients themselves cannot always accurately recall them (and may not feel it necessary to mention OTC/CAM medications) and partly because of poor communication from acute-care facilities and specialists. The best way to obtain an accurate list is to visit the patient's home and ask to see everything they use, or to ask them to put all the medications in a bag and bring them to your office.

Reduced compliance is common at all ages, but is particularly an issue in older people, who take more medications, may not hear or recall or be able to read instructions, may have difficulty opening packages and can be on complicated drug regimens. Fortunately, under-compliance may somewhat protect them from adverse drug reactions, but it does contribute to poorer disease control.

Drug–drug reactions and adverse drug reactions increase with age and with increasing numbers of medications used. Some 3% of all admissions to hospital are primarily due to adverse drug reactions and, if this is expanded to include poor disease control from suboptimal prescribing and compliance, the proportion of admissions rises to over 30%. Drug–drug interactions are almost unavoidable if a person is prescribed more than eight medications, and can cause adverse drug reactions and poor drug efficacy. The problem may be compounded by drug–nutrient or herb–drug interactions, particularly if the ingestion of herbs or nutrients is unknown to the doctor.

AETIOLOGY

A large part of the problem older people have with medication is that their bodies deal with drugs differently (altered pharmacokinetics) and may have a different response from younger people to the same drug concentration (altered pharmacodynamics). Absorption is relatively unaffected by age (much built-in reserve, to meet nutritional needs) but liver metabolism (so-called 'first pass' and oxidative cytochrome P-450 metabolism) is reduced, as is renal excretion. Drug distribution is also changed with age—relatively less body water and more body fat affects the peak level and elimination half-life of drugs, which tend to be either predominantly fat soluble (e.g. the benzodiazepines) or water soluble (e.g. digoxin). Protein binding is reduced in the unwell elderly person, leading to more free drug, but this free drug is consequently more available for metabolism and excretion.

Examples of altered pharmacodynamics include a less effective cardiovascular response to low blood pressure, increasing risk of postural hypotension and falls due to medications, and reduced beta-adrenergic receptors reducing the response to and efficacy of beta-blocking agents (older people are effectively already partly beta-blocked).

ASSESSMENT

Always ask older people about their medications and problems they may be experiencing with them. Older people do recognise minor adverse effects well (even though such effects can present atypically) but, surprisingly, have more difficulty recognising more serious adverse events. Sometimes more formal assessment of medication compliance and handling can be useful—pill counts, measuring blood levels of the drug and involving the pharmacist in this process. Poor disease control (e.g. ongoing fitting, depression or hypertension) may indicate poor compliance, and this should be excluded before increasing the medication dose or adding a new medication.

MANAGEMENT

Along with regular medication reviews, there should be a sustained intention to minimise the number of medications an older person takes, but also to ensure that all conditions are being treated effectively. 'De-prescribing' is both possible and beneficial, and the basic steps are shown in Box 57.1.[1] Unnecessary medications may include analgesics and laxatives no longer needed, or an antipsychotic for behavioural symptoms that are no longer complicating dementia. Additionally, many prophylactic medications (e.g. statins, bisphosphonates) may no longer be necessary as death approaches (palliative care, end-stage dementia). High-risk medications include anticholinergics (benztropine and benzhexol) and long-acting benzodiazepines.

In residential and acute-care settings, medication audits are another approach to improving medication outcomes—for example, the appropriateness of benzodiazepine prescribing can be audited against an evidence-based algorithm and these results then fed back to the prescribing team. Pharmacist and GP can also work as a team to review an individual's medication in residential and community settings—indeed, annual medication review is now required for those in residential care. Other approaches include academic detailing, and programs such as the National Prescribing Service GP education program in Australia.

IMPORTANT PITFALLS

It is all too easy to become complacent about the number and type of medications older people take, especially when many are commenced in hospital, by other doctors or earlier in life when the medication may well have been appropriate. Such complacency may not serve the patient well.

Also, when a medication is ceased the patient may reintroduce it if not supported and reviewed

BOX 57.1 De-prescribing principles[1]

1. Establish an accurate list of all current medications.
2. In partnership with the patient and carer, plan a de-prescribing regimen.
3. Cease all unnecessary medications and, if possible, those causing adverse effects.
4. Cease, if possible, medications with a high likelihood of causing adverse effects.
5. Review and support the patient (and carers) regularly.
6. Update medication list and consider repeating the cycle.

(e.g. temazepam—cessation in hospital is almost always followed by recommencement after discharge).

Finally, the original condition may re-emerge once a medication is ceased—for example, hypertension may recur if a calcium channel blocker causing swollen legs is ceased. The patient should therefore be monitored, often for up to a year, for this.

PATIENT EDUCATION

The GP may want to have available notices and pamphlets on the importance of correct use of medication and the hazards of unnecessary medications. More detailed brochures can alert patients that any new symptoms may be due to their medications, and to always discuss their medication with their doctor.

CONFUSIONAL STATES: DELIRIUM AND DEMENTIA

DELIRIUM

Background and prevalence

Delirium is an acute-onset confusional state characterised by impairment of cognition—especially attention—with marked fluctuations. There is a hypoactive form, more prevalent in older people, and a hyperactive form, where a person may have difficulty sleeping and may be physically active or even aggressive. Hallucinations (usually visual) and paranoia are common. Delirium affects about 30% of hospitalised elderly people at any one time, with 20% having delirium on admission and up to another 20% developing delirium during their hospitalisation. Prevalence in the community is less, but it must always be considered when there is a sudden change in cognitive status.

Aetiology

Delirium always has a medical cause.[2] The most common causes include infections, metabolic disturbances (e.g. electrolyte deficiencies, hyperglycaemia, hypercalcaemia) and drugs (adverse effects or drug withdrawal). Other causes include pain, intracerebral lesions, myocardial infarction, organ ischaemia, faecal impaction and epilepsy.

Diagnosis

The diagnosis of the clinical syndrome of delirium is frequently missed, especially as lucid periods tend to coincide with morning contact with the doctor. Screening in hospital is worthwhile—the Confusion Assessment Method is more accurate than the Mini-Mental State Examination (MMSE). Once the syndrome is suspected, it must be differentiated from dementia, although they can coexist. The differential characteristic of delirium is its acute onset, although dementia may begin acutely (e.g. often after a stroke). A collaborative (informant) history is essential here. The other major differential is depression, and again they may coexist. Depression usually lacks the fluctuations.

Once the clinical syndrome is diagnosed, a cause must be sought. After physical examination, investigations are usually required and include urea and electrolytes, full blood count, random blood glucose, oxygen saturation, calcium/phosphorus, liver function tests and mid-stream urine (or dipstick). Other investigations that may be indicated, or can be used if no cause is yet apparent, include EEG, chest X-ray, CT brain, drug levels, ECG and cardiac enzymes, lumbar puncture, X-ray of painful areas, joint aspiration and so on. It is usually necessary to hospitalise a delirious person as the syndrome indicates significant underlying illness.

Management

The cause must be treated—for example, antibiotics for infection, correction of electrolyte disturbances, ceasing an offending medication or relief of faecal impaction. General management includes a safe environment with minimal disruptions and a minimal number of new care staff (not the norm in hospitals!). Hydration is essential, and glasses and hearing aids should be on and working. If agitation or physical aggression cannot be managed non-pharmacologically, haloperidol or newer antipsychotic agents such as olanzapine can be used, in low dose and for a short period only—e.g. 0.5 mg haloperidol once, or olanzapine wafer 2.5 mg once. Benzodiazepines may be more effective for delirium induced by drug or alcohol withdrawal.

Complementary therapies are not well researched for delirium but those that are effective for behavioural disturbance in dementia (e.g. lavender oil and other aromatherapy) may be tried in addition to the above approaches.

Prevention of delirium can be achieved—in a seminal study, Inouye and colleagues[3] reduced the incidence by 40% through the multifactorial approach outlined in Box 57.2.

Pitfalls

Although delirium affects cognition, it is not usually primarily due to brain disease. Routine CT of the brain is therefore an inappropriate investigation.

Not listening to nursing staff/family's description of the person being confused when you are not there can lead to delays in the diagnosis.

Using chemical restraint (antipsychotics) too early and in too high a dose can lead to unnecessary complications, such as falls and fractures. Similarly, physical restraint has almost no place in delirium management, and can lead to patient injury and even death.

BOX 57.2 Prevention of delirium

1. Maintain hydration.
2. Reduce noise and other disturbances.
3. Avoid hypno-sedatives—encourage sleep with a back rub and relaxing music. Check other medications for delirium as a side effect before prescribing for the elderly, and seek alternative treatments.
4. Ensure glasses and hearing aids are working/clean and used.
5. Orientation to time and place with an orientation board in the room.
6. Aggressively manage pain.
7. Treat/prevent dehydration.
8. Encourage mobility.

Under-investigating delirium can worsen the outcome—delirium is a sign that something serious is underlying.

Prognosis

Most recover at least partially from delirium, within 1–4 weeks. Unfortunately, at least 50% can be shown to have cognitive deficits up to 6 months after the onset, suggesting that delirium itself may damage brain function. Some of these cases are due to pre-existing cognitive impairment not diagnosed before the episode of delirium.

Patient education

Most people retain some memory of the episode of delirium—and these may be very frightening memories. The person should be reassured that they are not 'mad' but have simply suffered from an illness that also affected their brain function.

During the episode, family members require similar reassurance that the person is not going 'mad', and also should be taught ways in which they can assist (e.g. bring in relaxing music, offer drinks, fix hearing aids). They should also be told that too many visitors—even close family—can be detrimental.

DEMENTIA

Dementia is a chronic, progressive impairment of cognition, including memory, which is usually irreversible and always causes some impairment of function. It affects 5% of those over age 60, but the incidence doubles every 5 years, with around 30% affected by age 80. The average GP is likely to have 5–10 patients with dementia, but this will vary depending on how many elderly patients he/she has.

Aetiology

It is not known why one individual develops dementia and another does not. There are genetic mutations that nearly always cause dementia, but this early-onset dementia (in the forties or fifties) is very rare. Risk factors for the much more common late-onset dementia include older age, family history of dementia, apolipoprotein E4 (a carrier of cholesterol), previous head injury, less formal education, lower socioeconomic status and cardiovascular risk factors (hypertension, diabetes, smoking, atrial fibrillation, past cardiac surgery). There are also protective factors, including active leisure activities, physical activity, social contact and marriage, moderate alcohol use, exposure to non-steroidal anti-inflammatory agents, omega-3 fatty acids and use of vitamins E and C. It is also becoming apparent that attentional training, such as mindfulness-based practices, is associated with cell maintenance and neurogenesis in the prefrontal cortex and hippocampus.[4]

The most common cause of dementia is Alzheimer's disease (AD), usually mixed with cerebrovascular pathology. Pure vascular dementia (that is, with no AD pathology) is uncommon. The emerging concept of 'cerebral reserve' may explain this synergism and some protective factors—those with a lesser number of synapses (e.g. from less education or a past head injury) are more prone to the clinical syndrome of dementia once AD pathology develops, especially if they also have cerebrovascular damage (e.g. lacunar infarcts or extensive white matter changes).

Other relatively frequent causes of dementia include dementia with Lewy bodies (DLB) and frontotemporal dementia (FTD). In DLB there is a combination of cognitive impairment, fluctuations, parkinsonism, visual hallucinations and sleep disturbances—but not all features have to be present for the diagnosis to be made. The hallucinations are often of small animals or creatures just outside or coming into the room. Sleep disturbance affects the REM sleep component, with a failure to paralyse muscles during dreams, leading to violent movements. DLB is in the same spectrum as Parkinson's disease with dementia (PDD)—the main difference is that in PDD the motor changes precede the cognitive changes.

Frontotemporal dementia usually begins with behavioural or language changes with relative preservation of memory initially. The behavioural changes reflect frontal lobe impairment and include disinhibition, apathy, lack of insight, and impaired judgment and reasoning. Language changes can occur with all forms of FTD but there are two language-specific forms, called *semantic dementia* (language is fluent but the meaning of words is lost) and *primary progressive aphasia* (language is simply lost, with mutism occurring early in the dementia).

There are over 200 other causes of dementia but these are uncommon. A few are occasionally at least partially reversible (e.g. hypothyroidism, vitamin B_{12} deficiency, syphilis) and explain why investigations for these are performed. Normal pressure hydrocephalus (characterised by dementia, urinary incontinence and gait disturbance) is also potentially reversible, although many neurosurgeons are reluctant to perform the required shunt, as results are often disappointing.

Pathology

Alzheimer's disease is characterised by amyloid plaques and neurofibrillary tangles, which begin in the hippocampal/limbic region of the brain and progress throughout the cerebral cortex as the disease progresses. The plaques are composed of the amyloid beta (Ab) peptide, which is a fragment of the amyloid precursor protein (APP), a transmembrane protein whose function is not well understood. This fragment is cleaved off by two enzymes (beta and gamma secretase), and mutations in a component of the gamma secretase as well as mutations in APP cause most of the (rare) early-onset AD. The tangles are composed of hyperphosphorylated tau, a protein which normally stabilises the microtubules that neurons use to transport protein from their nucleus, down axons to the synapse. Which of these two main pathological processes is key to the development and severity of AD is hotly debated—probably both are.

In vascular dementia the pathology is brain tissue damage due to cerebral ischaemia and this can affect any region of the brain, although frontal lobe dysfunction is common, even if the damaged area is distant to the frontal region. There is a spectrum of pathology that can contribute to vascular dementia—a single large critical infarct, multiple large-vessel infarcts, multiple lacunar infarcts, extensive white matter lesions and multiple haemorrhages. Usually this vascular pathology coexists with AD pathology.

Dementia with Lewy bodies (DLB) is characterised by cortical Lewy bodies, which contain alpha-synuclein. Abnormal folding of this protein is thought to be a key precipitant of DLB.

Frontotemporal dementia has a range of pathology, including Pick bodies in one subtype. AD pathology is not found. Recently, a mutation of the progranulin gene has been found in a large proportion of FTD cases—progranulin appears to be a neuronal growth factor. This is associated with an abnormal form of the protein TDP 43 and this can be identified in (post mortem) diagnostic tests.

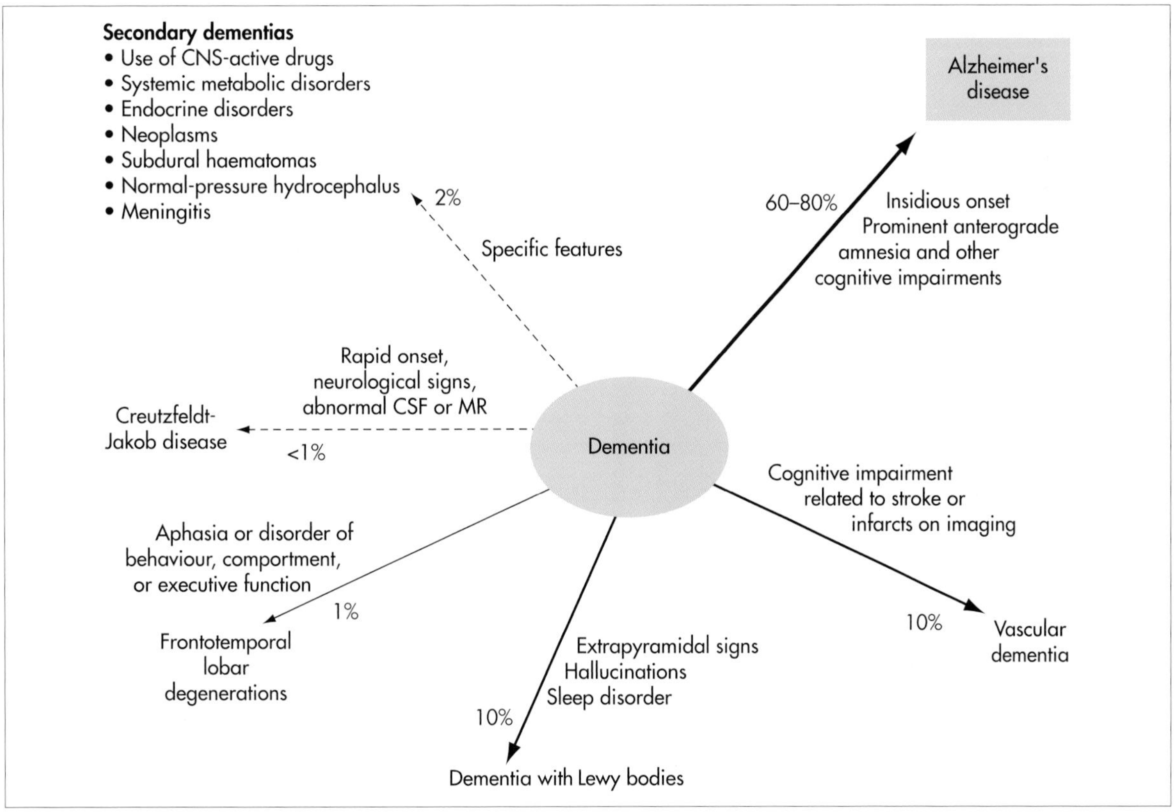

FIGURE 57.1 Differential diagnosis of dementia and Alzheimer's disease

Diagnosis

History

The key to diagnosing the dementias is the clinical history, combined with judicious use of specific investigations. AD is characterised by an insidious onset of memory loss—usually at least 1–2 years before presentation—and progressive decline. (Ask: 'Has there been definite decline in the past 6 months?') Specific questions may include:

- Does he/she repeat information or questions?
- Does he/she frequently misplace objects or put items away in unusual places?
- Doe he/she forget to turn things off/close things?
- Does he/she forget appointments/arrangements?
- Does he/she forget names of family members?

It is also important to establish whether the cognitive changes are affecting function (e.g. unable to manage finances, unable to operate appliances previously used independently, unable to fix broken items around the house). Cognitive impairment with no effect on function suggests mild cognitive impairment (MCI), which is not dementia, although it is increasingly recognised as a prodromal state.

In vascular dementia there will usually be a history of more sudden episodes of decline associated with other features of cerebral ischaemia events—but not always (e.g. in progressive white matter damage). The history of DLB, FTD and the rarer dementias is driven by enquiring about the specific features described above.

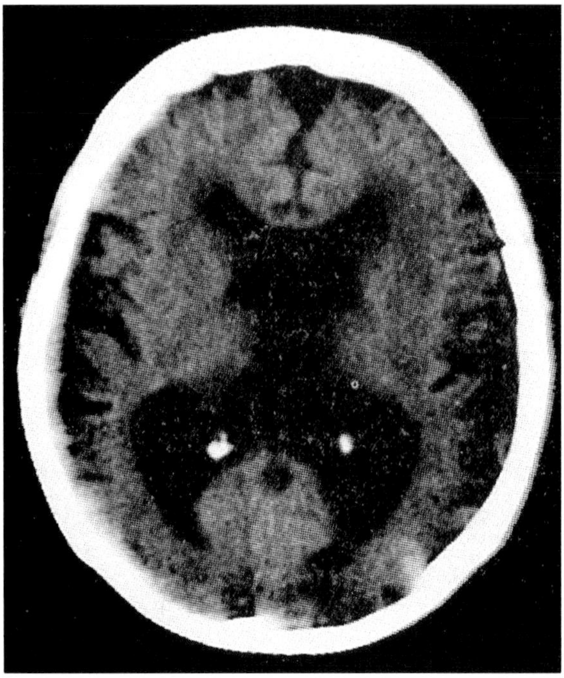

FIGURE 57.2 Brain scan showing Alzheimer's disease

Examination

Physical examination is necessary and should concentrate on neurological signs—such as parkinsonism in DLB and focal signs in some vascular dementias. The most important reason for performing the physical examination is to detect rarer, potentially reversible, causes of dementia (e.g. thyroid disorders) and comorbidities. Cognitive assessment is essential. The best known screening tool is the MMSE, a 30-item questionnaire that is useful in screening for AD but has less utility with the other dementias. The clock drawing test (CDT) is also useful—the patient is asked to draw a large circle (or the circle can be provided), place the numbers of a clock and then show a requested time with the hands (e.g. 11:10 or 1:50). Errors include incorrect number placement and inability to show the time. Combining the MMSE and the CDT achieves around 90% sensitivity for cognitive impairment—that is, an MMSE score below 26 and an abnormal CDT indicates a 90% chance that the person has significant cognitive impairment.

More-detailed assessment is required in order to characterise the dementia type. In FTD, questioning should concentrate on executive function (e.g. similarities, problem solving) and language (e.g. describe a complex task, name objects, read a paragraph). In DLB there are prominent visuo-spatial deficits, so assessment should include drawing a cube to supplement the CDT and the intersecting pentagons in the MMSE. For vascular dementia, assessment of frontal lobe function is useful but cognitive changes are influenced by the site and extent of the lesions—for instance, if they are in the dominant temporoparietal cortex there may be language changes.

More-detailed neuropsychological assessment usually requires referral to a specialist (geriatrician, psychogeriatrician or neurologist), who may use the expertise of a neuropsychologist.

Investigations

Routine blood tests and neuroimaging should be performed as shown in Box 57.3—mainly to rule out potentially reversible causes of dementia and comorbidities. Increasingly, specialists are ordering tests to 'rule in' a diagnosis of dementia and to characterise the type.

The MRI of the brain is moving towards this identification of dementia—for instance, hippocampal atrophy is seen in AD, and frontal atrophy in FTD. The PET scan is only available in a few centres but can be most useful. The FDG PET shows a characteristic pattern in AD (bilateral temporoparietal hypometabolism with sparing of occipital metabolism), whereas sparing of the posterior cingulate metabolism is very much against a diagnosis of AD. In DLB, occipital metabolism is reduced and in FTD frontal and temporal metabolism is down, with characteristic patterns in the language variants. Another PET technique available in even fewer centres is amyloid imaging using PIB or other agents. Absence of amyloid excludes AD, and its presence excludes FTD. Amyloid is frequently found in DLB and vascular dementia. Combining both PET techniques achieves very high diagnostic accuracy.

Management

Prevention

To what extent dementia can be prevented is not fully known, but individual risk reduction is achievable through attention to risk and protective factors. Alzheimer's Australia has an excellent program that outlines this ('Mind Your Mind') and it can obtained from their website or by contacting them directly. Much of the focus is on diet, lifestyle and cardiovascular risk factors—'what is good for your heart is also good for your mind'. All newly diagnosed people should be advised to follow the recommendations of the program, as should family members. Those with MCI should be particularly encouraged to pursue these practices, although they have not been proved to prevent progression to dementia. At this time, no medication is recommended as a preventative strategy, although two large trials, of *Ginkgo biloba* (United States and Europe—'GEM' and 'GUIDANCE') examined this.

BOX 57.3 Investigations for dementia

Routine
- blood tests:
  - U&E
  - Ca/P
  - RBG (or FBG)
  - LFT
  - B_{12} & folate
  - TFTs
  - syphilis serology
- neuroimaging:
  - CT brain (non-contrast acceptable)

Additional, as indicated
- EEG
- LP
- MRI brain scan
- 'Rule in' investigations
- PET scan
  - with the radiotracer fluorodeoxyglucose (FDG)
  - with the ^{11}C-labelled Pittsburgh Compound-B (11C-PIB)

General supportive measures

It is important to diagnose the presence and type of dementia in the early stages—this can allow planning for the course of the disease and assists the family/caregivers in understanding symptoms. For instance, the sexually explicit repetitive joking of a person with FTD, while not pleasant, can be understood and arrangements made to avoid contact with younger relatives and friends. In later stages, dementia type is less relevant—the very dependent high-level care resident with severe AD has similar symptoms and care needs to the person with severe DLB or FTD.

Not initiating treatment with medication is also a valid option, as current therapies (see below) are only modestly effective. However, pharmacological therapy is becoming a standard of practice (for those dementias responsive to it), with over 50% of people diagnosed with AD receiving such therapy.

For FTD and most of the rarer dementias there is no specific drug therapy, and 'general supportive measures' in that therapeutic domain are valid. As described above, for normal pressure hydrocephalus it is not uncommon for the specialist team to elect to not shunt.

Self-help and lifestyle

The preventative strategies described in 'Mind Your Mind' are still appropriate in early dementia and should be encouraged. These include physical exercise, engaging in social and leisure activities, a well-balanced diet (rich in omega-3 fatty acids and vitamins C and E, with only modest amounts of saturated fat) and avoiding cardiovascular risk factors (e.g. cease smoking and control diabetes well).

General practitioners can be a powerful motivating force in encouraging individuals to pursue these sage approaches. An individual program can be constructed. This could include:

- walking for 40 minutes
- dining with others at least five times a week
- attending the elderly citizens' club (or similar) twice a week
- recommencing knitting as a leisure activity
- doing three sudokus a week
- eating a freshly prepared salad five times a week
- moderate use of alcohol—3–5 drinks a week
- taking a daily multivitamin/mineral and omega-3 supplement
- going on an (accompanied) country trip, for a week, within the next year.

Pharmacological

The great advance in dementia therapy has been the development of acetylcholinesterase inhibitors (AChEIs).[5] In AD, and also in DLB and vascular dementia, there is a deficiency of acetylcholine (ACh). This is due to damage either to the central nucleus (nucleus basilis of Meynert) that produces the enzyme that makes ACh (in AD and DLB) or to the axons within which this enzyme is transported (vascular dementia). The AChEIs boost ACh levels by inhibiting another enzyme, at the synapse, which degrades ACh. These agents include donepezil (Aricept®), galantamine (Reminyl® or Razadyne®) and rivastigmine (Exelon®). They differ somewhat in action, with galantamine also stimulating nicotinic receptors and rivastigmine also inhibiting another enzyme that breaks down ACh (butyrylcholinesterase), but no study has convincingly demonstrated that one agent is superior to others. At this time, only rivastigmine is given more than once daily, but a once-daily patch preparation is marketed in many countries. These agents have predictable cholinergic side effects, including nausea, vomiting, abdominal pain, diarrhoea, anorexia and weight loss. Such symptoms can be significant in about 20% of patients but usually attenuate over 1–2 weeks. More serious and rarer adverse effects include bradycardia, peptic ulceration and precipitation of asthma, so they should not be used in patients with such conditions until the illness is well controlled (e.g. *Helicobacter* eradication or insertion of a pacemaker).

The efficacy of the AChEIs is significant but modest. On average, there is a stabilisation of cognition for 6–12 months, then a continued decline that would be worse if the agent was ceased. Some do show a clinically apparent improvement and, indeed, the Australian Pharmaceutical Benefits Schedule (PBS) requires that this be demonstrated for subsidised supply to be continued beyond the first 6 months. The scheme requires that these agents only be used in those with mild to moderate AD and that the initial MMSE be above 9 (but lower MMSE is acceptable if due to a non-cognitive cause such as aphasia). The MMSE must improve by two points or more within the first 6 months for subsidised supply to continue. For those with an initial MMSE score above 24, it is harder to show a two-point improvement (ceiling effect), so a baseline ADAS-Cog (another cognitive scale with scores ranging from 0 to 70 and used mainly in research settings) is recommended, with a four-point improvement required. The ADAS-Cog can be performed by some medical specialists and memory clinics, or by some psychologists. Once sufficient initial improvement on one of these scales has been demonstrated, no further scores are required by the PBS (or the DVA equivalent, the RSPB) but the prescriber must confirm, each time a new script is authorised, that the patient still has mild to moderate AD. It is not inappropriate to continue these agents until the end stages of dementia, especially as trials have suggested that they may also have beneficial effects on behaviour and function. Recently, donepezil has gained marketing approval for severe AD, based on recently published trials where it was initiated in those with severe AD.

The other drug with marketing approval for AD is memantine (Ebixa®). It only has marketing approval for moderately severe AD, based on trials where it was used as monotherapy rather than as add-on therapy (to an AChEI). There is trial data, however, to support its use in milder AD and as add-on therapy and, indeed, it is increasingly being used this way. The agent works on a different neurotransmitter system (the glutamatergic system), which is also affected by AD. It has remarkably few side effects. Efficacy has been demonstrated on cognition and behaviour.

None of these agents (AChEIs or memantine) has approval in Australia for other dementias, but in some countries memantine has approval for vascular dementia. There are trial data to support AChEI use in DLB (and in PDD), where there is a cholinergic deficit and where AD pathology is usually also present. No agent has yet proved beneficial in preventing progression from MCI to dementia.

The other pharmacological area of management is the use of atypical antipsychotic agents for the behavioural disturbances ('challenging neuropsychiatric symptoms') that can complicate dementia.[6] Several trials have demonstrated modest efficacy of low doses of risperidone for agitation, aggressive and psychosis complicating more severe dementia, and there is also some (but less) data to support olanzapine and haloperidol. As these agents are usually used for weeks and months rather than days, side-effect profiles must be considered, and the extrapyramidal effects of haloperidol make it usually an inappropriate choice. While quetiapine has some support due to it almost completely lacking extrapyramidal adverse effects, there are almost no data to support its efficacy for this syndrome.

The antipsychotic agents should only be used when non-pharmacological approaches have failed. Adverse effects include an increased risk of cerebrovascular events and death, which affects all agents recommended for these symptoms (all antipsychotics including older agents, and the benzodiazepines). The agents should therefore be used in low doses (risperidone 0.25 mg b.i.d. up to 1 mg b.i.d., olanzapine 2.5 mg daily up to 10 mg daily) and they should be back-titrated and ceased as soon as possible (e.g. target symptom controlled for 1–2 months). Because of their risks, consent for their use should be sought from family and, if feasible, the patient.

Other agents for behavioural disturbance have much less supportive efficacy data and include benzodiazepines (some role for anxiety), antidepressants (appropriate for depression, which not infrequently complicates dementia) and mood stabilisers (e.g. valproate). A psychogeriatrician or geriatrician can be a useful resource if behavioural disturbances are proving difficult to manage.

Complementary therapies

A number of products are purported to have efficacy in those with dementia (usually the dementia type is not specified, or merely for 'memory problems'). These include:

- *Ginkgo biloba*—this herbal preparation from the bark of a tree does have some trial evidence of efficacy in dementia. The preparation used in one trial was Egb 761, at doses of 120–240 mg/day. The product is marketed as Tebonin® and efficacy was about half that of the cholinesterase inhibitors. There was no significant toxicity. Other ginkgo preparations vary in content and efficacy has been inadequately trialled.
- *brahmi*—this preparation has no positive published trial evidence but is often used. It is derived from an Indian plant and recommended dosing is 400 mg daily. Adverse effects include nausea, fatigue and urinary frequency but are insignificantly more frequent than with placebo.
- *Curcumin*—this component of turmeric, an Indian spice, may be beneficial—consumption was found to be associated with a lower risk of having AD, and in vitro studies support efficacy. There is no significant toxicity but there is no recommended dose.
- *polyphenols*—these antioxidants are found in a wide range of plant products including berries, tea and also wine. Highest concentrations are in thin-skinned berries (they have a 'sunscreen' effect) such as blueberries and pinot noir grapes. Epidemiological studies have associated higher consumption with reduced risk of developing dementia but no prospective study has established therapeutic benefit. A number of commercial preparations include polyphenols.
- *vitamins*—consumption of vitamins E and C, as food or tablets, has been associated with a lower risk of developing dementia. There is less, but some, evidence for consumption of B-group vitamins including B_6 and folate. One study in severe dementia[7] showed that high doses of vitamin E (2000 IU/day) reduced risk of progression to greater dependency or nursing home care, but this has not been replicated. Vitamin E was not effective, in another trial,[8] in preventing conversion of MCI to dementia, and in the Heart Protection Study[9] multivitamin supplements did not prevent cognitive decline.

  High doses (above 400 IU/day) of vitamin E have been shown in a meta-analysis[10] to be associated with increased mortality and other adverse events, so daily doses should not exceed this.
- *aromatherapy*—there is some support in the literature for this for behavioural problems, especially lavender oil. This can be rubbed on or administered as a vapour but be sure that it cannot be inadvertently consumed.
- *other environmental therapies*—bright light, music, pets and other approaches have been successfully used to modify agitation and aggression, and improve sleep in those with dementia. Music is more effective if items that the person has liked are used (i.e. individualised), and light seems more effective in the morning, or all day, than in the afternoon. One recent study in a residential care facility[6] demonstrated that bright light in common areas improved sleep more in those with more severe dementia, adding 16 minutes of sleep each night, on average. This compared very favourably with 4.5 minutes of sleep added by the use of temazepam in one study of older people.

Ongoing review/monitoring

Ongoing review/monitoring is important for all those with dementia. The disease inevitably progresses and both carers and the patient face new challenges as this occurs. Progress can be quantified with the MMSE repeated 3–6 monthly but other issues should also be enquired about—behaviour, function, comorbidity, medications, caregiver stress, support services. It is helpful to interview the caregiver and the person with dementia separately. Eventually, most people with dementia require residential care, and an aged care assessment team (ACAT) referral is needed to allow this. The ACAT should also be involved earlier to facilitate extra home supports such as through community aged care packages and extended aged care at home (dementia).

Important pitfalls

- In diagnosis, it is easy to incorrectly diagnose vascular dementia because an infarct/lacune is seen on neuroimaging. The history is vital—if it suggests AD, the ischaemic lesion is probably incidental.
- A low MMSE does not diagnose dementia—other causes include poor education, very old age (a normal MMSE at 90 can be 20 or 21) and coming from a culturally and linguistically diverse background. When in doubt, seek a specialist opinion.

- AChEIs should only be used when dementia is diagnosed—not for other cognitive disorders.
- Memantine may not be offered because the doctor feels the family and/or patient cannot afford it.
- Antipsychotic agents are often used too early, without a trial of non-pharmacological management, or for too long (sometimes years). Behavioural disturbances do not usually persist in those with dementia and attempts to cease the agent need to be frequent.
- Caregiver stress is not always adequately recognised or addressed. A well supported caregiver can delay institutionalisation of the person with dementia, improving their quality of life. National Alzheimer's disease associations are a valuable source of information to assist caregivers, and all caregivers should be aware of them.

Prognosis

The average time course of dementia, from first symptoms to death, is less than 10 years (around 7–8 years for AD, more variable for vascular dementia and shorter for DLB and FTD) but there is much variability. If the diagnosis is correct, sustained improvement is extremely rare—it is only transient when there is a response to an AChEI.

New therapies on the horizon offer great promise for those with AD. These include immunotherapies to remove amyloid inhibitors of the secretases that cleave off Ab and agents to solubilise amyloid. It is likely that these agents will be truly disease modifying or even curative if used early enough.

Patient education

Most Alzheimer's associations offer a range of fact sheets on their websites (see the Resources list for an example). These cover most of the issues relevant to the person with dementia and their caregivers, and are updated regularly.

INSOMNIA

Insomnia is a subjective lack of sleep associated with daytime tiredness. Poor sleep is a common complaint of older people, with up to 50%, in community surveys, saying they regularly sleep poorly. Sleep does change with age, towards less refreshing and more interrupted sleep, with daytime napping, but insomnia is not inevitable. Poor sleep is even more common in residential and acute-care settings.

BOX 57.4 Conditions that may cause insomnia

- Advanced sleep phase
- Alcohol (initially promotes sleep, then rebound insomnia)
- Antidepressants (some—e.g. SSRIs)
- Anxiety disorders
- Arthritis and other musculoskeletal pain
- Bedding/bed
- Behavioural factors
- Beta-blockers
- Caffeine
- Circadian rhythm sleep disorders
- CNS stimulants
- Constipation
- Corticosteroids
- Daytime napping
- Delayed sleep phase
- Delirium
- Dementia, including DLB
- Depression
- Diet
- Early retirement to bed
- Environmental factors, especially in institutions
- Gastro-oesophageal reflux
- Lack of exercise
- Lack of exposure to sunlight
- Medications & other substances
- Nicotine
- Nocturia, urinary retention
- Nocturnal angina
- Nocturnal breathlessness
- Noise, light, ambient temperature
- Other painful conditions
- Parkinson's disease
- Peptic ulceration
- Periodic limb movements
- Physical illness
- Pruritus
- Psychiatric and cognitive disorders
- REM sleep disorders
- Restless legs syndrome
- Sleep apnoea
- Sleep disorders
- Stroke
- Sympathomimetics
- Thyroid disorders
- Time zone change syndrome
- Use of bed for other activities
- Withdrawal from medication (e.g. benzodiazepines)

AETIOLOGY

There are changes in circadian rhythm with ageing that tend to move older people to earlier retirement to bed, then many hours spent awake in the morning before rising. Thus, sleep time may be normal but the longer time in bed can be perceived as insomnia. Most insomnia in older people is accompanied by pain and/or physical illness and other comorbidities, although it is arguable as to whether these are the cause of the insomnia.

BOX 57.5 Sleep hygiene techniques

- Maintain regular sleep hours.
- Avoid excessive time in bed.
- Avoid daytime naps.
- Use bed for sleep (and sexual activity) only.
- Regular pre-retirement routine.
- Schedule time to relax before bed, and discuss relaxation routine.
- Encourage physical activity by day.
- Ensure exposure to sunlight.
- Make the bedroom quiet, comfortable, correct temperature, adequately dark and secure.
- Minimise stimulants, especially after 5 pm.
- Avoid large or late evening meal.
- Provide information about normal sleep patterns.

Common conditions associated with insomnia are shown in Box 57.4. The main aetiological factor behind insomnia, however, is probably the sleep changes that occur with ageing. It should also be remembered that sleep quality and mental health are intimately related. Although depression is a common cause of insomnia, insomnia is a common cause of depression. Therefore, the assessment of sleep problems should never ignore mental health issues, and the management of mental health issues should always involve behavioural approaches to improve sleep.

DIAGNOSTIC APPROACH

The main aim is to establish that the person does indeed have insomnia. This can be established most accurately by having the person keep a sleep diary, detailing time to bed, (estimated) delay in falling asleep, awakening times and naps by day. Occasionally a more formal sleep study is useful—this requires referral to a sleep centre/specialist. A medication review is also important, as prescribed medicines (such as antidepressants and steroids) may cause insomnia.

History and examination

Comorbid conditions should be sought through history and examination, which may need to be quite directive (e.g. 'Do you drink caffeine later in the day?' is less useful than 'Do you drink tea/coffee/chocolate after 4 pm?').

The examination needs only to be limited—areas to be assessed include tenderness (pain), cardiac (congestive cardiac failure), respiratory (chronic obstructive airways disease) and cognitive function.

MANAGEMENT[11]

Prevention, self-help and lifestyle

Insomnia can be both prevented and managed by a range of sleep hygiene techniques as outlined in Box 57.5. The individual should be persuaded to go to bed at a comfortable time (e.g. 11 pm) and rise at a regular time that allows sufficient but not excessive sleep (e.g. 7 am). Long hours spent reading or watching TV in bed should be discouraged. If there is regular daytime napping, this could be reduced by engaging in other activities—e.g. a walk after lunch rather than a nap. Preparation for bed can include a hot (non-caffeinated) beverage and listening to relaxing music (before, not in, bed). At least 30 minutes daily of moderate activity (e.g. a walk), preferably in sunlight, should be encouraged. Often people are relieved to know that if they feel refreshed by 6½ hours sleep nightly, that is all they need—not 8–10 hours, as some of their friends may be requiring. Patients need to be reassured that sleep requirement may change with age.

Insomnia can be transient but if it persists (certainly beyond 2–4 weeks) it should be addressed, especially as it has been associated with adverse health outcomes (see 'Prognosis' below).

Pharmacological

When sleep hygiene fails, pharmacological therapy for insomnia should be considered—as an add-on rather than an alternative. There are a range of prescribed hypnosedatives including the benzodiazepines and the benzodiazepine-like 'Z' drugs (e.g. zopiclone, zolpidem). All other prescribed drugs (e.g. antidepressants, antipsychotics) and many OTC drugs (antihistamines) are *not* recommended, because of adverse effects and limited efficacy.

If a benzodiazepine is felt necessary, the preferred agents have relatively short half-lives (e.g. temazepam rather than nitrazepam or flunitrazepam) and should not be used in high dosages (e.g. temazepam 10 mg only—not repeated overnight). This is mainly due to concerns about adverse effects which, for all benzodiazepines, include falls, fractures, motor vehicle accidents and cognitive impairment. The agents are only modestly effective—one study found only 4.5 additional minutes of sleep with temazepam and another no difference from placebo, but most show about 30 minutes per night of extra sleep. Few studies with significant numbers of elderly people have extended beyond 2 weeks and these drugs are only approved for short-term management of insomnia. The patient should be warned of adverse effects when they are begun, and agree to a clear plan to cease them after a short period.

The 'Z' drugs have not been demonstrated to be safer and have their own additional adverse effects—zolpidem, for instance, has been associated with abnormal nocturnal activities, including eating and even driving, while asleep. There have been fatal accidents. Again, they should be used only in the short term.

Complementary therapies

Valerian has modest efficacy for insomnia, and is almost devoid of adverse effects. It can be taken as a tablet or a tea.

Melatonin is also useful for insomnia. It may work by re-establishing circadian rhythms, but this is not proven. Adverse effects are rare, although coronary vasospasm has been reported. Dose is 1–2 mg nocte.

Bright light therapy is also useful—see the section on dementia.

ONGOING REVIEW AND MONITORING

The main purpose of ongoing review and monitoring is to ensure that hypnosedative agents are ceased, and to support the patient who (incorrectly) feels certain that they require medication in order to sleep.

IMPORTANT PITFALLS

A complaint of poor sleep alone does not make a diagnosis of insomnia—additional information should be sought.

Sleeping tablets are begun too easily, without the patient (and sometimes the prescriber) being aware of their risks, and the difficulties that can occur in attempting to cease them. Sleep hygiene should always be tried first, and continued even when a hypnosedative is prescribed.

PROGNOSIS

Insomnia is not entirely benign—studies have shown increased mortality in those with chronic insomnia. Bad sleeping habits, once established, can certainly be difficult to change.

DIABETES AND THYROID DISORDERS

These are discussed in detail in other sections of this book (see Chs 26 and 29) —the following discussion will briefly cover areas unique to older people.

DIABETES

Diabetes is diagnosed in about 20% of people aged over 65 years, and undiagnosed in up to a further 20%. It is usually type 2, largely due to insulin resistance.

Diagnosis usually follows reporting of symptoms or routine checking of fasting and random glucose levels. Older people may present newly with very high blood sugar levels but rarely with ketoacidosis. Lacticacidosis and non-ketotic coma need to be considered in an unwell elderly person even if diabetes has not yet been diagnosed. Other rarer initial presentations, which can also complicate established diabetes, include malignant cachexia (extreme muscle wasting), femoral neuropathy with marked proximal lower limb weakness and peripheral neuropathy. Diabetes is also a risk factor for dementia.

Management is directed at controlling sugar levels without significant risk of hypoglycaemia, which is poorly tolerated in older people, especially if recurrent. Therefore, target glucose levels may be a little higher (e.g. 8–12 mmol/L). Although the oft-cited UK diabetes study supported some benefits of tighter sugar control, it did not include a population typical of the older diabetic and was not conducted in ways that mimicked usual clinical practice.

Pharmacological management is indicated when diet and other lifestyle changes fail to control sugar levels, and initial therapy is usually with a sulforylurea and/or metformin.[12] Only shorter-acting sulforylureas should be used (e.g. gliclazide)—even glibenclamide (gliburide) has too long a half-life, and therefore too high a risk of inducing hypoglycaemia, in older people. If maximal doses of these fail to achieve control, consideration should be given to adding a 'glitazone' such as rosiglitazone, but recent concerns about increased mortality and cardiac adverse events from these agents should be considered. These agents should be avoided if there is heart failure, and the patient should be monitored for fluid accumulation. If oral therapy is failing, insulin should be added. Initially, once-daily longer-acting insulin should be trialled. There is synergism with metformin, which can therefore be continued, but not with the sulfonylureas, which should be ceased. If hypoglycaemia occurs despite insulin dosage adjustments, one of the newer semi-synthetic insulins (e.g. insulin glargine) should be substituted, as these have less risk of causing severe hypoglycaemia.

Other complementary therapies are discussed in the diabetes chapter (Ch 26).

Diabetic complications should be carefully monitored—the patient should see an eye specialist regularly and urine should be checked for microalbumin. Peripheral sensation should be assessed—a monofilament is useful for this. Older people may have reduced flexibility, impairing regular feet checks—this may require a carer or, less satisfactorily, regular podiatry visits. Diabetic leg ulcers require urgent and comprehensive management, which may include referral to a wound management specialist or a wound/diabetic 'high-risk foot' clinic. Cognitive symptoms should lead to an MMSE or other screening tool, and referral to a memory clinic or other memory specialist if indicated.

At the end of life, diabetic control may be less important, although uncontrolled hyperglycaemia does not lead to a quality death and usually some therapy is continued.

THYROID DISORDERS[13]

In older people, hypothyroidism is usually due to autoimmune thyroid disease (Hashimoto's thyroidism) but may be due to past radioactive iodine (^{131}I) therapy, lithium toxicity or to amiodarone—other causes are rare. Hyperthyroidism is usually due to a toxic multinodular goitre or autoimmune (Graves') disease; again, amiodarone and other sources of iodine should be considered.

The diagnosis can be difficult—often there is only a single major clinical manifestation (e.g. rapid atrial fibrillation or confusion) and the signs of hypothyroidism can be confused with ageing. Unusual presentations are not uncommon (e.g. depression, paranoia or leg ulceration). Fortunately, specific, sensitive blood tests are now available, and are frequently performed. An elevated TSH is usually diagnostic of hypothyroidism (but this is best confirmed with a low free T_4) and a low TSH is usually diagnostic of hyperthyroidism (again, best confirmed with either an elevated free T_4 or free T_3). Autoantibody test results rarely affect clinical management. A thyroid ultrasound can be useful in distinguishing a toxic multinodular goitre from autoimmune thyroiditis.

Referral to an endocrinologist is usually appropriate for further diagnostic tests as well as an initial management plan. Management of both is rarely urgent—occasionally severely unwell patients (e.g. myxoedema coma or 'madness') require hospitalisation. Any offending agent (e.g. amiodarone) should be ceased/avoided where possible, but this may not be sufficient to achieve control. Hypothyroidism requires thyroxine therapy but it is vital to start in low doses, to avoid cardiac complications, and increase slowly, using the TSH and symptoms to monitor effectiveness. A starting dose of 25 μg daily, increased by 25 μg every 2–4 weeks, is usually sufficient. Larger initial doses can precipitate coronary ischaemia and death. Hyperthyroidism is usually initially managed with medication—carbimazole or propylthiouracil along with a beta-blocker if there is sympathetic activation. Longer-term management with ^{131}I is often appropriate in older people, as delayed hypothyroidism is less of a risk in those already of advanced age, and the risks of polypharmacy (see above) lead prescribers to prefer non-drug therapy. Surgery is rarely indicated—except where there is superior mediastinal pressure on the trachea or oesophagus.

Ongoing monitoring is essential—for hypothyroidism the TSH should be checked and the thyroxine dose adjusted, and for thyrotoxicosis (especially after ^{131}I) emergent hypothyroidism needs to be detected early and treated (with thyroxine).

Thyroid cancer is usually euthyroid and more commonly presents as a mass or as metastatic disease, but should be considered in older people with a neck mass and thyroid dysfunction. Early diagnosis and treatment is vital.

WOUNDS

The management of wounds requires a holistic approach as there are usually many contributing factors to the non-healing wound. Chronic ulcers (wounds present for more than 4 weeks) are particularly troublesome. Not only are they expensive for the individual and the community, but they cause significant psychological and physical morbidity.

IMPORTANT CONDITIONS

Common types of acute wounds include: surgical (not discussed here), traumatic (such as skin tears in the elderly) and burns (not discussed here).

Skin tears are very common in the elderly. The most common cause of chronic leg ulcers is chronic venous insufficiency.

Pressure ulcer incidence is reported to be up to 38% in acute care.[14] In 2006 the Pressure Ulcer Point Prevalence Study (PUPPS) found a prevalence of 26% in public hospitals.

Approximately 15% of individuals with diabetes will develop an ulcer at some point.

AETIOLOGY

Common chronic wounds, according to aetiology, include:

- vascular insufficiency—venous, arterial or vasculitis
- pressure—decubitus ulcers or bedsores
- diabetes related.

PATHOLOGY

- Chronic venous insufficiency causing venous hypertension results in leg oedema, haemosiderin staining and lipodermatosclerosis.
- Peripheral atherosclerosis results in decreased blood supply to the extremities.
- Direct pressure, friction and shear forces and moisture combined in the immobile patient increase the risk of pressure ulcers.
- Patients with diabetes frequently have neuropathy leading to unrecognised trauma, often combined with poor arterial supply and a less effective immune system.

DIAGNOSTIC APPROACH

History

History should aim to identify the aetiology of the wound and current barriers to healing. Factors suggestive of chronic venous insufficiency include varicose veins, previous deep vein thrombosis, surgery or trauma to the limb, obesity, long periods of standing (enquire about employment history) and increased intraabdominal pressure. These wounds frequently commence spontaneously. Risk factors for peripheral vascular disease are as for cardiovascular disease: hypertension, hyperlipidaemia, smoking, family history and diabetes. Enquire about previous amputations. Patients with foot lesions should be questioned regarding causes of neuropathy. Patients with diabetic foot wounds generally have peripheral neuropathy, a history of initiating trauma and often poor arterial supply or infection.

Patients with pressure areas will have reasons for immobility or inability to reduce pressure or neuropathy. Common examples include fractured neck of femur, stroke and spinal lesions. Patients with severe dementia or inability to communicate are also at high risk. Other risk factors for pressure areas include incontinence, temperature abnormality, poor nutritional intake and multiple medical comorbidities.

Skin tears occur in those with frail skin (check for steroid use, warfarin and nutritional status) and are initiated by trauma. Common causes include wheelchair footplates and screws on walking frames.

Pain is common in chronic wounds. This may be background pain or associated with dressing changes or particular dressing products.

Nutritional and hydration status should be reviewed. Adequate vitamin C, zinc and protein are needed for wound healing, and it can be delayed by psychological stress.

Enquire about the current dressing regimen and who applies them. Ideally, gain further history from this person. Also note which dressings have been tried so far and the effects of each.

Examination

General examination should include the cardiovascular system, including peripheral pulses and fluid status.

The common sites of pressure areas if the patient is supine are heels and sacrum. Grade the pressure area (1–4).

- Grade 1 indicates non-blanchable erythema of intact skin.
- Grade 2 is a loss of epidermis and dermis.
- Grade 3 is full thickness skin loss, which may extend to fascia.
- Grade 4 is full thickness skin loss and tissue necrosis down to bone or joint capsule.

The appearance of the surrounding skin often gives an indication of aetiology. Chronic venous insufficiency causes haemosiderin (brown) staining of the lower third of the leg, lipodermatosclerosis, venous eczema and scaly skin. Deformities of the feet and areas of callus indicate areas of pressure.

The wound itself should be described, including: location, dimensions (including depth), edge, the presence of slough or necrotic tissue, signs of infection or inflammation and the volume and type of exudates.[15]

Skin tears may be graded according to the amount of skin lost; the STAR tool by the Silverchain group is useful.[16]

Review footwear if implicated in wound formation.

INVESTIGATIONS

Consulting room

An ankle brachial index (using Doppler ultrasound) compares the blood pressure in the dorsalis pedis or posterior tibialis to that in the brachial artery. An index of 1.0 indicates normal arterial supply. A ratio higher than this may indicate calcification of the vessels. A result lower than 0.8 means reduced arterial supply and implies that any application of compression should proceed with caution.

Pathology

Inflammatory markers, electrolytes, renal function, liver function and albumin may be warranted. Blood sugar level (BSL) and glycosylated haemoglobin are measured in those with diabetes.

A biopsy of the edge of the wound will help determine whether malignancy is present. Culture of biopsy tissue will give more accurate information regarding organisms causing infection. A wound swab will provide information regarding the types of organisms on the surface of the wound, but not necessarily those deeper in the tissue.

Special tests

Vascular imaging of veins and arteries may clarify the aetiology of the wound and outline potential surgical options.

If osteomyelitis is suspected, the best test is MRI—however, the initial starting point is more likely to be X-ray or bone scan.

INTEGRATIVE MANAGEMENT

Prevention

Compression hosiery is not only comfortable, but will reduce the risk of further venous ulcers in those with chronic venous insufficiency.

Peripheral vascular disease may be minimised through control of cardiovascular risk factors.

Pressure area prevention is the cornerstone of management. Braden, Norton and Waterlow scales will stratify the risk of pressure areas. Air mattresses and cushions, gel cushions, bed cradles and orthotic devices have become part of pressure care of the immobile patient. Nursing care such as turning patients and adequate nutrition is still vital.[14]

Diabetic patients must be educated regarding footwear, blood sugar level management, and the benefits of regular podiatric care and early recognition of foot trauma.

Non-surgical management

Many wounds will heal eventually if nothing is done other than protective dressings. However, wounds which are due to untreated arterial insufficiency, unrelieved pressure and undiagnosed malignancy are unlikely to heal without intervention.

Self-help/lifestyle

Lifestyle factors such as smoking cessation and ensuring adequate diet and hydration[17] help wound healing. Exercise is beneficial for venous leg wounds in particular.

Pharmacological

Analgesia may be required. Some medications are known to cause wounds (such as hydroxyurea) or to affect wound healing (such as prednisolone). The indication for these medications should be reviewed.

An appropriate wound dressing should be chosen to prepare the wound bed for healing. A plan for long-term management should then be developed. This will encompass the likelihood of healing or other surrogate goals.

Surgical

Vascular surgery for chronic venous insufficiency and peripheral vascular disease may be required. Skin grafts and flaps may be needed. Occasionally amputation is the only option.

Other medical

Specialist wound clinics generally contain a multidisciplinary team with up-to-date knowledge of the latest wound products and research. Further referral to hyperbaric oxygen may be recommended.

Paramedical

Chronic wounds in the elderly frequently require a multidisciplinary approach. Nursing care is often required for dressing changes, pressure care or diabetic education. Podiatric involvement is vital in the management of diabetic feet and in footwear advice. Dieticians are of particular benefit to those with pressure areas, patients with diabetes and those who are undernourished or obese. Pharmacists with an interest in wound care will be able to advise on wound dressings and costs. Specialised physiotherapists may advise on massage techniques for lymphoedema.

Complementary therapies

Wound dressings are a fast-growing industry.[15] Complementary therapies are also becoming more 'mainstream'. For example, manuka honey is being developed in new and more user-friendly preparations. Although research is somewhat lacking regarding the true mechanism of action, it is thought to have antimicrobial activity due to the slow release of hydrogen peroxide.[15]

Dietary supplements are also now considered virtually mainstream in the management of pressure areas. Commercial products containing arginine (an amino acid), vitamin C and zinc have been proved to aid the healing of pressure areas.[18] Caution is required with the supplementation of zinc, as its benefit is probably only in those with deficiency and the appropriate dosage is not established. High-dose zinc may be associated with nausea and may result in copper deficiency (which can cause anaemia).[19] However, topical zinc oxide preparations may be helpful.[20]

Horse chestnut is thought to be useful in chronic venous insufficiency. Liver function tests and coagulation profile should be monitored.[21]

Ongoing review/ monitoring

The risk of future wounds due to chronic venous insufficiency can be reduced with surgical correction of varicose veins or lifelong use of correctly fitted compression stockings.

Patients with arterial insufficiency should avoid trauma.

Patients with pressure areas frequently have irreversible predisposing conditions. Constant review of pressure areas and scrupulous pressure care are therefore required.

Patients with peripheral neuropathy (diabetes being the most common cause) must inspect their feet daily (or have someone inspect their feet for them). Any trauma must be addressed quickly. Particular attention must be paid to footwear and callus formation (ulcers may form under callus). Regular podiatry review is recommended.

IMPORTANT PITFALLS

Failure to identify the aetiology of the wound, or barrier to healing, is the most important pitfall. For example, if osteomyelitis is present, the overlying ulcer will not heal. Mixed venous and arterial disease is common in the elderly and limits the use of compression. The arterial component is often under-recognised. The principles of moist wound healing do *not* apply to the dry eschar of digits or heels in ischaemic limbs. These wounds are best kept dry, to limit the risk of infection. Cheaper wound dressings may need to be applied more frequently and slow wound healing, thus increasing the overall cost.

PROGNOSIS

Prognosis is governed by the ability to address the underlying aetiology. Healing may not be possible; substitute goals such as pain relief and exudate management may be more achievable.

PATIENT EDUCATION

Educate regarding wound dressings or compression therapy and the benefits of smoking cessation.

CONTINENCE

Urinary or faecal incontinence is the involuntary or inappropriate loss of urine or faeces. Over 50% of residents of aged care facilities suffer from incontinence and it is one of the major reasons for admission to such a facility. Bladder control problems are thought to treble the cost of care in nursing homes and take up approximately 60% of nursing time. Seventy per cent of incontinence suffers are women, with problems arising after pregnancy and childbirth. Lower urinary tract symptoms increase with age. Incontinence in the elderly frequently has a multifactorial origin. Most importantly, incontinence affects self-esteem, motivation, independence and dignity.

IMPORTANT CONDITIONS

Urinary incontinence:

- *Stress incontinence* is the leakage of urine with physical exertion such as coughing, laughing, walking or lifting. It commonly affects older women who have oestrogen deficiency or have had children. Being overweight, constipation and chronic cough are also risk factors. Men may have stress incontinence following prostate surgery.
- *Urge incontinence* occurs when the patient develops a sudden strong urge to urinate; they may not get to the toilet in time. Benign prostatic hypertrophy may cause urge incontinence, but is also associated with detrusor failure (atonic bladder). Detrusor failure is loss of elasticity and may occur with ageing and lower motor neuron lesions. These patients generally have a high residual volume and low voiding pressure.
- *Overflow incontinence* is the leakage of an overly full bladder that is unable to empty completely. Symptoms include straining to pass urine, a weak stream, feeling that the bladder is not completely empty, no warning to passing urine, passing urine while asleep and frequent urinary tract infections. It may be due to constipation, prostate enlargement, prolapse, damaged innervation of the bladder (such as in stroke, Parkinson's disease and multiple sclerosis) and medications.

Other:

- *Constipation* is hardening of faeces and decreased frequency of bowel motions.
- *Faecal incontinence* is the involuntary loss of faeces. It is commonly associated with constipation, weakened pelvic floor muscles or inadequate sphincter.

BACKGROUND/AETIOLOGY

Continence requires the individual to know where to toilet, be able to get there, be able to hold on to get there and be able to undress and then re-dress. Older people have a reduced bladder capacity, lessened sphincter strength and reduced ability to defer, but environmental factors are often also significant.

The normal bladder empties approximately every 3–4 hours. It has a capacity of 400–600 mL, but feels full at about 200–300 mL. One episode of nocturia is considered normal. A normal bladder does not leak and empties completely.

Normal bowel motions only require a small push to pass. The frequency is from up to three times per day to once every three days.

PATHOLOGY

Sensory urgency is due to a small-capacity bladder or recurrent urinary tract infections.

Overactive bladder (detrusor instability and hyperreflexia) results from spontaneous reflexic detrusor contractions and results in urge incontinence (associated with a sudden strong urge to pass urine). It is often associated with neurological conditions such as Parkinson's disease, stroke and dementia. Symptoms include urinary frequency and nocturia.

Reduced bladder capacity may result in frequency, nocturia, urgency and urge incontinence (detrusor instability). Hesitancy, slowed stream and terminal dribble may be due to underactive bladder (detrusor failure) or outlet obstruction.

Stress incontinence is due to weakened pelvic floor musculature or intrinsic sphincter failure.

Comorbidities are likely to contribute in the elderly patient. General poor health, frailty, poor mobility, cognitive deficits or renal or cardiac dysfunction may affect continence. Cortical micturition centres exert an inhibitory effect on the sacral reflex arc and may be damaged in neurological and dementing illnesses.

It is generally thought that there is no reduction in bowel movement frequency with normal ageing. The elderly community probably overestimates constipation. However, severe constipation is the most common cause of faecal incontinence, with watery stool flowing around the hard faeces. Constipation has many potential causes; those common in the elderly include inadequate fluid or dietary fibre, immobility, medication, bowel pathology, neurological conditions such as stroke and Parkinson's disease causing slow-transit bowel and poor toileting habits. Inadequate sphincter function due to poor pelvic floor or neurological condition may also result in faecal incontinence.

DIAGNOSTIC APPROACH

History

Enquire about lower urinary tract symptoms: frequency, urgency, nocturia, voiding difficulties, dysuria, haematuria, urge incontinence, stress incontinence, overflow incontinence and functional incontinence.

Consider reversible causes: delirium, urinary tract infection, atrophic vaginitis in women, psychological (severe depression, neurosis), pharmacological, excess fluid intake or output, restricted mobility or environment, stool impaction.[22]

Medical conditions that may affect continence include neurological conditions (especially multiple sclerosis, stroke and Parkinson's disease), dementia, diabetes, cardiac failure and those that impair mobility. Gynaecological and urological history (including surgery), obstetric and menstrual history, sexual history and previous continence assessments should be taken.

Regarding constipation and faecal incontinence, the history should include the relevant past surgical history. Diet, fluid intake, mobility, duration of constipation, frequency of bowel actions, character of the stool, pain, straining and laxative use are also vital.[23]

Consider impact on quality of life—for example, limitation of social activities, sleep disturbance.

Examination

Abdominal examination including per rectal examination: note the size and texture of the prostate in men, and anal tone. The vaginal examination in women should check for urine excoriation, senile changes, infection, prolapse and pelvic floor strength.

Stress incontinence can be checked by asking the patient to stand and cough (ensure there is adequate protection on the floor, to prevent embarrassment). This can also be checked in the supine position when examining.

Check mobility and cognitive function.

INVESTIGATIONS

Consulting room:
- urine dipstick
- urine residual volume (bladder scan).

Pathology:
- urine cytology and culture
- renal function, potassium, glucose level, calcium level and prostate marker if relevant
- consider faecal occult blood.

Special tests:
- urodynamics—indicated in cases not responding to conventional treatment or pre-surgery
- abdominal X-ray
- cystoscopy.

INTEGRATIVE MANAGEMENT

Prevention

Avoid urinating 'just in case'. Avoid deferring bowel movements, prolonged use of irritant laxatives and constipation.

General measures

The patient may manage urinary incontinence—for example, more frequent or regular voiding, use of continence aids. Laxatives are also available over the counter—many patients may self-medicate. Unfortunately, continence problems may worsen if no changes are made.

Self-help

Eating adequate fibre (fruit, vegetables, lentils and high-fibre breakfast cereal) and fluid (approximately 2 L per day if there are no contraindications) can help avoid constipation. Stopping smoking (reduces coughing) and losing weight also help to reduce incontinence.

If caring for a confused incontinent person, consider labelling the toilet with a sign or picture, keep a light on in the toilet, keep a regular daily routine for eating, walking and toileting. Offer the toilet at predicted toileting times (for example, after breakfast) or times of unsettled behaviour. Ensure that clothing is easy to remove. Encourage double voiding. Restrict fluids after 7 pm.

An occupational therapy assessment of toilet facilities may help with issues such as aids to sitting and standing to void.

Lifestyle

- Exercise and weight reduction.
- Reduce or eliminate caffeine.
- Lifestyle can be inhibited by incontinence—ensuring that the patient is 'socially continent' with the use of continence aids is valuable.

Pharmacology

A medication review should be undertaken and altered as appropriate. Drugs may induce urinary incontinence.
- Alpha-blockers reduce urethral resistance.
- Opioids result in constipation.

- Anticonvulsants may cause confusion and ataxia.
- Calcium channel blockers may cause constipation and urinary retention.
- Loop diuretics increase urgency.[22]

Cholinesterase inhibitors (donepezil, galantamine, rivastigmine) are reported to increase urinary frequency and perhaps urinary incontinence. There is now evidence that anticholinergic treatment for urinary incontinence in this situation may be helpful—although it does seem illogical.[22]

Topical oestrogen (cream applied to the vaginal entrance or using vaginal applicators) may improve symptoms of urgency and stress incontinence and help prevent future episodes of cystitis.

Antibiotics should be used to treat urinary tract infections and should be accompanied by probiotic support.

Detrusor instability is best managed with anticholinergics, such as oxybutynin. Newer agents such as solifenacin succinate are claimed to be more specific to muscarinic receptors in the bladder and thus have fewer of the systemic anticholinergic side effects, such as confusion and dry mouth. Anticholinergics should not be used in those with previous closed angle glaucoma or atonic bladder, or those with any cause of increased post-void residual volume.

Botulinum A toxin injections into the bladder neck or detrusor have also been reported to manage detrusor instability.

Benign prostatic hypertrophy may be managed with alpha-1 blockers; androgen blockade is used in cases with clinically enlarged prostate.[22]

Sensory urgency may benefit from a urine alkaliniser, which helps reduce the irritability of the urine.

Treatment of autonomic dysfunction is appropriate if present in nocturnal polyuria. Desmopressin is reported to help, but is not generally recommended in the elderly, due to the risk of hyponatraemia.

Aperients can be used in the short-term to manage constipation. Options include stimulants such as senna, psyllium, bulking agents and osmotic agents. Enemas and suppositories may be needed for impaction.

Surgical/other medical

Referral to a specialist continence clinic for multidisciplinary assessment is appropriate, especially if lower urinary tract symptoms have not responded to conventional treatment such as bowel management, bladder training, pelvic floor exercises and anticholinergic medication. Geriatricians, physiotherapists, urologists, urogynaecologists, gynaecologists, gastroenterologists and colorectal surgeons may be needed. Surgical opinion may be required if other measures have failed. Operations include prostate surgery, surgical correction of prolapse and sphincter repair.

Paramedical

- Continence physiotherapy for training of the pelvic floor—may use aids such as electrostimulation, pressure biofeedback or weighted vaginal cones.
- Continence nursing for education and advice regarding continence aids such as pads, pants, bedpads and chairpads, protective bedding, condom drainage and catheters; also skin care and odour management.
- Occupational therapists may advise regarding raised toilet seats, commodes and urinals.
- Dietician for dietary advice.

Complementary therapies

- Therapies centered on dietary regulation of bowel habit.
- Cranberry juice or tablets for frequent urine infections.

ONGOING REVIEW

Review management strategies and aetiology if not responding to management as expected. Monitor residual volume and renal function, especially in those with unresolved obstruction.

IMPORTANT PITFALLS

- Differentiating prostatic obstruction from atonic bladder or detrusor hyperreflexia with impaired contractility.
- Failure to exclude polyuria as a cause of frequency.
- Faecal impaction causing faecal incontinence being mistaken for diarrhoea.
- Urinary incontinence due to overflow from urinary retention.
- Applying too much barrier cream or talcum powder—will transfer to the continence pad, restricting absorption.

PROGNOSIS

Not all cases of incontinence may be treatable, but many will be manageable. An incontinent individual may be able to be 'socially continent' or 'dependently' continent.

PATIENT EDUCATION

- Bladder retraining is aimed at increasing the storage capacity of the bladder for management of urge incontinence.
- Pelvic floor exercises.

- Intermittent self-catheterisation or managing a permanent indwelling catheter, for management of overflow incontinence.
- Appropriate defecation techniques and normal bowel habit—for example, when sitting on the toilet, place the elbows on the knees, lean forward with a straight back and put feet on a stool. Passing a bowel action should take less than one minute. Wipe from front to back. The strongest urge to defecate will occur approximately 30 minutes after eating, particularly breakfast. A hot drink may also stimulate a bowel movement.

CARDIOVASCULAR

Important cardiac conditions in the elderly include ischaemic heart disease, heart failure, valvular heart disease and arrhythmia, especially atrial fibrillation.

BACKGROUND/AETIOLOGY

Important risk factors for ischaemic heart disease are: age, gender, hypertension, dyslipidaemia, smoking, poor mental health and diabetes mellitus. Heart failure can be divided into ischaemic and non-ischaemic causes. Common non-ischaemic causes are hypertension and valve disease.

PATHOLOGY

Ischaemic heart disease (IHD) results from coronary atherosclerosis and usually becomes symptomatic once a stenosis occupies 70% or more of the vessel lumen. Elderly patients often have significant vessel calcification, which can increase the difficulty of interventional procedures.

Heart failure may be caused by:

- systolic dysfunction—characterised by reduced left ventricular contraction
- diastolic dysfunction—characterised by impairment of left ventricular relaxation and raised left atrial pressure
- a combination of systolic and diastolic dysfunction.

Risk factors for diastolic heart failure are increasing age, female gender, hypertension and diabetes mellitus.

Degenerative valvular disease is a common finding in the elderly. Calcific, degenerative aortic stenosis (AS) is the most common valvular disease. Mitral valve disease is also common and may result from degenerative processes causing prolapse and flail leaflets, ischaemic papillary muscle dysfunction or dilatation of the mitral annulus due to cardiac enlargement.

Atrial fibrillation (AF) is frequently found in elderly patients. Left atrial enlargement, left ventricular hypertrophy and left ventricular dysfunction are associated with an increased likelihood of AF. Sinus node and atrioventricular (AV) node dysfunction increase with age due to degeneration of the conduction system. AV node blocking agents such as beta-blockers, calcium channel blocker and digoxin can exacerbate AV node disease.

DIAGNOSTIC APPROACH

History

History is vital; however, elderly patients frequently present atypically. While the classic IHD presentation may occur, elderly patients may present without pain or with dyspnoea alone. A comprehensive cardiac history should still include questions regarding chest pain, 'indigestion', breathlessness, exercise tolerance and classic symptoms of cardiac failure, palpitations, syncope and presyncope. Questions regarding concomitant acute illness, such as pneumonia, are important as these are frequent precipitants of acute cardiac presentations such as heart failure or AF.

Examination

Full cardiovascular examination including pulse (rate and rhythm), fluid status and heart sounds. Postural blood pressure and heart rate are also relevant. The blood pressure and heart rate should be taken initially when lying or sitting and then on standing. After waiting for 3–5 minutes, the blood pressure and heart rate should be repeated. A blood pressure drop of more than 15–20 mmHg is significant. The heart rate should increase to compensate for the initial drop in blood pressure.

INVESTIGATIONS

Consulting room:

- 12-lead electrocardiogram.

Pathology:

- Full blood count (anaemia and platelet count), electrolytes and renal function, cardiac enzymes (creatine kinase and troponin) if suspect acute coronary syndrome.
- Thyroid function tests.

Special tests:

- Further investigations may be appropriate, such as a stress test (exercise or pharmacological ECG, echocardiogram or nuclear myocardial perfusion scan) to investigate ischaemia. An echocardiogram will identify cardiac function and valve pathology. A Holter monitor will record any arrhythmia, but sensitivity is low.

INTEGRATIVE MANAGEMENT

Prevention

Modification of cardiovascular risk factors

Self-help/lifestyle

Exercise, weight loss, dietary modification, etc (see Ch 25).

Pharmacology
Therapies available for elderly patients in the management of IHD are the same as those for younger patients: antiplatelet therapy (aspirin and/or clopidogrel), statin, beta-blocker, angiotensin-converting enzyme inhibitor or angiotensin II receptor blocker, nitrates.

Medications for heart failure include ACE inhibitors (angiotensin receptor blockers), beta-blockers if euvolaemic (carvedilol, bisoprolol, metoprolol XL), diuretics (for symptom control only).

There is currently no effective pharmacological management for chronic valvular disease.

The best management of AF includes management of the cause. A rate control strategy (beta-blocker or non-dihydropyridine calcium channel blocker ± digoxin) is generally sufficient as it is safer than rhythm control and has similar outcomes. Patients over the age of 75 years with an additional risk factor, such as left ventricular systolic dysfunction, hypertension, diabetes mellitus or previous stroke, benefit from the addition of warfarin therapy. The CHADS2 score helps to assess risk.[24] The benefits of anticoagulation must be considered in the context of the patient's comorbidities. Some studies have suggested that the rate of severe bleeding complication is not as significant as perhaps perceived.[25]

Complementary therapies
See Ch 25, Cardiovascular.

Surgical
Several interventions are available for cardiac disease, including percutaneous intervention (angioplasty/stenting) or coronary artery bypass surgery for IHD; revascularisation for ischaemic cardiac failure and biventricular pacemakers for those with dyssynchronous ventricular contraction.

Aortic valve replacement is the only effective treatment for symptomatic severe aortic stenosis. Age is not a barrier to treatment. Surgery should be considered for severe symptomatic mitral regurgitation. Valve repair is preferred over replacement.

Paramedical
Coronary care units are beneficial to the elderly in the acute coronary syndrome setting. Multidisciplinary cardiac rehabilitation and chronic disease community nursing are especially helpful in the management of heart failure. Advice from a dietician may assist with coronary risk factors such as hyperlipidaemia or obesity.

ONGOING REVIEW
Monitoring of symptomatic status, cardiac risk factors, fluid balance and tolerance of medications is necessary. Review patients for the appropriateness of new technologies and drugs.

IMPORTANT PITFALLS
Elderly people may not always present with classic symptoms of ischaemic chest pain. They may present with dyspnoea, syncope or confusion.

Digoxin should be considered a second-line or add-on therapy in the rate control of AF. This is due to the narrow therapeutic range and significant side effects.

Vasodilators such as calcium channel blockers and ACE inhibitors should be used with caution in severe aortic stenosis. Caution should be exercised with beta-blockers in severe aortic stenosis.

Non-steroidal anti-inflammatory drugs may exacerbate heart failure, an additional reason to avoid these agents in the elderly.

Ankle oedema has many potential aetiologies in the elderly, including dependent oedema, venous insufficiency, hypoproteinaemia and heart failure. Unless other signs of heart failure are present, diuretics should be avoided as side effects may outweigh benefit. Leg elevation and compression therapy may be more appropriate.

PROGNOSIS
The goal of therapy in many elderly individuals with cardiac disease is symptom control. There is limited evidence for most treatments specific to the very elderly population.

PATIENT EDUCATION
Some patients with heart failure may be able to follow a management plan based on regular weigh-ins and adjustment of diuretics. Patients taking anginine should be informed of how to take it safely and to sit down when doing so, to avoid problems with hypotension.

PAIN IN THE ELDERLY POPULATION
Pain is an 'unpleasant sensory and emotional experience associated with actual or potential tissue damage, or described in terms of such damage. The inability to communicate verbally does not negate the possibility that a patient is experiencing pain and is in need of appropriate pain relieving treatment' (International Association for the Study of Pain). Up to 50% of older community dwellers and 80% of those in residential care suffer from persistent pain.[26]

Chronic pain is 'without apparent biological value and persists beyond normal tissue healing time' (IASP). Conditions common in the elderly include arthropathy, postherpetic neuralgia (PHN), polymyalgia rheumatica, peripheral vascular disease and cancer.

BACKGROUND/AETIOLOGY

Nociception is the sensation evoked by noxious stimulation of the neural system. Older patients have higher pain thresholds, which may mean they present later for conditions such as acute myocardial ischaemia and peritonitis. However, pain tolerance decreases with age. Older adults appear to be more vulnerable to developing severe and persistent pain. This implies that those older patients who do have pain are more likely to have severe and persistent pain.

PATHOLOGY

Animal and human studies suggest a reduced plasticity of the nocioceptive system and prolonged dysfunction following tissue injury, inflammation or nerve injury in the elderly. Older patients therefore will not recognise mild pain until there is significant damage and will be less likely to recover from it.

Cell-mediated immunity is impaired with ageing, placing the elderly at risk of reactivation of *Herpes zoster* and development of PHN.[27]

DIAGNOSTIC APPROACH

Identify and treat the cause of the pain and associated symptoms, if possible. Select the appropriate modes of therapy for pain relief. Review and modify therapy.

History

Identify the onset, cause and time frame, factors that increase and decrease the pain, severity and impact on lifestyle.[28] Gain an understanding of which treatment modalities have already been tried, and their effectiveness. Watch for 'red flags' indicating serious underlying pathology, such as thoracic pain, pain associated with incontinence or gait disturbance or back pain in someone with known malignancy.

Examination

Use a pain intensity scale to quantify the pain. Examples include verbal descriptor scale and numeric rating scale. Pain scales for those with dementia, or those who cannot verbalise, include: pain assessment in advanced dementia (PAINAD) and the Abbey pain scale. Although these scales are not particularly useful when comparing patients, they are useful for assessing management strategies in an individual.

Look for a zoster-type rash if indicated.

INVESTIGATIONS

These will be guided by the history and examination. Consider inflammatory markers and prostate-specific antigen (in men) in new-onset back pain—serious pathology would be malignancy or discitis. Arrange or review imaging of the area. For example, MRI spinal cord if 'red flags' for spinal cord compression are present.

INTEGRATIVE MANAGEMENT

Prevention

Appropriate treatment of acute pain syndromes and acute illness may help reduce the risk of a pain syndrome becoming chronic. Prevention of *Varicella zoster* virus infection and immunisation against *Herpes zoster* may decrease the incidence of this condition in the future.[27]

General measures

General supportive measures, such as meditation, may be an option in the chronic pain setting, if this suits the patient (see Ch 38, Pain management).

Self-help

Patients may find ways to limit their pain by adjusting their activity.

Lifestyle

In many cases, pain cannot be completely eliminated, although self-help and lifestyle strategies can help a person to cope better with it.[28] Lifestyle may have to be adjusted to allow best function for the majority of the time.

Pharmacology

For mild to moderate pain, simple analgesics such as paracetamol are preferred.[28] Glucosamine and paracetamol may provide enough relief for many patients suffering from osteoarthritis pain. Long-term use of non-steroidal anti-inflammatory agents is best avoided in the elderly due to the side-effect profile (gastrointestinal upset, renal failure, fluid retention, hypertension). COX-2 inhibitors have similar issues.

For moderate to severe pain, agents such as codeine or tramadol may be considered. However, side effects including constipation and confusion should be taken into consideration in the elderly. Tramadol is generally avoided in the elderly population due to the incidence of delirium.

Newer transdermal patches of fentanyl or buprenorphine have the advantages of steady-state medication delivery and less frequent dosing[28]; however, side effects including delirium may limit their use. Initiation at low dose, and slow titration, are appropriate in the elderly.

Opioids such as oxycodone and morphine may be required in the elderly patient with severe pain. Constipation, nausea and confusion are common unwanted effects. A long-acting oxycodone for background relief and a short-acting oxycodone for breakthrough pain are usually prescribed. A low dose should be used initially in the elderly, due to pharmacokinetic and pharmacodynamic changes related to ageing, caused by altered organ function and volumes of distribution. Initially the dose should be reviewed frequently.[29] Aperients are generally prescribed at the same time as opioids, to avoid constipation.

In neuropathic pain syndromes, such as PHN, the combination of opioid and gabapentin or pregabalin is often helpful; tricyclic antidepressants (TCA) and tramadol have also been shown to be of use.[30] However, these agents may cause confusion in the elderly and the TCAs have undesirable potential cardiac side effects. Topical capsaicin and lignocaine also show promise.[27,30]

Surgical
This is largely dependent on the underlying pathology, but may be appropriate in some cases, such as spinal cord compression.

Other medical
Pain clinic assessment may be required for resistant severe pain. Anaesthetists may be able to offer minimally invasive techniques and alternative approaches for delivery of analgesic preparations.

Paramedical
Physiotherapy (heat, cold, hydrotherapy, ultrasound, massage, stretching) and transcutaneous electrical nerve stimulation are worth considering. Psychological input may be required, as associated symptoms of fear, anxiety and depression are common in those with chronic pain. Relaxation and biofeedback may be useful.

Complementary therapies
Acupuncture and massage for a range of pain syndromes, and glucosamine for osteoarthritis, are complementary therapies but have almost become 'mainstream' on the back of consistent evidence of their safety and efficacy. These will be useful adjuncts to offer patients to help manage pain and also to reduce the dosage of analgesic medication required to restore quality of life.

ONGOING REVIEW
Ongoing review of the patient's pain and response to therapy is necessary. The person's ability to function and their pain score should be reassessed. Adjustment of analgesia is frequently required in the initial period. Side effects are very troublesome in the elderly and often limit the use of various analgesic preparations.

IMPORTANT PITFALLS
Patients often expect to have complete relief of symptoms—this is less likely in chronic pain states. Although acute pain is well managed with medications, a much more multifaceted approach is needed for chronic pain.

PATIENT EDUCATION
Patients need to learn what triggers their pain, and to avoid this if possible. Some patients need to come to terms with the idea of regular analgesia to prevent pain, and 'top-ups' or 'breakthrough' analgesia at times of worsening pain.

FALLS
In the elderly the consequences of falls are significant—they include fractures, bruising and developing a fear of falling. Approximately one-third of people aged over 65 years and living in the community will experience one or more falls per year; the number is higher in institutions. Less than 10% of falls result in fracture, but 20% require medical attention.[31]

Hip fracture is the most serious fall-related injury in older people. Fifteen per cent die in hospital and a third do not survive beyond one year.[32] However, other fractures, intracranial hemorrhage and the development of fear of falling are also important.

BACKGROUND/AETIOLOGY
The aetiology of falls in most elderly patients is multifactorial. Extrinsic factors (environment and accidents) and intrinsic factors play a part. Intrinsic factors include gait disturbances, cardiovascular disease, neurological disorders, sensory impairment, foot abnormalities and de-conditioning.

PATHOLOGY
The underlying intrinsic pathology commonly involves the neurological and cardiovascular systems. Gait disturbance may include parkinsonism, stroke, normal-pressure hydrocephalus, peripheral neuropathy, cerebellar disease or orthopaedic disorders. Significant cardiovascular disorders include postural hypotension (this is particularly common in the elderly), arrhythmia, vaso-vagal episodes, myocardial ischaemia and aortic stenosis. Autonomic dysfunction is present in most elderly patients to some degree, and in some patients it is more significant. It may manifest as nocturnal hypertension and morning postural hypotension. Epilepsy is not infrequent, especially following stroke.

DIAGNOSTIC APPROACH
Identify and correct as many contributing factors as possible, through comprehensive evaluation of history, physical examination and medication review.

History
Discuss the history of the falls in detail—for example, where and when they occurred, during what activity

and any perceived warning signs. Quantify the number of falls in recent months. Identify the significance of trauma caused by the fall. Ideally, confirm the history of falls with an eye witness.

Identify extrinsic factors, such as footwear, uneven footpath, use of gait aid, use of visual aids or poor nocturnal lighting.

Enquire about loss of consciousness, postural dizziness, palpitations and blood sugar control. A patient's self-report of perceived loss of consciousness or lack of loss of consciousness is often unreliable. Medication use, both prescribed and OTC, and the initiation and compliance of medications should be documented. Identify intrinsic causes, such as neurological and cardiovascular history.

Features of autonomic dysfunction include nocturnal polyuria, lack of increased heart rate on standing and lack of sweating.

Examination

- Examine for signs of trauma.
- Cardiovascular examination, in particular heart rate and rhythm, blood pressure, cardiac murmurs and carotid bruits.
- Limb examination, including gait pattern, joints, deformities and amputations.
- Neurological examination, including proprioception and sensation.
- Assess visual acuity.
- The gait aid appropriateness and patient's technique for using it should be reviewed, as should the footwear.

INVESTIGATIONS

Consulting room

- Check lying, then standing, heart rate and blood pressure. The standing blood pressure should be measured initially and then 3 minutes after standing. A fall in systolic pressure of greater than 20 mmHg or 15 mmHg in diastolic pressure may be classed as postural hypotension.
- Romberg's test for balance.
- Electrocardiogram.

Pathology

- Creatine kinase may be elevated in those who have recently fallen, resulting in muscle damage.
- Full blood count, as acute blood loss may contribute to postural hypotension. Elevated white cell count may reveal infection.
- Hypoglycaemia and electrolyte disturbance may need to be excluded on the acute setting. Cardiac enzymes and troponin may be indicated, depending on history.
- Vitamin D will indicate deficiency, identifying those at risk of further fracture.

Special tests

- X-ray limbs if fracture suspected.
- CT brain if cerebrovascular accident is suspected.
- Consider 24-hour Holter monitor (arrhythmia), tilt table testing or echocardiograph (ventricular function, valve pathology) if a cardiac cause is implicated.
- Bone mineral density.

INTEGRATIVE MANAGEMENT

Prevention

Prevention is based on multidisciplinary assessment and intervention. In the residential care setting, subacute and acute hospital measures such as mat, chair and bed alarms may be needed, to alert staff when a patient is on the move. Hip protectors should be placed on the patient. A hospital bed that can be lowered to the floor limits the amount of damage a patient may do, should they roll out. Rails near shower and toilet will help with activities of daily living. Designing facilities with corridors and doorways wide enough to allow the use of gait aids is also important. Access ramps may also be beneficial. Physical restraint in the confused patient is rarely helpful, as the individual tends to struggle more and then risks harming themselves. Equally, chemical restraint should be limited as much as possible due to the inevitable effect on gait and balance.

General supportive measures

The elderly frequently choose this option. However, the risk of morbidity, increased dependency and mortality is significant and warrants intervention.

Self-help

Review and modify the home: avoid slippery floors, loose rugs, clutter, poor lighting, poor footwear. Consider a personal alarm if home alone, or a mobile or portable phone.

Lifestyle

Modify behaviour: use a gait aid if advised, avoid climbing ladders, wear glasses, wear shoes. Exercise, including resistance training, to strengthen and improve gait and balance.

Evidence suggests that some psychosocial factors have an independent protective effect on hip fracture risk. These include: currently married, living in present residence for 5 years or more, proactive coping strategies, having a higher level of life satisfaction and engagement in social activities in older age.[33]

Pharmacology

- Reduction in the total number of medications is advisable.
- Aim to withdraw psychotropic medication.[33]
- Antihypertensives, antiparkinsonian medications, anticholinergics and medications with cardiac arrhythmia side effects should all be reviewed, as they may all contribute to postural hypotension.
- Addition of vitamin D and calcium for bone and muscle strength.[34]
- Consider whether the patient would benefit from a bisphosphonate or other anti-osteoporosis medication.

Surgical

Cataract surgery.

Other medical

- Multidisciplinary falls and balance clinics.
- Cardiology opinion regarding pacing for those with cardioinhibitory carotid sinus hypersensitiy.[31]

Paramedical

- Physiotherapy regarding gait, strength and balance, and gait aid and hip protector prescription.[31,35] Hip protectors come in a variety of designs and should be fitted to the individual.[34]
- Occupational therapy to review and advise on environment and activities of daily living.[31]
- Podiatry regarding footwear and foot care.
- Psychology if there is a significant 'fear of falling'.
- Optometry if the patient has an inappropriate prescription. Initiation of bifocal glasses is probably best avoided in the elderly.

Complementary therapies

T'ai chi has been shown to aid balance and thus help to reduce falls.[31]

ONGOING REVIEW

Few studies have evaluated the longer-term effects of interventions, so ongoing review and further identification and modification of risk factors as they arise is warranted.

IMPORTANT PITFALLS

- Inaccurate history due to lack of eye witnesses.
- Patients with cognitive impairment may be difficult to manage, due their inability to remember gait aids, assess risk and use a personal alarm.

PROGNOSIS

Prevention of falls can be difficult in the elderly. Success is determined by the ability to reverse extrinsic and intrinsic factors. In many cases the falls can only be minimised. Potential trauma may be reduced by osteoporosis and vitamin D deficiency treatment, and items such as hip protectors.[32] Falls are one of the most common reasons for institutionalisation of the elderly.

PATIENT EDUCATION

Patients should be educated on:

- intrinsic and extrinsic risk factors for falls and the need to improve as many risk factors as possible
- how to get up from the floor
- fitted, lace-up or Velcro shoes with adequate non-slip soles
- correct use of gait aids
- how to de-clutter the house
- appropriate dressing techniques
- turning on lights and wearing visual aids when going to the toilet at night.

RESOURCES

Alzheimer's Australia, http://www.alzheimers.org.au/

REFERENCES

1. Woodward M. De-prescribing: achieving better health outcomes for older people through reducing medications. J Pharm Pract Res 2003; 33:323–328.
2. Moran JA, Dorevitch MI. Delirium in the hospitalised elderly. J Pharm Pract Res 2001; 31:35–40.
3. Inouye SK, Bogardus ST, Charpentier PA et al. A multicompartment intervention to prevent delirium in hospitalized patients. N Engl J Med 1999; 340:669–676.
4. Holzel BK, Ott U, Gard T et al. Investigation of mindfulness meditation practitioners with voxel-based morphometry. Soc Cogn Affect Neurosci 2008; 3(1):55–61.
5. Hecker JR, Snellgrove AA. Pharmacological management of Alzheimer's disease. J Pharm Pract Res 2003; 33:24–29.
6. Woodward M. Pharmacological treatment of challenging neuropsychiatric symptoms of dementia. J Pharm Pract Res 2005; 35:228–234.
7. Sano M, Ernesto C, Thomas RG et al. A controlled trial of selegiline, alpha-tocopherol, or both as treatment for Alzheimer's disease. N Engl J Med 1997; 336:1216–1222.
8. Petersen RC, Thoma RG, Grundman M et al. Vitamin E and donepezil for treatment of mild cognitive impairment. N Engl J Med 2005; 352:2379–2388.
9. MRC/BHF Heart Protection Study of antioxidant vitamin supplementation in 20 536 high-risk individuals: a randomised placebo-controlled trial. Lancet 2002; 360(9326):23–33.
10. Miller ER III, Pastor-Barriuso R, Dalal D et al. Meta-analysis: high-dosage vitamin E supplementation may

increase all-cause mortality. Ann Intern Med 2005; 142(1):37–46.
11 Woodward MC. The management of insomnia in older people. Aust J Hosp Pharm 1996; 26:462–465.
12 Crandall J, Barzilai N. Treatment of diabetes mellitus in older people: oral therapy options. J Am Geriatr Soc 2003; 51:272–274.
13 De Luise MA. Thyroid diseases in the elderly. J Pharm Pract Res 2003; 33:228–230.
14 Reddy MM, Gill SS, Rochon PA. Preventing pressure ulcers: a systematic review. JAMA 2006; 296:974–984.
15 Weller C, Sussman G. Wound dressings update. J Pharm Pract Res 2006; 36:318–324.
16 Carville K, Lewin G, Newall N et al. STAR: a consensus for skin tear classification. Primary Intention 2007; 15(1):18–28.
17 Posthauer ME. Hydration: does it play a role in wound healing? Adv Skin Wound Care 2006; 19:74–76.
18 Desneves KJ, Todorovic BE, Cassar A et al. Treatment with supplementary arginine, vitamin C and zinc in patients with pressure ulcers: a randomised controlled trial. Clin Nutr 2005; 24(6):979–987.
19 McClain CJ, McClain M, Barve S et al. Trace metals and the elderly. Clin Geriatr Med 2002; 18:801–818.
20 Agren MS. Studies on zinc in wound healing. Acta Derm Venereol Suppl (Stockh) 1990; 154:1–36.
21 Moses G. Complementary and alternative medicine use in the elderly. J Pharm Prac Res 2005; 35:63–68.
22 Bird MR. Urinary incontinence in the elderly. J Pharm Prac Res 2004; 34:319–321.
23 Woodward MC. Constipation in older people: pharmacological management issues. J Pharm Prac Res 2002; 32:37–43.
24 Gage BF, Waterman AD, Shannon W et al. Validation of clinical classification schemes for predicting stroke. Results from the National Registry of Atrial Fibrillation. JAMA 2001; 285:2864–2870.
25 Johnson CE, Lim WK, Workman BS. People aged over 75 in atrial fibrillation on warfarin: the rate of major haemorrhage and stroke in more than 500 patient-years of follow-up. J Am Geriatr Soc 2005; 53:655–659.
26 Gibson SJ, Weiner DK. Older people's pain. Pain: Clinical Updates 2006; 14:1–4.
27 Christo PJ, Hobelmann G, Maine DN. Post-herpetic neuralgia in older adults: evidence-based approaches to clinical management. Drugs Aging 2007; 24:1–19.
28 Katz B. Pharmacological management of pain in older people. J Pharm Pract Res 2007; 37:63–68.
29 Wilder-Smith OHG. Opioid use in the elderly. Europ J Pain 2005; 9:137–140.
30 Hempenstall K, Nurmikko TJ, Johnson RW et al. Analgesic therapy in postherpetic neuralgia: a quantitative systematic review. PLoS Medicine 2005; 2:628–644.
31 Gillespie LD, Gillespie WJ, Robertson MC et al. Interventions for preventing falls in elderly people. Cochrane Database Syst Rev 2003; 4:CD000340.
32 McClure R, Turner C, Peel N et al. Population-based interventions for the prevention of fall-related injuries in older people. Cochrane Database Syst Rev 2005; 1:CD004441.
33 Peel NM, McClure RJ, Hendrikz JK. Psychosocial factors associated with fall-related hip fractures. Age Ageing 2007; 36:145–151.
34 Minns RJ, Marsh A-M, Chuck A et al. Are hip protectors correctly positioned in use? Age Ageing 2007; 36:140–144.
35 Howe TE, Rochester L, Jackson A et al. Exercise for improving balance in older people. Cochrane Database Syst Rev 2007; 4:CD004963.

APPENDIX: COMPREHENSIVE GERIATRIC ASSESSMENT

Past history
Medications:
- Prescribed, OTC and CAM
- Vaccination (flu, pneumococcal, tetanus, *Herpes zoster*)

History
Including:
- Cognition/memory symptoms
- Mobility/falls
- Sensory changes
- Swallowing and nutrition
- Continence and constipation
- Sexual
- Sleep
- Depression/anxiety/other psychiatric symptoms
- Alcohol/smoking/other drugs

An informant/caregiver history should also be sought.

Physical examination
Comprehensive and should include:
- Weight
- Postural BP change
- Oral/dentition
- Skin
- Eyes/ears—including vision and hearing
- PR/gynaecological if relevant symptoms
- Feet (and footwear)
- Joints
- Full neurological assessment

Cognitive assessment
Screening:
- MMSE
- Clock drawing test

Targeted as indicated:
- Executive function (judgment, reasoning, insight)
- Visuo-spatial function
- Language

Functional status
Personal activities of daily living (ADLs):
- Mobility assessment (e.g. Get up and go test)

Domestic ADLs
Community ADLs:
- Including driving

Psychological/mood
- Depression screening (e.g. Geriatric Depression Scale)
- Other assessment as indicated

Behaviour
- Challenging behaviours such as wandering, vocalisation, physical aggression, sexually inappropriate

Social/environment
Current residential arrangements
Family/informal supports
Formal supports
Had an aged care assessment team assessment?
- Including assessment of home for safety

Financial
- Including Power of Attorney

Advanced care planning
- e.g. respecting patient choices
- Will

chapter 58

Ageing

INTRODUCTION AND OVERVIEW

The global population trends of ageing reported by the US government show that the world population nearly quadrupled during the twentieth century, and is projected to grow by roughly 50% before stabilising during the late twenty-first century.[1] This transition is expected to leave the population much larger and, on average, older than it was previously, with significant health and socioeconomic implications.

Before the demographic transition of populations began,[2,3] fertility and mortality were both high throughout the world. Children often died in infancy, and people who reached adulthood tended to have many children and die relatively young. Famines and epidemics could rapidly and suddenly kill many people, causing large fluctuations in rates of mortality. As a consequence, most people were young, and very few lived to old age.[2]

The pattern of population mortality change has a number of recognised stages (listed below) and links with the epidemiological transition that began in Europe in the 1700s (Fig 58.1).[3]

- *Stage I*—improvements in living standards led to a decline in the death toll from plagues and famines, and to less dramatic fluctuations in mortality.
- *Stage II*—during the 1800s, continued improvements in living standards and sanitation led to a gradual decline in mortality rates and a rise in average life expectancy, mainly in Europe and

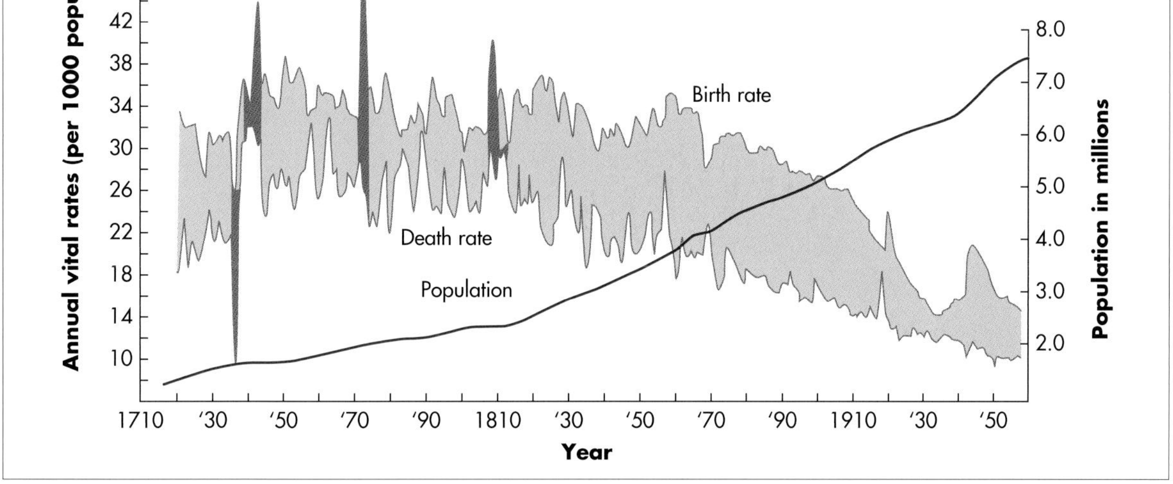

FIGURE 58.1 Population transition in Sweden (adapted from Omran 1971[3] and Vielrose 1965[4])

in regions (such as the United States) settled by Europeans.

- *Stage III*—beginning around 1900, medical advances contributed to a rapid decline in mortality rates, especially infant mortality. As a result, life expectancy at birth rose by roughly one-third of a year per year for much of the twentieth century.
- *Stage IV*—since around 1960, further medical advances have reduced mortality among the elderly, leading to improvements in life expectancy for those who have already reached advanced age.

At present, people born in one of the developed countries can expect to live well into their mid-seventies, or longer if current mortality rates prevail, and even longer if those rates continue to fall. Life expectancy at birth in these countries is therefore projected to rise continuously well into the future. This trend is exemplified in the growth of the world's population (Fig 58.2).

Significant gains have occurred through reductions in death rates among the middle-aged and elderly, especially from artery disease (heart disease and stroke), over the past few decades. In Australia, males aged 30 in 2001 could expect to live to 78 years and females to 82.8 years.[7] This is about 12 years longer than the respective life expectancies during 1901–1910. Males aged 65 years in 2001 could expect to live to 81.6 years and females to 85.2 years, about 6 years longer than for those in 1901–1910.[1–3,7] Similar trends can be observed with the populations from other developed countries, such as the United States.[1]

Ninety per cent of all healthcare dollars are spent on extraordinary care in the last 2–3 years of life.[2,3] The leading causes of death have undergone a profound shift, primarily due to improvements in sanitation and infection control since the turn of the twentieth century. The most common causes of death are now cardiovascular disease (heart disease and stroke) and cancer, and these diseases consume approximately 50% of the healthcare budget.[7] In the United States, the reported leading causes of death include heart disease, malignant neoplasms, cerebrovascular diseases (stroke), chronic lower respiratory diseases, accidents (unintentional injuries), diabetes mellitus and Alzheimer's disease.[8] Nearly 80% of people aged 65 years or older in the United States have at least one chronic condition, such as heart disease, diabetes, arthritis or depression, and half have at least two chronic conditions.[2,8] These trends are also applicable to other developed countries.[1,9] In the United States, chronic diseases account for 16.2% of the nation's gross domestic product, and this is among the highest of all industrialised countries.[9]

In order to make an impact on healthcare, there must be a focus on preventing degenerative diseases of ageing that are lifestyle-related.[9] There needs to be an emphasis on preventing, delaying or reversing the diseases associated with ageing. In the past 10 years, fewer Australians have died from heart attacks, strokes and cancer. The life expectancy of Australians continues to increase; however, there are a number of areas where we

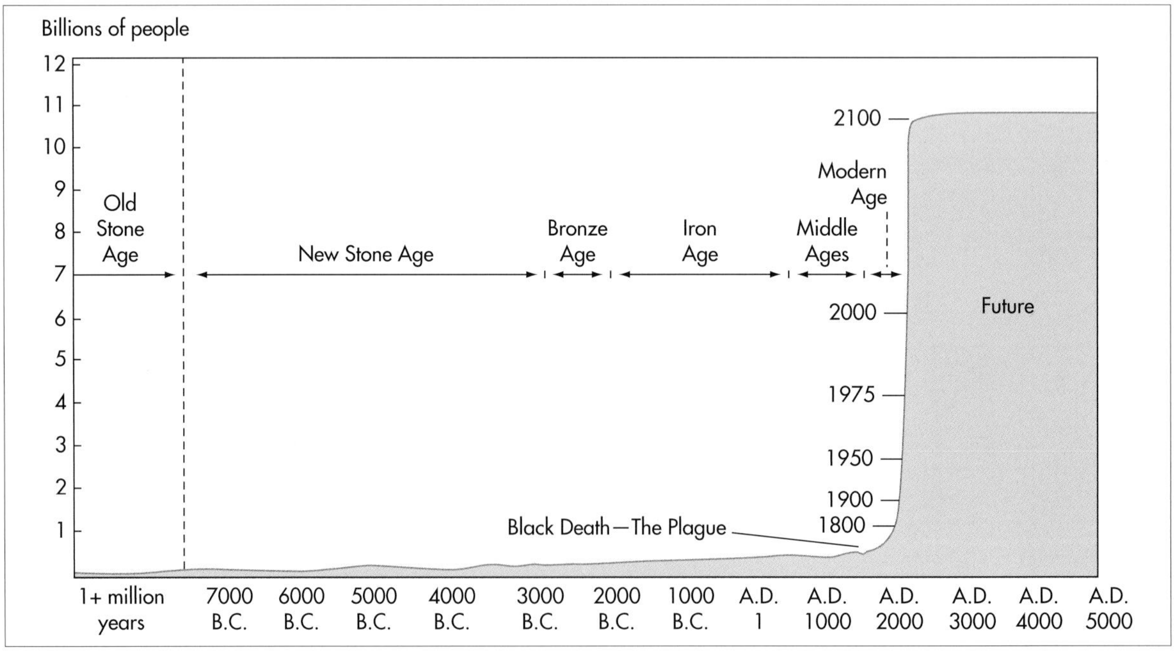

FIGURE 58.2 World population growth throughout history (adapted from Population Reference Bureau[5] and United Nations 1998[6])

can do better. For example, Australians are getting fatter and exercising less, which has serious implications for the health of our population and potentially could reduce life expectancy in the future.[7] Recently, an international Chronic Disease Action Group was established that will encourage, support and monitor accomplishments on the implementation of evidence-based efforts to promote global, regional and national actions to prevent and control the development of chronic diseases.[10]

LIFE EXPECTANCY

A French Canadian woman who died at the age of nearly 123 years, as based on her birth certificate, is thought to have lived longer than any other human on record. A Japanese man who died before his 121st birthday had held the longevity record before her.

Japan has the highest life expectancy of any nation. Approximately one-third of those aged over 110 years worldwide are living in the Okinawa region of Japan.[11–13] It is clear that the Japanese rural lifestyle and diet are important in determining their longevity.

When the Japanese move to the United States, their life expectancy is reduced to that of the local population by the second generation. Japanese who migrate to the United States develop breast cancer at the same rate as locals after one generation, but with bowel cancer a similar rate occurs by the second generation.[14]

Considerable attention has also been focused on populations from three other geographical areas in the world: Abkhazia, in Georgia; Hunza, in Northern Pakistan; and Vilcabamba, in Ecuador. Life expectancy in these regions is considered to be much higher than average.[13–19] In these areas, several observations have been made indicating that these people live in an area that is reasonably isolated and has little pollution. Some of the features of long-lived populations such as those documented from Okinawa are that families are closely knit, couples report having happier relationships, the elderly are respected within their communities, in general their diets would be considered healthy, and their level of physical activity is high. It is of great significance that not only do these groups live to an above-average life expectancy, but they are also healthy most of the time when they are elderly.[15–17]

PHYSIOLOGICAL CHANGES WITH AGEING

The ageing process is characterised by a number of factors that can reduce human mean life expectancy, and these changes are summarised in Table 58.1.

TABLE 58.1 Body changes with ageing

System	Major changes
Musculoskeletal / Body composition	Loss of muscle mass and strength[I] Increased fat[II] Joints—loss of cartilage and flexibility Loss of bone mass Loss of height
Nervous	Neuronal mass loss Decreased sensory and motor functions (e.g. smell, taste, hearing) Loss of balance
Ocular	Degeneration of lens and retina
Ears	Decreased ossical function
Cardiovascular	Artery disease Decreased cardiac output Decreased endurance Increased hypertension, irregular rhythms Increased varicosities
Immunity	Reduced cell-mediated immunity and increased auto-antibodies
Endocrine	Decrease in some hormones
Renal	Decreased number and function of glomeruli
Respiratory	Lung fibrosis Decreased cough reflex, cilia activity
Digestive	Decreased digestive secretions and motility
Skin	Loss of elasticity, sensitivity Increased sun-related pigmentation

Level of evidence: I = strong, II = moderate.

MOLECULAR BIOLOGY OF LONGEVITY

CELL DIVISION, CHROMOSOMES AND TELOMERES

During cell division, replication of DNA molecules occurs and must be meticulous and without error. Error in replication can lead to a mutant protein and, depending on how vital this protein may be, this could have a major influence on body function.

The ends of chromosomes are called *telomeres* (Fig 58.3). In most animal cells the enzyme responsible for replication of the ends of the chromosomes is telomerase.[20–22]

If the telomeres of the chromosomal DNA are lost, cell cycle or cellular functions are lost, resulting in reduction of cell proliferation and re-differentiation. DNA nucleotides are added to the tip of the strand by the reverse transcriptase enzyme called *telomerase*. Telomerase hence adds DNA sequence repeats (i.e. TTAGGG in all vertebrates) to the 3' end of DNA strands in the telomere regions. These regions are found at the ends of eukaryotic chromosomes, stabilising the structure and function of the entire chromosome. Normal human somatic cells undergo a finite number of cell divisions before they reach a non-dividing or senescence state. Each time a cell divides, the telomeres shorten due to the end of replication. As a consequence, this is reflected by the ever-shortening telomeres during organismal ageing, which is documented to occur in most animals.[20–22] The absence of telomere shortening has led to the hypothesis of telomere length and cell longevity.[24, 25]

It is possible to influence the length of telomeres of human cells *in vitro* by adding telomerase. This has subsequently been reported to decrease the rate of cellular ageing.[25] Cancer cells do not seem to lose their telomerase activity and hence do not undergo cell death, indicating that cancer and longevity may have common properties.

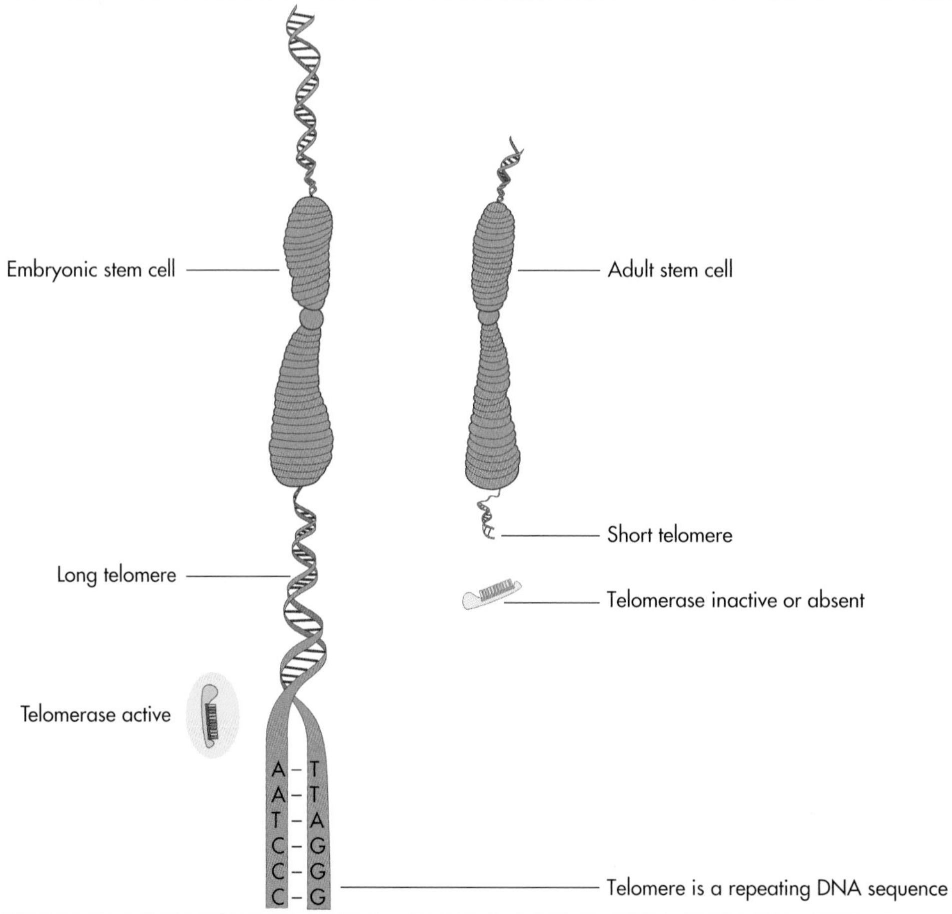

FIGURE 58.3 Diagrammatic representation of the spatial relationship between chromosome, telomeres and telomerase activity in embryonic stem cells and adult stem cells

A gene called longevity assurance or LAG-1 gene has been discovered in yeast cells.[24] The LAG-1 gene can influence the number of yeast cell divisions and the cell's longevity. The function of this gene is unknown, but it is believed to result in the synthesis of a protein found in the cell membrane. Attempts to clone a similar human gene are under way to ascertain whether it may influence longevity of the human cell.

In 1987, Denham Harman proposed that oxygen free radicals cause much of the damage associated with ageing.[26] Oxygen free-radicals are molecules with an unpaired highly reactive electron produced normally as the body converts food and oxygen into energy. In an attempt to stabilise the free-radical, oxygen molecules take up an electron from another molecule, which then becomes unstable and starts a chain reaction. Some of these free-radicals are harmful to proteins, DNA, cell membranes and other cell structures such as mitochondria. In the normal cell most oxidative damage can be prevented by enzymes such as superoxide dismutase (SOD), catalase, glutathione, peroxidase and antioxidants such as vitamins C, E and beta-carotene, but the damage to the cells is felt to be cumulative. SOD levels and other antioxidants have been correlated with lifespan in at least 20 species.

Genetic engineering techniques could be employed to extend the life cycles of human cells and thereby extend the human lifespan. Ageing is likely to result from accumulated cellular damage by external and environmental factors or a program of internal biological clocks. Cell damage can be caused by genetic mutations in somatic cells, faulty protein production resulting in loss of self-control or malfunction. Damage can also be caused by wear and tear of replicating cells.

MITOCHONDRIA AND FREE-RADICALS

That mitochondria have a pivotal role in the effective provision of energy to eukaryotic cells is an undisputed scientific fact. Cellular mechanisms regulating energy utilisation must function properly to sustain life. With increased ageing, there is a decrease in mitochondrial energy output.[27] Hence, in aerobic animals, mitochondrial health for effective energy provision is central to life.

The free-radical theory of ageing, as formulated by Denham Harman,[26] is supported by observations that the lifespan of most organisms is roughly proportional to their metabolic rate and thus due to the rate at which the organism generates mitochondria-derived reactive oxygen species (ROS). This view, however, may require modification within the confines of ageing. Cellular-generated ROS contributing to the overall production of ROS are apparently traced back to the mitochondria.[27] ROS have been viewed as mostly deleterious to health and hence ageing. Reports that show that in a wide spectrum of animal species, dietary antioxidants or caloric restriction as well as chemical antioxidants or increased expression of antioxidant proteins can lower mitochondrial ROS production, which translates into an extension of the lifespan of these species, serve to support the free-radical theory of ageing.[28–31] However, it is known that ROS are generated in multiple cellular compartments and by multiple enzyme systems within the cell and have cellular signalling functions that are critical for the normal physiological function of the cell.[32–34]

ROS produced by mitochondria have been demonstrated to have important and specific roles in cellular signalling.[34] The notion that the mitochondria are the sole most abundant site of ROS formation is currently subject to much discussion and debate.[33–38]

The disruption of mitochondrial functions has been implicated in more than 40 known diseases, including atherosclerosis, ischaemic heart disease, cancer, diabetes and neurodegenerative diseases such as Alzheimer's disease, Parkinson's disease, Huntington's disease and amyotrophic lateral sclerosis.[39–41] Together these data indicate that mitochondrial health is an important factor for health and ageing. Current and future research would aim to further improve and preserve mitochondrial function. Although further research is warranted, recent reports show that supplementation with coenzyme Q10 shows promise in maintaining the health of mitochondria.[42,43]

The internal biological clock may be reflected by the ageing–hormonal changes, which produce a decline in immunity and influence regulatory genes by switching them on or off.

ENDOCRINOLOGY OF AGEING

The loss of muscle strength resulting in frailty is the limiting factor for an individual's chances of living an independent life until death. During normal ageing, there is a decrease in three hormonal systems:

- oestrogen (in menopause) and testosterone (in andropause)
- dehydroepiandrosterone (DHEA) and its sulfate (in adrenopause)
- the growth hormone/insulin-like growth factor I axis (in somatopause).

It is possible that the physical changes associated with ageing are physiological, but there is some evidence to suggest that a decline in hormonal activity plays an important role. As a result, studies have looked at the role of hormonal replacement strategies, so as to increase blood hormone levels. Unfortunately, the use of hormone replacement therapy (HRT) was not an overall success. There may be specific reasons for this failure, and hence more studies are necessary in order to establish whether hormone replacement can be both of benefit and safe.

PHYSICAL FRAILTY WITH AGEING

Physiological functions gradually decline with ageing. Such decline in functions includes diminished capacity for cellular protein synthesis, a decline in immune function, an increase in fat mass, a loss of muscle mass and strength and a decrease in bone density. People die from old age and it is mostly from cardiovascular disease, cancer or dementia. The characteristics of ageing include generalised weakness, impaired mobility and balance and poor endurance.[44,45]

Associated with physical frailty are falls (contributing to 40% of admissions to nursing homes), fractures that impair daily activities of everyday living and loss of independence.[46]

Experts on ageing define the characteristic aspect of ageing as a loss of muscle strength.[33,37] A decline in muscle strength results from a sedentary lifestyle and decreased physical activity, as well as ageing of muscle fibres and their innervation, osteoarthritis and chronic debilitating diseases.[47]

A study utilising 100 frail nursing home residents with an average age of 87 years investigated supervised resistance exercise training, and found a doubling of muscle strength and a significant increase in their walking and climbing power. The investigation demonstrated that these muscle changes of ageing are not irreversible and that they can be reduced and possibly prevented. Prevention of frailty can be achieved by exercise, which is difficult to institute in an ageing population and, hence, there are very high numbers of dropouts from these programs.[48] Muscle resistance exercises can also improve insulin sensitivity.[49] A cultural change where exercise becomes a routine part of life may make a difference.

Changes in the endocrine system may be responsible for part of the ageing process that affects the body composition, including loss of muscle size and strength, loss of bone and increase in fat mass.[50]

PHYSICAL ACTIVITY AND AGEING

One of the common traits of the elderly is sarcopenia, which gives them the appearance of frailty due to loss of skeletal muscle mass. In a study with a representative North American population sample, it was reported that sarcopenia increased from 24% in those aged less than 70 years of age to over 50% in those aged over 80 years of age.[51] The age-related sarcopenia that results in loss of skeletal muscle mass has been associated with a decrease in muscle fibre area, especially type II fibre.[52] There are numerous consequences related to this reduction in muscle mass, including a decline in muscle strength and function, and impaired functional capacity. Sarcopenia also results in a reduction in the body's major protein pool. Adequate dietary protein to replace obligatory nitrogen loss and to support protein turnover is essential for maintaining muscle mass, and therefore nutritional options are equally important in order to reduce and significantly slow the progression of loss of skeletal muscle mass. It is usually recommended that protein requirements in older people should be maintained above 1 g/kg/day. An inactive lifestyle may contribute to the loss of skeletal mass in elderly people. Physical activity can significantly assist in reversing this deficit and may improve the regeneration potential of muscle fibres.[52]

HORMONES AND AGEING

PANCREAS AND THYROID FUNCTION

The reduction of pancreas and thyroid function is clinically the most important change in endocrine activity with ageing. Approximately 40% of those aged 65–74 years and 50% of those aged over 80 years old have diabetes mellitus and nearly half are undiagnosed.[53,54] Apart from insulin secretion by the beta cells, there is also insulin resistance related to stress, poor diet, lack of exercise, increased abdominal fat mass and decreased lean body mass.[55–57]

Age-related thyroid dysfunction is also common in the elderly.[58,59] Lowered thyroxine (T_4) and increased thyroid thyrotropin-stimulating hormone (TSH) occur in approximately 5–11% of elderly hospitalised men and women.[60–62] Dysfunction is mainly the result of autoimmunity and is not a consequence of ageing.[63–65] Ageing is accompanied by a decrease in TSH release and a decline in conversion of T_4 to the more active triiodothyronine (T_3).[65] A study has found that T_3 and T_4 lead to improvements in cognition, depression, fatigue and general wellbeing.[66]

MENOPAUSE

(See also Ch 53, Menopause.)

The evidence that both the brain and the ovary are key pacemakers in menopause is compelling.[67,68] Menopause does not result only from exhaustion of ovarian follicles.

Whereas menopause occurs quite abruptly, the changes in the hypothalamic–pituitary–gonadal axis in males are slower and more subtle (andropause, see below). There is a gradual decline of testosterone with ageing.[69,70] This andropause is characterised by a decrease in testicular Leydig cell numbers and a decrease in gonadotropin secretion.[69,70]

In most women, the period of decline in oestrogens is accompanied by vasomotor reactions, depressed mood and changes in skin and body composition (increase in body fat and decrease in muscle mass). Menopause is associated with the increased incidence of cardiovascular disease, loss of bone mass and cognitive impairment.[71,72] With increasing life expectancy, the time a woman spends after menopause is more than a third of her life.

It was initially thought that long-term therapy with oestrogens in combination with progestins would provide an overall benefit. Benefits from HRT included relief of hot flushes and mood changes, and reduction of skin and reproductive tract atrophy (i.e. dryness of the vagina and urinary incontinence).

A large prospective study on HRT, the Women's Health Initiative, found that HRT helped in reducing hip fracture and bowel cancer but had negative effects in increasing heart deaths, thrombosis (embolic disease) and breast cancer. This study proved that the form of HRT being used was an overall failure.[73] The results of this study were confirmed by the Million Women Study.[74]

The use of other forms of HRT as well as other modes of administration could relieve the symptoms of menopause as well as delaying or preventing the associated changes and avoiding side effects.

The significant adverse effects that have been documented with the long-term use of HRT have elicited caution in relation to the long-term use of other forms of HRTs, such as natural oestrogens (e.g. oestradiol valerate extracted from soya beans), synthetic oestrogens (e.g. ethinyloestradiol), tibolone (a synthetic hormone that has some oestrogen-like and some progesterone-like activity), skin patches and oestrogen gels, oestrogen implants, vaginal oestrogen, phyto-oestrogens, progesterone treatments (e.g. tablets: dydrogesterone, levonorgestrel/norgestrel, medroxyprogesterone; patches) and testosterone replacement.[72–74]

ANDROPAUSE

There is a gradual decline in testosterone levels with ageing. Variability exists among the aged. Of those men aged over 65 years, two-thirds have testosterone levels below the normal values of men aged between 30 and 35 years.[75] Impotence increases in men aged 60–70 years, to over 50%.[76–78] There is an association between decline in free testosterone levels and increase in impotence.[79] Overall, testosterone replacement therapy is not effective for the treatment of impotence in elderly males. Other factors such as artery disease, diabetes, excessive alcohol consumption, smoking and quality of the relationship seem to be more important.[80,81]

Although it has been shown that testosterone has anabolic effects,[82–85] it is not clear whether the decline in muscle mass and muscle strength with ageing is related to the decrease in free testosterone levels. In mid-adult hypogonodal men who have muscle weakness, anaemia, decreased bone mass and mood disturbances, there is a rapid normalisation with testosterone replacement therapy.[83,84] Pharmacological doses of testosterone therapy combined with exercise or weight training have been shown to increase muscle mass and strength in eugonadal adult men.[84] An early study demonstrated that testosterone supplementation for 6 months in older men with a low normal testosterone concentration did not affect functional status or cognition but increased lean body mass and had mixed metabolic effects.[85]

There are limited long-term data on testosterone replacement therapy but in general there is a positive effect on muscle mass and strength as well as on cognition and sense of wellbeing.[86,87] An adverse effect on lipid profiles has been reported with testosterone treatment.[87] There are inadequate studies on testosterone replacement therapy in the elderly to ascertain who benefits and whether prostate disease and artery disease negate these benefits. Androgenic compounds with variable biological actions in different organs (antiandrogenic in the prostate) are currently being investigated.[88] Moreover, a recent review concluded that on current evidence the studies in elderly men with lower than normal testosterone that have reported improvement in features of the metabolic syndrome, bone mineral density, mood and sexual functioning have provided no definitive proof. The beneficial effects of restoring testosterone levels to normal in elderly men, with regard to clinical parameters, requires further rigorous research.[88]

ADRENOPAUSE

With age there is a gradual decline in dehydroepiandrosterone (DHEA), resulting in adrenopause.[89,90] Adrenal secretion of DHEA gradually decreases over time, whereas adrenocorticotropin (ACTH) secretion, which is physiologically linked to plasma cortisol levels, remains largely unchanged. The decrease in DHEA is due to a decrease in production from the adrenal cortex and is not due to a hypothalamic pacemaker.

Males over 90 years of age with the lowest DHEA levels have the lowest levels of activities of daily living.[90] DHEA levels at age 30 are approximately five times higher than at age 85.[90]

Peripheral tissues contain a number of DHEA-metabolising enzymes capable of converting DHEA to androgenic and oestrogenic hormones in peripheral tissues. DHEA levels have been shown to be constantly consistently low in patients with Alzheimer's disease, osteoporosis, inflammatory bowel disease and chronic fatigue syndrome.

In animal studies with very low levels of DHEA, its administration prevents obesity, diabetes mellitus, cancer and heart disease, while enhancing immune function.[91–94] Supportive data in humans are few and highly controversial. Higher DHEA levels are associated with some reduced risk of cardiovascular deaths in males.[91]

DHEA has been shown to be beneficial in two randomised placebo-controlled studies.[95,96] Twenty adults aged between 40 and 70 years were given 50 mg of DHEA daily over a 3-month period, with an increase in DHEA levels similar to those in young adults, resulting in increased androgen and insulin-like growth factor (IGF-1) concentrations. There was also a significant increase in physical and psychological wellbeing without an effect on libido in both sexes.[96]

Another study using 100 mg of DHEA for 6 months showed an increase in lean body mass in both sexes, but muscle strength was increased in men only.[97]

Recent short-term and long-term studies investigating the administration of an oral low dose (25 mg/day) of DHEA have demonstrated that DHEA increased serum DHEA, DHEAS, androstenedione and oestradiol levels of participants in the older group to the same level as that of younger participants.[98] Further, it has been shown that DHEA was capable of modifying circulating levels of androgens and progestins in both early- and late-postmenopausal women by modulating the age-related changes in adrenal function.[99]

Further studies are required prior to the routine use of DHEA for delaying or preventing the physiological consequences of ageing. The major concern with DHEA supplementation is prostate disease and polycythaemia.

SOMATOPAUSE

The growth hormone (GH) / insulin-like growth factor I (IGF-1) is the third endocrine system that gradually declines with ageing.[100,101] There is a progressive fall in circulating IGF-1 levels in both sexes with ageing.[102] The triggering pacemaker appears to be localised in the hypothalamus and is linked with a decrease in GH.[103] It is not known whether changes in gonadal function (menopause and andropause) are interrelated with adrenopause and somatopause, which occur in both sexes.

Changes such as muscle size and function, fat and bone mass, progression of atherosclerosis and changes in cognitive function have not been related to the changes in GH/IGF-1 endocrine activity. Some effects of normal ageing resemble features of isolated hormonal deficiency (i.e. hypogonadism and GH deficiency), which in mid-adult patients are reversed by replacement therapy with the appropriate hormone.[104] Ageing is not simply the result of various hormone deficiencies.

The biological consequences of somatopause are poorly understood.[105] A number of catabolic processes that are central in the biology of ageing can be reversed with GH administration. The IGF-1 levels in elderly individuals can be increased to those seen in the young after 3–6 months of GH administration.[106] GH also significantly increased muscle mass, skin thickness and bone mineral, and reduced fat mass.[107] Muscle strength and maximal oxygen consumption were not improved with GH therapy.[108] GH therapy did not give any additional benefit to that of resistance exercise training in relation to muscle mass and muscle strength.[109] An association between maximum aerobic capacity and circulating IGF-1 levels has been demonstrated.[108,109]

In summary, GH replacement therapy in GH-deficient adults has been shown to increase:

- muscle mass
- muscle strength
- bone mass
- quality of life.

In addition, lipid profile was improved and fat mass decreased.[106–109]

If GH is given to those over 65 years old with hip fracture, there is an earlier return to independent living.[110]

Several other similar studies have investigated the role of GH in the treatment of acute catabolic states in the frail elderly. Hypothalamic peptide growth hormone releasing hormone (GHRH), when given subcutaneously over 2 weeks to healthy 70-year-old men, increased GH and IGF-1 levels to those of 35-year-olds.[111] Long-term oral non-peptide analogues of GH-releasing peptides have even more powerful GH-releasing effects, restoring IGF-1 secretion in the elderly to those of young adults.[112] Long-term administration in the elderly increased lean body mass but not muscle strength.[113] These non-peptide analogues may be important in the prevention of frailty and reversing acute catabolism. Studies of the long-term use of these analogues are not available. There is concern about tumour growth, as IGF-1 receptors are present in most human solid cancers. The concerns related to GH have recently been reviewed.[114]

LIFESTYLE

Willet emphasised that genetic and environmental factors, including diet and lifestyle, both contribute to cardiovascular diseases, cancers and other major causes of mortality and that numerous lines of evidence indicate that environmental factors are the most important in disease prevention (Fig 58.4).[115] Hence, environmental factors may certainly have the strongest influence on life expectancy and hence lifespan (Fig 58.2).[115,116] It should be noted that life expectancy is a statistical projection of the length of time a human being is expected to live, based upon probabilities and assumptions of genetic predispositions, living conditions, medical discoveries and advances, natural disasters and other environmental factors, compared with lifespan defined as the characteristic observed age of death for its very oldest individuals.[117] Intertwined with nutritional practices and lifestyle is life stressor modification.[116]

Evidence continues to accumulate that strongly suggests that the state of the human mind—which associates psychosocial factors with emotional states such as depression and with behavioural dispositions that include hostility and psychosocial lifestyle stresses—can directly and significantly influence human physiological function and, in turn, health outcomes.

Stressors and negative stress-related reactions have been documented and recognised as having multiple ill-health-related sequelae, and exposure to chronic social stress has been associated with many systemic and mental disorders.[118] These have significant deleterious outcomes that significantly reduce life expectancy.

Different research groups support the notion that health consequences are more likely to occur when unpredictable stressors of a social nature chronically induce physiological and behavioural adjustments that may create wear and tear on underlying physiological functions. When stressors challenge an organism's integrity, a set of physiological reactions is elicited to counteract the possible threat and adjust the physiological setting of the organism to the new situation. This has become known as the stress response.[119]

Stressors and lifestyle choices can be a significant trigger for disease through immunomodulation of the immune system enhancing disease susceptibility, which can then affect life expectancy.[119] Immune function modulation influenced and expressed by stressful life experiences has a significant correlate with Willett's[115] environmental trigger view of disease initiation.

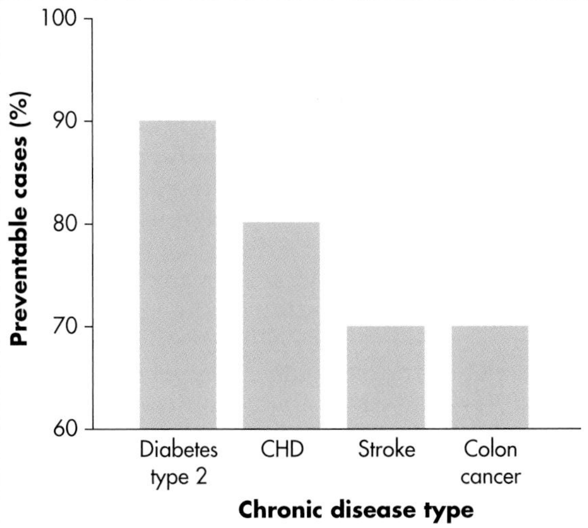

FIGURE 58.4 Chronic disease prevention (adapted from Willett 2002[115])

Psychoneuroendocrinology and psychoneurocardiology have also been established, to help explain the mechanisms of health and disease.

Some recent research is now suggesting that psychological factors such as chronic stress and pessimism[120] may have a direct effect on telomere length and telomerase activity, thus giving plausible mechanisms to explain the relationship between mental health and ageing. There is now also research to suggest that psychological strategies such as mindfulness techniques may help to slow the ageing process through their effects on stress, cognition and, consequently, telomerase activity.[121]

NUTRITION

Triggers for adverse and inappropriate nutritional practices in childhood have been shown to have psychosocial correlates in adult life, with an increase in risk for disease.[122]

Obesity in humans, influenced by poor dietary choices and inactivity, is significantly associated with an increased risk of chronic diseases such as diabetes, high blood pressure, high cholesterol, cardiovascular diseases, asthma, arthritis, some cancers and overall poor health status, which can significantly reduce an individual's life expectancy.

Calorie restriction (CR) is linked to nutritional choices. CR with nutritionally poor foods (e.g. consuming half the quantity of a fast food) is still an unbalanced nutritional choice, albeit in smaller portions, and provides no health advantage.

Recently it was reported, and further confirmed, that a greater adherence to a traditional Mediterranean diet was associated with a significant reduction in total all-cause mortality.[123] Meyer and colleagues have demonstrated that associating a CR diet with adherence to a Mediterranean-type diet that consisted of whole grains, beans, fish, fruit, olive oil and many different kinds of vegetables was beneficial for heart health.[124] Hence, when optimal nutritional choices are coupled with CR, an increase in life expectancy is made possible. Such nutritional practices can serve to further extend the human lifespan.

CALORIC RESTRICTION

Optimising nutrition relates food intake to the benefits of prudent CR. That is, CR refers to a dietary regimen low in calories without under-nutrition that would lead to increased disease risk due to nutritional deficits. Following the pioneering work of McCay and colleagues over 70 years ago, CR was then first noted to significantly extend the lifespan of rodents.[125] Since that time, the increase in longevity has been demonstrated to result from the limitation of total calories derived from carbohydrates, fats or proteins to 25–60% below that of control animals fed ad libitum.[29,126,127] The extension in lifespan can approach 50% in rodents.[125,128] Moreover, CR has been shown to extend the lifespan in a broad range of organisms including yeast, rotifers, spiders, worms, fish, mice and rats.[126] Emerging data show that its effect may also apply to non-human primates.[129] CR has also been reported to delay a wide spectrum of diseases in different experimental animals such as kidney disease,[129] a variety of neoplasias,[130–132] autoimmune disease[133,134] and diabetes,[135] and it reduces age-associated neuronal loss in most mouse models of neurodegenerative disorders such as Parkinson's disease[136] and Alzheimer's disease.[137,138] The CR regimen also prevents age-associated decline in psychomotor and spatial memory tasks[139] and loss of dendritic spines necessary for learning,[140] and improves the brain's plasticity and ability to self-repair.[137]

Numerous biomarkers of CR have been identified in rodents, such as temperature, and DHEAS, insulin and glucose levels.[141] Roth and colleagues have recently observed that body temperature and insulin and DHEAS levels were also altered in primates that had been subjected to CR, hence validating the usefulness of these biomarkers in longer-lived species.[141] More importantly, they have also shown that these parameters were altered in longer-lived men. Together these findings support the role of these factors as biomarkers of longevity in humans.

Recently, a trial on the effect of a 6-month CR diet on metabolic biomarkers such as energy expenditure, and oxidative stress in humans was completed.[142] The report showed that prolonged CR significantly reduced two biomarkers of longevity, namely, fasting insulin level and body temperature. This is the first human study to show that CR, in addition to significantly reducing well known biomarkers of ageing, also caused a metabolic adaptation in CR individuals and a reduction in DNA fragmentation that reflected less DNA damage.[142]

Plant factors such as resveratrol have been shown to increase longevity in several organisms by regulating genes.[143] In mammals, there is growing evidence that resveratrol can prevent or delay the onset of cancer, heart disease, ischaemic and chemically induced injuries, diabetes, pathological inflammation and viral infection. These effects are observed despite extremely low bioavailability and rapid clearance of resveratrol from the circulation.[143] Resveratrol has been suggested to be associated with the prevention of age-related diseases such as cancer because of its regulation of transcription factors that control tumour cell survival.[144,145]

NON-DRUG INTERVENTIONS IN CHRONIC DISEASES

The role of non-drug interventions in chronic diseases is summarised in Tables 58.2 and 58.3.

HEALTHY AGEING

Throughout most of recorded human history, it has been recognised that poor socioeconomic and nutritional status are strongly associated with decreased life expectancy, a trend that is also very much evident today.[146]

The Alameda County Study highlights the importance of an overall plan for health maintenance and disease prevention that can lead to enhanced survival. The Human Population Laboratory, known as the Alameda County Study, quantified health risk practices and lifestyle issues such as exercise, diet, sleep, smoking and alcohol consumption, and defined their relationship to mortality.[147] The first cohort participated in a health survey in 1965 and this has been followed with subsequent surveys to the present day. Health behaviours including seven health habits were considered and were reported to be strongly associated with most (current) or subsequent morbidity and mortality. This study emerged from efforts in the 1950s to measure health—physical, mental and social wellbeing—in accordance with the WHO definition of health, and asked questions about common health-related habits.

Lifestyle and future health issues were investigated and it was reported that there was a disparity of good health practices in 1965 between those with good health and those with poor health practices. Those with an intermediate level of health practices experienced about two-thirds the relative disability risk of those with poor health practices.[148]

Subsequent studies from the Alameda County Study showed that greater personal control over one's biopsychosocial health after retirement was beneficial to health, providing a greater survival advantage.[149,150]

Many factors can influence longevity and scientists are beginning to discover methods that can manipulate cell longevity, including stem cell research, therapeutic cloning and nanotechnology (the science and technology of building miniscule devices for manipulating single atoms and molecules).

Restoration of telomerase activity, isolation and deciphering the activity of longevity genes, protection against environmentally induced free-radicals (e.g. excessive UV radiation) and supplementation with beneficial hormones, nutrients and herbs may increase longevity. We need to learn more about why people from certain countries have a greater life expectancy. Individuals who live to be 100 years of age or more also require further study to show how they may be

TABLE 58.2 Chronic diseases (by system) and non-drug interventions and supplements

System/disorder	Non-drug interventions and supplements* and strength of evidence
Musculoskeletal / Body composition	
Bone	Physical activity—repetitive and resistance exercises[I]
Joints	Vitamin D[I] and other supplements (antioxidants, vitamin K, magnesium[I], boron[II])
	Glucosamine[II], chondroitin[II], fish fats[II]
Nervous	
Cognitive decline	Mental exercises[II]
	Folate[I] and various supplements (vitamins C, E, B_3, B_6, B_{12}, phosphatidyl serine, acetyl L-carnitine, glutamine, lipoic acid[II])
	Ginkgo biloba[II]
	Pinebark *(Pinus radiata)* extract[II], *Bacopa monnieri*[II]
	Lithium[III]
Ocular	
Cataract and macular disease	Sunglasses—protection of lens and retina
	Multivitamin/mineral[III]
Ears	
Decreased hearing	Various supplements may assist
Decreased balance	Avoid loud noise, e.g. music and machinery
	Specific exercises
	Coenzyme Q10[I], vitamin D[II], *Ginkgo biloba*[II]
Cardiovascular	
Hypertension	Coenzyme Q10[I]
Abnormal lipids	Cocoa—dark chocolate[I]
Elevated homocysteine	Fish fats, red rice[II], artichoke[II]
	Folate, B_6, B_{12} supplements[I]
Immunity	Normalised digestive tract flora[I]
	Various supplements (vitamins D, C, E, A; minerals: zinc, selenium)[II]
	Fish fats[I]
	Mushroom extracts[I], *Astragalus*[I], olive leaf extract[II], *Curcumin*[II]
Endocrine deficiency	Avoid excess weight gain[I]
	Can prevent:
	• type 2 diabetes
	• decreased growth hormone and testosterone[II]
Respiratory	
COPD	Avoid polluted air, smoking[II]
	Supplements such as vitamin C[II] can help, selenium[II], fish[II], magnesium[II]
Skin	
Loss of elasticity/ pigmentation	Avoid sunburn, use sunblock[I]
	Vitamins A and C[II] can assist repair, zinc[II]

* Progression halted by lifestyle changes including diet, stress reduction, exercise, relaxation techniques and adequate sunlight exposure.

Level of evidence: I = strong, II = moderate, III = weak.

TABLE 58.3 Chronic diseases and non-drug interventions and supplements

Disorder	Non-drug interventions and supplements* and strength of evidence
Metabolic syndrome	Prevent excess weight gain[I] Exercise[I] Adhere to Mediterranean diet[I] Increase insulin sensitivity with herbs (e.g. cinnamon, fenugreek, *Gymnema sylvestre*)[I]
Chronic inflammation: can involve most body systems	Fish fats are antiinflammatory[I] Herbs (e.g. curcumin, devil's claw, *Boswellia*)[II]
Cancer	Prevent smoking[I] Exercise[I] Diet, especially fish fats[I], selenium[I], other: vitamins E, C, A[II], minerals (zinc[II]) Note: • beta-carotene and vitamin A can reverse oral dysplasia[II] • folate can reverse cervical dysplasia[I]
Behavioural	Ensure adequate folate and vitamin D[I], fish fats[I] Sunlight exposure[II]—serotonin[II]
Pain	Pain relief with acupuncture[I], antiinflammatory herbs (see above)
Urinary problems	Saw palmetto[II], other herbs: stinging nettle (*Urtica dioica*)[II], pygium[II]
Sleep apnoea	Weight loss[I] Sleep position[I] Stress reduction[II]

* Progression halted by lifestyle changes including diet, stress reduction, exercise, relaxation techniques and adequate sunlight exposure.

Level of evidence: I = strong, II = moderate, III = weak.

different from others with an average life expectancy. Increasing knowledge should help us to postpone or prevent the advent of chronic and disabling diseases, as well as resetting the internal biological clocks that control longevity.

Can we live happily ever after?

RESOURCES

Duke University Center for the Study of Aging and Human Development, http://www.geri.duke.edu/resource/resource.html

National Academy of an Aging Society, http://www.agingsociety.org/agingsociety/index.html

National Institute on Aging (NIH), http://www.grc.nia.nih.gov/branches/blsa/blsanew.htm

Resource Centre on Aging, University of California, Berkeley, http://socrates.berkeley.edu/~aging/Web.html

Rosenthal Centre, Information Resources for Research on Aging, http://www.rosenthal.hs.columbia.edu/Aging_resources.html

Sheffield Institute for Studies on Ageing, http://www.sheffield.ac.uk/sisa/

REFERENCES

1 Congress of the United States, Congressional Budget Office. Global population ageing in the 21st century and its economic implications; 2005. Online. Available: http://www.cbo.gov/ftpdocs/69xx/doc6952/12–12–Global.pdf

2 United Nations. World population prospects; 2004 revision. Online. Available: http://www.un.org/esa/population/publications/WPP2004/2004Highlights_finalrevised.pdf

3 Omran A. The epidemiologic transition: a theory of the epidemiology of population change. Milbank Quarterly 1971; 49:509–538.

4 Vielrose E. Elements of the natural movement of populations. Oxford: Pergamon Press; 1965.

5 Population Reference Bureau. 2009 World population data sheet. Online. Available: http://www.prb.org/pdf09/09wpds_eng.pdf

6 United Nations, Population Division of the UN Secretariat. World population projections to 2100; 1998.

7 World Health Organization. Data on longevity in Australia. Online. Available: http://www.who.int/countries/aus/en/

8 Kung HC, Hoyert DL, Xu JQ et al. Deaths: final data for 2005. National Vital Statistics Reports 2008;56(10). Online. Available: http://www.cdc.gov/nchs/data/nvsr/nvsr56/nvsr56_10.pdf

9 Centers for Medicare and Medicaid Services, Office of the Actuary, National Health Statistics Group, National Health Care Expenditures Data, January 2010.

Online. Available: http://www.cms.hhs.gov/nationalhealthexpenddata/01_overview.asp?
10 Beaglehole R, Ebrahim S, Reddy S et al. Chronic Disease Action Group. Prevention of chronic diseases: a call to action. Lancet 2008; 370(9605):2152–2157.
11 Willcox DC, Willcox BJ, Sokolovsky J et al. The cultural context of 'successful ageing' among older women weavers in a northern Okinawan village: the role of productive activity. J Cross Cult Gerontol 2007; 22(2):137–165.
12 Willcox DC, Willcox BJ, Todoriki H et al. Caloric restriction and human longevity: what can we learn from the Okinawans? Biogerontology 2006; 7(3):173–177.
13 Willcox BJ, He Q, Chen R et al. Midlife risk factors and healthy survival in men. JAMA 2006; 296(19):2343–2350.
14 Maskarinec G, Noh JJ. The effect of migration on cancer incidence among Japanese in Hawaii. Ethn Dis 2004; 14(3):431–439.
15 Willcox BJ, Willcox DC, Ferrucci L. Secrets of healthy aging and longevity from exceptional survivors around the globe: lessons from octogenarians to supercentenarians. J Gerontol A Biol Sci Med Sci 2008; 63(11):1181–1185.
16 Dodge HH, Kita Y, Takechi H et al. Healthy cognitive aging and leisure activities among the oldest old in Japan: Takashima study. J Gerontol A Biol Sci Med Sci 2008; 63(11):1193–1200.
17 Mazess RB, Forman SH. Longevity and age exaggeration in Vilcabamba, Ecuador. J Gerontol 1979; 34(1):94–98.
18 Grigorov IG, Kozlovskaia SG, Semesko TM. Characteristics of nutrition in persons of older age groups in areas with different patterns of longevity. Vopr Pitan 1991; (5):24–32.
19 Vlahchev T, Zhivkov Z. Hunza—a healthy and a long living people. Asklepii 2002; 15:96–97.
20 Gilley D, Herbert BS, Huda N et al. Factors impacting human telomere homeostasis and age-related disease. Mech Ageing Dev 2008; 129:27–34.
21 Hayflick L, Moorhead PS. The serial cultivation of human diploid cell strains. Exp Cell Res 1961; 25:585–621.
22 Nakamura TM, Cech TR. Reversing time: origin of telomeres. Cell 1998; 92:587–590.
23 Weinrich SL, Pruzan R, Ma L et al. Reconstitution of human telomerase with the template RNA component hTR and the catalytic protein subunit hTR. Nat Genet 1997; 17(4):498–502.
24 Bodnar A, Ouellette M, Frolkis M et al. Extension of life-span by introduction of telomerase into normal human cells. Science 1998; 279:349–352.
25 Wright WE, Shay JW. Telomere biology in aging and cancer. J Am Geriatr Soc 2005; 53:S292–S294.
26 Harman D. Ageing: a theory based on free radical and radiation chemistry. J Gerontol 1956; 11(3):298–300.
27 Lenaz G, Bovina C, D'Aurelio M et al. Role of mitochondria in oxidative stress and ageing. Ann NY Acad Sci 2002; 959:199–213.
28 Orr WC, Sohal RS. Extension of life-span by overexpression of superoxide dismutase and catalase in *Drosophila melanogaster*. Science 1994; 263:1128–1130.
29 Sohal RS, Weindruch R. Oxidative stress, caloric restriction, and ageing. Science 1996; 273:59–63.
30 Parkes TL, Elia AJ, Dickinson D. Extension of *Drosophila* lifespan by overexpression of human SOD1 in motorneurons. Nat Genet 1998; 19:171–174.
31 Sun J, Tower J. FLP recombinase–mediated induction of Cu/Zn–superoxide dismutase transgene expression can extend the life span of adult *Drosophila melanogaster* flies. Mol Cell Biol 1999; 19:216–228.
32 Linnane AW, Kios M, Vitetta L. The essential roles of superoxide radical and nitric oxide formation for healthy ageing. Mitochondrion 2007; 7(1/2):1–5.
33 Linnane AW, Kios M, Vitetta L. Healthy ageing: regulation of the metabolome by cellular redox modulation and prooxidant signaling systems. The essential roles of superoxide anion and nitric oxide. Exp Gerontol 2007; 8(5):445–467.
34 Linnane AW, Kios M, Vitetta L. Coenzyme Q10—its role as a prooxidant in the formation of superoxide anion/hydrogen peroxide and the regulation of the metabolome. Mitochondrion 2007; Suppl 1:S51–S61.
35 Rhee CG, Chang TS, Bae YS et al. Cellular regulation by hydrogen peroxide. J Am Soc Nephrol 2003; 14(8 Suppl 3):S211–S215.
36 Balaban RS, Nemoto S, Finkel T. Mitochondria, oxidants, and ageing. Cell 2005; 120:483–495.
37 Linnane AW, Eastwood H. Cellular redox poise modulation: the role of coenzyme Q10, gene and metabolic regulation. Mitochondrion 2004; 4(5/6):779–789.
38 Moldovan L, Moldovan NI. Oxygen free radicals and redox biology of organelles. Histochem Cell Biol 2004; 122(4):395–412.
39 Schon EA. Mitochondrial genetics and disease. Trends Biochem Sci 2000; 25:555–560.
40 McKenzie M, Liolitsa D, Hanna MG. Mitochondrial disease: mutations and mechanisms. Neurochem Res 2004; 3:589–600.
41 Wallace DC. A mitochondrial paradigm of metabolic and degenerative diseases, ageing, and cancer: a dawn for evolutionary medicine. Ann Rev Genet 2005; 39:359–407.
42 Kagan T, Davis C, Lin L et al. Coenzyme Q10 can in some circumstances block apoptosis, and this effect is mediated through mitochondria. Ann NY Acad Sci 1999; 887:31–47.

43 Crestanello JA, Doliba NM, et al. Effect of coenzyme Q10 supplementation on mitochondrial function after myocardial ischemia reperfusion. J Surg Res 2002; 102(2):221–228.

44 Buchner DM, Wagner EH. Preventing frail health. Clin Geriatr Med 1992; 8(1):1–17.

45 Cobon GS, Verrills N, Papakostopoulos P et al. The proteomics of ageing. Biogerontology 2002; 3(1/2): 133–136.

46 Tinetti ME, Speechley M, Ginter SF. Risk factors for falls among elderly persons living in the community. N Engl J Med 1988; 319(26):1701–1707.

47 Kallman DA, Plato CC, Tobin JD. The role of muscle loss in the aged-related decline of grip strength: cross-sectional and longitudinal perspectives. J Gerontol 1990; 45(3):M82–M88.

48 Rakowski W, Mor V. The association of physical activity with mortality among older adults in the Longitudinal Study of Ageing (1984–1988). J Gerontol 1992; 47(4):M122–M129.

49 Dela F, Kjaer M. Resistance training, insulin sensitivity and muscle function in the elderly. Essays Biochem 2006; 42:75–88.

50 Konerman SG. Endocrine aspects of ageing. New York: Elsevier; 1982.

51 Baumgartner RN, Koehler KM, Gallagher D et al. Epidemiology of sarcopenia among the elderly in New Mexico. Am J Epidemiol 1998; 147(8):755–763.

52 Bonnefoy M, Constans T, Ferry M. Influence of nutrition and physical activity on muscle in the very elderly. Presse Med 2000; 29(39):2177–2182.

53 Pierson RN Jr. Body composition in ageing: a biological perspective. Curr Opin Clin Nutr Metab Care 2003; 6(1):15–20.

54 Tonino RP, Minaker KL, Rowe JW. Effect of age on systemic delivery of oral glucose in men. Diabetes Care 1989; 12(6):394–398.

55 Harris MI. Epidemiology of diabetes mellitus among the elderly in the United States. Clin Geriatr Med 1990; 6(4):703–719.

56 Hales CN. Non-insulin-dependent diabetes mellitus. Br Med Bull 1997; 53(1):109–122.

57 Hu FB, Manson JE, Stampfer MJ et al. Diet, lifestyle, and the risk of type 2 diabetes mellitus in women. N Engl J Med 2001; 345(11):790–797.

58 Chuo AM, Lim JK. Thyroid dysfunction in elderly patients. Ann Acad Med Singapore 2003; 32(1): 96–100.

59 Mariotti S, Franceschi A, Cossarizza A et al. The ageing thyroid. Endocr Rev 1995; 16(6):686–715.

60 Weissel M. Disturbances of thyroid function in the elderly. Wien Klin Wochenschr 2006; 118(1/2):16–20.

61 Livingston EH, Hershman JM, Sawin CT et al. Prevalence of thyroid disease and abnormal thyroid tests in older hospitalized and ambulatory patients. J Am Geriatr Soc 1987; 35:109–114.

62 Vanderpump MPJ, Tunbridge WMG, French JM et al. The incidence of thyroid disorders in the community: a twenty year follow-up of the Whickham survey. Clin Endocrinol 1995; 43:55–68.

63 Rose NR. Thymus function, ageing and autoimmunity. Immunol Lett 1994; 40(3):225–230.

64 Prelog M. Ageing of the immune system: a risk factor for autoimmunity? Autoimmun Rev 2006; 5(2):136–139.

65 Bunevicius R, Kazanavicius G, et al. Effects of thyroxine as compared with thyroxine plus triiodothyronine in patients with hypothyroidism. N Engl J Med 1990; 340:424–429.

66 Hall JE. Neuroendocrine changes with reproductive ageing in women. Semin Reprod Med 2007; 25(5):344–351.

67 Wise PM, Krajnak KM, Kashon ML. Menopause: the ageing of multiple pacemakers. Science 1996; 273(5271):67–70.

68 Ginsberg TB. Ageing and sexuality. Med Clin North Am 2006; 90(5):1025–1036.

69 Lambert SM, Masson P, Fisch H. The male biological clock. World J Urol 2006; 24(6):611–617.

70 Lobo RA. Postmenopausal hormones and coronary artery disease: potential benefits and risks. Climacteric 2007; 10(Suppl 2):21–26. Review.

71 Vitale C, Miceli M, Rosano GM. Gender-specific characteristics of atherosclerosis in menopausal women: risk factors, clinical course and strategies for prevention. Climacteric 2007; Suppl 2:16–20.

72 Barrett-Connor E, Grady D, Stefanick ML. The rise and fall of menopausal hormone therapy. Ann Rev Pub Health 2005; 26:115–140.

73 Faber A, Bouvy ML, Loskamp L et al. Dramatic change in prescribing of hormone replacement therapy in The Netherlands after publication of the Million Women Study: a follow-up study. Br J Clin Pharmacol 2005; 60(6):641–647.

74 Moskowitz D. A comprehensive review of the safety and efficacy of bioidentical hormones for the management of menopause and related health risks. Altern Med Rev 2006; 11(3):208–223.

75 Schatzl G, Madersbacher S, Temml C et al. Serum androgen levels in men: impact of health status and age. Urology 2003; 61(3):629–633.

76 Anawalt BD, Merriam GR. Neuroendocrine ageing in men. Andropause and somatopause. Endocrinol Metab Clin North Am 2001; 30(3):647–669.

77 Harman SM, Tsitouras PD. Reproductive hormones in ageing men. II. Basal pituitary gonadotropins and gonadotropin responses to luteinizing hormone-releasing hormone. J Clin Endocrinol Metab 1982; 54(3):547–551.

78 Chahal HS, Drake WM. The endocrine system and ageing. J Pathol 2007; 211(2):173–180. Review.
79 Chew KK, Stuckey B, Bremner A et al. Male erectile dysfunction: its prevalence in Western Australia and associated sociodemographic factors. J Sex Med 2008; 5(1):60–69.
80 Fink RI, Kolterman OG, Olefsky JM. The physiological significance of the glucose intolerance of ageing. J Gerontol 1984; 39(3):273–278.
81 Spark RF. Testosterone, diabetes mellitus, and the metabolic syndrome. Curr Urol Rep 2007; 8(6):467–471. Review.
82 Morley JE. Testosterone and behavior. Clin Geriatr Med 2003; 19(3):605–616. Review.
83 Alexander GM, Swerdloff RS, Wang C et al. Androgen behavior correlations in hypogonadal and eugonadal men: cognitive abilities. Horm Behav 1998; 33:85–94.
84 Urban RJ, Bodenburg YH, Gilkison C et al. Testosterone administration to elderly men increases skeletal muscle strength and protein synthesis. Am J Physiol 1995; 269:E820–E826.
85 Tenover JS. Androgen administration to ageing men. Endocrinol Metab Clin North Am 1994; 23:877–892.
86 Emmelot-Vonk MH, Verhaar HJ, Nakahi Pour HR et al. Effect of testosterone supplementation on functional mobility, cognition, and other parameters in older men: a randomized controlled trial. JAMA 2008; 299(1):39–52.
87 Vigna GB, Bergami E. Testosterone replacement, cardiovascular system and risk factors in the ageing male. J Endocrinol Invest 2005; 28:69–74.
88 Gooren LJ. Androgens and male aging: current evidence of safety and efficacy. Asian J Androl 2010; 12(2):136–151.
89 Herbert J. The age of dehydroepiandrosterone. Lancet 1995; 345:1193–1194.
90 Ravaglia G, Forti P, Maioli F et al. The relationship of dehydroepiandrosterone sulfate (DHEAS) to endocrine: metabolic parameters and functional status in the oldest-old. Results from an Italian study on healthy free-living over-ninety-year-olds. J Clin Endocrin Metab 1996; 81(3):1173–1178.
91 Barrett-Connor E, Goodman-Gruen D. The epidemiology of DHEAS and cardiovascular disease. Ann NY Acad Sci 1995; 774:259–270.
92 Wolf OT, Kirschbaum C. Actions of dehydroepiandrosterone and its sulfate in the central nervous system: effects on cognition and emotion in animals and humans. Brain Res Rev 1999; 30(3):264–288.
93 Brooke AM, Kalingag LA, Miraki-Moud F et al. Dehydroepiandrosterone improves psychological well-being in male and female hypopituitary patients on maintenance growth hormone replacement. Clin Endocrinol Metab 2006; 91(10):3773–3779.
94 Watson RR, Huls A, Araghinikuam M et al. Dehydroepiandrosterone and diseases of ageing. Drugs Ageing 1996; 9(4):274–291.
95 Yen SS, Morales AJ, Khorram O. Replacement of DHEA in ageing men and women. Potential remedial effects. Ann NY Acad Sci 1995; 774:128–142.
96 Morales AJ, Nolan JJ, Nelson JC et al. Effects of replacement dose of dehydroepiandrosterone in men and women of advancing age. J Clin Endocrinol Metab 1994; 78(6):1360–1367.
97 Morales AJ, Haubrich RH, Hwang JY et al. The effect of six months treatment with a 100 mg daily dose of dehydroepiandrosterone (DHEA) on circulating sex steroids, body composition and muscle strength in age-advanced men and women. Clin Endocrinol (Oxf) 1998; 49(4):421–432.
98 Yamada Y, Sekihara H, Omura M et al. Changes in serum sex hormone profiles after short-term low-dose administration of dehydroepiandrosterone (DHEA) to young and elderly persons. Endocr J 2007; 54(1):153–162.
99 Genazzani AR, Pluchino N, Begliuomini S et al. Long-term low-dose oral administration of dehydroepiandrosterone modulates adrenal response to adrenocorticotropic hormone in early and late postmenopausal women. Gynaecol Endocrinol 2006; 22(11):627–635.
100 Clayton P, Gleeson H, Monson J et al. Growth hormone replacement throughout life: insights into age-related responses to treatment. Growth Horm IGF Res 2007; 17(5):369–382.
101 Corpas E, Harman SM, Blackman MR. Human growth hormone and human ageing. Endocr Rev 1993; 14(1):20–39.
102 Sievers C, Schneider HJ, Stalla GK. Insulin-like growth factor-1 in plasma and brain: regulation in health and disease. Front Biosci 2008; 13:85–99.
103 Blackman MR. Pituitary hormones and ageing. Endocrinol Metab Clin North Am. 1987; 16(4):981–994.
104 Merriam GR, Schwartz RS, Vitiello MV. Growth hormone-releasing hormone and growth hormone secretagogues in normal ageing. Endocrine 2003; 22(1):41–48.
105 Lamberts SW. The somatopause: to treat or not to treat? Horm Res 2000; 53(Suppl 3):42–43.
106 Rudman D, Feller AG, Nagraj HS et al. Effects of human growth hormone in men over 60 years old. N Engl J Med 1990; 323(1):1–6.
107 Papadakis MA, Grady D, Black D et al. Growth hormone replacement in healthy older men improves body composition but not functional ability. Ann Intern Med 1996; 124(8):708–716.
108 Taaffe DR, Pruitt L, Reim J et al. Effect of recombinant human growth hormone on the muscle strength

response to resistance exercise in elderly men. J Clin Endocrinol Metab 1994; 79(5):1361–1366.
109 Vittone J, Blackman MR, Busby-Whitehead J et al. Effects of single nightly injections of growth hormone-releasing hormone (GHRH 1-29) in healthy elderly men. Metabolism 1997; 46(1):89–96.
110 Bach MA, Rockwood K, Zetterberg C et al. The effects of MK-0677, an oral growth hormone secretagogue, in patients with hip fracture. J Am Geriatr Soc 2004; 52(4):516–523.
111 Poehlman ET, Copeland KC. Influence of physical activity on insulin-like growth factor in healthy younger and older men. J Clin Endocrin Metab 1990; 71(6):1468–1473.
112 Corpas E, Harman SM, Pineyro MA et al. Growth hormone (GH)-releasing hormone (1-29) twice daily reverses the decreased GH and insulin-like growth factor-I levels in old men. J Clin Endocrin Metab 1992; 75(2):530–535.
113 Merriam GR, Buchner DM, Prinz PN et al. Potential applications of GH secretagogs in the evaluation and treatment of the age-related decline in growth hormone secretion. Endocrine 1997; 7(1):49–52.
114 Perls TT, Reisman NR, Olshansky SJ. Provision or distribution of growth hormone for 'antiageing': clinical and legal issues. JAMA 2005; 294(16):2086–2090.
115 Willett W. Balancing lifestyle and genomics research for disease prevention. Science 2002; 296:695–698.
116 Vitetta L, Anton B, Cortizo F et al. Mind–body medicine: stress and its impact on overall health and longevity. Ann NY Acad Sci 2005; 1057:492–505.
117 Vitetta L, Anton B. Lifestyle and nutrition, caloric restriction, mitochondrial health and hormones: scientific interventions for anti-aging. Clin Interv Aging 2007; 2(4):537–543.
118 Hassed C. New frontiers in medicine: the body as the shadow of the soul. Melbourne: Michelle Anderson Publishing; 2000.
119 Selye H. The stress of life. New York: McGraw-Hill; 1987.
120 Lin J, Dhabhar FS, Wolkowitz O et al. Pessimism correlates with leukocyte telomere shortness and elevated interleukin-6 in post-menopausal women. Brain Behav Immun 2009; 23(4):446–449.
121 Epel E, Daubenmier J, Moskowitz JT et al. Can mediation slow rate of cellular aging? Cognitive stress, mindfulness and telomeres. Ann NY Acad Sci 2009; 1172:34–53.
122 Jackson AA. Integrating the ideas of life course across cellular, individual, and population levels in cancer causation. J Nutr 2005; 135(Suppl 12):S2927–S2933.
123 Trichopoulou A, Costacou T, Bamia C et al. Adherence to a Mediterranean diet and survival in a Greek population. N Engl J Med 2003; 348(26):2599–2608.
124 Meyer TE, Kovacs SJ, Ehsani AA et al. Long-term caloric restriction ameliorates the decline in diastolic function in humans. J Am Coll Cardiol 2006; 47(2):398–402.
125 McCay CM, Cromwell MF, Maynard LA. The effect of retarded growth upon the length of life span and upon the ultimate body size. J Nutr 1935; 10:63–79.
126 Weindruch R, Keenan KP, Carney JM et al. Caloric restriction mimetics: metabolic interventions. J Gerontol A Biol Sci Med Sci 2001; 56(Spec No 1): 20–33.
127 Weindruch R, Sohal RS. Seminars in medicine of the Beth Israel Deaconess Medical Center. Caloric intake and ageing. N Engl J Med 2001; 337:986–994.
128 Holloszt JO. Mortality rate and longevity of food-restricted exercising male rats: a reevaluation. J Appl Physiol 1997; 82(2):399–403.
129 Lane MA, Black A, Handy A et al. Caloric restriction in primates. Ann NY Acad Sci 2001; 928: 287–295.
130 Fernandes G, Yunis EJ, Good RA. Suppression of adenocarcinoma by the immunological consequences of calorie restriction. Nature 1976; 263:504–507.
131 Fernandes G, Good RA. Inhibition by restricted calorie diet of lymphoproliferative disease and renal damage in MRL/lpr mice. Proc Natl Acad Sci 1984; 81: 6144–6148.
132 Kubo C, Day NK, Good RA. Influence of early or late dietary restriction on life span and immunological parameters in MRL/Mp–lpr/lpr mice. Proc Natl Acad Sci USA 1984; 81:5831–5835.
133 Engelman RW, Day NK, Chen RF et al. Calorie consumption level influences development of C3H/Ou breast adenocarcinoma with indifference to calorie source. Proc Soc Exp Biol Med 1990; 193:23–30.
134 Sarkar NH, Fernandes G, Telang NT et al. Low-calorie diet prevents the development of mammary tumors in C3H mice and reduces circulating prolactin level, murine mammary tumor virus expression, and proliferation of mammary alveolar cells. Proc Natl Acad Sci USA 1982; 79:7758–7762.
135 Everitt AV, Le Couteur DG. Life extension by calorie restriction in humans. Ann NY Acad Sci 2007; 1114:428–433.
136 Duan W, Mattson MP. Dietary restriction and 2-deoxyglucose administration improve behavioral outcome and reduce degeneration of dopaminergic neurons in models of Parkinson's disease. J Neurosci Res 1999; 57:195–206.
137 Zhu H, Guo Q, Mattson MP. Dietary restriction protects hippocampal neurons against the death-promoting action of presenilin-1 mutation. Brain Res 1999; 842:224–229.
138 Mattson MP. Neuroprotective signaling and the ageing brain: take away my food and let me run. Brain Res 2000; 886:47–53.

139 Ingram DK, Weindruch R, Spangler EL et al. Dietary restriction benefits learning and motor performance of aged mice. J Gerontol 1987; 42:78–81.

140 Moroi-Fetters SE, Mervis RF, London ED et al. Dietary restriction suppresses age-related changes in dendritic spines. Neurobiol Ageing 1989; 10:317–322.

141 Roth GS, Lane MA, Ingram DK et al. Biomarkers of caloric restriction may predict longevity in humans. Science 2002; 297:811.

142 Heilbronn LK, de Jonge L, Frisard MI et al. Effect of 6-month calorie restriction on biomarkers of longevity, metabolic adaptation, and oxidative stress in overweight individuals: a randomized controlled trial. JAMA 2006; 295(13):1539–1548.

143 Baur JA, Sinclair DA. Therapeutic potential of resveratrol: the in vivo evidence. Nat Rev Drug Discov 2006; 5(6):493–506.

144 Guarente l, Kenyon C. Genetic pathways that regulate ageing in model organisms. Nature 2000; 408:255–262.

145 Howitz KT, Bitterman KJ, Cohen HY et al. Small molecule activators of sirtuins extend *Saccharomyces cerevisiae* lifespan. Nature 2003; 425: 191–196.

146 Kirkland JL. The biology of senescence: potential for prevention of disease. Clin Geriatr Med 2002; 18(3):383–405.

147 Wiley J, Camacho T. Lifestyle and future health: evidence from the Alameda County Study. Prevent Med 1980; 9:1–21.

148 Seeman T, Kaplan G, Knudsen L et al. Social network ties and mortality among the elderly in the Alameda County Study. Am J Epidemiol 1987; 126: 714–723.

149 Breslow L, Breslow N. Health practices and disability: some evidence from Alameda County. Prevent Med 1993; 22:86–95.

150 Vaillant G, Mukamal K. Successful ageing. Am J Psych 2001; 158(6):839–847.

part SEVEN

Social conditions

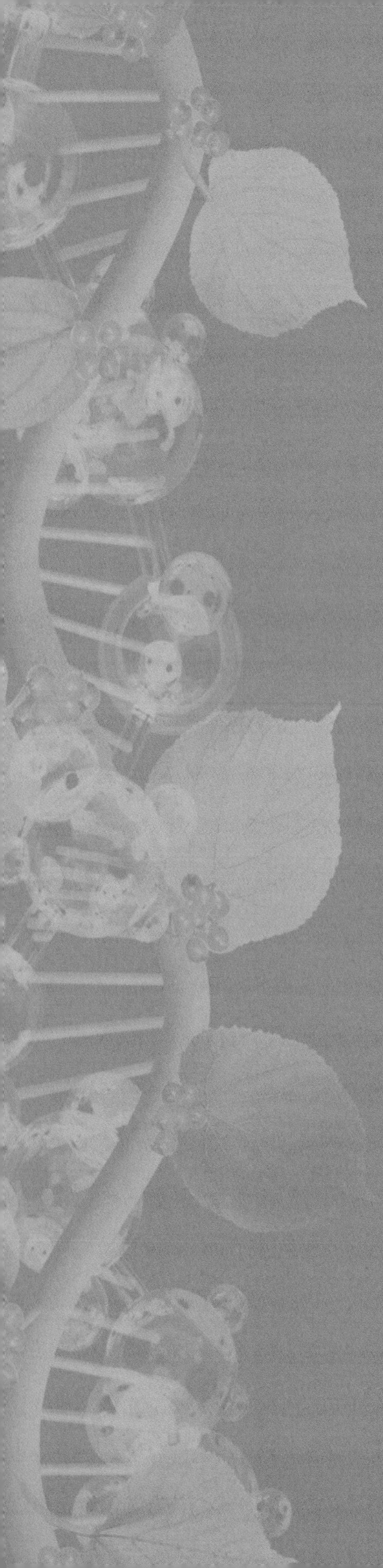

chapter 59

Domestic violence

INTRODUCTION AND OVERVIEW

In the past decade, domestic violence has been recognised as a health problem resulting in significant morbidity and mortality. It is a serious and widespread problem that affects all economic, educational, ethnic and regional groups. This chapter outlines the nature and prevalence of domestic violence, how it presents in clinical practice, how to ask about it and how to respond to it holistically.

WHAT IS DOMESTIC VIOLENCE?

In the community, domestic violence is usually taken to mean physical violence between partners, usually perpetrated by the husband on the wife, although men may be victims and abuse does occur in same-sex relationships. Sometimes the term is used to refer to abuse that occurs in any relationship within households and thus would include child, elder and sibling abuse. This chapter concentrates on *partner abuse* (marriage, de facto relationship, boyfriend or girlfriend), which is a complex pattern of behaviours that includes emotional, physical and sexual abuse, not just simple acts of violence (Fig 59.1).

The World Health Organization uses the term *intimate partner violence* and defines it as:

> Any behavior within an intimate relationship that causes physical, psychological or sexual harm to those in the relationship, includes: physical aggression, psychological abuse, forced intercourse & other forms of sexual coercion, various controlling behaviors.[1]

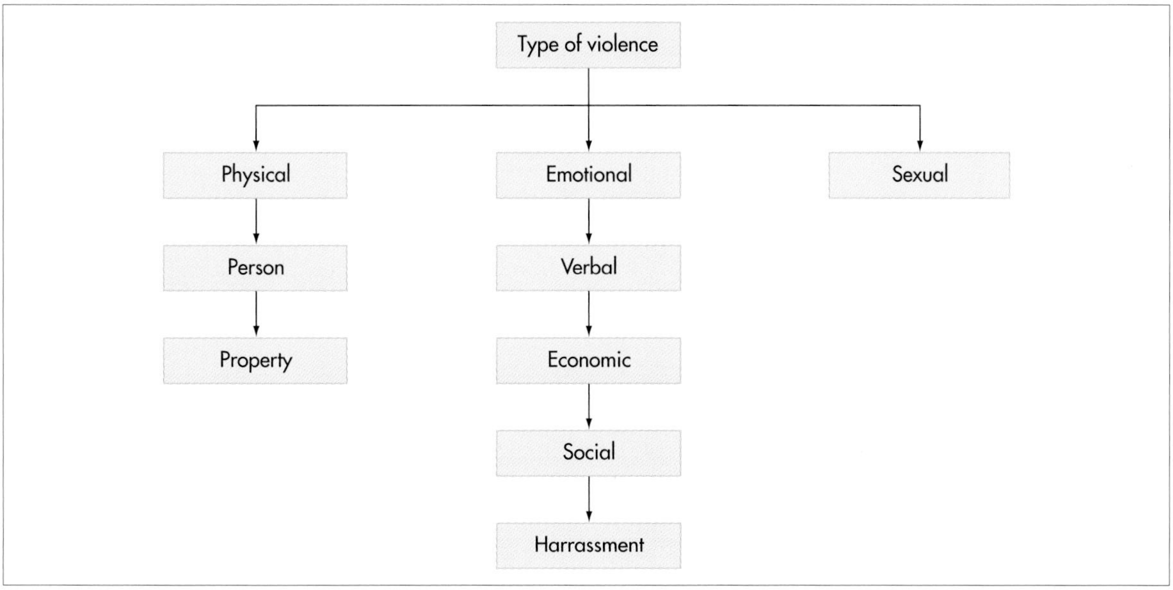

FIGURE 59.1 Types of abuse in partner violence

From a health perspective, domestic violence is best understood as a chronic syndrome characterised not by the episodes of physical violence that punctuate the problem but by the emotional abuse that the perpetrator uses to maintain control over the partner. Furthermore, as most victims of partner abuse report, the physical violence is the least-damaging abuse suffered. It is the relentless psychological abuse that cripples and isolates the victim and results in fear of the partner. Domestic violence against women is the focus of this chapter, because most abuse with serious health and other consequences is committed by men against their female partners.[2]

BACKGROUND AND PREVALENCE

Abuse of women by their partners or ex-partners is a worldwide phenomenon.[3] The World Health Organization *World Report on Violence and Health* revealed that in 48 population-based surveys around the world, 10–69% of women had been physically assaulted by their partners at some stage in their lives.[1] Clinical samples obtain higher rates than community surveys. For example, recent general practice studies in Australia, the United States, the United Kingdom and Ireland have found high lifetime physical abuse rates ranging from 23.3% to 41.0% of women, and 12-month rates from around 5% to 17%.[4] A full-time general practitioner probably sees at least one abused woman each week, although she may not be presenting with obvious signs or symptoms. Similar rates are found in emergency departments, mental health clinics, antenatal care and drug and alcohol clinics. Today, on average, one in fifty women presenting to the emergency department do so because of domestic violence.

Thus women experiencing domestic violence present very frequently to healthcare services and require wide-ranging medical services. The societal economic impact is great, with an Australian study estimating that in 2002/03 the cost to the community of domestic violence was in the order of AUD$8.1 billion, with the main contributors being pain, suffering and premature mortality.[5] The total cost of intimate partner violence to services and to the economy as a whole in the United Kingdom has been estimated at £3.1 billion and £5.7 billion a year, respectively.[6]

AETIOLOGY

Researchers have postulated that there are many causes of domestic violence at the individual, family, community and societal levels. Originally, people thought that abuse was caused by psychiatric illness. Once the prevalence of abuse in the community was recognised, however, it was realised that this explanation was unrealistic. Subsequently, researchers felt that conflict in the family was the major cause. Unfortunately for this theory, many women describe there being no conflict before abuse happening. Review of the evidence for societal risk factors shows that violence in the family of origin of victim and perpetrator, and unemployment of the perpetrator, were the only variables that had sound evidence of an association. It seems that the combination of environment, social and economic factors may contribute to domestic violence. However, feminist researchers have argued that patriarchy in today's society underlies much of the abuse of women. The World Health Organization certainly places domestic violence in the context of violence against women, which includes such issues as rape and genital mutilation.

HEALTH CONSEQUENCES

Domestic violence can have short-term and long-term negative health consequences for survivors, even after the abuse has ended.[7] Abused women experience many chronic health problems, with depression, post-traumatic stress disorder, chronic pain and gastro-intestinal and gynaecological problems being the most common (Box 59.1). It is also a very common cause of femicide, with over 50% of all female murders being committed by their partners or ex-partners, in the United Kingdom and the United States. In Australia, a far higher percentage of Indigenous than non-Indigenous women are murdered by their partners.

EFFECT ON CHILDREN AND ADOLESCENTS

Up to 60% of children witness their mother's abuse.[8] This witnessing includes:

- *seeing*—including homicide and non-fatal beatings
- *hearing*—heated arguments, humiliation and abusive language
- *being used*—in threats, as hostages, as a physical weapon, as a spy on a parent's activities
- *the aftermath*—injuries, removal to a shelter/refuge, trauma of removal of the perpetrator and, in some cases, the murder of a parent.

Children exposed to domestic violence in the home have a higher risk of physical, emotional, behavioural and educational problems that persist into adulthood. In adolescents, it may manifest as depression, running away from home, drug and alcohol abuse, criminal behaviour, self-harming and suicidal ideation.

A DIAGNOSTIC APPROACH

Intuitively, it would seem that early detection and intervention with women who have experienced domestic violence might improve health outcomes, but there is

BOX 59.1 Potential presentations of domestic violence in clinical practice

Psychological
- Insomnia
- Depression
- Suicidal ideation
- Anxiety symptoms and panic disorder
- Somatoform disorder
- Post-traumatic stress disorder
- Eating disorders
- Drug and alcohol abuse

Physical
- Obvious injuries, especially to the head and neck or multiple areas
- Bruises in various stages of healing
- Sexual assault
- Sexually transmitted diseases
- Chronic pelvic pain
- Chronic abdominal pain
- Chronic headaches
- Chronic back pain
- Chest pain
- Numbness and tingling from injuries
- Lethargy
- Miscarriages
- Unwanted pregnancy
- Antepartum haemorrhage
- Lack of prenatal care
- Low birth weight of infant

General
- Delay in seeking treatment or inconsistent explanation of injuries
- Multiple presentations
- Non-compliance with drug treatment and attendances
- Accompanying partner who is over-attentive or coercive
- Recent separation or divorce
- Past history of child abuse
- Age less than 40 years
- Abuse of a child in the family

Children
- Aggressive behaviour and language
- Anxiety or difficulty adjusting to change
- Psychosomatic illness
- Bedwetting

currently no empirical evidence for the effectiveness of routine screening. Although domestic violence is an important health problem, it fails to meet the most crucial criterion for screening—that early detection must enable early intervention, to reduce morbidity and/or mortality. Rather, opportunistic case finding in practice settings such as emergency departments, psychiatry clinics, antenatal clinics and general practices is appropriate with women who are presenting with the potential clinical indicators of domestic violence.[9]

HOW TO ASK ABOUT DOMESTIC VIOLENCE

Up to one-third of women disclose abuse to their GPs, particularly if asked in a non-judgmental, empathic way (Box 59.2). However, there are major internal and external barriers to women disclosing about domestic violence. Reasons given by women living in situations of domestic violence include fear, denial and disbelief, emotional bonds to partner, commitment to marriage, hope for change and staying for the sake of the children. Normalisation of violence (i.e. coming from a background where abuse was the norm) and women's isolation, depression and stress play a major role in their non-disclosure. Feeling that they will not be believed by health practitioners and that available services will not be able to help or maintain confidentiality may reflect negative experiences in the past.

INTEGRATIVE MANAGEMENT

Managing partner abuse does not really follow the simple line of history taking, examination, diagnosis and referral. Rather, there are simple communication skills that the healthcare professional should exercise that women in situations of violence and abuse say they expect and hope for from their healthcare practitioner.[10] Often women who feel supported see their GP as an advocate for them.

Women need emotional support from their healthcare practitioner, their multiple physical symptoms investigated and treated, their mental health issues managed, their injuries documented and their social and environmental situation acknowledged and validated. Apart from seeking help from doctors, many women in their attempts to heal look to alternative therapies (e.g. music therapy, art therapy), while others seek spiritual help from ministers and other religious leaders. Practitioners

BOX 59.2 Possible questions to ask if you suspect domestic violence

- Has your partner ever physically threatened or hurt you?
- Is there a lot of tension in your relationship? How do you resolve arguments?
- Sometimes partners react strongly in arguments and use physical force. Is this happening to you?
- Are you afraid of your partner?
- Have you ever been afraid of any partner? Violence is very common in the home. I ask many of my patients about abuse, because no one should have to live in fear of their partner.

need to be aware that these are often a great source of comfort for women at times of stress from the abuse.

PREVENTION

Practitioners do not have a major role in primary prevention of domestic violence (e.g. community campaigns and school programs). They can, however, play a role in prevention by modelling non-abusive workplace practices, by early intervention with children who are witnesses of domestic violence and by speaking out in public forums about this common social problem. Education at the undergraduate and postgraduate levels across the disciplines is necessary to provide an educated healthcare workforce (Fig 59.2), which is essential for interventions in the domestic violence area. Healthcare practitioners need to actively intervene, with this social condition that affects the health of women and their families.

INITIAL RESPONSE

All healthcare professionals need to be trained to be able to validate the experience of abuse, affirm that violence is unacceptable behaviour and express support, before any other response. Even if a woman does not choose to pursue other interventions or engage with other agencies, validation of her experience and the offer of support is an act that may in the long run contribute to her being able to change her situation (Box 59.3).

BOX 59.3 Possible validation statements if a woman discloses domestic violence

- Everybody deserves to feel safe at home.
- You don't deserve to be hit or hurt. It is not your fault.
- I am concerned about your safety and wellbeing .
- You are not alone. I will be with you through this, whatever you decide. Help is available.
- You are not to blame. Abuse is common and happens in all kinds of relationships. It tends to continue.
- Abuse can affect your health and that of your children in many ways.

BOX 59.4 Assessing the safety of women experiencing partner abuse

- What does she need in order to feel safe?
- Have the frequency and severity increased?
- Is he obsessive about her?
- How safe does she feel?
- Has she been threatened with a weapon?
- Does he have a weapon in the house?
- Has the violence been escalating?

In addition to offering support, the practitioner needs to make an initial assessment of the woman's safety (Box 59.4). This may be as simple as checking with the woman about whether it is safe for her (and

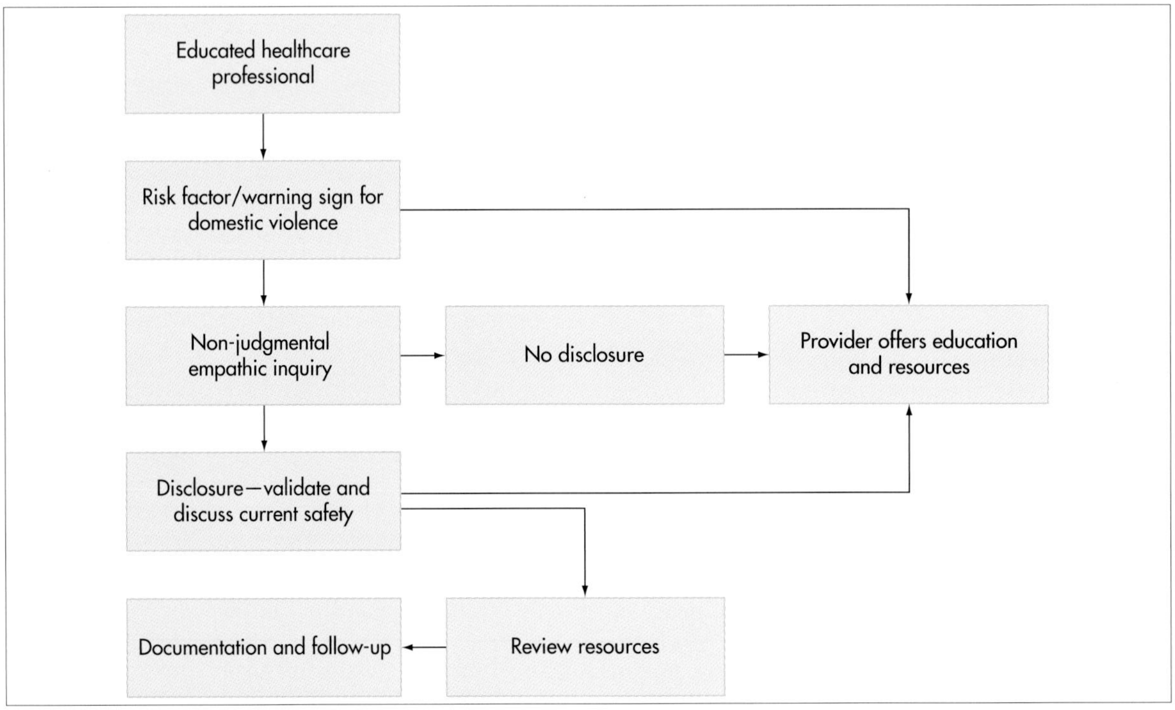

FIGURE 59.2 Clinical care pathway

her children) to return home. A more detailed risk assessment will include questions about escalation of abuse, the content of threats and direct and indirect abuse of the children.

REFERRAL TO EXTERNAL AGENCIES

In addition to assessing the woman's safety, a key step for clinicians to whom women disclose domestic violence, particularly if it is current or recent violence, is offer of referral to specialist domestic violence support. This is provided in a variety of ways, usually by a non-governmental organisation or a social service agency; or sometimes it is government funded. Domestic violence advocacy, particularly for women who have actively sought help from professional services or are in a refuge setting, is likely to be beneficial. It has been shown to reduce abuse, increase social support and quality of life and lead to increased use of safety behaviours and accessing of community resources. For women identified in healthcare settings, we are unsure whether advocacy works, because of the small number and relatively poor design of current studies.[11]

SELF-HELP

Resilience is a commonly used concept to describe the ability to bounce back after encountering difficulties, negative events or hard times. For women who have experienced abuse, recovery is seen not as returning to normal, but rather as constructing a self built on the experience of having survived. Resilience can be seen to include a sense of self-esteem, the ability to adapt and a belief that problems can be solved. The central process involved in building resilience is the training and development of adaptive coping skills. An important aspect of this is socially focused, such as emotional support from others, which is when women may start to be able to break away from the abuse.

The literature identifies varying numbers of stages (Fig 59.3) that women undergo in dealing with domestic violence, and women may move in either direction along the path. For example, a woman often has to leave an abusive partner a number of times before the relationship is finally ended, and the abuse might not end when the relationship does. In the final stage, which is generally considered to be a lack of violence in a woman's life, recovery is not returning to 'normal', but constructing a self built on the experience of having survived and left an abusive situation. Reclaiming the self may be a stage where women move from surviving to thriving. There are many self-help books, support groups and online support forums (chat rooms, bulletins and email groups) that women can access on this journey to recovery.

The importance of relating to other women who have shared experiences in order to reconstruct a self where abuse is no longer part of a woman's life cannot be underestimated. In Figure 59.3, the concept of a catalyst for change that propels women towards acting to end the violence is introduced. The 'turning point' moment connects the external and internal in a moment

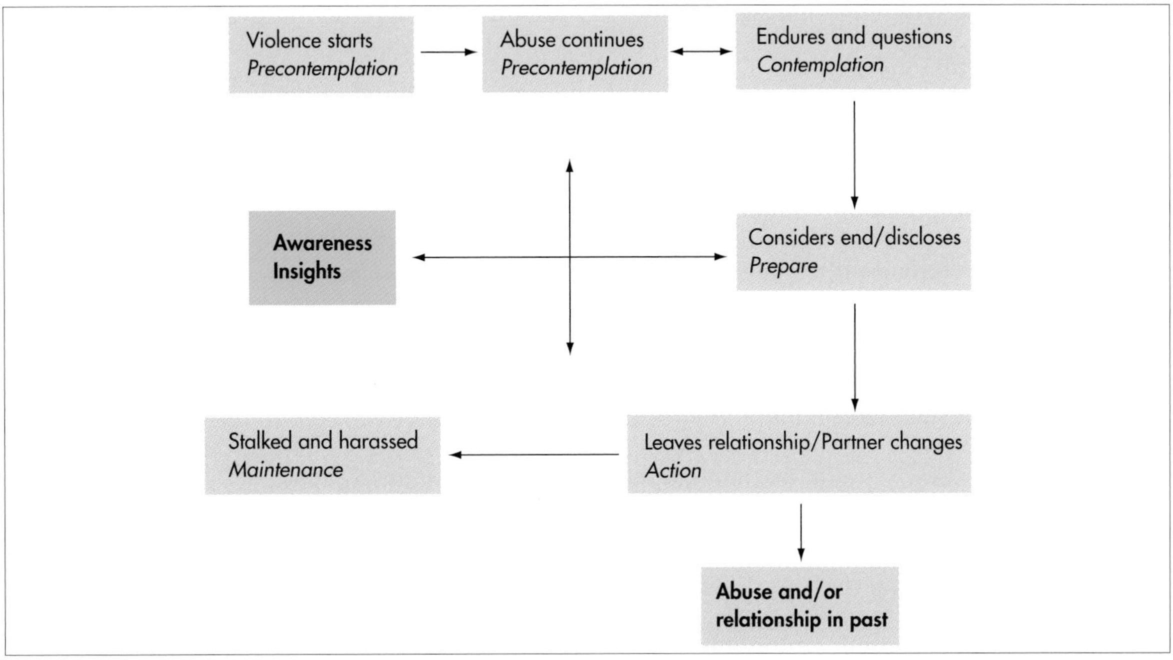

FIGURE 59.3 Stages of change[12]

of change. It generally coincides with an environmental shift (e.g. children becoming teenagers, getting a job, taking up study) and leads to an adjustment to the woman's sense of self.

LIFESTYLE AND OTHER INTERVENTIONS

Many women experiencing current abuse are socially isolated and prevented by their partner from seeking help in the community. They may find it difficult to access any of the above social support networks because of fear of their partner finding out. They may also find it difficult to become involved in any stress management activities (e.g. exercise, healthy diet, yoga or relaxation), as their activities are monitored and they are on constant alert. Their sleep may be affected to a great extent and they may then seek pharmacological management (e.g. sleeping tablets or antidepressants) to cope. Sometimes doctors will medicalise their condition without recognising the underlying hidden social problem, resulting in multiple diagnoses and medications (e.g. painkillers). However, the woman's access to medical, mental health and alternative healthcare practitioners may be limited or controlled by her partner.

PSYCHOLOGICAL THERAPY

There is evidence that cognitive behavioural therapy principles used in group or solo therapy may benefit survivors of abuse if delivered by therapists who have had additional training in dealing with domestic violence. They are not appropriate or even safe while a woman is still experiencing abuse from her partner.[11]

PERPETRATOR MANAGEMENT

Men who use violence in their relationships are at increased risk of depression, substance abuse or abuse in their childhood and it is unlikely that they will spontaneously disclose.[12] Current evidence suggests that clinicians should ask men general questions about how things are at home, but then ask specifically about what happens when the couple argue. Offering ongoing support if he is willing to attempt change, and referral to an accredited behaviour change program, is a key component of management. Assessing the patient's suicide risk and his family's safety is vital. Although the evidence for effective interventions for perpetrators is not strong and is based mostly on mandatory programs, evidence from their partners suggests that for those men who do remain in programs, their partners' quality of life improves.

COMPLEMENTARY THERAPIES

There is limited evidence about what type of other therapies might assist women, although individual women's stories describe hypnosis, meditation, touch, music and art therapy as key on their roads to recovery. The number of abused women who seek help from complementary therapists is unknown. We do know, however, that abused women experience a high level of chronic symptoms, including pain. It is likely that a high proportion of women attending chiropractors, osteopaths, naturopaths and acupuncturists will have experienced domestic violence.

IMPORTANT PITFALLS

The largest pitfall is that domestic violence is missed completely by the majority of practitioners. Practitioners need to be alert to the signs and symptoms of domestic violence and to train themselves in how to ask and respond appropriately.

PROGNOSIS

Allowing the woman to progress at her own therapeutic pace and understanding the chronicity of the problem is important in the ongoing relationship with the abused woman as the practitioner provides follow-up and continued support. Respecting the woman's wishes, even if this means she does not follow up on your referral, shows that you understand the nature of the effects of domestic violence. Women who did not disclose initially may disclose at a later date. The likelihood is that the pathway to recovery and wellness is long for women who have experienced domestic violence. Practitioners need to be prepared to walk the journey with them, acting as support and advocate in a woman-centered, holistic way.

RESOURCES

For healthcare professionals

Roberts G, Hegarty K, Feder G. Intimate partner abuse and health professionals: new approaches to domestic violence. London: Churchill Livingstone/Elsevier; 2006.

Taft A, Hegarty K, Feder G, on behalf of the Guidelines Development Group. Management of the whole family when intimate partner violence is present: guidelines for the primary care physician. Melbourne, Australia: Victorian Government Department of Justice; 2006, www.racgp.org.au/Content/NavigationMenu/ClinicalResources/RACGPGuidelines/Familywomenviolence/Intimatepartnerabuse/20060507intimatepartnerviolence.pdf

For patients and the public

Australian Domestic and Family Violence Clearinghouse, http://www.austdvclearinghouse.unsw.edu.au/

Family Violence Prevention Fund, http://endabuse.org/programs/healthcare

Women's Aid, http://www.womensaid.org.uk

REFERENCES

1 Krug E, Dahlberg L, Mercy J et al. World report on violence and health. Geneva, Switzerland: World Health Organization; 2002.

2 Taft A, Hegarty K, Flood M. Are men and women equally violent to intimate partners? Aust NZ J Public Health 2001; 25(6):498–500.

3 Watts C, Zimmerman C. Violence against women: global scope and magnitude. Lancet 2002; 359:1232–1237.

4 Hegarty K. What is domestic violence and how common is it? In: Roberts G, Hegarty K, Feder G, eds. Intimate partner abuse and health professionals: new approaches to domestic violence. London: Elsevier; 2006.

5 Partnerships Against Domestic Violence and Access Economics Pty Ltd. The cost of domestic violence to the Australian economy. Canberra: Australian Government, Office of the Status of Women, Commonwealth of Australia; 2004.

6 Walby S. The cost of domestic violence. London: Department of Trade and Industry; 2004.

7 Campbell J, Laughon K, Woods A. Impact of intimate partner abuse on physical and mental health: how does it present in clinical practice? In: Roberts G, Hegarty K, Feder G, eds. Intimate partner abuse and health professionals. London: Elsevier; 2006: 43–60.

8 Smith J. The impact of intimate partner abuse on children. In: Roberts G, Hegarty K, Feder G, eds. Intimate partner abuse and health professionals. London, UK: Elsevier; 2006.

9 Hegarty K, Feder G, Ramsay J. Identification of partner abuse in health care settings: should health professionals be screening? In: Roberts G, Hegarty K, Feder G, ed. Intimate partner abuse and health professionals. London: Elsevier; 2006.

10 Feder G, Hutson M, Ramsay J et al. Women exposed to intimate partner violence: expectations and experiences when they encounter health care professionals: a meta-analysis of qualitative studies. Arch Intern Med 2006; 166(1):22–37.

11 Ramsay J, Feder G, Rivas C. Interventions to reduce violence and promote the physical and psychosocial well-being of women who experience partner abuse: a systematic review. London: Department of Health; 2006.

12 Taft A, Shakespeare J. Managing the whole family when women are abused by intimate partners: challenges for health professionals. In: Roberts G, Hegarty K, Feder G, eds. Intimate partner abuse and health professionals: new approaches to domestic violence. London: Elsevier; 2006:145–163.

chapter 60

HIV management in general practice

INTRODUCTION AND OVERVIEW

Human immunodeficiency virus (HIV) infection has had, since the early 1980s, a global impact of unprecedented scale, including the decimation of some populations and the retardation of some nations' development. There have also been revolutions in our understanding of immunology and the pharmacology of anti-retroviral treatments. Researchers in all the sciences have had to change the way they investigate and communicate with affected communities. There have been changes, too, in the way communities are harnessed to prevent and to care, but also in how they can be stigmatised and blamed.

Globally, in 2007, it was estimated that 30–36 million people were living with HIV infection, with a death toll to that point of 1.8–2.3 million.[1]

General practitioners have always had a central role in the delivery of healthcare to communities (especially marginalised groups) and they have played a key role here as well. Their skills in chronic disease management, their teamwork, their holistic view of health and their long-term relationships with patients and communities all contribute to the care they can bring to the HIV-infected patient.

The HIV epidemic continues to grow and change around the world, influenced by many factors, including but not confined to:

- patterns of behaviour (especially sexual and IV drug use)
- the prevalence of sexually transmitted infections (STIs) in communities—these are important because they aid the transmission of HIV
- politically driven responses that can help or hinder infection rates
- the burgeoning number of new antiviral medications of increasing effectiveness and safety
- the continuing paucity of resources in those very countries with the highest prevalence rates
- the inability so far to develop an effective vaccine.[2]

How many HIV-infected patients are managed in general practice? The BEACH study in Australia counted 80 consultations per 100,000 and this low figure would probably be seen in other similar developed countries, where it is a predominantly gay male population that is affected.[3]

However, within all capital cities there are general practice clinics that have a special interest in sexual health and which would see a vastly greater number of HIV-infected patients. In countries where the prevalence of HIV is much higher and health resources are much more scarce, the GP will be seeing many cases of HIV every day. In those countries HIV is high on the differential diagnosis for any chronic health complaint.

For the GP, therefore, different roles are possible, from sole management, through shared care, to early referral. The role chosen will depend on the setting, the interest of the doctor and the resources available.

In resource-poor communities where there are limited antiviral agents available there will be a higher involvement of primary care / general practice and more reliance on traditional healing and so on. However, even here the number of people with HIV who are taking antiviral medications is growing, with the primary care being delivered in a variety of ways.[4]

In resource-rich communities there is greater complexity of choices and an interest in complementary/integrative measures. Here there will be more centralisation of care to specialist doctors and clinics. Yet even so there is a large burden of poverty within the HIV-affected community and consequent difficulties in gaining access to best care.[5]

Other important aspects of this disease are:

- the importance of guarding confidentiality and of working *with* risk groups
- the importance of harm minimisation principles
- the importance of a holistic approach—despite a burgeoning 'HIV industry', the GP has to also manage the rest of the patient's biopsychosocial issues
- the importance of research that can be done at primary care level—this also includes research into psychosocial aspects. Many anti-retrovirals have been trialled with the help of primary care, as this is where the majority of potential participants can be recruited.

HIV AND THE IMMUNE SYSTEM

This disease has a long lead-time, with decline of immunity as the central but not the only aspect. Many comorbidities are possible along the way:

- sexually transmitted infections, hepatitis B, hepatitis C, tuberculosis and other infections (including the opportunistic infections associated with immune deficiency)
- substance abuse problems, including alcohol and/or illicit drug use
- mental health issues, especially depression, but also including cognitive changes later in the evolution of the illness.[6]

Optimising immune health is therefore an important primary care task, especially among HIV-infected patients. This is important not just from the perspective of improving outcomes and slowing the rate of progression of HIV, but also because of its potential to improve quality of life at the same time. Measures include:

- improving lifestyle in terms of nutrition and exercise
- minimising the use of alcohol, drugs and smoking
- maintaining family and community involvement and the supports they can provide
- promoting a positive outlook, self-esteem and maintenance of hope
- controlling side effects of medications and optimising adherence
- treating depression
- early detection and treatment of STIs
- controlling herpes simplex virus outbreaks
- regular Pap smears
- use of complementary therapies (see below).[7]

PRIMARY PREVENTION IN GENERAL PRACTICE

HIV transmission is mainly the result of certain behaviours. General practice is well placed therefore to tackle the following:

- reducing at-risk behaviours—this includes promoting safer sex and safer IV use, and antenatal care such as anti-HIV medication prior to delivery
- case-finding and treating other STIs, because the presence of these will enhance transmission of HIV
- education at an individual and population level—not only about how HIV is or is not transmitted (Box 60.1), but also about how health can be optimised
- in resource-rich settings there may be the option of using post-exposure prophylaxis (PEP for occupational or n-PEP for non-occupational exposure)—this is a two or three anti-retroviral drug treatment for 4 weeks following an episode of moderate to severe risk. In the occupational setting this is usually a sharps injury; in the non-occupational setting it usually involves a sexual contact or intravenous drug use
- advocating for change—for example, policy responses to intravenous drug use (needle exchange programs), provision of clean syringes in prisons, and education, regulation and empowerment of sex industry workers.

SECONDARY PREVENTION

HIV infection must now be considered whenever there is uncertainty about the clinical presentation. It is another of those diseases with protean symptoms and signs. Yet early diagnosis is important in order to intervene while immune function is well preserved. Early intervention is also important because patients are most infective in the early stages of the disease, when their viral load is high. The GP's role may therefore include:

BOX 60.1 Transmission of HIV

Transmission possible:
- Sexual intercourse without condoms
- Needlestick injury
- Sharing injecting equipment
- Mother to infant (vertical transmission)
- Transfusion

Transmission risk very low:
- Kissing
- Oral sex
- Sexual intercourse with condoms

Transmission not possible:
- Social contact, embracing
- Sneezing/coughing
- Touch (skin surfaces intact), toilet seats
- Exposure to tears, sweat, faeces or urine
- Sharing of eating utensils

Sources: ASHM 2009[8] and *Australasian Contact Tracing Manual* 2006[9]

- case-finding of new HIV infections—this may be in the setting of the vague illness of primary infection, or of opportunistic screening of an asymptomatic person. In some cases of established HIV infection there will be presentations with symptoms of severe immune depletion
- working with risk-groups—after all, they will not agree to testing if testing leads to discrimination, and confidentiality needs to be assured
- opportunistic screening of asymptomatic people in novel settings such as in brothels, on the streets, at injection venues and at male saunas
- screening in the more traditional settings of antenatal and sexual health clinics.

TERTIARY PREVENTION

Once the patient is known to have HIV infection, the role of the GP may include:

- timely introduction of treatment (highly active anti-retroviral therapy) to reduce decline of immunity
- contact tracing (Box 60.2) and the optimisation of safe sexual practices
- optimising immune health (as above)
- vaccinations against influenza and pneumococcal disease
- use of prophylactic antibiotics when immune function is very low
- reducing risk of treatment-related morbidities—diabetes, osteoporosis, renal disease, cardiovascular disease, lipodystrophy, peripheral neuropathy and diarrhoea
- addressing issues of adherence—non-adherence leads to early resistance and treatment failure; repeated treatment failures eventually exhaust even the extensive pharmacology now available (Box 60.3)
- managing other comorbidities:
  - hepatitis B and hepatitis C
  - tuberculosis
  - cognitive decline
- managing treatment failure (often in conjunction with specialist centres)
- providing information about treatment and other trials that are available
- advocating for patients' rights, including access to adequate care
- assisting in the provision of palliative care.

COMPLEMENTARY THERAPIES

The use of complementary and alternative medicine (CAM) among HIV-positive people is widespread. On average, some 60% use CAM to treat HIV-related concerns.[10] However, this proportion differs markedly

BOX 60.2 Contact tracing

Recent court decisions have re-emphasised the responsibility that all healthcare professionals have for the health and welfare of their patients' sexual or drug-using partner(s), when the patient has been diagnosed with an infectious disease. This extends to partners or contacts who are not themselves patients or clients of the healthcare worker. However, these responsibilities are exercised with respect for the human rights, dignity and autonomy of the patient; and seek to balance sometimes competing interests.

In the setting of a new HIV diagnosis, often in a male who has sex with other men, the recent sexual contacts may have been anonymous and contact tracing is inappropriate or impossible. The GP can encourage and advise the patient to notify their own contacts (if known) and/or may liaise with contact tracers at the relevant sexual health clinic. These highly trained and experienced professionals can work with the patient (the index case) to trace contacts that may have been at risk.

Very rarely would more onerous sanctions be applied to a patient who continued to expose others to risk. These cases are deeply troubling for doctors, who would be well advised to seek the assistance of their medical defence organisation in deciding their actions.

Source: *Australasian Contact Tracing Manual* 2006[9]

BOX 60.3 Broad principles of HIV treatment

- Eradication of HIV from the infected patient is not achievable with currently available antiretroviral agents, and management must focus on attempting to control HIV replication with chronic suppressive therapy.
- The first antiretroviral agent (zidovudine) was introduced in 1987. Since then many more drugs have been developed, now grouped in six classes. The agents in each class are designed to interrupt the viral replication at a particular step of that process.
- The standard treatment now is to use at least three agents, from at least two of the classes. Such combination therapy (cART) has been made simpler by the development of tablets and capsules that include two or even three agents. Once-a-day dosing regimens have also helped.
- The broad aim of treatment is to achieve an undetectable viral load—in which setting it can be expected that the CD4 lymphocyte count will gradually rise. With such suppression, the ability of the virus to develop resistance is much reduced.
- The most common reason for viral replication to increase again is the development of resistance, and this is often due to difficulties in maintaining the strict adherence required. A key role for the treating doctor or general practitioner then is to enquire about difficulties with adherence and to help resolve those difficulties. This may include control of side effects, or reminder systems, or using some other drug administration aid.

Source: ASHM 2009[8]

from study to study.[11] This is despite the effectiveness of current antiretroviral therapies, and despite the potential for certain types of CAM to compromise those therapies.[10,12,13] Some studies suggest that those people who are more likely to use CAM are also more likely to refuse anti-retroviral therapies.[11]

Published research suggests that those who are more likely to use CAM are Caucasian, men who have sex with men, more educated and of higher income.[10] They are also more likely to have AIDS (than just HIV infection), to have symptoms related to HIV (and those symptoms to be more severe) and to have longer disease duration and a higher degree of disability.[10]

It is not surprising therefore that the reason for CAM use is more often to relieve symptoms and alleviate side effects of treatment, thereby improving quality of life.[10]

The types of CAM used are varied—Table 60.1 lists rates of use for various types of CAM.

Reviews of the evidence supporting CAM have pointed to methodological flaws and limited trial numbers and therefore lack of evidence for efficacy. However, stress management did appear to increase quality of life.[14]

There are other particular recommendations regarding optimising immune health, which include aspects of stress management, diet and supplements. However, data on the efficacy of herbal medicines has been assessed as insufficient to make firm recommendations.[15]

TABLE 60.1 Rates of CAM

Type of CAM	% using
Drug or diet therapies	71
Psycho-spiritual therapies	66
Meditation	54
Massage	39
Herbs	34
Faith healing	33
Megavitamins*	28
Chiropractor	25
Visualisation	24

*The most frequently reported of these have been vitamin C, vitamin E, garlic and multiple vitamin and mineral supplements.[12]

Source: Bormann et al 2009[11]

MIND–BODY

HIV progression to AIDS and speed of AIDS progression has been consistently linked with a range of psychosocial factors. For example, a study controlling for a range of relevant variables, including treatment, showed that increased stressful life events, coping by means of denial, low social support and high serum cortisol (a marker of chronic stress) significantly predicted disease progression.[16] The increased risk for progression from HIV to AIDS was two to three times at 5 years follow-up.[17] The high cortisol levels associated with chronic stress are also found to be associated with low white cell count and higher dehydroepiandrosterone sulfate (DHEAS) concentrations, both markers of poor prognosis.[18] Other studies have also confirmed the findings of social isolation and pessimism being poor prognostic factors[19] and 'active confrontational coping style' being associated with better prognosis, probably because of both improved compliance and immunological mechanisms described by psychoneuroimmunology.[20] Promising findings from a randomised controlled trial also suggest that reducing stress through cognitive-behavioural stress management, relaxation training and increasing social support is associated with reduced anxiety. This finding corresponded with changes in important physiological markers such as reduced catechol output, increased white cell counts,[21] reduced cortisol, DHEA-S and herpes simplex virus type 2 antibody titres (a common infection in gay men).[22] In another arm of the same study it was also found that the relaxation training on its own was associated with reductions in cortisol levels, depending on the level of compliance.[23] This research has now gone further to demonstrate that mind–body interventions like mindfulness meditation can buffer $CD4^+$ T-lymphocyte decline in HIV-1 infected adults.[24] Religious coping and religious behaviour (church attendance, prayer, spiritual discussion, reading religious literature) have also been found to be associated with reduced scores for depression and better immune parameters such as higher white cell count, independent of symptom status.[25,26]

It is therefore important to consider the role of psychosocial factors and mind–body therapies in any complete approach to HIV therapy.

SUMMARY

The role of general practice in caring for HIV-positive patients is well established. The increased complexity of care in resource-rich countries may argue for a more specialist-centric approach, but it is in general practice that the broadest approach can be taken, looking after patients where they are—in their communities. It is also the GP who can draw together a multiplicity of understandings about health and health optimisation.

RESOURCES

Australian Government, Health Insite, Complementary medicines, http://www.healthinsite.gov.au/topics/Complementary_Medicines

National Association of People Living with HIV/AIDS, http://www.napwa.org.au
National Institutes of Health, National Center for Complementary and Alternative Medicine (US), http://www.nccam.nih.gov

REFERENCES

1 UNAIDS. Report on the global AIDS epidemic. Executive summary; 2008. Online. Available at: unaids.org/en/KnowledgeCentre/HIVData/GlobalReport/2008
2 UNAIDS. Report on the global AIDS epidemic. Ch 4: Preventing new HIV infections: the key to reversing the epidemic; 2008. Online. Available at unaids.org/en/KnowledgeCentre/HIVData/GlobalReport/2008
3 Fahridin S, Miller G. Management of HIV/AIDS. Aust Family Physician 2009; 38(8):573.
4 UNAIDS. Report on the global AIDS epidemic. Ch 5: Treatment and care; 2008. Online. Available: http://unaids.org/en/KnowledgeCentre/HIVData/GlobalReport/2008
5 Grierson J, Thorpe R, Pitts M. HIV futures five. The Living with HIV Program at the Australian Research Centre in Sex, Health and Society. Melbourne: La Trobe University; 2006. Online. Available: http://www.latrobe.edu.au/hiv-futures/
6 Australasian Society for HIV Medicine. HIV, viral hepatitis and STIs: a guide for primary care. Darlinghurst, New South Wales: ASHM; 2008.
7 Hassed C. The essence of health. The seven pillars of wellbeing. Sydney: Ebury Press / Random House; 2008.
8 Australasian Society for HIV Medicine. HIV Management in Australasia. A guide for clinical care. Darlinghurst, New South Wales: ASHM; 2009:37–39.
9 Australasian Contact Tracing Manual. Australian Government Department of Health and Ageing; 2006. 3rd edn.
10 Littlewood RA, Vanable PA. Complementary and alternative medicine use among HIV-positive people: research synthesis and implications for HIV care. AIDS Care 2008; 20(8):1002–1018.
11 Bormann JE, Uphold CR, Maynard C. Predictors of complementary/alternative medicine use and intensity of use among men with HIV infection from two geographic areas in the United States. J Assoc Nurses AIDS Care 2009; 20(6):468–480.
12 Ernst E. The dark side of complementary and alternative medicine. Int J STD AIDS 2002; 13:797–800.
13 Hennessy M, Kelleher D, Spiers JP et al. St John's wort increases expression of P-glycoprotein: implications for drug interactions. Br J Clin Pharmacol 2002; 53:75–82.
14 Mills E, Wu P, Ernst E. Complementary therapies for the treatment of HIV: in search of the evidence. Int J STD AIDS 2005; 16(6):395–403.
15 Liu JP, Manheimer E, Yang M. Herbal medicines for treating HIV infection and AIDS. Cochrane Database Syst Rev 2005; 3:CD003937.
16 Leserman J, Petitto JM, Golden RN et al. Impact of stressful life events, depression, social support, coping, and cortisol on progression to AIDS. Am J Psychiatry 2000; 157(8):1221–1228.
17 Leserman J, Jackson ED, Petitto JM et al. Progression to AIDS: the effects of stress, depressive symptoms, and social support. Psychosom Med 1999; 61(3): 397–406.
18 Petitto JM, Leserman J, Perkins DO et al. High versus low basal cortisol secretion in asymptomatic, medication-free HIV-infected men: differential effects of severe life stress on parameters of immune status. Behav Med 2000; 25(4):143–151.
19 Byrnes DM, Antoni MH, Goodkin K et al. Stressful events, pessimism, natural killer cell cytotoxicity, and cytotoxic/suppressor T cells in HIV+ black women at risk for cervical cancer. Psychosom Med 1998; 60(6):714–722.
20 Mulder CL, Antoni MH, Duivenvoorden HJ et al. Active confrontational coping predicts decreased clinical progression over a one-year period in HIV-infected homosexual men. J Psychosom Res 1995; 39(8):957–965.
21 Antoni MH, Cruess DG, Cruess S et al. Cognitive-behavioral stress management intervention effects on anxiety, 24-hr urinary norepinephrine output, and T-cytotoxic/suppressor cells over time among symptomatic HIV-infected gay men. J Consult Clin Psychology 2000; 68(1):31–45.
22 Cruess S, Antoni M, Cruess D et al. Reductions in herpes simplex virus type 2 antibody titers after cognitive behavioral stress management and relationships with neuroendocrine function, relaxation skills, and social support in HIV-positive men. Psychosom Med 2000; 62(6):828–837.
23 Cruess DG, Antoni MH, Kumar M et al. Reductions in salivary cortisol are associated with mood improvement during relaxation training among HIV-seropositive men. J Behav Med 2000; 23(2):107–122.
24 Creswell JD, Myers HF, Cole SW et al. Mindfulness meditation training effects on CD4+ T-lymphocytes in HIV-1 infected adults: a small randomized controlled trial. Brain Behav Immun 2009; 23(2):184–188.
25 Woods TE, Antoni MH, Ironson GH et al. Religiosity is associated with affective and immune status in symptomatic HIV-infected gay men. J Psychosom Res 1999; 46(2):165–176.
26 Dalmida SG, Holstad MM, Diiorio C et al. Spiritual well-being, depressive symptoms, and immune status among women living with HIV/AIDS. Women Health 2009; 49(2/3):119–143.

chapter 61

Sexual health

O Rose, thou art sick!
The invisible worm
That flies in the night,
In the howling storm,
Has found out thy bed
Of crimson joy
And his dark secret love
Does thy life destroy.

William Blake

INTRODUCTION AND OVERVIEW

Sexual health medicine is generally thought of as primarily concerned with the management of sexually transmissible infections (STIs). While STIs are an important facet, sexual health also includes a wide range of other topics including fertility and contraception, sexuality and gender, sexual problems and various dermatological and gynaecological conditions. Sexual health physicians are also involved with the public health aspects of STIs, particularly the reporting, monitoring and control of infectious diseases.

The vast majority of sexual health should (and does) take place in primary care—a point agreed on by sexual health physicians, general practitioners (GPs) and their professional bodies alike. GPs are well placed to provide the majority of sexual health services, and are the favoured first point of contact for most of the community. Sexual health is an important part of providing holistic care.

Specialised sexual health services are best utilised for the management of more complex STIs and genital syndromes, and for servicing high-risk populations and those who experience barriers to accessing primary care. Sexual health services can provide GPs with clinical advice and formal medical education, as well as useful information about local epidemiology, and can assist in the management of disease clusters.

The integrative approach is well suited to primary care management of sexual health. Preventive counselling and holistic lifestyle approaches resonate particularly well with best practice in the assessment and management of sexual difficulties, STI prevention and the management of chronic viral infections.

COMMUNICATING WITH PATIENTS ABOUT SEX

We are exposed to a constant stream of sexualised messages. Advertisers use sex to sell almost every conceivable type of product. The print media is littered with stories about sex, whether about sex crimes, advice on how to improve one's sex life or appraisals of a celebrity's sexiness. Electronic media are packed with messages about how we should look, how our relationships should work and how interested we should be in sex. Radio advertising tells us how much happier we would be if sex lasted longer, penises were harder and libidos were higher. As well as showing us what our genitals should look like, the internet even tells us which particular facial expressions should be worn during intercourse. Novels, television shows, music lyrics and video clips, newspapers, graffiti, unsolicited emails, magazines, movies, ring-tones, train platforms, pop-up spam and bus stops: messages containing sex are everywhere.

Despite the constant stream of sexualised messages, talking meaningfully and frankly about an individual's personal sexual matters remains difficult for many patients and healthcare professionals. Open, confident and personal communication about sexual matters

BOX 61.1 Sexual health history*

- Presenting condition
- Targeted symptom search: dysuria, frequency, discharge, lumps, rashes, ulcers
- Past medical and surgical history
- Medication
- Allergy
- Recreational drug use: cigarettes, alcohol, illicit drugs (especially in relation to sex)
- History of injecting drug use, shared injecting equipment, tattooing, body piercing, medical procedures
- History of incarceration
- Menstrual history
- Obstetric history
- Pap smear history
- Contraceptive history
- Previous STIs, treatments and outcomes
- Previous sexual health testing
- Vaccination for hepatitis B (and hepatitis A, for men who have sex with men)
- Last sexual activity
- Number of partners in the previous 3 and 6 months
- Are partners male/female/both?
- Are partners symptomatic, from overseas, sex workers?
- Type of sex: oral, vaginal, anal
- Condom use
- Sexual assault

*Not all these questions are appropriate to ask asymptomatic patients in low-risk settings.

is not well entrenched in most societies, and may be more difficult with individuals from some cultural and religious backgrounds. Despite this, facilitating effective communication about sex is professionally rewarding to the provider, can be a therapeutic intervention in its own right and is appreciated by anxious patients.

The exhaustive list of questions to ask during a full sexual health history is shown in Box 61.1. Such a history is really only suitable for sexual health clinics and special circumstances such as symptomatic or otherwise high-risk patients. There is growing appreciation that a full sexual history for all patients in all scenarios is unnecessary and intrusive, and yields false responses from a significant proportion of patients—an observation that would probably not surprise most experienced GPs.

A recent Australian study illustrates this point well.[1] The authors examined the attitudes of women to chlamydia testing in general practice. Acceptance of age-based chlamydia testing was high, but women did not want to be asked to provide a sexual history as part of being asked to have a chlamydia test. Some reported that they would lie if asked how many partners they had had. The authors conclude that chlamydia

BOX 61.2 Sexual health history: clinical pearls

Introduce sexual health with normalising statements.

- 'I routinely offer everyone in your age group a sexual health check.'
- 'I routinely offer a sexual health check at the same time as doing a Pap smear.'
- 'Many diabetic men experience problems with erections, so I routinely ask about it. Has that been a problem for you?'

Start with less intrusive questions.

- 'Are you sexually active?'
- 'Do you have a regular partner?'
- 'Have you had any symptoms you've been concerned about?'
- 'Have you had any sex you've been concerned about?'

If in doubt, play the wild card.

- 'Is there anything else I should know?'
- 'Have you been concerned about something in particular?'

screening in general practice needs to be normalised and destigmatised.

That having been said, there is still a place for more detailed sexual histories. In some settings, such as sexual health clinics, patients expect to be asked about their sexual histories and are not surprised or unwilling to offer a response. Similarly, patients who present with genital symptoms or have previously had an STI might reasonably expect to be asked about their sexual history.

The aims of sexual history taking depend on the clinical scenario. For patients presenting for sexual health testing, the history should focus on the presence of symptoms and the risk of STI acquisition. The history will help to determine which tests to take, and tailor the extent of pre-test counselling. A history for sexual problems is often more wide-ranging and includes assessment of relationships, stressors, mood, sexuality, physical problems, medications and so on.

An asymptomatic patient attending a general practice setting, or one whose symptoms are not obviously related to sexual health, might be more surprised by a line of questioning directed at their sexual history. A patient who presents to the GP with a maculopapular rash, for example, might not suspect syphilis as the cause.

It falls to the person taking a sexual history to employ non-intrusive strategies that distinguish low-risk from high-risk settings, and then alter the direction of the history accordingly. This is a complex task, and it is reasonable to initially find the process daunting. The task, however, gets easier with experience and practice. In turn most patients will read the comfort level of the interviewer and respond in kind: the interviewer who can respectfully and confidently collect an intimate history provides an obvious cue for the patient to respond with similar openness and confidence (see Box 61.2, for example).

Doctor–patient power dynamics can lead to the patient feeling it necessary to please their healthcare provider. Sensitivity in history-taking, and listening to cues from the patient, will avoid the assumption of heterosexuality. Simple clarification of partners as male, female or both will facilitate disclosure.

Patients might expect that unsafe sex will be displeasing or disappointing to healthcare professionals and minimise the risks they report. Providing a non-threatening space for the patient to honestly disclose an accurate sexual history is better than an authoritarian, judgmental response. Similarly, focusing on finding tailored solutions is more effective than focusing on the problems.

Patients who are diagnosed with an STI should be counselled on the route of transmission, strategies for prevention and (where applicable) partner management.

SAFER SEX AND STI PREVENTION

The World Health Organization ranks unsafe sex as the world's fifth most prevalent cause of mortality.[2,3] This includes mortality from HIV infection, consequences of pregnancy (predominantly lack of access to safe abortion and contraception), cervical and anal cancers and bacterial STI. Disease acquired through sexual activity accounts for 0.5% of the burden of disease in Australia.[4] Lower rates in developed countries are attributable to education, access to contraception (particularly condoms) and safe abortion, cervical screening and better healthcare for those who acquire STIs.

Condoms have become an integral part of safer sex strategies. Used consistently, they provide excellent protection against HIV transmission, as well as other STIs spread through infected secretions, such as gonorrhoea, chlamydia and trichomoniasis. Protection against those infections transmitted via skin and mucous membrane contact, including herpes virus infection and human papillomavirus, appears to be less. Condoms are also reasonably effective as a contraceptive method. Compared with most other contraceptives, they are readily available, inexpensive and safe.

Between 16% and 20% of Australian couples reported using condoms with their regular partner in the previous 3 months, and condom use was higher with casual partners than with regular partners. Gay men reported higher rates of condom use than heterosexuals. Condom use has increased significantly among people having sex for the first time.[5]

Common problems with condoms include slippage, breakage, loss of erection and reduced spontaneity. The most common problem, however, is simply not using them. Problems of slippage and breakage are usually related to lubricant: either using an oil-based lubricant, or not using any lubricant. Storing condoms in hot places, using expired condoms or not applying condoms correctly can also contribute. Ill-fitting condoms, either too tight or too loose, might break or slip more readily. For those with latex allergy, polyurethane condoms are available. Not only are these condoms as effective as latex, they transmit heat and sensation better than latex, and are less likely to degrade with heat.

Abstinence, like condoms, is effective only if used consistently. While celibacy is a valid personal choice for some people, there is incontrovertible evidence that it is ineffective as a public health strategy to reduce STIs or unintended pregnancies.[6]

Primary care presents many opportunities for introducing safer sex messages. Consultations about contraception, Pap smears, sexual health checks, STIs, genital dermatology and so on can lead to a discussion about safer sex. In the safety of a confidential consultation, patients respond well to being presented with an opportunity to ask questions about safer sex, and this can segue into assessing their understanding of safe sex. A combination of verbal and printed information gives patients the opportunity to review information later.

Identifying problems with consistent condom (or other contraceptive) use represents a golden opportunity to engage in preventive activities. The topic can be introduced with non-threatening questions that give patients permission to report problems. For example: 'Have you had any problems with condoms?' can lead to identification of specific problems.

The urges that humans experience to engage in sex (including unsafe sex) are powerful, and not always amenable to rational thinking strategies. Sometimes, however, unsafe sex can be a symptom of other underlying problems—mental health problems such as depression or mood elevation, low self-esteem and issues of dependence, alcohol or recreational drug use or sexual abuse are worth considering when patterns of unsafe sexual behaviour are identified.

SEXUALLY TRANSMISSIBLE INFECTIONS

Sexually transmissible infections are caused by a diverse group of organisms. They range in size from viruses, usually measured in micrometres, to ectoparasites such as pubic lice, which are visible to the human eye. Their life cycles differ enormously, and may include stages of latency, asymptomatic carriage, systemic spread, immune evasion or neural invasion. Some are extraordinarily well adapted to coexist with humans and

BOX 61.3 Populations at risk of STI

- People aged 15–29 years
- People with a past history of STI
- Men who have sex with men
- Contacts of a person with an STI
- People who have had sex overseas
- People who don't use a barrier method consistently with casual contacts
- People with multiple sexual partners
- People who have recently changed sexual partners
- Neonates born to mothers with an STI

cause their host such little damage that they are spread widely from person to person. Some cause disease so severe that they damage their own chances of onward transmission by causing disabling symptoms, or even remove their host from the population altogether.

What these organisms share is the exploitation of normal human behaviour: sex. For STIs, sex represents a way to breach the gap from host to host without having to deal with the extremes of temperature, desiccation, ultraviolet radiation and sheer distances that usually separate one host from another. For some pathogens, this is further facilitated by transport directly to target sites of the new host within warm, buffered, nutrient-rich media such as semen and other genital secretions.

Current treatments for STIs are, wherever possible, single high-dose treatments in order to ensure adherence and minimise the induction of resistance in other flora.

Below is a brief description of the sexually transmissible organisms that are more commonly encountered in most affluent countries.

CHLAMYDIA

Chlamydia trachomatis is a common bacterial pathogen that infects the epithelial cells of the genital tract and can lead to urethritis or cervicitis and facilitates the polymicrobial infection of pelvic inflammatory disease. It can also cause proctitis and conjunctivitis. Despite such a wide range of disease in which chlamydia is implicated, most infections (about 85%) are asymptomatic. Many countries are experiencing an epidemic of chlamydia infection, and risk groups include younger age groups, Indigenous populations and men who have sex with men (MSM). Globally, chlamydia infections have a worldwide distribution and are prevalent in almost all human populations. The treatment of choice for chlamydia is the macrolide-like antibiotic azithromycin. Fortunately, resistance to azithromycin is rare.

GONORRHOEA

Neisseria gonorrhoeae is a bacterial pathogen that can cause urethritis or cervicitis and facilitate the polymicrobial infection of pelvic inflammatory disease. It can also cause proctitis, pharyngitis and conjunctivitis. Gonorrhoea is frequently asymptomatic in the cervix, throat and rectum, but is usually symptomatic in the male urethra. Gonorrhoea has been epidemic for many years, although rates are only about one-tenth of that of chlamydia. Risk groups include MSM and Indigenous populations. Internationally, gonorrhoea has remained endemic in most of the world's populations. Gonorrhoea is infamous for its ability to acquire resistance to antimicrobial agents, and (with the exception of some rural Indigenous populations) there is no oral first-line agent available in Australia. The treatment of choice for gonorrhoea is ceftriaxone.

SYPHILIS

Treponema pallidum infections have made a spectacular resurgence in urban communities in recent years. Globally, syphilis remains endemic in most of the world's population. Primary syphilis presents at the site(s) of inoculation with an ulcer. Secondary syphilis presents weeks to months later with truncal rash, rash on palms and soles, malaise and occasional involvement of the eye, meninges, liver and other organs. Tertiary syphilis occurs after many years (sometimes sooner, in immunosuppressed patients) and represents an immunological reaction against organisms in the brain, spinal cord, blood vessels and heart, skin, bones, joints and many other soft tissues. The recent urban epidemic of syphilis has centred on MSM. Syphilis is epidemic among many rural Indigenous communities, and the few cases of congenital syphilis in recent times have arisen from here. It is diagnosed by serological tests and by polymerase chain reaction (PCR) (where available). Syphilis is treated with injections of penicillin G, to which it remains sensitive.

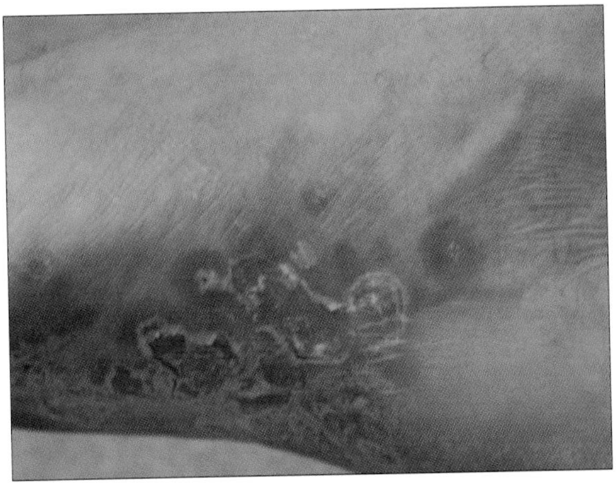

FIGURE 61.1 Secondary syphilis on the sole of the foot

TRICHOMONAS

Trichomonas vaginalis is a protozoan parasite that infects the vagina and male urethra. It causes vaginitis, or sometimes cervicitis, in women, but is usually asymptomatic in men. Trichomoniasis is rarely seen in urban Australia, but is highly prevalent in some rural Indigenous communities. Internationally, trichomonas can be found at high prevalence wherever a sexually active population has poor access to healthcare. Trichomoniasis can be seen as a marker of health service equity: it requires no eradication program, but disappears from communities upon the instigation of good-quality, accessible general health services. It is diagnosed by microscopy of vaginal swabs or PCR, and can be visualised in Pap smears (although only in about 60% of cases). Treatment is with metronidazole or tinidazole.

HERPES SIMPLEX VIRUSES

Genital herpes is caused by the two herpes simplex viruses: type 1 (HSV-1) and type 2 (HSV-2). The prevalence of HSV-2 in the general Australian population is 12%, but the prevalence in women is double that of men. The prevalence of HSV-1 is 76%, but it is not possible to determine how much of this infection represents genital infection, and how much is oro-labial. Globally, herpes simplex viruses are the most common cause of genital ulceration. In the past, HSV-1 was observed to be restricted to the face, where it caused herpes labialis or cold sores; HSV-2 was thought to be restricted to the genitals, where it caused genital herpes. This situation has changed in recent years, and HSV-1 has become a much more common cause of genital herpes in younger generations.

MOLLICUTES

Mycoplasma genitalium is a sexually transmissible organism of emerging significance. It has been associated with male urethritis, cervicitis and pelvic inflammatory disease. Testing, treatments and contact management are yet to be standardised, although the regimens used to treat non-specific urethritis will effectively treat most infections. Liaison with a sexual health physician is recommended advice.

Ureaplasma urealyticum is a sexually transmissible organism that is associated with male urethritis. It is usually managed successfully by the agents used to treat non-specific urethritis.

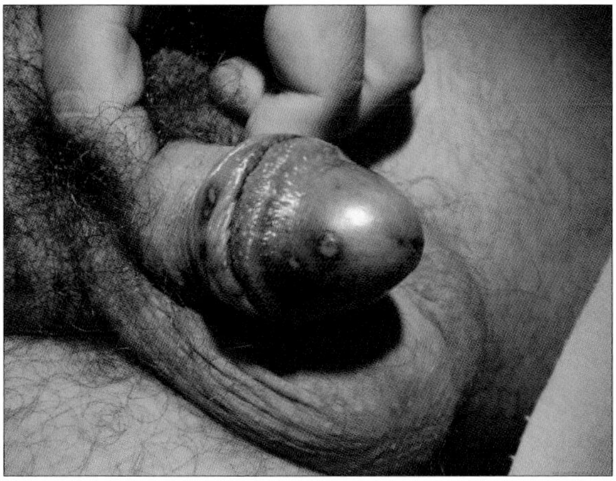

FIGURE 61.2 Primary herpes

HUMAN IMMUNODEFICIENCY VIRUS

HIV is covered in Chapter 60.

ASYMPTOMATIC SEXUAL HEALTH CHECKS

Chlamydia, gonorrhoea, syphilis, HIV and hepatitis B are frequently asymptomatic, but nevertheless can be transmitted to others. These particular infections also carry significant public health implications.

Screening strategies are justifiable when a condition is common, has serious consequence, can be readily tested for or can be managed effectively. STIs share these features to varying degrees.

STIs are not evenly distributed throughout the population. Several groups in the community experience higher than average rates of STI. Focusing screening strategies on those at highest risk makes testing more cost-effective and lessens the chance of yielding excessive false-positive tests in low-risk populations.

The sexual health history is the tool by which primary care providers can determine whether an asymptomatic individual is suitable for screening, and helps to determine which tests to perform.

Urogenital:

- women:
  - endocervical swab for chlamydia and gonorrhoea
  - first-catch urine for PCR for chlamydia and gonorrhoea
- men:
  - first-catch urine for PCR for chlamydia and gonorrhoea.

Serology:

- HIV antibody
- hepatitis B surface antigen and core antibody
- hepatitis A total antibody
- hepatitis C antibody (if at risk, e.g. intravenous drug user)
- syphilis serology—most laboratories use enzyme immunoassay (EIA) for screening.

'Window periods' exist for serological tests, and tests may need to be repeated once the window period has elapsed, to completely exclude infection after a particular exposure:

- HIV—12 weeks
- hepatitis B—24 weeks
- hepatitis A—4 weeks
- hepatitis C—24 weeks
- syphilis—12 weeks.

GENITAL SYNDROMES

Several sexually transmissible agents can affect one anatomical site and induce similar pathological processes, or syndromes. Rather than discuss organisms separately, it seems sensible to group them together by the nature of the syndromes they cause. This approach has the added advantage of better matching the way patients present.

URETHRITIS

Urethritis is characterised by urethral discharge, meatal erythema, dysuria or urethral irritation. Chlamydia and gonorrhoea represent the most important causes of urethritis; they carry significant public health implications, including consequences for partners such as pelvic inflammatory disease, chronic pelvic pain and tubal factor infertility. Complications such as epididymo-orchitis and dissemination of gonococci may arise from these infections.

Chlamydia urethritis typically presents as a mucoid discharge, urinary frequency or urethral irritation. It is important to again note, however, that most urethral infections in men will be asymptomatic. Chlamydia urethritis is treated with azithromycin 1 g orally statim. Other regimens include doxycycline 10 mg b.i.d for 7 days, or roxithromycin 150 mg b.i.d. for 10 days.

Gonococcal urethritis typical presents as a profuse purulent discharge. Less than 10% of men with urethral gonorrhoea are asymptomatic, but there is an over-representation of dissemination and epididymo-orchitis among these cases. Coexistent pharyngeal and rectal infections are common among MSM, but are usually asymptomatic. Chlamydia coinfection is very commonly seen among men with gonorrhoea. Gonococcal urethritis is best treated with 500 mg ceftriaxone IMI as a single dose dissolved in 2 mL of 1% lignocaine. Treatment for chlamydia coinfection is recommended.

Non-specific urethritis (NSU) represents the syndrome of urethritis caused by agents other than chlamydia or gonorrhoea. Its clinical features are very similar to chlamydial urethritis, and unless a specific cause can be found, the treatment for NSU is (fortuitously) the same as for chlamydia.

Patients who present with urethritis should be treated clinically, rather than withholding treatment until test results are available. For urban heterosexual men with a scant, clear discharge, empiric treatment with azithromycin will cover chlamydia and non-specific urethritis; gonorrhoea treatment can be withheld until tests are received. In settings where gonorrhoea is more likely—for example, purulent urethral discharge in a returned traveller—empiric treatment for both gonorrhoea and chlamydia should be given.

For around half the cases of urethritis, no easily identifiable cause is found. For most men with NSU, empiric treatment is sufficient to alleviate symptoms; those who do not respond may require further assessment to exclude important pathology.

Sexually transmissible agents implicated in NSU include herpes simplex viruses and *Trichomonas vaginalis*. The role of *Mycoplasma genitalium* as a sexually transmissible agent of public health significance is currently being investigated. While this organism is responsible for a substantial proportion of NSU, testing is not widely available and optimal treatment regimens are yet to be determined. Specialist liaison is recommended for treatment options. Viral agents such as adenovirus and herpes simplex viruses are sometimes distinguished by intense perimeatal erythema, inguinal adenopathy, but scant mucoid discharge. Adenovirus urethritis may be accompanied by conjunctivitis and coryzal symptoms.

Other organisms include *Ureaplasma urealyticum*, anaerobes and various organisms which, when inoculated into the male urethra, may cause localised mucosal irritation. However, these same organisms can be found in asymptomatic men. Specific diagnostic tests for these organisms are not routinely recommended, as their detection is difficult and would not alter the management of uncomplicated urethritis.

Non-infective causes of urethritis include trauma from, for example, vigorous sexual activity, urethral

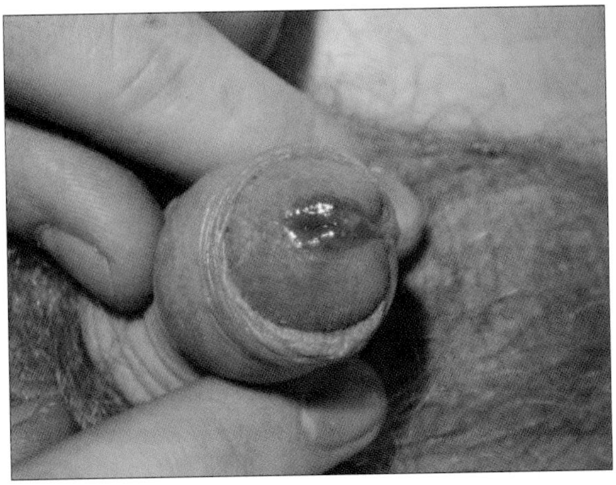

FIGURE 61.3 Viral urethritis

stricture (fortunately rare these days), foreign body and Reiter syndrome. The anxious patient who 'milks' his urethra in search of discharge will, if he is diligent enough, cause a traumatic urethritis.

VAGINAL DISCHARGE

The most common causes of vaginal discharge are candidiasis and bacterial vaginosis. Although these are not sexually transmissible, concomitant STI should be excluded by collecting an endocervical nucleic acid amplification test (NAAT) (e.g. PCR) for chlamydia and gonorrhoea. Bacterial vaginosis and candidiasis can be diagnosed on microscopy of the high vaginal swab.

Bacterial vaginosis is an overgrowth of the anaerobic species that usually make up a minority of the bacterial populations in the healthy vagina. It can arise spontaneously, or be induced by altering the physicochemical environment of the vagina (e.g. with frequent sexual intercourse, or douching). Bacterial vaginosis is not an invasive process and seldom leads to an inflammatory response. Asymptomatic women who present with bacterial vaginosis reported on a high vaginal swab do not require treatment (unless they are in a high-risk pregnancy or about to undergo cervical instrumentation). Bacterial vaginosis typically presents with a thin, malodorous, homogenous, greyish discharge. Symptoms are often worse after sex or during menstruation. Treatment with metronidazole or clindamycin is effective, but relapse is common. Recurrences might be reduced by stopping douching, or avoiding semen in the vagina. Probiotic therapy has not been successful in treating bacterial vaginosis or preventing recurrence.

Candida species are normal vaginal flora, and do not require treatment unless symptomatic. Candidiasis represents overgrowth of the endemic *Candida albicans* population, either through an increase in their trophic factors (e.g. oestrogen-containing oral contraceptives or HRT), reduction in their inhibitory factors (e.g. removal of bacterial flora through antibiotics or douching) or immunosuppression (e.g. diabetes or HIV). Candidiasis typically presents with a clumping, thick, white or yellowish discharge, often accompanied by vulval erythema. Topical and oral azoles are equally effective at eradicating *Candida albicans*. Topical preparations work faster, but oral fluconazole is less messy and more convenient. Longer courses of topical azoles are more effective than shorter courses. Women with disordered glucose metabolism will often notice candidiasis symptoms promptly after ingesting a sugar load; they certainly benefit from good glycaemic control. The role of sugar in the diets of women with normal glucose metabolism, however, is less clear. Similarly, yeast-free diets are an evidence-free zone. Yoghurt and other probiotics are lacking in evidence of efficacy, but topical yoghurt on a tampon may provide symptomatic relief through its emollient properties. Less messy is the insertion of a probiotic (*Lactobacillus*) capsule per vagina daily for one week. It can also be done several days premenstrually if candida exacerbations occur with periods.

Recurrent candidiasis (four or more microbiologically confirmed episodes per year) is more difficult to treat. Weekly oral fluconazole for up to 6 months may help to reduce the bowel carriage of *Candida* from which recurrences are thought to arise. Alternatively, doubling the duration of standard doses may help. Attention to predisposing factors is recommended. Care should be taken to ensure that the *Candida* species recovered by the laboratory are *albicans*, as non-*albicans* species such as *C. glabrata* and *C. krusei* are often resistant to azoles. Liaison with a sexual health physician, gynaecologist or microbiologist is recommended. The available evidence for use of probiotics for prevention of recurrent vulvovaginal candidiasis is limited. There are some small clinical trials supporting the effectiveness of oral or intravaginal administration of lactobacilli, particularly the strains *acidophilus*, *rhamnosus* GR-1 and *fermentum* RC-14. In vitro studies have shown that lactobacilli inhibit the growth of *C. albicans* and its adherence to the vaginal epithelium. A recent review of probiotics for recurrent vulvovaginal candidiasis concluded that there is limited beneficial evidence, but as adverse effects are rare, it may be recommended.[7]

Garlic has antifungal properties, and wrapping a single clove in unbleached gauze may be effective in treating candidiasis. Side effects, however, include local irritant and allergic reactions, as well as odour.[8] Tea tree oil is ineffective for vulvovaginal candidiasis, and can lead to severe contact reactions.[8] Gentian violet has antifungal properties, but there are no randomised controlled trials of its efficacy, and side effects include vulval irritation and staining of clothes.[8]

Douching is not a recommended treatment of candidiasis. Douching can in fact be quite harmful and has no place in women's hygiene practices. It may remove the normal vaginal bacteria, leading to an overgrowth of pathogenic species and a predisposition to STIs, such as *Neisseria gonorrhoeae* or *Chlamydia trachomatis*. The pressurised fluid can force pathogens upwards from the lower genital tract into the cervix, uterus, uterine tubes and abdominal cavity, potentially causing pelvic inflammatory disease. Douching is also linked to vulval dermatitis and chemical burns, ectopic pregnancy and bacterial vaginosis.[9]

Cervicitis is most frequently caused by chlamydia, but gonorrhoea and trichomoniasis are less common causes. Cervicitis may present with vaginal discharge, dyspareunia, abnormal menstrual bleeding, postcoital bleeding or intermenstrual bleeding. Chlamydia cervicitis is treated with azithromycin 1 g orally statim. Alternatively, doxycycline (100 mg b.i.d. for 7 days) can be used in women with macrolide allergy.

Involvement of the normally sterile upper genital tract can result from chlamydial or gonorrhoeal cervicitis facilitating polymicrobial infection to ascend from the vagina. The result is pelvic inflammatory disease (PID). Treatment of PID involves a longer course of antibiotic therapy: doxycycline 100 mg b.i.d. and metronidazole 400 mg b.i.d., both for 14 days. Ceftriaxone 500 mg IMI should be added where gonorrhoea is suspected or proven, particularly in areas where gonorrhoea is prevalent in women (e.g. remote Indigenous communities). The role of azithromycin as a replacement for doxycycline is evolving an evidence base, and most would agree that adding a stat dose of azithromycin at the beginning of the course is good practice. For more severe PID, refer to a gynaecologist.

Trichomoniasis causes a vaginal discharge that resembles bacterial vaginosis, but may show inflammatory features (e.g. vaginitis, vulvitis or cervicitis). Trichomoniasis is treated with tinidazole or metronidazole 2 g orally statim. As it is an STI, partner treatment is recommended.

Other causes of vaginal discharge include foreign body, physiological discharge, pregnancy, ectopic pregnancy and malignancy of the cervix or vagina. Some dermatological conditions (e.g. lichen planus) can also affect the vaginal mucosa and present with discharge.

PROCTITIS

Anal problems are common, but the history and examination is often non-specific. STIs are often forgotten causes of anorectal symptoms, and it is not unusual for sexual health clinics to 'inherit' patients who have delayed and arrived by circuitous routes to the correct diagnosis.

Proctitis can present with anal discharge, or irritation of the perianal skin from constant exposure to discharge. Painful spasm (tenesmus) and a feeling of incomplete emptying with defecation may be reported. Bowel habit may be altered and vary, from diarrhoea, to constipation, to alternating diarrhoea and constipation. Systemic symptoms are sometimes seen in more severe cases, and the patient may be quite unwell.

Examination may show inguinal adenopathy, discharge at the anal verge. Proctoscopy must be performed very gently and carefully, and sometimes requires the instillation of lignocaine jelly to relieve the pain and spasm enough to allow examination. Discharge, oedema, ulceration, fissures or haemorrhoids should be noted. NAAT (e.g. PCR) swabs for chlamydia and herpes should be collected, as should cultures for gonorrhoea. Syphilis can cause proctitis, and serology should be collected, as might a syphilis PCR where it is available.

Proctitis is caused by chlamydia, gonorrhoea, herpes and, less frequently, syphilis. As patients can be quite ill, and deteriorate quickly, it is recommended that treatment be commenced immediately, rather than waiting for tests to come back. Treatment is recommended to cover chlamydia, gonorrhoea and herpes. Empiric treatment with doxycycline 100 mg b.i.d. for 10 days, ceftriaxone 500 mg IMI and valaciclovir 500 mg b.i.d. for 5 days is recommended.

Asymptomatic carriage of chlamydia and gonorrhoea is common among MSM who have anal sex, but should be considered in anyone who has anal sexual practices. It should be noted that penile–anal intercourse is not the only way to transmit STIs to the anus: digital play has been implicated with infection too.

Lymphogranuloma venereum (LGV), caused by invasive strains of chlamydia, has been reported in MSM from many cities. Presentation is usually with severe proctitis or proctocolitis. Chlamydia PCR tests will be reactive for LGV, and further testing should be discussed with a local sexual health physician or microbiologist. LGV is usually treated with prolonged courses of doxycycline, but azithromycin will probably have a role here in the future.

GENITAL LUMPS

Warts are overwhelmingly the most common cause of genital lump. The causative agent, human papillomavirus (HPV) is acquired by up to 80% of sexually active adults, yet only about 5% of those exposed will develop warts. Most warts are caused by the non-oncogenic strains of HPV, primarily HPV6 and HPV11, although there are approximately thirty other genotypes that show a tropism for genital skin.

Treatments for genital warts are not very well studied; this is perhaps surprising for such a common condition. There are few well-designed, randomised trials, and those that exist vary greatly in their duration of follow-up and methodology. Unfortunately, this makes intelligent comment comparing various treatments impossible. The situation is complicated further by the high rate of response to placebo, a feature that has led to erroneous conclusions being drawn from substandard trials. The H_2 blocker, cimetidine, is probably the best example of this: non-comparative studies using cimetidine reported encouragingly high rates of wart resolution. In placebo-controlled trials, however, cimetidine performed no better than placebo. The use of cimetidine for wart treatment is an ideal study in medical quackery.

Medical treatments for warts include imiquimod and podophyllotoxin, both of which can be applied by the patient at home. Practitioner-applied medical therapy includes podophyllin resin and trichloroacetic acid, but training is required for the use of these. Commercially available over-the-counter preparations for warts are not suitable for genital warts as the concentrations of salicylic acid, podophyllin derivatives and other ingredients are too high. Care should be taken to avoid using imiquimod or podophyllin/toxin in pregnant women.

Ablative therapies include liquid nitrogen or nitrous oxide cryotherapy. These are easy to use, widely available and can be used as adjunctive therapy with medical treatments when they fail to resolve warts.

More invasive ablative therapy such as electrocautery, scissor excision or laser ablation requires local, or even general, anaesthaesia and is probably no more effective than other modalities. It should, ideally, be reserved for warts that have failed to respond to more sensible treatments.

Zinc supplementation has been examined in one double-blind randomised controlled trial[10] and showed a significantly greater response to zinc than to placebo. The dose of zinc studies was reasonable high, and side effects included gastrointestinal symptoms such as nausea, vomiting and abdominal pain.

Lifestyle modification may be useful in managing warts, particularly those that are difficult to treat. Smoking and stress are likely contributors to ongoing genital warts. Hypnosis was found to be an effective treatment for warts in one trial.[11] In this study, hypnosis resulted in greater wart regression than placebo or salicylic acid.

MOLLUSCUM CONTAGIOSUM

Normal anatomical features are commonly misdiagnosed as warts. Clinicians should be aware of the appearance of features such as pearly penile papules, vestibular papillae, Fordyce spots and Tyson glands.

Other causes of genital bumps include skin tags (acrochordon), seborrhoeic keratoses and tumours.

GENITAL ULCERS

Ulcers on genital skin and mucosal membranes are a common presentation in primary care. The causes of genital herpes are listed in Box 61.4. Almost all genital ulcers in developed communities are caused by the herpes simplex viruses. Other causes of genital ulcers are important because of their public health implications, and the seriousness of their complications if left untreated.

Herpes is the most common cause of genital ulceration worldwide.

Herpes infection can present either as an initial infection or as a recurrence. An initial infection may be more severe in its manifestation, with bilateral ulceration, larger and deeper lesions, adenopathy and extragenital manifestations such as fever, headache, radiculopathy and meningism. Primary infection, in which the newly infected person has not been previously infected by either HSV-1 or HSV-2, is associated with the most severe presentations. Previous exposure to HSV-1 does not protect people from acquiring HSV-2 (or vice versa), but does tend to reduce the severity of the clinical manifestations if the other virus is acquired later.

BOX 61.4 Common causes of genital ulcer disease

Infectious:
- herpes simplex viruses (HSV-1, HSV-2)
- syphilis
- donovanosis
- lymphogranuloma venereum

Non-infectious:
- trauma
- Behçet's disease
- aphthous ulceration
- tumours
- Crohn's disease
- lichen planus

Recurrences are the hallmark of herpes simplex viruses. HSV rapidly establishes latency in the lumbo-sacral dorsal root ganglia during initial infection. After latency is established, virions are continuously transported to the skin or mucosal surface via sensory neurons. Sub-epithelial lymphocytes destroy viruses, leaving the neuron, and limit viral replication. When neuronal production of virus increases or the function of these lymphocytes is disturbed, recurrences occur. In this way, recurrences can be seen as having virological and/or immunological triggers.

Triggers for recurrence are poorly understood, and may vary widely among individuals. Commonly described triggers include sunburn or windburn, concomitant infections such as URTIs, sleep deprivation, changes in nutrition (e.g. skipping meals) and physical or psychological stress. Recurrences are more frequent early in the course of infection, and tend to become less frequent and less severe as time goes on. This is particularly true of HSV-1 genital infections, where it is uncommon to see clinical recurrences after the first 6–12 months. Recurrences are seen with greater frequency and severity in the immunosuppressed.

Virtually all patients who have herpes infections will experience virological recurrence, whereby there is viral replication and shedding of virus from the skin. The 'classic' clinical appearance of a recurrence is of grouped vesicles on an erythematous base that burst to form painful ulcers. These recurrences are very easy to recognise clinically, but only about one-fifth of people with genital herpes will experience these classic recurrences. Another fifth will periodically shed virus, but remain completely asymptomatic. The other 60% will have 'atypical' recurrences and have a wide variety of clinical manifestations. Atypical lesions include fissures, painless ulcers, erythema or altered sensation without any visible changes. Unsurprisingly, most people with herpes simplex infections on their genitals remain unaware of the infection.

Transmission of herpes is predominantly through asymptomatic or subclinical shedding of virus—that is, production of virus from skin or mucosa that has few, if any, signs or symptoms.

Transmission can be reduced by consistent condom use, avoiding sexual contact when symptoms are present, and suppressive use of valaciclovir (the efficacy of other antivirals in interrupting transmission remains to be determined).

Although initial infections can be severe, the psychosocial consequences are by far the most significant source of morbidity from herpes, and the GP will need to provide advice on coping with the emotional and social impact of the virus.

Treatment approaches

Drug therapy

Antiviral therapy—three agents are licensed for the suppressive and episodic treatment of genital herpes: aciclovir and the pro-drugs valaciclovir and famciclovir. All three drugs are highly effective and well tolerated as described in many well-designed, randomised trials.

Lysine has demonstrated some efficacy in reducing the frequency of recurrences in randomised trials if used in high enough doses. Evidence for its effect in reducing the severity of recurrences is weaker.

Herbal therapy

Echinacea has demonstrated in vitro antiherpetic activity, but firm evidence supporting its use is lacking.

Dietary advice

Lysine is readily absorbed from dietary sources (red meat, soy products) and lysine-rich diets may reduce the frequency of recurrences. Decreasing dietary arginine may play a role in reducing recurrences further.

Topical therapy

Aciclovir ointment has demonstrated small but statistically significant improvements in healing in well-designed randomised trials.

Bee products or honey have shown early promising results in randomised clinical trials.

Zinc has shown in vitro antiherpetic activity, but can cause stinging if applied to inflamed tissues.

Tea tree oil is antiseptic if applied to herpes sores, but also causes inflammation.

Lifestyle advice

Stress reduction and relaxation techniques are useful strategies, particularly when stress is identified as a trigger. For some, recurrences can be used as tools to help identify stressors that might have otherwise remained unapparent.

Accessing support groups and online communities can assist with coming to terms with a new diagnosis, getting on with life and significant life events such as starting a relationship.

People with herpes respond positively to information about herpes. Verbal, printed and online resources can be useful.

Pregnant women who are infected with HSV-1 or HSV-2 have a higher risk of miscarriage, premature labour, retarded fetal growth or transmission of the herpes infection to the infant during vaginal delivery. Herpes infection in the newborn can be life-threatening or cause disability. Delivery by caesarean section should be discussed with the woman's obstetrician.

SYPHILIS

Syphilis has made something of a comeback in recent years, with an epidemic among MSM. Other risk factors include HIV seropositivity, and attendance at sex clubs, sex parties and other venues where high rates of partner change can be facilitated. Finding partners over the internet has also been linked with syphilis acquisition.

Early diagnosis, prompt treatment, contact tracing and opportunistic screening for those at risk are the main public health strategies for controlling the current syphilis epidemic.

Unfortunately, clinicians' unfamiliarity with syphilis has led to delays in treatment and the risk of ongoing transmission in many cases. While a detailed description of the clinical spectrum of syphilis is beyond the scope of this book, the key clinical features of early syphilis are listed in Box 61.5.

Treatment of syphilis is best done in conjunction with a sexual health physician, or other specialist with training in syphilis management.

Contact management of syphilis is a crucial part of management. Contacts should be treated on presentation, rather than awaiting tests that may still be negative in the incubation period.

SPECIAL POPULATIONS

YOUTH

Young people have a number of factors that predispose them to acquiring STIs. The comparatively high rate of partner change experienced by young people still

BOX 61.5 Key clinical features of syphilis

Primary syphilis:
- Incubation period is 9–90 days.
- Painless ulcer is common, although ulcers are occasionally painful.
- Ulcer may be missed if hidden, e.g. anal, pharyngeal.
- Ulcer is often indurated: like a button under the skin.
- If ignored, the lesion slowly disappears.
- Primary lesions are teeming with organisms and are highly infectious.

Secondary syphilis:
- Appears a few weeks after the primary lesion has gone.
- Sometimes primary lesion is still present.
- Wide spectrum of clinical manifestations.
- Non-itchy maculopapular rash involving the trunk, palms and soles.
- Systemic symptoms often present: fatigue, malaise.
- Adenopathy, hepatomegaly and splenomegaly are common.
- Sometimes neurological and eye involvement: stroke-like signs, uveitis.
- Patients with secondary syphilis are highly infectious.

Tertiary syphilis:
- Rarely seen nowadays.
- Inflammatory lesions of bone, brain, heart, skin, eye, viscera.
- Very wide spectrum of clinical manifestations.
- Patient is no longer infectious.

learning about relationships, sex and themselves provides an epidemiological opportunity for disease acquisition. Biological factors such as cervical ectropion may predispose younger women, and those using oestrogen-containing contraceptives may be at increased risk of chlamydia acquisition. Young people have a greater chance of encountering new pathogens to which they have not mounted immunological defences, further predisposing them to new infections.

Opportunistic screening is recommended for people aged between 15 and 29 years.

ABORIGINALS AND TORRES STRAIT ISLANDERS

Some Aboriginals and Torres Strait Islanders (ATSI), particularly in rural and remote areas, have higher rates of bacterial infections such as gonorrhoea, chlamydia and syphilis. There are also higher rates of herpes and hepatitis B infections. HIV infection rates are comparable to those of the general population. ATSI in the remote northern parts of Australia are among the few populations in which donovanosis is still seen. *Trichomonas vaginalis* remains common in rural and remote ATSI, despite being rarely seen in the general population. Vaccination for hepatitis B is recommended.

MEN WHO HAVE SEX WITH MEN

Some MSM, particularly in large urban centres, have higher rates of bacterial infections such as gonorrhoea, chlamydia and syphilis. There are also higher rates of herpes, hepatitis A, hepatitis B and HIV infection. STIs are associated with higher rates of HIV transmission. Vaccination for hepatitis A and B is recommended.

In addition to the testing listed for asymptomatic men above, rectal swabs for chlamydia (NAAT) and gonorrhoea (NAAT or culture) and throat swabs for gonorrhoea (NAAT or culture) are strongly encouraged as a routine part of screening MSM.

WOMEN WHO HAVE SEX WITH WOMEN

STIs can be transmitted between women through the sharing of cervical, vaginal and anal secretions. Reported rates of most STIs among women who have sex with women (WSW) are probably no less than rates among heterosexual women. Rates of HIV, hepatitis B, hepatitis C and syphilis, however, are reported at very low rates. Bacterial vaginosis is more commonly found among WSW and, unlike heterosexual contact, it appears that bacterial vaginosis can be sexually transmitted. Cervical abnormalities are reported as frequently as in women in general, but uptake of screening among younger women is suboptimal. Healthcare practitioners play an important role in encouraging WSW to participate in cervical screening. Lesbians need Pap smears even if they have never had sex with a man.[12]

Safer sex between women:[13]
- Acknowledge risk of STI transmission via body fluids and skin-to-skin contact
- Hepatitis B vaccination
- Regular STI testing when changing partners
- Latex dams are not popular, but other helpful strategies include:
  - ensuring adequate lubrication
  - keeping fingernails short
  - using condoms on sex toys and changing between partners, or washing toys between partners
  - using latex gloves for penetrative sex and avoiding oral sex during menstruation if BBV status is unknown or if there is risk of BBV transmission.

COMMERCIAL SEX WORKERS

In the early days of the HIV epidemic, commercial sex workers (CSW) in Australia were pivotal in preventing the spread of HIV into the general community. Sex worker organisations vigorously promoted safer sex practices, and CSW incorporated condoms for all penetrative services with an outstanding level of uniformity and consistency. Consequently, STIs are infrequently seen in CSW, and when they do occur they have often been acquired from private, rather than professional, life.

RETURNED TRAVELLERS

Those who have sex in countries with high rates of endemicity are at high risk of acquiring STIs. The risk is particularly high after unprotected sex with sex workers. Clinicians should be aware of the higher risk of unusual conditions, including HIV, syphilis, LGV and chancroid.

MANAGING PARTNERS

Contact tracing is a necessary part of managing STIs of public health significance. Responsibility for contact tracing is considered an intrinsic part of testing for, diagnosing and managing patients with an STI. As many people with STI are asymptomatic, infected partners are usually unaware of the infection. Ensuring they are diagnosed and treated is important from ethical, public health and personal health aspects. It also prevents reinfection of the index case.

Partners can be notified in two main ways: provider referral, in which the clinician contacts the partner; and patient referral, in which the patient notifies the partner. Provider referral is the preferred strategy for uncommon or serious conditions such as syphilis or HIV, and many state or local authorities will have contact tracers to assist in these cases. Sexual health clinics can assist in these cases too, and can further assist in the counselling, treatment and follow-up of these patients. Partners can be contacted by telephone, letter or, in some instances, personal visit.

Patient referral is much less labour-intensive, and is more appropriate for common conditions, such as chlamydia.

Email and text messages are another way for partners to be contacted. The website of the STI in Gay Men Action Group (see Resources list) was created to assist gay men to notify their contacts via a text message or an ePostcard.

A common pitfall in the management of contacts is not treating them on presentation. Where there is an established risk of contact with a treatable STI, treatment should be offered immediately, rather than waiting for test results. Testing should still occur, but should not delay treatment. Box 61.6 summarises the management of partners.

The *Australasian Contact Tracing Manual*[14] contains more information about contact tracing and such useful additions as patient handouts, case studies, privacy legislation considerations and sample contact tracing letters.

BOX 61.6 Management of contacts of patients with STI

- *Chlamydia*—priority of contact tracing is high. Contacts from the previous 6 months (or as determined by symptoms or testing history) should be offered presumptive therapy with azithromycin 1 g orally statim.
- *Gonorrhoea*—priority of contact tracing is high. Contacts from the previous 6 months (or as determined by symptoms or testing history) should be offered presumptive therapy with ceftriaxone 500 mg IMI statim, dissolved in 2 mL of 1% lignocaine. Ciprofloxacin 500 mg orally statim may be used only if the isolate is known to be sensitive.
- *Syphilis*—priority of contact tracing is high. Consultation with a sexual health physician is recommended in all cases.
- *Trichomoniasis*—priority of contact tracing is medium (easily contactable partners only). Contacts from the previous 3 months (or as determined by symptoms or testing history) should be offered presumptive therapy with metronidazole or tinidazole 2 g orally statim.
- *HIV*—priority of contact tracing is high, and referral to a sexual health clinic or other HIV specialist is recommended. Contacts who may have been exposed in the previous 3 days may be eligible for post-exposure prophylaxis.
- *Genital herpes*—priority of contact tracing is low. Contacts should present if they become symptomatic, or require information or counselling. Post-exposure prophylaxis or other presumptive therapy is not recommended.
- *Genital warts*—contact tracing is not recommended, but partners may be seen for information.
- *Candidiasis*—contact tracing is generally not recommended, but regular partners might be considered for treatment if they are symptomatic, or in recurrent candidiasis.
- *Bacterial vaginosis*—is not sexually transmissible (except perhaps in women who have sex with women).

Adapted from the *Australasian Contact Tracing Manual*[14]

GENITAL DERMATOLOGY

A complete discussion of genital dermatology is beyond the scope of this chapter. Genital skin differs from other skin. It is thin skin that is usually under conditions approaching those of occlusion. The microbiology includes colonisation with yeasts, coliform and various organisms that thrive in dark, moist environments. Genital skin is often sweaty and moist, and might be exposed to urine, genital secretions or faecal matter. Perhaps most importantly, the range of irritants that this delicate skin is exposed to is mind-boggling.

Soaps, detergents and over-washing are the most frequent irritants. Increasing one's washing habits is, unfortunately, a common reaction to irritation or rash on genital skin. Over-the-counter preparations, such as antifungals, tea tree oil, paw-paw ointment and antiseptics can all be potent irritants, especially when applied to non-intact skin. Often, by the time patients present, the clinical picture has become complicated.

Skin conditions affecting the genitals may appear different from extragenital skin. Psoriasis, for instance, is often less well demarcated and has less scale. A careful history and extragenital skin examination will often give the clinician the diagnosis before the genitals are even visualised.

Treatment of dermatological conditions is described in Chapter 42, Skin. Similar treatment strategies can be employed in the genitals, but care should be taken to account for the occluded conditions and thinness of genital skin. Tar solutions and salicylic acid concentrations should not exceed 3%, and care should be taken with the use of calcipotriol. Ointments are better tolerated than creams on genital surfaces, and provoke less irritation.

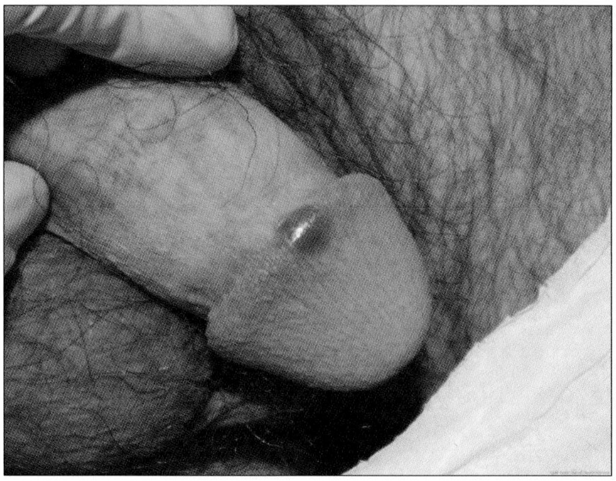

FIGURE 61.4 Psoriasis of the glans penis

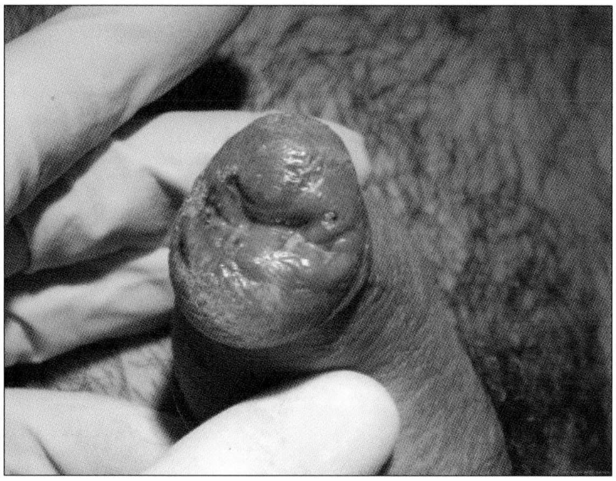

FIGURE 61.5 Severe balanoposthitis (see Ch 46)

Both vulvitis and balanitis are more commonly associated with irritant exposure than most clinicians appreciate. Other causes, such as candida infection and bacterial superinfection, may complicate the picture, but care should be taken to address any underlying irritant dermatitis. Combination preparations that include corticosteroid, antifungal and antibacterial in an ointment base are useful.

SEXUAL DIFFICULTIES

It is not possible to give a detailed account of sexual difficulties here, but some of the common themes and problems are introduced. Erectile dysfunction is covered separately in Chapter 49, reflecting the recent increase in research and availability of newer treatments in recent times.

Delayed ejaculation

In delayed ejaculation, there is a very prolonged time from arousal to ejaculation despite appropriate stimuli. This may be caused by medication (SSRIs are the most common), pathological causes (diabetes, prostatectomy, neurological disorders) and psychological causes (depression and anxiety). Exploring patient expectations is worthwhile, as some (usually males) have unrealistic expectations of their ability to perform sexually. Organic causes are usually associated with delayed ejaculation all the time, whereas psychogenic causes are associated with a fluctuating course.

Anorgasmia

Anorgasmia is failure to reach orgasm during sexual activity. Anorgasmia is more common in women, and can be an extension of the same processes that cause delayed ejaculation. Individuals vary greatly in the time it takes to reach orgasm and, for many women, orgasm is not routinely experienced during 'missionary position' penetrative sex. It is worth exploring the perceptions of 'failure' in anorgasmia and perhaps redefining success for both partners. For many, orgasm is not the sole goal of every act of intercourse. Helping partners appreciate each other's turn-ons and turn-offs through counselling and sensate focus can help.

Dyspareunia

Pain during sex is known as dyspareunia. It is much more common in women, and seldom seen in men. It can arise from multiple causes including vaginismus (see below), pelvic pathology, postmenopausal vaginal dryness, dermatological problems and penetration when the woman is not aroused. See also Ch 52.

Vaginismus

Vaginismus is caused by involuntary spasm of the muscles that encircle the vagina, leading to pain on penetration or attempted penetration. While most cases are attributed to psychological causes, painful pathology of the vulva, vagina or pelvis may contribute. Sometimes vaginismus persists after the original physical cause has resolved. Sensate focus and counselling can help once physical causes have been excluded or managed.

Low libido

Low libido was recently noted to be the most commonly reported sexual difficulty, but it remains difficult to define. Exploring patients' expectations can be useful. Depression, anxiety, hypothyroidism, hypogonadism and almost any chronic medical condition can be associated with loss of libido. Relationship problems, sexuality issues and a wide variety of inter- and intra-personal issues can be involved. External stressors, such as work pressures, family pressures, financial problems and many others, can be implicated. Often the problem is not low libido per se, but a desire mismatch between partners. Education about desire discrepancy can help, as can counselling.

Premature ejaculation

In premature ejaculation there is a very short time from arousal to ejaculation. Exploring what the client means by 'too early' and identifying unrealistic expectations can be useful. Premature ejaculation is most frequently reported by young men who are becoming sexually active, or entering their first relationship. Many men find that the problem decreases as they settle into a new relationship, and become more sexually experienced and more confident. For some men, the biological threshold for ejaculation is set very low, and does not settle with time. Strategies for treating premature ejaculation that is problematic include: using a condom; numbing creams (e.g. EMLA); SSRIs in low doses, e.g. sertraline 25 mg daily, titrated up if necessary. Exercises aimed at 'desensitising' the premature ejaculator, such as Seman's exercises and stop-start and squeeze techniques, are options for those who don't want SSRI therapy, but the acceptability and efficacy of these techniques in clinical practice is doubtful.

It does not take much time in general practice to gain an awareness of how common sexual difficulties are. The prevalence of sexual difficulties was illustrated in the landmark Study of Health and Relationships[5] and confirms that sexual difficulties are common, perhaps surprisingly so. Table 61.1 describes the frequency of various sexual difficulties.

TABLE 61.1 Sexual difficulties for at least one month in the previous year

Sexual difficulties	Men (%)	Women (%)
Lacked interest in having sex	25	55
Came to orgasm too quickly	24	12
Worried during sex that body looked unattractive	14	36
Unable to orgasm	6	29
Felt anxious about ability to perform	16	17
Did not find sex pleasurable	6	27
Physical pain during intercourse	2	20
Vaginal dryness	–	24
Trouble keeping erection	10	–
Used treatment to aid erections	2	–

Adapted from Richters & Rissel 2005,[5] p 85

Sexual function is a complex process that involves coordination of emotional, cognitive and physical factors. Not surprisingly, many facets of client's lives, including relationship issues, physical health, mental health and the social milieu in which this all occurs, can affect sexual function.

Client expectations are a necessary part of assessing sexual difficulties. Given that 55% of women report a lack of interest in having sex, one might conclude that it is normal. Alternatively, one might question whether the messages that women are given about how much sex they should want are realistic. Given the high levels of sexual difficulties reported by women generally, the final conclusion is that the type of sex that women in contemporary society are getting is simply not the sort of sex they want. Similar arguments might apply to the 24% of men who reported coming to orgasm too quickly. How quickly is 'too quickly'? What are clients expecting of themselves?

Although pathological processes are well described as causes of sexual difficulty, it is always pertinent to remember that the vast majority of sexual dysfunction includes psychosocial factors. To further complicate matters, sexual problems that start from a purely physical cause are prone to be complicated by secondary psychological reactions, such as performance anxiety or loss of libido.

Relationship issues can be complex in the setting of sexual difficulty. Relationship dysfunction can lead directly to sexual difficulty, but loss of the ameliorating and bonding effects of sex can have a negative impact on relationships in return.

RESOURCES

Al-Gurairi FT, Al-Waiz M, Sharquie KE. Oral zinc sulphate in the treatment of recalcitrant viral warts: randomized placebo-controlled clinical trial. Br J Dermatol 2002; 146:423–431.

Australian Herpes Management Forum, http://www.ahmf.com.au

Bradford D, Russell D. Talking with clients about sex: a health professional's guide. Melbourne: IP Communications; 2006.

Cunningham AL, Taylor J. Prevalence of infection with herpes simplex virus types 1 and 2 in Australia: a nationwide population-based survey. Sex Trans Infect 2006; 82:65–68.

dialog, a comprehensive Australian website addressing healthcare for lesbian, bisexual and same-sex attracted women, with many links to other sites, research and specific resources, http://www.dialog.unimelb.edu.au

girl2girl, a website for patient-orientated information regarding sexual activity, http://www.girl2girl.info

Perfect MM, Bourne N, Ebel C et al. Use of complementary and alternative medicine for the treatment of genital herpes. Herpes 2005; 12:2.

Russell D, Bradford D, Fairley C. Sexual health medicine. Melbourne: IP Communications; 2005.

Scarlet Alliance: Australian Sex Workers' Association, http://www.scarletalliance.org.au

Spanos NP, Williams V, Gwynn MI. Effects of hypnotic, placebo, and salicylic acid treatments on wart progression. Psychosom Med 1990; 52:109–114.

STI in Gay Men Action Group, http://www.whytest.org

STIGMA Guidelines, http://www.ashm.org.au/uploads/STIGMA_STI_Testing_Guidelines_for_MSM.pdf

Temple-Smith M, Gifford S. Sexual health: an Australian perspective. Melbourne: IP Communications; 2005.

Tomblin FA, Lucas KH. Lysine for the management of herpes labialis. Am J Health-Syst Pharm 2001; 58(4): 298–304.

Venereology Society of Victoria and Australasian Chapter of Sexual Health Medicine, Royal Australasian College of Physicians. National management guidelines for sexually transmissible infections. Melbourne: Venereology Society of Victoria; 2008.

REFERENCES

1 Pavlin NL, Parker R, Fairley CK et al. Take the sex out of STI screening! Views of young women on implementing chlamydia screening in general practice. BMC Infectious Disease 2008; 8:62.

2 World Health Organization. Gender and reproductive health. Sexuality. Online. Available: www.who.int/reproductive-health/gender/sexual_health.html#2.

3 World Health Organization. Reducing risks, promoting healthy life; 2002.

4 Australian Institute of Health and Welfare. Australia's Health 2006. AIHW Cat. no. AUS 73. Canberra: AIHW; 2006:146.

5 Richters J, Rissel C. Doing it down under: the sexual lives of Australians. Crows Nest, New South Wales: Allen & Unwin; 2005.

6 Mindel A, Sawleshwarkar S. Condoms for sexually transmissible infection prevention: politics versus science. Sexual Health 2007; 5(1):1–8.

7 Falagas ME, Gregoria IB, Athanasiou S. Probiotics for prevention of recurrent vulvovaginal candidiasis: a review. J Antimicrobial Chemotherapy 2006; 58(2): 266–272.

8 Watson C, Calabretto H. Comprehensive review of conventional and non-conventional methods of management of recurrent vulvovaginal candidiasis. Aus NZ J Obstet Gynaecol 2007; 47:262–272.

9 Martino JL, Vermund SH. Vaginal douching: evidence for risks or benefits to women's health. Epidemiol Rev 2002; 24(2):110–116.

10 Al-Gurairi FT, Al-Waiz M, Sharquie KE. Oral zinc sulphate in the treatment of recalcitrant viral warts: randomized placebo-controlled clinical trial. Br J Dermatol 2002; 146:423–431.

11 Spanos NP, Williams V, Gwynn MI. Effects of hypnotic, placebo, and salicylic acid treatments on wart regression. Psychosom Med 1990; 52(1): 109–114.

12 Marrazzo JM, Koutsky LA, Kiviat NB et al. Papanicolaou test screening and prevalence of genital human papilloma virus among women who have sex with women. Am J Pub Health 2001; 91:947–952.

13 Martin S. Lesbian sexual health needs. Medical Observer 2009; 9 October. Online. Available: http://www.medicalobserver.com.au/news/lesbian-sexual-health-needs

14 Australian Government, Department of Health and Ageing. Australasian Contact Tracing Manual, 3rd edn; 2006. Online. Available: http://www.ashm.org.au/images/publications/aust-contact-tracing.pdf

chapter 62

Substance (drug and alcohol) misuse

INTRODUCTION AND OVERVIEW

We define a drug (substance) as a chemical entity, self-administered (non-medically) for its psychoactive effect. The effect usually includes a change in mood, arousal or perception, thinking (cognition) and/or behaviour. It may vary according to which drug is used, the amount used, the route of administration, the mixture of drugs used, the expectations of effect by the user, the setting of use and the personal characteristics of the user such as weight, gender and previous drug experience.

Drugs can be classified according to their physiological effects:

- *depressants*—lower inhibitions and impair consciousness, coordination and concentration
- *opioids*—are strong analgesics with euphoric properties that impair consciousness
- *cannabinoids*—have a mixture of mild hallucinogenic and depressant properties
- *stimulants*—increase nervous energy and suppress sleep and appetite
- *hallucinogens*—distort perception of reality.

In this chapter we briefly consider the more important drugs in most of the categories, and for each we consider the drug and its mode of action, use and clinical effects, and current medical and integrative treatments.

WHY PEOPLE USE DRUGS

Although there is no easy explanation for why people use drugs, the aim of using drugs may be broadly considered to be the pleasurable alteration of consciousness. The neural circuits that underlie the experience of pleasure clearly have high evolutionary value, as there is powerful survival value in repeating adaptive behaviour associated with pleasure or the relief of suffering. The 'reward centre' is the brain pathway responsible for the subjective experience related to natural reinforcers such as sexual activity and eating. These cells arise in the midbrain and extend to the nucleus accumbens, the amygdaloid nucleus, hippocampus, olfactory bulb and parts of the prefrontal cortex. Dopamine is released in anticipation of reinforcing activity and it facilitates approach behaviour (that is, feeling drawn to the things we find attractive or pleasurable). Dopamine release is necessary for associative conditioning, essentially enabling emotionally tagged information to be acquired and retained efficiently—in essence, dopamine has distinct motivational properties and important survival value in signalling reinforcement and in facilitating incentive learning. Anticipatory release of dopamine may assume an attentional role and be the biological basis of drug-related craving. Drugs of abuse may be thought of as increasing dopamine release (e.g. amphetamines), inhibiting post-synaptic dopamine reuptake (e.g. cocaine) or interfering with interneuron inhibition of dopaminergic pathways (e.g. opioids).

Not all effects of drugs on brain function are due to dopamine: dopamine modulates the presynaptic release of glutamate (the major excitatory neurotransmitter) and gamma aminobutyric acid (GABA, the major inhibitory neurotransmitter), both of which are implicated in reward pathways. Generally, the more efficiently a drug alters neurochemical function, the stronger its potential reward or reinforcing effect. And vice versa—with opioids, for example, use of a partial agonist (e.g. buprenorphine) or an antagonist (e.g. naltrexone) that blocks opioid receptors can be beneficial in treatment.

The collective impact of drugs of abuse is that neurotransmitter release is occurring as a result of direct stimulation of brain pathways, rather than their stimulation by sensory input. The ease, reliability, intensity and rapidity of such effects go a large way towards explaining the potential for such drugs to lead to abuse. The underlying brain structures and processes responsible for drug-related reinforcement are at least partially under genetic control. For example, studies suggest that the heritability of liability to alcohol abuse is 50%.

Studies also suggest that there are a myriad psychosocial influences on drug use patterns. For example, risk factors for heavy adolescent substance abuse include social environmental factors (e.g. high unemployment and liberal, cultural norms of use), family factors (e.g. family disruption), peer factors (e.g. greater attachment to peers than to parents) and individual factors (e.g. low self-esteem and depression).

The influence of genes is not static and can be expressed differently in the presence of differing environmental conditions.

DRUG USE AND HEALTH

The health effects of tobacco and alcohol dwarf those of all illicit drugs combined. Up to 25% of hospital medical admissions are directly due to the effects of excessive alcohol consumption, and an estimated 15–20% of all general practice attendees consume harmful amounts of alcohol. Alcohol-related injuries account for 3–4% of the annual global burden of disease and injury, and tobacco smoking is the major cause of preventable death and disability worldwide.

DOCTORS AND SUBSTANCE ABUSE

- Medical practitioners are well placed to influence, assess, diagnose and treat people whose drug and alcohol consumption contributes to their health problems.
- Doctors are particularly prone to the excesses of alcohol and drugs, and this is the most common cause of disciplinary measures in the profession.
- Doctors are also a major source of street or illicit prescription drugs that can be misused.

MEDICAL AND PSYCHOSOCIAL PROBLEMS

Drug and alcohol use is not an all-or-nothing phenomenon. It exists as a spectrum extending from abstinence through intermittent non-hazardous and sometimes beneficial use to risky, hazardous use, or harmful use, to dependence. There are four core diagnoses.

- *Hazardous or risky use* is a repetitive pattern of use that confers a risk of harmful physical and psychological consequences. Hazardous substance abuse is also definable in terms of at-risk behaviours, such as bingeing to severe intoxication or sharing intravenous needles. Brief interventions that provide information and advice are effective in reducing many forms of hazardous use.
- *Harmful use* is use that is actually causing physical or psychological harm to the individual, e.g. over 40 grams of alcohol per day for women.
- *Substance abuse* is use that disrupts prevailing social norms, which vary with culture, gender and generation.
- *Dependence* is present when there are any three of the following features:
  - impaired control over use of a psychoactive substance
  - a strong desire or craving to take it
  - a priority given to substance use over other activities
  - a stereotyped or predicable pattern of use, tolerance and withdrawal
  - continued use despite harm. Severe dependence is typically associated with drug withdrawal on cessation of use.

SPECIFIC SUBSTANCE ABUSE

ALCOHOL

Excessive alcohol consumption is a major risk factor for morbidity and mortality. The WHO estimates that, worldwide in 2002, alcohol caused 3.2% of deaths (1.8 million) and 4.0% of the burden of disease.[1] In Australia, for example, it has been estimated that harm from alcohol was the cause of 5.3% of the burden of disease for males and 2.2% for females.[2] In Australia in 1998–99, the total tangible cost attributed to alcohol consumption (which includes lost productivity, healthcare costs, road accident-related costs and crime-related costs) was estimated at $5.5 billion. Nevertheless, some benefits are thought to arise in the longer term from low to moderate alcohol consumption, largely through reduced risk of stroke and ischaemic heart disease. The net harm associated with alcohol consumption, after taking these benefits into account, was around 2.0% of the total burden of disease in Australia in 2003.[3]

In most developed countries, around 10% of the population drink at levels considered low risk for long-term harm. Around one-third of people drink above safe limits for short-term harm. Groups with higher than average consumption include young people, people in rural and remote areas and certain occupational groups such as miners and hospitality workers.

Alcoholic beverages are made by yeast fermentation of sugars from different plant sources to give a variety of drinks. The alcoholic strength (expressed by volume) varies from 2–5% for beers to 10–15% for table wines, to 35–55% for spirits. A standard drink contains approximately 10 g alcohol. Compared with most other drugs, alcohol has low potency, and large doses are required to produce its toxic effects.

The effects of alcohol on the central nervous system (CNS) vary according to the blood alcohol concentration, starting with mild euphoria, muscle relaxation and pleasure, possibly through release of noradrenaline, dopamine and endogenous opioids; then impairment of performance, especially of complex tasks; then ataxia and slurred speech, intellectual impairment and amnesia; and finally, profound depression and progressive loss of consciousness, respiratory failure and death.

Alcohol enhances the effects of the inhibitory neurotransmitter GABA at the GABA-A receptor to produce anxiolytic, muscle-relaxant and sedative effects. Alcohol also blocks the NMDA receptors (*N*-methyl *d*-aspartate receptors), probably causing the amnesic and cerebral depressant effects. Alcohol dilates blood vessels, irritates the gastrointestinal tract and damages the liver and other organs.

Regular intake of alcohol results in the development of tolerance, with larger amounts required to produce the same degree of intoxication. Tolerance develops in parallel with physical dependence.

A compulsive desire to use alcohol is attributed in part to its strong reinforcing properties—avoiding withdrawal symptoms and stimulation of the brain reward system with reduced anxiety and euphoria. Alcohol increases the firing of dopamine neurons in the ventral tegmental area and the release of dopamine in the nucleus accumbens. The alcohol-induced euphoria and stimulant effect in humans is antagonised, and craving for alcohol in chronic users is reduced by drugs that block the synthesis of catecholamines and deplete brain dopamine. Alcohol appears to increase endogenous opioid activity, and opioid receptor antagonists such as naltrexone decrease animal intake in both humans and animals and reduce the alcohol high and the number of relapses.

Clinical effects

Just as alcohol intake depresses the nervous system, its withdrawal produces over-excitation of the CNS. A mild acute withdrawal (hangover) can develop following a single intoxicating dose of alcohol or a short period of drinking, and manifests as headache, nausea, dehydration, tremulousness, lethargy and sleep disturbance.

Minor withdrawal syndrome

Minor withdrawal may cause symptoms within 24 hours of the last drink, including tremor, tachycardia, hypertension, sweating, nausea, diarrhoea, reduced appetite, anxiety, restlessness, headache, difficulty sleeping and bad dreams. The syndrome peaks on days 2–3 of abstinence and the major symptoms subside by day 4–5 or within a week. Fifteen per cent of withdrawing chronic alcohol users will experience withdrawal seizures 1–3 days after their last drink, and usually in the first 48 hours. These are usually grand mal in type, and between one and four seizures may occur.

Major withdrawal (delirium tremens)

Major withdrawal occurs 3–10 days after the last drink. Fewer than 5% of chronic alcohol patients (rarely under age 30 years) can suffer from agitation, disorientation, high fevers, sweating, paranoia and visual hallucinations. The patient gives a history of heavy alcohol use for at least 5 years and a recent episode of heavy drinking for two or more weeks.

Protracted withdrawal

Protracted withdrawal may be present, with symptoms of anxiety, irritability, hostility, depression, insomnia, fatigue and craving most severe in the first 5 days following the last drink. These may last for weeks or months following cessation of drinking and may be the major trigger for relapse.

Acute alcohol toxicity

The manifold manifestations of acute alcohol toxicity include acute alcohol hallucinosis or paranoia, pathological or idiosyncratic alcohol intoxication, blackouts, sleep disturbances, alcohol overdose, decreased myocardial contractility, peripheral vasodilatation with drop in blood pressure then systolic hypertension, atrial or ventricular arrythmias, oesophagitis, gastritis, subepithelial haemorrhages, increased small bowel motility and decreased water and electrolyte absorption, increased red cell volume, mild anaemia and leucopenia, hyperplasia of the bone marrow, mild thrombocytopenia and decreased platelet aggregation.

Chronic alcohol intoxication

Chronic alcohol use may affect almost every body system, and most of these effects are detrimental. Regular consumption of two drinks per day for men and one for women has been shown to be beneficial through decreased risk of atherosclerosis due to increased concentrations of circulating high-density lipoprotein cholesterol and inhibition of blood coagulation.

- Studies have linked high comorbidity of chronic alcohol dependence with mental disorders, especially anxiety disorders (25%), depression (20–40%) and alcohol-induced hallucinosis.
- Wernicke–Karsakoff syndrome is a neuropsychiatric condition found in the presence of ongoing carbohydrate load where thiamine is deficient.

  Wernicke's encephalopathy is an acute, reversible condition, seen in chronic alcohol-dependent individuals, characterised by ataxia, ophthalmoplegia and confusion. Not all of the classical triad of signs need be present for the diagnosis to be made. Indeed, it is underdiagnosed by up to a factor of 80% on this basis. Thiamine is required to act as an enzyme co-factor for pyruvate kinase, at the conclusion of glycolysis in the cytosol. It is mandatory for the production of high levels of ATP, produced via the Krebs cycle in mitochondria. Its absence causes significant under-utilisation of carbohydrates in the form of anaerobic over aerobic metabolism. Essentially the brain is starved of energy despite a high carbohydrate load. Despite the enormous variance of alcohol detoxification protocols and choice of detoxification agents used across the world, the single most important drug and the one common theme to all protocols is thiamine. In the absence of signs, parenteral (IV or IM) thiamine 100 mg q8h is thought to be sufficient prophylaxis.

Korsakoff syndrome (or Korsakoff's psychosis) is the irreversible sequel to Wernicke's, where thiamine is not administered quickly enough or in sufficient doses, and is characterised by inability to form new memories, loss of short-term memory and eventually long-term memory, confabulation and hallucinations. Treatment is with parenteral thiamine and is currently thought to require at least 500 mg per day, although resolution of symptoms is likely to be incomplete.

- Pancreatitis—inflammation of the pancreas (see Ch 30, Gastroenterology).
- Hepatic inflammation and cirrhosis (see Ch 30).
- Bones—chronic alcoholism is associated with other risk factors such as poor nutrition, leanness, liver disease, malabsorption, vitamin D deficiency, hypogonadism, haemosiderosis, parathyroid dysfunction and tobacco use, and these may contribute to the pathogenesis of bone disease related to alcoholism.[4] Alcohol-related low bone density requires comprehensive lifestyle management in addition to alcohol reduction or abstinence in order to slow or prevent the development of osteoporosis.
- Poor immune function—alcohol has a deleterious effect on many immune system functions, and chronic alcoholism is associated with increased susceptibility to bacterial and viral infection. Assess immunisation status and arrange appropriate immunisation (e.g. influenza and pneumococcus, tuberculosis, hepatitis A and B).

Current guidelines[5]

- *Low risk*—less than 2 standard drinks per day on average for women and 4 per day for men, with 2 alcohol-free days per week in the long term. No more than 4 drinks for women and 6 for men on any one occasion, with consumption above long-term low-risk levels on more than 3 days per week. The guidelines suggest low-risk levels of < 25 g alcohol per day for women and up to 25–45 g per day for men.
- *Hazardous*—3–4 standard drinks for women and 5–6 for men per day in the long term. No more than 5–6 drinks per day for women and 7–10 for men on any one occasion.
- *Harmful*—5 or more standard drinks for women and 7 or more for men in the long term. More than 7 for women and 11 for men on any one occasion.
- No level is safe in pregnant women.

Without systematic screening, GPs are likely to miss up to 75% of risky drinking. A useful approach is to screen all patients annually and infrequent attenders opportunistically. The assessment should include:

- the level, frequency and pattern of alcohol consumption
- symptoms of alcohol dependence
- physical, psychological and social problems related to drinking.

Tools to assess alcohol intake:

- The WHO's Alcohol Use Disorders Identification Test (AUDIT) is one of the most reliable to use.
- Another simple tool is the quantity–frequency index—on how many occasions in the past 30 days has the patient consumed more than 7 (women) or 10 (men) standard drinks?
- Physical examination and laboratory tests are not useful for identifying harmful drinking, and may be normal in alcohol dependence.

Management

1. *Brief interventions*—even as short as 5 minutes—have been shown to be effective. Compared to those receiving no intervention, those receiving any brief intervention show a 20–30% reduction in drinking and are at least twice as likely to modify their drinking. Brief interventions of 1–4 sessions can have an impact on drinking behaviour.
2. *Follow-up* is useful to reinforce changes and assess the need for further treatment.
3. Some patients find *Alcoholics Anonymous* (AA) helpful. A meta-analysis of AA and other 12-step programs found similar outcomes to other standard treatments including cognitive behaviour therapy (CBT).[6]
4. *Motivational interviewing* aims to motivate change in drinking behaviour by creating a discrepancy between the patient's goals and their current actions. Evidence suggests that it is useful in risky and dependent drinkers.

5 *Dependence and withdrawal management*—patients who are physically dependent will require inpatient or outpatient withdrawal treatment, the latter being more common these days.
   - Acamprosate (333 mg two tablets t.d.s. for patients < 60 kg and 4 tablets per day for patients > 60 kg) and naltrexone (50 mg daily) are generally well tolerated and can be continued if the patient is drinking. They are modestly effective in reducing relapse, delaying return to drinking and reducing drinking days.
   - Disulphiram (Antabuse®) (200 mg daily) causes patients to become intensely unwell if they drink alcohol. It can be effective in patients when dosage is closely supervised. As reactions can be life threatening, it is not recommended as a first-line therapy.
   - Psychosocial interventions have been shown to be effective in combination with anti-craving medications (acamprosate and naltrexone), and weekly follow-up may increase the effectiveness of pharmacotherapy.

Integrative approaches

Herbal medicines[7]

Herbal treatments such as St John's wort (*Hypericum perforatum*), kudzu extracts (*Pueraria lobata*), panax ginseng, dried roots of *S. militorrhiza* (a Chinese medicine used for insomnia) and ibogaine (from a Central African root bark) may reduce alcohol consumption.[8] While the mechanisms of action remain to be clarified, they probably act through several neurotransmitter systems. St John's wort may provide some relief from comorbid depression.

Silybum marinarum (milk thistle)—silymarin, the flavonoid extracted from milk thistle, has been studied for treating all types of liver disease. Silymarin has the ability to block fibrosis, a process that contributes to the eventual development of cirrhosis in people with inflammatory liver conditions secondary to alcohol abuse.[9]

Nutrition

Nutritional deficiencies are common in people who chronically ingest excessive alcohol and may require dietary management and nutritional supplementation. Common deficiencies include vitamin B_1, vitamin A, vitamin D, selenium, folate, riboflavin, zinc and vitamin B_6.

Dietary advice

- Include foods high in B vitamins and iron, such as whole grains, dark leafy greens (such as spinach and kale) and sea vegetables.
- Include fruits (such as blueberries, cherries and tomatoes) and vegetables.
- Protein—alcohol causes both whole-body and tissue-specific changes in protein metabolism, resulting in loss of lean tissue mass. Clinical studies in alcoholic patients without overt liver disease show reduced rates of skeletal muscle protein synthesis. Ensure adequate protein with food sources (meat, chicken, fish, soy foods) and/or supplementation.
- Eliminate simple sugars and increase complex carbohydrates.
- Increase essential fatty acids, including omega-3 supplementation.
- Avoid caffeine.
- Recommend a multivitamin daily.

Acupuncture

Studies provide some evidence that acupuncture is more effective than placebo in:
- reducing alcohol intake over the subsequent 3 months and reducing the desire to drink
- reducing re-admissions for alcohol detoxification.

The studies have substantial methodological weaknesses, however, and there have been problems in finding appropriate control groups in blinded studies.[7]

It is claimed that complementary therapies may be effective in specific subgroups of alcohol abuse patients and that, in any case, acupuncture integrated with conventional treatment could represent a valid support treatment for some patients.

There are very few data on the effectiveness of homeopathy for alcohol dependence. Researchers generally agree on the need for more well-conducted studies.

TOBACCO

Smoking remains the most prevalent behavioural risk factor for disease and premature death. Daily smoking varies widely in different countries. For example, it is reported by nearly three-quarters of the male population in some Middle Eastern countries and by just over one-sixth of the population in Australia. A number of groups within the community, such as Indigenous Australians, those from specific ethnic groups, those with a mental health problem and those with other drug use problems have much higher rates. Nearly three-quarters of smokers report that they want to stop smoking, but the success rate of unaided attempts is low.

The process of drying, curing and ageing the tobacco leaf increases the concentration of the alkaloid nicotine and other constituents that contribute to the toxicity of tobacco. Substances added during manufacture to improve flavour, control burning and enhance nicotine delivery result in a complex cocktail of hundreds of biologically active substances in tobacco smoke.

Nicotine is selective for the nicotinic acetylcholine receptor. There are two major types of these receptors: at the skeletal neuromuscular junction, and at acetylcholine receptors in the brain and autonomic ganglia.

Nicotine increases arousal and attentiveness, and improves reaction time and psychomotor performance. It appears that nicotinic receptors have an important role in modulating higher brain functions; their effects on memory and learning are less clear. Nicotine can improve mood by relieving anxiety, and it reduces appetite. Autonomic effects include nausea and vomiting, tachycardia, vasoconstriction, increased blood pressure and cardiac output, and decreased gastrointestinal motility. It increases antidiuretic hormone secretion, reduces urine flow and suppresses the immune system via decreased T-cell activity. Smoking accelerates atherosclerosis and increases the risk of cardiovascular disease including angina, myocardial infarction and stroke.

The fastest route of absorption is by inhalation, which delivers a bolus of nicotine to the brain in about 10 seconds, leading to reinforcement. The rapid reinforcement probably contributes to the highly addictive nature of tobacco smoking. Absorption from nicotine gum is much slower, with a peak plasma level after 30 minutes of chewing compared with 5–10 minutes after smoking. Transdermal patches are even slower, with a peak level reached after 3–12 hours.

Smoking induces many liver enzymes responsible for the metabolism of nicotine itself and other drugs. There are therefore significant interactions, and nicotine seems to reduce the sedative effects of alcohol, possibly explaining their common consumption together.

Tolerance

Repeated exposure to nicotine results in neuronal adaptations that are reflected in tolerance, sensitisation and withdrawal. Tolerance of the cardiovascular and behavioural effects of nicotine develops during the course of one day, and smokers lose the tolerance overnight while sleeping and regain it the next day on resumption of smoking.

Dependence and withdrawal

Cessation of nicotine intake causes withdrawal: the symptoms can affect behaviour and provide strong motivation to continue smoking. Withdrawal symptoms start within a few hours of cessation and peak around 24–72 hours after the last cigarette. The DSM-IV criteria for nicotine withdrawal include four or more of eight symptoms and signs:

- dysphoria or depressed mood
- insomnia
- irritability, frustration, anger
- anxiety
- difficulty concentrating
- breathlessness
- decreased heart rate
- increased appetite or weight gain.

Craving, while not a diagnostic criterion, is an important element in withdrawal.

Smokers commonly maintain blood nicotine levels of 10–40 ng/mL. Withdrawal symptoms are believed to be mainly due to decreased nicotine concentration. Stress and anxiety affect nicotine tolerance and dependence because cortisol reduces the effect of nicotine. Elevated levels of cortisol mean that more nicotine needs to be consumed to achieve the same effect. Part of the reinforcement of smoking comes from relief of nicotine withdrawal (negative reinforcement). Nicotine also produces pleasurable effects that are important in positive reinforcement in that the smoker feels alert, yet relaxed. Nicotine activates the brain reward system with increased extracellular dopamine. Inhaled nicotine gets to the brain rapidly and each puff produces some discrete reinforcement.

Toxicity

The acute fatal dose of nicotine for an adult is about 60 mg of base. The average intake from a cigarette is 1–3 mg. The typical smoker obtains 20–40 mg nicotine per day. Acute tobacco poisoning results in symptoms of nausea, vomiting, dizziness and general weakness. Severe poisoning can result in convulsions, unconsciousness and possible death. Chronic tobacco exposure affects many organ systems. Nicotine, smoke tar and carbon monoxide play important roles in leading to atherosclerosis and cardiovascular disease, chronic obstructive airways disease, peptic ulceration, gastrointestinal tract cancers, impaired fertility, abortion, premature birth, low birth weight, SIDS, myopathy and osteoporosis.

Helping smokers to quit

There is good evidence that brief advice from healthcare providers to quit has a small effect: 2–3% of quitters one year later. This effect can be increased by adding other strategies including pharmacotherapy, active follow-up, and referral to quit-smoking services. The 5 A's approach[10] is recommended:

- Ask—being aware of who the smokers are in practice is important for effective management of chronic diseases. About one in three smokers attending their GP have not been correctly identified.
- Assess—assessment of interest in quitting is helpful in tailoring relevant advice to help motivate a quit attempt. Nicotine dependence can be rapidly assessed by asking about time to first cigarette after waking, the number of cigarettes smoked per day, and whether the patient had cravings or withdrawal

symptoms in previous attempts to quit. Yes to any of these suggests nicotine dependence.
- Advise—brief assessment and advice to quit, often taking as little as three minutes, acts as a prompt to quit attempts and has a measurable effect on quit rates.
- Assist—all smokers interested in quitting should be given counselling and support by a GP or a trained practice nurse. A quit kit and referral to a Quitline should be provided.
- Arrange—a follow-up visit one week and one month after quit date to check for relapse has been shown to increase the likelihood of successful long-term abstinence.

Pharmacotherapy
Several drugs have been shown to assist smoking cessation but they are not a substitute for motivational and professional counselling support. Three pharmacotherapy agents have been licensed for smoking therapy: nicotine replacement therapy (NRT), bupropion and varenicline.

Nicotine replacement therapy
All forms of NRT are effective in aiding cessation, nearly doubling the cessation rate at 12 months compared to placebo. Combination therapy (patch and gum) should be recommended to smokers who are not able to quit or who experience craving when using one form of NRT. NRT can also help smokers who are unwilling or unable to stop smoking to reduce their nicotine consumption. Some of these smokers will go on to attempt to quit. Some points to note:
- More than one form of NRT can be used concurrently.
- NRT can be used by pregnant and lactating women.
- All forms of NRT can be used by patients with cardiovascular disease.
- All forms of NRT can be used by smokers aged 12–17 years.
- There is a high likelihood of persistent addiction to NRT.

Bupropion
The mode of action of this antidepressant is not known but may be due to inhibition of reuptake of dopamine and noradrenaline. Bupropion doubles the cessation rate at 12 months compared with placebo. It has been shown to be effective in patients with chronic conditions—depression, cardiac disease, pulmonary disease and schizophrenia. It is not as effective as varenicline and should be used if the latter is contraindicated. The dose is 150 mg once a day for 3 days, then b.i.d.

Varenicline
Varenicline is a partial agonist of the alpha-4 beta-2 nicotinic acetylcholine receptor, where it acts to alleviate symptoms of craving and withdrawal. At the same time it blocks nicotine from binding to the alpha-4 beta-2 receptor, reducing the intensity of the rewarding effects of smoking. A 12-week course of varenicline produced a continuous abstinence rate of nearly one-quarter at 12 months, significantly more effective than bupropion and placebo. The main adverse effects include nausea (30%) and abnormal dreams (13%).

People should set a date to stop smoking. Start varenicline 1–2 weeks before their quit date.[11] Titrate the dose as follows:
- days 1–3: 0.5 mg daily
- days 4–7: increase to 0.5 mg twice daily
- continue with 1 mg twice daily from day 8 to the end of a 12-week treatment course.

Nortryptyline
This antidepressant drug is not registered for smoking cessation but a 12-week course appears to double cessation rates compared with placebo. Its use is limited by its potential to produce serious side effects including arrythmias in those with cardiovascular disease, and it can be dangerous in overdose.

Integrative approaches
Acupuncture and hypnotherapy are used in some patients to aid smoking cessation but only a limited number of studies have tested these approaches. In controlled trials, acupuncture does not increase quit rates over sham acupuncture.

CANNABIS
Cannabis, used for over 4000 years, is the most popular drug used worldwide after caffeine, alcohol and tobacco. There is a popular perception that it is a soft drug and perhaps less addictive than harder drugs such as stimulants and opioids.

Australia has the highest rate of use in the OECD countries, with 10% of adult males current users and 4% of adult females. Twenty-five per cent of adolescents have used cannabis and nearly 20% of these exposures occurred before the age of 12 years. Earlier onset of cannabis use predicts greater addiction severity and morbidity.

Cannabis sativa (hemp) produces a resin with about 60 cannabinoids, of which one, tetrahydrocannabinol (THC), is principally responsible for the psychoactive effects of cannabis. The drug is usually smoked, to deliver the vaporised THC and other pyrolysis products rapidly to the lungs, blood and brain. Lipophilic THC is taken up by the body lipids and the metabolites are excreted slowly in the urine over the next several days.

There are two types of cannabinoid receptors: CB1 (brain and peripheral tissues such as testes and endothelial cells) and CB2 (in the immune system, especially T-cells). The CB1 receptors mediate most of the well-known effects of cannabis, and among these is the facilitation of mesolimbic dopaminergic pathways.

Cannabis produces a feeling of euphoria, relaxation and wellbeing, perceptual distortions such as apparently sharpened senses, and psychomotor and cognitive impairment. Peripheral effects include tachycardia, vasodilatation (especially in the conjunctivae), hypotension, reduced intraocular pressure, and bronchodilation. It stimulates the appetite and is antiemetic, being used in some countries to treat nausea from cancer chemotherapy. Blood concentrations of THC do not correlate well with effects, and the presence of THC metabolites in urine may not necessarily reflect recent usage.

Tolerance, dependence and withdrawal syndromes occur with cannabis, and there is concern that dependence may develop rapidly in some younger people and that it may be more severe than previously thought. Two joints a day for 3 weeks is sufficient to induce withdrawal symptoms after cessation in some people. Symptoms of withdrawal include:

- anxiety
- anorexia
- disturbed sleep and vivid dreams
- nausea
- salivation
- increased body temperature
- tremor
- weight loss
- irritability
- stomach pain.

Acute toxicity is characterised by:

- anxiety, panic attacks, delusions (persecutory), visual hallucinations, overt psychotic reactions in vulnerable people
- impairment of short-term memory and attention
- impairment of motor skills, reaction time and ability to perform skilled activities
- a shortlived psychotic state—has been reported associated with high-dose use
- slight increase in heart rate.

Chronic toxicity is characterised by:

- impairment of short-term memory, attention and the organisation and integration of complex information
- effects on major mental illnesses, such as precipitation and relapse of schizophrenia
- chronic respiratory disease
- effect on pregnancy—low birth weight
- other problems possibly related to chronic cannabis use—precipitation and aggravation of chronic psychosis; amotivational syndrome; reduced fertility; respiratory cancers; impaired immune function.

Cannabis and psychosis:

- Cannabinoids increase dopamine release.
- Cannabis precipitates relapses of schizophrenia.
- Heavy use can cause an acute toxic psychosis.
- There is little evidence for chronic toxic psychosis.

Patient assessment

Patient assessment should focus on:

- form of cannabis and method of administration
- amount used and money spent each week
- number of hours per day spent using, being intoxicated and recovering from use
- activities undertaken while intoxicated
- withdrawal symptoms
- age when first tried and started to use regularly
- other substances used
- comorbid—physical and mental health
- insight and motivation to change.

Medical treatment

- Develop therapeutic rapport—cannabis dependence rarely occurs in isolation from other drug use.
- Cognitive behavioural therapy (CBT) interventions that include motivational interviewing techniques are effective in reducing problematic cannabis use (see below).
- Treatment of overdose is rarely required.
- Provide information handouts.
- Set a 'quit date'.
- 'Detoxification'.
- Although there are no specific pharmacological treatments, associated psychological conditions may benefit from symptomatic treatment:
  - bupropion valproate—exacerbate withdrawal symptoms
  - antidepressant—side effects may limit use (e.g. SSRIs exacerbate insomnia)
  - benzodiazepines—risk of abuse; use temazepam 10–20 mg nocte, maximum 1 week
  - mirtazapine—30 mg nocte; may help with sleep disturbance. Initial reports suggesting reduced cannabis intake have not been supported with one small clinical trial to date
  - rimonabant—20 mg mane; possible role in abstinence-based treatment.
- Antipsychotic drugs are occasionally needed for cannabis-induced psychotic states—these states

are usually shortlived and resolve within a week of cessation of cannabis use:
  - drug abstinence, rehydration, sleep hygiene, regular review
  - olanzapine 5–10 mg nocte *or* quetiapine 50–100 mg nocte for the first 2 nights, then 100–200 mg nocte depending on degree of sedation, *or* temazepam 10–20 mg nocte, up to 1 week
  - admission when uncooperative and risk to self or others.
- Other medication may be required for coexisting conditions such as depression, anxiety or phobias (see below).
- Relapses are not uncommon—treat as an opportunity to learn, rather than as a failure.

Psychological interventions

Most interventions have been developed from those used for alcohol.

- Usually follow brief intervention format, including motivational interviewing.
- Psychological interventions—even one session of CBT has been shown to be of value compared with no treatment. No difference has yet been demonstrated between CBT, motivational therapy and social support sessions.
- CBT includes management of withdrawal symptoms, motivational interviewing, cognitive restructuring, coping skills training, lifestyle modification and relapse prevention, including management of urges and triggers.
- Marijuana Anonymous exists in some countries.

Cannabis and mood disorders

- Pre-existing symptoms may initially be alleviated through self-medication with cannabis (poor evidence).
- Cannabis use is more common in certain social groups that are also at a higher risk of depression (good evidence).
- Cannabis use may carry a direct risk for depression and anxiety (good evidence).

Amotivational syndrome:

- Described in chronic users—may be due to chronic intoxication.
- Loss of ambition, drive, motivation.
- Affective restriction.
- Reduced capacity to complete complex tasks, including those at school or work.

Cannabis and physical health

The effects of cannabis are difficult to differentiate from the effects of smoking. They include:

- carcinoma of head and neck, respiratory and upper digestive tracts
- chronic airways disease
- coronary artery disease
- hypertension
- infertility in men and women.

Key points

- Cannabis use is common, and cannabis dependence is relatively uncommon.
- There is good evidence for the efficacy of psychological treatment (especially CBT).
- In managing cannabis abuse, it is important to treat comorbidity (e.g. psychosis, other drug-use disorders).

PHARMACEUTICALS

Benzodiazepines

Benzodiazepines were discovered in 1954. Chlordiazepoxide (Librium®) was the first patented benzodiazepine drug, in 1960. Diazepam (Valium®) was introduced in 1963, and was found to be not only sedative but also a useful muscle relaxant. Other agents followed, from the mid-1960s with nitrazepam (Mogadon®), through to the 1980s with alprazolam (Xanax®). Benzodiazepines rapidly became popular because they were superior to barbiturates in having decreased tissue toxicity and a vastly improved safety profile in overdose.

Indications

Benzodiazepines are primarily used as anxiolytic, sedative/hypnotic, anticonvulsant, antispasmodic, anaesthesia and amnesia agents for medical procedures and for drug and alcohol withdrawal.

Prevalence

Benzodiazepines such as temazepam, diazepam, oxazepam and nitrazepam tend to rate as some of the most widely prescribed medications.

Mode of action

Benzodiazepines appear to modulate the effect of gamma-aminobutyric acid (GABA), the main inhibitory neurotransmitter of the CNS, via the GABA receptor complex. The GABA receptor complex includes binding sites for benzodiazepines, barbiturates and steroids.

Short-term effects

Low-dose benzodiazepines cause loss of motor coordination, drowsiness, lethargy, fatigue, cognitive impairment, memory loss, confusion, depression, blurred vision, slurred speech, vertigo, tremors and respiratory depression. High doses can cause extreme drowsiness. In high-dose intoxication, the above symptoms may be observed as well as mood swings, hostile, violent and erratic behaviour, and euphoria.

Long-term effects

Because some benzodiazepines have long half-lives, exceeding 24 hours, and as a result of their lipid solubility, accumulation may occur in body fat stores. The symptoms of over-sedation may not appear for several days. These include: cognitive impairment, memory loss, poor judgment, disorientation, delirium, confusion, slurred speech, muscle weakness and lack of coordination.

Tolerance

Long-term benzodiazepine use can result in neuro-adaptation and dependence. The mechanism is unclear but may be due to altered sensitivity of GABA NMDA or other receptors. Benzodiazepine dependence may also be due to the unfixed sensitivity of the GABA receptor to various neurotransmitters. In this model, the set-point where drugs can bind but are not effective appears to shift with long-term use.

Common benzodiazepine withdrawal symptoms include: perceptual distortions, sense of movement, depersonalisation, derealisation, hallucinations (visual, auditory), distortion of body image, tingling, numbness, altered sensation, formication, sensory hypersensitivity (light, sound, taste, smell), muscle twitches, jerks, fasciculation, tinnitus. In addition, rapid withdrawal from high doses has been associated with psychosis, delirium and convulsions.

Dependence

Time from first dose to the development of dependence is based on the dosage, potency and duration of habit. For example, in someone who is taking a high dosage of alprazolam, dependency can develop within one to two months. Short-acting benzodiazepines are popular among opiate-dependent individuals as they have a rapid onset of sedation. As dependence develops, increased doses are required to invoke and maintain a therapeutic effect.

Detoxification

Detoxification regimens are broadly divided into two main scenarios:

- those where a client's daily intake is either at or near a therapeutic dose—such clients can usually be managed as outpatients with a modest detoxification program
- those where a client's daily intake is extremely high and very erratic—this is often seen in the context of poly-drug use with heroin, for example, where benzodiazepines are used between heroin injections to manage withdrawal and insomnia. These clients may at times be managed as outpatients, but may also require inpatient management.

In assessing suitability for home or ambulatory detoxification, the following points should be considered:

- The patient is not 'doctor shopping'.
- There is no evidence of severe and high dose dependence.
- There is no history of seizures.
- Doses are either therapeutic or only slightly above.
- There is no psychiatric or medical comorbidity.
- There has been no previous treatment failure in this setting.
- The home environment is stable and there is a carer.
- There is no poly-substance abuse/dependence.
- The patient is highly motivated.

Patients considered unsuitable for home detoxification and therefore possibly requiring inpatient specialist unit care may exhibit the following:

- previous complicated withdrawal
- moderate–severe dependence
- ingestion of non-therapeutic, high doses of benzodiazepines
- chaotic ingestion patterns
- significant use of other psychotropic drugs
- physical or psychiatric comorbidity
- absence of care or an unstable household
- access/exposure to benzodiazepines in the home environment.

Ambulatory/home detoxification

For low (therapeutic) dose dependence, home detox can be considered. This has been adapted from Queensland Health Detoxification Protocols.[12]

- 2 days diazepam 5–10 mg at 6 am, midday and 6 pm, and 10 mg at bedtime
- 2 days diazepam 5 mg at 6 am, midday and 6 pm, and 10 mg at bedtime
- 2 days diazepam 5 mg at lunchtime and at bedtime
- then diazepam 5 mg at bedtime for one night.

The doses required to begin the detoxification should not exceed those admitted by the patient. It may be necessary to reduce doses much slower than suggested by weeks or even months, particularly at the lower end of the dose scale.

Symptomatic therapy can include metoclopramide for nausea, antacids for reflux, antidiarrhoeals, and paracetamol for headache.

Inpatient detoxification

Patients who have been on high doses of benzodiazepines for long periods are more likely to experience withdrawal reactions than those on lower doses, particularly if withdrawal is abrupt.

Patients should be commenced on a dose of diazepam which safely prevents seizures and delirium, and then steadily reduced over time. There is avid debate regarding the cases for and against structured detoxification from benzodiazepines on several grounds. Safety is the most notable issue, but efficacy is also questionable, with high relapse rates described. If undertaken, current recommendations suggest management of patients at a dose which prevents withdrawal seizures, between 40 and 60 mg per day in divided doses. Reductions should be gradual and should not exceed 10% of the total dose per week. This is particularly important at the lower end of the dose range and towards the conclusion of the detoxification, where flexibility is essential. Given the high relapse rate of patients to uncontrolled benzodiazepine use in this group, it is useful to explore other mental health comorbidity and other addictions, e.g alcohol and opioids, which may be drivers of ongoing chaotic substance use among this group of patients.

There is evidence to support the use of brief interventions. In addition, evidence is quite strong for the use of CBT in this setting.

Self Management and Recovery Training (SMART) has been shown to be of benefit as a self-help strategy. It is a group-based therapy based on the principles of CBT and rational emotive therapy.

Integrative approaches

The first step in the integrated management of benzodiazepine use is to assess the underlying reasons for the drug abuse. It is also important to exclude adverse drug reactions from other prescribed and illicit drugs—for example, SSRIs can cause anxiety and patients may be using benzodiazepines to manage that side effect.

Management of underlying anxiety

Vitamin and mineral supplements that may assist include thiamine, magnesium, phosphate, folate, zinc and vitamins A, C, D, E and B group.

While there have been case reports and uncontrolled series involving auricular acupuncture, there is a lack of randomised trials and systematic reviews to support its use widely.

Neither valerian nor melatonin has been found to have a significant effect on benzodiazepines consumed by those trying to detoxify, nor have they had a reproducible effect on sleep quality among those who have successfully stopped using benzodiazepines.

PRESCRIPTION OPIATES AND OVER-THE-COUNTER MEDICATIONS

A prescription is written by an approved medical, dental, optometric or nursing practitioner, and medications are dispensed to the consumer or patient at hospitals, pharmacies or clinics. Doctors occasionally dispense drugs to patients directly, in the form of samples, in remote areas in lieu of a dispensing chemist or via the doctor's bag.

There are a number of other avenues by which people may obtain prescription medications. Online outlets have become popular in the past 5–10 years. In some cases, highly addictive and dangerous drugs are available via the internet without medical assessment or prescription. In a number of cases, drugs may not have been formally approved for sale in the country of purchase. An example of this is oxycodone (Endone®), an opioid analgesic, commonly marketed in many countries as a sustained-release preparation (e.g. OxyContin® in Australia). In the United States, oxycodone is available in combination with paracetamol in an over-the-counter (OTC) formulation.

The range of agents in the opiate category is very broad, ranging from codeine available OTC, to morphine available on prescription. Recently, hydromorphone (Dilaudit®) has become popular again after a long absence. These opiate preparations are all highly addictive and their long-term use results in significant problems for both the prescriber and the patient.

In addition to these narcotics, a number of other drugs have significant abuse and dependence potential. Table 62.1 provides a list of the classes and names of drugs that may be addictive or have potential for abuse. Use of these drugs has increased dramatically in the past decade.

In the United States, it is currently estimated that 20% of the population have at some time in their lives used a prescription drug for indications not recommended by the prescriber. A US national survey on drug use[13] found that 6.4 million Americans over the age of 12 years, or 2.6% of the population, had used a psychotherapeutic drug for non-medical reasons in the previous month, with the main three categories being analgesics, tranquillisers and stimulants. Retail sales of opioid medications in the United States had increased from 1997 for various medications listed in Table 62.1. Methadone was the most common, with a 933% increase in sales over the eight-year period. Over the same time, retail sales of oxycodone increased by 588%. The US Department of Justice reported that pharmaceutical drug abuse exceeded that of all other drugs except cannabis and accounted for the high annual number of pharmaceutical deaths.

In many countries there have been reports of increased prescribing of opiates for non-cancer pain. For example, in Australia, the Department of Health and Ageing reported a rise of greater than 800% in the use of oxycodone between 2001 and 2006.[14] In 5 years, oxycodone has moved from being insignificant to being

TABLE 62.1 Common prescription and OTC drugs, classified by organ system, action and name, and matched to adverse effects

Organ system	Action and drug name	Adverse effect/dependence
Gastrointestinal	Antispasmodics • Hyoscine	Drowsiness, intoxication
Cardiovascular	Beta-blockers • Propanolol	Reduce tremor, calmative
	Caffeine • coffee, cafergot, No-doze	Increase alertness, stay awake, performance enhancing, dependence
	Diuretics • Frusemide	Short-term weight loss, Masking agent
Neurological	Sedative/anxiolytics • Benzodiazepines	Intoxication, withdrawal, self-medication, respiratory depression, overdose, death
	Anticonvulsants • Clonazepam • Phenobarbitone	As above, cardiac, respiratory and renal failure, death
Neurological, other	Movement disorders • Benztropine	Drowsiness, intoxication
	Travel sickness • Antihistamines	Drowsiness, intoxication
Analgesics	Narcotic analgesics Oxycodone, morphine, pethidine, codeine, hydromorphone	Drowsiness, intoxication, respiratory depression, death, dependence
Endocrine	Human growth hormone • Erythropoietin • Anabolic steroids	Performance enhancement in sport, increased strength and stamina, improved recovery
Genitourinary	Erectile dysfunction • Tadalafil • Sildenafil • Vardenafil	Crushed and injected at dance parties with psychostimulants and hallucinogens; no actual benefit from this technique; causes embolism, increases BBV
Paediatric	Treatment of ADD/ADHD Psychostimulants • Methylphenidate • Dexamphetamine	CNS and CVS hyper-stimulation, mood changes, psychosis, dependence
Dietary	Anorectics • Phentermine • Diethylpropion	As for psychostimulants
Respiratory	Antitussives • Codeine • Dextromethorphan	As for narcotics
	Antihistamines • Chlorphenphiramine	Drowsiness, intoxication
	Decongestants • Pseudoephedrine	As for psychostimulants

in the top ten fastest-rising rates of prescription drug, and it was seventh for volume of drug and sixteenth for cost.

US internet suppliers of prescription drugs sell to consumers worldwide. Although the sale of opioids is controlled in the United States and in Australia, this is difficult to enforce, because a third-party country where such laws do not exist is often used to supply the drugs. Internet providers rarely give detailed warnings regarding use, contraindications and precautions while taking medication. This is particularly true of warnings about addiction.

Treatment options

A careful history, examination and review of previous investigations is required. If prescriptions were given previously by other doctors, try to locate the source of the original diagnosis and verify the presence or absence of the condition for which the patient claims to need the drug in question.

Be completely transparent with the patient in an empathic, non-judgmental way. If their diagnosis cannot be confirmed, it is reasonable to establish the diagnosis by referrals and special tests, as long as they can be justified on clinical grounds. Too many investigations can have the effect of magnifying the patient's concerns, while too few may leave an important diagnosis undiscovered.

Once dependence has been established, use treatments for the same class of illicit drug—for example methadone or buprenorphine for opioid dependence. This will not be possible in all cases, and may be prohibited in certain jurisdictions. This is particularly relevant for psychostimulants, where specialist evaluation is necessary. It may be worthwhile to consider other treatments depending upon the patient's mental state, such as antidepressants and CBT.

Where no direct drug-receptor combination and effect exists, brief intervention, CBT and long-term follow-up are required, as relapse is common. Factors affecting relapse include lack of desire to change, hyperalgesia and the ready availability of prescription and OTC drugs.

It is important to remember that there is no compelling evidence to support the long-term use of opiates for chronic back pain or chronic headache.

Opiate and stimulant prescribing patterns by doctors are monitored by state health regulatory bodies. If they are found to be abnormal, action can be brought against the doctor to counsel and ameliorate such practices. In some cases medical boards limit or prohibit prescribing privileges.

Integrative approaches

As with other drug groups, it is important to assess the cause of opiate use and abuse, and this includes appropriate pain management. Psychosocial interventions such as those mentioned above can help to treat dependence on prescription or OTC preparations.

OPIOIDS

It is estimated that there are over 74,000 dependent heroin users in Australia. Use of illicit opioids is associated with a substantially higher mortality and morbidity than use of prescription opioids. Complications of intravenous use of opioids include infectious conditions: hepatitis B, C, HIV, bacterial endocarditis and tetanus. Users may suffer injection site infections and vascular and nerve damage. Environmental factors including poor living conditions, exposure to violence and accidents increase the likelihood of poor health, with regular illicit opioid injectors having 13 times the mortality rate of the general population.

Opium is named after the juice of the opium poppy; morphine is the major active ingredient of the poppy. Morphine and codeine are derived from the poppy juice. Opioids are a class of substances with morphine-like effects that can be reversed by the specific antagonist naloxone. Some opioids are semi-synthetic chemical derivatives of morphine (e.g. heroin, acetylated morphine) and some, such as pethidine and methadone, are fully synthetic and share a common core structure that enables them to bind to opioid receptors. Opioid peptides and their receptors are widely distributed in the brain and spinal cord and in many non-neuronal tissues including the gastrointestinal tract. The endogenous opioid system is activated by stress, and is involved in the modulation of pain perception and mood and in the regulation of physiological systems such as respiration and immune function.

The principal effects of morphine include miosis, drowsiness, contentment, euphoria, analgesia (through altered perception of pain), respiratory depression, cough suppression, nausea and vomiting, constipation and increased bladder and urethral tone. Morphine activates receptors in the reward pathway, causing increased dopamine release. Tolerance develops after the first dose. Strong agonists such as morphine and methadone activate opioid receptors to elicit a full response, whereas partial agonists such as buprenorphine do not elicit a full response. Antagonists such as naloxone occupy the receptors and block agonist effects.

The acute toxic effects of opioids involve many body systems: pruritis, constipation, nausea, vomiting, confusion, delirium, stupor, miosis, urine retention, hypothermia, pulmonary oedema, hypotension, coma and death due to respiratory depression.

Tolerance is characterised by a shortened duration and reduced intensity of the euphoric, analgesic and sedative effects. There is marked variation between individuals in the development of tolerance, perhaps due to genetic variation in receptor characteristics.

Opioid withdrawal is unpleasant but not life threatening. It is characterised by insomnia, irritability, restlessness, malaise, bone and joint pain, fatigue and increased gastrointestinal motility.

Clinical assessment

A non-judgmental interviewing style should be used, and observation for signs of intoxication or withdrawal and their timing in relation to last dose of the drug is vital. The patient may appear malnourished and underweight.

The psychosocial history is often complex, with substantial disadvantage, and the assessment should include personality, comorbid psychopathology, employment and treatment history, and history of illegal activities.

Physical examination should include inspection of limbs for increased pigmentation, track marks, thrombosed veins and injection site abscesses. It is important to check for sexually transmitted infections, HIV infection and hepatitis C, endocarditis and tuberculosis.

Investigations should include tests to exclude the above. Urine drug screens for opioids and metabolites are often performed.

Treatment

Treatment for opioid use takes many forms. It is most important that clinicians treating opioid-dependent patients adopt a non-judgmental attitude and a treatment philosophy that incorporates the principles of harm reduction or harm minimisation.

Opioid overdose is a medical emergency that should be treated immediately with cardiopulmonary resuscitation, clearance and maintenance of airways, and urgent call for paramedical services. Naloxone 0.4–1.2 mg should be given IV or IMI titrated to support respiratory function. Treatment for the impact of other sedative drugs may also be required for complicated opioid overdose.

Opioid dependence is a chronic relapsing disorder. While opioid withdrawal can be effectively treated with well-researched agents, relapse is common. Pharmacotherapies for opioid withdrawal management include:

- oral methadone—tapering by 1–2 mg/day from an initial dose of 30–40 mg per day; the rate of reduction should be slowed towards the end
- buprenorphine—given sublingually at least 6 hours after the last heroin dose and 24 hours after last methadone dose, in a dose of 4, 8, 12, 12, 12 mg on days 1–5 sequentially and then stopped or reduced by 2 mg per day.
- adrenergic agonists and adjunctive medications—can be used, such as clonidine (75–150 μg t.d.s.) to reduce withdrawal symptoms and then tapered over 1–2 weeks. Other agents that are sometimes used for symptom relief include: benzodiazepines or hypnotics to reduce anxiety or the former in tapering regimen for coexisting benzodiazepine dependence; loperamide for diarrhoea; quinine sulfate for cramps; non-steroidal anti-inflammatories for pain management; metoclopramide for nausea; and neuroleptics for agitation and insomnia
- psychological therapies—can improve the effectiveness of pharmacotherapies and be used in the treatment of those who do not wish to undertake such treatments. Only a minority of patients will participate in psychological therapy for extended periods.

Integrative approaches

Studies comparing acupuncture to methadone detoxification found that acupuncture produced comparable clinical outcomes or superior outcomes relative to methadone detoxification regimens. One study also found acupuncture plus methadone detoxification produced greater alleviation of withdrawal symptoms than methadone detoxification alone. Some studies provide evidence that acupuncture has clinical value as a component of detoxification treatment for opiate abuse. Correct site acupuncture appears to have greater therapeutic effect than incorrect site acupuncture. Reported studies have methodological problems, however, and reveal conflicting results, making interpretation difficult.[11]

Meta-analyses have not demonstrated a significant efficacy of other complementary therapies, including pharmacological and biological treatments such as herbal therapies, dietary supplements, natural hormones, health and healing practices (e.g. hypnosis, meditation, yoga, biofeedback, exercise, chiropractic or massage therapy) or acupuncture.

PSYCHOSTIMULANTS AND OTHER DRUGS

Psychostimulants are the group of chemicals that affect the CNS monoamine transmitters, such as dopamine, noradrenaline and serotonin. Although they have greatest effect on dopamine, most have some effect on the other two, which often results in complications and significant health risks.

Psychostimulants are a heterogeneous collection of chemicals including cocaine, amphetamines, ecstasy and 'club' or 'party' drugs. In many ways, these names are misplaced, as all drugs can be taken at parties, but these are also often taken alone, in solitude and under very dangerous conditions. It is important to remember that alcohol and nicotine are also party drugs, and kill more people per year than all other drugs combined.

Cocaine is an alkaloid derived from the leaves of the plant *Erthroxylan coca*. It is not as common in Australia as other stimulants. Cocaine blocks the reuptake of dopamine into the terminal neuronal bouton, causing increased concentrations to be present in the synapse for longer periods of time. This results in a pleasurable experience for the user. It has a very short half-life, about 60 minutes, which results in binge use of the drug. It is commonly inhaled intranasally, but is also very effective if injected.

In 1927 Gordon Alles discovered that amphetamine ameliorated fatigue and improved nasal and airway passages. It was marketed as Benzedrine in the 1930s, during which time it became extremely popular. Soon after, other compounds such as methamphetamine were developed.

Amphetamines promote the release of dopamine, noradrenaline and serotonin from the terminal boutons of neurons. With repeated use, they lead to an exhaustion of endogenous monoamine neurotransmitters, causing reduced effects and a 'crash' depression. They can be used in a variety of ways owing to their chemistry, including orally, intranasally, smoked and injected. While there are differences in bioavailablity and absorption with different methods of administration, the effects are fairly similar.

Ecstasy, or 3,4-methylenedioxy-methamphetamine (MDMA), first became apparent as a recreational drug in the late 1960s but did not come to prominence until the 1990s. The methylenedioxy side-chain has the effect of raising its boiling point, and therefore this chemical is usually not smoked but taken orally, usually in tablet form. It can, however, be injected, although this is rarely done.

More recent side-chain variation has resulted in a variety of drugs being illicitly produced and marketed as stimulants. Among these has been para-methoxyamphetamine (PMA), also known as 'red Mitsubishi' as it is a red-coloured tablet. A more recent addition, 4-bromo-2,5-dimethoxy-phenethylamine (2CB) has a side-chain bromine substation and is a powerful hallucinogen. It is usually swallowed as a red or white tablet. One of the more worrying trends with MDMA is that it may contain varying levels of impurities or other stimulants such as these, creating powerful and unwanted effects. In addition, these tablets may contain caffeine, pseudoephedrine or ketamine. Indeed, it is estimated that at least 10% of ecstasy tablets may not contain any MDMA.

A number of other drugs are often associated with psychostimulants and party drugs, and also have varying degrees of hallucinogenic effect. These include gamma-hydroxybutyrate (GHB), ketamine and LSD. Most of these agents are either sedative or depressant drugs, rather than stimulants, and all have the potential to be hallucinogenic. They can be quite dangerous and, along with benzodiazepines, are associated with sex-based crimes, such as 'date rape'.

The typical age of first use of these types of drugs is quite late compared with other drugs. On average, adolescents start to smoke when aged between 15 and 16 years, and drink alcohol when aged between 16 and 17 years. Psychostimulants and other drugs are mostly first used by people when aged in their twenties, rather than in their teens.

Clinical effects

The effects, both wanted and unwanted, are essentially driven by increased, prolonged agonistic monoamine activity in the synapse. There is no simple drug–receptor reaction as is seen with opiates. As a result, withdrawal and detoxification is more complex, and not simply driven by replacement therapy, as is the case with heroin and methadone or buprenorphine.

The popular (positive) effects sought by stimulant users are: euphoria, increased energy; improved social interaction; increased confidence; perceived improvement in sexual performance/prowess; improved concentration, productivity and creativity; and reduced fatigue and anorexia.

The negative effects of stimulants include anxiety, anger, agitation, impaired judgment and hypervigilance. In addition, users often experience stereotyped or repetitive behaviours, nausea, vomiting, confusion, psychosis or convulsions. Bingeing is associated with poor sleep and self-care, irritability, paranoia and strong cravings. Users often report an inability to achieve the original high, causing frustration and unstable behaviour. Increased violence, crimes and accidents are common among heavy amphetamine users.

With ongoing binge use, dopamine levels are exhausted and higher doses of stimulants are taken, in a vain attempt to increase or prolong the desired effect. Without endogenous monoamine neurotransmitters, psychostimulant drugs have little capacity for augmenting the euphoria, causing frustration to the user. As the dose of drugs increases, so does the danger of unwanted effects.

Stimulants may impair the thermoregulatory system, leading to increased body temperature. This is a major component of a condition known as *serotonin syndrome*. It is a constellation of signs present after the ingestion of a serotonergic agent. Autonomic signs include tremor, fever and sweats. Agitation is usually present. In addition there is a neuromuscular component, consisting of hypertonia, hyperreflexia and clonus. This is a medical emergency, requiring urgent resuscitation and transfer to hospital. Patients will require advanced life support. In severe cases, rhabdomyolysis, elevated creatine kinase and metabolic acidosis may ensue, along with multi-organ failure. The mortality from this condition is about 11%.

Stimulant withdrawal, amphetamines in particular, can be separated into three phases—crash phase, acute phase and chronic phase—and these may blend into one another. The 'crash' occurs after depletion of dopamine stores in the presynaptic bouton and lasts from a few hours to 2–3 days. It occurs more frequently after prolonged or heavy binge use and is characterised by excessive sleeping, eating, and depression and irritability. It is described as a separate entity from acute withdrawal and is thought to be more like a hangover, as seen with alcohol use. The acute phase lasts for 5–7 days. Common complaints include mood swings, emotional lability, anger, aggression and intense cravings. The chronic phase can last for weeks to months. Symptoms include depression, dysphoria, lethargy and cravings. Relapse is common in this group as symptoms of depression and boredom are set in a context of fairly ready availability of this class of drugs.

Treatment options

Mood disorders and dysphoria count heavily among the symptoms seen in stimulant users. Depression follows binge or heavy use. It is reasonable to use an antidepressant such as an SSRI to assist. Mirtazapine has been trialled in 15–30 mg doses at night to assist with night-time anxiety in short periods of up to 4 weeks. Early results are promising.

Psychosis can occur with heavy or binge-style use and requires urgent treatment. The hallucinations that occur in this context are often referred to as 'pseudo-hallucinations' as the patient is aware of the difference between fantasy and reality. It is common for such patients to have hallucinations about their drug use and getting caught. If mild, treatment can be initiated as an outpatient using an atypical antipsychotic. If the psychosis is severe, or if harm is likely to the patient or others, admission to a psychiatric emergency facility should be undertaken for stabilisation.

While some patients will require long-term treatment with antipsychotics, they are in the minority, as drug-induced psychosis is usually a self-limiting condition. Those requiring permanent treatment may have had previously undiagnosed schizophrenia. This group will usually require lifelong care.

As drinking alcohol is often associated with stimulant use, there is good evidence to demonstrate that using aversive drugs such as disulfiram (Antabuse®), as well as anti-craving medications such as naltrexone, will concomitantly reduce alcohol and stimulant use. It is vital that adequate counselling be given to the patient prior to prescribing. If the patient has recently drunk alcohol or has some while taking disulfiram, profound vomiting, headache, hypotension and loss of consciousness will almost certainly ensue. If opiates are taken in significant amounts by an opiate-dependent individual, withdrawal may be precipitated by naltrexone.

Psychosocial interventions are the mainstay of treatment in this group. There is good evidence to support the use of CBT and brief interventions in the management of stimulant dependence. CBT-based interventions indicate that the retention rate of patients in treatment, urine test results and self-reported drug use are all significantly better than self-help strategies.

Integrative approaches

There is no evidence for effectiveness of treatment by herbal treatments or acupuncture for stimulant use or dependence.

FUTURE DIRECTIONS

Vaccines for cocaine are being trialled, on the pretext of making antibodies to cocaine and thus reducing the available free drug for the brain. Replacement therapy for amphetamines has been trialled with dexamphetamine in fairly modest doses. The results remain inconclusive, possibly because limits must be placed on therapeutic doses to prevent unwanted side effects, such as psychosis in treatment.

A newer form of medication—modafinil—used in sleep apnoea and narcolepsy is in trial at the moment. This drug improves wakefulness without euphoria or positive reinforcement for abuse potential. It has been used successfully off-licence for shift work sleep–wake disturbance in France and the United States, and is currently under evaluation for this condition in amphetamine use. Results of this and other trials are eagerly awaited.

RESOURCES

General

Amphetamines, http://www.drugtext.org/library/books/recreationaldrugs/amphetamines.htm

Cochrane Library, http://www3.interscience.wiley.com/cgi-bin/mrwhome/106568753/HOME

Freudenmann RQ, Bernschneider-Reif S. The origin of Ecstasy. Addiction 2006; 101(9):1241–1245. Abstract online, http://www.mdma.net/merck/origin.html

SMART Recovery, http://www.smartrecovery.org

Tiller JWG. Management of insomnia. Australian Prescriber 2003; 26:78–81. Online. Available: http://www.australianprescriber.com/magazine/26/4/78/81/

Cameron C. Serotonin syndrome precipitated by an over-the-counter cold remedy. Australian Prescriber 2006; 29:71. Online. Available: http://www.australianprescriber.com/magazine/29/3/artid/802/

Alcohol

Australian Institute of Health and Welfare 2003. Statistics on drug use in Australia, 2002. AIHW Cat. No. PHE 43. Canberra: AIHW (Drug Statistics Series No. 12).

Australian Institute of Health and Welfare 2006. Australia's Health, 2006. AIHW Cat No. AUS 73. Canberra: AIHW:158.

Hulse G, White J, Cape G. Management of alcohol and drug problems. UK: Oxford University Press; 2002.

Lee NK. Alcohol intervention. What works? Aust Fam Physician 2008; 37(12):16–19.

World Health Organization. The ICD-10 Classification of mental and behavioural disorders: diagnostic criteria for research. Geneva: WHO; 1993.

Tobacco

Australian Institute of Health and Welfare 2006. Australia's Health 2006. AIHW Cat No. AUS 73. Canberra: AIHW:158.
Hulse G, White J, Cape G. Management of alcohol and drug problems. UK: Oxford University Press; 2002.
Zwar N. Smoking cessation: what works? Aust Fam Physician 2008; 37(1/2):10–14.

Cannabis

Australian National Council on Drugs. Cannabis: answers to your questions, http://www.ancd.org.au/publications/index.htm
Montebello ME. Cannabis-related disorders. Medical Observer 2006; 19 May:27–30.
ANCD. Evidence-based answers to cannabis questions—a review of the literature, http://www.ancd.org.au/publications/index.htm
Hulse G, White J, Cape G. Management of alcohol and drug problems. UK: Oxford University Press; 2002.

Benzodiazepines

Cockayne L. Detoxification from benzodiazepines. PowerPoint presentation, http://www.sdf.org.uk/sdf/files/Benzos%20Conf%2007%20Lucy%20Cockayne.ppt
Morin CM, Bastien C, Guay B et al. Randomized clinical trial of supervised tapering and cognitive behavior therapy to facilitate benzodiazepine discontinuation in older adults with chronic insomnia. Am J Psychiatry 2004; 161:332–342. Online. Available: http://ajp.psychiatryonline.org/cgi/reprint/161/2/332
Benzodiazepines, http://nawrot.psych.ndsu.nodak.edu/Courses/465Projects06/Benzo/Index.htm
Ashton CH. The diagnosis and management of benzodiazepine dependence. Curr Opinion Psychiatry 2005; 18(3):249–255.
Longo LP, Johnson B. Addiction: Part I. Benzodiazepines: side effects, abuse risk and alternatives. Am Family Physician 2000; 61(7):2121–2127.
Oude Voshaar RC, Couvee JE, Vanbalkom AJLM et al. Strategies for discontinuing long-term benzodiazepine use. Br J Psychiatry 2006; 189:213–220.
Peles E, Hetzroni T, Bar-Hamburger R et al. Melatonin for perceived sleep disturbances associated with benzodiazepine withdrawal among patients in methadone maintenance treatment: a double-blind randomized clinical trial. Addiction 2007; 102(12):1947–1953.

Prescription and OTC

Australian Institute of Health and Welfare. Statistics on drug use in Australia, 2004. Canberra: AIHW; 2005:18.
Bell JR. Australian trends in opioid prescribing for chronic non-cancer pain, 1986–1996. Med J Aust 1997; 167(1):26–29.
New drugs. Australian Prescriber 1999, 22(5):125–127; 2001, 24(2):43–47; 2004, 27(1):21–23.
NSW Therapeutic Assessment Group. Low back pain. Rational use of opioids in chronic or recurrent non-malignant pain, http://www.ciap.health.nsw.gov.au/nswtag/publications/guidelines/LowBackPain41202.pdf
US Department of Health and Human Services. Results from the 2005 National Survey on Drug Use and Health: National Findings, http://www.oas.samhsa.gov/nsduh/2k5nsduh/2k5Results.pdf

Psychostimulants

Baker A, Kay-Lambkin F, Lee NK et al. A brief cognitive behavioural intervention for regular amphetamine users. Australian Government Department of Health and Ageing, 2009.
Khong E. The growing challenge of party drugs in general practice. Aust Family Physician 2004; 33:709–713.
Sidis A, Haber P. Psychostimulants and party drugs. Australian Doctor, March 2005: 25–32.

REFERENCES

1 World Health Organization. Management of substance abuse: Alcohol. Online. Available: http://www.who.int/substance_abuse/publications/alcohol/en/index.html
2 Mathers CD, Vos ET, Christopher E et al. The burden of disease and injury in Australia. Bull World Health Org 2001; 79(11). Online. Available: http://www.scielosp.org/scielo.php?pid=S0042-96862001001100013&script=sci_arttext&tlng=en
3 Australian Institute of Health and Welfare. Burden of disease and injury in Australia. Executive summary. Online. Available: http://www.aihw.gov.au/publications/hwe/bodaiia03/bodaiia03-c01.pdf
4 Kim MJ, Shim MS, Kim MK et al. Effect of chronic alcohol ingestion on bone mineral density in males without liver cirrhosis. Korean J Intern Med 2003; 18(3):174–180.
5 Australian Government, Department of Health and Ageing. Australian guidelines to reduce health risks from drinking alcohol. Online. Available: http://www.health.gov.au/internet/alcohol/publishing.nsf/Content/guidelines. Last updated 2010.
6 Kownacki RJ, Shadish WR. Does Alcoholics Anonymous work? The results from a meta-analysis of controlled experiments. Subst Use Misuse 1999; 34(13):1897–1916. Online. Available: http://www.ncbi.nlm.nih.gov/pubmed/10540977
7 Linde K, Vickers A, Hondras M et al. Systematic reviews of complementary therapies—an annotated

bibliography. Part 1: Acupuncture. BMC Comp Altern Med 2001; 1:3. Online. Available: http://www.biomedcentral.com/1472-6882/1/3

8 Carai MA, Agabio R, Bombardelli E et al. Potential use of medicinal plants in the treatment of alcoholism. Fitoterapia 2000; 71(Suppl 1):S38–S42.

9 Schuppan D, Strösser W, Burkard G et al. Legalon® lessens fibrosing activity in patients with chronic liver diseases. Zeits Allgemeinmed 1998;74:577–584.

10 Zwar N. Smoking cessation: What works? Aust Fam Physician 2008; 37(1/2):10–14.

11 Hays JT, Ebbert JO, Sood A. Efficacy and safety of varenicline for smoking cessation. Am J Med 2008; 121(Suppl 1):S32–S42. Online. Available: http://www.ncbi.nlm.nih.gov/pubmed/18342165

12 Saunders JB, Yang J. Clinical protocols for detoxification. Alcohol and Drug Services, Royal Brisbane Hospital and Prince Charles Hospital Health Service Districts; 2002. Online. Available: http://www.health.qld.gov.au/atod/documents/24904.pdf

13 United States Department of Health and Human Services. National Survey on Drug Use and Health; 2007. Online. Available: http://www.icpsr.umich.edu/icpsrweb/SAMHDA/studies/23782/detail;jsessionid=E775EAA4F9D3824AE281A26F3FA7DAD0

14 Australian Government, Department of Health and Ageing. Hydromorphone hydrochloride. PBS public summary document; 2005. Online. Available: http://www.health.gov.au/internet/main/publishing.nsf/Content/pbac-psd-hydromorphone

appendix 1

Herb/nutrient–drug interactions

NOTES

ASSUMPTIONS

The following assumptions were made when collating and assessing information for this table:

- The clinical significance of many interactions is still unknown because controlled trials are lacking in most cases. In these instances, interactions are based on evidence of pharmacological activity and case reports, and have a sound theoretical basis, although remain to be tested.
- All information refers to oral dose forms unless otherwise specified.
- Information is correct at the time of writing; however, because of the ever-expanding knowledge base developing in this area, new research is constantly being published.
- The interaction table is provided as a guide only and should not replace the use of professional judgment. It has been developed to assist clinicians when advising patients.

USING THIS GUIDE IN PRACTICE

- Commonly used prescription and over-the-counter medications are organised by therapeutic class and subclass and are listed alphabetically.
- Common names have been used when referring to herbs.

RECOMMENDATIONS

Avoid—There may be insufficient information available to be able to advise using the two substances safely together, so avoid until more is known. The drug may have a narrow therapeutic index and there is sufficient evidence to suggest that the interaction may be clinically significant. Consider an alternative treatment that is unlikely to produce an undesirable interaction.

Avoid use unless under medical supervision—Harmful effects of the potential interaction can be avoided if doses are altered appropriately under professional supervision or the patient is closely monitored. Some of these interactions can be manipulated to the advantage of the patient. Changes to the dosage regimen may be required for safe combined use.

Exercise caution—The possibility exists of an interaction that may change effects clinically; be aware and monitor. It is prudent to tell patients to be aware and seek advice if they are concerned.

Observe—Interaction may not be clinically significant at the usual recommended doses and may be theoretical; however, the clinician should be alert to the possibility of an interaction.

Beneficial interaction possible—Prescribing the interacting substance may improve clinical outcomes; for example, reducing drug requirements, complementing drug effects, reducing drug side effects, counteracting nutritional deficiencies caused by drugs, alleviating drug withdrawal symptoms, and enhancing patient wellbeing.

Drug	Herb or supplement	Potential outcome	Recommendation	Evidence/Comments
ALLERGIC DISORDERS				
Antihistamines				
Antihistamines and mast-cell-stabilising drugs	Albizia	Has additive effects.	Beneficial interaction possible.	Both in vitro and in vivo tests have reported significant mast-cell-stabilisation effects similar to those of cromoglycate—clinical significance unknown.
	Baical skullcap	Additive effects.	Beneficial interaction possible.	Luteolin and baicalein have been shown to inhibit IgE antibody-mediated immediate- and late-phase allergic reactions in mice—clinical significance unknown.
	Perilla	Additive effects.	Observe—drug dose may need modification.	Perilla seed extract has been shown to inhibit histamine release from mast cells in a dose-dependent manner—clinical significance unknown
ANALGESIA				
Narcotic analgesics				
Codeine	Adhatoda	Additive effects.	Beneficial interaction possible.	Theoretically will increase antitussive effects of drug.
	Kava kava	Additive effects.	Exercise caution.	Increased CNS depression theoretically possible.
Morphine	Kava kava	Additive effects.	Exercise caution—may be beneficial under professional supervision.	Increased CNS depression theoretically possible.
	Tyrosine	Additive effects.	Observe—potential beneficial interaction under professional supervision.	Tyrosine potentiates morphine-induced analgesia by 154% in mice.
	Withania	Reduced morphine tolerance/ dependence.	Beneficial interaction possible with professional supervision.	In animal studies, repeated administration of withania (100 mg/kg) inhibited morphine tolerance and dependence, so it is sometimes used in opiate withdrawal.
Simple analgesics and antipyretics				
Simple analgesics and antipyretics	Meadowsweet	Additive effects.	Observe—beneficial interaction possible.	Additive anti-inflammatory and analgesic effects theoretically possible.

(continues)

Drug	Herb or supplement	Potential outcome	Recommendation	Evidence/Comments
ANALGESIA (continued)				
Simple analgesics and antipyretics (continued)	Vitamin E	Additive effects.	Beneficial interaction possible. Drug dosage may require modification.	Vitamin E may enhance the pain-modifying effects of drug in RA.
	Willowbark	Additive effects.	Observe—beneficial interaction possible.	Additive anti-inflammatory and analgesic effects theoretically possible.
Aspirin	Andrographis	Increased bruising and bleeding.	Observe.	Herb inhibits platelet aggregation, observed in animal and clinical studies.
	Bilberry	Increased bruising and bleeding.	Exercise caution with high-dose (> 170 mg) anthocyanadins unless under medical supervision.	Dose is extremely high and not relevant to clinical practice.
	Evening primrose oil	Increased bruising and bleeding.	Observe, although beneficial interaction possible.	Theoretically concomitant use may enhance anti-inflammatory and antiplatelet effects—clinical significance unknown.
	Feverfew	Increased bruising and bleeding.	Interaction unlikely but observe.	Feverfew inhibits platelet aggregation in vitro and in vivo, no effects were seen in clinical study; however, contradictory evidence exists.
	Fish oils	Additive effects.	Observe—beneficial interaction possible.	No haemorrhagic effects were seen in a clinical study—theoretical concern only if increased bruising or bleeding. Pharmacological activity of fish oils may have benefits for some patients taking aspirin for CVD prevention or for its anti-inflammatory properties.
	Garlic	Increased bruising and bleeding.	Interaction unlikely at usual doses. Observe when using higher doses (> 7 g).	Theoretically, a pharmacodynamic interaction is possible when using garlic at high doses (> 7 g) in excess of usual dietary amounts; however, results from clinical studies cast doubt on this proposition.

Drug	Herb or supplement	Potential outcome	Recommendation	Evidence/Comments
ANALGESIA (continued)				
Aspirin (continued)	Ginger	Increased bruising and bleeding.	Interaction unlikely at usual doses. Exercise caution at high dose (> 10 g) unless under professional supervision.	Inhibits platelet aggregation at very high doses—dietary intake appears safe.
	Ginkgo biloba	Increased bruising and bleeding.	Interaction unlikely.	Pharmacodynamic interaction theoretically possible because of platelet-activating-factor inhibitor activity; however, clinical trials show no significant change to bleeding or platelet activity, so interaction unlikely to be significant.
	Grapeseed extract	Increased bruising and bleeding.	Observe.	Theoretically may enhance antiplatelet activity and anti-inflammatory activity of aspirin and may increase risk of bleeding.
	Guarana	Increased bruising and bleeding.	Observe.	Theoretically possible as in vitro and in vivo research has identified antiplatelet activity—clinical significance unknown.
	Meadowsweet	Increased bruising and bleeding.	Observe—beneficial interaction possible.	Theoretically may enhance anti-inflammatory and antiplatelet effects.
	Myrrh	Increased bruising and bleeding.	Observe with myrrh preparations. Exercise caution with guggul preparations.	Guggul inhibited platelet aggregation in vitro and in a clinical study, so concurrent use may theoretically increase the risk of bleeding—implications for *Commiphora molmol* use unclear.
	Policosanol	Increased bruising and bleeding.	Observe.	Doses > 10 mg/day may inhibit platelet aggregation.
	Turmeric	Increased bruising and bleeding.	Observe with concentrated extracts.	Curcumin inhibits platelet aggregation in vitro and in vivo—clinical significance is unclear and likely to be dose dependent.

(continues)

Drug	Herb or supplement	Potential outcome	Recommendation	Evidence/Comments
ANALGESIA (continued)				
Aspirin (continued)	Vitamin C	Decreased vitamin C effects.	Observe.	Aspirin may interfere with both absorption and cellular uptake mechanisms for vitamin C, thereby increasing vitamin C requirements, as observed in animal and human studies. Increased vitamin C intake may be required with long-term therapy.
	Willowbark	Increased bruising and bleeding.	Exercise caution with high dose (> 240 mg/day).	Theoretically may enhance anti-inflammatory and antiplatelet effects. Although a clinical study found that consumption of salicin 240 mg/day produced minimal effects on platelet aggregation, higher doses may have a significant effect.
Paracetamol	Andrographis	Reduced side effects.	Beneficial interaction possible	Andrographis may exert hepatoprotective activity against liver damage induced by paracetamol.
	Garlic	Reduced side effects.	Beneficial interaction possible.	Garlic may exert hepatoprotective activity against liver damage induced by paracetamol.
	Quercetin	Reduced side effects.	Beneficial interaction possible.	Quercetin may exert hepatoprotective activity against liver damage induced by paracetamol.
	St Mary's thistle	Reduced side effects.	Beneficial interaction possible under professional supervision.	St Mary's thistle may exert hepatoprotective activity against liver damage induced by paracetamol.
	SAMe	Reduced side effects.	Beneficial interaction possible.	SAMe may exert hepatoprotective activity against liver damage induced by paracetamol.
	Schisandra	Reduced side effects.	Beneficial interaction possible.	Schisandra may exert hepatoprotective activity against liver damage induced by paracetamol.
CARDIOVASCULAR SYSTEM				
Anti-angina agents				
Nitroglycerin/ glyceryl trinitrate (e.g. anginine)	Arginine	Additive hypotensive effects.	Caution.	Theoretically, additive vasodilation and hypotensive effects may occur.

Drug	Herb or supplement	Potential outcome	Recommendation	Evidence/Comments
CARDIOVASCULAR SYSTEM (continued)				
Nitroglycerin/ glyceryl trinitrate (continued)	Vitamin E	Prevention of drug tolerance.	Beneficial interaction possible.	Oral vitamin E prevented nitrate tolerance when given concurrently with transdermal nitroglycerin (10 mg/24 h) according to one randomised placebo-controlled study
Anti-impotence				
Phosphodiesterase-5 inhibitor (e.g. Sildenafil)	Arginine	Additive effects.	Exercise caution.	Theoretically, additive vasodilation and hypotensive effects may occur.
Anti-arrhythmic agents				
	Astragalus	Additive effects.	Observe.	Additive effects are theoretically possible with IV administration of astragalus, based on positive inotropic activity identified in clinical studies; the clinical significance of these findings for oral dose forms is unknown.
	Devil's claw	Additive effects.	Observe.	Devil's claw has demonstrated anti-arrhythmic activity, but interaction is theoretical and clinical significance is unclear.
	Hawthorn	Additive effects.	Observe.	Hawthorn has demonstrated anti-arrhythmic activity in vitro and in vivo, but interaction is theoretical and clinical significance is unclear.
	Magnesium	Additive effects.	Observe.	High-dose oral magnesium has demonstrated anti-arrhythmic activity according to one clinical trial.
Amiodarone	Vitamin B_6 (pyridoxine)	Increased drug side effects.	Exercise caution.	Vitamin B_6 may increase risk of drug-induced photosensitivity.
Anticoagulants, antiplatelets Monitor bleeding time and signs and symptoms of excessive bleeding				
Anticoagulants (e.g. warfarin)	Andrographis	Increased bruising and bleeding.	Exercise caution—monitor bleeding time.	Andrographolide and other constituents of andrographis are clinically confirmed to inhibit platelet-activating-factor-induced platelet aggregation.

(continues)

Drug	Herb or supplement	Potential outcome	Recommendation	Evidence/Comments
CARDIOVASCULAR SYSTEM (continued)				
Anticoagulants (continued)	Baical skullcap	Increased risk of bruising and bleeding.	Exercise caution.	Baical flavonoids have been shown to inhibit platelet aggregation in vitro—clinical significance unknown.
	Carnitine	Increased bruising and bleeding.	Observe.	According to one case report, L-carnitine 1 g/day may potentiate the anticoagulant effects of acenocoumarol. Further investigation required to confirm interaction.
	Celery	Increased bruising and bleeding.	Observe with high dose extracts.	Although celery contains naturally occurring coumarins, interaction is unlikely.
	Chamomile	Increased bruising and bleeding.	Observe.	According to one case report, internal haemorrhage occurred in elderly patient taking warfarin and topical and oral chamomile preparations. Further investigation required to confirm interaction.
	Chondroitin	Increased bruising and bleeding.	Observe.	Theoretical risk; not observed in clinical trials.
	Coenzyme Q10	Reduced drug effects.	Interaction unlikely with standard doses. Observe patients taking high doses.	A double-blind crossover study found that oral CoQ10 100 mg/day had no significant effect on INR or warfarin levels; however, in vivo tests using 10 mg/kg/day CoQ10 decreased serum concentrations of warfarin by increasing drug metabolism.
	Cranberry	Increased bruising and bleeding.	Exercise caution—due to potential seriousness of interaction.	Clinical investigations are conflicting. However a recent study suggests a pharmocodynamic interaction is likely. Monitor INR closely.
	Devil's claw	Increased bruising and bleeding.	Observe until clinical studies can confirm interaction.	Case reports suggest possible anticoagulant activity but most are inconclusive. Further investigation required to confirm interaction.

Drug	Herb or supplement	Potential outcome	Recommendation	Evidence/Comments
CARDIOVASCULAR SYSTEM (continued)				
Anticoagulants (continued)	Dong quai	Increased bruising and bleeding.	Observe with oral supplements.	A controlled trial using an IV preparation of dong quai found that it prolonged prothrombin times, but it is unknown whether this effect occurs with oral dose forms.
	Evening primrose oil	Increased bruising and bleeding.	Exercise caution—monitor bleeding time, signs and symptoms.	Gamma-linoleic acid in evening primrose oil affects prostaglandin synthesis, leading to inhibition of platelet aggregation—clinical significance is unknown.
	Fenugreek	Increased bruising and bleeding.	Interaction unlikely.	While it contains naturally occurring coumarins, a placebo-controlled study found no effect on platelet aggregation, fibrinogen or fibrinolytic activity.
	Feverfew	Increased bruising and bleeding.	Interaction unlikely. Observe.	Although feverfew inhibits platelet aggregation in vitro and in vivo, no effects were seen in a clinical study.
	Fish oils	Increased bruising and bleeding.	Interaction unlikely at usual therapeutic doses. Exercise caution with very high doses (> 12 g) unless under medical supervision.	A review of clinical studies concluded there was no clinically significant effect on bleeding with usual therapeutic doses. According to one clinical study, bleeding time may be increased at high doses of 12 g/day.
	Garlic	Increased bruising and bleeding.	Interaction unlikely at usual dietary intake. Exercise caution with use of high dose (> 7 g) supplements.	Theoretically, a pharmacodynamic interaction is possible when using garlic at high doses (> 7 g) in excess of usual dietary amounts; however, results from clinical studies cast doubt on this proposition.
	Ginger	Increased bruising and bleeding.	Observe at usual therapeutic doses. Exercise caution at high dose (> 10 g).	Inhibits platelet aggregation at high doses.

(continues)

Drug	Herb or supplement	Potential outcome	Recommendation	Evidence/Comments
CARDIOVASCULAR SYSTEM (continued)				
Anticoagulants (continued)	Ginkgo biloba	Increased bruising and bleeding.	Interaction unlikely based on clinical trials. Observe high risk patients—due to potential seriousness of interaction.	Theoretically ginkgo may increase bleeding and there have been several case reports of haemorrhage; however, evidence from clinical studies does not support this. Ginkgo has no effect on pharmacokinetics, pharmacodynamics or clinical effects of warfarin. This is supported by a recent systematic review.
	Ginseng—Korean	Possibly increased bruising and bleeding.	Observe.	Two case reports have indicated ginseng reduced antithrombotic effects of warfarin. In vitro and in vivo ginseng has demonstrated inhibition of platelet aggregation; however, a recent open-label study found no effect of ginseng on warfarin in healthy males.
	Ginseng—Siberian	Increased bruising and bleeding.	Observe.	In vivo study demonstrated that an isolated constituent in Siberian ginseng has anticoagulant activity and a clinical trial found a reduction in blood coagulation induced by intensive training in athletes—whether these effects also occur in non-athletes is unknown. A recent combination study of Siberian ginseng, andrographis and warfarin produced no significant effects on drug pharmacokinetics and pharmacodynamics.
	Glucosamine		Exercise caution until interaction can be confirmed.	Case reports suggest a possible interaction with warfarin.
	Goji	Increased bruising and bleeding.	Exercise caution until interaction confirmed clinically.	Two case reports of interaction between goji and warfarin producing altered INR. Further investigation required to confirm interaction.
	Grapeseed extract	Increased bruising and bleeding.	Exercise caution until interaction confirmed clinically.	Inhibits platelet aggregation in vitro and ex vivo—clinical significance unknown.

Drug	Herb or supplement	Potential outcome	Recommendation	Evidence/Comments
CARDIOVASCULAR SYSTEM (continued)				
Anticoagulants (continued)	Green tea	Reduced drug effects.	Exercise caution with high doses.	A case report of excessive intake (2.25–4.5 L green tea daily) was reported to inhibit warfarin activity and decrease INR. Further investigation required to confirm interaction.
	Guarana	Increased bruising and bleeding.	Exercise caution until interaction confirmed clinically.	In vitro and in vivo research has identified antiplatelet activity—clinical significance unknown.
	Horseradish	Increased bruising and bleeding risk.	Interaction unlikely.	Although it contains coumarins, interaction unlikely.
	Licorice	Increased bruising and bleeding.	Exercise caution until interaction confirmed clinically.	Isoliquiritigenin inhibits platelet aggregation, and glycyrrhizin inhibits prothrombin, according to in vitro and in vivo tests—clinical significance unknown.
	Meadowsweet	Increased bruising and bleeding.	Observe until interaction confirmed clinically.	In vitro tests have indicated anticoagulant activity—clinical significance unknown.
	Myrrh	Increased bruising and bleeding.	Observe with myrrh preparations. Exercise caution with guggul preparations.	Guggul inhibited platelet aggregation in vitro and in a clinical study, so concurrent use may theoretically increase the risk of bleeding—implications for *Commiphora molmol* use unclear.
	Policosanol	Increased bruising and bleeding.	Exercise caution with doses > 10 mg daily.	Current evidence is contradictory, as one study failed to detect an interaction between policosanol and warfarin, but others have found that doses > 10 mg/day may inhibit platelet aggregation.
	Psyllium	Decreased drug absorption.	Separate doses by at least 1 hour.	

(continues)

Drug	Herb or supplement	Potential outcome	Recommendation	Evidence/Comments
CARDIOVASCULAR SYSTEM (continued)				
Anticoagulants (continued)	Red clover	Increased bruising and bleeding.	Interaction unlikely.	Theoretically, coumarin content could exert anticoagulant activity; however, dicoumarol produced by micro-organisms in poorly dried sweet clover has established anticoagulant effects. Interaction unlikely from extracts prepared from properly dried red clover.
	Rosemary	Increased bruising and bleeding.	Exercise caution with concentrated extracts until interaction confirmed clinically.	Rosemary demonstrates antithrombotic activity in vitro and in vivo—clinical significance unknown.
	St John's wort (unlikely to relate to low-hyperforin-containing products)	Decreased drug effects.	Exercise caution—monitor for signs of reduced drug effectiveness and adjust dose if necessary. Prothrombin time or INR should be closely monitored with addition or withdrawal of St John's wort.	Metabolism of warfarin is chiefly by CYP2C9, and a minor metabolic pathway is CYP3A4, so theoretically it may interact with St John's wort. A clinical study found no change to INR or platelet aggregation, but there are case reports suggesting St John's wort may lower the INR.
	Slippery elm	Decreased drug absorption.	Separate doses by at least 2 hours.	Theoretical interaction—clinical significance unknown.
	Turmeric	Increased bruising and bleeding.	Exercise caution with concentrated extracts until interaction confirmed clinically.	Curcumin inhibits platelet aggregation in vitro and in vivo—concomitant use with high dose turmeric may theoretically increase risk of bleeding.
	Vitamin E	Increased bruising and bleeding.	Exercise caution with high-dose supplements (> 1000 IU daily). Until clinical significance can be established, prothrombin time or INR should be closely monitored with addition or withdrawal of high-dose vitamin E supplements.	Clinical studies have produced conflicting results: several found no effects of platelet aggregation or coagulation, although others found an increased bleeding risk. Clinical study of 1200 IU/d for 28 days had no effects on platelet aggregation; another of 900 IU/d for 12 weeks did not alter coagulation activity. Alternatively 50 mg/d increased gingival bleeding. Overall, it appears people with reduced levels of vitamin K may be more susceptible to the effects of vitamin E potentiating warfarin activity.

Drug	Herb or supplement	Potential outcome	Recommendation	Evidence/Comments
CARDIOVASCULAR SYSTEM (continued)				
Anticoagulants (continued)	Willow bark	Increased bruising and bleeding.	Exercise caution with high dose (> 240 mg/day).	Theoretically, may enhance anti-inflammatory and antiplatelet effects. Although a clinical study found that consumption of salicin 240 mg/day produced minimal effects on platelet aggregation, higher doses may have a significant effect.
Antiplatelet drugs (e.g. aspirin)	Andrographis	Increased bruising and bleeding.	Observe.	Herb inhibits platelet aggregation, observed in animal and clinical studies.
	Bilberry	Increased bruising and bleeding.	Exercise caution with high-dose (> 170 mg) anthocyanadins unless under medical supervision.	Dose is extremely high and not relevant to clinical practice.
	Evening primrose oil	Increased bruising and bleeding.	Observe, although beneficial interaction possible.	Theoretically, concomitant use may enhance anti-inflammatory and antiplatelet effects—clinical significance unknown.
	Feverfew	Increased bruising and bleeding.	Observe.	Feverfew inhibits platelet aggregation in vitro and in vivo; no effects were seen in clinical study; however, contradictory evidence exists.
	Fish oils	Additive effects.	Observe—beneficial interaction possible.	No haemorrhagic effects were seen in a clinical study—theoretical concern. Pharmacological activity of fish oils may have benefits for some patients taking aspirin for CVD prevention or for its anti-inflammatory properties.
	Garlic	Increased bruising and bleeding.	Interaction unlikely.	Theoretically, may enhance platelet aggregation. Recent clinical investigation found garlic had no effect on platelet function.
	Ginger	Increased bruising and bleeding.	Interaction unlikely at standard intake. Exercise caution at high dose (> 10 g) unless under professional supervision.	Inhibits platelet aggregation at very high doses.

(continues)

Drug	Herb or supplement	Potential outcome	Recommendation	Evidence/Comments
CARDIOVASCULAR SYSTEM (continued)				
Antiplatelet drugs (continued)	Ginkgo biloba	Increased bruising and bleeding.	Interaction unlikely.	Theoretically possible because of platelet-activating-factor inhibitor activity. There are rare case reports of haemorrhage and haematoma; however, clinical trials show no significant change to bleeding or platelet activity. This is confirmed in a recent systematic review.
	Grapeseed extract	Increased bruising and bleeding.	Observe.	Theoretically, may enhance antiplatelet activity.
	Guarana	Increased bruising and bleeding.	Observe.	Theoretically possible, as in vitro and in vivo research has identified antiplatelet activity—clinical significance unknown.
	Meadowsweet	Increased bruising and bleeding.	Observe—beneficial interaction possible.	Theoretically may enhance anti-inflammatory and antiplatelet effects.
	Myrrh	Increased bruising and bleeding.	Observe with myrrh preparations. Exercise caution with guggul preparations.	Guggul inhibited platelet aggregation in vitro and in a clinical study, so concurrent use may theoretically increase the risk of bleeding—implications for *Commiphora molmol* use unclear.
	Policosanol	Increased bruising and bleeding.	Observe.	Doses > 10 mg/day may inhibit platelet aggregation.
	Turmeric	Increased bruising and bleeding.	Observe with concentrated extracts.	Curcumin inhibits platelet aggregation in vitro and in vivo—clinical significance is unclear and likely to be dose dependent.
	Vitamin C	Decreased vitamin C effects.	Observe.	Aspirin may interfere with both absorption and cellular uptake mechanisms for vitamin C, thereby increasing vitamin C requirements, as observed in animal and human studies. Increased vitamin C intake may be required with long-term therapy.

Drug	Herb or supplement	Potential outcome	Recommendation	Evidence/Comments
CARDIOVASCULAR SYSTEM (continued)				
Antiplatelet drugs (continued)	Willow bark	Increased bruising and bleeding.	Interaction unlikely at usual doses. Exercise caution with high dose (> 240 mg/day)	Theoretically, may enhance anti-inflammatory and antiplatelet effects. Although a clinical study found that consumption of salicin 240 mg/day produced minimal effects on platelet aggregation, higher doses may have a significant effect.
Antihypertensive agents				
Antihypertensive drugs	Arginine	Additive hypotensive effects.	Exercise caution.	Theoretical concern.
	Essential fatty acids—omega-3 and omega-6	Increased drug effects.	Observe—beneficial interaction possible.	Both omega-3 and omega-6 fatty acids exhibit mild antihypertensive activity.
	Evening primrose oil	Additive effects.	Observe—monitor drug requirements (interaction may be beneficial).	Evening primrose oil has been shown to enhance the effects of several antihypertensive drugs, including dihydralazine, clonidine and captopril in rats under experimental conditions.
	Garlic	Additive effects.	Observe—beneficial interaction possible.	Clinical trials have shown garlic to reduce blood pressure, which may lead to reduced drug requirements.
	Hawthorn	Additive effects.	Observe—beneficial interaction possible.	Mild antihypertensive activity has been reported with long-term use of hawthorn, which may lead to reduced drug requirements.
	Licorice	Reduced drug effect.	Exercise caution—monitor blood pressure when high-dose licorice preparations are taken for more than 2 weeks.	High-dose glycyrrhizin taken long-term can lead to increased blood pressure.
	Oats (oat-based cereals)	Additive effects.	Observe—monitor drug requirements (interaction may be beneficial).	A clinical trial has shown that ingestion of oat-based cereals decreased blood pressure in 73% of hypertensive patients and reduced drug requirements. Patients taking oats, oat milk and oat bran should be monitored.

(continues)

Drug	Herb or supplement	Potential outcome	Recommendation	Evidence/Comments
CARDIOVASCULAR SYSTEM (continued)				
Antihypertensive drugs (continued)	Olive leaf and olive oil	Additive effects.	Possible beneficial interaction possible under professional supervision.	Theoretical, as hypotensive effects have been observed with olive oil and olive leaf extracts.
	Stinging nettle	Additive effects.	Observe.	Additive effects are theoretically possible.
Hydralazine (e.g. Apresoline, Alphapress)	Coenzyme Q10	Reduced CoQ10 serum levels.	Beneficial interaction possible.	Increased CoQ10 intake may be required with long-term therapy.
	Vitamin B_6 (pyridoxine)	Reduced vitamin B_6 absorption.	Separate doses by at least 2 hours.	A clinical trial has shown that the drug may induce B_6 deficiency, so increased intake may be required with long-term therapy.
Methyldopa (e.g. Aldomet)	Coenzyme Q10	Reduced CoQ10 serum levels.	Beneficial interaction possible.	Increased CoQ10 intake may be required with long-term therapy.
ACE inhibitors (e.g. captopril, enalapril)	Iron	Reduced drug effect.	Separate doses by at least 2 hours.	Reduced absorption of ACE inhibitors. A small clinical trial found that concomitant iron administration reduced area-under-the-curve plasma levels of unconjugated captopril by 37%.
	Zinc	Reduced zinc levels.	Monitor for zinc efficacy and zinc status.	These drugs increase urinary excretion of zinc. Increased zinc intake may be required with long-term therapy.
Verapamil	St John's wort	Reduces drug levels via increased metabolism.	Monitor and adjust dose as necessary	Decreases drug serum levels via CYP induction.
Beta-adrenergic-blocking agents	Coenzyme Q10	Reduced CoQ10 serum levels.	Beneficial interaction possible.	Increased CoQ10 intake may be required with long-term therapy.
	Calcium	Reduced drug effects.	Separate doses by at least 2 hours.	Simultaneous use can reduce both agents. Separate doses by 2 hours.
Propranolol	Myrrh	Reduced drug effect.	Observe.	A clinical trial has shown that guggulipid reduces bioavailability of propranolol. It is uncertain what implications this has for use of *Commiphora molmol*.

Drug	Herb or supplement	Potential outcome	Recommendation	Evidence/Comments
CARDIOVASCULAR SYSTEM (continued)				
Propranolol (continued)	Vitamin E	Reduced drug effect.	Observe.	According to in vitro research, vitamin E inhibits drug uptake in human cultured fibroblasts—clinical significance unknown.
Calcium-channel blockers (e.g. verapamil)	Calcium	Reduced drug effect.	Avoid high-dose supplements unless under medical supervision.	Calcium may reduce antihypertensive effect of drug.
	Magnesium	Additive effects.	Observe—monitor drug requirements (interaction may be beneficial).	A meta-analysis of 20 randomised trials showed that magnesium has a modest antihypertensive activity and may enhance the activity of calcium-channel blockers.
	Vitamin D	Reduced drug effect.	Exercise caution unless under medical supervision.	Vitamin D may reduce effectiveness of these drugs.
Felodipine	Peppermint oil	Increased drug effects.	Exercise caution.	Peppermint oil has been shown to increase the oral bioavailability of felodipine in animal studies.
Nifedipine	Ginseng—Korean	Increased drug effects.	Exercise caution.	
	St John's wort	Reduced drug effect.	Monitor for signs of reduced drug effectiveness—adjust dose where necessary.	St John's wort has been shown to induce nifedipine metabolism.
Diltiazem	Myrrh	Reduced drug effect.	Observe.	A clinical trial has shown that guggulipid reduces bioavailability of diltiazem. It is uncertain what implications this has for use of *Commiphora molmol*.
	Quercetin	Increased drug effects.	Exercise caution under professional supervision; drug dose may need adjustment.	Increased drug bioavailability observed in vivo—clinical significance unknown.
Antimigraine preparations				
Antimigraine preparations	Coenzyme Q10	Additive effects.	Beneficial interaction possible.	CoQ10 demonstrated migraine-prevention activity in a clinical study.
	Feverfew	Additive effects.	Beneficial interaction possible.	Feverfew demonstrated migraine-prevention activity in several clinical studies.

(continues)

Drug	Herb or supplement	Potential outcome	Recommendation	Evidence/Comments
CARDIOVASCULAR SYSTEM (continued)				
Antimigraine preparations (continued)	Vitamin B_2 (riboflavin)	Additive effects.	Beneficial interaction possible.	Vitamin B_2 has demonstrated migraine-prevention activity in several clinical studies.
Clonidine (e.g. Catapres)	Coenzyme Q10	Reduced CoQ10 serum levels.	Beneficial interaction possible.	In vivo study indicates that clonidine reduces serum CoQ10 levels. Increased CoQ10 intake may be required with long-term therapy.
Cardiac inotropic agents				
Cardiac glycosides	Calcium	Additive effects.	Exercise caution.	Concurrent use of high-dose calcium can act synergistically and may induce arrhythmias and potentiate their toxicity.
Cardiac glycosides	Hawthorn	Additive effects.	Exercise caution—monitor drug requirements (interaction may be beneficial).	Theoretical interaction, as in vitro and in vivo studies indicate that hawthorn has positive inotropic activity. Small clinical study found interaction not clinically significant when digoxin 0.25 mg taken with hawthorn (WS1442) 450 mg twice daily.
	Psyllium	Reduced drug absorption.	Separate doses by at least 1 hour.	Soluble fibre may decrease the bioavailability of cardiac glycosides.
Digoxin (e.g. Lanoxin) Adverse effects of high-dose digoxin include: nausea, vomiting, diarrhoea, confusion, fainting, palpitations, irregular heartbeat, visual disturbances.	Aloe vera	Increased drug toxicity.	Avoid long-term use of high-dose preparations.	Long-term oral use of aloe can deplete potassium levels and reduced potassium status lowers the threshold for drug toxicity.
	Ginseng—Korean	Interferes with therapeutic drug monitoring for digoxin.	Exercise caution—drug assay may produce false positive and negative results.	There are no confirmed clinical case reports of actual interaction.
	Guarana	Increased drug toxicity.	Avoid long-term use of high-dose preparations.	Long-term guarana use can deplete potassium levels and reduced potassium status lowers the threshold for drug toxicity.

Drug	Herb or supplement	Potential outcome	Recommendation	Evidence/Comments
CARDIOVASCULAR SYSTEM (continued)				
Digoxin (continued)	Licorice	Increased drug toxicity.	Avoid long-term use of high-dose preparations (> 100 mg glycyrrhizin daily > 2 weeks) unless under medical supervision.	Long-term use of licorice can induce hypokalaemia, which can increase sensitivity to cardiac glycoside drugs, thereby reducing the threshold for drug toxicity. One case report exists of digitalis toxicity in an elderly man taking licorice-containing Chinese herbal laxative.
	Quercetin	Increased drug toxicity.	Avoid concurrent use owing to seriousness of interaction.	Increased drug bioavailability possible, observed by in vivo study.
	St John's wort	Reduced drug effects.	Avoid unless under medical supervision. Monitor for signs of reduced drug effectiveness and adjust dose if necessary. When St John's wort is started or ceased, monitor serum levels and alter drug dosage as required.	St John's wort induces CYP enzymes and P-glycoprotein. A clinical trial shows that St John's wort significantly decreases serum levels of drug within 10 days of concomitant use. More recently herb drug interaction was found to be clinically significant.
	Slippery elm	Decreased drug absorption.	Separate doses by at least 2 hours.	Theoretical interaction—clinical significance unknown.
	Withania	Interferes with therapeutic drug monitoring for digoxin.	Exercise caution—drug assays may be modestly altered.	
Diuretics				
Diuretics	Dandelion leaf	Additive effects.	Observe.	Theoretically, increased diuresis is possible—clinical significance is unknown.
	Elder	Additive effects.	Observe.	Theoretically, increased diuresis is possible with concomitant use; clinical significance is unknown.
	Green tea	Additive effects.	Observe.	Theoretically, increased diuresis possible owing to caffeine content of herb—clinical significance is unknown.
	Guarana	Additive diuretic effects but decreased hypotensive effects of drug.	Exercise caution. Monitor potassium status.	Theoretically, increased diuresis and decreased hypotensive effects are possible—clinical significance is unknown.

(continues)

Drug	Herb or supplement	Potential outcome	Recommendation	Evidence/Comments
CARDIOVASCULAR SYSTEM (continued)				
Diuretics (continued)	Licorice	Increased potassium excretion.	Avoid long-term use unless under medical supervision. Monitor potassium status.	Potassium loss may become significant when licorice is used in high doses (> 100 mg glycyrrhizin daily) for longer than 2 weeks.
Loop diuretics	Magnesium	Increased magnesium excretion.	Monitor magnesium efficacy and status—beneficial interaction possible.	Increased magnesium intake may be required with long-term therapy.
	Stinging nettle	Additive effects.	Observe.	Theoretically, increased diuresis is possible—clinical significance is unknown.
	Vitamin B_1 (thiamin)	Reduced B_1 levels.	Monitor B_1 efficacy and status—beneficial interaction possible.	Chronic use may result in lowered vitamin status. Increase intake of vitamin B_1-containing foods or consider long-term supplementation.
	Zinc	Increased urinary zinc excretion.	Monitor zinc efficacy and status—beneficial interaction possible.	Increased zinc intake may be required with long-term therapy.
Potassium-sparing diuretics	Magnesium	Increased magnesium effects.	Observe.	
Thiazide diuretics	Calcium	Decreased urinary calcium excretion.	Observe. Monitor serum calcium and look for signs of hypercalcaemia.	
	Magnesium	Increased magnesium excretion.	Monitor magnesium efficacy and status—beneficial interaction possible.	Increased magnesium intake may be required with long-term therapy.
	Zinc	Increased urinary zinc excretion.	Monitor zinc efficacy and status—beneficial interaction possible.	Increased zinc intake may be required with long-term therapy.
Hydrochlorothiazide (e.g. Diclotride)	Coenzyme Q10	Reduced CoQ10 serum levels.	Beneficial interaction possible.	Increased CoQ10 intake may be required with long-term therapy.
	Vitamin B_{12} (cobalamin)	Reduces drug-induced hyper-homocysteinaemia.	Beneficial interaction possible in conjunction with folate.	Hydrochlorothiazide may increase homocysteine levels.

Drug	Herb or supplement	Potential outcome	Recommendation	Evidence/Comments
CARDIOVASCULAR SYSTEM (continued)				
Hypolipidaemic agents				
Hypolipidaemic agents	Chromium	Additive effects.	Observe. Monitor drug requirements—interaction may be beneficial.	Clinical trials indicate that chromium reduces total cholesterol levels.
	Evening primrose oil	Additive effects.	Observe—interaction may be beneficial.	Several animal studies have demonstrated EPO's lipid-lowering effects—clinical significance unknown.
	Fenugreek	Additive effects.	Observe. Monitor drug requirements—interaction may be beneficial.	Clinical trials indicate that fenugreek exerts a lipid-lowering activity in diabetics with elevated lipids.
	Garlic	Additive effects.	Observe. Monitor drug requirements—interaction may be beneficial.	A meta-analysis of 13 clinical trials concluded that garlic significantly reduces total cholesterol levels—effects are described as modest.
	Myrrh	Additive effects.	Observe. Monitor drug requirements—interaction may be beneficial for guggul preparations.	Guggul has demonstrated cholesterol-lowering activity in several clinical studies.
	Oats (oat-based cereals)	Reduced drug absorption. Additive effects.	Separate doses by 2–3 hours. Beneficial interaction possible—monitor drug requirements.	Clinical trials indicate that oat-based cereals reduce total cholesterol levels. However, two case reports exist of a reduced effect of lovastatin in patients taking 50–100 g oat bran daily. This effect is probably due to the fibre content inhibiting the absorption of the drug.
	Policosanol	Additive effects.	Interaction uncertain	Pharmacodynamic interaction previously thought possible; however, recent clinical studies cast doubt on this.
	Psyllium	Additive effects.	Beneficial interaction possible	Recent meta-analysis confirmed the capacity of psyllium to exert a time- and dose-dependent cholesterol-lowering effect.
	Red yeast rice	Additive effects.	Observe—beneficial interaction possible. Drug dose may require modification.	Red yeast rice contains low levels of naturally occurring statins, which exert clinically significant lipid-lowering activity.

(continues)

Drug	Herb or supplement	Potential outcome	Recommendation	Evidence/Comments
CARDIOVASCULAR SYSTEM (continued)				
Hypolipidaemic agents (continued)	Vitamin B_3 (niacin)	Additive effects.	Beneficial interaction possible—caution with sustained-release form.	Several clinical trials confirm the cholesterol-lowering activity of niacin and the safety of niacin with statins; however, the sustained-release form may be less safe.
Cholestyramine (e.g. Questran Lite, colestipol [e.g. Colestid])	Fat-soluble vitamins (A, D, E, K, beta-carotene)	Reduced vitamin absorption.	Separate doses by at least 4 hours and monitor vitamin status.	Increased dietary intake may be required or consider vitamin supplementation with long-term therapy.
	Folate	Reduced folate absorption.	Separate doses by at least 4 hours and monitor iron status.	Increased vitamin intake may be required with long-term therapy.
	Iron	Reduced iron absorption.	Separate doses by at least 4 hours and monitor iron status	Investigations have shown that cholestyramine and colestipol bind to iron citrate. Increased iron intake may be required with long-term therapy.
	Lutein and zeaxanthin	Reduced vitamin absorption.		Increased vitamin intake may be required with long-term therapy.
	Lycopene	Reduced vitamin absorption.	Separate doses by at least 2 hours and monitor vitamin status.	Drugs that reduce fat absorption may also reduce lycopene absorption. Increased vitamin intake may be required with long-term therapy.
	Vitamin D	Reduced vitamin absorption.	Separate doses by at least 1 hour prior to or 4–6 hours after drug ingestion.	Such drugs may compromise the absorption of all fat-soluble vitamins.
	Vitamin E	Reduced vitamin absorption.	Separate doses by at least 4 hours and monitor vitamin status.	Increased vitamin intake may be required with long-term therapy.
Chitosan	Vitamin C	May increase cholesterol-lowering effect.	Beneficial interaction possible.	According to preliminary animal study, concomitant use may provide additional benefit in lowering cholesterol.
Fibric acid derivatives (e.g. gemfibrozil)	Coenzyme Q10	Reduced CoQ10 serum levels.	Beneficial interaction possible—separate doses by 4 hours.	Increased CoQ10 intake may be required with long-term therapy.

Drug	Herb or supplement	Potential outcome	Recommendation	Evidence/Comments
CARDIOVASCULAR SYSTEM (continued)				
Fibric acid derivatives (continued)	Beta-carotene	Improved drug effects.	Beneficial interaction possible	In clinical studies, a positive interaction was established between fibrate and beta-carotene, generating significantly increased HDL-cholesterol levels.
HMG-CoA reductase inhibitors (statins)	Carnitine	Additive effects.	Beneficial interaction.	Human studies have demonstrated the addition of L-carnitine to statin therapy lowers serum lipoprotein (a) levels in patients with type 2 diabetes.
	Coenzyme Q10	Reduced CoQ10 serum levels.	Beneficial interaction possible.	Clinical study indicates several statin drugs reduce CoQ10 levels—increased CoQ10 intake may be required with long-term therapy.
	Vitamin A	Increased vitamin A activity.	Observe.	A clinical trial has reported increased serum levels of vitamin A—clinical significance unclear.
	Vitamin B_3 (niacin)	Additive effects.	Beneficial interaction possible—caution with sustained-release form.	Several clinical trials confirm the cholesterol-lowering activity of niacin and the safety of niacin with statin; however, the sustained-release form may be less safe.
	Vitamin D	Increased vitamin effects.	Monitor nutrient status	Through unknown mechanisms long-term use of statins is associated with increased 25(OH)-D level—clinical significance is unknown.
Pravastatin (e.g. Pravachol)	Fish oils	Additive effects.	Beneficial interaction possible.	A clinical trial suggests improved lipid-lowering effects when used concurrently. In particular, fish oils will lower triglycerides.
Simvastatin (e.g. Lipex, Zocor)	Peppermint oil	Additive effects.	Observe. Monitor drug requirements—interaction may be beneficial.	Peppermint oil has been shown to increase the oral bioavailability of simvastatin in animal studies—clinical significance unknown.
	St John's wort	Reduced drug effects.	Monitor for signs of reduced drug effectiveness and adjust the dose if necessary.	St John's wort increases metabolism of simvastatin (interaction not expected with pravastatin).

(continues)

Drug	Herb or supplement	Potential outcome	Recommendation	Evidence/Comments
CENTRAL NERVOUS SYSTEM				
Anticonvulsants				
Anticonvulsants	Carnitine	Reduced side effects.	Beneficial interaction possible.	L-Carnitine deficiency may cause or potentiate valproic acid toxicity, and supplementation is known to reduce the toxicity of valproate as well as symptoms of fatigue—concurrent use is recommended, as a beneficial interaction is possible.
	Folate	Reduced side effects.	Monitor for drug effectiveness. Beneficial interaction possible.	Requires close supervision to ensure that drug efficacy is not substantially reduced.
	Ginkgo biloba	Reduced drug effects.	Observe.	Based on case reports—further investigation required.
	Psyllium	Reduced drug absorption.	Separate doses by 1–1.5 hours before or after drug.	Absorption of drug concomitantly with psyllium may be delayed.
	St John's wort	Reduced drug effects.	Avoid unless under medical supervision to alter doses appropriately. When St John's wort is started or ceased, monitor serum levels and alter drug dosage as required.	St John's wort may increase drug metabolism, resulting in reduced drug efficacy.
Carbamazepine (e.g. Tegretol) NTI: signs of overdose include CNS and respiratory depression, hypotension, vomiting, fluid retention.	St Mary's thistle	Increased drug effects.	Exercise caution—monitor drug requirements.	May reduce metabolism of drug resulting in increased serum levels and adverse effects (difficult to evaluate evidence).
	Vitamin B_{12} (Cobalamin)	Decreased B_{12} levels.	Observe for signs and symptoms of B_{12} deficiency. Beneficial interaction possible.	In studies with children, long-term carbamazepine use led to a decrease in vitamin B_{12} levels. Increased intake may be required with long-term therapy.
Phenobarbitone	Celery	Prolonged action.	Exercise caution	Celery juice has been found to prolong the action of phenobarbitone in rats—clinical significance unknown.

Drug	Herb or supplement	Potential outcome	Recommendation	Evidence/Comments
CENTRAL NERVOUS SYSTEM (continued)				
Phenobarbitone (continued)	Withania	Increased sedation.	Observe, although beneficial interaction possible under professional supervision.	
Phenobarbitone and phenytoin	Kava kava	Increased sedation.	Exercise caution.	
	St John's wort	Decreased drug effects (increased drug metabolism).	Avoid—monitor drug requirements. When St John's wort is started or ceased, monitor serum levels and alter drug dosage as required.	St John's wort may increase drug metabolism, resulting in reduced drug efficacy.
	Vitamin B_{12} (cobalamin)	Increased serum B_{12} levels.	Observe.	One clinical study reported that combined long-term use of phenobarbital and phenytoin resulted in significantly increased serum B_{12} levels—clinical significance unknown.
Phenytoin	Vitamin B_6 (pyridoxine)	Reduced drug effects.	Exercise caution—monitor for reduced drug effectiveness.	Vitamin B_6 supplements may lower plasma levels and efficacy of drug and decrease seizure control.
	Slippery elm	Decreased drug absorption.	Separate doses by at least 2 hours.	Theoretical interaction—clinical significance unknown.
Phenytoin and valproate	Vitamin D	Reduced nutrient effects.	Beneficial interaction possible.	Anticonvulsants induce catabolism of vitamin D through liver induction—prolonged use is associated with increased risk of developing rickets and osteomalacia; therefore, increased intake may be useful with long-term therapy.
Valproate	Beta-carotene	Reduced nutrient status.	Observe.	Epileptics who gain weight on valprolate were found to have reduced plasma concentrations of beta-carotene and other fat-soluble vitamins—which is reversible after valproate withdrawal. Increased intake may be necessary with long-term therapy.

(continues)

Drug	Herb or supplement	Potential outcome	Recommendation	Evidence/Comments
CENTRAL NERVOUS SYSTEM (continued)				
Antidepressants				
Antidepressants including SSRIs, SNRIs, tricyclics and MAOIs	Albizia	Additive effects.	Observe.	Increased risk of serotonergic syndrome is theoretically possible, as the herb increases serotonin levels, according to in vivo studies—clinical significance unknown.
	Ginkgo biloba	Reduced side effects.	Beneficial interaction possible.	Initial open study produced significant improvement in SSRI-induced sexual dysfunction; however, more recent investigations have been inconclusive. Clinical significance difficult to ascertain.
	Lavender	Additive effects.	Observe—beneficial interaction possible	Lavender may have additive effects.
	St John's wort	Additive effects.	Avoid unless under medical supervision to monitor dose requirements.	Risk of serotonergic syndrome if combined use is not carefully monitored; however, increased antidepressant activity is also possible with appropriate doses.
	SAMe	Additive effects.	Exercise caution.	Theoretically may increase risk of serotonergic syndrome, and a case report exists; however, an experimental study found that brain SAMe levels were significantly reduced after chronic treatment with imipramine, so may be useful adjunctive therapy.
	Tyrosine	Additive effects.	Avoid unless under medical supervision.	Tyrosine is a precursor for several neurotransmitters, which theoretically increases risk of serotonin syndrome.
	Zinc	Improved drug efficacy.	Beneficial interaction possible.	Clinical study has shown 25 mg/d zinc for 2 weeks improves the efficacy of SSRIs and tricyclic antidepressants.
MAOIs	Tyrosine	Increased side effects.	Avoid—unless under medical supervision.	Some tyrosine may be metabolised to tyramine. Concurrent use with MAOIs may lead to hypertensive crisis.

Drug	Herb or supplement	Potential outcome	Recommendation	Evidence/Comments
CENTRAL NERVOUS SYSTEM (continued)				
MAOIs (continued)	Rhodiola	Additive effect.	Observe.	Recent in vitro data suggests inhibition of MAO A by rhodiola extracts. A theoretical interaction exists with MAOI antidepressants. Clinical significance yet unknown.
Tricyclic antidepressants	Andrographis	Reduced side effects.	Beneficial interaction possible.	Andrographis may exert hepatoprotective activity against liver damage induced by tricyclic antidepressants.
	Coenzyme Q10	Reduced CoQ10 serum levels.	Beneficial interaction possible.	Increased CoQ10 intake may be required with long-term therapy.
	St John's wort (reduction in drug plasma levels)	Additive effects.	Avoid unless under medical supervision.	Although St John's wort decreases drug plasma levels of tricyclic antidepressants, it may increase available serotonin.
	St Mary's thistle	Reduced side effects.	Beneficial interaction possible.	St Mary's thistle may exert hepatoprotective activity against liver damage induced by tricyclic antidepressants.
	Vitamin B_2 (riboflavin)	Reduced nutrient absorption.	Monitor for signs and symptoms of B_2 deficiency—beneficial interaction possible.	Tricyclic antidepressants may reduce the absorption of riboflavin. Increased vitamin B_2 intake may be required with long-term therapy.
Amitryptyline	Vitamin B_2 (riboflavin)	Increased nutrient excretion.	Monitor for signs and symptoms of deficiency.	Amitryptyline has been found to increase the renal excretion of riboflavin. Increased dietary intake may be required with long-term therapy.
Imipramine	Vitamin B_3 (niacin)	Additive effects.	Beneficial interaction possible.	A combination of imipramine with L-tryptophan 6 g/day and niacinamide 1500 mg/day has been shown to be more effective for people with bipolar disorder than imipramine alone.
Lithium	Psyllium	Reduced drug absorption.	Separate dose by 1 hour or after drug.	Soluble fibre may decrease bioavailability of drug.
	Slippery elm	Decreased drug absorption.	Separate doses by at least 2 hours.	Theoretical interaction—clinical significance unknown.

(continues)

Drug	Herb or supplement	Potential outcome	Recommendation	Evidence/Comments
CENTRAL NERVOUS SYSTEM (continued)				
Lithium (continued)	Vitamin B_{12} (cobalamin)	Reduced nutrient status.	Monitor B_{12} status.	Lithium administration is shown to decrease serum B_{12} concentrations—clinical significance unclear.
Antipsychotic agents				
Haloperidol (e.g. Serenace)	Ginkgo biloba	Increased drug effects and reduced side effects.	Observe—beneficial interaction possible under professional supervision.	Three clinical trials demonstrate that ginkgo increases drug effectiveness.
	Iron	Reduced iron effect.	Monitor iron status.	May cause decreased blood levels of iron—clinical significance unclear. Increased iron intake may be required with long-term therapy.
	Quercetin	Reduced drug side effects.	Beneficial interaction possible. under professional supervision.	According to in vivo studies, co-administration with quercetin dose-dependently reduced haloperidol-induced chewing movements and tongue protrusions.
	Withania	Reduced drug side effects.	Beneficial interaction possible under professional supervision.	According to in vivo studies, withania is beneficial in the treatment of drug-induced dyskinesia—reduced chewing movements and tongue protrusions possible with concurrent use.
Phenothiazines (e.g. chlorpromazine, trifluoperazine)	Evening primrose oil	Reduced drug effects.	Avoid concomitant use.	Several case reports suggest that evening primrose oil may reduce seizure threshold and reduce drug effectiveness in patients with schizophrenia treated with phenothiazines.
	Coenzyme Q10	Reduced drug-induced side effects.	Beneficial interaction.	Coenzyme Q10 reduces adverse effects of this drug class on CoQ10-related enzymes NADH-oxidase and succinoxidase.
Chlorpromazine (e.g. Largactil)	Vitamin E	Reduced drug effects.	Observe.	According to in vitro research, vitamin E inhibits drug uptake in human cultured fibroblasts—clinical significance unknown.

Drug	Herb or supplement	Potential outcome	Recommendation	Evidence/Comments
CENTRAL NERVOUS SYSTEM (continued)				
Atypical anti-psychotic agents				
Olanzapine (e.g. Clozapine)	Ginkgo	Enhanced drug effects.	Beneficial interaction possible under professional supervision.	According to placebo-controlled trial, ginkgo may enhance drug effect on negative affect refractory schizophrenic patients.
CNS agents				
Cholinergic drugs (tacrine [e.g. Cognex])	Brahmi	Additive effects.	Observe—beneficial interaction possible under professional supervision.	Cholinergic activity has been identified for brahmi, so increased drug activity is theoretically possible.
	Ginkgo biloba	Additive effects.	Observe—beneficial interaction possible.	Cholinergic activity has been identified for ginkgo, so increased drug activity is theoretically possible.
	Lemon balm	Additive effects.	Observe—beneficial interaction possible.	Cholinergic activity has been identified for lemon balm, so increased drug activity is theoretically possible.
	St Mary's thistle	Reduced side effects.	Beneficial interaction possible.	St Mary's thistle may exert hepatoprotective activity against liver damage induced by tacrine.
CNS stimulants	Green tea	Additive effect.	Observe.	Theoretical increase of CNS-stimulant effects of drugs such as nicotine and beta-adrenergic agonists—clinical significance is unknown.
	Guarana	Additive effects.	Exercise caution.	Herb has demonstrated CNS-stimulant activity.
	Tyrosine	Additive effects.	Exercise caution.	Tyrosine is a precursor for several neurotransmitters.
Amphetamines	Tyrosine	Increased side effects.	Observe.	Tyrosine (200 and 400 mg/kg) has been shown to increase side effects of anorexia caused by ephedrine and amphetamine in a dose-dependent manner in rats—clinical significance unknown.
Methylphenidate	Zinc	Improved drug efficacy.	Beneficial interaction possible.	Clinical study of ADHD children with co-administration of 15 mg zinc for 6 weeks demonstrated improved drug efficacy.

(continues)

Drug	Herb or supplement	Potential outcome	Recommendation	Evidence/Comments
CENTRAL NERVOUS SYSTEM (continued)				
Movement disorders				
L-Dopa (levodopa)	Calcium	Reduced drug absorption.	Separate doses by 2 hours.	L-dopa can form an insoluble complex with calcium.
	Iron	Reduced drug effect.	Separate doses by 2 hours.	May reduce bioavailability of carbidopa and L-dopa, which can form an insoluble complex with iron.
	Kava kava	Reduced drug effects.	Avoid unless under medical supervision.	Theoretical interaction, as dopamine antagonist effects have been reported for kava kava.
	Magnesium	Reduced drug absorption.	Separate doses by 2 hours.	L-dopa can form an insoluble complex with magnesium.
	SAMe	Reduced drug effectiveness.	Observe.	Theoretical interaction, as SAMe methylates levodopa. Interaction not observed clinically.
	Tyrosine	Decreased drug and tyrosine effect.	Avoid unless under medical supervision.	L-Dopa competes with tyrosine for uptake, so concurrent use may decrease uptake of both substances, thereby reducing efficacy.
	Vitamin B_6 (pyridoxine)	Increased nutrient requirements.	Observe—beneficial interaction possible under medical supervision.	L-dopa can cause hyperhomocysteinaemia in Parkinson's disease (PD) patients, relative to vitamin B status. Vitamin B requirements are higher in L-dopa treated patients, as such supplementation may be warranted in PD patients.
	Vitamin C	Reduced side effects.	Beneficial interaction possible.	A case report of co-administration with vitamin C suggests this may reduce drug side effects.
	Zinc	Reduced drug absorption.	Separate doses by 2 hours.	L-Dopa can form an insoluble complex with zinc.
L-Dopa with carbidopa	Iron	Reduced drug effect.	Separate doses by at least 2 hours.	May reduce bioavailability of carbidopa and L-dopa, which can form an insoluble complex with iron.

Drug	Herb or supplement	Potential outcome	Recommendation	Evidence/Comments
CENTRAL NERVOUS SYSTEM (continued)				
Sedatives, hypnotics				
CNS sedatives	Eucalyptus	Additive effects.	Exercise caution.	Theoretical interaction, as oral ingestion of eucalyptus has been associated with CNS depression.
	Green tea	Additive effects.	Observe.	Theoretically, high intakes can decrease the CNS-depressant effects of drugs such as benzodiazepines—clinical significance is unknown.
	Guarana	Reduced drug effects.	Observe.	Theoretically, guarana may reduce the sedative effects of drug via its CNS-stimulant effects; however, an in vivo study found no interaction with pentobarbital.
	Hops	Additive effects.	Observe.	Additive effects theoretically possible, generating increased sedation; interaction may be beneficial in benzodiazepine withdrawal.
	Kava kava	Additive effects.	Exercise caution. Monitor drug dosage—beneficial interaction possible under medical supervision.	May be useful in benzodiazepine withdrawal.
	Lavender	Additive effects.	Observe—beneficial interaction possible under professional supervision.	Theoretically, lavender may potentiate the effects of sedatives.
	Passionflower	Additive effects.	Exercise caution. Beneficial interaction possible under medical supervision—monitor drug dosage.	Increased sedation; interaction may be beneficial in benzodiazepine withdrawal.
	Valerian	Additive effects.	Observe—beneficial interaction possible under medical supervision.	Increased sedation; interaction may be beneficial in benzodiazepine withdrawal.

(continues)

Drug	Herb or supplement	Potential outcome	Recommendation	Evidence/Comments
CENTRAL NERVOUS SYSTEM (continued)				
Midazolam (e.g. Hypnovel)	St John's wort	Reduced drug effects.	Exercise caution. Monitor for signs of reduced drug effectiveness and adjust the dose if necessary.	St John's wort may increase drug metabolism and so reduce serum levels of drug.
Barbiturates	Albizia	Additive effects.	Exercise caution—beneficial interaction possible under medical supervision.	Potentiating of phenobarbitone-induced sleeping was observed in vivo—clinical significance unknown.
	Andrographis	Additive effects.	Observe—beneficial interaction possible under medical supervision.	Potentiating effects observed in vivo—clinical significance unknown.
	Folate	Reduced drug effects.	Exercise caution. Monitor for signs of reduced drug effectiveness.	Concomitant folic acid use can reduce seizure control—supervision may be required.
	Kava kava	Additive effects.	Exercise caution. Beneficial interaction possible under medical supervision—monitor drug dosage.	Increased sedation effects.
	Lemon balm	Additive effects.	Observe—beneficial interaction possible under medical supervision.	Increased sedation effects; one animal study found increased sedative effects from co-administration of lemon balm and pentobarbital—clinical significance unknown.
	Passionflower	Additive effects.	Exercise caution. Beneficial interaction possible under medical supervision—monitor drug dosage.	Additive CNS sedation is theoretically possible.
	St John's wort (may not relate to low-hyperforin-containing products)	Reduced drug effects.	Avoid—monitor drug requirements. When St John's wort is started or ceased, monitor serum levels and alter drug dosage as required.	St John's wort induces CYP enzymes and P-glycoprotein, so can reduce drug serum levels.

Drug	Herb or supplement	Potential outcome	Recommendation	Evidence/Comments
CENTRAL NERVOUS SYSTEM (continued)				
Barbiturates (continued)	Slippery elm	Decreased drug absorption.	Separate doses by at least 2 hours.	Theoretical interaction—clinical significance unknown.
	Valerian	Additive effects.	Observe—beneficial interaction possible under medical supervision.	Increased sedation; interaction may be beneficial in benzodiazepine withdrawal.
	Vitamin B_6 (pyridoxine)	Reduced plasma levels and drug effects.	Caution. Monitor for drug effectiveness.	Concomitant B_6 use can reduce seizure control—supervision may be required.
	Withania	Additive effects.	Observe—beneficial interaction possible under medical supervision	Theoretically may increase sedation.
Benzodiazepines	Chamomile	Additive effects.	Observe — beneficial interaction possible under medical supervision.	Theoretically, an additive effect can occur with concurrent use.
	Kava kava	Additive effects.	Exercise caution. Beneficial interaction possible under medical supervision—monitor drug dosage.	Combination has been used to ease symptoms of benzodiazepine withdrawal under medical supervision.
	Passionflower	Additive effects at high doses.	Exercise caution. Beneficial interaction possible under medical supervision—monitor drug dosage.	May be useful in benzodiazepine withdrawal.
	St John's wort	Decreased drug effects.	Exercise caution—monitor for signs of reduced drug effectiveness.	St John's wort induces CYP enzymes and P-glycoprotein, so can reduce drug serum levels.
	Valerian	Additive effects.	Observe—beneficial interaction possible under medical supervision.	Combination has been used to ease symptoms of benzodiazepine withdrawal under medical supervision.

(continues)

Drug	Herb or supplement	Potential outcome	Recommendation	Evidence/Comments
CENTRAL NERVOUS SYSTEM (continued)				
Benzodiazepines (continued)	Withania	Additive effects.	Observe—beneficial interaction possible under medical supervision.	Increased sedative effect theoretically possible.
CONTRACEPTIVE AGENTS				
Combined oral contraceptive agents				
Oral contraceptive pill (OCP)	Chaste tree	Reduced herb effects.	Observe.	There has been speculation as to whether chaste tree is effective when OCP is being taken. Several clinical studies conducted in women taking OCP have confirmed that chaste tree still reduces symptoms of premenstrual syndrome.
	Folate	Reduced folate levels.	Beneficial interaction possible.	Folate levels are reduced with long-term use. Increased intake may be required with long-term therapy.
	Licorice	Increased side effects.	Observe. Exercise caution with high-dose licorice (> 100 mg/day glycyrrhizin) or long-term use (> 2 weeks). Monitor patients closely.	Increased risk of side effects such as hypokalaemia, fluid retention and elevated blood pressure have been noted in case reports.
	St John's wort	Reduced drug effects.	Exercise caution—avoid use with low-dose OCP.	Breakthrough bleeding has been reported in 12 cases, which may indicate decreased effectiveness. Caution related to hyperforin content. Recent investigations demonstrate low hyperforin extracts appear safe with OCP use.
	Vitamin A	Increased vitamin A levels.	Exercise caution with large doses of retinol.	OCP increases serum vitamin A levels due to longer storage in the liver.
	Vitamin B_2 (riboflavin)	Reduced vitamin B_2 levels.	Beneficial interaction possible.	OCP may increase demand for vitamin B_2. Increased intake may be required with long-term therapy.
	Vitamin B_3 (niacin)	Reduced vitamin B_3 levels.	Beneficial interaction possible.	Increased intake may be required with long-term therapy.
	Vitamin B_5 (pantothenic acid)	Reduced vitamin B_5 levels.	Beneficial interaction possible.	Increase dietary intake of foods rich in vitamin B_5 or consider supplementation.

Drug	Herb or supplement	Potential outcome	Recommendation	Evidence/Comments
CONTRACEPTIVE AGENTS (continued)				
Oral contraceptive pill (OCP) (continued)	Vitamin B_6 (pyridoxine)	Reduced vitamin B_6 levels.	Beneficial interaction possible.	OCP may induce pyridoxine deficiency. Increase dietary intake of foods rich in vitamin B_6 rich or consider supplementation.
	Vitamin B_{12} (cobalamin)	Reduced vitamin B_{12} levels.	Observe for signs and symptoms of B_{12} deficiency—beneficial interaction possible.	OCP users showed significantly lower concentrations of cobalamin than controls in a clinical study; however, this may be due to an effect upon B_{12}-binding proteins. Increased intake may be required with long-term therapy.
ENDOCRINE AND METABOLIC DISORDERS				
Adrenal steroid hormones				
Corticosteroids	Calcium	Reduced side effects. Reduced nutrient status.	Beneficial interaction possible.	Through inhibiting vitamin D-mediated calcium absorption, overall levels may be decreased. Increased calcium intake may be required with long-term therapy.
	Chromium	Reduced side effects.	Beneficial interaction possible.	Corticosteroids increase urinary losses of chromium, and chromium supplementation has been shown to aid in recovery from steroid-induced diabetes mellitus.
	Licorice	Additive effects.	Beneficial interaction possible but patients should be monitored closely for corticosteroid excess.	Concurrent use of licorice preparations potentiates the effects of topical and oral corticosteroids (e.g. prednisolone) as glycyrrhizin inhibits the metabolism of prednisolone. Some practitioners use licorice to minimise requirements for, or to aid in withdrawal of, corticosteroid medications.
	Vitamin B_{12} (cobalamin)	Reduced nutrient status.	Monitor nutrient status—beneficial interaction possible.	Decreased B_{12} levels have been identified in serum and cerebrospinal fluid of multiple sclerosis patients following high-dose 1000 mg/10 days IV methylprednisolone. Supplementation may be indicated.

(continues)

Drug	Herb or supplement	Potential outcome	Recommendation	Evidence/Comments
ENDOCRINE AND METABOLIC DISORDERS (continued)				
Corticosteroids (continued)	Vitamin C	Reduced vitamin C effects.	Beneficial interaction possible.	May increase requirement for vitamin C based on in vitro and in vivo data. Increased intake may be required with long-term therapy.
	Vitamin D	Reduced nutrient status.	Beneficial interaction possible.	Decreases levels of active vitamin D via an unknown mechanism. During long-term therapy of oral or inhaled corticosteroids, vitamin D supplementation should be considered.
Betamethasone	Carnitine	Additive effects.	Beneficial interaction possible.	RCT has shown that a combination of low-dose betamethasone (2 mg/day) and L-carnitine (4 g/5 days) was more effective in preventing respiratory distress syndrome (7.3% vs 14.5%) and death (1.8% vs 7.3%) in preterm infants than high-dose betamethasone given alone (8 mg/2 days).
Agents affecting calcium and bone metabolism				
Alendronate (e.g. Fosamax) and etidronate (e.g. Didronel)	Calcium	Reduced drug absorption.	Separate doses by at least 2 hours.	Calcium may reduce drug absorption; however, adequate calcium is required for optimal drug effects.
	Iron	Reduced drug absorption.	Separate doses by at least 2 hours.	
	Magnesium	Reduced drug absorption.	Separate doses by at least 2 hours.	Magnesium may reduce drug absorption; however, adequate magnesium is required for optimal drug effects.
	Zinc	Reduced drug absorption.	Separate doses by at least 2 hours.	
Gonadal hormones				
Oestrogen	Chromium	Improved nutrient status.	Beneficial effects.	Women receiving HRT appear to have improved chromium status. Combination therapy has been suggested to inhibit IL-6.
	Hops	Additive effects.	Observe.	Theoretical interaction, based on mild oestrogenic effect of hops.

Drug	Herb or supplement	Potential outcome	Recommendation	Evidence/Comments
ENDOCRINE AND METABOLIC DISORDERS (continued)				
Oestrogen (continued)	Red clover	Reduced drug effects.	Observe.	Theoretically, if taken in large quantities phyto-oestrogens may compete with synthetic oestrogens for receptor binding; however, a review considered 2 mg/kg of red-clover-derived isoflavones to be a safe dose for most patients.
Oestrogen and progesterone	Calcium	Additive effects.	Beneficial interaction possible.	Possible beneficial interaction on bone mineralization.
	Licorice	Increased side effects.	Observe. Exercise caution with high-dose licorice or long-term use (> 2 weeks).	OCP can increase sensitivity to glycyrrhizin side effects such as hypertension, fluid retention, hypokalaemia.
Testosterone	Licorice	Altered testosterone effect.	Observe. Monitor testosterone levels.	Contradictory evidence suggests possible effects on testosterone levels.
	Saw palmetto	Reduced drug effectiveness.	Observe. Monitor drug efficacy.	Theoretically may reduce effectiveness of therapeutic androgens.
Haemopoietic agents				
Erythropoietin	Ginseng—Korean	Enhanced drug effects.	Beneficial interaction possible.	The total saponin fraction has been shown to promote haemopoiesis—clinical significance for total herb unknown.
	Iron	Additive pharmacological effect.	Beneficial interaction possible.	IV iron supplementation demonstrated improved success of darbepoetin in chemotherapy-related anaemia without iron deficiency without increasing toxicity.
	Withania	Enhanced drug effects.	Beneficial interaction possible.	Animal studies indicate herb increases haematopoiesis—clinical significance unknown.
Antidiabetic agents				
Thioglitazones (e.g. rosiglitazone & pioglitazone)	Quercetin	Enhanced drug effects.	Exercise caution.	Due to potential for toxicity careful monitoring of hepatic and cardiac function is required.
Sulfonylurea antidiabetic (e.g. gliclazide)	St John's wort	Reduced drug effects.	Avoid—unless under professional supervision—monitor drug effectiveness.	St John's wort found to induce significant clearance of gliclazide.

(continues)

Drug	Herb or supplement	Potential outcome	Recommendation	Evidence/Comments
ENDOCRINE AND METABOLIC DISORDERS (continued)				
Hypoglycaemic agents				
Hypoglycaemic (e.g. metformin) agents. Adverse effects associated with increased hypoglycaemic effects include sweating, hunger, depression, tremor and headaches.	Aloe vera	Additive effects.	Observe.	Oral aloe vera may have hypoglycaemic activity, so additive effects are theoretically possible.
	Andrographis	Additive effects.	Exercise caution—blood glucose levels should be checked regularly—beneficial interaction possible under professional supervision.	Andrographis has hypoglycaemic activity comparable to that of metformin in vivo, so additive effects are theoretically possible.
	Bilberry	Additive effects.	Observe.	Animal study identified that the constituent myrtillin exerts hypoglycaemic actions—relevance for bilberry unclear.
	Bitter melon	Additive effects.	Exercise caution. Monitor drug requirements—possible beneficial effect under professional supervision.	
	Chromium	Additive effects.	Exercise caution. Monitor drug requirements—beneficial interaction possible under professional supervision.	Clinical studies have shown that chromium has hypoglycaemic activity in some individuals.
	Cinnamon	Additive effects.	Observe—potentially beneficial interaction under professional supervision.	Clinical studies have produced contradictory results.
	Damiana	Additive effects.	Observe.	Theoretically possible—clinical significance is unknown.
	Elder	Additive effects.	Observe.	Hypoglycaemic effects demonstrated in vitro—clinical significance is unknown.

Drug	Herb or supplement	Potential outcome	Recommendation	Evidence/Comments
ENDOCRINE AND METABOLIC DISORDERS (continued)				
Hypoglycaemic agents (continued)	Eucalyptus	Additive effects.	Exercise caution—monitor blood glucose levels.	If used orally in combination with glucose-lowering agents may contribute to hypoglycaemia.
	Fenugreek	Additive effects.	Exercise caution—blood glucose levels should be checked regularly. Beneficial interaction possible under professional supervision.	
	Ginseng—Siberian	Additive effects.	Observe.	Speculation is based on IV use in animal studies and has not been observed in humans with oral dose forms.
	Green tea	Additive effects.	Observe.	High intake of caffeine-containing drinks can increase blood sugar; however, green tea is reported to be hypoglycaemic, which may negate this effect—clinical significance of combination uncertain.
	Gymnema sylvestre	Additive effects.	Exercise caution. Interaction may be beneficial—reduction in drug dose may be achieved.	Gymnema may theoretically enhance blood-glucose-lowering effects of insulin and hypoglycemic agents.
	Horse chestnut	Additive effects.	Observe—monitor blood glucose levels.	Horse chestnut exerts a hypoglycaemic activity. Concurrent use with hypoglycaemic agents required monitoring of blood glucose levels—clinical significance is unclear.
	Myrrh	Additive effects.	Exercise caution—blood glucose levels should be checked regularly. Beneficial interaction possible.	Myrrh has been shown to increase glucose tolerance in both normal and diabetic rats—clinical significance unknown.
	Oats	Additive effects.	Exercise caution—beneficial interaction possible under medical supervision. Insulin requirements should be monitored.	In an uncontrolled pilot study, an oatmeal intervention reduced insulin requirements by 42.5%.

(continues)

Drug	Herb or supplement	Potential outcome	Recommendation	Evidence/Comments
ENDOCRINE AND METABOLIC DISORDERS (continued)				
Hypoglycaemic agents (continued)	Olive leaf extract	Additive effects.	Beneficial interaction possible under professional supervision—drug dose may need modification.	Olive leaf has demonstrated a hypoglycaemic activity in animal models. Theoretically an interaction is possible, though speculative.
	Psyllium	Additive effects.	Beneficial interaction possible under professional supervision. Drug dose may need modification.	Psyllium has clinically demonstrated a capacity to slow the absorption of glucose and modulate glucose response.
	Vitamin B_3 (niacin)	Increased drug requirement.	Exercise caution. Monitor drug effectiveness	Niacin may affect glycaemic control and increase fasting blood glucose levels, so medication doses may need to be reviewed.
Metformin	Vitamin B_{12} (Cobalamin)	Decreased vitamin B_{12} levels.	Observe—monitor for signs and symptoms of deficiency.	In patients with type 11 diabetes, metformin has been shown to reduce B_{12} levels and increase homocysteine. Supplementation may be beneficial.
Sulfonylureas (e.g. glibenclamide)	Coenzyme Q10	Reduced drug side effects.	Beneficial interaction	Co-administration reduces side effects of this drug class on CoQ10 related enzymes NADH-oxidase.
Thyroid hormones and antithyroid agents				
Levothyroxine (e.g. Oroxine)	Aloe vera	Decreased drug levels.	Observe.	Reduced serum levels of T3 & T4 have been reported in one IV study. Single case report of depressed thyroid hormones in patient ingesting 10 mL of aloe juice daily for 11 months. Hormone levels returned to normal after discontinuing aloe.
	Calcium	Reduced drug absorption.	Separate doses by 2–4 hours.	Calcium and thyroxine form an insoluble complex.
	Celery	Decreased drug effect.	Observe	One case report suggests that celery extract may reduce drug effects. Clinical significance unknown.
	Horseradish	Increased drug requirement.	Observe. Monitor thyroid function. Dose may need to be adjusted.	Isothiocyanates may inhibit thyroxine formation and be goitrogenic, although this has not been demonstrated clinically.

Drug	Herb or supplement	Potential outcome	Recommendation	Evidence/Comments
ENDOCRINE AND METABOLIC DISORDERS (continued)				
Levothyroxine (continued)	Iron	Reduced drug effect	Observe—monitor thyroid function and L-thyroxine dose may need alteration. Separate doses by 2–4 hours.	Iron supplements may decrease absorption of thyroid medication; however, iron deficiency may impair the body's ability to make thyroid hormones.
	Magnesium	Reduced drug absorption.	Separate doses by 2–4 hours.	Magnesium and thyroxine form an insoluble complex together
	Psyllium	Reduced drug absorption.	Separate dose by 1–½ hour. Dose may need to be adjusted under medical supervision.	Soluble fibre may decrease drug bioavailability.
	SAMe		Exercise caution. Drug monitoring may be warranted.	
	Tyrosine	Additive effects.	Observe.	Additive effects theoretically possible, as tyrosine is a precursor to thyroid hormones.
	Withania	Additive effects.	Observe.	An in vivo study reported that daily administration of *Withania somnifera* root extract enhanced serum T4 concentration. One case report of withania induced thyrotoxicosis exists—further investigation required to confirm.
	Zinc	Reduced drug absorption.	Separate doses by 2–4 hours.	Zinc and thyroxine form an insoluble complex together.
EYE				
Glaucoma preparations				
Timolol eye drops	Coenzyme Q10	Reduced side effects.	Beneficial interaction possible.	A clinical trial of people with glaucoma found that oral CoQ10 reduced cardiovascular side effects of timolol eye drops without affecting intraocular pressure.
GASTROINTESTINAL SYSTEM				
Digestive supplements				
Pancreatin	Folate	Reduced folate absorption.	Separate doses by 2–3 hours.	Monitor for folate efficacy and folate status.

(continues)

Drug	Herb or supplement	Potential outcome	Recommendation	Evidence/Comments
GASTROINTESTINAL SYSTEM (continued)				
Anti-emetic drugs				
Metoclopramide	Shatavari	Additive effect possible.	Exercise caution.	In animal studies shatavari root exerts similar effects on gastric emptying to those of metoclopramide; therefore, additive effects are possible.
Hyperacidity, reflux and ulcers				
Aluminium-based antacids	Vitamin C	Increased aluminium absorption.	Separate doses by at least 2 hours.	Vitamin C increases the amount of aluminium absorbed.
Antacids	Folate	Reduced folate absorption.	Separate doses by 2–3 hours.	
	Iron	Reduced iron absorption.	Separate doses by at least 2 hours.	Reduced iron effect.
Anti-ulcer drugs				
Sucralfate (e.g. Carafate, Ulcyte)	Vitamin E	Reduced vitamin absorption.	Separate doses by at least 4 hours. Monitor vitamin status.	Increased vitamin intake may be required with long-term therapy.
	Calcium	Reduced calcium absorption.	Monitor calcium status.	Calcium supplementation may be required.
Gastric-acid inhibitors (proton-pump inhibitors [e.g. omeprazole], H_2-receptor antagonists [e.g. ranitidine])	Cranberry	Adjunct to treatment.	Beneficial interaction possible.	Concurrent use increased vitamin B_{12} absorption.
	Folate	Reduced folate absorption.	Separate doses by 2–3 hours.	
	Iron	Reduced effect of iron.	Monitor for iron efficacy and iron status.	Drug reduces gastric acidity and therefore iron absorption.
	Licorice	Adjunct treatment.	Beneficial interaction.	May enhance ulcer healing.
	St John's wort	Reduced drug effectiveness.	Monitor for signs of reduced drug effectiveness—adjust dose if necessary.	St John's wort decreases levels via CYP induction.
	Vitamin B_{12} (cobalamin)	Reduced B_{12} absorption.	Beneficial interaction possible. Monitor B_{12} status.	Studies show that omeprazole acutely decreases cyanocobalamin absorption in a dose-dependent manner. Supplementation may be required with long-term therapy.
Helicobacter pylori triple-therapy	Garlic	Additive effects.	Observe—interaction may be beneficial.	Garlic inhibits growth of *H. pylori* in vitro and in vivo, and two studies have shown a synergistic effect with omeprazole.

Drug	Herb or supplement	Potential outcome	Recommendation	Evidence/Comments
GASTROINTESTINAL SYSTEM (continued)				
Laxatives				
Helicobacter pylori triple-therapy (continued)	Aloe vera	Additive effects.	Exercise caution.	Anthraquinones have significant laxative activity and may increase adverse effects of griping.
GENITOURINARY SYSTEM				
Bladder function disorders				
5-alpha-reductase inhibitors (e.g. finasteride [e.g. Proscar])	Pygeum	Additive effects.	Beneficial interaction possible—drug requirements may need to be modified.	Exerts only a weak inhibition of 5-alpha-reductase.
	Saw palmetto	Additive effects.	Beneficial interaction possible—drug requirements may need to be modified	Additive effect theoretically possible. Meta-analyses show that herb is beneficial for BPH and in vitro tests show it may also inhibit 5-alpha-reductase activity—clinical significance is unknown
	Stinging nettle root	Additive effects.	Beneficial interaction possible—drug requirements may need to be modified.	Clinical studies show nettle root improves symptoms of BPH.
IMMUNOLOGY				
Immune modifiers				
Cyclosporin	Baical skullcap	Reduced drug effects.	Avoid.	*S. Baicalensis* decreased plasma levels in animal model—clinical significance unknown.
	Peppermint oil	Additive effects.	Avoid concurrent use unless under medical supervision.	Peppermint oil has been shown to increase the oral bioavailability of cyclosporin in animal studies—clinical significance unknown.
	Echinacea	Decreased drug effects.	Exercise caution.	Theoretically, the immunostimulant activity of the herb may reduce drug effects—clinical significance unknown.
	Goldenseal	Increased drug effects.	Exercise caution.	RCT found berberine 0.2 g tds 3 m increased blood concentrations of cyclosporine A in renal transplant patients by 29.3% to that of cyclosporine A. Clinical significance of oral ingestion of goldenseal is unknown.

(continues)

Drug	Herb or supplement	Potential outcome	Recommendation	Evidence/Comments
IMMUNOLOGY (continued)				
Cyclosporin (continued)	Quercetin	Reduced drug effects.	Avoid.	Significant decrease in drug bioavailability demonstrated in animal studies.
	St John's wort	Reduced drug. effects.	Avoid.	Decreases plasma levels significantly within 3 days of concomitant use. Recent clinical study found effect is not significant when low hyperforin products are used.
	St Mary's thistle	Reduced drug side effects but possible increase of drug effects.	Exercise caution.	Decreases hepatotoxicity; however, herb may reduce drug metabolism, leading to increased effects—clinical significance unknown.
Interferon	Baical skullcap	Increased side effects.	Exercise caution.	There have been reports of acute pneumonitis due to a possible interaction between Sho-saiko-to preparation (containing baical skullcap) and interferon, which appears to be due to an allergic–immunological mechanism rather than direct toxicity.
Interferon-alpha	Carnitine	Reduced side effects.	Beneficial interaction possible under professional supervision.	Clinical trials with patients being treated with interferon-alpha for hepatitis C found a reduction in fatigue associated with treatment when carnitine 2 g/day was co-administered.
Tacrolimus (e.g. Prograf)	St John's wort	Reduced drug effects.	Avoid unless under medical supervision—monitor for signs of decreased drug effectiveness.	Decreased drug serum levels via CYP induction.
Vaccines				
Cholera	Zinc	Immunoadjuvant effect.	Beneficial interaction possible.	In a clinical study co-administration with zinc acetate improved seroconversion of vibriocidal antibodies in children in both faecal and serum titres.
Diphtheria, tetanus, pertussis (DTP) vaccine	Shatavari	Immunoadjuvant effect.	Beneficial interaction possible.	Animal model demonstrated improved antibody titres and immunoprotection on challenge.

Drug	Herb or supplement	Potential outcome	Recommendation	Evidence/Comments
IMMUNOLOGY (continued)				
Influenza virus vaccine	Ginseng—Siberian	Reduced side effects.	Beneficial interaction possible.	May reduce the risk of post-vaccine reactions
INFECTIONS AND INFESTATIONS				
Antibiotics	Probiotics	Reduced side effects.	Beneficial interaction possible.	Reduces gastrointestinal and genitourinary side effects. A meta-analysis of nine studies found that *Lactobacilli* and *Saccharomyces boulardii* successfully prevent antibiotic-induced diarrhoea. Increase intake with antibiotic therapy.
	Soy	Reduced phyto-oestrogen effect.	Inhibits metabolism of isoflavones to equol through inhibition of intestinal microflora.	
	Vitamin B_1 (thiamin)	Reduced endogenous vitamin production.	Beneficial interaction possible.	Increase dietary intake or consider supplementation with long-term therapy.
	Vitamin B_2 (riboflavin)	Reduced endogenous vitamin production.	Beneficial interaction possible.	Increase dietary intake or consider supplementation with long-term therapy.
	Vitamin B_5 (pantothenic acid)	Reduced endogenous vitamin production.	Beneficial interaction possible.	Increase dietary intake or consider supplementation with long-term therapy.
	Vitamin B_6 (Pyridoxine)	Reduced endogenous vitamin production.	Beneficial interaction possible.	Increase dietary intake or consider supplementation with long-term therapy.
Aminoglycosides (e.g. gentamicin)	Magnesium	Decreased magnesium absorption.	Exercise caution. Monitor for signs and symptoms of magnesium deficiency.	Aminoglycosides may deplete magnesium levels and result in neuromuscular weakness. Increased magnesium may be required with long-term therapy.
Glycopeptide antibiotics (e.g. vancomycin)	Ginseng—Korean		Beneficial additive effect possible.	In animal studies, co-administration of Korean ginseng and vancomycin treated for *Staphylococcus aureus* demonstrated 100% survival compared with 67% of animals treated with Korean ginseng or 50% of animals treated with vancomycin. Clinical human studies required.

(continues)

Drug	Herb or supplement	Potential outcome	Recommendation	Evidence/Comments
INFECTIONS AND INFESTATIONS (continued)				
Quinolone antibiotics (e.g. norfloxacin [e.g. Noroxin])	Calcium	Reduced drug absorption.	Separate antibiotic dose by at least 2 hours before or 4 hours after oral calcium.	
	Dandelion	Reduced drug absorption.	Separate doses by at least 2 hours.	Reduced drug absorption observed in an experimental study.
	Iron	Reduced drug absorption.	Take drug 2 hours before or 4–6 hours after iron dosing—monitor patient for antibiotic efficacy.	
	Magnesium	Reduced drug absorption.	Separate antibiotic dose by taking at least 2 hours before or 4 hours after oral magnesium.	
	Quercetin	Reduced drug effect.	Exercise caution.	Theoretical concern based on in vitro studies as quercetin may compete for bacterial binding site with antibiotics.
	Zinc	Reduced drug and zinc absorption.	Separate doses by at least 2 hours.	Complex formation between zinc and quinolones results in reduced absorption of both substances, with potential reduction in efficacy.
Tetracycline antibiotics (e.g. minocycline [e.g. Minomycin], doxycycline)	Calcium	Reduced drug and calcium absorption.	Separate doses by at least 2 hours.	Tetracyclines form insoluble complexes with calcium, thereby reducing its absorption.
	Iron	Reduced drug effect.	Separate doses by at least 4 hours.	Initial studies indicated tetracyclines form insoluble complexes with iron, thereby reducing its absorption. More recent investigations have found no effect on erythrocyte iron uptake. Monitor iron efficacy during long-term tetracycline use.
	Magnesium	Reduced drug and magnesium absorption.	Separate doses by at least 2 hours.	Tetracyclines form insoluble complexes with iron, thereby reducing its absorption.
	Vitamin A	Increased side effects.	Avoid.	Concomitant use may increase side effects such as headaches. Long-term use increases the risk of pseudotumour cerebri.

Drug	Herb or supplement	Potential outcome	Recommendation	Evidence/Comments
INFECTIONS AND INFESTATIONS (continued)				
Tetracycline antibiotics (continued)	Vitamin B_{12} (cobalamin)	Reduced drug absorption.	Separate doses by at least 2 hours.	B complexes containing B_{12} may significantly reduce the bioavailability of tetracycline hydrochloride.
	Zinc	Reduced drug and zinc absorption.	Separate doses by at least 2 hours.	Complex formation between zinc and tetracycline results in reduced absorption of both substances, with potential reduction in efficacy.
Other antibiotics and anti-infectives (trimethoprim [e.g. Triprim])	Folate	Reduced folate levels; reduced drug toxicity.	Exercise caution—beneficial interaction possible under medical supervision.	Monitor folate status; increased folate intake may be required with long-term or high-dose therapy.
Anthelmintic drugs				
Albendazole	Ginseng—Korean	Reduced drug effects.		In animal studies, co-administration found to accelerate intestinal clearance of anthelmintic; clinical significance unknown.
Antileishmanial drug				
Stibanate	Quercetin	Improved drug effect.	Beneficial interaction possible.	Concurrent use with quercetin appears to improve drug efficacy and reduce condition side effects of anaemia and parasitaemia.
Antimalarials				
Chloroquine (e.g. Chlorquin)	Vitamin E	Reduced drug effects.	Observe.	According to in vitro research, vitamin E inhibits drug uptake in human cultured fibroblasts—clinical significance unknown.
Pyrimethamine (e.g. Daraprim)	Folate	Reduced folate effects.	Beneficial interaction possible with folinic acid.	Impaired folate utilisation occurs with drug use—supplementation may be required.
Antituberculotics and antileprotics				
Cycloserine and isoniazid	Vitamin B_6 (pyridoxine)	Reduced B_6 levels.	Beneficial interaction possible.	Drug may induce pyridoxine deficiency. Increased dietary intake of vitamin B_6 rich foods or supplementation may be required with long-term therapy.

(continues)

Drug	Herb or supplement	Potential outcome	Recommendation	Evidence/Comments
INFECTIONS AND INFESTATIONS (continued)				
Isoniazid	Vitamin B_3 (niacin)	Reduced B_3 levels.	Beneficial interaction possible.	Prolonged isoniazid therapy (the drug replaces niacinamide in NAD) may induce pellagra. Increased vitamin intake may be required with long-term therapy.
	Vitamin E	Reduced vitamin absorption.	Separate doses by at least 4 hours and monitor vitamin status.	Increased vitamin intake may be required with long-term therapy.
Rifampicin and isoniazid	Vitamin D	Reduced vitamin D levels.	Beneficial interaction possible.	Drugs reported to induce catabolism of vitamin D. May be a concern for subjects already at risk of compromised vitamin status. Increase vitamin D intake with long-term therapy.
Antiviral agents				
Antiretroviral drugs	Vitamin B_3 (niacin)	Reduced drug side effects.	Beneficial interaction under professional supervision.	Extended release niacin may improve the dyslipidaemia associated with antiretroviral therapy and is considered a safe and effective therapeutic option.
HIV drugs (e.g. zidovudine [AZT, e.g. Retrovir])	Carnitine	Reduced carnitine levels.	Beneficial interaction possible.	In vitro studies indicate prevention of muscle damage due to carnitine depletion. Increased intake may be required with long-term therapy.
	Ginseng—Korean	Delayed viral resistance.	Beneficial interaction possible.	Long intake of Korean ginseng in HIV-1 infected patients demonstrated delay in resistance mutation to zidovudine.
HIV non-nucleoside transcriptase inhibitors	St John's wort	Reduced drug effects.	Avoid.	St John's wort increases drug metabolism, thereby reducing drug serum levels.
HIV protease inhibitors	St John's wort	Reduced drug effects.	Avoid.	St John's wort increases drug metabolism, thereby reducing drug serum levels.
Saquinavir	Garlic	Reduced drug effects.	Avoid until safety can be established.	Clinical studies have generated conflicting results: one clinical study found that garlic reduces serum levels of saquinavir and therefore drug efficacy, whereas a subsequent study found no significant effect on drug pharmacokinetics.

Drug	Herb or supplement	Potential outcome	Recommendation	Evidence/Comments
INFECTIONS AND INFESTATIONS (continued)				
Saquinavir (continued)	Quercetin	Possible reduced drug effects.	Exercise caution.	Co-administration does not appear to alter saquinavir; however, owing to substantial subject variability of drug concentrations caution should be exerted until more is known.
MUSCULOSKELETAL SYSTEM				
Non-steroidal anti-inflammatory drugs				
NSAIDs	Celery seed extract	Reduced side effects.	Beneficial interaction possible.	Gastroprotective activity seen in animal model.
	Chamomile	Reduced side effects.	Interaction is beneficial.	Gastroprotective activity seen in animal model.
	Chondroitin	Additive effects.	Beneficial interaction possible. Drug dosage may require modification.	May enhance the anti-inflammatory effects of the NSAID.
	Colostrum	Reduced side effects.	Interaction is beneficial.	Has gastroprotective activity.
	Devil's claw	Additive effects.	Beneficial interaction possible. Drug dosage may require modification.	May enhance the anti-inflammatory effects of the NSAID.
	Fish oils	Additive effects.	Beneficial interaction possible. Drug dosage may require modification.	May enhance the anti-inflammatory effects of the NSAID.
	Ginger	Additive effects.	Beneficial interaction possible. Drug dosage may require modification.	May enhance the anti-inflammatory effects of NSAIDs at high doses.
	Glucosamine	Additive effects.	Beneficial interaction possible. Drug dosage may require modification.	Theoretically may enhance the anti-inflammatory effects of the NSAID.
	Glutamine	Reduced side effects.	Beneficial interaction possible.	May ameliorate the increased intestinal permeability caused by indomethacin.

(continues)

Drug	Herb or supplement	Potential outcome	Recommendation	Evidence/Comments
MUSCULOSKELETAL SYSTEM (continued)				
NSAIDs (continued)	New Zealand green-lipped mussel	Additive effects.	Beneficial interaction possible. Drug dosage may require modification.	Anti-inflammatory activity reported in a clinical study—may enhance the anti-inflammatory effects of the NSAID.
	Stinging nettle	Additive effects.	Beneficial interaction possible. Drug dosage may require modification.	Anti-inflammatory activity reported in a clinical study—may enhance the anti-inflammatory effects of the NSAID.
	SAMe	Additive effects.	Beneficial interaction possible. Drug dosage may require modification.	Anti-inflammatory activity reported in a clinical study—may enhance the anti-inflammatory effects of the NSAID.
	Vitamin E	Additive effects.	Beneficial interaction possible. Drug dosage may require modification.	May enhance the pain-modifying effects of the NSAID when used in high doses for RA.
	Willow bark	Additive effects.	Beneficial interaction possible. Drug dosage may require modification.	May enhance the anti-inflammatory effects of the NSAID.
	Zinc	Reduced absorption.	Separate doses by at least 2 hours.	
Diclofenac sodium (topical)	Licorice	Additive effects.	Beneficial interaction possible.	In vitro studies have shown that the addition of glycyrrhizin enhanced the topical absorption of diclofenac sodium—significance for licorice unknown.
Sulfasalazine (e.g. Salazopyrin)	Folate	Reduced drug absorption.	Separate doses by 2–3 hours.	
	Iron	Reduced drug and iron effects.	Separate doses by at least 2 hours.	May bind together and reduce absorption of both.
NEOPLASTIC DISORDERS				
Chemotherapy	Ginseng—Korean	Reduced side effects. May improve drug response.	Beneficial interaction possible under medical supervision but further research required to confirm.	Preliminary evidence suggests Korean ginsengmay reduce nausea and vomiting associated with chemotherapy and radiation by antagonising serotonin receptors. Ginseng may also sensitise cancer cells to chemotherapeutic agents.

Drug	Herb or supplement	Potential outcome	Recommendation	Evidence/Comments
NEOPLASTIC DISORDERS (continued)				
Chemotherapy (continued)	Ginseng—Siberian	Reduced drug effects—improved treatment tolerance.	Exercise caution—possible beneficial interaction under medical supervision but further research required to confirm.	Increased tolerance for chemotherapy and improved immune function demonstrated in women with breast and ovarian cancer. Theoretically, co-administration may reduce drug effects; however, improves immune function.
	L-Glutamine	Reduced side effects.	Beneficial interaction possible under medical supervision.	Number of clinical trials have demonstrated that glutamine supplementation improves side effects such as oral pain and inflammation, increased gut permeability and reduced lymphocyte count.
	Rosemary	Increased drug effects of P-gp substrates.	Exercise caution with concentrated extracts until clinical significance determined.	Inhibits P-glycoprotein, so may affect the bioavailability of P-gp substrates.
	Vitamin A	May improve drug response.	Beneficial interaction possible under medical supervision but further research required to confirm.	Adjunctive treatment may improve drug response; consider individual patient characteristics, form and presentation of cancer, and drugs before administration.
	Vitamin C	May enhance anti-tumour activity.	Beneficial interaction possible.	Controversial—further research required.
	Withania	Reduced side effects.	Observe. Beneficial interaction possible under medical supervision but further research required to confirm.	Animal studies suggest a potential role for withania as an adjunctive treatment during chemotherapy for the prevention of drug-induced bone marrow suppression—clinical significance unknown.
Myelosuppression	Echinacea	Reduced side effects.	Beneficial interaction possible under professional supervision.	Use of echinacea between chemotherapy treatment cycles theoretically may improve white cell counts and reduce dose limiting toxicities on myelopoeisis.
Anti-oestrogen (e.g. Tamoxifen)	Hops	Reduced drug effects.	Exercise caution until confirmed clinically.	Theoretically hops may alter the effectiveness of these drugs owing to the herb's oestrogenic activity.

(continues)

Drug	Herb or supplement	Potential outcome	Recommendation	Evidence/Comments
NEOPLASTIC DISORDERS (continued)				
Anti-oestrogen (continued)	Soy	May enhance drug effect.	Potential beneficial interaction under professional supervision.	Recent large prospective study found soy isoflavones consumed at comparative levels to those in Asian populations may reduce the risk of cancer recurrence in women receiving tamoxifen therapy and does not appear to interfere with tamoxifen efficacy. In vivo studies indicate soy isoflavone daidzein may enhance tamoxifen activity against breast cancer burden and incidence—usual dietary intake appears safe but the safety of concentrated extracts is yet to be established.
	Vitamin B_3 (Niacin)	Improved drug activity and mitochondrial function.	Beneficial interaction possible under professional supervision.	The adjunct of B_2, B_3 & CoQ10 to tamoxifen therapy demonstrated both improved mitochondrial antioxidant status and antitumour activity. Exact mechanism of niacin is unclear; however, combination therapy may be advantageous.
	Vitamin C	Enhanced drug effects.	Beneficial interaction possible under professional supervision.	In vivo study indicated vitamin C enhanced tamoxifen antitumour activity—potentially beneficial but difficult to assess.
Proteasome inhibitor (e.g. Bortezomib, velcade)	Green tea	Reduced drug effects.	Avoid.	In vitro and in vivo green tea extract almost completely blocked the effects of Bortezomib.
	Vitamin C	Reduced drug effects.	Avoid.	Vitamin C inactivated drug activity in vitro.
Topoisomerase enzyme inhibitor (e.g. Irinotecan)	St John's wort	Reduced drug effects.	Exercise caution. Monitor for signs of reduced drug effectiveness and adjust the dose if necessary.	St John's wort may increase drug metabolism and so reduce serum levels of drug.
Topoisomerase enzyme inhibitor (e.g. Etoposide)	Vitamin C	Enhanced drug effects.	Beneficial interaction possible under medical supervision.	Vitamin C enhanced the antitumour activity of etoposide in vitro—potentially beneficial but difficult to assess.

Drug	Herb or supplement	Potential outcome	Recommendation	Evidence/Comments
NEOPLASTIC DISORDERS (continued)				
Alkylating agents				
Cyclophosphamide	Astragalus		Possibly beneficial under professional supervision.	
	Echinacea	Increased drug effects.	Avoid in autoimmune disease.	Echinacea appears to increase the immunostimulatory effect of low-dose cyclophosphamide—clinical significance unknown.
	Rhodiola	Enhanced drug effects and reduced drug-side effects.	Beneficial interaction under professional clinical supervision.	In animal models combination therapy has demonstrated enhanced antitumour and antimetastic action. In addition reduced drug-toxicity in bone marrow was observed.
	Turmeric	Reduced drug effects.	Avoid until confirmed clinically.	Animal studies indicate reduced drug efficacy.
	Withania	Reduced drug effects. Reduced side effects/toxicity.	Exercise caution.	The ability to stimulate stem-cell proliferation has led to concerns that withania could reduce cyclophosphamide-induced toxicity and therefore reduce its usefulness in cancer therapy, although preliminary animal studies indicate a potential role as a potent and relatively safe radiosensitiser and chemotherapeutic agent. Theoretically it may also decrease the effectiveness of other immunosuppressant drugs.
	Vitamin C	Enhanced drug effects.	Beneficial interaction possible under professional supervision.	In vivo study demonstrated enhanced drug effects; potentially beneficial but difficult to assess.
	Herbs with immunostimulant properties (e.g. echinacea, andrographis, astragalus, baical skullcap, garlic, Korean ginseng, pelargonium, Siberian ginseng)	Reduced drug effects.	Observe.	Theoretically, immunostimulating agents may reduce drug effectiveness; however, clinical significance is unknown.

(continues)

Drug	Herb or supplement	Potential outcome	Recommendation	Evidence/Comments
NEOPLASTIC DISORDERS (continued)				
Antibiotic cytotoxics				
Doxorubicin (e.g. Adriamycin)	Black cohosh	Increased drug cytoxicity.	Avoid until safety can be confirmed.	Black cohosh increased the cytotoxicity of doxorubicin in experimental model; clinical significance unknown.
	Carnitine	Reduced side effects.	Beneficial interaction possible. Use only under professional supervision.	Animal and human studies suggest that long-term carnitine administration may reduce the cardiotoxic side effects of adriamycin—further research required.
	Coenzyme Q10	Reduced side effects.	Beneficial interaction possible.	Animal and human studies suggest that the cardiotoxic side effects of adriamycin are reduced with CoQ10 supplementation—further research required.
	Ginkgo biloba	Reduced side effects.	Beneficial interaction possible.	Animal studies suggest ginkgo reduces hyperlipidaemia and proteinuria associated with adriamycin-induced nephropathy, which may enhance drug therapeutic index. Clinical trials have not been conducted to confirm this activity.
	Ginkgo biloba	Reduced side effects.	Beneficial interaction possible.	In vivo research suggests that ginkgo can prevent doxorubicin-induced cardiotoxicity, although no human studies are available to confirm this activity.
	Quercetin	Reduced side effects.	Beneficial interaction.	In an animal study, administration of quercetin has exerted a protective effect against the cardiotoxic effects of adriamycin; no human studies available. In human breast cancer cells, quercetin appears to inhibit the formation of cardiotoxic doxorubicinol.
	Rhodiola	Reduced drug side effects.	Beneficial interaction under clinical supervision.	Rhodiola is shown to reduce liver dysfunction without altering adriamycin's antitumour effects

Drug	Herb or supplement	Potential outcome	Recommendation	Evidence/Comments
NEOPLASTIC DISORDERS (continued)				
Doxorubicin (continued)	St Mary's thistle	Increased drug effectiveness and reduced drug side effects.	Beneficial interaction—under professional supervision.	Silymarin reduces cardiotoxicity and possibly chemosensitises resistant cells to anthracyclines.
	Vitamin C	Reduces side effects and enhances therapeutic action.	Beneficial interaction possible.	Vitamin C enhanced the therapeutic drug effect and reduced drug toxicity in vivo. Potentially beneficial but difficult to assess.
	Vitamin E	Reduced side effects.	Beneficial interaction possible.	One study found that oral DL-alpha-tocopheryl acetate (1600 IU/day) prevented doxorubicin-induced alopecia; however, the same dosage failed to prevent alopecia after doxorubicin treatment post-mastectomy for breast cancer and also failed to prevent alopecia in second study.
	Withania	Reduced drug side effects.	Beneficial interaction possible.	In withania-pretreated animals, attenuation of doxorubicin-induced cardiocytoxic side effects occurred.
Bleomycin	Ginkgo	Reduced side effects.	Beneficial interaction possible.	Animal studies suggest ginkgo reduces drug induced oxidative stress and improves drug tolerance. Clinical studies are necessary to confirm this.
Antimetabolites				
Docetaxel	Black cohosh	Increased drug effects.	Exercise caution.	Increased cytotoxicity of docetaxel observed in experimental model—clinical significance unclear.
Methotrexate	Folate	Reduced side effects but may reduce drug response.	Exercise caution in cancer treatment. Observe in other conditions—medical supervision advised.	Methotrexate is a folate antagonist drug; supplementation may reduce toxicity. This action may be problematic in cancer treatment and reduce drug response, but may be beneficial in other uses.
Paclitaxel	Licorice	Additive effects.	Observe. Beneficial interaction may be possible under medical supervision—further research required.	A constituent of licorice has been demonstrated to significantly potentiate the effects of paclitaxel in vitro—clinical significance for licorice unknown.

(continues)

Drug	Herb or supplement	Potential outcome	Recommendation	Evidence/Comments
NEOPLASTIC DISORDERS (continued)				
Paclitaxel (continued)	Quercetin	Increased drug effects.	Exercise caution. Drug doses may need adjustment—further research required.	Increased drug bioavailability seen in animal study.
	Withania	Potentiates chemotherapeutic effect.	Beneficial interaction possible under medical supervision—further research required.	Co-administration in animal studies has demonstrated enhanced chemotherapeutic effects through modulation of protein-bound carbohydrates and marker enzymes. Combination therapy has shown potential in treatment of benzo(a)pyrene-induced lung cancer through increased antioxidant capacity and attenuation of cell proliferation.
Immunosuppressant drugs				
Immunosuppressant drugs	Andrographis	Reduced drug effects.	Exercise caution.	Immunostimulant activity has been demonstrated in vivo.
	Astragalus	Reduced drug effects.	Exercise caution.	Due to known immunostimulant effects observed clinically.
	Baical skullcap	Reduced drug effects.	Exercise caution.	Due to known immunostimulant effects observed clinically.
	Echinacea	Reduced drug effects.	Exercise caution.	Due to known immunostimulant effects observed clinically.
	Garlic	Reduced drug effects.	Exercise caution.	Due to known immunostimulant effects observed clinically.
	Ginseng—Korean and Ginseng—Siberian	Reduced drug effects.	Exercise caution.	Due to known immunostimulant effects observed clinically.
Cisplatin	Black cohosh	Reduced side effects.	Beneficial interaction may be possible under professional supervision—further research required.	In an experimental breast cancer model, black cohosh decreased the cytotoxicity of cisplatin—clinical significance unknown.

Drug	Herb or supplement	Potential outcome	Recommendation	Evidence/Comments
NEOPLASTIC DISORDERS (continued)				
Cisplatin (continued)	Carnitine	Reduced side effects.	Beneficial interaction possible under professional supervision.	Treatment with carboplatin results in marked urinary losses of L-carnitine. Research into the use of L-carnitine 4 g/day for 7 days showed reduced fatigue from treatment with cisplatin.
	Ginger	Reduced side effects.	Beneficial interaction possible under professional supervision—further research required.	Pretreatment with ginger has restored testicular antioxidant parameters and sperm motility in cisplatin-induced damage—clinical significance unknown.
	Ginkgo biloba	Reduced side effects.	Beneficial interaction possible under professional supervision.	Ginkgo has been indicated in two in vivo studies to reduce nephrotoxic effects of cisplatin. Animal models have indicated the use of ginkgo in protecting against cisplatin-induced cytotoxicity. Clinical trials are required to confirm clinical significance.
	Pelargonium	Reduced drug effectiveness.	Avoid.	Avoid until safety can be established.
	Quercetin	Increased drug effects.	Beneficial interaction theoretically possible under professional supervision.	Pretreatment may sensitise human cervix carcinoma cells to drug according to preliminary research—further research required.
	St John's wort	Reduced side effects.	Beneficial interaction. Monitor under professional supervision.	Clinical study found St John's wort inhibited cisplatin-induced kidney histological abnormalities. St John's wort did not alter serum drug concentrations.
	St Mary's thistle	Increased drug effects. Reduced side effects.	Beneficial interaction possible under professional supervision.	Preliminary research has shown that this combination may reduce toxicity effects yet enhance antitumour activity—further research required.
	Selenium	Reduced side effects.	Beneficial interaction possible under professional supervision.	In vitro and in vivo studies indicate that selenium may reduce drug-associated nephrotoxicity, myeloid suppression and weight loss—further research required.

(continues)

Drug	Herb or supplement	Potential outcome	Recommendation	Evidence/Comments
NEOPLASTIC DISORDERS (continued)				
Cisplatin (continued)	Vitamin C	Increased drug effects—reduced side effects.	Beneficial interaction possible under professional supervision.	In vitro and in vivo studies indicate that vitamin C enhanced the antitumour activity of cisplatin and reduce drug toxicity—potentially beneficial but difficult to assess.
	Vitamin E	Reduced side effects.	Beneficial interaction possible under professional supervision.	A review of 4 clinical trials with concomitant use of vitamin E and cisplatin demonstrated significant reduction in chemotherapy-induced peripheral neuropathy in all trials.
	Withania	Reduced drug effects.	Exercise caution—beneficial interaction may be possible under professional supervision.	The ability to stimulate stem cell proliferation has led to concerns the *W. somnifera* could reduce the effectiveness of immunosuppressant drugs.
Interleukin-2-immunotherapy	Carnitine	Reduced side effects.	Beneficial interaction possible under professional supervision.	Clinical trials using L-carnitine (1000 mg/day orally) found that it may successfully prevent cardiac complications during IL-2-immunotherapy in cancer patients with clinically relevant cardiac disorders.
Vinca alkaloids				
Vinblastine	Licorice	Has additive effects.	Observe. Beneficial interaction possible under medical supervision.	A constituent of licorice has been demonstrated to significantly potentiate the effects of vinblastine in vitro—clinical significance unknown.
Vincristine	Vitamin C	Has additive effects.	Beneficial interaction possible under medical supervision.	Vitamin C enhanced drug's effect in vivo—potentially beneficial but difficult to assess.
Radiotherapy				
	Zinc	Reduced plasma nutrient status.	Beneficial interaction under professional supervision.	Radiotherapy reduces plasma zinc levels.
NUTRITION				
Anorectics and weight-reducing agents				
Orlistat (e.g. Xenical)	Lutein and zeaxanthin	Reduced vitamin absorption.	Long-term administration may reduce plasma levels.	Increased vitamin intake may be required with long-term therapy.

Drug	Herb or supplement	Potential outcome	Recommendation	Evidence/Comments
NUTRITION (continued)				
Orlistat (continued)	Lycopene	Reduced vitamin absorption.	Separate doses by at least 2 hours. Monitor vitamin status.	Drugs that reduce fat absorption may reduce lycopene absorption. Increased vitamin intake may be required with long-term therapy.
	Vitamin A	Reduced vitamin absorption.	Separate doses by at least 4 hours. Monitor vitamin status.	Increased dietary intake of food rich in vitamin A or consider supplementation with long-term therapy.
	Vitamin D	Reduced vitamin absorption.	Separate doses by at least 4 hours either side of drug. Monitor vitamin status.	Concurrent supplementation of multivitamin with vitamin D is advised.
	Vitamin E	Reduced vitamin absorption.	Separate doses by at least 4 hours. Monitor vitamin status.	Increased vitamin intake may be required with long-term therapy.
	Vitamin K	Reduced vitamin absorption.	Separate doses by at least 4 hours. Monitor vitamin status.	Increased vitamin intake may be required with long-term therapy.
POISONING, TOXICITY AND DRUG DEPENDENCE				
Agents used in drug dependence				
Methadone	Kava kava	Has additive effects.	Exercise caution.	Increased sedation theoretically possible.
	St John's wort	Reduced drug effects.	Avoid.	Decreases serum levels via CYP induction.
Detoxifying agents, antidotes				
Penicillamine (e.g. D-penamine)	Calcium	Reduced drug effects.	Separate doses by 2 hours.	Combination forms insoluble complex.
	Iron	Reduced drug and iron effects.	Separate doses by at least 2 hours. Do not suddenly withdraw iron.	Sudden withdrawal of iron during penicillamine use has been associated with penicillamine toxicity and kidney damage.
	Magnesium	Reduced drug effects.	Separate doses by 2 hours	Combination forms insoluble complex.
	Vitamin B_6 (pyridoxine)	Reduced B_6 effect.	Beneficial interaction possible.	Drug may induce pyridoxine deficiency—increase intake of vitamin B_6 rich foods or consider supplementation.
	Zinc	Reduced drug effects.	Separate doses by 2 hours.	Combination forms insoluble complex.

(continues)

Drug	Herb or supplement	Potential outcome	Recommendation	Evidence/Comments
RESPIRATORY SYSTEM				
Broncospasm relaxants				
Ephedrine	Tyrosine	Increased side effects.	Observe.	Tyrosine (200 and 400 mg/kg) has been shown to increase side effects of anorexia caused by ephedrine and amphetamine in a dose-dependent manner in rats—clinical significance unknown.
Theophylline	St John's wort	Reduced drug effects.	Monitor for signs of reduced drug effectiveness and adjust the dose if necessary.	Decreased drug serum levels.
	Vitamin B_6 (pyridoxine)	Reduced B_6 levels	Beneficial interaction possible.	Drug may induce pyridoxine deficiency. Increased intake may be required with long-term therapy.
Expectorants, antitussives, mucolytics and decongestants				
	Adhatoda	Increased drug effects.	Observe.	Results from animal studies show that *Adhatoda vasica* extract exerts considerable antitussive activity when administered orally and is comparable to codeine when cough is due to irritant stimuli.
Phenylpropanolamine (found in Neo-Diophen)	Tyrosine	Increased side effects.	Observe.	Tyrosine (200 and 400 mg/kg) has been shown to increase side effects of anorexia caused by phenylpropanolamine in a dose-dependent manner in rats—clinical significance unknown.
SKIN				
Acne, keratolytics and cleansers				
Isotretinoin (e.g. Roaccutane)	Vitamin A	Has additive effects.	Avoid.	Isotretinoin is a vitamin A derivative, so adverse effects and toxicity may be increased.
Psoriasis, seborrhoea and ichthyosis				
Ketoconazole (e.g. Nizoral)	Vitamin D	Reduced vitamin D effects.	Compromised vitamin status.	Ketoconazole reduces the conversion of vitamin D to its active forms. Increased intake may be required with long-term therapy.

Drug	Herb or supplement	Potential outcome	Recommendation	Evidence/Comments
SKIN (continued)				
Topical corticosteroids				
Topical corticosteroids (e.g. hydrocortisone)	Aloe vera (topical)	Has additive effects.	Beneficial interaction possible.	In addition to its own anti-inflammatory effects, animal studies have shown that aloe vera increases the absorption of hydrocortisone by hydrating the stratum corneum, inhibits hydrocortisone's antiwound-healing activity and increases wound tensile strength.
OTHER				
Alcohol	Andrographis	Reduced side effects.	Beneficial interaction possible.	May reduce hepatic injury.
	Ginseng—Korean	Reduced side effects.	Beneficial interaction possible.	May reduce hepatic injury.
	Kava kava	Has additive effects.	Observe.	Potentiation of CNS sedative effects have been reported in an animal study; however, one double-blind placebo-controlled study found no additive effects on CNS depression or safety-related performance.
	Magnesium	Reduced vitamin status.	Monitor for deficiency.	Chronic alcohol ingestion may lead to nutrient deficiency—consider increased intake.
	St Mary's thistle	Reduced side effects.	Beneficial interaction possible.	May reduce hepatic injury.
	SAMe	Reduced side effects.	Beneficial interaction possible.	May reduce hepatic injury caused by such agents as paracetamol, alcohol and oestrogens.
	Schisandra	Reduced side effects.	Beneficial interaction possible.	May reduce hepatic injury.
	Vitamin B_1	Reduced vitamin status.	Monitor for deficiency.	Chronic alcohol ingestion may lead to nutrient deficiency—consider increased intake.
	Vitamin B_2	Reduced vitamin status.	Monitor for deficiency.	Chronic alcohol ingestion may lead to nutrient deficiency—consider increased intake.

(continues)

Drug	Herb or supplement	Potential outcome	Recommendation	Evidence/Comments
OTHER (continued)				
Colchicine	Vitamin A	Reduced Vitamin A effects.	Monitor for deficiency—beneficial interaction possible.	Colchicine may interfere with vitamin A absorption and homeostasis.
Dopamine antagonists	Chaste tree	Reduced drug effects.	Observe.	Anatagonistic action theoretically possible.
Hepatotoxic drugs	Andrographis	Reduced side effects.	Beneficial interaction possible.	May exert hepatoprotective activity against liver damage induced by drugs such as paracetamol and tricyclic antidepressants.
	Garlic	Reduced side effects.	Beneficial interaction possible.	May exert hepatoprotective activity against liver damage induced by drugs such as paracetamol.
	Quercetin	Reduced side effects.	Interaction is beneficial.	Exerts hepatoprotective activity.
	St Mary's thistle	Reduced side effects.	Beneficial interaction possible.	May exert hepatoprotective activity against liver damage induced by drugs such as paracetamol.
	SAMe	Reduced side effects.	Beneficial interaction possible.	May exert hepatoprotective activity against liver damage induced by drugs such as paracetamol.
	Schisandra	Reduced side effects.	Beneficial interaction possible.	May exert hepatoprotective activity against liver damage induced by drugs such as paracetamol.
Lipophilic drugs	Chitosan	Reduced drug absorption.	Separate doses by at least 2 hours.	Binds to dietary fats and reduces their absorption and so can also affect the absorption of lipophilic drugs.
PUVA therapy	Celery	Has additive effects	Exercise caution.	While celery has been found to contain psoralens, celery extract does not seem to be photosenitising even after ingestion in large amounts; however, it may increase the risk of phototoxicity with concurrent PUVA therapy.
	St John's wort (hypericin component)	Has additive effects.	Exercise caution.	Hypericin may increase sensitivity to UV radiation.

Picture credits

Chapter 6

6.1 Adapted from Rozanski. Impact of psychological factors on the pathogenesis of cardiovascular disease and implications for therapy. Circulation 1999; 99: 2192–2217

Chapter 7

7.1 Prochaska, J.O. & DiClemente, C. Transtheoretical therapy: toward a more integrative model of change. Psychotherapy: Theory, Research, and Practice 1982; 19: 276–288

Chapter 8

8.1 Hassed C. The essence of health: the seven pillars of wellbeing. Sydney: Random House; 2008

Chapter 9

9.1 Frontera WR. Essentials of physical medicine and rehabilitation. 2nd ed. St Louis: Saunders; 2008; 9.2 Jurca R, Lamonte MJ et al. Association of muscular strength with incidence of metabolic syndrome in men. Med Sci Sports Exerc 2005; 37(11): 1849.1855; 9.3 Myers J, M Prakash et al. Exercise capacity and mortality among men referred for exercise testing. NEJM 2002; 346(11): 793–801

Chapter 16

Figures for Progress of Medicine box provided by E. Fries, and shows 'Progress of Medicine' artwork from the entrance to the medical building at the University of Melbourne; 16.1 Adapted from Silverman J, Kurtz S, Draper J. Skills for communicating with patients. Oxford: Radcliffe Medical Press Ltd; 1998

Chapter 21

21.1 Krouse HJ, Derebery MJ, Chadwick, SJ. Managing the allergic patient. Philadelphia: Saunders; 2008; Fig 21.2 Habif TP. Clinical dermatology: a color guide to diagnosis and therapy. 5th ed. St Louis: Mosby; 2010

Chapter 22

22.1, 22.9, 22.13 McPherson SS, Pincus N. Henry's clinical diagnosis and management by laboratory methods. 21st ed. Philadelphia: Saunders; 2006; 22.2 Marx J: Rosen's emergency medicine, 7th ed. St Louis: Mosby; 2009; 22.3, 22.4 Rakel D. Textbook of family medicine, 7th ed. Philadelphia: Saunders; 2007; 22.5, 22.10, 22.12 Hoffman R. Hematology: basic principles and practice. 5th ed. St Louis: Churchill Livingstone; 2008; 22.6 Katz VL. Comprehensive gynecology. 5th ed. St Louis: Mosby; 2007; 22.7 DeLee JC. DeLee and Drez's orthopaedic sports medicine. 3rd ed. Philadelphia: Saunders; 2009; 22.8, 22.11 Kumar V. Robbins and Cotran pathologic basis of disease. 8th ed. Philadelphia: Saunders; 2009

Chapter 23

Nguyen ND, Frost SA, Center JR et al. Development of prognostic nomograms for individualizing 5-year and 10-year fracture risks. Osteoporos Int 2008; 19(10): 1431–1444

Chapter 25

25.2 Rozanski A, Blumenthal JA, Kaplan J. Impact of psychological factors on the pathogenesis of cardiovascular disease and implications for therapy. Circulation 1999; 99:2192–2217; 25.3 Jackson R. Updated New Zealand cardiovascular disease risk–benefit prediction guide. Editorial. BMJ 2000; 320:709–710; 25.4 Wilson PWF, D'Agostino RB, Levy D et al . Prediction of coronary heart disease using risk factor categories. Circulation 1998; 97:1837–1847; 25.5 Baker T. Practical cardiology. 2nd ed. St Louis: Churchill Livingstone; 2008; 25.6 Fulde GWO. Emergency medicine. 5th ed. Sydney: Churchill Livingstone; 2009; 25.7 Hampton JR. The ECG made easy. 6th ed. St Louis: Churchill Livingstone; 2008; 25.8 Goldberger Al. Clinical electrocardiography: a simplified approach. 7th ed. St Louis: Mosby; 2006; 25.9 Rakel D. Textbook of family medicine, 7th ed. Philadelphia: Saunders; 25.10 Libby P. Braunwald's heart disease: a textbook of cardiovascular medicine. 8th ed. St Louis: Saunders; 2007

Chapter 26

26.1 Kumar V. Robbins and Cotran pathologic basis of disease. 8th ed. Philadelphia: Saunders; 2009; 26.4 Bornet FRL. Glycaemic index concept and metabolic diseases. International Journal of Biological Macromolecules 21 (1997) 207–219

Chapter 27

27.1 Talley NJ, O'Connor S. Clinical examination: a systematic guide to physical examination. 6th ed. Sydney: Churchill Livingstone; 2009; 27.2, 27.3 Roberts, JR, Hedges JR. Roberts: Clinical procedures in emergency medicine, 5th ed. Philadelphia: Saunders; 2009; 27.4 Auerbach PS. Wilderness medicine. 5th ed. St Louis: Mosby; 2007; 27.5 Goldman

L. Cecil medicine. 23rd ed. Philadelphia: Saunders; 2007; 27.6, 27.8, 27.9 Flint PW. Cummings otolaryngology: head and neck surgery. 5th ed. St Louis: Mosby; 2010; 27.7 Rakel D. Textbook of family medicine. 7th ed. Philadelphia: Saunders; 27.11 DeLee JC. DeLee and Drez's orthopaedic sports medicine. 3rd ed. Philadelphia: Saunders; 2009

Chapter 28

28.1 Adapted from Gates, P. Clinical neurology: a primer. Sydney: Churchill Livingstone; 2010; 28.2 Talley NJ, O'Connor S. Pocket clinical examination. 3rd ed. Sydney: Churchill Livingstone; 2008; 28.4, 28.5, 28.7, 28.8, 28.9, 28.10, 28.11, 28.14, 28.15, 28.16, 28.18 Kanski JJ. Clinical diagnosis in ophthalmology. St Louis: Mosby; 2006; 28.6, 28.17 Webb LA. Manual of eye emergencies: diagnosis and management. 2nd ed. London: Butterworth-Heinemann; 2004; 28.13, 28.19, 28.20, 28.24 Batterbury M, Bowling B. Ophthalmology. 2nd ed. St Louis: Churchill Livingstone; 2005; 28.25 Schapira AHV, Byrne E. Neurology and clinical neuroscience. Philadelphia: Mosby; 2007

Chapter 29

29.1 Patton KT, Thibodeau GA. Anatomy and physiology. 7th ed. St Louis: Mosby; 2010; 29.2 Kronenberg HM. Williams textbook of endocrinology. 11th ed. Philadelphia: Saunders; 2008; 29.3, 29.4 Ferri FF: Practical guide to the care of the medical patient. 7th ed. Philadelphia: Mosby; 2007

Chapter 30

30.1 Townsend CM. Sabiston textbook of surgery. 18th ed. Philadelphia: Saunders; 2007. 30.2 Auerbach PS. Wilderness medicine. 5th ed. St Louis: Mosby; 2007; 30.3 Brown D, Edwards H. Lewis's medical-surgical nursing. 2nd ed. Sydney: Mosby; 2008; 30.3, 30.4 Fordtran M. Sleisenger and Fordtran's gastroinstestinal and liver disease. 9th ed. St Louis: Saunders; 2010; 30.5 Klatt EC. Robbins and Cotran atlas of physiology. 2nd ed. St Louis: Saunders; 2010; 30.6 Kumar V. Robbins and Cotran pathologic basis of disease. 8th ed. Philadelphia: Saunders; 2009

Chapter 31

31.1, 31.3, 31.4 Huether SE, McCance KL. Understanding physiology. 4th ed. St Louis: Mosby; 2008; 31.2, 31.6, 31.7 Barlow-Stewart K. The Australasian genetics resource book. Sydney: Centre for Genetics Education, Royal North Shore Hospital; 2007

Chapter 33

33.1 Rakel D. Textbook of family medicine, 7th ed. Philadelphia: Saunders; 2007; 33.2 DeLee JC. DeLee and Drez's orthopaedic sports medicine. 3rd ed. Philadelphia: Saunders; 2009; 33.3 Green NE, Browner BD. Skeletal trauma in children. 4th ed. Philadelphia: Saunders; 2008; 33.4, 33.5, 33.6, 31.13 Marx J: Rosen's emergency medicine, 7th ed. St Louis: Mosby; 2009; 33.7, 33.9 Ferri FF. Ferri's clinical advisor 2010. St Louis: Mosby; 2010; 33.8 Mettler FA. Essentials of radiology. 2nd ed. Philadelphia: Saunders; 2005; 33.10 Frontera WR. Essentials of physical medicine and rehabilitation. 2nd ed.Philadelphia: Saunders; 2008; 31.11, 31.12 Canale ST, Beaty JH. Campbell's operative orthopaedics. 11th ed. St Louis: Mosby; 2007; 31.14 Adam A. Grainger and Allison's diagnostic radiology. 5th ed. St Louis: Churchill Livingstone; 2008; 31.15 Cummings CW. Otolaryngology: head & neck surgery. 4th ed. St Louis: Mosby; 2005; 31.16 Firestein GS. Kelley's textbook of rheumatology. 8th ed. Philadelphia: Saunders; 2008

Chapter 34

34.2, 34.3, 34.3, 34.5, 34.6 Adapted from Talley NJ, O'Connor S. Clinical examination: a systematic guide to physical examination. 6th ed. Sydney: Churchill Livingstone; 2009; 34.9 Watson P. The recovergram. Australasian Musculoskeletal Medicine 2000; 5(2):24–28; Appendix 1 McGuirk B, King W, Govind J et al. The safety, efficacy and cost-effectiveness of evidence-based guidelines for the management of acute low back pain in primary care. Spine 2001; 26:2615–2622; Appendix 2 Blomberg S. A pragmatic strategy for low back pain—an integrated multimodal programme based on antidysfunctional medicine. In: Hutson M, ed. Textbook of musculoskeletal medicine. Oxford University Press; 2005:1–20

Chapter 35

35.1 Habif TP. Clinical dermatology: a color guide to diagnosis and therapy. 5th ed. St Louis: Mosby; 2010

Chapter 36

36.1, 36.2, 36.3 Gates, P. Clinical neurology: a primer. Sydney: Churchill Livingstone; 2010; 36.4, 36.5, 35.6 Bradley GW. Neurology in clinical practice. 5th ed. St Louis: Butterworth-Heinemann; 2008

Chapter 37

37.1 Ogden CL, Carroll MD, McDowell MA et al. Obesity among adults in the United States—no change since 2003–2004. NCHS data brief no 1. Hyattsville, MD: National Center for Health Statistics; 2007.

Chapter 38

38.3 Fordtran M. Sleisenger and Fordtran's gastroinstestinal and liver disease. 9th ed. St Louis: Saunders; 2010; 38.4 Walsh TD. Palliative medicine. Philadelphia: Saunders; 2009; 38.4, 38.5 Litscher G. Modernization of traditional acupuncture: using multimodal computer-based high-tech methods—recent results of blue laser and teleacupuncture from the Medical University of Graz. J Acupunct Meridian Stud 2009;2(3):202–209; 38.6 Casanelia L, Stelfox, D. Foundations of massage. Sydney: Churchill Livingstone; 2010

Chapter 41

41.1, 41.2, 41.4 Mason RJ. Murray & Nadel's textbook of respiratory medicine. 4th ed. Philadelphia: Saunders; 2005; 41.3 National Asthma Council Australia (NACA). Asthma management handbook 2006. Melbourne: NACA; 2006; 41.5 Ferri FF. Practical guide to the care of the medical patient. 7th ed. Philadelphia: Mosby; 2007; 41.6 GOLD (Global Initiative for Chronic Obstructive Lung Disease); 41.7 Mettler FA. Essentials of radiology. 2nd ed. Philadelphia: Saunders; 2005; 41.8 Goldman L. Cecil medicine. 23rd ed. Philadelphia: Saunders; 2007; 41.9 Kliegman R. Nelson textbook of paediatrics. 18th ed. Philadelphia: Saunders; 2007; 41.10 Talley NJ, O'Connor S. Clinical examination: a systematic guide to physical examination. 6th ed. Sydney: Churchill Livingstone; 2009; 41.11 Mettler FA. Essentials of radiology. 2nd ed. Philadelphia: Saunders; 2005

Chapter 42

42.1 Long CC, Findlay AY. The rule of hand. Arch Dermatol 1992; 128:1129–1130; 42.2 Mackarness R. Chemical victims. London: Macmillan; 1980

Chapter 46
46.1 Walsh TD. Palliative medicine. Philadelphia: Saunders; 2009

Chapter 49
49.2 Cancer Control. H Lee Moffitt, Cancer Center & Research Institute Inc. 2006.

Chapter 50
50.1 Abeloff MD. Abeloff's clinical oncology. 4th ed. St Louis: Churchill Livingstone; 2008; 50.2 Walsh PC, Rettic AB, Stamey CA, Vaughan ED Jr. Campbells's textbook of urology, 6th ed. Philadelphia: Saunders; 1992; 50.3 C Stewart, Bradley, Leibovich, Weaver, Lieber. Prostate cancer diagnosis using a saturation needle biopsy technique after previous negative sextant biopsies. J. Urol. 166:1, 2001; 50.4 Kumar V. Robbins and Cotran pathologic basis of disease. 8th ed. Philadelphia: Saunders; 2009; 50.5, 50.6 Wein AJ. Campbell-Walsh urology. 9th ed. Philadelphia: Saunders; 2007

Chapter 51
51.1, 51.2, 51.4 Adam A. Grainger and Allison's diagnostic radiology. 5th ed. St Louis: Churchill Livingstone; 2008; 51.3 Mettler FA. Essentials of radiology. 2nd ed. Philadelphia: Saunders; 2005; 51.5 Abeloff MD. Abeloff's clinical oncology. 4th ed. St Louis: Churchill Livingstone; 2008

Chapter 52
52.1 Herlihy B. The human body in health and illness. 3rd ed. Philadelphia: Saunders; 2007; 52.2 Hacker NF. Hacker and Moore's essentials of obstetrics and gynaecology. 5th ed. Philadelphia: Saunders; 2010; 52.3, 52.9, 52.10, 52.11, 52.13, 52.14 Katz VL. Comprehensive gynecology. 5th ed. St Louis: Mosby; 2007; 52.4 Habif TP. Clinical dermatology: a color guide to diagnosis and therapy. 5th ed. St Louis: Mosby; 2010; 52.5 Adapted from Pairman S. Midwifery: preparation for practice. 2nd ed. Sydney: Churchill Livingstone; 2010; 52.6 Kumar V. Robbins and Cotran pathologic basis of disease. 8th ed. Philadelphia: Saunders; 2009; 52.7, 52.8 Kronenberg HM. Williams textbook of endocrinology. 11th ed. Philadelphia: Saunders; 2008; 52.12 Adam A. Grainger and Allison's diagnostic radiology. 5th ed. St Louis: Churchill Livingstone; 2008; 52.15 Goldman L. Cecil medicine. 23rd ed. Philadelphia: Saunders; 2007

Chapter 53
53.1 MacLennan AH. HRT: a reappraisal of the risks and benefits. Med J Aust 2007; 186(12):643–646

Chapter 54
54.1 Brenner BM. Brenner and Rector's the kidney. 8th ed. Philadelphia: Saunders; 2007; 54.2, 54.3 Pairman S. Midwifery: preparation for practice. 2nd ed. Sydney: Churchill Livingstone; 2010

Chapter 55
55.2 My Asthma Management Plan © Commonwealth of Australian, produced with permission

Chapter 56
56.1, 56.2, 56.3 Tanner JM. Growth at adolescence. Oxford: Blackwell Science; 1962

Chapter 57
57.1 Goldman L. Cecil medicine. 23rd ed. Philadelphia: Saunders; 2007; 57.2 Richter RW. Rapid reference to Alzheimer's disease. St Louis: Mosby; 2002

Chapter 58
58.1 Omran A. The epidemiologic transition: a theory of the epidemiology of population change. Milbank Quarterly 1971; 49:509–538; 58.2 Population Reference Bureau and United Nations, World Population Projections to 2100 (1998); 58.4 Willett W. Balancing lifestyle and genomics research for disease prevention. Science 2002; 296: 695–698

Chapter 59
59.1 Krug E, Dahlberg L, Mercy J, Zwi A, Lozano R. World report on violence and health. Geneva, Switzerland: World Health Organisation, 2002; 59.3 Taft A, Shakespeare J. Managing the whole family when women are abused by intimate partners: challenges for health professionals. In: Roberts G, Hegarty K, Feder G. Intimate partner abuse and health professionals: new approaches to domestic violence. London: Elsevier; 2006

Index

Page numbers followed by 'f' denote figures; those followed by 't' denote tables; and those followed by 'b' denote boxes